# Textbook of Nuclear Medicine

# Textbook of Nuclear Medicine

### Editor

**Michael A. Wilson, M.D.**
*Chief of Nuclear Medicine*
*Professor of Radiology and Medicine*
*University of Wisconsin Hospital and Clinics*
*Madison, Wisconsin*

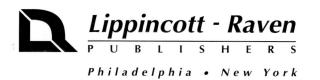

**Lippincott - Raven**
PUBLISHERS

*Philadelphia • New York*

Acquisitions Editor: Joyce-Rachel John
Developmental Editor: Julia Benson
Manufacturing Manager: Dennis Teston
Associate Managing Editor: Kathleen Bubbeo
Production Editor: Jenn Nagaj, Silverchair Science + Communications, Inc.
Cover Designer: Karen Quigley
Indexer: Linda Hallinger
Compositor: Lisa Cunningham, Silverchair Science + Communications, Inc.
Printer: Courier Westford

Printed in the United States of America

9 8 7 6 5 4 3 2 1

Library of Congress Cataloging-in-Publication Data

Texbook of nuclear medicine / [edited by] Michael A. Wilson
    p.   cm.
    Includes bibliographical references and index.
    ISBN 0–7817–0303–4
    1. Radioisotope scanning.   2. Nuclear medicine.   I. Wilson,
Michael Andrew, 1943– .
    [DNLM: 1. Nuclear Medicine--methods.  2. Radiobiology.  WN 440
T3546 1997]
RC78.7.R4T49   1997
616.07'575--dc21
DNLM/DLC
for Library of Congress                                       97–34815
                                              CIP

*To the three girls in my life: Mollie, Pat, and Judy*

# Contents

## Section III. Fundamentals of Nuclear Medicine

## Section IV. Appendices

# Contributors

**Hussein M. Abdel-Dayem, M.D.**
*Professor of Radiology*
*New York Medical College*
*Director of Nuclear Medicine*
*St. Vincent's Hospital and Medical Center*
*153 West 11th Street*
*New York, New York 10011*

**Hani Abdel-Nabi, M.D., Ph.D.**
*Professor of Clinical Nuclear Medicine*
*State University of New York at Buffalo*
*105 Parker Hall*
*3435 Main Street*
*Buffalo, New York 14214*

**W. Earl Barnes, Ph.D.**
*Physicist, Nuclear Medicine Service*
*Veterans Affairs Hospital*
*Hines, Illinois 60141*

**Joseph Bellissimo, M.D., M.S.**
*Assistant Professor of Medicine*
*University of Wisconsin Hospital and Clinics*
*Director of Nuclear Cardiology*
*Physicians Plus Medical Group*
*345 West Washington Avenue*
*Madison, Wisconsin 53703*

**Jesus A. Bianco, M.D.**
*Professor of Radiology*
*Nuclear Medicine Section, E3/311*
*University of Wisconsin Hospital and Clinics*
*600 Highland Avenue*
*Madison, Wisconsin 53792-3252*

**Ronald R. Bresell, M.S.**
*Radiation Safety Officer, Safety Department*
*University of Wisconsin*
*30 North Murray Street*
*Madison, Wisconsin 53715*

**David L. Bushnell, M.D.**
*Associate Professor of Radiology*
*University of Iowa*
*Chief of Diagnostic Imaging/Radioisotope Therapy*
  *Service*
*Veterans Affairs Medical Center*
*Highway 6 West*
*Iowa City, Iowa 52246*

**Ian H. Carlson, Ph.D.**
*Professor of Pathology and Laboratory Medicine*
*University of Wisconsin Hospital and Clinics*
*600 Highland Avenue*
*Madison, Wisconsin 53792*

**Rosinda De La Pena, M.D.**
*3020 Aspen Drive*
*Paris, Texas 75462*

**Onofre T. DeJesus, Ph.D.**
*Associate Professor of Medical Physics*
*University of Wisconsin Hospital and Clinics*
*1300 University Avenue*
*Madison, Wisconsin 53706*

**Janet Endorf-Olson, R.N., B.S.N.**
*Quality Improvement Specialist*
*Utilization and Quality Management*
*Bryan Memorial Hospital*
*1600 South 48th Street*
*Lincoln, Nebraska 68506-1299*

**John F. Fowler, D.Sc., Ph.D.**
*Professor of Human Oncology and Medical*
  *Physics, Emeritus*
*University of Wisconsin Hospital and Clinics*
*150 Lambeth Road*
*London SE1 7DF*
*United Kingdom*

**Richard J. Hammes, B.S., M.S., B.C.N.P.**
*Associate Clinical Professor of Pharmacy*
*Department of Radiology and Nuclear Medicine*
*University of Wisconsin Hospital and Clinics*
*600 Highland Avenue*
*Madison, Wisconsin 53792-3252*

**Kristine M. Leahy-Gross, R.N., B.S.**
*Quality Improvement Analyst*
*University of Wisconsin Hospital and Clinics*
*600 Highland Avenue*
*Madison, Wisconsin 53792*

**Richard B. Mazess, Ph.D.**
*Professor of Medical Physics, Emeritus*
*University of Wisconsin Hospital and Clinics*
*President, Lunar Corporation*
*313 West Beltline Highway*
*Madison, Wisconsin 53713*

**Scott B. Perlman, M.D., M.S.**
*Director, PET Program*
*Associate Professor of Radiology*
*University of Wisconsin Hospital and Clinics*
*600 Highland Avenue*
*Madison, Wisconsin 53792-3252*

**Robert W. Pyzalski, Ph.D.**
*Senior Scientist, Department of Radiology*
*University of Wisconsin Hospital and Clinics*
*600 Highland Avenue*
*Madison, Wisconsin 53792*

**James E. Seabold, M.D.**
*Professor of Radiology*
*University of Iowa Hospitals and Clinics*
*200 Hawkins Drive*
*Iowa City, Iowa 52242*

**Richard M. Shore, M.D.**
*Assistant Professor of Radiology*
*Children's Memorial Hospital*
*Northwestern University Medical School*
*2300 Children's Plaza*
*Chicago, Illinois 60614*

**Donald J. Stallman, M.D.**
*Department of Radiology*
*Meritcare Medical Center*
*737 Broadway*
*Fargo, North Dakota 58123*

**Charles K. Stone, M.D.**
*Associate Professor of Medicine*
*University of Wisconsin Hospital and Clinics*
*600 Highland Avenue, H6/317*
*Madison, Wisconsin 53792-3248*

**Raymond K. Tu, M.S., M.D.**
*Medical Director and Director of PET Imaging*
*HealthSouth Diagnostics*
*Chief of Radiology*
*Whitman Walker Clinic*
*Assistant Professor of Radiology and Nuclear*
  *Medicine*
*Uniformed Services University*
*George Washington University School of*
  *Medicine*
*5454 Wisconsin Avenue, Suite 1765*
*Chevy Chase, Maryland 20815*

**G. John Weir, M.D.**
*Clinical Professor of Radiology*
*University of Wisconsin Hospital and Clinics*
*Director of Nuclear Medicine*
*Marshfield Clinic and St. Joseph's Hospital*
*1000 North Oak Street*
*Marshfield, Wisconsin 54449*

**Michael A. Wilson, M.D.**
*Chief of Nuclear Medicine*
*Professor of Radiology and Medicine*
*University of Wisconsin Hospital and Clinics*
*600 Highland Avenue*
*Madison, Wisconsin 53792*

**Louis V. Zager, B.S.**
*Nuclear Medicine Manager*
*University of Wisconsin Hospital and Clinics*
*600 Highland Avenue*
*Madison, Wisconsin 53792-3252*

# Preface

With the recent economic changes in health care, there are no longer limitless financial resources for medicine. Patients must be diagnosed and managed with fewer imaging procedures, and imaging specialists must ensure that only appropriate studies are performed for each patient.

Because nearly 70% of all nuclear imaging is performed by physicians not certified in nuclear medicine, this textbook is primarily designed to assist them. The text is divided into three sections. The first 10 clinical chapters provide current utilization rates, a brief history, the common system procedures and their clinical indications, and necessary basic radiopharmaceutical and dosimetry information. The next 10 chapters include specialized applications that represent subdisciplines in nuclear medicine—for example, pediatrics, organ transplantation, acquired immunodeficiency syndrome, and positron emission tomography.

The third section is designed for non–nuclear medicine physicians and describes basic scientific knowledge required for the practice of nuclear medicine. The description of radioactive decay is quantum in nature and the radiation detection discussion emphasizes the photon-crystal interaction. There is a simplified look at single photon emission computed tomography reconstruction techniques and a very detailed description of radiopharmaceuticals. This section also describes quality improvement procedures and application for a Nuclear Regulatory Commission license and ends with individual protocols that readers can modify to suit their own clinical practice, whims, other recommendations, and other protocol sources.

The appendices include weight nomograms, a description of Système Internationale units, and common abbreviations.

The *Textbook of Nuclear Medicine* is primarily intended for trainees in radiology and those general radiologists practicing nuclear medicine, but it is also designed to be a solid and concise clinically oriented text for all nuclear medicine practitioners.

# Acknowledgments

I wish to express my extreme gratitude to the authors who contributed to this textbook. To them I am indebted. Although many are colleagues or past trainees here at the University of Wisconsin, three individuals are known to me primarily through their work in their respective fields: Drs. James Seabold, Hani Abdel-Nabi, and Hussein Abdel-Dayem. I am extremely grateful for the good humor and demeanor of all of the authors when their contributions were drastically changed or modified.

I am very thankful for the University of Wisconsin Radiology Department for funding the production of figures and graphs required. Without such generous support, the book would not have been possible.

I am indebted to my physician, technologist, and secretarial staff for their unflagging support in the last few years as they have worked on the text, have supplied superior images, and were tireless in their efforts to bring this book to fruition. I am especially grateful for the secretarial and editorial assistance provided by Mrs. Judy Imhoff. I could not have completed this project without her efforts.

Last, I am very grateful for the comments of other university nuclear medicine colleagues who reviewed the chapter drafts I wrote and offered constructive criticism of various chapters: David Collier, M.D.; Howard Dworkin, M.D.; Alexander Gottschalk, M.D.; Peter Kirchner, M.D.; Conrad Nagle, M.D.; James Seabold, M.D.; and Brahm Shapiro, M.D.

# SECTION I

# General Clinical Nuclear Medicine

*Textbook of Nuclear Medicine,*
edited by Michael A. Wilson.
Lippincott–Raven Publishers, Philadelphia © 1998.

CHAPTER 1

# Musculoskeletal System

Michael A. Wilson

Bone scanning represents approximately one-third of all radionuclide imaging studies in most hospital practices. A decade ago, 95% of bone scans requested were for the detection of metastases, but now the indications are those described in Table 1-1. Excellent reviews of the current applications of bone scanning are available (1–4).

## RADIOPHARMACEUTICALS

### History

Radiotracers established bone as a metabolically active organ in the 1940s. Although calcium 47 (Ca-47) has been used for metabolic studies, there is no calcium radionuclide with a suitable imaging gamma ray emission for bone scanning. As a consequence, other radionuclides from the same column in the periodic table have been used. Strontium 85 (Sr-85) was first used for imaging in 1961, but was restricted to known cancer patients because of the high dose of radiation it imparted. The development of Sr-87m, eluted from an yttrium generator, broadened the patient population considerably. The cyclotron-produced positron emitter fluorine 18 (F-18) as fluoride, which readily exchanges with the hydroxyl ion of hydroxyapatite (HAP), was used where available. Many of the current applications were developed by the centers using F-18; one paper outlined the role of bone scanning in extraordinary detail and is prescient in its applications (5).

The technetium-labeled polyphosphates (phosphates linked by oxygens) introduced in 1972 revolutionized nuclear medicine, moving it from a primarily thyroid-oriented to a more general specialty, and causing the replacement of thicker-crystalled rectilinear scanners designed for iodine 131 (I-131) with thin-crystal gamma cameras suitable for technetium 99m (Tc-99m). The first phosphate radiopharmaceutical marketed in the United States was the two-phosphate version of polyphosphate (pyrophosphate), although initial agents linked phosphate molecules in chains of 40 to 60 units. This particular tracer remains a U.S. Food and Drug Administration (FDA)–approved

drug because of two nonskeletal approved uses: the rarely indicated acute myocardial infarct imaging agent (because of the grading scale established) and in vivo red blood cell labeling (because of the large amount of stannous ion in the kit).

The diphosphonate (two phosphates linked by a carbon atom) molecules, introduced in 1973, are the bone-seeking radiopharmaceuticals of choice. They were initially investigated as potential therapeutic agents. Etidronate and others are currently used in the treatment of myositis ossificans, Paget's disease, hypercalcemia of malignancy, and osteoporosis. The acute intravenous use of etidronate (ethylene hydroxydiphosphonate [EHDP]) actively competes with the routinely used diphosphonate bone-scanning agents and results in the nonvisualization of normal skeleton, although skeletal metastases may be seen (6). This effect occurs within a day or so of a single intravenous dose and lasts up to 2 weeks. This can also occur with chronic low-dose oral administration of etidronate (7).

Currently, imaging departments use either methylene diphosphonate (MDP) or hydroxymethylene diphosphonate (HMDP) for bone scanning, with the choice primarily dictated by cost. Three diphosphonates (EHDP, MDP, and HMDP) and pyrophosphate are New Drug Application (NDA)–approved drugs for bone-scanning purposes, but currently only MDP and HMDP are marketed as bone-scanning agents (Table 1-2). The newest agents include dicarboxypropane diphosphonate (DPD) and dimethylamino diphosphonate (DMAD) Other phosphate molecules have been used in bone scanning, including monofluorophosphate and trimetaphosphate, but they have no current clinical role. The excellent clinical characteristics of MDP and HMDP make the successful introduction of a new bone radiopharmaceutical highly unlikely.

### Physiology of Tracer Uptake

Many mechanisms of tracer uptake by the skeleton have been proposed, and many factors play a role. Tracer must be delivered by blood, and the early phase of deposition occurs at the rapid calcifying front of bone where the calcium-to-

**TABLE 1-1.** *Bone scan use*

| | |
|---|---|
| 40% | Follow-up metastatic cancer therapy |
| 20% | Diagnosis of metastatic disease |
| 20% | Orthopedic applications |
| 5% | Primary bone tumors |
| 5% | Infection diagnosis |
| 10% | Miscellaneous |
| | Paget's disease, fibrous dysplasia, viability, myositis ossificans, metabolic disease, frostbite assessment, osteonecrosis, other |

phosphorus molar ratio is low and where the region is well hydrated by bone extracellular fluid (ECF). Bone has an immense surface area, and 10% of the total ECF is skeletal. The tracer must first pass through the osteoid tissue matrix to gain access to the new bone at the growing surface of trabeculae. Immature amorphous calcium phosphate takes up the tracer in this reactive new bone formation phase. The immature amorphous calcium triphosphate $(Ca_3[PO_4]_2 \cdot [OH]_2)$ then matures into HAP. A similar process occurs in soft-tissue uptake of bone tracer, as in acute myocardial infarction, in which tracer is taken up into the myocyte mitochondrion, and electron microscopy shows fluffy, amorphous calcium triphosphate and spicules of HAP.

The calcium and phosphate of mature bone is present as HAP, whose formula is $Ca_{10}(PO_4)_6(OH)_2 \cdot 2H_2O$, arranged in sheets of calcium and hydroxyl ions with phosphate bridges linking them (Fig. 1-1). Various radionuclides have replaced different components of HAP for imaging and in other disease processes. The painters of luminous watch dials ingested radium by licking their fine paint brush tips when applying luminescent materials to watch dials and subsequently developed osteonecrosis and bone tumors. Other anions incorporated into HAP include strontium, barium, lead, thorium, and gallium. Fluoride ions have been used to replace hydroxyl ions, and the ease of this substitution is evidenced by the success of fluoridated toothpaste (such as Crest), where fluoroapatite is formed in lieu of HAP by the simple exchange of fluoride with hydroxyl ions in preformed HAP of dentine (Fig.

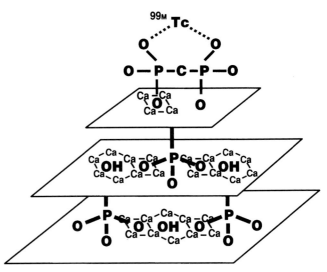

**FIG. 1-1.** An idealized structure of hydroxyapatite with sheets of calcium and hydroxyl ions (six OH around each Ca) with phosphate molecules linking these sheets. The Tc-diphosphonate molecule shown at the top is being incorporated into this structure and will result in distortion of the structure. It is not known if the Tc-99m atom disassociates itself from the diphosphonate molecule and becomes entrapped in the formation or if the entire Tc-diphosphonate complex gets incorporated into the structure.

1-2). This simple substitution explains the use of F-18 fluoride ion as a measure of skeletal blood flow because quantitative extraction occurs with a single passage of tracer. These various substitutions result in either altered chemical or physical properties, such as toothpaste-strengthened tooth enamel with fewer cavities or a spread HAP lattice that results from substituting larger ions (e.g., strontium, lead, barium) for calcium.

### Bone Blood Flow

Bone blood flow is a major determinant of tracer uptake: When flow decreases, skeletal tracer uptake decreases;

**TABLE 1-2.** *Diphosphonate types and availability*

| Diphosphonate | $R_1$ radical | $R_2$ radical | Year introduced | NDA approval | Available in United States |
|---|---|---|---|---|---|
| EHDP | OH | $CH_3$ | 1973 | + | − |
| MDP | H | H | 1975 | + | + |
| HDP | OH | H | 1980 | + | + |
| DPD | $N(CH_3)_2$ | H | 1981 | − | − |
| DMAD | $CHCH_2(COOH)_2$ | H | 1982 | − | − |

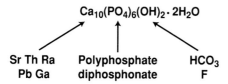

$$Ca_{10}(PO_4)_6(OH)_2 \cdot 2H_2O$$

Sr Th Ra   Polyphosphate   HCO₃
Pb Ga   diphosphonate   F

**FIG. 1-2.** The chemical formula of HAP and the possible substitutions that can occur. The fluoride ion can freely exchange with the hydroxyl ion in preformed HAP, whereas the other tracers must be incorporated during bone formation, often resulting in minor physical changes; for example, $Sr^{++}$ causes further separation of the sheets of calcium and hydroxyl ions due to its larger atomic size.

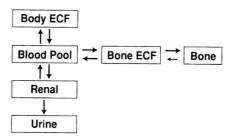

**FIG. 1-3.** A five-compartment model that helps explain physiology of in vivo tracer distribution. The smaller arrow returning from the bone compartment to the bone ECF indicates that most tracer reaching the bone remains in the skeleton. (Modified from ND Charkes. Skeletal blood flow: implications for bone-scan interpretation. J Nucl Med 1980;21:91–98.)

when bone blood flow increases, skeletal tracer uptake increases. With hyperemia alone, two- to threefold increases in bone uptake can occur, in contrast to 15- to 20-fold increases in uptake that result from increased osteoblastic activity. This general hyperemic process occurs clinically in local soft-tissue inflammation (e.g., cellulitis), postsympathectomy, and after hemiplegia. The role of perfusion is important because at rest approximately 15% of the cardiac output goes to the skeleton. The nutrient artery carries the majority of bone blood flow, and approximately one-fourth of the flow comes from synovial and periosteal sources (8).

### Model of Tracer Uptake

All osteocytes and osteoblasts at the bone surface receive nutrients from capillaries, but the capillaries are not in direct contact with the cellular or osteoid surface. Between the blood pool and the bone mass is the large-bone ECF space. From this knowledge, a model (Fig. 1-3) can be constructed (8). Tracer that is incorporated into immature woven bone is tightly bound, whereas there is more exchange between HAP and the bone tracer. This may explain why lesions due to reactive bone formation (e.g., tumor, infection, and trauma) show progressive increases in uptake relative to normal bone over 24 hours—the so-called fourth phase of the bone scan. Twenty percent of the tracer that reaches the kidney is filtered and excreted. This model rationalizes the three-phase bone scan: The first phase represents vascular supply, the second "blood pool" or "post-

flow" phase represents the combined vascular and ECF distributions, and the delayed phase represents osteoblastic activity of new bone formation.

### Bone Radiopharmaceuticals

The amount of tracer taken up by the skeleton determines the *appearance* of the bone scan; the higher the uptake, the *better looking* the scan. The attempts at improvement in scan appearance are reflected by the numbers of new tracers introduced over a decade (see Table 1-2). The initial agents, polyphosphate and pyrophosphate (introduced in 1971 and 1972), had <20% of the injected dose concentrate in the skeleton. Normal images were relatively poor, and these tracers were rapidly eclipsed by the introduction of the diphosphonates, with their higher skeletal uptake.

The earliest diphosphonate used clinically, EHDP, was established as better at lesion detection than either pyrophosphate or F-18, but similar comparisons have not shown advantages over the current NDA-approved diphosphonates. Each new agent produced better-looking scans as the skeletal uptake and ratio of bone to soft tissue increased (Table 1-3), but improvements in ratios of lesion to normal bone or lesion detection rates were never established except for a diphosphonate (DMAD) reported to show poor ratio of normal bone to soft tissue (12% skeletal uptake). This agent is not available in the United States.

**TABLE 1-3.** *Diphosphonate imaging characteristics*

| Agent type | 24-hr skeletal uptake | Lesion-to-bone ratio | Ratio of bone to soft tissue |
|---|---|---|---|
| EHDP | 21% | ++ | ++ |
| MDP | 33% | ++ | ++/+++ |
| HDP | 39% | ++ | +++ |
| DPD | 43% | ++ | +++ |
| DMAD | 12% | +++ | + |

+, least; ++, moderate; +++, excellent.

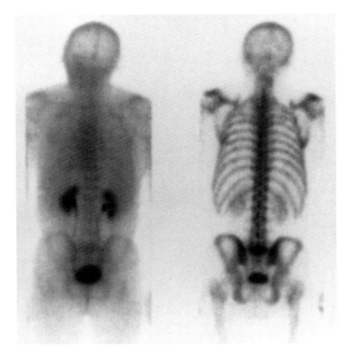

**FIG. 1-4.** The left image shows bone scan tracer (Tc-99m MDP) distribution at 5 to 10 minutes postinjection, the right image tracer localization at 3 hours. Although it appears that there is little tracer in bone in the early image, this impression is created by the moderate soft tissue and very high renal tracer activity. The degenerative joint disease of lumbosacral junction is apparent on both early and late images.

Thirty-three percent of MDP sequesters in the skeleton at 24 hours; the remainder is excreted renally (9). Sixty percent of the tracer that ultimately localizes in the skeleton does so within 5 to 10 minutes. Routine images are delayed until 2 to 3 hours later so that the ECF and blood activity is cleared, increasing the ratios of bone to soft tissue and improving skeletal images (Fig. 1-4).

## Quality Control of Radiopharmaceuticals

The labeling of diphosphonates with Tc-99m uses the reduction of the Tc-99m pertechnetate (Tc-99m-Tc-[VII]$O_4^-$) from the VII state to a lower and more reactive oxidation state (III, IV, or V), which then attaches to the bone-seeking diphosphonate ligand. The reducing agent used is stannous ion, the same used in the preparation of most other Tc-99m radiopharmaceuticals. Before the $TcO_4^-$ eluate is used to prepare the diphosphonate, it must by law be tested for $Al^{+++}$ (from the alumina column) and molybdenum 99 (Mo-99) breakthrough (molybdenum attached to the alumina column is insoluble in the NaCl eluate). The $Al^{+++}$ is tested with a colorimetric paper tape, and 10 ppm or 10 µg/ml is the maximum allowable in eluate. Molybdenum breakthrough is tested using differential absorption by lead of the respective Mo-99 (740 and 780

**TABLE 1-4.** *Radiopharmaceutical QC summary*

| Assayed component | Migrates with | Component effect on image |
| --- | --- | --- |
| Free $TcO_4$ | Acetone and saline | Stomach, thyroid, and salivary gland seen |
| Desired Tc-MDP | Saline only | Normal bone uptake and renal excretion |
| Reduced $TcO_2$ | Stays at origin | Produces colloid with hepatic visualization |

keV with half-value layer [HVL] 6 mm in lead) and Tc-99m (140 keV with 0.2 mm HVL in lead) photons. This is accomplished by the use of the dosimeter's manufacturer-supplied lead container (approximately 6 mm thick) equivalent to 35 HVLs for a 140-keV photon and 1 HVL for a 740-keV photon. The maximum allowed Mo-99 breakthrough is 15 µCi/mCi.

The radiopharmaceutical should be prepared exactly as specified in the manufacturer's package insert. Bone radiopharmaceuticals represent simple "shake-and-bake" procedures, in which a volume of oxidant-free sodium Tc-99m pertechnetate is added to the vial, the vial is shaken for 1 minute, and then allowed to stand for 1 or 2 minutes before use. Before patient use, chromatographic electrophoresis quality control (QC) testing should be performed. The vial of prepared radiopharmaceutical can only contain free pertechnetate, the desired radiopharmaceutical, reduced or hydrolyzed technetium ($TcO_2$), and unreacted stannous ion. The first three species must be assayed to confirm that adequate purity of the radiopharmaceutical is present (Table 1-4). We average 99.4% purity of the radiopharmaceutical, the U.S. Pharmacopeia lower limit being 90%.

Sporadic visualization of the stomach, thyroid, and salivary glands can occur and presumably is due to free pertechnetate (Fig. 1-5). The radiopharmaceutical may have acceptable QC parameters at the time of preparation, but over the period of expected use of a multidose vial (6 hours), a progressive increase in the percent of patients with gastric visualization can increase from a trivial incidence to as much as 67% after 2 hours (10). Not only may the scan be impaired by the nonskeletal organ visualization due to free pertechnetate, but the scan quality as judged by visualization of normal skeletal structures can be reduced, presumably due to the production of various species of technetium diphosphonate (10). This sporadic problem is probably due to the inadvertent introduction of an oxidant between drawings from a multidose vial and is remedied by the routine use of an antioxidant (e.g., ascorbic acid), a practice now incorporated in most manufacturers' products (e.g., MDP Squibb). In general, the order of unwanted organ visualization with increasing amounts of free pertechnetate is thyroid, gastric, and salivary gland.

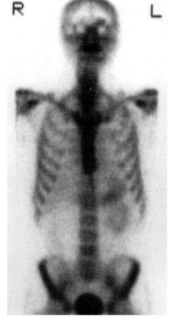

**FIG. 1-5.** This anterior whole-body image shows faint left upper quadrant activity, due to free pertechnetate in the stomach. Incidental note is made of the solitary left kidney and a benign left supraorbital lesion.

**TABLE 1-5.** *Dosimetry for bone scans*

| Target organ | Dose (rads/20 mCi) (cGy/740 MBq) |
| --- | --- |
| Total body | 0.13 |
| Bone total | 0.70 |
| Red marrow | 0.56 |
| Kidneys | 0.80 |
| Liver | 0.06 |
| Bladder wall* | |
|    2-hr void | 2.60 |
|    4.8-hr void | 6.20 |
| Ovaries (2-hr void) | 0.24 |
| Testes (2-hr void) | 0.16 |

*Critical organ.

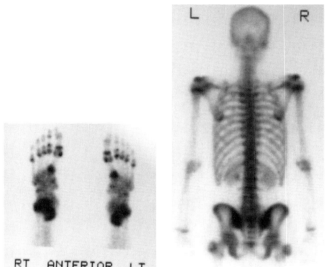

**FIG. 1-6. (A)** The detail of these feet images in this teenager is excellent. These images look like pages from *Gray's Anatomy* showing the growth plates. **(B)** The detail in the sacrum in the posterior body image is also excellent. Note the cross-hatching of the ribs due to modest photon attenuation of the anterior ribs by air-filled lungs that result in their "shine through" in this image.

## THE SCANNING PROCESS

### Protocol

#### *Radiopharmaceutical Injection*

The radiopharmaceutical is injected intravenously after proper identification of the patient. Because Tc-99m MDP is distributed throughout the entire body, a dose of 20 to 30 mCi (740 to 1,110 MBq) is injected to permit high-quality images in a reasonable time frame, thus limiting patient motion, which degrades the image quality. This produces high-count images in relatively short acquisition times. Increased doses are often given for overweight individuals or for single photon emission computed tomography (SPECT) imaging. The patient is advised to drink four 8-oz glasses of fluid and to void frequently from the time of injection to imaging. This encourages renal excretion of tracer, clears the ECF, and lowers the bladder and gonadal dose (Table 1-5).

As a rule, nuclear medicine radiopharmaceuticals do not cause patient reactions because very small doses are used. Each multidose vial contains 10 to 20 mg MDP, from which 10 individual doses can be drawn. Reactions to MDP have been reported; the most common is itching and a rash that appear 4 to 24 hours after injection, with an incidence of 1 in 10,000. This can be associated with chills, nausea, and vomiting. No specific therapy is required, but most nuclear medicine physicians discount patient complaints as unlikely to be due to the injected tracer, so the true incidence may be underreported.

#### *Effect of Patient Age*

Age affects the bone scan in two distinctly different ways. First, in young individuals the bone scan demonstrates no uptake before the development of ossification centers (the tarsal navicular may not be visualized until 3 years of age) and the growth plate shows increased activity that persists beyond radiographic evidence of closure. These growth plates appear between the first and fifth year of life as intense linear regions of increased uptake and disappear between puberty and age 20 (Fig. 1-6). Age also has a significant effect on bone scan quality, as judged by identification of

**TABLE 1-6.** *Comparison of multiple spot views versus whole-body scan*

| Multiple spots | Whole body |
|---|---|
| Care needed to overlap regions | Little technologist intervention required |
| Collimator closer in anterior view | Feet and head increase collimator separation |
| Slower to complete than whole body scan | Faster whole-body scanning process |
| Normalization of images difficult | Intrascan and interscan correlation easier |

normal bony structures, especially the visual separation of lumbar vertebrae and the identification of the pedicles and spinous processes of the lumbar and thoracic vertebrae (11).

### Technical Factors in Scan Quality

Technical factors have an even more significant potential effect in decreasing scan quality. These factors include

- Radiopharmaceutical used (percentage uptake, i.e., ratio of bone to soft tissue)
- Time from injection to imaging (bone-to-soft-tissue ratio inversely related to injection-to-imaging interval)
- Extravasation of dose (bone-to-soft-tissue ratio inversely related to injection-to-imaging interval)
- Increased ECF localization (obesity, renal impairment, ascites, and pleural effusions)
- Oxidation of the radiopharmaceutical after preparation and before use
- Technical imaging parameters (especially collimator-to-patient distance)

### Dosimetry

With diphosphonates, the critical organ is the rather radioresistant bladder wall. Doses to the bladder and gonads are decreased by encouraging the patient to void frequently. Patients visiting the radiology department are away from home and familiar bathrooms, and they tend to not seek out the rest rooms unless the technologist staff actively informs them of the benefit of frequent voiding. The halving of the bladder dose associated with a 2- versus 4.8-hour void should provide adequate incentive for frequent voiding if the information is provided in a positive manner. Dosimetry is described in Table 1-5, and comes from the manufacturer's package insert (a readily available and reliable source of dosimetry data).

### Image Acquisition

Whole-body and dual-head gamma cameras are increasingly being used, so excellent-quality scans can be obtained in 15 to 20 minutes. Presently a ⅜-in.–thick gamma camera crys-

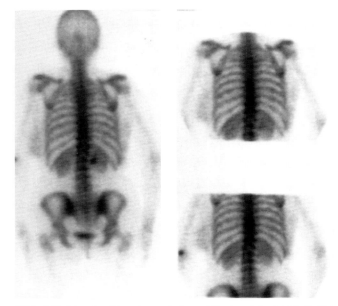

A,B

**FIG. 1-7.** No significant resolution difference is seen in the posterior views of **(A)** the whole-body and **(B)** multiple-spot formats. These images highlight the wasteful overlap that can occur with spot views. The same time was used for image acquisition in each image set, yet more of the skeleton was imaged by the whole-body format.

tal is the standard, but if the device is dedicated to bone scanning, then ¼-in.–thick crystal will provide a 20% increase in resolution with only a 6% decrease in efficiency. If the scanner is to be used for other radionuclides (e.g., gallium 67, indium 111 [In-111], or I-131), thicker crystals are preferred for their improved stopping power of the higher-energy photons.

There is some minor controversy over whether multiple spot images are preferable to whole-body imaging. Those advocating spot films indicate that, provided care is taken to include the entire skeleton by overlapping regions sufficiently, the best possible image resolution comes from spot films because the detector can be closer to the patient. They also claim that clinically important sites can have more counts collected, resulting in improved ratios of lesion to normal bone. The best argument for spot films is that, in the anterior view, the distance from the body to the collimator can be minimized for each body part; this distance is the most critical element in image resolution (Table 1-6).

Others suggest that the whole-body image can be acquired without the requirement of "stepping" from one spot view to the next. This saves time and ensures that no regions are missed. The whole-body format allows for comparison of abnormal regions within the entire skeleton and enables comparisons of regions in each patient scan and between repeat scans in the same patient. This helps in the detection of subtle interval changes. In the posterior view there is no difference in collimator-to-patient distance, and provided sufficient counts are collected, there is no difference between stepped images and the whole-body format (Fig. 1-7). Sev-

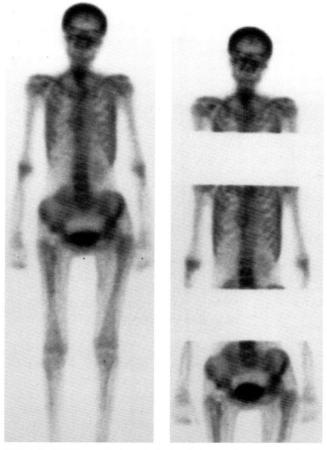

A,B

**FIG. 1-8. (A)** The anterior whole-body image is compared with **(B)** spot views taken for a comparable time. The spot views demonstrate the photopenic coin artifact on the right anterior pelvis view (lower) and the skeleton (ribs, middle) better, the result of reduced collimator-to-patient distance.

**TABLE 1-7.** *Bone scan protocols and indications*

| Protocol | Indication |
|---|---|
| Limited scans | Sports injuries |
| Whole body | Metastatic disease |
| TPBS | Osteomyelitis, RSD, bone tumors, osteoid osteoma, joint scanning |
| Triple-phase and WBC scans | Osteomyelitis in presence of local ulcers or infection, past trauma, and surgery |
| SPECT scans | Spine, hip, knee, and TMJ Subtle focal lesions |

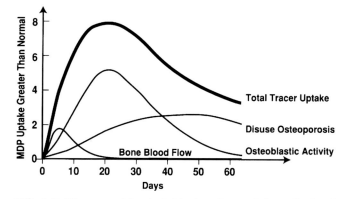

**FIG. 1-9.** Diagram of the individual and cumulative effects of hyperemia, osteoblastic repair, and disuse osteoporosis on the total tracer uptake that combine to provide the scan image.

eral modern gamma cameras allow either mode to be used, and some even combine the stepped images to produce a whole-body format with appropriate normalization between each spot view. The most significant recent change in imaging devices is the use of modern materials for imaging tables that can hold patients weighing up to 350 lb with only 6% attenuation of the 140-keV Tc-99m photon. Previously 10% to 14% attenuation was the standard.

We prefer whole-body imaging with a single automated motion. We have spent much effort in attempting to standardize the display format to allow us to detect subtle between-scan changes. We have done this in an automated fashion using software, which was developed at the University of Wisconsin Hospital and Clinics to eliminate technologist personal bias (12), that searches the upper half of the body (to exclude renal activity) for the maximal pixel count. Strict QC of formatters is required. In the anterior view, however, the technology does not exist to allow the camera to scan as closely as possible to the patient during automated whole-body imaging modes, so resolution is degraded (Fig. 1-8).

### Individual Scan Protocols

A multitude of bone-scanning protocols exist (see Chapter 30). The patient should be scheduled for the most effective imaging protocol for his or her clinical presentation (Table 1-7). The patient receives the same radiation dose regardless of regions imaged, and the imaging service should thus ensure that adequate prescan clinical information is obtained to determine the most appropriate procedure. If a whole-body study is obtained, but excellent detail images of a painful or clinically relevant site are not available, then the test is suboptimal. Special note should be made of the need to delay the final imaging when the clinical site is the feet. Five- or 6-hour postinjection images improve the bone-to–soft-tissue activity. This is probably helped by encouraging movement (e.g., flexion-extension of the ankle) that may improve lymphatic drainage of the soft-tissue ECF.

### Scan Interpretation

The concept presented in Fig. 1-9 is important in understanding the effect of noxious stimuli on bone scan images. The first two effects are hyperemia and the osteoblastic production of immature new bone as part of the repair process (both processes were discussed earlier). If there is significant

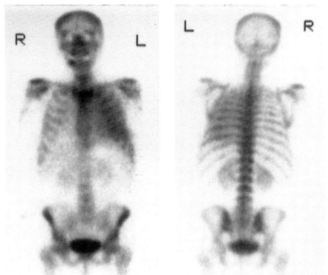

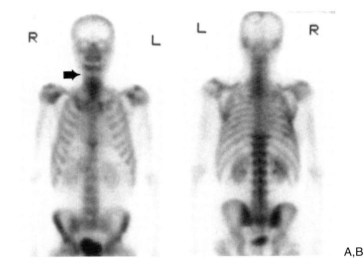

A,B

A,B

**FIG. 1-10.** The **(A)** anterior and **(B)** posterior images demonstrate a huge left pleural effusion with tracer within the outline of the chest cavity, as seen on a CXR. The effusion does extend more inferiorly in the posterior view, but as the volume of fluid is less, this is not well visualized. Incidental note is made of right mandibular dental disease.

**FIG. 1-11. (A)** This anterior view shows effects of irradiation in the sternum with sparing of the sternoclavicular joints. Incidental note is made of jaw and soft-tissue attenuation of upper cervical spine in the anterior view (*arrow*). **(B)** In the posterior view, the effects of irradiation are seen in the midthoracic spine.

local impairment of function, there will be an uptake of tracer associated with disuse osteoporosis, which may also be seen radiographically. All these effects are additive, so that the overall uptake is a combination of these various contributions. If there is considerable pain associated with the pathology, then the disuse osteoporosis may be a very significant contributor to overall uptake and will continue to be important well after the initial hyperemic effect has ended. This effect may be even more important than the osteoblastic repair process, in conditions such as Sudeck's atrophy.

The normal scan at 2 to 3 hours postinjection shows most of the tracer activity in the skeleton, some in the urinary system (kidneys and bladder), and some in the soft-tissue ECF. The skeleton should have a similar bone-to-soft-tissue uptake ratio as that of previous studies, and if this is not the case, a technical explanation should be sought (short injection-to-image time, tracer extravasation at injection site, or concurrent competing medication, e.g., etidronate). If considerable interval impairment in renal function has occurred, this would explain a change in normal bone-to-soft-tissue uptake.

If there is no ECF in a region (e.g., distended stomach after meal), reduced tracer is present. Similarly, if there is a regional increase in ECF, then more tracer may be present, as with ascites, lymphedema, and pleural effusions (Fig. 1-10), especially malignant effusions (13).

### Photopenic Lesions

The effective scan reader must develop a system for quickly screening bone scans. The most frequently missed

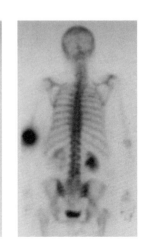

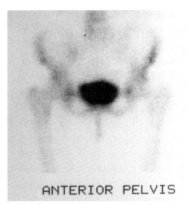

ANTERIOR PELVIS

A–C

**FIG. 1-12. (A)** The anterior upper body image shows injection site extravasation, right renal pelvis visualization, and significant asymmetry of the region of the anterior superior and anterior inferior iliac spines. **(B)** The iliac crest asymmetry confirmed in the posterior view suggests pelvic rotation. **(C)** An anterior spot film of the pelvis once the patient is straightened shows symmetry of the anterior iliac spine regions. The patient's generous abdominal soft tissue was attenuating the right iliac bone when this was dependent.

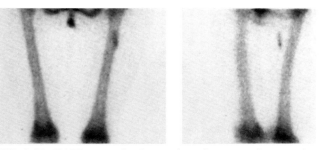

A,B

**FIG. 1-13. (A)** The anterior femur view shows uptake over the proximal left femur. **(B)** This is established as soft-tissue contamination on the LAO view. The groin activity is due to urine, the source of contamination.

lesions are photopenic. The most obvious photopenic lesions are caused by external artifacts: coins (see Fig. 1-8) or keys in pockets, belt buckles, snaps on trousers, earrings, necklaces, and pacemakers. Less obvious photopenic defects include a generalized decrease from x-ray therapy (XRT) (Fig. 1-11).

Focal defects can result from absent blood supply due to osteomyelitis or tumor involvement and are usually the consequence of

• Large masses completely displacing bone
• Rapid bone destruction without sufficient repair
• Absent perfusion due to tense marrow lesions preventing normal blood flow

Some regions of reduced tracer uptake can be explained by normal attenuation: The upper cervical region on the anterior view may show a marked decrease from attenuation by the jaw and oral soft tissues (Fig. 1-12; see also Fig. 1-11). If the patient is slightly rotated and has considerable lower abdominal soft tissue, there may be marked asymmetry of right and left superior and inferior anterior iliac spines with decreased activity due to overlying soft-tissue attenuation on the dependent side. This can occur frequently and is established by confirming rotation by asymmetry of outline of the hemipelvis, and repeating the view without rotation (see Fig. 1-12).

*Soft-Tissue Uptake*

After considering photopenic lesions, the reader should examine the scan for soft-tissue sites. Visualization of female breast tissue is normal and especially prominent if the patient is pregnant or lactating. Visualization of the stomach, thyroid, and salivary glands suggests free pertechnetate, whereas stomach and lung visualization suggests marked hypercalcemia. Urine contamination can mimic skeletal lesions, and additional orthogonal views should be obtained (Fig. 1-13). Focal hepatic visualization suggests dystrophic calcification of hepatic metastases, which can occur with all tumor types, especially large adenocarcinomas—as many as 40% of such lesions demonstrate this uptake (14). Diffuse hepatic uptake suggests either diffuse hepatic metastatic disease (Fig. 1-14),

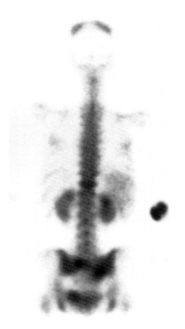

**FIG. 1-14.** This posterior image shows a large focal region of hepatic uptake of bone tracer due to an hepatic metastasis. Incidental note is made of sacral and T-11 skeletal metastases, injection site extravasation, and hyperostosis interna frontalis.

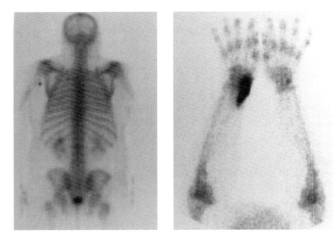

A,B

**FIG. 1-15. (A)** The posterior upper body image shows a soft-tissue focus in the axilla due to **(B)** extravasation in left wrist.

a QC problem with hydrolyzed technetium, or, very rarely, increased aluminum ion in the Tc-99m $TcO_4^-$ eluate.

Intense localization of tracer in soft tissues is seen with tumoral calcinosis, synovial sarcomas, myositis ossificans and heterotopic new bone formation, and malignant neoplasms (see later).

Unusual patterns of soft-tissue uptake include extravasation of injected dose, and there may be associated lymph node uptake (Fig. 1-15). Routine quality assurance evaluations at the University of Wisconsin Health Center indicate that 30% of whole-body bone scans show evidence of extravasation at

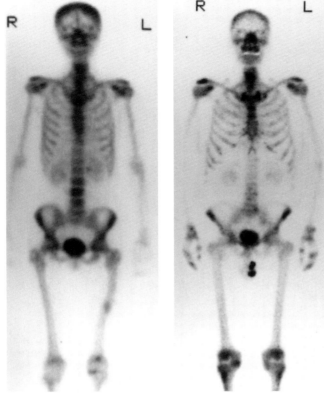

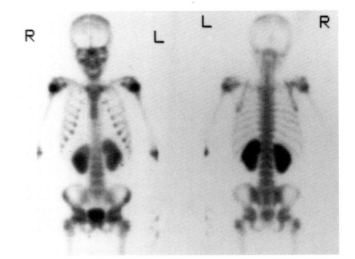

**FIG. 1-17.** The kidney uptake is enhanced due to chemotherapy.

A,B

**FIG. 1-16. (A)** The left anterior whole-body scan shows hyperostosis interna frontalis in the skull vault, prominent L3 due to normal lumbar lordosis, and uptake at stress site associated with a 30-year-old misaligned left femur fracture with associated degenerative joint disease (DJD) of the left medial tibial plateau. **(B)** The right scan shows left ethmoid sinusitis, DJD of right acromioclavicular along with sternoclavicular joint, L5/S1, hands, and the right medial tibial plateau as well as calcification of the costal cartilages.

the injection site; of these, very few are significant, and only very rarely are lymph channels or lymph nodes visualized.

Next, the scan should be searched for pathologic extraskeletal tracer activity. Infarcts can show intense uptake in the myocardium, brain, spleen, and gastrointestinal tract.

Damage to muscle can be associated with abnormal uptake and is seen in the following situations:

- Extreme exercise or dancing
- Long-distance running
- Repeated intramuscular injections
- Electrical shock

### Benign Variants

Benign variants of increased uptake include normal regional increases of sacroiliac (SI) joints, sacral tubercle, coracoid processes, sternal joints, L3–4 prominence in anterior view due to the lumbar lordosis (Fig. 1-16), prominent deltoid tuberosities, and iliocostalis insertions (both seen in 7% of all scans).

Common benign disease processes seen in more than half the scans include

- Dental disease and erupting teeth in children
- Frontal, ethmoid (see Fig. 1-16B), and maxillary sinusitis
- Old misaligned fractures of long bones (see Fig. 1-16A)
- Costal cartilage calcification (see Fig. 1-16B)

Degenerative joint disease should not be mistaken for significant disease processes. Typical sites include the following (see Fig. 1-16):

- Shoulder girdle (acromioclavicular joint, first rib to sternum joint, sternoclavicular joint)
- Base of first metacarpals
- Medial tibial plateau and patellae
- Facet joints of vertebrae
- Hands and feet

Renal tract assessment can provide important information: Renal parenchymal asymmetry equates with asymmetric function of any etiology, but visualization of renal pelves or calyces is normal and occurs in 8% of males and females; right-sided renal pelvis visualization occurs in 22% of females (15). Intense visualization of the kidneys can occur in patients receiving chemotherapy (Fig. 1-17) such as doxorubicin (Adriamycin), vincristine, and cyclophosphamide (16) or recent iron load.

### TUMOR APPLICATION

#### Historical Overview

For two decades the bone scan has been accepted as the premier imaging modality for skeletal metastatic disease. A memorable lecture in 1971 by Galasko, an orthopedic surgeon, placed the test in clinical context and highlighted features now considered the standard of bone-scanning practice

(5). The sensitivity of the scan was established when 83% of breast cancer patients with scan abnormalities subsequently developed radiographic lesions of tumor. He went on to report that bone pain was present in 65% of patients with metastases, pathologic fractures occurred in 10%, and 3% developed cord compression. The same researcher described the regional distribution of metastases (17) and noted that the microscopic skeletal reaction to tumor was nonspecific and that large quantities of new immature bone were produced in response to metastatic cancer (18). He demonstrated these occurrences in virtually all tumor types and likened this response to the callus formation that occurs with a fracture.

**Secondary Tumors**

Bone scanning is the accepted initial investigation of skeletal metastases and has a sensitivity in excess of 95%. The sensitivity of the technique results from the very early osteoblastic reaction that occurs even when microscopic tumor is present. In animal models, clumps of tumor cells as small as 25 cells wide are seen 24 hours after marrow inoculation with tumor cell suspensions. These stimulate regional osteoclasts, which erode nearby trabeculae, and a significant proliferation of osteoblasts occurs on the opposite side of the same trabecula and in any fibrous stroma that develops about the tumor. While destruction is occurring on one side of an individual trabecula, new bone formation occurs on the opposite side. Within weeks there is significant destruction of the existing trabeculae and very prominent production of immature new bone in the surrounding medullary cavity.

In studies of patients who died from a variety of malignant diseases, new bone formation can be measured by the amount of immature woven bone present near metastatic sites. Woven bone accounts for <1% of bone present in normal vertebral bodies, but in patients with vertebral metastases, 40% of the bone present can be immature woven bone (18). This explains the very high uptake of bone radiopharmaceutical that occurs as a result of osteoblastic activity. The stromal and reactive bone formation occurs in both osteolytic and osteoblastic radiographic lesions. In the case of osteolytic lesions the actual bone destruction outweighs the mass of new bone formed, but because the repair process is very active, this results in 10- to 15-fold increases in tracer uptake compared to normal bone. Similar amounts of new bone production occur in both lytic and blastic processes, and the bone scan appearances are similar in both types of metastases.

This universal marked new bone formation occurs in all tumors except myeloma (Fig. 1-18), some lymphomas, and leukemias, and is said to occur in other malignant (e.g., thyroid) and benign (e.g., eosinophilic granuloma) tumors.

Large, highly anaplastic tumor masses associated with rapid bone destruction and very slowly growing large tumor masses with little residual adjacent normal bone do not induce significant bone formation because few regional osteoprogen-

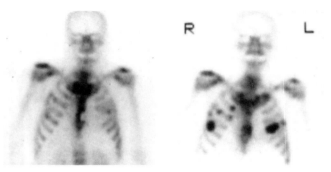

A,B

**FIG. 1-18. (A)** This unusual scan shows photopenic defects in the left side of the sternum and the left fourth rib medially, correlating with radiographic lesions of myeloma. **(B)** Four months later, these lesions were "hot," and additional lesions also appeared in the interim.

itor cells are present in and around these lesions. These unusual lesions can result in photopenic bone scan lesions, sometimes with a surrounding rim of increased uptake at the interface of the mass and normal surrounding bone.

*Pathophysiology of Metastatic Spread*

Metastatic cancer usually reaches the bone via hematogenous spread. Primary tumors shed individual cells and cell clumps at a massive rate, and the vast majority of these cells do not develop into metastases. Suitable conditions are required for the establishment of a metastasis, and the bone marrow is a favorable site. The marrow receives approximately 15% of the cardiac output at rest, and the red marrow of the axial skeleton and proximal ends of femora receive twice as much blood as the appendicular yellow marrow. This explains the axial predominance of skeletal metastases. This rich blood supply, together with the relatively slow flow of blood through the marrow cavity, provides an excellent opportunity for the metastatic seeding of the bone by tumor cells, which must migrate out of the blood vessels for implantation.

In 1940, Batson proposed that the vertebral venous plexus provided the opportunity to explain the predilection for the spine and pelvis for metastatic disease in certain cancers. He established that the vertebral plexus provided an alternative valveless plexiform network, which runs parallel to and communicates with the superior and inferior vena cava. This plexus extends the entire length of the vertebral column, from the cranial dural sinuses to the pelvic prostatic plexus. Batson classified the veins of the human body into two principal groups: those within the pressure chamber of the thoracoabdominal cavity and those of the paravertebral plexus. He "suggested that it is possible to explain most cases of aberrant malignant metastases, aberrant pyogenic metastases, and aberrant embolism following air injections by the demonstrated role of the vertebral vein system" (19). This concept was largely unchallenged until the 1950s, when

**TABLE 1-8.** *Regional distribution of metastases*

| Regional site of metastases | Patients with lesions | Percent of all lesions |
| --- | --- | --- |
| Thoracic[a] | 83% | 37 |
| Vertebral[b] | 65% | 26 |
| Pelvic[c] | 52% | 16 |
| Limbs | 52% | 15 |
| Skull | 34% | 6 |

[a] Thoracic region: rib, clavicle, sternum, scapulae.
[b] Vertebral region: cervical, thoracic, lumbar spine.
[c] Pelvic region: ilium, ischium, pubis, sacrum, SI joint
Source: Adapted from Wilson MA, Calhoun FW. The distribution of skeletal metastases in breast and pulmonary cancer: concise communication. J Nucl Med 1981;22:594–597.

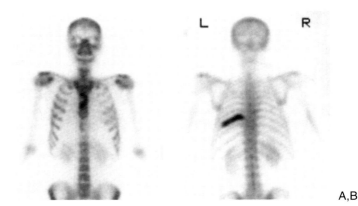

A,B

**FIG. 1-19. (A)** The anterior thorax scan shows a solitary metastasis on the right side of the sternum with a photopenic center, resulting from local invasion from the internal mammary lymphatic chain. **(B)** The posterior thorax scan shows a solitary rib abnormality involving a significant portion of the bone. Both of these lesions were confirmed as solitary metastases.

Wiley and Trueta (20) demonstrated that, although there are these two routes for the spread of disease processes to the vertebral marrow, the nutrient arteries of the systemic system provide easy access, whereas the paravertebral venous system is represented by minute twigs in the metaphysis. Furthermore, they suggested that the vertebral plexus was a drainage system and fills retrogradely only under conditions with increased pressure. In their study of osteomyelitis there was no evidence of spread via this plexus.

When tumor cells were injected into the femoral vein of animals while abdominal pressure was raised, there was a preponderance of tumor foci in the distribution of the paravertebral plexus, and many animals also developed cord compression (21). The bone was invaded from the plexus through the anterolateral surface of the vertebra, and there was direct extension of the tumor into the vertebral canal, causing cord compression. Under normal conditions this plexus probably does not form an important means of tumor spread.

The distribution of metastases throughout the skeleton has been reported to differ with tumor type, but there is no large series with statistical evaluation to confirm this. A different incidence of rib metastases has been reported in breast and lung cancer (22,23), and the explanation provided was the difference in delivery of these lesions, that is, systemic circulation for lung cancer, and paravertebral venous system for breast and prostate cancer. In a larger study looking at the regional distribution of metastases no statistical difference was seen in rib metastases in breast, lung, and other tumors either in the number of patients with metastases, total number of rib lesions, or the average number of rib lesions per patient (24). The regional distribution of metastases in the skeleton is shown in Table 1-8.

### Scan Diagnosis of Metastatic Disease

Multiple, random, intense, focal bone scan abnormalities away from joints suggest metastatic disease. The largest number of lesions would be expected in the axial skeleton and proximal long bones because of the increased blood supply associated with red marrow.

Unusual patterns of metastases include solitary lesions. Two rare patterns of solitary lesions are highly suggestive of metastatic disease. Three-fourths of solitary sternal lesions in breast cancer patients have a malignant etiology (Fig. 1-19), and are thought to occur secondary to internal mammary lymph node involvement. These have a predominance in the upper half of the sternum (25), and because in 15% of patients the internal mammary chain is unilateral, this scan finding is not always a localizing sign of the primary tumor. Another unusual pattern seen in the ribs is involvement of a significant length of bone (see Fig. 1-19) in contrast to the more usual discrete focal lesions of metastases at other sites (26).

The incidence of solitary skeletal metastases has been reported at approximately 6% to 8% (23), and studies using modern radiopharmaceuticals and gamma cameras suggest that approximately 11% to 21% of patients with breast cancer can present with a solitary metastasis (27,28). About half these patients will be confirmed as having metastatic disease with plain-film correlation and even more with computed tomography (CT) and magnetic resonance imaging (MRI). Combining data in several reports on breast cancer (27–29) suggests that only 5% of solitary rib lesions are metastatic, whereas 31% of solitary thoracolumbar spine lesions prove to be metastatic. One report (27) provides regional estimates of the probability that newly detected bone scan lesions in breast cancer patients are due to metastases:

- Five or more new lesions (100% probability of metastatic disease)
- Two to four new lesions (35%)
- Solitary thoracic spine lesion (30%)
- Solitary lesion elsewhere (10%)

In some cases biopsy will be needed for a definitive diagnosis, and preoperative localization of rib lesions is impor-

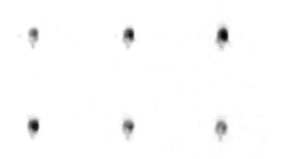

**FIG. 1-20.** SPECT images in this cancer patient show the vertebral lesion to extend from the body into the lamina, a finding typical of metastatic disease. We have found this technique increasingly useful in evaluating suspicious lesions in the spine.

tant. Postoperative imaging of the resected rib can confirm that the entire lesion has been removed (30).

Bone scanning is a nearly ideal tumor-seeking modality because of its sensitivity and ability to screen the entire body for the same radiation burden. With the increased use of MRI, there are reports of patients with normal bone scans but MRI evidence of marrow metastases (31,32). Such studies show up to a 65% increase in the number of detectable lesions in the thoracolumbar spine by MRI (31). MRI also identifies associated soft-tissue tumor extension and compressive myelopathy. Although *lesion* detection is increased with MRI, *patient* identification is not increased, because time and cost concerns make whole-body imaging with MRI impossible. Generally, SPECT improves the visualization of spinal lesions if applied to appropriate clinical populations, such as known cancer patients with back pain, or equivocal scans. SPECT patterns in the spine that suggest benign lesions in 87% to 100% of patients include

- Osteophytes that project beyond the vertebral body
- Diffuse or focal uptake confined to the vertebral body
- Lesions involving both body and posterior elements but with normal intervening pedicle

Individual lesions showing uptake in both the lamina and body of the vertebra (Fig. 1-20) are usually (83%) malignant (33).

Monoclonal antibody imaging with antigranulocytic agents (currently only available in Europe) result in >50% improvement in the number of metastatic lesions in breast cancer patients when compared to conventional bone scanning (34). It is probable that this may be as sensitive as MRI.

### Follow-Up of Metastatic Disease

The bone scan is now regularly used in the therapeutic management of patients with skeletal metastases. Prominent lesions in weight-bearing long bones should be radiographed

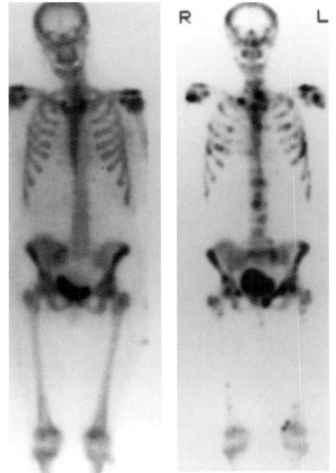

A,B

**FIG. 1-21.** This patient has a renal transplant (right iliac fossa) and breast cancer. These anterior whole-body scans were taken 1 year apart and show marked interval progression from **(A)** normal to **(B)** extensive metastatic disease.

to predict the likelihood of imminent pathologic fracture. This is also suggested for lesions of the upper limb long bones, but because patients will not become bedridden as a result of pathologic fracture this is not so important clinically. If bones have considerable cortical destruction seen on x-ray, prophylactic local irradiation or surgical fixation can be undertaken to prevent fracture.

The onset of metastases or appearance of new lesions in a patient on therapy would be an indication for the oncologist to consider the introduction of a change in therapy. These patients may have bone pain, but the scan may be the only evidence of status change. It is prudent to suggest progression in metastatic disease only when there is an increase in the number of lesions (Fig. 1-21) rather than rely on an increase in intensity of lesion. Technical factors can cause an apparent generalized increase in ratios of lesion to bone or lesion to soft tissue, such as technologist display of hard copy or changes in injection-to-scan time. The same care should be given to the determination of lesion regression (Fig. 1-22).

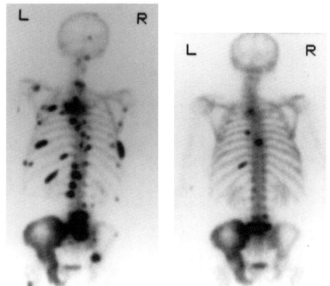

**FIG. 1-22.** These posterior scans of the same patient were obtained 1 year apart. They show Paget's disease of the left hemipelvis. All other lesions are metastatic, although the L5 lesion simulates Paget's, but with subsequent improvement after therapy, a malignant etiology was established. **(A)** Some rib, spinal, pelvic, femoral, and calvarial lesions have regressed completely over this treatment period **(B)**.

The flare phenomenon is a bone scan phenomenon that may occur in the first 3 to 6 months after introduction of hormonal or chemotherapy, and can cause problems in interpretation. This is represented by an increase in intensity of lesions and the development of additional lesions, which represent osteoblastic repair activity in response to therapy (35). By 6 months, all these responders should demonstrate improved bone scans. This is common in breast cancer patients but also occurs in prostate and lung cancer and has been reported to occur in patients with initial photopenic lesions, such as myeloma (see Fig. 1-18). This response in the osteoblastic repair process can be paralleled by biochemical markers, such as serum alkaline phosphatase bone isoenzyme and osteocalcin, which have been used to suggest a favorable therapeutic response. Scan readers should recognize that an immediate increase in intensity or number of lesions may result from either progression of disease or exuberant osteoblastic response to therapy. Although this represents a favorable response to therapy, it is not associated with significantly increased patient survival (35).

Care should be taken in correlating x-rays with scans because many patients with radiographic evidence of presumed osteoblastic metastases have normal bone scan uptake in those areas, suggesting that radiographic findings represent sclerosis of healing rather than true osteoblastic metastases (36).

Successful radiotherapy causes a reduction in the increased uptake of metastatic lesions to levels similar to adjacent normal bone. The bone response depends on the amount of radiation and the time over which it is delivered. Soon after delivery of XRT, hyperemia occurs and uptake increases, but this effect

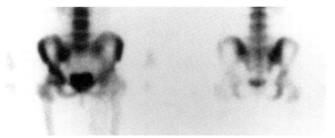

**FIG. 1-23.** The images show the XRT effect on the left hip region. Decreased uptake is seen involving the lower half of the left sacroiliac joint, the acetabular region, and the ischium.

is temporary. With significant irradiation there is associated osteocyte death and depression of skeletal bone tracer uptake. The rapidity of onset of this phase depends on the dose the bone receives. With 2,000 rads (20 Gy), it occurs in months and may be transient. With 3,000 rads (30 Gy), it occurs in weeks. With large doses (e.g., 6,000 rads [60 Gy]), uptake is permanently decreased (Fig. 1-23; see Fig. 1-11) due to irreversible osteonecrosis (37).

### Secondary Tumor

A decade ago all patients with common primary tumors had bone scans to determine the presence of metastases, a fact that could alter initial management. With recent changes in patient management, such as lumpectomy and lymph node sampling versus mastectomy in breast cancer patients, the pretherapy identification of metastases is not as important as was previously thought. With staging of tumors by conventional techniques (size, presence of nodes, etc.) the relative yield of bone scanning can be predicted. In some stages of some tumors this is sufficiently low to preclude the need for routine screening. Bone pain is an excellent predictor of the presence of skeletal metastases, and bone scanning can often be deferred until this symptom appears. In general, current indications for bone scans are as follows:

- Evidence of progressive disease (e.g., prostate-specific antigen [PSA] rise) in an otherwise asymptomatic patient
- Restaging of patient with local tumor recurrence
- Investigation of bone pain
- Examination of lesions detected by other modalities

### Breast Cancer

Approximately 70% of patients with breast cancer eventually develop skeletal metastases. In 50% of patients, the first recurrence is to the skeleton, and in 20% the skeleton only is involved. The stage of the tumor correlates with the incidence of skeletal metastases (Table 1-9). Although the presence of skeletal metastases indicates a fourfold increase in mortality, there is no overwhelming indication for a screening bone scan for staging when the diagnosis is

**TABLE 1-9.** *Skeletal metastases*

| Tumor stage | Incidence of skeletal metastases | |
| --- | --- | --- |
| | Breast cancer | Prostate cancer |
| I | 5% | 8% |
| II | 8% | 10% |
| III | 27% | 20% |
| IV | 60% | 60% |

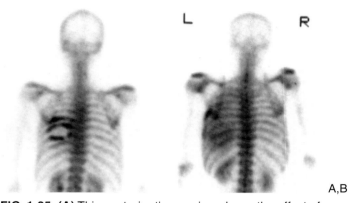

FIG. 1-25. **(A)** This posterior thorax view shows the effect of a posterior pulmonary mass eroding three adjacent ribs. **(B)** Bone tracer uptake in the periphery of a known non–small cell carcinoma and lateral rib changes from a thoracotomy 6 months earlier.

- Lymphedema (excellent lateralizing sign)
- Visualization of one breast only
- Better rib visualization on mastectomy side
- Presence of attenuating breast prosthesis
- Early postoperative edema in lumpectomy patient
- Solitary sternal lesion (internal mammary lymph chain) (see Fig. 1-19)

### Lung Cancer

The incidence of skeletal metastases in lung cancer patients is considerably lower than that of breast cancer (30% to 50%). In lung cancer, bone pain is a frequent and excellent indicator of skeletal metastases. The presence of skeletal metastases indicates a very poor prognosis. Despite the overall lower incidence of skeletal metastases and the frequent association of bone pain and skeletal metastases, the morbidity and mortality of elective surgical resection is significant, and all patients considered for an attempt at curative surgery warrant a bone scan to prevent unnecessary surgery.

The following patterns are suggestive of lung cancer in a bone scan patient:

- Postirradiation changes in spine (see Fig. 1-11)
- Local invasion of ribs
- Uptake into dystrophic regions of the primary tumor
- Effect of thoracotomy (Fig. 1-25)
- Pancoast tumor (Fig. 1-26)
- Pulmonary osteoarthropathy (Fig. 1-27)

The scan findings of hypertrophic pulmonary osteoarthropathy (HPOA) are most commonly caused by lung cancer, but in up to 15% of patients other etiologies, such as lung metastases, infectious lung disease, and congenital heart disease, exist. Although there are 20 potential causes of HPOA, the vast majority are the result of lung cancer. As

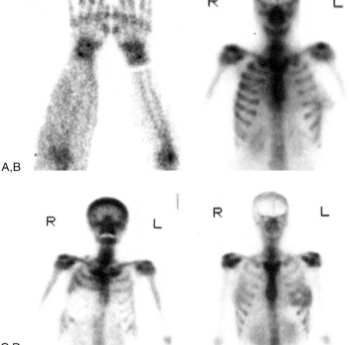

FIG. 1-24. **(A)** The presence of lymphedema is an excellent localizing sign for treated breast cancer. The distended limb confirms proximal lymphatic obstruction and axillary nodal dissection. Anterior upper thorax views demonstrate **(B)** visualization of one breast only and better visualization of ribs on the mastectomy side due to decreased tissue attenuation, **(C)** photopenic defect of right breast prosthesis, and **(D)** evidence of soft-tissue edema due to recent lumpectomy.

made. This results from the recent trend to lumpectomy and local irradiation regardless of tumor stage. When disfiguring curative operations, such as radical and modified radical mastectomy, were used, it was important to identify metastases to modify the surgical procedure. The scan is now reserved to investigate patients with symptoms suggestive of metastases, such as bone pain, and to follow systemic therapies.

Several nonskeletal scan patterns (Fig. 1-24) suggest the diagnosis of breast cancer:

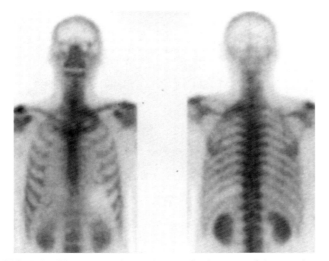

**FIG. 1-26.** These anterior and posterior images of thorax show increased uptake in the left first rib (Pancoast syndrome).

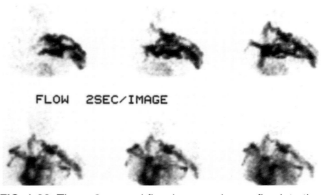

FLOW 2SEC/IMAGE

**FIG. 1-28.** These 2-second flow images show reflux into the right jugular and left axillary veins with extensive collaterals but with flow maintained into the SVC, suggesting partial SVC obstruction.

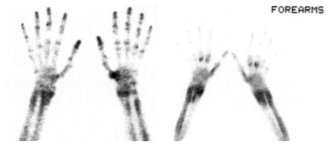

FOREARMS

A,B

**FIG. 1-27. (A)** Forearm and hand views show periosteal new bone formation corresponding with plain-film findings of HPOA. Increased uptake in distal phalanges corresponds with clubbing and distal long bone uptake. **(B)** The forearm periosteal new bone ("tram tracking") shows up more dramatically in the distal forearm bones and midulna.

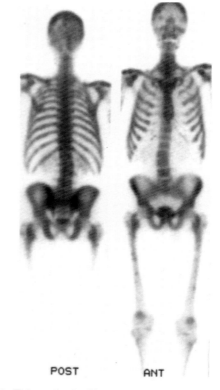

POST          ANT

**FIG. 1-29.** This patient with prostate cancer presents with a Superscan. The scan has excellent skeletal uptake for a patient of this age and reduced soft-tissue, renal, and bladder tracer. Important additional clues to Superscans include minor focal lesions identified in skull vault and long bones, as seen here.

many as 10% of end-stage lung cancer patients present with the clinical and scan features of HPOA. HPOA typically involves the long bones of forearm distally (see Fig. 1-27) and the knee region. The scan usually indicates a more extensive and symmetric involvement of the skeleton than is demonstrated radiographically (38). These patients complain of bone pain that corresponds to sites of periosteal new bone formation seen on the scan or plain-film radiographs. The symptoms of HPOA usually respond to surgery or XRT, even when palliative in nature.

Patients with lung cancer and hilar lymph node involvement may have partial or complete superior vena caval obstruction diagnosed at the time of radiopharmaceutical injection (Fig. 1-28).

### Prostate Cancer

Approximately 85% of patients with prostate cancer eventually develop skeletal metastases, and 35% have metastases at

the time of diagnosis. Half the patients with bone metastases are asymptomatic, in contrast to lung cancer patients, in whom pain is frequently present. As in breast cancer, a correlation between skeletal metastases and tumor size exists (see Table 1-9). Because of the relatively slow growth rate of prostate

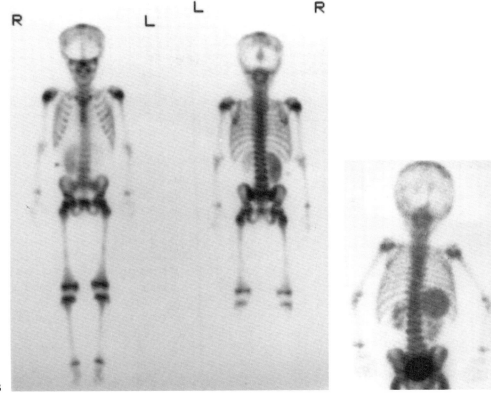

A,B

**FIG. 1-30. (A)** This image shows a patient with neuroblastoma treated with XRT. The scan shows hypertrophy of the right kidney, the left being affected by the XRT to the neuroblastoma. There are minor asymmetries of the femoral shafts and skull vault suspicious for marrow metastases. **(B)** The pretreatment image of another patient shows tracer uptake in the patient's known right neuroblastoma but no evidence of metastatic disease.

skeletal metastases and their responsiveness to hormonal manipulation, an important management role exists for bone scanning if radical prostatectomy is planned. Prostate cancer has a propensity for osteoblastic lesions, and patients may present with the atypical scan finding of involvement of a large portion of long bones in patterns that simulate Paget's disease. Prostate cancer patients may also present with a Superscan, which probably reflects the long-term survival of such patients with very slow progression of skeletal metastases (Fig. 1-29).

PSA has assumed an important role in prostate cancer management: When the PSA level is normal, the scan is usually normal. When PSA rises in the presence of a normal bone scan, local recurrence rather than skeletal metastases is suggested (39). When the bone scan is abnormal in the presence of normal PSA levels, x-rays can often establish a benign etiology for the scan finding. If the PSA is <8 ng/ml, usually no skeletal metastases are present (40). A rising PSA with abnormal bone scan confirms skeletal metastases and the need for systemic therapy (39,40). In patients treated with orchiectomy or with antiandrogen therapy, PSA evaluations are less reliable. Patients may show progressive abnormal bone scan findings that precede PSA elevations.

### Neuroblastoma

Neuroblastoma is one of the common malignancies of childhood, with a peak incidence in 2 to 3 year olds. These tumors are highly malignant with a tendency to metastasize to bone, especially the long bone metaphyses, skull vault, vertebrae, ribs, and pelvis. Prognosis is best in those children diagnosed when <1 year of age (by which time 40% already have distant metastases). Seventy percent of older children have distant metastases at diagnosis. Bone scan tracer is taken up by 35% to 60% of the primary neuroblastomas. Some skeletal metastases are photopenic, and the typical metaphyseal metastases may be technically difficult to identify by scan, giving a 10% false-negative rate. The scan is more sensitive than are plain films, in which 30% to 70% of the lesions may be missed. A subset of patients with disease confined to the liver, skin, and bone marrow (stage IV-S) do well. In this subset of patients, care must be taken not to confuse marrow disease with bone metastases (Fig. 1-30). NDA-approved radiopharmaceuticals that can be used in neuroblastoma include I-131–meta-iodobenzylguanidine for diagnosis and therapy, and In-111–octreotide for diagnosis (but not treatment).

### Primary Bone Tumors

#### Malignant Bone Tumors

Primary malignant bone tumors are rare, representing only 0.3% of total cancers. They have a bimodal age presentation: a peak in the younger age group with another

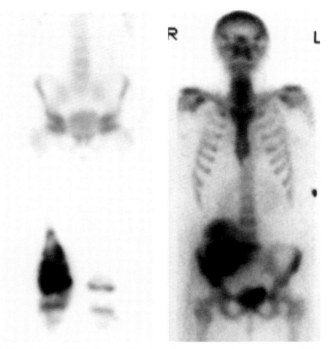

A,B

**FIG. 1-31. (A)** Patient with classic osteogenic sarcoma. This image is displayed to demonstrate the typical variability of tracer uptake within the lesion. **(B)** A pelvic extraosseous osteosarcoma is shown in the right pelvis.

peak extending into the sixth decade. These tumors present with similar symptoms: pain, swelling, and sometimes fracture at the tumor site. In all primary tumors except myeloma, the bone scan is very abnormal. In myeloma, the scan is abnormal in approximately half of the lesions detected by x-ray, although most patients have some scan lesions. The myeloma patient does not excite an osteoblastic response (see Fig. 1-18) to the marrow infiltration with tumor cells, which accounts for the reduced sensitivity.

The three common bone sarcomas can develop in pre-existing benign disease conditions:

- Osteosarcoma—Paget's and irradiated bone
- Chondrosarcoma—enchondromas, chondrodysplasia, and Paget's
- Fibrosarcoma—fibrous dysplasia

The role of bone scanning is limited diagnostically in these primary malignant tumors of bone because they produce nonspecific findings at the primary tumor site, that is, intense uptake of tracer corresponding to the clinical mass (Fig. 1-31). The lesion site and radiographic features usually classify tumor type sufficiently accurately. The extent of disease beyond the obvious mass can be misleading on bone scanning because tumor-associated hyperemia can suggest tumor extension beyond the true tumor margin.

There are numerous histologic forms of osteosarcomas, which have significant clinical differences; three-fourths are the conventional type that affect tubular bones and involve

the typical younger age group. Some appear to start beyond the bone (parosteal) and some are extraskeletal in origin (see Fig. 1-31). A childhood form with multiple sites (2% total tumors) may represent either a true multifocal primary lesion or metastases appearing synchronously with the primary lesion.

Bone scans are now part of the routine osteosarcoma patient follow-up for the detection of skeletal, soft-tissue, lymph node, and pulmonary metastases. Recent advances in treatment have increased the life expectancy of these patients. Bone scanning was limited to patients with known lung metastases and bone pain because skeletal spread rarely preceded lung metastases. With adjuvant therapy, patients are now found who have bone as the first site of recurrence.

Ewing's sarcoma is more difficult to specifically identify radiographically from other etiologies of painful masses. A triple-phase bone scan (TPBS) can exclude some of the common differential diagnoses, including myeloma, lymphoma, and eosinophilic granuloma. The latter lesions all have a relatively normal TPBS study. In Ewing's sarcoma there may be bone and pulmonary metastases at presentation, so bone scanning is indicated in all patients. In approximately one-third of patients, the skeleton is either the first or the only site of metastasis, and bone scanning is more sensitive than x-rays for detecting metastases. Survival is limited to those who receive prompt therapy, and regular and repeated bone scan screening is routinely performed on these patients.

### Benign Bone Tumors

Benign bone tumors generally do not elicit as much reactive new bone formation as malignant tumors and are not very "hot" on bone scans. Bone islands, enchondromas, exostoses (osteochondromas), and chondroblastomas are benign lesions with increase in tracer uptake varying from none to some. In multiple exostoses, the lesions with tracer uptake that exceeds that of neighboring bone may have an increased risk of malignant transformation, especially if located in the axial skeleton. The benign tumor exceptions with increased uptake include osteoid osteomas and osteoblastomas, aneurysmal bone cysts, and benign giant cell tumors.

### Osteoid Osteomas

The osteoid osteomas are the second most common benign bone tumor after enchondroma and are particularly suited to bone scan examination. The lesion is composed of osteoid and woven bone and is commonly located in the cortex of long bones. A dense reactive sclerosis occurs in the common subset called *cortical osteoid osteoma*. Patients are young and male and present with pain, which may be referred to another site, hence the advantage of the bone scan to image a large area around the symptomatic region.

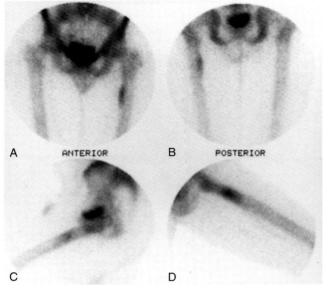

**FIG. 1-32.** Left femoral cortical osteoid osteoma. **(A)** The anterior and **(B)** posterior views demonstrate the cortical site. **(C)** The lateral view demonstrates the nidus, **(D)** the medial view the surrounding target zone sclerosis.

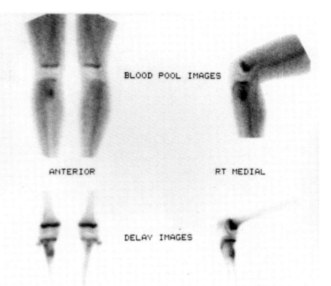

**FIG. 1-33.** An unusual case of BCD with increased perfusion, increased blood pool, and increased delayed uptake. The patient is a teenager and the lesion is undergoing sclerosis, explaining this visualization.

Other types of osteoid osteoma include the cancellous or medullary forms and the rare subperiosteal form, which have either mild or no reactive sclerosis and which occur at intra-articular or juxta-articular sites, most commonly in the hip. Fifty percent of osteoid osteomas occur in the long bones of the leg, and 30% occur in either the neural arch of the lumbar spine, the hand, or the foot (41).

All three stages of the TPBS are abnormal, and delayed images demonstrate a target lesion in the cortical subtypes (Fig. 1-32), with the most intense bull's-eye abnormality corresponding to the vascular nidus and the lesser uptake of the target zone corresponding to the radiographic and histologic sclerosis. The scan is very sensitive, and a normal scan effectively rules out the diagnosis of osteoid osteoma. The natural history of this lesion is for ultimate spontaneous remission if treatment is not required for pain. Osteoblastomas are large (>1.5 cm), less painful osteoid osteomas that have a natural history of progressive growth rather than spontaneous remission.

*Cystic Lesions*

Cystic lesions, such as benign cortical defects (BCDs), simple or unicameral bony cysts, aneurysmal bone cysts, and giant cell tumors, represent a spectrum of bone scan lesions. The flow and delayed image uptake seen on TPBS ranges from normal (BCDs) to intense (giant cell tumors). BCDs have no increase in flow or uptake, except during the normal sclerosing phase that occurs in adolescence (Fig. 1-33). Simple bone cysts show abnormalities only when complicated by incidental fractures, whereas aneurysmal

bone cysts show a slight flow and static abnormality at the rim of the lesion, and giant cell tumors show intense flow and static tracer abnormalities throughout the entire lesion.

*Histiocytosis X*

Histiocytosis X is a group of rare diseases that vary from monostotic eosinophilic granuloma to a neoplastic form called *Letterer-Siwe disease*. The most common form is the benign unifocal eosinophilic granuloma, which occurs in children, usually involves the skull or rib, is asymptomatic until fracture or bone erosion occurs, and remits spontaneously. Hand-Schüller-Christian disease is known as *multifocal eosinophilic granuloma* and involves children <5 years of age; 30% have associated exophthalmos or diabetes insipidus, and 50% have involvement of the liver, spleen, or lymph nodes. Letterer-Siwe disease is the most malignant form, affects infants and involves all organs, and requires chemotherapy with vinblastine and prednisone. The bone scan is not as sensitive as radiographs in the characterization of these lesions.

## ORTHOPEDIC INDICATIONS

### Trauma and Athletic Injuries

The scan in athletes provides functional information that influences management by confirming the presence of a significant injury with significant associated repair. The ability to screen large areas of the body without additional radiation exposure is exploited when there is the possibility that referred pain is present, as in lower back, hip, and knee conditions. When looking for lower limb stress fractures in this population exposed to repeated trauma, the entire lower limbs should be imaged to detect additional sites and provide a baseline for future scans. Occasionally, the scan is used to make a clinical diagnosis rather than assess the severity of the process; the point tenderness associated with fracture of the os trigonum is a nearly identical clinical presentation to that in Achilles tendonitis, yet the former scan has a small focal medial os calcis abnormality and the latter a diffuse posterior process.

### Stress Fractures and Periosteal Reactions

These injuries result from repetitive trauma associated with prolonged exercise, especially in individuals who are not physically conditioned or when an exercise program is changed to involve unaccustomed bones and muscles. The classic example is the march fracture of boot camp trainees, in which 1% to 30% of recruits have been reported to develop hot spots on bone scan at the symptomatic site, while the x-ray is normal. If stress continues, bone resorption continues and microfractures develop, indicating that the repair process is not able to keep up with the resorptive process. This ultimately progresses to cortical disruption, and the lesion becomes radiographically visible as a lucent line and may ultimately fracture. If the patient rests and the stress decreases, the repair continues, and the pain abates. The bone scan findings develop earlier than the x-ray changes and have been graded according to size of the increased cortical activity and whether this becomes sufficiently large and fusiform to appear larger than the cortex on the scan image. Typical sites for athletic stress fractures include the following (Fig. 1-34):

- Tibial and fibular shaft
- Medial aspect of femoral neck
- Inferior pubic ramus
- Metatarsals and os calcis
- Navicular and tarsal sesamoids

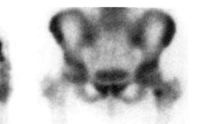

A,B

**FIG. 1-34. (A)** Intense focal uptake in the distal portion of the third metatarsal. Note the moderate increase in the entire third metatarsal indicating mild associated hyperemia to the bone. **(B)** The pelvis shows osteitis pubis and a stress fracture of the left femoral neck.

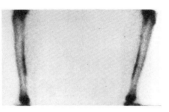

**FIG. 1-35.** Classic shin splints where the abnormality involves a long portion of the posteromedial tibia in contrast to the more focal stress fracture.

There is evidence that at-risk populations show scan abnormalities in both symptomatic and asymptomatic individuals, suggesting that the scan is too sensitive. The incidence of stress fractures is high in recruits even on arrival at boot camp before training begins (42). A possible explanation for this high incidence of scan stress fractures may be preparatory exercise in unaccustomed individuals before arrival at camp.

### Periostitis

Shin splints are a very common athletic disorder, representing a periostitis associated with the unaccustomed use of the soleus muscle when the heel is pronated. This results in increased uptake associated in the posteromedial aspect of the tibia (Fig. 1-35). These lesions extend over long regions of the tibia in contrast to the very focal nature of the stress fracture. The shin splints syndrome is but one of a series of conditions due to injuries of muscle, tendon, or ligamentous insertions to bone that elicit a periostitis detected by scan. Other typical conditions include

- Osteitis pubis (see Fig. 1-34)
- Plantar fasciitis
- Achilles tendonitis
- Patellar tendonitis (43)
- Trochanteric bursitis
- Muscle insertions in the femur
- Inflammation of sesamoid bones

### Fracture

The general description of the bone scan appearance of fractures is documented; in the young population, bone scans are usually abnormal on the day of fracture, but in the elderly, the appearance of a scan abnormality is delayed (Fig. 1-36). Initially this delay in bone scan abnormality appearance was presumed to be related to patient age (44), but investigators have suggested the difference in time of appearance of scan lesion is more likely related to the fracture site (45).

Early scans show an increase in tracer to much of the fractured bone, suggesting hyperemia, whereas later images demonstrate osteoblastic activity at the fracture site (45), as evidenced by

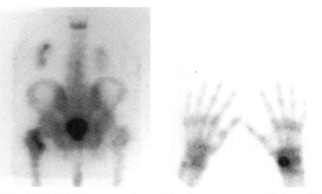

A,B

FIG. 1-36. (A) This posterior pelvis view shows an 11-day-old unsuspected intertrochanteric fracture that was subsequently pinned. Incidental note is made of an unsuspected fracture of the T11 vertebra. (B) The hand views show a 6-week-old (scan abnormality maximum at this time) carpal navicular fracture imaged through the cast.

TABLE 1-10. *Time for fracture scan abnormality to normalize*

|  | 1 year | 2 years | 3 years |
| --- | --- | --- | --- |
| Vertebra | 60% | 90% | 97% |
| Long bones | 65% | 90% | 95% |
| Ribs | 80% | 90% | 100% |
| Other bones | 60% | 90% | 95% |

Source: Adapted from Matin P. The appearance of bone scans following fractures, including immediate and long-term studies. J Nucl Med 1979;20:1227–1231.

- Regional hyperemia within 24 hours
- Extent and intensity of uptake depend on the bone involved and are greatest adjacent to joints; some axial and long bone shaft sites may take 10 to 12 days to become abnormal
- Increased uptake over the next 2 to 3 weeks
- Maximal uptake 2 to 5 weeks after trauma
- Irrelevance of patient age and gender

The scan abnormality then regresses over the next 3 years, with the minimum time to normal being 6 months and most (~97%) becoming normal by 3 years (Table 1-10). If open reduction and fixation are required, then only half of patients have a normal scan at 3 years. An uncommon but important medicolegal indication for a bone scan is dating fractures to work-related episodes. If a patient presents with a radiographic vertebral compression fracture and dates it to an episode 2 months earlier, yet the scan is normal, it suggests that the radiographic finding is not of recent origin.

Particular scan patterns of the ribs, vertebrae, and sacrum suggest trauma. Rib fractures typically occur in rows involving the adjacent ribs that were subject to the trauma. Solitary traumatic rib lesions are rare except in gymnasts, who suffer solitary posterior rib lesions beneath the scapula. Single costovertebral and costochondral lesions do occur with lesser trauma that causes disruption of the anterior and posterior rib attachment sites. In lateral rib fractures when the arc of

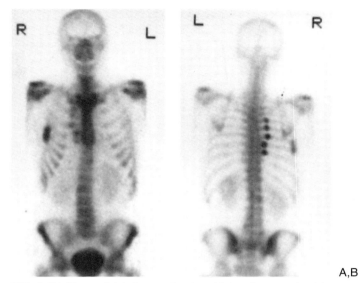

A,B

FIG. 1-37. Three right ribs are fractured laterally, seen best in (A) the anterior view, and (B) five costovertebral junctions have popped about these same ribs. Note the "shine through" of the posterior costovertebral junction abnormalities in the anterior image due to modest attenuation by air in the lungs.

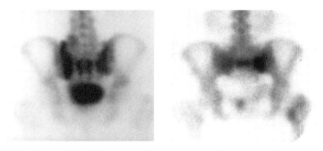

A,B

FIG. 1-38. (A) This is the Honda sign with unusual vertical sacral fractures. Note the disruption of both sacroiliac joints. (B) The half Honda sign of a sacral horizontal linear fracture with only one sacroiliac joint involved. In this instance the pelvis must be fractured elsewhere. The opposite symphysis pubis was fractured, and this is just discernible in this posterior view but is very obvious in the anterior view. Incidental note of right intertrochanteric trauma.

the rib is long and the ribs flexible, there is often associated costovertebral or costochondral junction disruption involving the same and adjacent ribs (Fig. 1-37). A classic example is cardiopulmonary resuscitation that causes ribs 1 through 3 to fracture in their anterolateral aspects, their shorter radii making them more susceptible to fracture along the arc. The lower ribs "pop" at the costochondral or costovertebral junctions. Vertebral fractures can involve just the superior or inferior plate, and occasionally several vertebral fractures can be associated with popped neighboring costovertebral junctions.

Sacral fractures are usually associated with SI joint disruptions, and if this SI disruption is unilateral, pelvic fractures must be associated (Fig. 1-38).

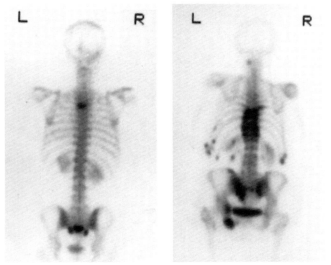

A,B

**FIG. 1-39. (A)** This image shows an unsuspected lower sacral and upper thoracic vertebra fracture in a patient being imaged for skeletal metastases. **(B)** This image shows, in another patient, multiple unsuspected trauma sites with a Honda sign of sacral-sacroiliac fractures, and associated pelvic brim, rib, and vertebral fractures. This patient had had a history of seizure and fall.

### Occult Fractures

The detection of occult fractures (fractures not obvious by conventional radiography) is an excellent use of the bone scanning technique. Such fracture sites include sacrum and coccyx (Fig. 1-39), carpal navicular (see Fig. 1-36), sternum, nondisplaced femoral neck in the elderly (see Fig. 1-36), tarso-metatarsal region, patella, pelvis, sesamoid, vertebrae (see Fig. 1-36), and other unusual fracture sites, such as the neural arch. In each situation, the scan can either establish the diagnosis or localize the site for additional imaging modalities, such as conventional tomography or thin-slice CT.

### Physical Abuse

The bone scan is frequently asked to confirm physical abuse, especially in the pediatric population, where the diagnosis should be considered in as many as 10% of childhood emergency room visits. The routine workup in this situation should include a skull view to identify fractures or spread sutures in an infant, because 25% of abused children may have subdural hematomas. A whole-body bone scan demonstrates rib fractures with exquisite sensitivity; these children often have multiple lesions with differing intensities, suggesting different ages and recurrent injuries, thus providing good evidence of physical abuse. The views of the long bones may demonstrate shaft fractures but sometimes even large amounts of old bone seen on radiographs may not be visualized on the scan because the healing process may already be complete. This discrepancy in itself can be useful if the patient has a scan lesion at another site because it would suggest repeated trauma. If the skull films and bone scan appear normal, the next investigation is plain films of the limbs to identify fractures near the epiphyses, especially of the knee, elbow, and wrist. At these sites the bone scan can be difficult to interpret without excellent image acquisition technique and exact symmetry of limbs to allow subtle differences in uptake at the growth plate regions to be identified (see Chapter 11). Nuclear medicine departments of children's hospitals are able to do this well with experienced personnel. In some instances, the pediatric sedation team may be required to assist, especially if multiple imaging procedures or other invasive tests are also required.

Abuse is not limited to children. The findings of trauma, especially linear arrays of rib fractures, can suggest spousal or elderly abuse when scans are obtained for other indications. It is common to identify alcoholism, epilepsy, or neurologic disability as the reason for repeated fractures in adults (see Fig. 1-39).

### Unexplained Pain or Limp

In children with a persistent limp or hip pain, the bone scan can identify many likely etiologies. These children require investigation of the entire lower limbs and lower back because they frequently present with referred pain. The acutely sick child of 2 to 10 years of age who is unwilling to move the hip likely has a septic arthritis or osteomyelitis; the workup is a medical emergency with x-ray and joint aspiration required. Nuclear medicine staff may be asked to investigate these patients after the initial investigation and intervention.

In patients with a long history of "irritable" hip, the workup includes a bone scan soon after the x-ray. If the bone scan is normal, the patient usually does not have a significant disease process but rather a benign transient synovitis or irritable hip syndrome. If the scan is abnormal, the differential diagnosis includes Legg-Calvé-Perthes disease, chronic osteomyelitis, osteoid osteoma, stress fracture, monoarticular rheumatoid arthritis, slipped femoral epiphysis, or avascular necrosis.

Adult chronic low back pain is a common complaint and can be due to spondylolysis, fractures, osteoid osteoma, degenerative joint disease, or sacroiliitis. All can be diagnosed by bone scan, but SPECT imaging is often required in addition to planar views of the pelvis, hips, and thoracolumbar spine (Fig. 1-40). The most common etiology in the young is spondylolysis, which becomes symptomatic at the time of the growth spurt. Spondylolysis is precipitated by repeated extension and lateral flexion of the back, as occurs with dancers, gymnasts, rowers, divers, weight lifters, swimmers, and other athletes. There is a familial tendency in approximately 60% of patients, and this tendency combined

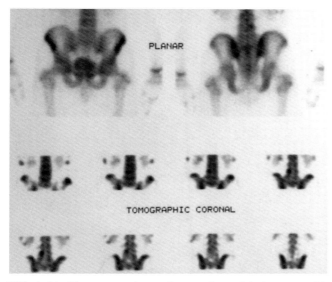

**FIG. 1-40.** Planar anterior and posterior pelvis images with minimal right-sided L4 abnormality seen. On SPECT images the spondylolysis is more apparent.

with stress results in an overall incidence of approximately 3% to 7%. Most involve the L5 vertebra. The patients do not develop neurologic deficits, such presentation being more typical of degenerative disease. The lesion starts as a stress injury to the pars interarticularis and can progress to a fracture (i.e., defect). Once a defect occurs, the process has passed from a stress fracture to spondylolysis, and participation in sports and strenuous activity will be limited. With a lesion on one side of the vertebra, stress occurs on the opposite side, leading to radiographic sclerosis. On the bone scan, bilateral abnormalities are common, and this distinguishes spondylolysis from other etiologies, such as osteoid osteoma. The use of SPECT doubles the sensitivity of the bone scan technique and is thus mandatory (46).

In older patients, chronic undiagnosed back pain is a frequent indication for bone scanning when plain films are normal. SPECT imaging can localize abnormalities to the vertebral body, pedicle, facet joints, pars interarticularis, lamina, or spinous process with careful inspection, and this can result in diagnostic information or indicate where thin-slice CT should be performed to obtain a specific diagnosis.

### Infection

Infection is discussed in detail in Chapter 8. In hematogenous osteomyelitis the TPBS is both sensitive and specific (>90%) provided the pattern of an intense focal uptake is seen in the delayed images with a blood pool abnormality and a very early flow abnormality present at the identical site. In secondary osteomyelitis—that is, infection complicating a prosthesis—past surgery or trauma, known previous scan abnormality, Charcot's joint, soft-tissue infection or ulcer, a dual study with labeled white blood cell (WBC) scan

is required to achieve sensitivities and specificities of 85% to 90% in acute osteomyelitis. Two WBC scan methods are available: In-111 WBC scanning can be performed simultaneously with the bone scan, or Tc-99m WBC scanning can be done 2 days after the bone scan. Similar specificities are obtained in acute and chronic osteomyelitis if the process is appendicular (47). The presence of chronic osteomyelitis in the central skeleton is more difficult to diagnose because labeled leukocytes accumulate in active bone marrow. False negatives do occur in central sites, where the WBC scan can display a photopenic defect (48). In these situations and when infection about a prosthesis is suspected, marrow imaging agents combined with WBC scans have been more helpful (49). It is possible that Tc-99m WBC scans may be useful in this condition because it behaves like both a marrow scan (1-hour images) and a WBC scan (4-hour images).

Detection of septic arthritis or discitis hinges on the ability to demonstrate abnormalities on both sides of the infected joint or disc. When cellulitis is present in a limb, the generalized increase in tracer uptake due to hyperemia is not marked, so an additional intense focal osteoblastic response within a region of slight diffusely increased uptake makes the diagnosis of osteomyelitis likely. In neonatal osteomyelitis, there may be considerable false-negative studies in the first 40 days of life.

### Viability

Viability includes such diverse conditions as graft viability, frostbite injury, and avascular necrosis. These are infrequent clinical indications for a scan, but the presence of tracer uptake into a graft, into the bone of a frostbitten digit or limb, or into bone suspected of avascular necrosis indicates viability.

### *Graft Viability*

Allografts to the limb, axial skeleton, and corallin hydroxyapatite ocular implants can show vascularization of the graft by the demonstration of uptake of bone agent. Initially these grafts appear as photopenic defects, but with vitalization there is uptake of tracer as a result of vascularization and osteoblastic repopulation of the grafted bone. In grafts with vascular supply transposed at the time of operation, the graft can show uptake from the time of grafting.

### *Frostbite Injury*

In frostbite injury, a TPBS at 48 hours is an excellent indicator of viability of the involved bone. If the bone is viable, as demonstrated by uptake in the delayed images (Fig. 1-41), limb or digit amputation is not required. The study does not alter the ultimate outcome but does allow the physician to be more accurate in prognostication (50).

2 days after injury          2 days later

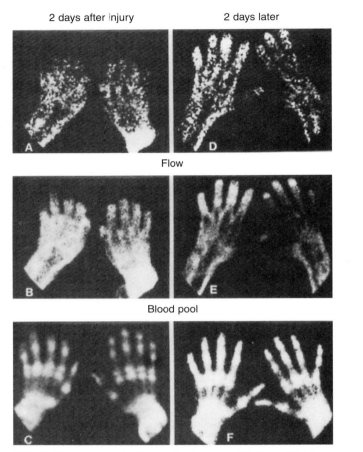

Flow

Blood pool

**FIG. 1-41.** Scans of both hands showing **(A)** flow, **(B)** blood pool, and **(C)** delayed images 2 days after exposure. The delayed images show uptake in all bones confirming deep tissue viability despite flow abnormality. The follow-up studies show **(D)** hyperemia, **(E)** increased blood pool, and **(F)** normal bone uptake. These digits required debridement only. (Reprinted with permission from Mehta RC, Wilson MA. Frostbite injury: prediction of tissue viability with triple-phase bone scanning. Radiology 1989;170:511–514.)

### Osteonecrosis

Osteonecrosis results from death of the marrow cells and osteocytes due to underlying vascular insufficiency from interruption of blood supply (traumatic disruption, nitrogen bubble formation, sickle-cell disease [Fig. 1-42]) or swelling of the marrow contents (steroid treatment, Legg-Calvé-Perthes disease). The bone marrow compartment is unusual because of the bone surroundings, so that swelling within this rigid compartment results in increasing ischemia and subsequent infarction. In the acute ischemic stage, a surgical core decompression procedure can prevent necrosis. Prolonged non–weight bearing of affected joints can prevent secondary degenerative changes of the infarcted region and allow bone repair. For either form of therapy to be effective early diagnosis of the disease must be made. In the very early stages of the disease, the scan demonstrates a photon-

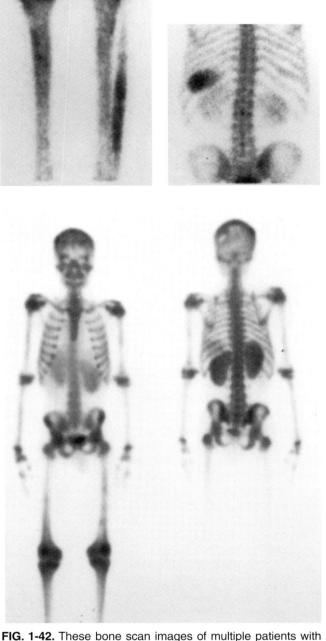

**FIG. 1-42.** These bone scan images of multiple patients with sickle-cell disease show **(A)** a fibular and tibial abnormality due to repair of long bone infarction and **(B)** splenic infarction with associated tracer uptake. The lower images show other features of sickle cell disease and expanded bone marrow **(C)** with subtle long bone lesions and large "hot" kidneys (especially at symptomatic times) with subtle splenic visualization in the posterior view. In the posterior image a photopenic skull vault lesion of recent infarction is apparent.

deficient region of ischemia (51), and within 4 to 8 weeks a very active osteoblastic response occurs. Lesions involving the long bone shafts, sites common in dysbaric osteonecrosis (caisson disease), do not result in important clinical sequelae.

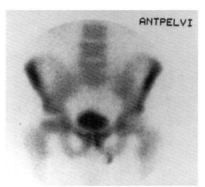

FIG. 1-43. Delayed anterior bone scan images in young patient with early osteonecrosis of right femoral head, shown as decreased uptake compared to left femoral head.

Bone scanning is exquisitely sensitive at the early stage of disease (Fig. 1-43), whereas radiographic modalities usually only demonstrate the late findings. Bone marrow edema is present on MRI in the early stage of osteonecrosis and is equivalent to the photopenic stage of bone scanning.

## Postsurgical Changes

Postsurgical changes occur with a similar time course to that of trauma. This is especially important to account for when complications of surgery are being sought and when the normal postsurgical repair can be confused with the complication; examples include osteomyelitis of the sternum post-coronary artery bypass graft versus the effect of sternotomy. Four separate processes require further explanation: nonunion, pseudoarthrosis, loosening of prosthetic joints, and reflex sympathetic dystrophy (RSD).

### Nonunion

Nonunion is defined as failure of fracture healing within 6 to 8 months, and it occurs most often in weight-bearing bones. The scan can show nonunion either with an increase in tracer uptake (reactive nonunion) or with the absence of tracer uptake (atrophic nonunion). Reactive nonunion may respond to conservative management with electrical stimulation but atrophic nonunion requires surgical intervention. Appropriate profiling of the fracture site may display a photopenic region and correctly identify the problem as atrophic nonunion and the need for surgery.

### Pseudoarthrosis

Pseudoarthrosis development in patients after fusion procedures of the lumbar spine, knee, hind foot, and wrist is usually signified by abnormally intense tracer localization in a small portion of the fusion site at a time when the remainder of the fusion site has returned to normal. This occurs in

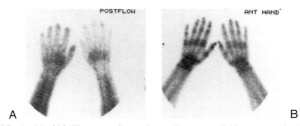

FIG. 1-44. (A) The postflow view show a mild increase in the right side (left) when compared to the left side. (B) The delayed view shows a mild but typical pattern of periarticular uptake in the right wrist and hand (marker side).

10% to 30% of patients (52). SPECT imaging may be helpful in explaining the pain and in separating fusion failure (hot spot in fusion site) from changes that frequently occur above and below the fusion level that may be the effect of the initial disease process.

### Reflex Sympathetic Dystrophy

RSD is a little-understood complication of a minor injury that represents a major problem because many patients develop permanent disability and do not resume prior activities. The precipitant is usually trivial; for example, 7% to 35% of patients with Colles' fracture develop this complication. There is agreement that the condition is caused by an abnormal sympathetic system. Classically, RSD has been divided into three stages: a warm phase of 2 to 3 months, a phase of vascular instability that lasts for several months, and a final cold phase (4). This universality of process has not been confirmed in a large study (53), where one-sixth of patients present with initial "cold" rather than hyperemic ("warm") symptoms. Several clinical signs and symptoms that either occur at rest or are elicited by exercise are required for the diagnosis of RSD. These include pain, edema, discoloration, temperature changes, and decreased function. With time, atrophic changes of the skin and soft tissues and a regional osteoporosis develop. In upper limb RSD, the typical scan appearance is of increased periarticular tracer uptake of all the joints of the hand and wrist in delayed images (Fig. 1-44). The flow and blood pool portion of the study is neither a sensitive nor specific indicator of the condition. Investigators have shown that with the hyperemic scan findings of RSD, corticosteroid therapy was more likely to be effective. A subset of patients have atypical scan findings with a decrease in flow blood pool and delayed uptake of tracer. This cold form of RSD occurs more frequently in the lower limb and younger patients.

### Prostheses

Prosthetic loosening is a very common long-term complication of joint replacement, and this diagnosis needs to be separated from osteomyelitis (54). Many modifications of the

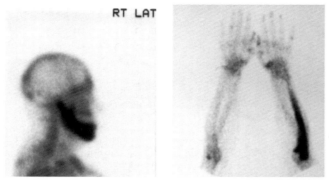

RT LAT

A,B

**FIG. 1-45. (A)** Paget's disease typically involves the entire bone, in this case the mandible. The abnormality may start from one end of a bone and eventually extend to the entire bone. **(B)** This is especially so in long bones with proximal involvement initially, here the ulna.

prosthesis itself (e.g., cementing, bonding agents, porosity) and the method of insertion have been attempted unsuccessfully to reduce the incidence of loosening. These procedural changes in themselves result in different scan appearances at various times after the surgery (54,55). Although the infected prosthesis classically has a positive TPBS and diffuse delayed bone scan abnormality involving the entire prosthesis and usually both sides of the prosthetic joint, this same pattern can also occur with loosening. Usually a loose prosthesis has only a mild abnormality on the TPBS, and focal abnormalities on the delayed images are classically limited to the tip of the prosthesis and in the region of the lesser trochanter. Serial imaging shows progression of the abnormality in loosening. The tip abnormality especially involving the lateral aspect is considered a more specific sign of loosening (55).

## MISCELLANEOUS APPLICATIONS

### Paget's Disease and Fibrous Dysplasia

Paget's disease is a common disease that is usually asymptomatic; it is rare in people under age 40. The incidence rises with age thereafter, and 10% of patients >90 have the condition. The disease is generally polyostotic (85%), and whole-body bone scanning (more sensitive than plain-film detection) is ideal for detection. There are examples of pagetic lesions seen on plain films not seen on bone scan, and although these were initially thought of as areas of "burnt-out" Paget's, they may occur in as many as 20% of x-ray–proven sites. When they occur, there is no evidence that they are the result of end-stage Paget's. Rather, they occur in Paget's disease of all typical x-ray stages. Decreases in bone scan abnormalities occur more often with treatment with diphosphonates (10% of lesions respond completely, 65% to some extent, and the remaining 25% not at all).

The distribution of pagetic bone in individual patients is as follows and reflects the polyostotic nature of the disease:

- Pelvis: 75%
- Lumbar spine and femur: 50% each site
- Thoracic spine, sacrum, and skull: 40% each site
- Tibia, femur, and scapula: 30% each site
- All other sites: 5% to 10% (56)

In men, seven sites are typically involved, five in women (56).

The general pattern of bone scan abnormality is intense tracer uptake involving the entire bone, although long bones may be often only partly involved, usually first involving the proximal epiphyses (Fig. 1-45). Paget's starts from one end of the bone and ultimately involves the entire bone. Although x-rays show expansion of bones, the apparent increase in bone size on the scan is due to septal penetration as a result of the intense local tracer uptake. The centimeter resolution of bone scanning precludes identification of the millimeter expansion of bone seen radiographically. The progression seen in the disease reflects an increase in the extent of involvement of individual bones rather than the spread from one bone to another. Distal involvement is unusual except in cancellous bone (e.g., os calcis).

Complications of Paget's include abnormal bone shape, compression of nerves, and malignant transformation. Although osteosarcoma is a rare complication of Paget's (<1%), it represents a common form of osteosarcoma in the elderly population.

Fibrous dysplasia is another benign skeletal disorder that may be confused radiographically with Paget's disease or osteoblastic metastases. This condition usually starts in early childhood and becomes quiescent once skeletal growth ends. The monostotic form occurs in 15% to 30% of patients, and when polyostotic, the lesions tend to be unilateral, often confined to a single limb, and associated with skin pigmentation and endocrine abnormalities (e.g., Albright's syndrome of precocious puberty with café-au-lait spots and polyostotic fibrous dysplasia). The order of skeletal involvement is ribs, tibia, femur, and craniofacial bones. Many patients develop pathologic fractures in the lesions. As in Paget's disease, a small number of these can transform into malignant tumors, usually fibrosarcomas.

Osteopoikilosis and melorheostosis are rare forms of benign sclerotic disease with striking x-ray findings: The bone scan is normal in osteopoikilosis and very abnormal (diffuse increase in tracer uptake) in melorheostosis.

### Diffuse Skeletal Scan Abnormalities

The classic metabolic bone diseases that cause scan abnormalities are renal osteodystrophy, hyperparathyroidism, hyperthyroidism, and osteomalacia; these are well described (57). In all patients there is very significant increase in the skeletal uptake of bone tracer, more than doubling the normal uptake. This process is generalized and results in excellent skeletal uptake with little renal and soft-tissue visualization. The increase is generalized so the

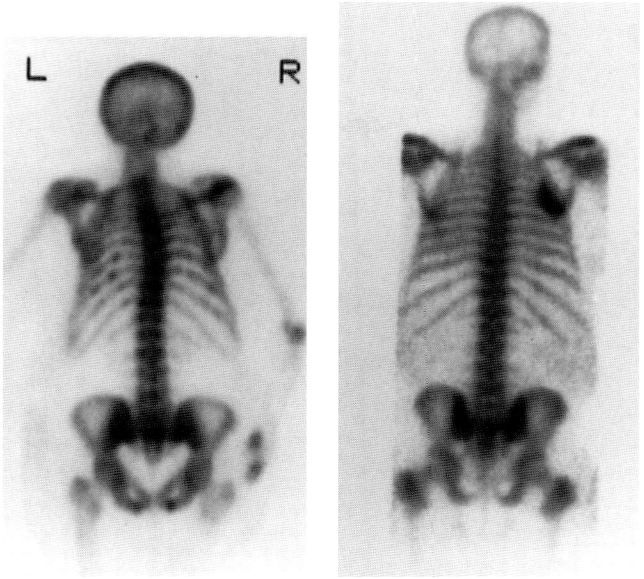

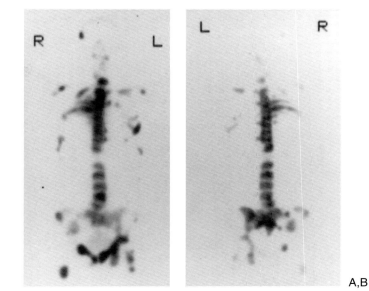

A,B

**FIG. 1-46. (A)** This posterior view shows no renal activity, reduced soft-tissue activity, and numerous rib and pelvic lesions typical of pseudofractures. These are the typical scan findings of osteomalacia. **(B)** Increased uptake through the entire posterior skeleton with brown tumor of the right scapula. The soft tissue and absent renal visualization confirm renal disease.

**FIG. 1-47.** All the tracer is taken up by metastatic sites with no soft-tissue renal or normal skeleton visualized. **(A)** Anterior view, **(B)** posterior view. If the disease was more diffuse this would have the appearance of a Superscan.

appendicular skeleton is seen as well as the axial skeleton. In addition, there may be particularly good visualization of the calvarium, mandible, costochondral junctions, and sternum. Other bone scan features can be superimposed: brown tumors in hyperparathyroidism, pseudofractures in osteomalacia (Fig. 1-46), and pulmonary and gastric visualization associated with hypercalcemia.

Other forms of diffuse involvement of skeleton include the Superscan. Here the scan is abnormal with excellent uptake into the axial skeleton. This was first described in a lymphoma patient and then identified in genitourinary tumors, especially prostatic cancer (58,59). The scans show axial predominance, reduced or absent renal visualization, absent appendicular uptake, and subtle asymmetries of the rib, skull vault, and proximal long bones (60) that indicate the true nature of the disease: extensive diffuse metastatic disease such that little or no soft tissue, renal, or normal bone is visualized (see Fig. 1-29). This condition should be considered when the bone scan appears to be of a quality that seems too good for the patient's stated age. A variant of this is in more focal but very extensive metastatic disease, in which all of the tracer is taken up into metastases, and soft tissue, renal, and normal skeleton are not visualized (Fig. 1-47). Another diffuse scan abnormality is that of HPOA already described with lung cancer (see Fig. 1-27).

The diffuse increased tracer uptake pattern is also seen in marrow expansion due to various blood dyscrasias, including myelofibrosis, sickle-cell disease, and neoplastic marrow infiltration (Fig. 1-48). These patterns of expanded marrow regions tend to be proximal limb abnormalities and to involve juxta-articular regions. Lymphoma has a predilection for asymmetric periarticular uptake (60). All these causes of marrow expansion are disease processes, but cytokines have been identified as showing similar patterns of scan abnormality in as many as 60% of recipients of colony-stimulating factor (61).

**Soft-Tissue Uptake**

This subject of soft-tissue uptake is well reviewed in *Radiographics* (62). Heterotopic ossification presents as a posttraumatic increase in tracer localization in the muscles and soft tissues (63). The clinical presentation can resemble a severe soft-tissue inflammation (i.e., abscess formation). It occurs commonly around regions of orthopedic surgery, especially prosthetic hip replacement, and was very common in paraplegia until etidronate was prescribed routinely. The scan finding is nonspecific but shows intense tracer localization in the region of the dystrophic calcification, with TPBS flow and blood pool abnormalities that cannot be separated from parosteal osteosarcomas, soft-tissue sarcomas, and synovial osteochondromatosis. The bone scan is more sensitive than plain film in the detection of early myositis ossificans (Fig. 1-49). When the scan is abnormal, active soft-tissue calcification is occurring, and surgery to remove calcification should be deferred until the process is quiescent to prevent extension of the myositis. Variants include fibrodysplasia ossificans progressiva, which was the first disease for which etidronate was prescribed before its introduction as a bone scanning agent.

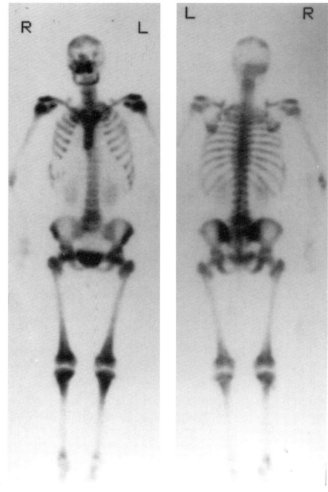

A,B

**FIG. 1-48. (A)** This anterior and **(B)** posterior whole-body scan shows a neutropenic patient with an expanded marrow cavity (note especially shoulders, hips, and knees). Incidental note is made of jaw reconstruction (graft is anterior portion of right seventh rib) and stable L5/S1 spinal fusion.

## SPECT

The role of SPECT is unrivaled in myocardial perfusion scans, liver scanning, brain scanning, and some orthopedic indications. The hip, knee, lumbar spine, and temporomandibular joints (TMJs) are accepted indications. SPECT increases the sensitivity of the scanning procedure by 25% to 50% despite a decrease in resolution that results from the tomographic nature of the technique, which eliminates overlying and underlying regions. The role of SPECT in low back pain has been discussed (64,65). The use of SPECT in examination of the hip is established, although the bladder activity artifact makes this technically difficult. The role in the knee is more controversial, but it appears that significant patellofemoral osteoarthritis, meniscal tears, synovitis, and intra-articular loose bodies result in an abnormal SPECT scan that would justify further expensive or invasive proce-

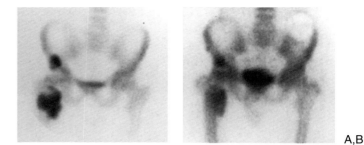

A,B

**FIG. 1-49.** Intense soft-tissue localization of tracer **(A)** about the right hip (acetabulum and intertrochanteric region) that 9 months later shows considerable regression **(B)**.

dures in a patient with chronic knee pain (66). The use in the TMJ is also established (67). SPECT does require very strict instrument QC.

## BONE MARROW IMAGING

Bone marrow scanning is done with Tc-99m sulfur colloid, of which only 5% to 8% goes to the marrow. Bone marrow scanning identifies significant reticuloendothelial function, and the red marrow is usually well demarcated. When antimony sulfide was available, the smaller colloid size made this the preferred agent for lymphoscintigraphy and bone marrow imaging. Because the agent is preferentially taken up in the liver and spleen, these organs obscure the adjacent marrow regions of the axial skeleton and, in effect, only the shoulder girdle, pelvis, and limbs are well visualized. The normal distribution of the red marrow varies with age and disease states, and considerable asymmetries can exist. When the femoral heads are examined with marrow imaging, there is normal bilateral visualization in all children and teens, but approximately one-half of adults do not demonstrate femoral head uptake (68). The initial major indication of marrow scanning was osteonecrosis of the femoral heads, but the inability to identify uptake in all patients limited the utility of the procedure except when asymmetry was present.

The scan can be used to assess the distribution of hemopoietic tissues, as in myeloproliferative disorders, but the conventional bone scan often shows increased uptake in regions of marrow expansion and so provides indirect evidence of this infiltrative process. Regions of marrow decrease can also be identified, such as radiotherapy fields, tumor replacement, myeloma, and infarction, but these also are identified on bone scan.

Sickle-cell disease presents a problem when the differentiation of acute sickle cell crisis and osteomyelitis is required. Here the marrow scan can be helpful as the underlying hematologic process causes an expansion of the red marrow into the distal appendicular skeleton. The marrow scan shows focally decreased uptake in the region of a marrow infarct. The bone scan shows a photopenic lesion somewhat smaller in extent during the acute phase (69). In osteomyelitis, the bone scan lesion will be hot, whereas the marrow scan may either show no abnormality or a photopenic defect. At the moment, the most established role for marrow imaging is in infection imaging on the prosthetic joint to rule out infection (48,49,70).

Other agents have been attempted for marrow imaging, including In-111–chloride and Tc-99m minimicrocolloid (71), but they have not received FDA approval. Labeled WBCs (In-111 or Tc-99m) show marrow uptake, and could be used for marrow uptake in specific circumstances. The Tc-99m–labeled monoclonal antibody to granulocyte precursors may ultimately prove to be an excellent marrow imaging agent and become a suitable replacement for the unavailable antimony colloid (34).

## REFERENCES

1. Brown ML, Collier BD Jr, Fogelman I. Bone scintigraphy: part 1. Oncology and infection. J Nucl Med 1993;34:2236–2240.
2. Collier BD Jr, Fogelman I, Brown ML. Bone scintigraphy: part 2. Orthopedic bone scanning. J Nucl Med 1993;34:2241–2246.
3. Fogelman I, Collier BD, Brown ML. Bone scintigraphy: part 3. Bone scanning in metabolic bone disease. J Nucl Med 1993;34:2247–2252.
4. Holder LE. Clinical radionuclide bone imaging. Radiology 1990;176: 607–614.
5. Galasko CSB. Skeletal metastases and mammary cancer. Ann R Coll Surg Engl 1972;50:3–28.
6. Sandler ED, Parisi MT, Hattner RS. Duration of etidronate effect demonstrated by serial bone scintigraphy. J Nucl Med 1991;32:1782–1784.
7. Krasnow AZ, Collier BD, Isitman AT, et al. False-negative bone imaging due to etidronate disodium therapy. Clin Nucl Med 1988;13:264–267.
8. Charkes ND. Skeletal blood flow: implications for bone-scan interpretation. J Nucl Med 1980;21:91–98.
9. Molloi S, Mazess R, Bendsen H, Wilson M. Whole body and regional retention of Tc-99m–labeled diphosphonates with a whole-body counter: a study with normal males. Calcif Tissue Int 1989;44:322–329.
10. Wilson MA, Pollack MJ. Gastric visualization and image quality in radionuclide bone scanning: concise communication. J Nucl Med 1981;22:518–521.
11. Wilson MA. The effect of age on the quality of bone scans using technetium-99m pyrophosphate. Radiology 1981;139:703–705.
12. Rowe B, Zager L, Fiers D, Wilson M. A technique for automatic scaling and display of dual intensity whole body bone scans [abstract]. J Nucl Med Tech 1993;21:115.
13. Sandler ED, Hattner RS, Parisi MT, Miller TR. Clinical utility of bone scan features of pleural effusion: sensitivity and specificity for malignancy based on pleural fluid cytopathology. J Nucl Med 1994;35:429–431.
14. Wilson MA, Liss LF, Studey CL. Uptake of technetium-99m MDP in hepatic metastases. Noninv Med Imag 1984;1:253–257.
15. Wilson MA, Calhoun FW. Right renal pelvis visualization in females: incidental detection in routine bone scanning. Urol Radiol 1980;2: 25–28.
16. Lutrin CL, McDougall IR, Goris ML. Intense concentration of technetium-99m pyrophosphate in the kidneys of children treated with chemotherapeutic drugs for malignant disease. Radiology 1978;128: 165–167.
17. Galasko CSB, Doyle FH. The detection of skeletal metastases from mammary cancer. A regional comparison between radiology and scintigraphy. Clin Radiol 1972;23:295–297.
18. Galasko CSB. The pathological basis for skeletal scintigraphy. J Bone Joint Surg Br 1975;57:353–359.
19. Batson OV. The function of the vertebral veins and their role in the spread of metastases. Ann Surg 1940;112:138.
20. Wiley AM, Trueta J. The vascular anatomy of the spine and its relationship to pyogenic vertebral osteomyelitis. J Bone Joint Surg 1959;41:796–809.
21. Coman DR, DeLong RP. The role of the vertebral venous system in the metastasis of cancer to the spinal column. Cancer 1951;4:610–618.
22. Krishnamurthy GT, Tubis M, Hiss J, Blahd WH. Distribution pattern of metastatic bone disease. JAMA 1977;237:2504–2506.
23. McNeil BJ. Value of bone scanning in neoplastic disease. Semin Nucl Med 1984;14:277–285.
24. Wilson MA, Calhoun FW. The distribution of skeletal metastases in breast and pulmonary cancer: concise communication. J Nucl Med 1981;22:594–597.
25. Kwai AH, Stomper PL, Kaplan WD. Clinical significance of isolated sternal lesions in patients with breast cancer. J Nucl Med 1988;29:324–328.
26. Harbert JC, George FH, Kerner ML. Differentiation of rib fractures from metastases by bone scanning. Clin Nucl Med 1981;6:359–361.
27. Jacobson AF, Stomper PC, Jochelson MS, et al. Association between number and sites of new bone scan abnormalities and presence of skeletal metastases in patients with breast cancer. J Nucl Med 1990;31:387–392.
28. Boxer DI, Todd CEC, Coleman R, Fogelman I. Bone secondaries in breast cancer: the solitary metastasis. J Nucl Med 1989;30:1318–1320.
29. Tumeh SS, Beadle G, Kaplan WD. Clinical significance of solitary rib lesion in patients with extraskeletal malignancy. J Nucl Med 1985;26:1140–1143.
30. Durzinsky DS, Messing EM, Myerowiz D, et al. Method for assuring accuracy of bone biopsy using technetium-99 bone scan. Cancer 1987;59:723–725.
31. Algra PR, Bloem JL, Tissing H, et al. Detection of vertebral metastases: comparison between MR imaging and bone scintigraphy. Radiographics 1991;11:219–232.
32. Gosfield E, Alavi A, Kneeland B. Comparison of radionuclide bone scans and magnetic resonance imaging in detecting spinal metastases. J Nucl Med 1993;34:2191–2198.
33. Evan-Sapir E, Martin RH, Barnes DC, et al. Role of SPECT in differentiating malignant from benign lesions in the lower thoracic and lumbar vertebrae. Radiology 1993;187:193–198.
34. Duncker CM, Carrio I, Berna L, et al. Radioimmune imaging of bone marrow in patients with suspected bone metastases from primary breast cancer. J Nucl Med 1990;31:1450–1455.
35. Janicek MJ, Hayes DF, Kaplan WD. Healing flare in skeletal metastases from breast cancer. Radiology 1994;192:201–204.
36. Hellman RS, Wilson MA. Discordance of sclerosing skeletal secondaries between sequential scintigraphy and radiographs. Clin Nucl Med 1982;7:97–99.
37. Hattner RS, Hartmeyer J, Wara WM. Characterization of radiation-induced photopenic abnormalities on bone scans. Radiology 1982;145:161–163.
38. Ali A, Tetalman MR, Fordham EW, et al. Distribution of hypertrophic pulmonary osteoarthropathy. AJR Am J Roentgenol 1980;134: 771–780.
39. Terris MK, Klonecke AS, McDougall IR, Stamey TA. Utilization of bone scan in conjunction with prostate-specific antigen levels in the surveillance for recurrence of adenocarcinoma after radical prostatectomy. J Nucl Med 1991;32:1713–1717.
40. Freitas JE, Gilvydas R, Ferry JD, Gonzalez JA. The clinical utility of prostate-specific antigen and bone scintigraphy in prostate cancer follow-up. J Nucl Med 1991;32:1387–1390.
41. Kransdorf MJ, Stull MA, Gilkey FW, Moser RP. Osteoid osteoma. Radiographics 1991;11:671–696.
42. "Hot" bone scans normal in military training. Radiology Today 1993;(August):12.
43. Kahn D, Wilson MA. Bone scintigraphic findings in patellar tendonitis. J Nucl Med 1987;28:1768–1770.
44. Matin P. The appearance of bone scans following fractures, including immediate and long-term studies. J Nucl Med 1979;20:1227–1231.
45. Spitz J, Lauer I, Tittel K, Weigand H. Scintimetric evaluation of remodeling after bone fractures in man. J Nucl Med 1993;34: 1403–1409.
46. Bellah RD, Summerville DA, Treves ST, Micheli LJ. Low-back pain in adolescent athletes: detection of stress injury to the pars interarticularis with SPECT. Radiology 1991;180:509–512.
47. Schauwecker DS. The scintigraphic diagnosis of osteomyelitis. AJR Am J Roentgenol 1992;158:9–18.
48. Palestro CJ, Kim CK, Swyer AJ, et al. Radionuclide diagnosis of vertebral osteomyelitis: indium-111-leukocyte and technetium-99m–

methylene diphosphonate bone scintigraphy. J Nucl Med 1991;32: 1861–1865.

49. Seabold JE, Nepola JV, March JL, et al. Postoperative bone marrow alterations: potential pitfalls in the diagnosis of osteomyelitis with In-111–labeled leukocyte scintigraphy. Radiology 1991;180: 741–747.

50. Mehta RC, Wilson MA. Frostbite injury: prediction of tissue viability with triple-phase bone scanning. Radiology 1989;170:511–514.

51. Wilson MA, Lin TF, Lehner CE, Lanphier EH. The early detection of avascular necrosis [abstract]. J Nucl Med 1994;34:143.

52. Lusins J. SPECT evaluation of lumbar spinal fusion: will it make the medal round [editorial]? J Nucl Med 1994;34:422–423.

53. Veldman PHJM, Reynen HM, Arntz IE, Goris RJA. Signs and symptoms of reflex sympathetic dystrophy: prospective study of 829 patients. Lancet 1993;342:1012–1016.

54. Utz JA, Lull RJ, Galvin EG. Asymptomatic total hip prosthesis: natural history determined using Tc-99m MDP bone scans. Radiology 1986;161:509–512.

55. Oswald SG, Van Nostrand D, Savory CG, Callaghan JJ. Three-phase bone scan and indium white blood cell scintigraphy following porous coated hip arthroplasty: a prospective study of the prosthetic tip. J Nucl Med 1989;30:1321–1331.

56. Meunier PJ, Salson C, Mathieu L, et al. Skeletal distribution and biochemical parameters of Paget's disease. Clin Orthop 1978;217: 37–44.

57. McAfee JG. Radionuclide imaging in metabolic and systematic skeletal diseases. Semin Nucl Med 1987;17:334–349.

58. Frankel RS, Johnson KW, Mary JJ, Johnston GS. "Normal" bone radionuclide image with diffuse skeletal lymphoma. Radiology 1974;111:365–366.

59. Sy WM, Patel D, Faunce H. Significance of absent or faint kidney sign on bone scan. J Nucl Med 1975;16:454–456.

60. Wilson MA, Calhoun FW, Gaines J, Goldsmith SJ. Patterns of diffusely increased skeletal radiopharmaceutical uptake. Australas Radiol 1981;25:177–180.

61. McAfee JG, Carrasquillo JA, Camera L, et al. Changes in skeletal images induced by granulocyte-macrophage colony–stimulating factor (GM-CSF) in patients with locally advanced and metastatic breast cancer [abstract]. J Nucl Med 1994;35:89P.

62. Peller PJ, Ho VB, Kransdorf MJ. Extraosseous Tc-99m MDP uptake: a pathophysiologic approach. Radiographics 1993;13:715–734.

63. Kransdorf JM, Meis JM. Extraskeletal osseous and cartilaginous tumors of the extremities. Radiographics 1993;13:853–884.

64. Ryan PJ, Evans PA, Gibson T, Fogelman I. Chronic low back pain: comparison of bone SPECT with radiography and CT. Radiology 1992;182:849–854.

65. Collier BD, Johnson RP, Carrera GF, et al. Painful spondylolysis or spondylolisthesis studied by radiography and single-photon emission computed tomography. Radiology 1985;154:207–211.

66. Collier BD, Johnson RP, Carrera GF, et al. Chronic knee pain assessed by SPECT: comparison with other modalities. Radiology 1985;157: 795–802.

67. Collier BD, Carrera GF, Messer EJ, et al. Internal derangement of the temporomandibular joint: detection by single-photon emission computed tomography. Radiology 1983;149:557–561.

68. Spencer RP, Lee YS, Sziklas JJ, et al. Failure of uptake of radiocolloid by the femoral heads: a diagnostic problem: concise communication. J Nucl Med 1983;24:116–118.

69. Gelfand MJ, Daya SA, Rucknagel DL, et al. Simultaneous occurrence of rib infarction and pulmonary infiltrates in sickle cell disease patients with acute chest syndrome. J Nucl Med 1993;34:614–618.

70. Flivik G, Sloth M, Rydholm U, et al. Technetium-99m-nanocolloid scintigraphy in orthopedic infections: a comparison with indium-111–labeled leukocytes. J Nucl Med 1993;34:1646–1650.

71. Datz FL, Morton KA. New radiopharmaceuticals for detecting infection. Invest Radiol 1993;28:356–365.

*Textbook of Nuclear Medicine*,
edited by Michael A. Wilson.
Lippincott–Raven Publishers, Philadelphia © 1998.

CHAPTER 2

# Myocardial Ischemia and Viability

Jesus A. Bianco and Michael A. Wilson

## OVERVIEW OF MYOCARDIAL PERFUSION IMAGING

Currently, one-fourth to one-third of all nuclear medicine studies are performed for cardiovascular disorders, and most are myocardial perfusion imaging (MPI) studies. In the United States, of these MPI studies, one-third of images use technetium 99m (Tc-99m) sestamibi and two-thirds use thallium 201 (Tl-201), but the proportion of Tc-99m sestamibi increases monthly. To put MPI in its proper perspective, some epidemiologic data on adult heart disease must be given. More than 60,000,000 Americans have hypertension, which is a major risk factor for the development of coronary artery disease (CAD). More than 6,000,000 Americans have CAD. Among individuals between the ages of 35 and 64, there are >1,500,000 acute myocardial infarctions (AMIs) and >600,000 deaths per year in the United States. The likelihood that an American male will experience AMI or death from CAD before age 65 is 20%.

Silent ischemia is increasingly recognized and has an unfavorable prognosis when occurring during exercise or dipyridamole testing or in patients with recent unstable angina (1). However, in the 40- to 55-year-old male group with high cholesterol and hypertension, two-thirds of these patients remain well during the subsequent 25 years (1). These data indicate that the burden to society from CAD is immense.

MPI has been performed clinically since 1976, and much has been learned about how it affects the diagnosis and management of patients with CAD. Review articles confirm the solid support for the clinical application of MPI. Seminal articles on MPI and its pathophysiologic basis (2–4), coronary flow reserve (5), and recent Tc-99m MPI agents (6) are worthy of review. The state of the art of cardiovascular nuclear medicine was discussed in the April 1994 issue of the *Journal of Nuclear Medicine*, and similar review articles are found in the *Journal of Nuclear Cardiology* since its first publication in January 1994. A recent competitor of MPI, stress echocardiography, does not yet have a similar track record (7), especially for forecasting prognosis of CAD.

### History

The following is a list of milestones in the development of MPI since 1954 (8):

- 1954: Myocardial accumulation of radioactive potassium and its analogs
- 1964: Potential clinical application of myocardial imaging with rubidium 86 (Rb-86) and cesium 131 (Cs-131)
- 1973: Myocardial imaging with nitrogen 13 (N-13) $NH_4^+$ and a positron camera
- 1973: Potassium 43 (K-43) for noninvasive patient assessment at rest, with stress, and during angina
- 1975: Tl-201 described for medical use (9)
- 1977: Tl-201 redistribution described (10)
- 1978: MPI and intravenous (IV) dipyridamole (11)
- 1983: Tl-201 used to determine patient prognosis (12)

### Indications for MPI

Patients should be referred for MPI for investigation of two issues: the detection of acute myocardial ischemia and the assessment of the potential recovery of left ventricular (LV) function by identifying scarred myocardium. This allows for the evaluation of the hemodynamic significance of angiographic CAD, risk stratification of patients for management purposes, and characterization of myocardial viability, all of which are useful to plan myocardial revascularization. These procedures are increasingly used to assess the effectiveness of medical or surgical interventions (Table 2-1). As technology advances, and the health care system is subject to more reform, it is important for the clinician to know the sensitivity and specificity of MPI and its relevance for patient outcome when compared to other diagnostic modalities.

### Pathophysiologic Basis of MPI

Figure 2-1 shows an illustration based on work done at Gould's lab in 1974 (13) and is the principle on which the

**TABLE 2-1.** *Indications for MPI (% average utilization)*

1. Diagnosis of CAD (~35%)
   (atypical chest pain and intermediate probability of
   presence of CAD)
2. Risk stratification (~35%)
   Post acute myocardial infarction
   Before vascular surgery (e.g., peripheral vascular disease, AAA, or carotid artery surgery)
   Before and after interventions (e.g., coronary artery
   bypass surgery, angioplasty, and thrombolysis)
   Assessment of myocardial perfusion when coronary
   angiography reveals minor lesions
3. Assessment of myocardial viability (15%)
4. Acute ischemic syndromes (10%)
   Myocardial stunning
   Myocardial salvage in acute myocardial infarction
5. Assessment of other diseases (5%)
   Hypertrophic cardiomyopathy
   Assessment of Kawasaki's disease
   Anomalous left coronary artery
   Corrected transposition of the great vessels

clinical application of MPI is based. In the presence of a coronary stenosis, resting baseline perfusion is normal. With exercise or pharmacologic stress (dipyridamole, adenosine, or dobutamine), the coronary blood flow (CBF) to normal segments increases

- Fourfold with adenosine or dipyridamole
- Threefold with dobutamine
- Twofold with exercise

However, because of the fall of radiopharmaceutical extraction that occurs at increased coronary flows, the actual stress-induced increase in myocardial uptake is not this large.

Segments supplied by stenotic coronary arteries have lesser stress increases in CBF than in normal segments. Quantitatively, this impairment in CBF reserve is inversely related to the degree of coronary arterial stenosis. For example, if an artery has a 90% coronary arterial stenosis, it is very likely that stress-induced coronary vasodilatation will produce a large flow dif-

ference between the nonstenotic and the stenotic myocardial zones and that this will appear as a scan defect on MPI (14).

### Radiopharmaceuticals

The K-43 method for investigating acute myocardial ischemia was described by Zaret and colleagues in 1973 (15). Their working hypotheses were as follows:

- In areas of myocardial infarction, perfusion to scarred regions would be reduced and nonviable cells would not take up tracer.
- In myocardial areas subserved by critically stenosed coronary arteries, resting perfusion would be maintained by antegrade flow and supplemented by retrograde collateral flow.
- During exercise, increased myocardial $O_2$ demand would not be met by increased CBF (i.e., ischemia).
- This would result in delayed and decreased myocardial tracer uptake.
- There would be differential washout of tracer from the nonischemic and ischemic regions.

These investigations validated (in normal, ischemic, and infarcted myocardium) a correlation between K-43 myocardial distribution and radioactive microspheres (the gold standard of perfusion), thus validating use of $K^+$ analogs as markers of myocardial perfusion.

### *Thallium 201*

MPI with Tl-201 is a very robust technology. A dose of 3.0 to 3.5 mCi (111 to 130 MBq) thallous chloride as Tl-201 is injected intravenously (IV) for single photon emission computed tomography (SPECT). The dose is adjusted for weight for patients <45 kg or >90 kg. Tl-201 decays by electron capture to mercury 201 (Hg-201) with a physical half-life of 73 hours, emitting 68 to 80 keV mercury characteristic x-rays, which are readily attenuated in soft tis-

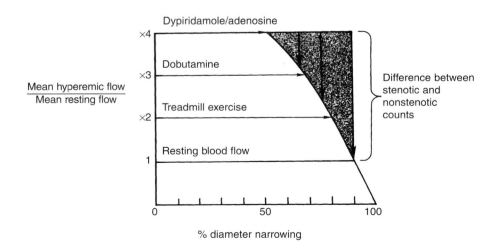

**FIG. 2-1.** A plot of the ratio of the mean hyperemic to resting myocardial blood flow versus percent diameter narrowing of a coronary artery. The vertical axis shows the increase in CBF with the various forms of stress (exercise and pharmacologic) when compared to rest. At rest, only stenoses >90% result in reduced resting CBF. With maximal stimulated coronary flow, a 50% stenosis results in reduced flow beyond the stenosis. The dark-shaded area is an indication of tracer heterogeneity resulting from decreased flow augmentation in stenosed coronary arteries. (Modified from Gould KL, Lipscomb K, Hamilton GW. Physiologic basis for assessing critical coronary stenosis. Am J Cardiol 1974;33:87–94.)

sue (Table 2-2). Tl-201 also has gamma rays that multipeak gamma cameras can utilize at 135 keV (3% abundance) and 167 keV (10% abundance). Removal of Compton scatter by "windowing" is very difficult because of the overlap of the three characteristic x-rays with the Compton scatter distribution. It is typical to find that 30% to 40% of Tl-201 photopeak events are due to Compton scatter.

After IV administration, Tl-201 clears rapidly from the blood, and the maximal myocardial accumulation occurs at 10 minutes. Tl-201 is a monovalent cation analogous to potassium, with a first-pass extraction fraction of nearly 90%. The major mechanism for cardiac uptake is the sodium-potassium–adenosine triphosphatase (Na-K-ATPase) sarcolemmal pump, and it indicates the presence of an intact cell membrane in a viable myocardial cell. Tl-201 distributes in the kidneys (critical organ), thyroid, liver, testes, ovaries, stomach wall and intestines, and assuming a biological half-life of 11 days (effective half-life of 2.4 days), the dosimetry is as in Table 2-3. In contrast, Tc-99m sestamibi kinetics are dominated by mitochondrial function, and Tc-99m sestamibi cardiac accumulation indicates cardiac viability (16). Optimal myocardial accumulation of tracer occurs in fasting patients, in the upright posture, and after brief ambulation because these actions can decrease hepatic and gastrointestinal Tl-201 accumulation. Table 2-4 describes the tracer kinetics of Tl-201 (17,18).

Compared to normal cell uptake, ischemic myocardial cell uptake of Tl-201 has the following characteristics:

- Smaller amount
- Slower uptake
- Slower washout

These features result in the typical scan findings of myocardial ischemia, a stress defect that improves (redistributes) in delayed imaging.

The tracer selection made by each imaging center is based on cost, convenience, imaging equipment available, and the clinical indications. As a generalization, Tl-201 imaging is often used for viability considerations and Tc-99m sestamibi for larger patients or when attenuation may be a problem. In situations in which slow myocardial tracer washout is an asset, as in delayed imaging after injection of tracer during acute ischemia in the emergency room (ER), Tc-99m sestamibi is the preferred agent.

*Stress and Rest Reinjection Protocol*

This protocol is used to establish myocardial ischemia. Tl-201 is injected IV 60 seconds before termination of adequate stress. The SPECT acquisition is performed 10 to 15 minutes later to avoid "upward creep" of the heart as the patient settles down after treadmill stress but early enough to anticipate redistribution, LV dilatation, and lung uptake (all important scan indicators of significant disease). The rest SPECT acquisition is obtained 4 hours later to determine which myocardial segments redistribute, such as

**TABLE 2-2.** *Comparison of physical characteristics of MPI radionuclides*

| Nuclide | Tc-99m | Tl-201 |
|---|---|---|
| Emission energy (keV) | 140 | 70–81 |
| Emission type | gamma ray | x-rays |
| Half-life (hrs) | 6.05 | 73 |
| Half-value layer (cm) | | |
| Lead | 0.03 | 0.001 |
| NaI crystal | 0.27 | 0.06 |
| Water | 4.50 | 3.95 |
| % scatter in photopeak* | 14–22 | 30–40 |

*Data from Berman DS, University of California, Cedars-Sinai Medical Center.

**TABLE 2-3.** *Radiation dosimetry of MPI nuclides injected at rest*

| | Rads/mCi | | Rads/dose[a] | |
|---|---|---|---|---|
| | Tl-201 | MIBI[b] | Tl-201 | MIBI[b] |
| Kidneys | 1.2 | 0.06 | 4.20 | 2.0 |
| Heart wall | 0.5 | 0.02 | 1.75 | 0.5 |
| Testes | 0.5 | 0.01 | 1.80 | 0.3 |
| Ovaries | 0.5 | 0.05 | 1.60 | 1.5 |
| Upper large intestine | 0.3 | 0.18 | 0.90 | 5.4 |
| Total body | 0.2 | 0.02 | 0.70 | 0.5 |

[a] 3.5 mCi Tl-201 dose, 30 mCi Tc-99m sestamibi dose.
[b] Tc-99m sestamibi.

**TABLE 2-4.** *Tracer (Tl-201 and Tc-99m sestamibi) kinetics*

| | Tl-201 | Tc-99m MIBI |
|---|---|---|
| Class | Cation | Isonitrile |
| Extraction fraction | 90% | 50% |
| Decreased extraction efficiency with flow | Yes | Yes |
| Cardiac uptake | 3–4% | 2% |
| Redistribution | Yes | Slow |
| Membrane transport | Active | Passive |
| Uptake mechanism | ATPase pump | Mitochondrial transport |

occurs in acute myocardial ischemia. If myocardial viability is an issue (when a fixed defect is seen in both stress and rest), another 1 mCi of Tl-201 may be injected IV, and a series of resting SPECT reinjection images is obtained 10 minutes later. If Tl-201 is taken up by the hypoperfused areas, the segment is viable.

*Rest and Redistribution Protocol*

The rest and redistribution protocol is the procedure of choice for determining presence of myocardial viability. Tl-201 is injected IV and resting SPECT images are obtained at 10 minutes. Another set of SPECT Tl-201 rest images is obtained 4 hours later. Delayed images can be obtained 12 to 24 hours later, preferably after IV injection of an additional 1 mCi of Tl-201 administered immediately after the rest images.

### Tc-99m Sestamibi

Tc-99m sestamibi is an isonitrile lipophilic complex with a positive charge. Structurally, it contains six isonitrile components around the central Tc-99m atom. In contrast to Tl-201, the cardiac membrane transport of Tc-99m sestamibi is passive. Uptake and retention of Tc-99m sestamibi requires an intact cell membrane and mitochondrial integrity because cardiac uptake is mediated by electromechanical gradients across sarcolemmal and mitochondrial membranes, and to a lesser extent an aerobic metabolism. Retention in the mitochondria results from the large negative transmembrane potential (16). The extraction efficiency of sestamibi (18) is approximately half that of Tl-201 (see Table 2-4), and the extraction fraction decreases as coronary flow increases (19). The dosimetry with 2-hour void is as shown in Table 2-3. Sestamibi is available in kit form, ensuring 24-hour availability. Because of the physical characteristics of decay of Tc-99m, doses of as much as 10 times that of Tl-201 can be given, resulting in improved images. Hammes and coworkers (20) have proposed an ethanol-based separation of impurities for improved quality control (QC) testing.

Myocardial uptake of Tc-99m sestamibi is proportional to regional blood flow at intermediate coronary arterial flow rates and redistributes at a very slow rate, although recently redistribution sestamibi scans have been proposed for assessment of myocardial viability (21). Because of slow redistribution of sestamibi, separate resting and exercise injections are needed to detect and differentiate myocardial ischemia from scar.

When Tc-99m sestamibi is injected at the time of a coronary occlusion it does not accumulate in the severely ischemic area at risk; instead, a photon-deficient area is seen. If Tc-99m sestamibi is injected during reperfusion, its uptake may be decreased as a consequence of microvascular injury and the no-reflow phenomenon, and the distribution reflects perfusion, microvascular injury, and myocyte viability. At very low coronary arterial flows, both Tl-201 and Tc-99m sestamibi overestimate myocardial blood flow as determined by microspheres.

Liver uptake of Tc-99m sestamibi is high, and although hepatobiliary clearance is relatively rapid, hepatic and bowel activity present at 1 hour postinjection may obscure the inferior myocardium. The heart-liver ratio is greater than 1:1 immediately after stress injection, and progressively increases over the next 3 hours. After rest injection the initial heart-liver ratio is 1:2 and progressively increases, so that by 2 hours the ratio is 1:1. Given these biodistributions, the optimal time to start cardiac SPECT imaging is 30 minutes postinjection for resting studies and 15 minutes postinjection for exercise studies.

### Ischemia Protocol

Twenty-five to 30 mCi (weight adjusted) of Tc-99m sestamibi is given IV at peak exercise stress, which is then continued for another 90 seconds and SPECT imaging is performed 15 minutes later. If these stress images are normal

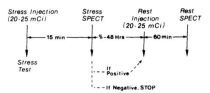

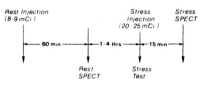

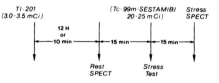

**FIG. 2-2.** Three Tc-99m sestamibi imaging protocols: 2-day study, same-day study, and dual isotope study (from top to bottom). Some workers perform the same-day Tc-99m sestamibi protocol with the reverse sequence: stress injection, 1- to 4-hour waiting period, then the rest injection study. The dual isotope study is extremely time efficient, whereas the 2-day study can result in considerable cost savings because up to one-half of patients do not need to return for the rest study.

and if the gated SPECT study is normal, no further imaging is necessary. If large areas of hypoperfusion are seen after stress and the gated SPECT study is normal, the patient may be directly referred for coronary angiography. If the images are not normal, the patient returns 24 to 48 hours later (4 to 8 half-lives) for the resting Tc-99m sestamibi images. The radiopharmaceutical dose is the same, but SPECT imaging at rest is done 30 minutes after IV administration of Tc-99m sestamibi. Figure 2-2 shows the different sestamibi imaging protocols in clinical use. Some centers prefer to accomplish this test in 1 day and the same day Tc-99m sestamibi protocol using 8 to 9 mCi of radiopharmaceutical for the first test and 20 to 25 mCi for the second test performed later in the same day. Taillefer et al. have compared Tc-99m sestamibi 1-day rest-stress to stress-rest protocols (22), and the stress-rest protocol tends to overestimate presence of the myocardial scar.

### AMI Protocol

In patients with suspected AMI (chest pain), a resting Tc-99m sestamibi study is obtained. Later, a risk-stratification stress Tc-99m sestamibi test may be obtained as a predischarge assessment. In some centers, dipyridamole or dobutamine MPI is used as early as 2 to 3 days after an acute chest pain syndrome.

### Dual Isotope Imaging

To assess myocardial perfusion and viability in patients with prior myocardial infarction, inpatients, and patients who live a distance from the imaging center, the separate acquisition dual isotope rest Tl-201/stress Tc-99m sestamibi 1-day MPI technique is used as a convenient and cost-effective alternative. In the dual isotope protocol, 3.0 to 3.5 mCi of Tl-201 is either injected the evening before or immediately before imaging, with imaging immediately before the stress test. The patient is then placed on a treadmill or administered pharmacologic stress, and 25 to 30 mCi of Tc-99m sestamibi is injected. SPECT stress images are acquired 15 minutes later. In patients with prior myocardial infarction, the clinical question is often the potential functional recovery of hypokinetic, akinetic, or dyskinetic segments. In these patients, the dual isotope 1-day MPI protocol is the best way to detect inducible ischemia and to determine the viability of a dysfunctional myocardial segment. This dual isotope protocol has been extensively used by the Berman group (23), who reported that in a group of 588 patients, a normal or equivocal dual isotope test indicates an excellent prognosis.

### Other MPI Agents

#### Tc-99m Teboroxime

Tc-99m teboroxime is a myocardial perfusion agent that has been temporarily withdrawn from the market for stability problems, although it was released by the U.S. Food and Drug Administration (FDA) the same day as Tc-99m sestamibi in 1991. It is a boronic adduct of technetium dioxime compound that is lipophilic and neutral, and diffuses passively into the myocardial cell without undergoing metabolism. Its extraction fraction is high (90%) and relatively stable at high coronary flows. However, myocardial washout is extremely rapid with fast and slow exponential components. This washout of teboroxime is faster from nonischemic than ischemic segments, and increases with increasing blood flow. Liver uptake is rapid (6-minute peak) and high, but excretion is slow. Because of the rapid washout, imaging must be accomplished quickly after injection and the protocol is technically demanding. Johnson has reviewed the clinical applications of Tc-99m teboroxime (24). The adenosine stress and rest SPECT protocol can be performed within 30 minutes using triple-detector cameras.

#### Tc-99m Tetrofosmin

Tc-99m tetrofosmin is a lipophilic compound that has good heart uptake and retention, with rapid clearance from liver,

lung, and blood. It was approved by the FDA in 1996. Whether faster liver washout will improve MPI is yet to be demonstrated. High-quality myocardial images can be obtained 5 minutes to several hours postinjection. A convenient 1-day Tc-99m tetrofosmin imaging protocol similar in duration to conventional Tl-201 imaging is feasible, but the more usual protocol is a 2-day protocol, such as with Tc-99m sestamibi. Tc-99m tetrofosmin does not appear to improve the sensitivity or specificity of MPI for detection of CAD; rather, it represents the manufacturer's need to compete in the MPI market (25).

#### Tc-99m Furifosmin

Gerson et al. (26) recently reported data on furifosmin, a Tc-99m diphosphine complex derived from a cationic mixed-ligand Tc-99 (III) complex that does not redistribute. Data showed that this compound accumulates in myocardium in direct relation to microsphere blood flow. At the time of this writing, release of this tracer appears likely.

#### Tc-99m N-NOET

Another Tc-99m agent undergoing evaluation is a nitrodo compound that has high cardiac uptake (3% to 5%), redistributes, and may provide throughput advantages.

### Clinical Efficacy of MPI

Reported data indicate that Tl-201 and Tc-99m sestamibi MPI provide similar information for detection of stress-induced transient myocardial ischemia in patients being investigated for CAD (6). Table 2-5 presents data for sensitivity, specificity, and normalcy rate (i.e., percentage of normal subjects with normal MPI) for Tl-201 SPECT (27–30). The overall sensitivity in these 1,169 patients was 99% for patients with myocardial infarction and 85% with no infarction (overall 90%). The sensitivity for detection of CAD (range, 82% to 95%) depends on the actual technique used (2). The specificity was 70% and the normalcy rate 90%, and varied depending on technical considerations (2). Note that the assumption is made that sensitivity and specificity of cardiac scintigraphy is constant over the whole range of CAD prevalence (see Referral Bias).

**TABLE 2-5.** Tl-201 and Tc-99m sestamibi SPECT in diagnosis of CAD

|  | Tl-201 | Tc-99m sestamibi |
|---|---|---|
| Sensitivity | 90% | 90% |
| Specificity | 70% | 88% |
| Normalcy rate* | 90% | 100% |
| Patient numbers | 1,169 | 125 |
| References | 24–27 | 28–30 |

*True negatives in subjects with <5% likelihood of CAD.

Table 2-5 also shows the reported sensitivities and specificities of Tc-99m sestamibi MPI for the detection of CAD (31–33). The similarity of diagnostic efficacy between Tc-99m sestamibi and Tl-201 extends to assessment of disease in individual coronary arteries, severity of perfusion defects, type of stressor, and defect reversibility.

## Imaging Limitations

### Relative Versus Absolute Uptake

Tl-201, Tc-99m sestamibi, and other radiopharmaceuticals used in MPI have a myocardial distribution proportional to regional perfusion, cardiac extraction efficiency, and viability of the perfused myocardium. These tracers measure relative myocardial perfusion. If perfusion to the three coronary arterial territories is decreased, the territory with the greatest coronary flow (least decrease) may appear to be normal on planar or SPECT imaging. This means that multivessel disease will be underestimated. For measurement of absolute flows, positron emission tomography (PET) scanning is required. However, the impact of measurement of absolute myocardial blood flow in clinical cardiology is unknown.

### Multivessel Disease

In a multicenter trial, Van Train et al. (34) investigated the accuracy of an automated quantitative analysis of same-day rest-stress Tc-99m sestamibi SPECT images for detection and localization of CAD. The automatic program included optimized acquisition, automatic feature extraction, comprehensive polar map analysis, gender-matched normal limits, and objective criteria for detection and localization of CAD. Of 161 individuals studied, 102 patients had ≥50% coronary arterial narrowing. Accuracy data for patient identification is shown in Table 2-6. Although the accuracy of Tc-99m sestamibi MPI for identifying CAD in individual patients was high, the overall accuracy for correctly identifying the number of diseased vessels only averaged 44% for single-, double-, and triple-vessel disease. Similar results have been reported with Tl-201 SPECT.

One reason for the reduced accuracy in detecting the correct number of abnormal vessels may be underestimation of disease because not all diseased vessels develop a relative flow reduction during peak exercise; that is, patients with multivessel disease who undergo stress may have their exercise capacity limited by the development of ischemia in the most severely diseased zone without ischemia in other vessel territories. Another factor contributing to the difficulty in localizing diseased vessels is related to the fixed territories that must arbitrarily be used in studies; for example, a stenosed coronary artery may produce a perfusion defect that extends outside of the usual designated territory, and a patient with single-vessel disease may be incorrectly interpreted as having double-vessel disease.

**TABLE 2-6.** *Multicenter trial of quantitative analysis of Tc-99m sestamibi MPI*

| | | |
|---|---|---|
| Overall detection of CAD | | |
|   87% sensitivity | | |
|   36% specificity | | |
|   81% normalcy* | | |
| No change in sensitivity occurs with: | | |
|   Equipment manufacturer | | |
|   Male or female patients | | |
|   Evidence of prior infarction | | |
|   70% or 50% coronary stenosis | | |
| Identification of individual vessel | | |
| Artery | Sensitivity | Specificity |
| LAD | 69% | 76% |
| LCX | 70% | 80% |
| RCA | 77% | 85% |
| Sensitivity vs. number of vessels | | |
|   Single, 84% | | |
|   Double, 91% | | |
|   Triple, 96% | | |
| Correct identification of vessel extent | | |
|   Single, 49% | | |
|   Double, 43% | | |
|   Triple, 38% | | |

*Normalcy rate: true negatives in subjects with <5% likelihood of CAD.
LAD, left anterior descending; LCX, left circumflex; RCA, right coronary.
Source: KF Van Train, EV Garcia, J Maddahi, et al. Multicenter trial validation for quantitative analysis of same-day rest-stress technetium-99-m-sestamibi myocardial tomograms. J Nucl Med 1994;35:609–618.

## Imaging Systems and Quantitation

### Planar Imaging

For 20 years, planar MPI with Tl-201 (and later Tc-99m sestamibi) has been used extensively (2,6). Planar imaging (Fig. 2-3) provides portability, provides efficacy in obese patients, and allows implementation of first-pass or gated studies. The key to a successful planar MPI study is proper patient positioning. It is best to first select the 45-degree shallow left anterior oblique (LAO) view. In this projection (the best septal view) the septum should be vertical and clearly separate the two ventricles from the base to apex. The two other views are the best septal view minus 45 degrees (the anterior view) and plus 45 degrees (the steep LAO or lateral view). Adherence to this positioning protocol ensures comparison between patients, and in the same patients between subsequent tests.

Common perfusion defect artifacts are the valve plane on the upper septum in the 45-degree LAO best septal view, and a "defect" in the inferobasal segment in the steep LAO (lateral) view. This latter defect can be eliminated with image acquisition in the right lateral decubitus position, which removes the diaphragmatic attenuation by the redistribution of abdominal contents.

In Tl-201 studies, a general purpose collimator, 64 × 64 acquisition matrix, and 400,000 counts per view are usual. In planar Tc-99m sestamibi studies (35), one uses the high-reso-

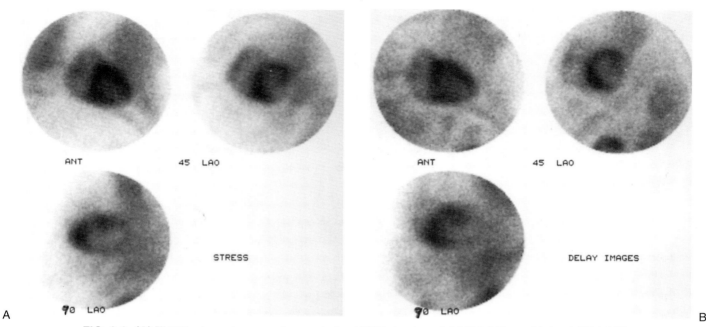

**FIG. 2-3. (A)** Tl-201 planar images show anterior (ANT), best septal (45 LAO), and lateral (90 LAO) views obtained at stress. A defect in uptake is seen in the inferoapical (ANT), apical and posterolateral (45 LAO), and the midinferior and inferobasal (90 LAO) segments. **(B)** These images were obtained at rest 4 hours later (delay) and demonstrate a virtually identical myocardial pattern, suggesting a myocardial infarct. The greater lung uptake in the stress images indicates stress-induced LV dysfunction.

lution collimator, $128 \times 128$ acquisition matrix, and the collection period is 5 to 8 minutes per view for one million counts.

In Tc-99m sestamibi and resting or postdipyridamole Tl-201 studies, visceral abdominal activity may be high. To deal with this problem, the heart image is scaled to the hottest pixel in the myocardium. The extracardiac activity can be suppressed by saturating these extracardiac pixels by overflow techniques.

### Planar Quantification

For quantitation of planar MPI defects, two procedures are available. The Virginia group (35) used four horizontal 1-cm myocardial count profiles plotted against time. In the commonly used circumferential distribution profile technique of Dr. Wackers (Yale University) (2), counts are sampled around the myocardial rim in each planar view (Fig. 2-4). After the center of the LV cavity and epicardial edge of the LV are located, a search is performed for the maximum count along radii from the LV center. A reference angle (usually the apex) is used to display these plots horizontally. Counts in the radii are plotted as a function of angle and count distribution in the myocardial walls obtained in a clockwise direction from the reference angle. Processed counts are compared with the tracer distribution (mean minus 2 SD) obtained in normal individuals. The exercise and the rest profiles are each normalized. The change in tracer distribution from the exercise to the resting state is an indication of defect size and defect reversibility.

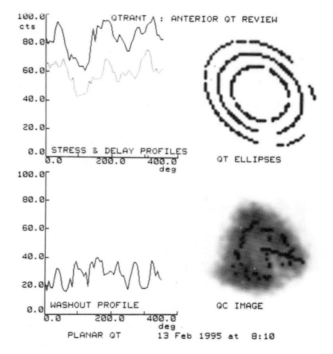

**FIG. 2-4.** A single anterior view of a quantitative planar Tl-201 plot is shown for the patient in Fig. 2-3. The stress and delay profiles (upper left) parallel each other, resulting in a normal washout profile (lower left). The QT ellipses (upper right) show a stress and washout defect in the inferior segment (i.e., fixed defect) and washout defects in the anterolateral and inferior segments (so-called reverse defects, not due to ischemia).

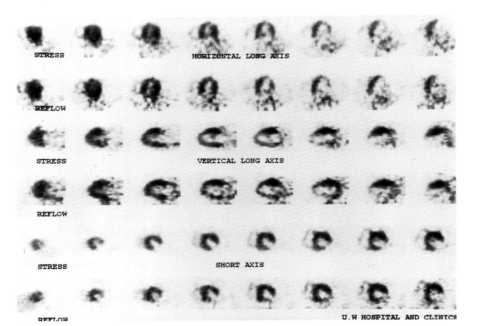

**FIG. 2-5.** This SPECT Tl-201 stress and redistribution image series is in the same patient as in Figs. 2-3 and 2-4. A fixed inferolateral wall defect of moderate size and severe decrease in counts is very clearly delineated. Note the improved statistics in the stress images when compared to the delayed images obtained 4 hours later when significant washout of Tl-201 has occurred. The rest count rate is typically 40% less than the stress images, but the image intensity is similar because of normalization of the stress and washout (reflow) images.

**FIG. 2-6.** The myocardial segments derived from the long-axis views of a SPECT study. (HLA, horizontal long-axis view; VLA, vertical long-axis view.) The named segments are AP, apical; DS, distal septum; PS, proximal (basal) septum; DL, distal lateral; PL, proximal (or basal) lateral; IAP, inferoapical; I, inferior; IB, inferobasal; DA, distal anterior; MA, middle anterior; PA, proximal (or basal) anterior.

### SPECT Imaging

A well-designed and accomplished QC program is necessary for optimal imaging (see Chapter 24). Many SPECT users employ the semicircular 180-degree arc (45 degrees right anterior oblique [RAO] to 45 degrees left posterior oblique [LPO]), with 32 increments taking 30 to 40 seconds each, in a 64 × 64-byte mode matrix using a 1.5 zoom. The images are displayed in the familiar echocardiographic standard horizontal long-axis, vertical long-axis, and short-axis views (Figs. 2-5 through 2-7). In MPI these are displayed in stress and rest pairs. It is critical in the comparison of rest and stress SPECT images that the operator aligns the heart axes identically to ensure that individual slices (36) are comparable. This point is important as the short-axis view is oriented 40 to 45 degrees to the left and slightly caudad in the human thorax. Significant technologist intervention is required to orient these views on the output display.

Various myocardial segmental descriptions are available: One is shown in Figs. 2-6 and 2-7, and numerous others exist (Fig. 2-8). The important thing is to select a system and be consistent, so the referring physician understands the report. Commercial gamma camera displays are not universal, with different orientation according to individual manufacturer's preferences (Fig. 2-9).

We use a three-detector system. Acquisition is in the stop-and-shoot configuration. For Tc-99m sestamibi rest and stress studies we use 15- to 20-second stops at 4-degree angles (30 stops or 120 degrees per detector head). For the resting Tl-201 studies the same acquisition parameters are used with 35 seconds per stop. When performing gated Tc-99m sestamibi stress images we use 6-degree angles, 50 heart beats per stop, and this usually takes 45 seconds. Processing of Tl-201 is done in 2-pixel-slice thickness, Tc-99m sestamibi in single pixel slices. However, Tc-99m sestamibi data are displayed by stacking several single pixel slices, so the overall thickness of the displayed slices is identical (Fig. 2-10). Rarely, the fundus of the stomach can be visualized behind the LV (Fig. 2-11).

Filtered back-projection is widely used in SPECT studies, but newer iterative methods are under development. At the time of writing there is no consensus as to which is the best filter to use in three-detector systems. Prereconstruction filters smooth the data but degrade the spatial resolution of images as the high-frequency components are eliminated. Projection data are filtered with a ramp filter. Reconstruction three-dimensional (3D) filtering of SPECT Tc-99m sestamibi studies (36) typically uses a Butterworth filter with a critical frequency of 0.4 cycle/cm and power of 10 for rest and gated stress images, and 0.52 cycle/cm with power of 5 for stress images. Tl-201 imaging typically uses a Butterworth filter with critical frequency of

# SHORT-AXIS

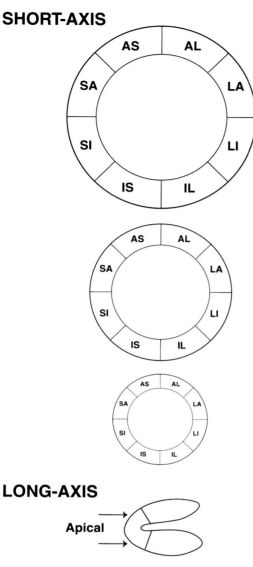

# LONG-AXIS

**Apical**

**FIG. 2-7.** Myocardial segments in the short-axis views. There are three short-axis slices: basal (upper), midventricular (middle), and apical (lower). Note that each short-axis slice is the composite of several SPECT slices, each 1 pixel thick. The lowest image is a long-axis view displaying the apical region. (AS, anteroseptal; SA, septoanterior; SI, septoinferior; IS, inferoseptal; IL, inferolateral; LI, lateroinferior; LA, lateroanterior; and AL, anterolateral.)

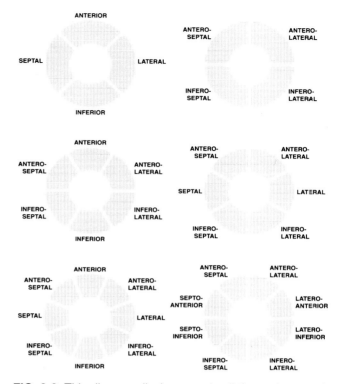

**FIG. 2-8.** This diagram displays nearly all the various methods published that describe myocardial segments in the short-axis views, including that of Fig. 2-7 (bottom right of this series). The terminology is similar in each method, but the identically named segments can vary significantly in size, for example, inferolateral segment can be a fourth, sixth, or eighth of the total slice. Note the vertical orientation of division on the right column where the anterior segment is divided, and the orientation of the left column with preservation of the anterior segment in all sized segments.

0.25 to 0.35 cycles/cm with a power of 10 (General Electric manufacturer guidelines).

The stress and rest images are each normalized to the maximum myocardial pixel count. There is no consensus on whether to use black-and-white or color display scales. We believe that all the data should be incorporated in interpretation of images, including a color scale, black-and-white scale, and polar plot. In general, color scales optimize the sensitivity of the method, whereas black-and-white scales optimize the specificity of the method. Color images are easier to interpret than black-and-white images, and, when suitably designed, can help differentiate relative degrees of radiopharmaceutical uptake.

## SPECT Quantitation

For quantitative evaluation of SPECT images, a bull's-eye or polar map is used (24,25) (Fig. 2-12). To construct the polar map one first uses LV short-axis slices of equal thickness from the apex to the base. The next step is to determine the location of the center of the LV cavity and the outer limit of the myocardium. Forty sectors are then constructed from the center of each slice radiating out across the myocardium. Maximal counts per sector are determined in a manner similar to the planar quantitative method and plotted in a polar coordinate profile as a bull's-eye plot. Gender-matched normal files consisting of patients with low likelihood of disease are used as the standard for comparison. There has been recent interest in distance and volume weighting of this two-dimensional (2D) plotting of the 3D chamber.

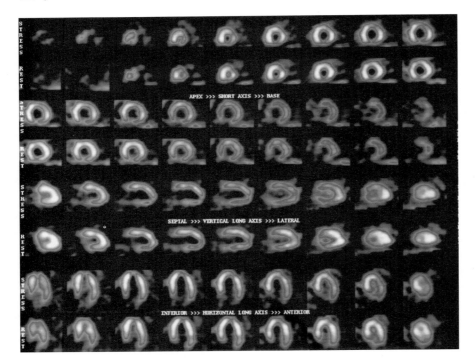

APEX >>> SHORT AXIS >>> BASE

SEPTAL >>> VERTICAL LONG AXIS >>> LATERAL

INFERIOR >>> HORIZONTAL LONG AXIS >>> ANTERIOR

**FIG. 2-9.** This multiheaded SPECT display is from a different gamma camera manufacturer than others used in this text. It displays all the short-axis slices (18 total) and nine slices in the long-axis views. The vertical long-axis view orientation is 180 degrees away from those of the scanners used in this text (see Figs. 2-5 and 2-10). The inferior-superior orientation is also different.

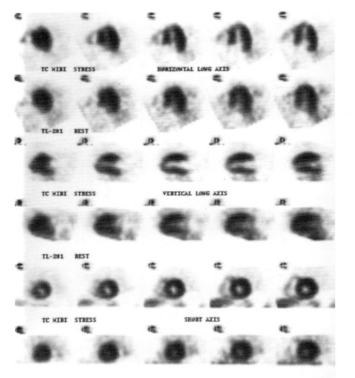

TC MIBI STRESS          HORIZONTAL LONG AXIS

TL-201 REST

TC MIBI STRESS          VERTICAL LONG AXIS

TL-201 REST

TC MIBI STRESS          SHORT AXIS

TL-201 REST

**FIG. 2-10.** This scan uses Tc-99m MIBI stress SPECT images and Tl-201 rest SPECT images. Note the better definition of the myocardium and higher heart-to-background ratio, with the high-count stress images using Tc-99m compared to the lower-count rest Tl-201 images. Note also the smaller ventricular cavity seen in the Tl-201 short-axis images due to increased scatter acceptance and poorer image resolution. Incidental note is made of the mild distal septal stress defect that normalizes in the rest images.

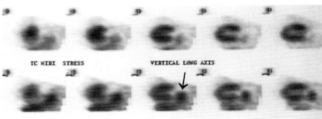

TC MIBI STRESS          VERTICAL LONG AXIS

TC MIBI REST

**FIG. 2-11.** Visualization of the fundus of the stomach (*arrow*) behind the LV in resting Tc-99m sestamibi images (lower panel) of this vertical long-axis stress and rest series. This patient had enterogastric reflux and a hiatal hernia confirmed on CT scan.

Because of the 2D display limitation and of the need to quantify Tc-99m sestamibi scintigrams, Van Train et al. (37) have developed a new approach for 3D investigation of Tc-99m sestamibi rest-stress SPECT studies to produce gender-matched rest-stress normal limits and criteria for abnormality. Tomograms were reconstructed at 1-pixel thickness (typically 6.4 mm), and adjacent slices were summed. After operator verification, maximum-count circumferential profiles were generated for all short-axis slices. The innovative portion of this technique is that a hybrid myocardial sampling technique was employed using spherical (sampling of the apical hemispheric portion of the LV) and cylindrical (sampling of the mid and basal portions of the LV) searches to give a true 3D representation of myocardial activity. Profile normalization in this technique is done by determining a scale factor that normalizes the patient data; then the most normal area of the patient's profile is normalized to the mean of the same area in

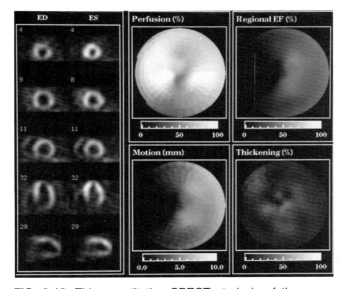

**FIG. 2-12.** This quantitative SPECT study is of the same patient obtained on the same scanner as in Fig. 2-9. In the left panel, the ED and ES Tc-99m sestamibi images of selected short-axis and long-axis slices demonstrate LV movement and thickening. The right panels demonstrates perfusion, regional ejection fraction, wall motion, and thickening parameters. The same output provided LV ED and ES volumes in milliliters and a ventricular volume curve.

the normal patient database. This is the present-day gold standard for quantitation of SPECT sestamibi MPI, and provides a "second reader" interpretation for MPI.

Quantitation of MPI SPECT studies is in its infancy. For proper quantitation of Tc-99m sestamibi image, attenuation, Compton scatter corrections, and compensation for depth-dependent collimator responses should be done. At the time of this writing, neither an accepted correction for image attenuation nor for Compton scatter has been accomplished (see Chapter 24). Tsui et al. (38) have presented an exhaustive discussion on possibilities for compensation for attenuation and Compton scatter in cardiac SPECT imaging; it deserves careful study and implementation for optimization of image quantitation of SPECT cardiac studies. Further studies are needed to extend these approaches to quantitation of Tc-99m sestamibi to pharmacologic stress, systems using three-detector units, and studies using dual isotope protocols.

## MYOCARDIAL STRESS TESTING

At the present, most MPI studies are performed using one of three stressors: exercise treadmill testing (ETT), dipyridamole (or adenosine) infusion, or dobutamine infusion. Many myocardial segments subserved by critically stenosed arteries maintain normal perfusion at rest via collateral channels (1,11,13,14). The purpose of stress testing is to demonstrate inducible ischemia under conditions of increased demand (see Fig. 2-1). The stress myocardial

tracer distribution of MPI mirrors stress-induced flow augmentation, whereas myocardial distribution at rest reflects resting perfusion and myocardial viability. These MPI tracers overestimate microsphere regional blood flows (the gold standard) in low-flow situations because of increased myocardial extraction and underestimate high microsphere flows of hyperemic zones because short residence times reduce myocardial extraction. These flow-related limitations, although important for absolute quantitation, are not critical for clinical application but merely serve to highlight the complicated nature of quantitative MPI.

### Electrocardiographic Treadmill Test

The ETT has been used to detect myocardial ischemia for nearly a quarter of a century. It is well known that the ETT is neither sensitive in patients with CAD nor specific in patients without CAD. This is why MPI has been performed in many individuals suspected of CAD since 1976.

Iskandrian et al. have correlated the effect of the exercise level during electrocardiographic (ECG) stress testing to the sensitivity and specificity of SPECT MPI in 461 patients (26). They found that the level of stress directly correlates with the Tl-201 imaging results in terms of localization of disease, evaluation of the extent of CAD, and detection of myocardial ischemia. Less demanding stress tests (e.g., submaximal exercise, arm ergometry, or supine bicycle exercise) may be performed if the patient cannot physically complete a Bruce protocol, but imaging results with these nonconventional stress tests may be less certain. Beta-blockers or calcium channel blockers should be tapered or withheld for 48 hours before the exercise test. Long-acting nitrates should be discontinued 12 hours before the study, although sublingual nitroglycerin may be given up to 2 hours before the test. If patients undergoing these diagnostic protocols cannot discontinue therapy or cannot exercise adequately, stressors such as dipyridamole, adenosine, or dobutamine should be used. In some patients (e.g., in prognostication) submaximal stress or exercise stress on therapy is preferred.

In the classic ETT, blood pressure, heart rate, duration of exercise, and symptoms (e.g., angina, shortness of breath, and fatigue) are recorded as the patient exercises using standard maximal or submaximal protocols. Exercise is continued for 60 (Tl-201) or 90 (Tc-99m sestamibi) seconds after injection of tracer, and imaging is begun within 5 to 10 minutes for Tl-201 and within 15 to 30 minutes for Tc-99m sestamibi.

Other parameters to document during ETT (besides cardiac symptoms and heart rate) include

- Estimated peak oxygen consumption in metabolic equivalent test units (METS) and that expected for presence or absence of cardiac disease, level of physical activity, and gender
- New York Heart Association functional class
- Pressure-rate (or double) product, a unitless parameter derived by multiplying systolic blood pressure by heart rate at maximal stress

**TABLE 2-7.** *ETT termination*

Desired stress end points
    Achievement of maximal predicted heart rate
    Symptom limitation by severe angina
Adequate stress
    ≥85% of the maximal predicted heart rate
    Double product of >25,000
    Achievement of appropriate estimated oxygen consumption (especially if on beta-blocker)
Early termination indicated
    4 mm ST-segment depression*
    Malignant arrhythmia
    >10 mm Hg decrease in systolic BP
    Nonanginal symptom (dyspnea or fatigue) limitation
Barely adequate stress
    75% maximal predicted heart rate

*When no baseline abnormalities present (e.g., LBBB, MI, LVH, digoxin effect).

These parameters are useful for the referring physician because detection of the presence, and assessment of the extent of CAD are linearly related to the work done by the heart during an ETT. When the patient achieves >85% of the maximal predicted heart rate, the test is considered adequate. The maximal predicted heart rate can be calculated by subtracting the patient's age from 220—for example, for a 50 year old, the maximum predicted heart rate is 170 (220 – 50). Otherwise, the test is designated submaximal, and the heart rate achieved during the ETT is specified. Heart rates in excess of 75% of the maximal predicted heart rate are considered barely adequate. Ischemic ECG changes are defined as horizontal or down-sloping ST-segment depressions of at least 1 mm during exercise or recovery, generally in contiguous leads, that were normal at rest. LV hypertrophy, concurrent administration of digoxin, prior myocardial damage, preexisting conduction defects (left and right bundle branch block [LBBB and RBBB]), rest repolarization abnormalities, valvular heart disease, and mitral valve prolapse decrease the specificity of ST-segment abnormalities. The various ETT end points are shown in Table 2-7.

## Pharmacologic MPI

The subject of pharmacologic vasodilatation has been extensively reviewed (39,40). It is widely thought that exercise and pharmacologic stress scintigraphy performed with either Tc-99m sestamibi or Tl-201 have equal diagnostic accuracy and predictive power for ischemic events. Exercise testing is universally favored because it provides additional important ECG and blood pressure data, which adds to the independent predictive value of stress scintigraphy, especially to medical practitioners such as cardiologists. With exercise testing, the aim is to induce myocardial ischemia; with dipyridamole and adenosine the aim often is to provoke myocardial perfusion heterogeneity.

One-third of patients referred for MPI cannot perform adequate treadmill exercise because of deconditioning, old age, low stress level (e.g., on propranolol), arthritis, peripheral vascular disease (PVD), aortic disease, orthopedic problems, muscular diseases, severe obesity, pacemakers, sick sinus syndrome, and arteriovenous (AV) block. Patients with aortic stenosis should be evaluated for the potential risk of exercise-induced syncope, and dipyridamole used if valvular stenosis is significant.

### *Dipyridamole*

Dipyridamole (Persantine) stress testing was first proposed by Gould in 1978 (41). Dipyridamole is a potent coronary vasodilator that increases local adenosine levels by inhibiting endothelial and red blood cell reuptake of adenosine, and inhibiting adenosine breakdown (via deaminase). The adenosine concentration builds up outside the cell and triggers vasodilation of coronary arterioles smaller than 150 μm. Adenosine effects are mediated by specific A2 receptors present on the cell membrane, which can be blocked by theophylline and caffeine. Vasodilation cannot occur in the arterial beds subtended by these critical coronary stenoses, and perfusion defects are induced.

Dipyridamole causes the vascular reserve in normal coronary arteries to increase four times above the baseline level and to twice that which occurs with exercise. There is no change of the pressure-rate product with pharmacologic (dipyridamole or adenosine) vasodilatation, and more than two-thirds of patients with CAD have perfusion defects induced without the development of myocardial ischemia. Myocardial regions that are collateral dependent may become ischemic from coronary steal phenomenon, as a result of adenosine-induced changes diverting flow from the stenotic to the nonstenotic vascular beds. This mechanism was confirmed when it was found that the angiographic presence of collaterals was the strongest predictor of ST-segment depression during adenosine vasodilatation. ST-segment depression during pharmacologic stress is a good marker of coronary steal and ischemia.

The clinical experience with dipyridamole MPI is substantial. The increase in CBF begins at the start of the infusion and continues for 4 minutes after infusion. The hemodynamic effects of dipyridamole are a slight increase in heart rate and slight decrease in blood pressure with no net change in pressure-rate product. Low-level treadmill exercise at the termination of the dipyridamole and before imaging may diminish splanchnic tracer content, which otherwise degrades image quality. Patients must be off caffeine, chocolate, and nicotine for 24 hours before the test. Aminophylline, theophylline (Slo-bid, Theo-Dur), and oral dipyridamole should also be discontinued. The test is contraindicated in patients with asthma, severe chronic obstructive pulmonary disease, and baseline hypotension; these patients should undergo dobutamine stress testing.

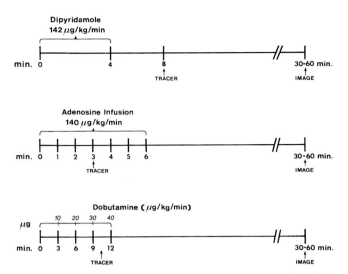

**FIG. 2-13.** Imaging protocols for pharmacologic vasodilatation. Schematics of time-related infusions of dipyridamole, adenosine, and dobutamine are shown with radiopharmaceutical injection and imaging times. (Modified from Iskandrian AS, Verani MS, Heo J. Pharmacologic stress testing: mechanism of action, hemodynamic responses, and results in detection of coronary artery disease. J Nucl Cardiol 1994;1:94–111.)

Figure 2-13 shows the protocol followed for dipyridamole MPI. Ranhosky and Kempthorne-Rawson reported data on 3,911 patients treated with IV dipyridamole (42). The rate of major adverse events was similar to what has been reported for routine treadmill stress testing. Common side effects (42) were chest pain (20%), headache (12%), dizziness (12%), ST-segment changes (8%), and ventricular premature contractions (VPCs, 5%). Most of these side effects are relatively minor. Very rarely acute subendocardial myocardial infarction, supraventricular tachycardia, and severe bronchospasm can occur. Bronchospasm requires IV injection of aminophylline (adenosine receptor antagonist). The biological half-life of dipyridamole is longer than desired, and it is our practice to give aminophylline, 100 mg slowly IV, 5 minutes after the injection of tracer to counteract its effect. Patients who develop severe chest pain or unstable angina with dipyridamole testing should be admitted to the hospital and treated with aminophylline, nitroglycerin, and other therapy as appropriate.

Overall, dipyridamole MPI has an average sensitivity of 90% and a specificity of 85% for the detection of CAD, similar to that of ETT. Just as with ETT stress MPI, the number of transient ischemic perfusion defects and large ischemic or nonreversible perfusion defects with either Tl-201 or Tc-99m sestamibi indicate a poor prognosis. With Tl-201, increased lung uptake and LV cavity dilatation are markers of poor prognosis in CAD (43).

### Adenosine

Adenosine has an ultrashort half-life of 2 seconds and kinetics that are many times faster than those of dipy-

ridamole, precluding the need for prophylactic aminophylline treatment or patient observation. Adenosine has the same imaging indications as dipyridamole but is more expensive. The side effect rate is greater than dipyridamole, but these subside within 2 to 3 minutes of discontinuing the infusion and include (40) flushing (37%), shortness of breath (35%), chest pain (35%), GI discomfort (15%), headache (14%), atrioventricular block (8%), and ST-segment depression (6%). Adenosine is contraindicated in patients with second- or third-degree AV block unless they have a functioning pacemaker in place.

Figure 2-13 shows the adenosine MPI protocol. Aminophylline and caffeine users should not undergo adenosine MPI for at least 12 hours after their last dose.

The sensitivity and specificity of adenosine MPI for detecting CAD are similar to that of ETT or dipyridamole MPI (39,40). The average sensitivity in patients with CAD is 88% (range, 83% to 98%), and specificity is 85% (range, 64% to 100%).

### Dobutamine

Dobutamine hydrochloride (44,45) is a synthetic catecholamine with a plasma half-life of 2 minutes that acts through the alpha$_1$- and beta$_2$-adrenoreceptors. Dobutamine stress is given to patients who cannot exercise and who suffer from bronchospasm and so cannot receive dipyridamole. Dobutamine mimics exercise physiology because it significantly increases the heart rate and blood pressure at doses >20 µg/kg per minute. Ischemia is provoked more frequently with dobutamine than with dipyridamole or adenosine. The threefold increase in coronary flow with dobutamine is less than the fourfold change seen with adenosine but more than the twofold increase that occurs with exercise testing. Rare hypersensitivity reactions occur, including skin rash, fever, bronchospasm, and eosinophilia. Side effects of dobutamine (39,40,44,45) are chest pain (31%), palpitation (29%), headache (14%), flushing (14%), dyspnea (14%), and other pain (14%).

The imaging protocol is shown in Fig. 2-13. Atropine (0.2 mg IV) may be needed after achieving a maximal dobutamine dose (40 µg/kg/min) if the increase in heart rate is submaximal (<85% of maximum predicted).

Pennell et al. (44) studied 50 patients with exertional chest pain and reported a sensitivity of 97% and specificity of 80% for dobutamine Tl-201 SPECT scintigraphy.

### Comparison of Drug Stress MPI and 2D Echocardiography

Marwick et al. (45) assessed prospectively in a consecutive series of patients the accuracy of adenosine (180 µg/kg/min) or dobutamine (40 µg/kg/min) stress in conjunction with Tc-99m sestamibi SPECT and 2D echocar-

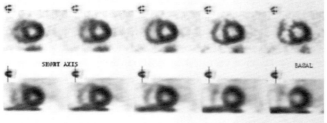

**FIG. 2-14.** Some of the short-axis views of a normal 1-day study using Tc-99m MIBI stress (upper row) and rest Tl-201 SPECT (lower row) scanning. Note the poorer resolution of Tl-201 with smaller LV cavity, and the more prominent RV visualization on the stress Tc-99m MIBI images.

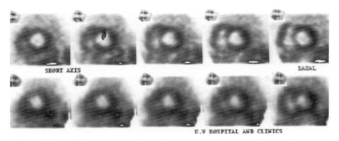

**FIG. 2-15.** These short-axis views show stress (upper) and rest (lower) Tc-99m sestamibi images through the basal portion of the heart. These images show poor uptake into the heart with high background activity and a defect involving the inferior right ventricle at stress that normalizes at rest.

diography. The sensitivities for detection of CAD were similar for Tc-99m sestamibi SPECT with either drug (80% to 86%) and dobutamine 2D echocardiography (85%) whereas the sensitivity for adenosine 2D echocardiography was only 58%.

**Normal Scans**

The stress and the rest MPI scans should contain a homogeneous radionuclide distribution. The resolution of the images depends on tracer used, dose, and the image acquisition and processing technique. The right ventricle (RV) is more commonly (and faintly) visualized in poststress Tc-99m sestamibi images than in Tl-201 scans, and is rarely imaged in rest images except in RV hypertrophy (Fig. 2-14). Occasionally, RV defects can be seen in stress images in inferior myocardial infarcts (Fig. 2-15).

Normal variants and technical considerations that might result in false-positive stress SPECT MPI tests (46,47) are shown in Table 2-8. Specific diseases that may cause scan abnormalities that emulate CAD include LBBB, cardiomyopathy, asymmetric septal hypertrophy, hypertension with intense septal activity, and sarcoidosis.

**TABLE 2-8.** *Causes of false-positive MPI*

| Patient | Technical |
|---|---|
| Dose infiltration | Low count studies |
| Patient or respiratory motion | Improper timing |
| Normal apical thinning | Camera nonuniformity |
| Prominent papillary muscle | Center of rotation errors |
| Diaphragmatic attenuation (inferoseptal in males) | Reconstruction errors |
| | Improper plane selection |
| Breast attenuation (anteroseptal for small and large breasts) | Count normalization (to "hotter" liver or GI tract activity) |

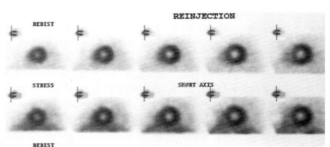

**FIG. 2-16.** Short-axis images of stress (upper row) and reinjection (lower row) Tl-201 SPECT scans of a patient with LBBB. The stress images show mild septal hypoperfusion that normalizes at rest. This is not due to CAD but is the result of LBBB.

Patients with LBBB should receive dipyridamole MPI because they often develop non-CAD transient septal defect (Fig. 2-16).

*Attenuation*

The most common artifact is attenuation. In men there is commonly a 10% to 15% reduction of counts in the inferoseptal region due to left diaphragmatic attenuation (Fig. 2-17) and in women there is a similar reduction of counts in the anterolateral or the anterior apical or septal region due to breast attenuation. The inferoseptal defect may be seen in any individual (male or female) with a protuberant abdomen, and can involve the inferolateral segment if the left diaphragm is elevated. The breast artifact depends on the shape and size of the breast, and some female normalization maps have tried to include this variable. If the breast is relatively small and firm, then the defect is seen in the distal anteroapical or anteroseptal segment. This defect can also be seen in men with gynecomastia. Breasts that are larger and more pendulous drape laterally in the supine position, and so the anterolateral wall is attenuated (Fig. 2-18). These attenuation defects should be equally well seen in the stress and rest images (i.e., fixed) unless imaging conditions are different (e.g., bra on and off). A fixed perfusion defect in the typical site with normal wall motion on gated SPECT imaging often indicates an attenuation artifact (see Figs. 2-17 and 2-18).

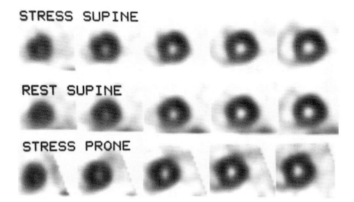

**STRESS SUPINE**

**REST SUPINE**

**STRESS PRONE**

**FIG. 2-17.** Short-axis views showing stress (upper row) and rest (middle row) supine Tc-99m sestamibi images and a mild persistent inferoseptal defect. This defect is not apparent on the prone stress image (lower row). Normal wall motion of all segments was seen in the gated SPECT images. This is typical of diaphragmatic attenuation. (Images provided by Dr. James Thomsen, Veterans Administration Medical Center, Madison, WI.)

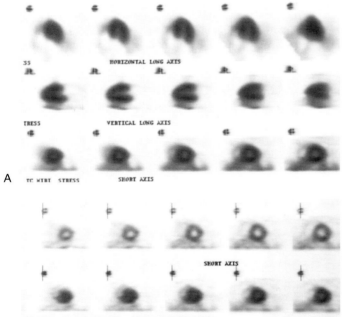

**A**  TC MIBI STRESS   SHORT AXIS

**B**  GATED MIBI ED & ES DISPLAY!

**FIG. 2-18. (A)** These three rows show the long- and short-axis views of Tc-99m sestamibi stress SPECT images and mild anterior decrease in counts. The same defect was seen at rest. **(B)** These two rows of gated SPECT short-axis views show the anterolateral segment to contract normally. These findings are typical of breast attenuation.

## Technical Artifacts

To optimize SPECT cardiac studies and minimize appearance of artifacts, SPECT detector QC is essential. Detector nonuniformities, misalignment of the center of rotation, and multidetector alignment errors are important. The technologist's reorientation of the heart image for display is critical to ensure appropriate stress and rest comparisons in short-axis views. Many users do not appreciate the extensive reorientation that occurs to get the images into the conventional display when the long axis of the ventricle is rotated 40 to 50 degrees.

### Radiopharmaceutical Artifact

Hepatic, bowel, and stomach (enterogastric reflux) activity in the rest studies can result in scattered photons mistakenly incorporated into the polar map with pseudonormalization of perfusion defects. Normalization between rest and stress and between the short-axis, horizontal, and vertical long-axis views is essential for valid comparisons. Visceral tracer localization is a common cause of normalization artifacts in rest or drug stress Tl-201 and rest-stress Tc-99m sestamibi images and results from gastrointestinal localization of tracer. This is particularly so with the hepatobiliary excretion of Tc-99m sestamibi, where small and large bowel activity and even enterogastric reflux and esophageal reflux can occur (see Fig. 2-11). Germano et al. (48) demonstrated that the incidence and severity of artifactual perfusion defects in Tc-99m sestamibi studies are directly proportional to the ratio of liver to cardiac activity.

### Patient Motion

It is probably not possible to retrospectively correct for motion in SPECT MPI studies, so the best strategy is to avoid patient motion (46). Motion artifacts are complex with the three-detector systems, and a successful correction technique of motion artifacts in patients imaged with three-detector imaging systems has not been published. The projection data of each SPECT MPI study should routinely be displayed as a sinogram in cine format to detect undesirable cardiac motion, which is manifested as a "jump" in the display. This usually indicates shifts of 2 or more pixels.

### Abnormal Scans

Perfusion defects on the stress study indicate that further imaging with the patient at rest is necessary to distinguish ischemia from infarction. If there are no poststress perfusion defects, no further studies are needed. Defects that improve or normalize on the Tc-99m sestamibi or Tl-201 myocardial slices obtained at rest are unequivocal evidence of acute reversible myocardial ischemia (Fig. 2-19). Defects that are similar in size on the poststress and rest, and that do not exhibit myocardial thickening on gated SPECT, indicate chronic myocardial infarction (see Figs. 2-3 and 2-5).

### Vessel Territories

The anteroseptal segment in the short-axis view (Fig. 2-20) is in the territory of the left anterior descending coronary artery.

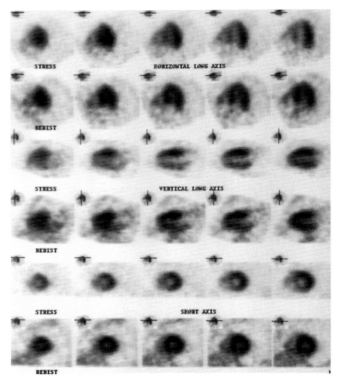

**FIG. 2-19.** This stress and rest redistribution Tl-201 scan shows a moderate-sized septal and inferoseptal stress abnormality of moderate degree that improves significantly on redistribution images, indicating ischemia.

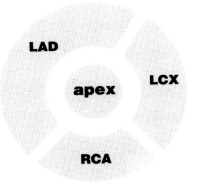

**FIG. 2-20.** This diagram shows the usual territories of the coronary arteries in the short-axis view.

The lateral segment in this and the horizontal long-axis view is in the territory of the left circumflex coronary artery (LCX). The inferoseptal segment in the short-axis view is supplied by the posterior descending artery (PDA) and is often an indication of the perfusion status of the right coronary artery (RCA). In 85% of patients, the PDA is a branch of the RCA, and in 15% of patients the PDA is a branch of the LCX. There is considerable overlap of the distribution of the coronary arteries, which is a confounding factor when attributing particular MPI defects to a particular coronary artery (34).

### Description of MPI Defects

*Size*

Defects are described arbitrarily as to size and degree of count depression. Most defects are called *small, moderate,* or *large* according to the extent of involvement of a myocardial segment as seen in more than one tomographic plane (defects that are not seen in the short-axis view are likely to be artifactual). Large defects involve two or more contiguous myocardial segments (see Fig. 2-8) in more than one tomographic view, moderate defects involve one myocardial segment in more than one tomographic view, and small defects involve less than one myocardial segment. The variability of segment nomenclature (see Fig. 2-8) makes a universal descriptive technique difficult.

*Degree*

To describe intensity of count depression, we follow the method of Bonow et al. (49). The normal reference area is the area with the maximum count in the entire myocardium. Any region with 85% to 100% of the normal reference area counts is considered nonpathologic and is commonly attributed to attenuation. A mild defect has 60% to 85% of the count density of the reference normal area, a moderate defect has a 50% to 60% relative decrease, and a severe defect has <50% of the reference activity. All mild or moderate defects with >50% of the counts of the reference region are considered viable myocardium.

*Reversibility of Defects*

Defects that are present on both stress and rest images are nonreversible or fixed (see Figs. 2-3 and 2-5). In contrast, reversible defects may have partial or complete reversibility. It is understood that partial reversibility is usually associated with segmental thinning on the gated wall-motion study, and the count density corresponds to 50% to 85% of the density in the normal reference regions. *Complete reversibility* refers to areas that have no myocardial thinning in rest images and that have resting count densities similar to that of the reference areas (see Fig. 2-19).

### CLINICAL APPLICATIONS

#### General Considerations

*Referral Bias*

When MPI was introduced it was primarily used for the diagnosis of CAD. With time, the referral population changed, so that CAD diagnosis now represents only 35% of total indications (see Table 2-1). Even in this population, the

**TABLE 2-9.** *Pretest MPI probability of CAD (%) subdivided by age, sex, and character of chest pain*

| Age | Nonanginal chest wall pain | | Atypical angina | | Typical angina | |
|---|---|---|---|---|---|---|
| | Men | Women | Men | Women | Men | Women |
| 30–39 | 5.2 | 0.8 | 22.2 | 4.2 | 69.7 | 25.8 |
| 40–49 | 14.1 | 2.8 | 46.1 | 13.3 | 87.3 | 55.4 |
| 50–59 | 21.5 | 8.4 | 58.9 | 32.4 | 92.6 | 79.4 |
| 60–69 | 28.1 | 18.6 | 67.1 | 54.4 | 94.3 | 90.6 |

Source: Reprinted with permission from Diamond GA, Forrester JS. Analysis of probability as an aid in the clinical diagnosis of coronary-artery disease. N Engl J Med 1979;300:1350–1358.

patients have changed to a more difficult diagnostic subset. Accordingly, the early sensitivity and specificity data for MPI do not apply today. The decreases in the sensitivity and specificity values for MPI do not reflect a change in the actual test performance, rather they result from changes in the referred patient population. The specificity of Tl-201 MPI is decreased if only the patients with abnormal scans have coronary angiograms. This type of bias (50) is responsible for the lower specificity found in recent prospective MPI SPECT studies. To avoid this problem, individuals of either sex should be considered normal in future studies if they have <5% pretest likelihood of CAD. This can be predicted (Table 2-9) from published probability tables, which yield estimated CAD probability based on age, sex, and character of chest pain (51). These individuals form a group from which the normalcy rate is derived: normal subjects with normal scans (see Table 2-5). The normalcy rate is a better parameter than the conventional specificity assessment to study diagnostic tests.

### *LV Function*

Concordance of myocardial perfusion and wall motion is designated as perfusion-work coupling. As an example, a soft-tissue artifact uncouples the perfusion (irreversible defect) from the function (good contractility). Other instances of discordant LV perfusion and wall motion data include the following:

- In breast or diaphragmatic attenuation, associated normal regional wall-motion data are useful to define a perfusion defect as artifactual.
- In "stunned" myocardium, perfusion may be normal but severe wall-motion abnormalities are present. These wall-motion abnormalities respond to catecholamine stimulation.
- In severe CAD, hibernating viable regions with normal or mild-to-moderate perfusion decreases may be severely hypocontractile.
- Segments may have normal coronary flow but reduced F-18 fluorodeoxyglucose (FDG) uptake and severe wall-motion abnormalities.
- In cardiomyopathy, valvular heart disease, small vessel disease, hypertension, sarcoidosis, myocarditis, and connective tissue diseases, there may be normal CBF in seg-

ments with wall-motion abnormalities, or the wall-motion abnormality may be worse than the perfusion defect.

### *Combined Perfusion and Contraction Data*

Tc-99m sestamibi imaging can provide useful MPI data together with assessment of global and regional LV function. Left ventricular ejection fraction (LVEF), wall motion, and wall thickening can be assessed using first-pass angiocardiography (52) or gated SPECT scans (53). For acquisition of gated Tc-99m sestamibi scans, data are acquired as for the regular myocardial perfusion SPECT studies, using 8 frames per cardiac cycle. With multidetector systems, 8 frames per cardiac cycle can be potentially acquired with a modest twofold additional acquisition time penalty, and increased processing time. Regional wall motion is assessed by evaluation of endocardial excursion. Regional wall thickening is assessed by image intensification from end-diastole to end-systole. More sophisticated analyses are possible from wall-motion studies, including regional ejection fractions (see Fig. 2-12).

### Diagnosis of CAD

MPI is more sensitive and specific than ETT in the detection of CAD. Since the work of Hamilton in 1978 and the probability study of Diamond and Forrester (51), the best policy for using Tl-201 MPI for diagnosing CAD is to select patients with chest pain who have an intermediate (15% to 85%) prescan probability of CAD (see Table 2-9). In this subclass, both positive and negative MPI scans have important diagnostic (and prognostic) implications. The following data are important information to identify: the post-test likelihood of disease, high-risk angiographic CAD patients, and the subsequent risk of cardiac events. Patients who have an uninterpretable ECG during exercise (LV hypertrophy, digoxin use) should also have MPI scans.

### *False-Positive Results*

Patients with low pretest probability of CAD, when subjected to MPI, are more likely to have false-positive test results (e.g., a 20-year-old athlete who has no CAD risk factors but presents with chest wall pain has a pretest probability of <5%). In an asymptomatic young male cohort of military air crew, MPI resulted in a high frequency of false-positive test results as expected by Bayes' probability theorem. It is now known that coronary angiograms underestimate lesion severity in coronary stenoses of intermediate severity, so this can also contribute to false-positive results.

### False-Negative Results

In contrast, patients with high pretest probabilities of CAD are likely to have false-negative MPI test results. The 55-year-old man with typical chest pain should go straight to coronary arteriography because his pretest probability exceeds 90% (see Table 2-9). False-negative MPI tests also occur with inadequate exercise, single-vessel disease, less than critical coronary stenosis, and drugs that impede increased cardiac work in ETTs (nitroglycerin, beta-blockers, and calcium channel blockers).

## Prognosis of CAD

A significant aspect of stress MPI is the use of scintigraphic patterns to identify advanced CAD, that is, to predict occurrence of hard coronary events, such as death, nonfatal myocardial infarction, recurrent angina, and revascularization procedures.

### High-Risk Scan Groups

Hard coronary events are predicted by the extent and severity of myocardial ischemia, as shown by stress Tl-201 scintigraphic features (3,43,54,55), including

- Size and number of reversible defects (predicts infarction or acute ischemia)
- Large nonreversible perfusion defects
- Multiple reversible defects, indicating two- or three-vessel disease
- Increased Tl-201 lung uptake (LV dysfunction)
- Transient exercise-induced LV dilatation

Note that lung uptake and transient exercise-induced LV dilatation are unlikely to be seen with Tc-99m sestamibi scans because these scan acquisitions routinely commence 15 minutes after stress is completed and require 5 to 10 minutes to complete.

### High-Risk Patient Groups

Patient groups in whom coronary angiography is contemplated are obvious candidates for MPI to help stratify risk:

- Chest pain syndromes (rule out AMI)
- Post–myocardial infarction
- Unstable angina
- Post–coronary revascularization
- Severe LV dysfunction (LVEF <50%)
- Those about to undergo major vascular noncardiac surgery

In these patient groups, a high-risk MPI result expedites referral for coronary angiography. In patients with typical angina and an abnormal ECG on stress testing and in patients with typical angina who are symptomatic or asymptomatic while receiving maximal medical therapy, an abnormal MPI test result yields incremental information regarding potential for future cardiac events (56).

### Low-Risk Scan Groups

All previous data are consistent with the observation that patients with one reversible defect (≤15% of LV mass) are a low-event risk group. An analysis of 23 clinical series including 5,285 patients shows (54) that a normal scintigraphic stress result predicts a very benign clinical patient outcome even in the presence of angiographic CAD and unstable angina (57) and that this is not affected by concurrent antianginal treatment or the degree of stress achieved. When the perfusion scans are low risk in the patients with typical angina, medical management is preferred.

## Post-AMI Risk Stratification

After an uncomplicated AMI, Gibson et al. (58) showed that presence of a single, small, fixed Tl-201 defect at discharge from hospital predicts a low rate of events. This is true for small fixed defects, just as in the prognosis of CAD generally, but not for moderate or large nonreversible defects. Conversely, patients with reversible ischemia, multiple defects, and lung uptake of Tl-201 had 14 times more cardiac events than did patients with a fixed single defect. Post-AMI patients who are asymptomatic or have nonanginal chest pain are candidates for MPI. A recent observation that has been thoroughly discussed is that MPI's predictive value for patients after an AMI may be less in those patients receiving thrombolytic therapy (59,60).

## Prediction of Perioperative Events

PVD often coexists with cerebrovascular disease and CAD. These patients are often older or diabetic and are at very high risk for perioperative cardiac events. This is especially so in patients with PVD and angina. Nearly half of all asymptomatic patients scheduled for PVD surgery have CAD. Patients with PVD often cannot exercise, and dipyridamole MPI has thus been extensively used in the last 10 years to assess the presence and functional significance of CAD. Reversible Tl-201 defects and ischemic ECG changes

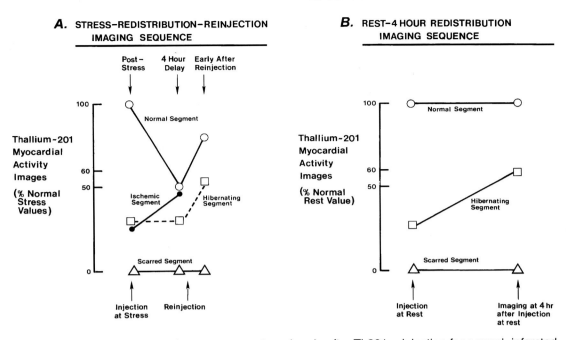

**FIG. 2-21. (A)** The Tl-201 uptake at stress, rest, and early after Tl-201 reinjection for normal, infarcted (scarred), ischemic, and hibernating segments when compared to normal stress uptake. **(B)** The Tl-201 uptake for normal, hibernating, and infarcted (scarred) segments compared to normal uptake at rest, in the rest–4-hour redistribution protocol.

during dipyridamole testing (61) identify patients at risk of perioperative cardiac events.

The presence of Q waves in the ECG, a history of ventricular ectopy, diabetes, age >70 years, and angina are strong clinical predictors for perioperative ischemic events in these patients (62). MPI with dipyridamole preoperatively is most efficacious in identifying CAD in these PVD patients who have one or two of these clinical predictors.

## Myocardial Viability

In patients with CAD, the presence of severe LV dysfunction (LVEF <30% and significant wall-motion abnormalities) increases cardiac morbidity and mortality during long-term medical therapy. In the Coronary Artery Surgery Survival study (63), coronary artery bypass surgery improved survival and functional status of these patients with severe LV dysfunction. There is uncertainty about selecting the most appropriate candidates for revascularization, because these patients also have unpredictable outcomes and represent high operative risks.

### Myocardial Hibernation

Rahimtoola (64) introduced the concept of myocardial hibernation to describe hypocontractile heart muscle that improves after coronary revascularization. This concept was based solely on clinical observations, and there is no experimental model for myocardial hibernation. No clear notion exists about the inter-relationship of chronic coronary hypoperfusion, myocardial metabolism, and damage in hibernating myocardial segments. Indeed, as of this writing, all recent quantitative investigations unexpectedly demonstrated that resting myocardial blood flow in dysfunctional LV segments is within normal limits.

In 1983, Gibson et al. (65) showed that approximately half of all patients with nonreversible defects on delayed Tl-201 scans had improved LV function after revascularization. This report was largely forgotten until studies using PET identified possible "hibernating cardiac regions" with impaired wall motion (akinesis, dyskinesis, or severe hypokinesis) that showed improved perfusion and contractility after coronary artery revascularization. PET scan evidence of enhanced glucose uptake by F-18 FDG scanning but decreased absolute regional perfusion by N-13 ammonia was designated as PET "mismatch" (66), with a positive predictive value of 78% to 85% and a negative predictive value of 78% to 92% for postrevascularization contractility improvement in a small number of patients. The hibernating segments that best respond to revascularization are in patients who have angina and chronically dysfunctional LV segments rendered ischemic during MPI.

The standard Tl-201 redistribution scan technique identifies ischemia well but underestimates the amount of viable myocardium. This limitation led to the introduction of the Tl-201 reinjection technique (67) where, if a defect is identified on the stress images, an additional 1 mCi Tl-201 is given 4 hours after the initial poststress images, and then the patient is imaged. The relative myocardial concentration of Tl-201 after reinjection (Fig. 2-21A) reflects a combination of the Tl-201

**TABLE 2-10.** *Characteristics of hibernating, stunned, and infarcted myocardium*

|  | Hibernating | Stunned | Infarcted |
|---|---|---|---|
| Tl-201 uptake (vs. normal) | >50% | Normal | <50% |
| Wall motion | Abnormal | Abnormal | Abnormal |
| FDG uptake | Preserved | Preserved | Absent |
| Dobutamine response | Yes | Yes | No |
| Improvement on revascularization | Yes | Yes | No |

uptake that occurred during stress, some washout, some redistribution uptake, and the additional uptake after rest reinjection. These reinjection images are therefore related to flow conditions, blood tracer concentrations present at rest, and the variable washout and redistribution rates of the myocardium as a result of the two injections.

Data now show (49) that the issue of myocardial viability arises only with severe stress or rest Tl-201 MPI defects (>50% to 60% reduction). MPI defects with lesser Tl-201 reductions are all viable. Half the regions with severe, nonreversible Tl-201 defects are also viable, as shown by uptake of Tl-201 after the reinjection procedure, FDG uptake by PET, and systolic wall thickening by gated MRI, and as established by postsurgical wall-motion improvement. In the vast majority of regions with severe fixed Tl-201 defects that have FDG uptake on PET scanning, Tl-201 reinjection scans show improved Tl-201 uptake, indicating viable and hibernating myocardium.

Ragosta et al. (68) similarly showed in CAD patients that rest-delay-rest Tl-201 MPI (Fig. 2-21B) identifies viability in one-half of hibernating segments. At Cedars-Sinai Hospital in Los Angeles, the initial and delayed resting Tl-201 images, obtained 4 to 12 hours or more apart, clearly show a significant increase in uptake in hibernating regions. These regions are expected to show improved function after coronary revascularization. Gutman et al. (69) showed that the time required for Tl-201 redistribution to occur in a segment correlates to the severity of stenosis. Thus, ample time (preferably several hours) must be allowed for Tl-201 rest redistribution studies to detect viability.

Table 2-10 shows the pathophysiologic characteristics of hibernating, stunned, and infarcted myocardium. It now appears that myocardial hibernation is the result of repeated episodes of myocardial stunning. It has been determined that the Tc-99m sestamibi scans can also identify myocardial viability (21,70).

### Myocardial Stunning

In stunned myocardium (67), postischemic coronary flow to a region is normal, but there may be marked segmental hypocontraction or akinesis, with a normal response to a catecholamine challenge (see Table 2-10). Conditions favoring stunned myocardium include

- Percutaneous transluminal coronary angioplasty (PTCA)
- Graft implantation
- Spontaneous postinfarction reperfusion
- Reperfusion after tissue plasminogen activator
- Post coronary vasospasm
- Post exercise-induced ischemia.

Return of wall motion in these patients may take hours, days, or weeks. Some believe that myocardial hibernation and myocardial stunning may coexist.

### Reverse Redistribution

Reverse redistribution is the worsening of a stress defect or the appearance of a new defect on Tl-201 redistribution images. Reverse redistribution has been associated with severe coronary stenosis, stable CAD, and thrombolytic therapy for AMI, as well as found in normal individuals. In patients with chronic stable CAD, most regions with reverse redistribution show viability by either normal wall motion or hypokinesis, increased Tl-201 content after the reinjection technique, FDG uptake, or absence of ECG Q waves.

### Selection for Revascularization

Patients with multivessel CAD and severe LV dysfunction often present with angina or heart failure and are appropriate surgical candidates for revascularization if it can be shown that more than two adjacent dysfunctional segments have inducible ischemia. Coronary anatomy is a key factor in the decision to operate, but MPI identifies these high-risk patients for angiography (56).

Tc-99m sestamibi allows assessment of the severity and extent of myocardial ischemia, identification of the culprit lesion, and estimation of the prognosis in patients with low-risk (Braunwald classification) unstable angina and those with acute chest pain (43,56). MPI is considered for unstable angina patients who respond to medical therapy and those with abnormal ECGs (including those on digoxin).

In patients who present to the ER with chest pain, MPI with Tc-99m sestamibi can help the clinician to select patients who need to be admitted to the hospital when the more usual tests, such as ECG, are inconclusive (71). Only 30% to 40% of patients with suspected unstable angina actually have CAD. The cost benefit of this triaging is potentially immense because less than one-third of the 5 million patients who present annually to the ER with chest pain have AMI. Logistically, this test is difficult because the tracer must be injected during or soon after the chest pain.

### Assessment of Infarct Size Reduction

It is known that during AMI, the ultimate size of the infarct depends on the size of the hypoperfused area at risk, the duration of the ischemia, and the adequacy of the collateral network.

Although we do not have a means of measuring collateral circulation using MPI, we can semiquantitatively assess the cardiac area at risk. The greatest amount of salvaged myocardium occurs when occlusion time is limited to 1 or possibly 2 hours, hence the emphasis on rapid thrombolytic therapy. At the present time, only 30% of AMI patients undergo adequate thrombolytic therapy. Tc-99m sestamibi traces flow and viability (21) independent of myocardial stunning, compensatory hyperkinesia, and loading. If Tc-99m sestamibi is given before thrombolytic therapy (because it redistributes very slowly), the image obtained hours later represents the area at risk. A subsequent image, obtained days later, can indicate the final extent of the defect, with the difference representing the salvaged area. Experimental data confirm the usefulness of Tc-99m sestamibi for semiquantitative measurement of the area at risk. However, these data are difficult to obtain in the clinical environment because precise measurements of the volumes of acutely infarcted and noninfarcted regions are difficult and because radiopharmaceutical logistics and cost to make Tc-99m sestamibi available for rapid injection at night or on weekends are prohibitive.

Gibson et al. (72) demonstrated that the sestamibi perfusion defect size and severity on early serial imaging is related to location and patency of the infarct artery. Patients who show a substantial change in defect size on serial imaging and develop symptoms need repeat urgent angiography to detect reocclusion. Sestamibi myocardial perfusion was used in a randomized trial that showed that in AMI, immediate angioplasty does not produce greater myocardial salvage than do thrombolysis and conservative therapy (73).

Although the clinical investigative data support use of Tc-99m sestamibi to measure infarct size, there are limitations to this approach: uncertainties about defining epicardial and endocardial boundaries in myocardial areas with large amounts of hypoperfusion, limited spatial resolution of SPECT (1.5-cm resolution vs. 2- to 3-mm [endocardial] and 7- to 8-mm [epicardial] thicknesses), photon attenuation, Compton scatter, and difficulties aligning serial perfusion studies.

### Other Uses of MPI

After PTCA, restenosis occurs in one-third to one-half of all patients. Stress MPI, preferably performed after discontinuation of anti-ischemic medications, is used 4 or more weeks after coronary angioplasty prognostically for the detection of residual myocardial ischemia or incomplete revascularization (74). Atypical or typical chest pain after angioplasty is an indication for repeat MPI. Because >50% of saphenous vein grafts occlude beyond the fifth year after surgery, MPI is also recommended at this time or for those patients who become symptomatic.

**TABLE 2-11.** *Problems with stress echocardiography*

Variable sensitivity with stress
  Maximum exercise 90%
  Submaximal exercise 42%
Semiquantitative nature
Underestimates myocardial viability
May miss entire vascular territory
Technically adequate in only 63% of patients
Reproducibility unknown
Difficult to interpret if other cardiac disease or LV wall-motion abnormalities are present

Reversible Tl-201 abnormalities during exercise stress are markers of myocardial ischemia in hypertrophic cardiomyopathy. MPI has been used to assess patients with anomalous left coronary artery originating from the pulmonary artery and with Kawasaki's disease.

### Other Modalities

In principle, stress echocardiography is similar to the stress radionuclide ventriculogram, with reported sensitivities of 45% to 97% and specificities of 64% to 100%. There are efforts to compare stress echocardiography to MPI for the detection of single-vessel CAD, assessment of the extent of CAD, and detection of disease in the LCX (75,76). At present, dobutamine echocardiography is as useful as MPI when the LVEF is normal and there are no major wall-motion abnormalities, whereas in patients with large or dysfunctional LVs, the scoring of wall motion and thickening for stress echocardiography has not been standardized.

Results of dobutamine echocardiography for identification of low- and high-risk CAD patients have not been as favorable as those for MPI. A normal MPI study predicts a mere 1.8% incidence of ischemic events, whereas a normal stress echocardiography predicts an 8% rate of cardiac events. Table 2-11 shows the limitations of stress and dobutamine echocardiography for the assessment of diagnosis and prognosis of CAD.

### IMAGING MYOCARDIAL INFARCTION

### Tc-99m Pyrophosphate

In 1974, Bonte et al. introduced the use of Tc-99m pyrophosphate (PYP) for the radionuclide detection of AMI (77). Although the sensitivity of Tc-99m PYP exceeds 90% for patients with acute transmural infarcts, the overall specificity for all acute infarcts was reported at 64% by a multicenter study. Tc-99m sestamibi has been found useful in the same clinical setting (72,73). The uptake of Tc-99m PYP in acutely infarcted muscle occurs because of calcium deposition within the mitochondria of damaged cells. Uptake of Tc-99m PYP in necrotic myocardium requires the presence of residual CBF. Infarct-avid imaging is valuable when serum enzymes and ECG are indeterminate in patients with suspected AMI, for example, with LBBB, immediately after cardiac surgery, postcardioversion, 12 hours after the onset of pain with nonspecific ECG, ECG showing previous infarcts, and ECG showing subendocardial infarcts.

Tc-99m PYP is also taken up into noninfarcted zones. Most investigators have similarly noted that localization of Tc-99m PYP occurs preferentially in the periphery of AMI. This is consistent with uptake of Tc-99m PYP in injured, but viable, myocytes. Our own observations (78), among others, indicate that Tc-99m PYP accumulates in acutely ischemic cardiac tissue and is maximal in myocardial regions with moderate (30% to 40%) reductions of coronary arterial flow. This is also the case for F-18 FDG and Tc-99m glucarate. This complex relationship of myocardial uptake and blood flow may be responsible in part for preferred accumulation of Tc-99m PYP in the periphery of infarcts.

### Antimyosin Antibody

Indium 111 (In-111) antimyosin monoclonal antibody (MOAB) binds to dead cells at sites of membrane disruption and directly to intracellular myosin (79,80), so it accumulates only in cells with histologic necrosis. This differs from Tc-99m PYP, which is maximal in regions of moderate flow reduction. Antimyosin MOAB localization occurs at the border of the necrotic zones, near vessels in the border zones in reperfused infarctions, and in the endocardium, probably due to intermediate zones of normal and necrotic myocytes accumulating high amounts of the MOAB. Delivery to acutely infarcted muscle appears to depend on the regional blood flow in the infarct territory via antegrade coronary arteries or retrograde collaterals.

We have extended these observations in animal experiments (81) and found that in coronary occlusion without reperfusion, no or minimal In-111 antimyosin MOAB enters the area at risk because the rabbit has no collateral circulation. In coronary occlusion with reperfusion, however, the MOAB accumulates heterogeneously (Fig. 2-22) in the area at risk during reperfusion.

### *Imaging Protocol*

For clinical imaging, 2 mCi In-111 MOAB is injected IV, and imaging is performed using a medium-energy collimator with dual (173- and 247-keV) photopeaks 24 and 48 hours after injection. The biological half-life of In-111 MOAB is 4 to 6 hours. The 48-hour image is especially important in disorders in which a diffuse uptake of antimyosin MOAB occurs, to distinguish it from activity in the blood pool. For SPECT imaging, 64 × 64 frames are obtained in 180-degree acquisition from RAO to LPO positions at 30 seconds per stop and 3-degree increments. The total time required is

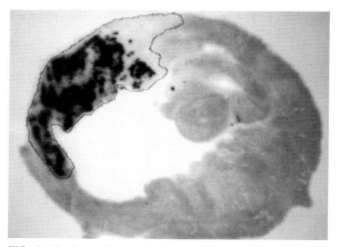

**FIG. 2-22.** Autoradiographic image of deposition of In-111 antimyosin antibody and perfusion agent (C-14 iodoantipyrine). In this image, the antibody (high density) is deposited heterogeneously in the reperfused myocardial infarct zone. The background density is myocardial perfusion as defined with C-14 iodoantipyrine.

approximately 30 minutes. In-111 antimyosin imaging has been approved for clinical use by the FDA.

### *Clinical Results*

The technique was sensitive (91%) and specific (95%) in a multicenter trial and did not localize in infarcts older than 4 weeks. The sensitivity was less in non–Q wave infarcts (76%), but uptake was seen also in 37% of unstable angina patients without clinical evidence of infarction. This indicates the heterogeneity of ischemic and infarcted myocardial cells in ischemia and infarction. The test appears to be indicated in identifying infarcts acutely (within 48 hours) in patients with equivocal ECG findings, RV infarcts, and infarcts after cardiac surgery.

### REFERENCES

1. Gould KL. Coronary Artery Stenosis. New York: Elsevier, 1991;1.
2. Zaret BL, Wackers FJ. Nuclear cardiology (I). N Engl J Med 1993; 329:775–783.
3. Beller GA. Current status of nuclear cardiology techniques. Curr Probl Cardiol 1991;16:450–535.
4. L'Abbate A. Pathophysiological basis for noninvasive functional evaluation of coronary stenosis. Circulation 1991;83(Suppl III):2–7.
5. Gould KL, Kirkeeide RL, Buchi M. Coronary flow reserve as a physiologic measure of stenosis severity. J Am Coll Cardiol 1990;15:459–474.
6. Kiat H, Berman DS, Maddahi J. Myocardial perfusion imaging using Tc-99m radiopharmaceuticals. Radiol Clin North Am 1993;31:795–815.
7. Verani M. Myocardial perfusion imaging versus two-dimensional echocardiography: comparative value in the diagnosis of coronary artery disease. J Nucl Cardiol 1994;1:399–414.
8. Strauss HW, Pitt B, James AE. Cardiovascular Nuclear Medicine. St. Louis: Mosby, 1974;182.
9. Lebowitz E, Greene MV, Fairchild R, et al. Thallium-201 for medical use. J Nucl Med 1975;16:151–155.
10. Pohost GM, Zir LM, Moore RH. Differentiation of transiently

ischemic from infarcted myocardium by serial imaging after a single dose of thallium-201. Circulation 1977;55:294–302.

11. Albro PC, Gould KL, Westcott RJ. Noninvasive assessment of coronary stenoses by myocardial imaging during pharmacologic coronary vasodilatation. III. Clinical trial. Am J Cardiol 1978;42:751–760.

12. Brown KA, Boucher CA, Okada RD. Prognostic value of exercise Tl-201 imaging in patients presenting for evaluation of chest pain. J Am Coll Cardiol 1983;1:994–1001.

13. Gould KL, Lipscomb K, Hamilton GW. Physiologic basis for assessing critical coronary stenosis. Am J Cardiol 1974;33:87–94.

14. Fintel DJ, Links JM, Brinker JA, et al. Improved diagnostic performance of exercise thallium-201 single photon emission computed tomography over planar imaging in the diagnosis of coronary artery disease: a receiver operating characteristic analysis. J Am Coll Cardiol 1989;13:600–612.

15. Zaret BL, Strauss HW, Martin ND, et al. Noninvasive regional myocardial perfusion with radioactive potassium: study of patients at rest, with exercise, and during angina pectoris. N Engl J Med 1973; 288:809–815.

16. Piwnica-Worms D, Kronauge JF, Chiu ML. Uptake and retention of hexakis (2-methoxyisobutyl isonitrile) technetium (I) in cultured chick myocardial cells: mitochondrial and plasma membrane potential difference. Circulation 1990;82:1826–1838.

17. Pohost GM, Alpert NM, Ingwall JS, Strauss HW. Thallium redistribution: mechanism and clinical utility. Semin Nucl Med 1980;10:76–93.

18. Marshall RC, Leidholdt EM, Zhang D-Y, Barnett CA. Technetium-99m hexakis 2-methoxy-2-isobutyl isonitrile and thallium-201 extraction, washout, and retention at varying coronary flow rates in rabbit heart. Circulation 1990;82:998–1007.

19. Leppo JA, Meerdink DJ. Comparison of the myocardial uptake of a technetium-labeled isonitrile analogue and thallium. Circ Res 1989; 65:632–639.

20. Hammes R, Kies S, Koblenski D, et al. A better method of quality control for technetium-99 sestamibi. J Nucl Med Tech 1991;19:232–235.

21. Dilsizian V, Arrighi JA, Diodati JG, et al. Myocardial viability in patients with chronic coronary artery disease. Comparison of Tc-99m sestamibi with Tl-201 reinjection and F-18 fluorodeoxyglucose. Circulation 1994;89:578–587.

22. Taillefer R, Gagnon A, Laflamme L, et al. Same day injections of Tc-99m methoxy isobutyl isonitrile (hexamibi) for myocardial tomographic imaging: comparison between rest-stress and stress-rest injection sequences. Eur J Nucl Med 1989;15:113–117.

23. Berman DS, Kiat HS, Van Train KF, et al. Myocardial perfusion imaging with technetium-99m-sestamibi: comparative analysis of available imaging protocols. J Nucl Med 1994;35:681–688.

24. Johnson LL. Clinical experience with technetium 99m teboroxime. Semin Nucl Med 1991;21:182–189.

25. Miller DD. The growing flood of technetium-99m myocardial perfusion agents. More water . . . or more mud? Circulation 1995;91:555–558.

26. Gerson MC, Millard RW, Roszell NJ, et al. Kinetic properties of Tc-99m-Q12 in canine myocardium. Circulation 1994;89:1291–1300.

27. DePasquale EE, Nody AC, DePuey EG, et al. Quantitative rotational thallium-201 tomography for identifying and localizing coronary artery disease. Circulation 1988;77:316–327.

28. Maddahi J, Van Train K, Prigent F, et al. Quantitative single photon emission computed thallium-201 tomography for detection and localization of coronary artery disease: optimization and prospective validation of a new technique. J Am Coll Cardiol 1989;14:1689–1699.

29. Iskandrian AS, Heo J, Kong B, Lyons E. Effect of exercise level on the ability of thallium-201 tomographic imaging in detecting coronary artery disease: analysis of 461 patients. J Am Coll Cardiol 1989;14:1477–1486.

30. Mahramian JJ, Boyce TM, Goldberg RK, et al. Quantitative exercise thallium–201 single photon emission computed tomography for the enhanced diagnosis of ischemic heart disease. J Am Coll Cardiol 1990;15:318–329.

31. Kiat H, Maddhi J, Roy LT, et al. Comparison of technetium 99m methoxy isobutyl isonitrile and thallium 201 for evaluation of coronary artery disease by planar and tomographic methods. Am Heart J 1989;117:1–11.

32. Kahn JK, McGhie I, Akers MS, et al. Quantitative rotational tomography with Tl-201 and Tc-99m 2-methoxy-isobutyl-isonitrile: a direct comparison in normal individuals and patients with coronary artery disease. Circulation 1989;79:1282–1293.

33. Iskandrian AS, Heo J, Kong B, et al. Use of technetium-99m isonitrile (RP-30A) in assessing left ventricular perfusion and function at rest and during exercise in coronary artery disease, and comparison with coronary arteriography and exercise thallium-201 SPECT imaging. Am J Cardiol 1989;64:270–275.

34. Van Train KF, Garcia EV, Maddahi J, et al. Multicenter trial validation for quantitative analysis of same-day rest-stress technetium-99m-sestamibi myocardial tomograms. J Nucl Med 1994;35:609–618.

35. Smith WH, Watson DD. Technical aspects of myocardial planar imaging with Tc-99m sestamibi. Am J Cardiol 1990;66:16E–22E.

36. Cullom SJ. Principles of Cardiac SPECT. In DePuey EG, Berman DS, Garcia EV (eds), Cardiac SPECT Imaging. New York: Raven, 1995;1–19.

37. Van Train KF, Areeda J, Garcia EV, et al. Quantitative same-day rest-stress technetium-99m-sestamibi SPECT: definition and validation of stress normal limits and criteria for abnormality. J Nucl Med 1993;34:1494–1502.

38. Tsui BMW, Zhao X, Frey EC, McCartney WH. Quantitative single-photon emission computed tomography: basic and clinical consequences. Semin Nucl Med 1994;24:38–65.

39. Verani MS. Pharmacologic stress myocardial perfusion imaging. Curr Probl Cardiol 1993;18:485–525.

40. Iskandrian AS, Verani MS, Heo J. Pharmacologic stress testing: mechanism of action, hemodynamic responses, and results in detection of coronary artery disease. J Nucl Cardiol 1994;1:94–111.

41. Gould KL. Noninvasive assessment of coronary stenoses by myocardial perfusion imaging during pharmacologic coronary vasodilatation. I. Physiologic basis and experimental validation. Am J Cardiol 1978;41:267–278.

42. Ranhosky A, Kempthorne-Rawson J. The safety of intravenous dipyridamole thallium myocardial perfusion imaging. Circulation 1990;81:1205–1209.

43. Guidelines for clinical use of cardiac radionuclide imaging. Special report. American Heart Association/American College of Cardiology/American Society of Nuclear Cardiology. Circulation 1995;91:1278–1303.

44. Pennell DJ, Underwood SR, Swanton RH, et al. Dobutamine thallium myocardial perfusion tomography. J Am Coll Cardiol 1991;18:1471–1479.

45. Marwick T, Willemart B, D'Hondt AM, et al. Selection of the optimal nonexercise stress for the evaluation of ischemic regional myocardial dysfunction and malperfusion: comparison of dobutamine and adenosine using echocardiography and Tc-99m MIBI single-photon emission computed tomography. Circulation 1993;87:345–354.

46. Botvinick EH, Zhu YY, O'Connell WJ, Dae MW. A quantitative assessment of patient motion and its effect on myocardial perfusion SPECT images. J Nucl Med 1993;34:303–310.

47. Wackers FTH. Artifacts in planar and SPECT myocardial perfusion imaging. Am J Card Imag 1992;6:42–58.

48. Germano G, Chua T, Kiat H, et al. A quantitative phantom analysis of artifacts due to hepatic activity in technetium-99m myocardial perfusion SPECT studies. J Nucl Med 1994;35:356–359.

49. Bonow RO, Dilsizian V, Cuocolo A, Bacharach SL. Identification of viable myocardium in patients with chronic coronary artery disease and left ventricular dysfunction: comparison of thallium scintigraphy with reinjection and PET imaging with F-18-fluorodeoxyglucose. Circulation 1991;83:26–27.

50. Rozanski A, Berman DS. The efficacy of cardiovascular nuclear medicine studies. Semin Nucl Med 1987;17:104–120.

51. Diamond GA, Forrester JS. Analysis of probability as an aid in the clinical diagnosis of coronary-artery disease. N Engl J Med 1979;300:1350–1358.

52. Borges-Neto S, Coleman RE, Potts JM, et al. Combined exercise radionuclide angiocardiography and single photon emission computed tomography perfusion studies for assessment of coronary artery disease. Semin Nucl Med 1991;21:223–229.

53. Mannting F, Morgan-Mannting MG. Gated SPECT with technetium-99m sestamibi for assessment of myocardial perfusion abnormalities. J Nucl Med 1993;34:601–608.

54. Brown KA. Prognostic value of thallium-201 myocardial perfusion imaging. Circulation 1991;83:363–381.

55. Machecourt J, Longere P, Fagret D, et al. Prognostic value of thallium-201 single-photon emission computer tomographic myocardial

perfusion imaging according to extent of myocardial defect. J Am Coll Cardiol 1994;23:1096–1106.

56. Berman DS, Hachamovitz R, Kiat H, et al. Incremental value of prognostic testing in patients with known or suspected ischemic heart disease: a basis for optimal utilization of exercise Tc-99m sestamibi myocardial perfusion single-photon emission computed tomography. J Am Coll Cardiol 1995;26:639–647.

57. Brown KA. Prognostic value of thallium-201 myocardial perfusion imaging in patients with unstable angina who respond to medical treatment. J Am Coll Cardiol 1991;17:1053–1057.

58. Gibson RS, Watson DD, Craddock GB, et al. Prediction of cardiac events after uncomplicated myocardial infarction: a prospective study comparing predischarge exercise thallium-201 scintigraphy and coronary angiography. Circulation 1983;68:321–336.

59. Haber HL, Beller GA, Watson DD, Gimple LW. Exercise Tl-201 scintigraphy after thrombolytic therapy with or without angioplasty for acute myocardial infarction. Am J Cardiol 1993;71:1257–1261.

60. Gimple LW, Bellar GA. Assessing prognosis after acute myocardial infarction in the thrombolytic era. J Nucl Cardiol 1994;1:198–209.

61. Boucher CA, Brewster DC, Darling RC, et al. Determination of cardiac risk by dipyridamole-thallium imaging before peripheral vascular surgery. N Engl J Med 1985;312:389–394.

62. Eagle KA, Coley CM, Newell JB, et al. Combining clinical and thallium data optimizes preoperative assessment of cardiac risk before major vascular surgery. Ann Int Med 1989;110:859–860.

63. Alderman EL, Fisher LD, Litwin P, et al. Results of coronary artery surgery in patients with poor left ventricular function (CASS). Circulation 1983;68:785–795.

64. Rahimtoola SH. Coronary bypass surgery for chronic angina—1981: a perspective. Circulation 1982;65:225–241.

65. Gibson RS, Watson DD, Taylor GJ, et al. Prospective assessment of regional myocardial perfusion before and after coronary revascularization surgery by quantitative thallium-201 scintigraphy. J Am Coll Cardiol 1983;1:804–815.

66. Tillisch J, Brunken R, Marshall R, et al. Reversibility of cardiac wall-motion abnormalities predicted by positron tomography. N Engl J Med 1986;314:884–888.

67. Dilsizian V, Bonow RO. Current diagnostic techniques of assessing myocardial viability in patients with hibernating and stunned myocardium. Circulation 1993;87:1–19.

68. Ragosta M, Beller G, Watson DD, et al. Quantitative planar rest-redistribution Tl-201 imaging in detection of myocardial viability and prediction of improvement in left ventricular function after coronary bypass surgery in patients with severely depressed left ventricular function. Circulation 1993;87:1630–1641.

69. Gutman J, Berman DS, Freeman M, et al. Time to complete redistribution of thallium-201 in exercise myocardial scintigraphy: relationship to the degree of coronary artery stenosis. Am Heart J 1983;106:989–995.

70. Udelson JE, Coleman PS, Metherall J, et al. Predicting recovery of severe regional ventricular dysfunction. Comparison of resting scintigraphy with Tl-201 and Tc-99m sestamibi. Circulation 1994;89:2552–2561.

71. Hilton TC, Thompson RC, Williams HJ, et al. Technetium-99m sestamibi myocardial perfusion imaging in the emergency room evaluation of chest pain. J Am Coll Cardiol 1994;23:1016–1022.

72. Gibson WS, Christian TF, Pellikka PA, et al. Serial tomographic imaging with Tc-99m–sestamibi for the assessment of infarct-related arterial patency following reperfusion therapy. J Nucl Med 1992;33:2080–2085.

73. Gibbons RJ, Holmes DR, Reeder GS, et al. Immediate angioplasty compared with the administration of a thrombolytic agent followed by conservative treatment for myocardial infarction. N Engl J Med 1993;328:685–691.

74. Miller DD, Verami MS. Current status of myocardial perfusion imaging after percutaneous transluminal coronary angioplasty. J Am Coll Cardiol 1994;24:260–266.

75. Marwick T, D'Hondt AM, Baudhuin T, et al. Optimal use of dobutamine stress for the detection and evaluation of coronary artery disease: combination of echocardiography or scintigraphy, or both? J Am Coll Cardiol 1993;22:159–167.

76. Quinones MA, Verani MS, Haighin RM, et al. Exercise echocardiography versus thallium-201 single photon emission computed tomography in evaluation of coronary artery disease. Circulation 1992;85:1026–1031.

77. Bonte FJ, Parkey RW, Graham KD, et al. A new method for radionuclide imaging of acute myocardial infarction. Radiology 1974;110:473–474.

78. Bianco JA, Kemper AJ, Taylor A, et al. Technetium-99m(Sn2+)pyrophosphate in ischemic and infarcted dog myocardium in early stages of acute coronary occlusion: histochemical and tissue-counting comparisons. J Nucl Med 1983;24:485–491.

79. Khaw BA, Strauss HW, Moore R, et al. Myocardial damage delineated by In-111 antimyosin Fab and technetium-99m pyrophosphate. J Nucl Med 1987;28:76–82.

80. Khaw BA, Beller GA, Haber E, Smith TW. Localization of cardiac myosin-specific antibody in myocardial infarction. J Clin Invest 1976;58:439–446.

81. Bianco JA, Hammes RJ, Sebree L, Wilson MA. Imaging of acute myocardial infarction and reperfusion. Cardiology 1995;86:186–196.

*Textbook of Nuclear Medicine,*
edited by Michael A. Wilson.
Lippincott–Raven Publishers, Philadelphia © 1998.

CHAPTER 3

# Gastrointestinal Tract

Michael A. Wilson

Since 1985, a dramatic change has occurred in the clinical use of gastrointestinal (GI) nuclear medicine imaging studies. This has resulted in a decreased role of liver-spleen (L/S) scanning for the detection of liver metastases and the coming of age of hepatobiliary imaging (Table 3-1). General and historic reviews (1–5) cover much of this imaging field.

## HEPATOBILIARY IMAGING

As recently as 1990, virtually all hepatobiliary scans were done to rule out acute cholecystitis. Now, the diagnosis of acalculous biliary disease (chronic acalculous cholecystitis, the cystic duct syndrome, and biliary dyskinesia) and the detection of bile leaks after surgical intervention account for half of all hepatobiliary scan indications. Other indications are infrequent but include evaluation of hepatic transplants (see Chapter 13), biliary obstruction, biliary atresia, choledochal cysts, trauma, and various other quantitative studies (4).

### Radiopharmaceuticals

Iminodiacetic (IDA) agents are now the sole hepatobiliary radiopharmaceutical; although previously other agents were used (e.g., pyridoxylidene glutamate and penicillamine). A whole family of IDA agents have been investigated that include these acronyms: HIDA, BIDA, PIPIDA, DISIDA, TMBIDA (or BRIDA). The relative proportion of renal to biliary excretion under different conditions of hepatic function varies with each IDA agent according to polarity, lipid solubility, molecular weight (300–1,000), and degree of protein binding (4,6).

The two U.S. Food and Drug Administration (FDA)-approved agents (and their approved names) are DISIDA (disofenin) and TMBIDA (mebrofenin) and individual nuclear medicine departments must select the tracer they desire (Table 3-2). One other agent was formerly available: HIDA (lidofenin), an older but more recently FDA-approved tracer, which is effective to serum bilirubin (BR) values of 5 to 8 mg/dl and has 15% renal excretion with normal hepatic function. HIDA was priced at about half the cost of DISIDA and TMBIDA, but production was discontinued in May 1995. Dosimetry for TMBIDA (the agent we use) is provided in Table 3-3.

### Physiology

IDA agents are removed from the blood pool by hepatocytes and compete with BR for transport binding sites, which explains why hepatic IDA uptake falls as BR rises. TMBIDA usually allows visualization of the biliary tree with BR levels in excess of 40 mg/dl. With intravenous (IV) injection of DISIDA or TMBIDA, there is rapid blood clearance, maximum uptake in the liver and hepatic function under normal conditions at 10 to 15 minutes, common bile duct (CBD) and gallbladder (GB) visualization at 15 to 30 minutes, and bowel visualization at 30 to 60 minutes (Table 3-4). Approximately 600 ml of bile is produced every day and, although the GB capacity averages only 60 ml, it concentrates bile 10-fold. Quantitative hepatobiliary studies show that, on average, 70% of the total daily production of bile produced passes into the GB for storage, and 30% passes directly into the small intestine. This proportion varies during the day according to whether the patient has fasted or eaten, that is, according to circulating levels of cholecystokinin.

### Hepatobiliary Protocol

#### *Routine Protocol*

Ten millicuries (370 MBq) of the radiopharmaceutical TMBIDA is injected IV, and continuous acquisition of images is made in 1-minute frames. We use TMBIDA because of the faster visualization of the biliary tree, lower renal excretion, and greater efficacy in elevated serum BR. For ease of review we acquire these images in 20-minute blocks, so that the earlier part of the study can be reviewed while the current acquisition is continuously monitored. The images are displayed and recorded in 5-minute frames for permanent storage (Fig. 3-1).

**TABLE 3-1.** *Typical use of GI studies in a university hospital*

| | |
|---|---|
| 45% | Hepatobiliary imaging |
| 35% | Gastrointestinal bleeding |
| 10% | Gastroesophageal studies |
| 3% | Gastric mucosa studies |
| 3% | Hepatic hemangioma |
| 3% | Liver/spleen imaging |
| 1% | Miscellaneous: salivary scan |

**TABLE 3-2.** *Approved IDA agents*

| Chemical acronym | DISIDA | TMBIDA/BRIDA |
|---|---|---|
| Generic name | Disofenin | Mebrofenin |
| Renal excretion | 9% | 1% |
| Effective to BR of | 10–30 mg/dl | 10–50 mg/dl |
| Blood clearance | 12.5 mins | 9.6 mins |
| Liver clearance | 23 mins | 16 mins |
| GB uptake | 29 mins | 23 mins |
| Bowel appearance | 40 mins | 29 mins |
| FDA approval | 1981 | 1987 |

DISIDA, diisopropyliminodiacetic acid; TMBIDA/BRIDA, Bromotrimethylphenylaminooxoethyliminobisacetic acid.

Sources: Package inserts from DuPont Nemours, Billerica, MA; and Squibb Diagnostics, Princeton, NJ.

**TABLE 3-3.** *TMBIDA dosimetry*

| | Rads/10 mCi (cGy/370 MBq) | |
|---|---|---|
| Organ | Normal patient | Severely jaundiced patient |
| Total body | 0.20 | 0.17 |
| Testes | 0.05 | 0.11 |
| Ovaries | 1.00 | 0.64 |
| Bladder wall | 0.29 | 2.42 |
| Liver | 0.47 | 0.81 |
| GB | 1.37 | 1.25 |
| Small intestine | 2.99 | 1.60 |
| Lower LI | 3.64 | 1.97 |
| Upper LI* | 4.74 | 2.48 |

*Critical organ.

**TABLE 3-4.** *TMBIDA: time at which organ is best visualized*

| | Bilirubin level | |
|---|---|---|
| Organ | Normal | Increased |
| Blood pool | 1–5 mins | 1–20 mins |
| Liver | 5–15 mins | 20–60 mins |
| GB, CBD | 15–30 mins | 1–4 hrs |
| Bowel | 30–60 mins | 4–12 hrs |

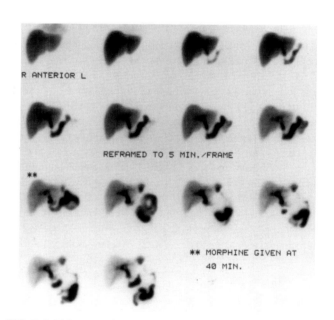

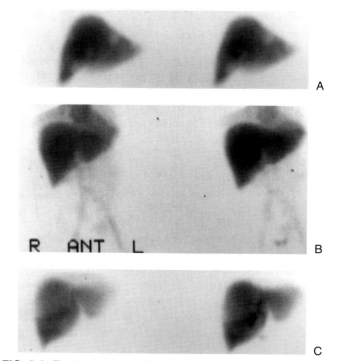

**FIG. 3-1.** This scan shows our routine hepatobiliary scan hardcopy format and demonstrates acute cholecystitis. In the first 5-minute frame, the cardiac blood pool is visualized, and blood clearance is nearly complete in the next frame. The falciform ligament, cardiac impression, and GB fossa are visible in these early frames. In the third frame, the common bile duct and small bowel are visualized. At 40 minutes (*double asterisk*), morphine is administered, and there is clearance of tracer from the duodenum with some enterogastric reflux seen on the next frame. The GB is not visualized, indicating acute cholecystitis. In the later frames there is a possible pericholecystic rim sign, that is, accentuation of tracer uptake in the region of the GB fossa.

**FIG. 3-2.** Each row shows the first two 5-minute frames of a hepatobiliary scan. **(A)** Large and small focal defects are seen in this patient with hepatic metastases from breast cancer. **(B)** Prolonged blood pool visualization in the heart and major vessels, indicating impaired hepatocellular function. **(C)** The effect of breast attenuation with an apparent relative decrease in liver uptake in the superior portion of the right lobe of the liver.

The initial images show liver architecture, and both normal and pathologic findings can be readily identified (Fig. 3-2).

### Augmented Hepatobiliary Scans

#### Cholecystokinin-8 "Augmentation"

To allow for GB filling, the GB should be neither full nor actively contracting at the time of radiopharmaceutical injection; this is achieved by requiring the patient to fast for 2 to 4 hours. If the patient is imaged too soon after eating, the presence of food in the duodenum and proximal small bowel results in the release of endogenous cholecystokinin, the chief hormone causing GB contraction. This hormone level can increase fivefold after ingestion of the commonly used medium chain triglyceride stimulant, Lipomul, and continued hormone secretion occurs for an hour.

Delayed filling or nonvisualization of the GB may occur if it has not been stimulated to contract for a long time because of prolonged fasting, total parenteral nutrition (TPN), severe illness, or chronic cholecystitis. In these cases there may be sludge present in the GB, a gelatinous material that can be difficult to evacuate. In these patient groups we routinely administer the synthetic terminal octapeptide cholecystokinin analog (CCK-8, or Kinevac) before the procedure. Because these are usually inpatients or ER patients, we often ask the referring service to administer CCK-8 before transportation to nuclear medicine, using the package insert suggestion of 0.02 µg/kg over a 3-minute slow IV injection. The use of CCK-8 does not actually augment the hepatobiliary scan, which is usually performed to demonstrate GB filling. Because CCK-8 empties the GB, the term *augmentation* is used loosely.

A word of caution is needed here because CCK-8 also acts on the sphincter of Oddi, causing muscle tone relaxation, and this effect can continue for up to 1 hour. It is perhaps most prudent to do the scan an hour after IV CCK-8 injection. When CCK-8 is administered before the scan, it can cause an increased proportion of the injected tracer to enter the GB and so delay visualization of the small bowel. Pretreatment with CCK-8 causes delayed visualization of the bowel in 49% of subjects versus 2% to 10% without CCK-8 (7), so care must be taken not to overdiagnose obstruction when CCK-8 is administered before hepatobiliary imaging.

#### Morphine Augmentation

The major indication for hepatobiliary scans is acute cholecystitis, and the nuclear medicine hallmark of this condition is GB nonvisualization due to obstruction of the cystic duct by a stone, edema, or inflammation. Delayed imaging was previously required in cases of chronic cholecystitis, where GB filling might may be normally delayed 2 to 4 hours. The introduction of morphine augmentation in

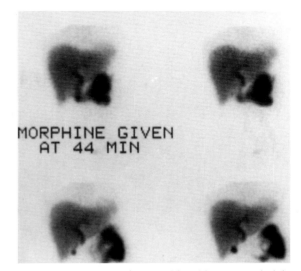

**FIG. 3-3.** Four 1-minute frames. Morphine was administered at 44 minutes (first frame). Very prompt visualization of the GB is seen in the next three frames (minutes), ruling out acute cholecystitis. The effect of morphine is confirmed by the rapid clearing of tracer from the duodenum. There is no enterogastric reflux of the biliary agent in this patient.

1984 shortened the duration of the test considerably (8). If at 40 minutes the GB is not visualized, and provided duodenal and hepatic activity are present, we administer IV morphine, 0.04 mg/kg (2.8 mg for 70-kg individual) slowly over 1 or 2 minutes. If the CBD, but not the duodenum, is visualized, we wait until the bowel is seen. The morphine causes increased tone of the sphincter of Oddi, raises the intraductal pressure severalfold, and fills the GB with tracer in normal individuals or patients with chronic cholecystitis (Fig. 3-3). Normal GB visualization occurs within 20 minutes of morphine administration, so the whole test is usually completed at 60 minutes (8). We keep morphine in our radiopharmacy for immediate access, stocked by the hospital pharmacy but under nuclear medicine control. Some services prefer to wait 60 minutes before deciding on augmentation, and then allow 30 minutes after augmentation for the GB to fill. Such practice often requires a supplemental dose of IDA (especially if the rapidly excreted TMBIDA is used) to ensure the presence of adequate tracer in the liver to demonstrate GB filling.

The adequacy of sphincter of Oddi contraction is confirmed by observing clearance of tracer from the duodenum. This results from normal anterograde passage from the duodenum into the small bowel associated with no flow from the CBD to refill the duodenum. The drug effect is confirmed by this duodenal clearance during the IV injection of morphine (Fig. 3-4; see also Figs. 3-1 and 3-3). Morphine also causes alterations in duodenal muscle activity and, in our experience, 60% of patients injected with morphine demonstrate enterogastric reflux (see Figs. 3-1 and 3-4), which is seen in only 15% of hepatobiliary scan patients who do not receive morphine.

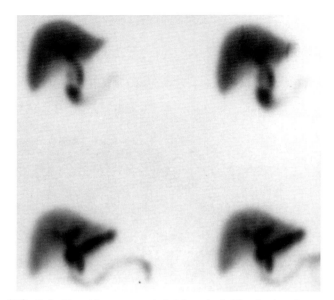

FIG. 3-4. Morphine was administered at 40 minutes (upper right, 5-minute image). The duodenum activity decreased significantly, and there is significant enterogastric reflux (lower left and right, 5-minute images), indicating physiologic effect of morphine. The GB is not visualized, demonstrating the typical findings of acute cholecystitis.

## Scan Interpretation

The hepatobiliary scan is a classic example of the physiologic nature of a nuclear medicine imaging test. The transit of a given tracer from the bloodstream to the bowel varies in rate (time to appearance) and proportion (e.g., biliary vs. renal excretion) depending on the presence of hepatic dysfunction and other disease processes. Images obtained immediately after injection demonstrate the heart, spleen, liver, and large-vessel blood pools. Over the next few minutes the blood pool (heart, spleen, and large vessels) activity decreases, and tracer accumulates in the hepatocytes. Tracer is then excreted into the bile canaliculi and the biliary tree, and the GB is visualized. If the CBD or proximal small bowel is not seen, it is unlikely that a normal GB will be visualized. Nonvisualization of the GB should only be considered abnormal when the small bowel is already well visualized (Fig. 3-5). This means that very delayed imaging may be required in severe hepatic dysfunction (see Table 3-4).

In the early images that reflect hepatocyte uptake, the scan reader should identify the GB fossa (Table 3-5). This helps identify GB filling in later images. In the early and late images the region adjacent to fossa is observed to determine whether there is increased tracer localization, the so-called rim sign (Fig. 3-6). Although the pathophysiologic explanation of this finding is not known, its clinical implication is severe GB inflammation, and half of the patients have acute gangrenous cholecystitis or GB perforation (9,10). A naive explanation of this finding is increased tracer delivery due to secondary regional hepatic hyperemia from the cholecystitis

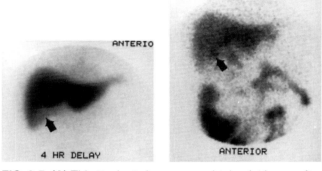

FIG. 3-5. (A) This 5-minute image was obtained 4 hours after tracer injection; GB fossa is identified by an arrow. The patient had been receiving morphine and meperidine for an infected pancreatic pseudocyst, and both drugs and the disorder may contribute to the delayed hepatic clearance. The CBD and SI are not visualized even in this delayed image, so the nonfilling of the GB is not diagnostic for acute cholecystitis. (B) The 5-minute image obtained at 24 hours shows minimal tracer in the GB (*arrow*) and good bowel visualization as well as considerable hepatic activity. This delayed study probably rules out acute cholecystitis.

**TABLE 3-5.** *Hepatobiliary scan review*

| Prescan data | BR level—dose and timing |
| --- | --- |
| | Is CCK-8 required? |
| | Role of morphine and dose |
| Early scan (0–10 mins) | Blood pool clearance |
| | Hepatic visualization |
| | GB fossa identification |
| Later scan (15 mins–12 hrs) | CBD visualization |
| | GB visualization |
| | Small bowel visualization |

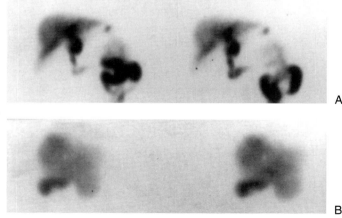

FIG. 3-6. (A) These two images show the last two 5-minute frames of a routine 1-hour hepatobiliary scan with absent GB but a rim sign in the GB fossa region. This suggests the diagnosis of gangrenous cholecystitis. (B) These two images show the first two 5-minute frames, with costal indentation and attenuation of the liver mimicking a rim sign. The GB filled at 20 minutes, excluding acute cholecystitis. Note the prominent left lobe of the liver and the photopenic defect over the right lobe due to an ECG lead.

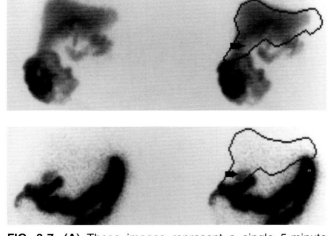

**FIG. 3-7. (A)** These images represent a single 5-minute image 60 minutes after IDA injection. The right-hand image has an ROI drawn about the liver. The GB fossa is seen (*arrow*), and there is much activity in the small intestine. **(B)** This row is a 5-minute image obtained 24 hours postinjection; the tracer is now in the large intestine with minimal hepatic activity. The GB is now visualized with tracer (*arrow*). This visualization is helped because the identical hepatic ROI used in the early image is reimposed and outlines the liver. Delayed imaging can help reduce the acute acalculous cholecystitis FP rate in critically ill patients (see also Fig. 3-5), but increased false-negative results can occur.

**TABLE 3-6.** *Hepatobiliary scan caveats*

| | |
|---|---|
| Morphine too late | Redose with IDA |
| Delayed bowel visualization | Morphine or CCK-8 vs. obstruction |
| Poor test performance | Acalculous disease, TPN, very ill patients, and nonindicated diseases |

morphine augmentation, and if these are not visualized, a further dose of radiopharmaceutical should be injected. This and other caveats are listed in Table 3-6.

## Clinical Applications

### Acute Calculous Cholecystitis

Acute cholecystitis is a common disease: 30% of ER presentations with right upper quadrant (RUQ) or epigastric pain have acute cholecystitis. The differential diagnosis of acute cholecystitis is large (Table 3-7), but the typical presentation is a dull constant epigastric pain initially localized to the right subcostal area that with peritoneal involvement radiates to the back and changes in character. Murphy's sign (tenderness in RUQ with inspiration) is a relatively specific but insensitive sign of acute cholecystitis. Nonspecific nausea and vomiting, fever, mild leukocytosis, and hyperbilirubinemia are often present. This group of patients should have a hepatobiliary imaging scan as the first test because of the high specificity compared to other imaging modalities, such as ultrasound (US). Other patients with less typical clinical presentations should have a US examination because it can detect other hepatic, renal, and pancreatic etiologies of RUQ pain.

In our own institution, most surgeons and internists seem to refer patients with RUQ pain initially for US, perhaps because >90% of patients have cholelithiasis, which is easily and rapidly detected by US. However, although cholelithiasis is readily diagnosed by US and acute cholecystitis is more common with cholelithiasis, cholelithiasis is not synonymous with acute cholecystitis. In fact, whereas two-thirds of patients with acute RUQ pain have cholelithiasis, only half of these patients have acute cholecystitis. Furthermore, only one-fifth of the patients with incidentally

and swelling of the liver about the severely inflamed GB, with trapping of the IDA agent in the hepatocytes due to bile canaliculi compression from the edematous liver. If flow images are obtained, this region may show marked hyperperfusion, confirming local hepatic inflammation. Patients with a marked rim sign or marked hyperperfusion generally have complicated acute cholecystitis (11). Although a typical patient with acute cholecystitis may be treated conservatively and the GB removed electively, those with the rim sign and nonvisualization of the GB after morphine should undergo acute surgical intervention. The rim sign is a contraindication to laparoscopic cholecystectomy in many institutions.

The pathognomonic hepatobiliary scan sign of acute cholecystitis is nonfilling of the GB due to obstruction of the cystic duct (see Fig. 3-1). Delayed filling of the GB occurs in 10% of patients with chronic cholecystitis, and to make the test specific for acute cholecystitis, nonvisualization of the GB on delayed imaging at 2 to 4 hours was formerly required. If the GB is visualized on delayed scans, acute cholecystitis is ruled out (Fig. 3-7). The introduction of morphine augmentation of hepatobiliary scanning has eliminated this prolonged imaging procedure by filling the GB earlier, making it a more clinically acceptable test (8,12,13). For morphine augmentation to work, however, sufficient tracer must still be excreted by the liver and there should be evidence of contraction of the sphincter of Oddi by morphine (see Figs. 3-1, 3-3, and 3-4). The scan should display activity still present in the liver and proximal bile ducts before

**TABLE 3-7.** *Differential diagnosis of RUQ pain*

| |
|---|
| GB: cholecystitis, biliary colic |
| Hepatic: abscess, hepatitis, hepatoma |
| Peptic ulcer disease |
| Pancreatitis |
| Renal: colic or pyelonephritis |
| Appendicitis |
| Cardiac: pericarditis, CHF, infarction |
| Lung: pleuritis, pneumonia, empyema |
| Others: herpes zoster |

**TABLE 3-8.** *IDA sensitivity and specificity*

| Criteria | Sensitivity (%) | Specificity (%) |
|---|---|---|
| Strict criteria[a] | 98 | 91 |
| Liberal criteria[b] | 95 | 99 |
| ≤1-hr images | 100 | 90 |
| ≤2.5-hr images | 100 | 93 |
| ≤4-hr images | 98 | 97 |
| Strict criteria and 1-hr scan | 100 | 85 |
| Liberal criteria and 4-hr scan | 95 | 99 |

[a] Strict pathologic criteria: transmural inflammatory exudates.

[b] Liberal pathologic criteria: GB wall edema along with various clinical criteria, postcholecystectomy relief, fever, pain, and leukocytosis.

Source: Freitas JE, Coleman RE, Nagle CE, et al. Influence of scan and pathologic criteria on the specificity of cholecystitis: concise communication. J Nucl Med 1983;24:876–879.

detected gallstones go on to have acute biliary colic in the next two decades.

Hepatobiliary imaging is the best means of diagnosing acute cholecystitis. The sensitivity and specificity for this diagnosis is excellent, but different reports using slightly different scan or pathologic criteria yield different results. Combining two variables (time to GB visualization and pathologic criteria) illustrates the variability that occurs in different studies (14): Strict pathologic and early scan criteria gave 100% sensitivity and 85% specificity, whereas liberal pathologic and delayed scan criteria gave 95% sensitivity and 99% specificity (Table 3-8). A meta-analysis published in 1994 in the *Archives of Internal Medicine* establishes hepatobiliary imaging as the preferred diagnostic test for evaluation of acute cholecystitis, with a sensitivity of 97% and specificity of 90% (15). This meta-analysis did not include studies with the now accepted morphine augmentation technique, which improves the specificity by reducing the false-positive (FP) rate due to chronic cholecystitis (8,12,13). The scan variability has been decreased by the introduction of the morphine augmentation scan, but the pathologic criteria variabilities persist.

Understanding the clinical presentation helps explain the pathologic findings. Acute cholecystitis develops as a result of cystic duct obstruction, and the lithogenic bile is concentrated by normal GB function, resulting in vascular congestion, GB wall edema, and raised intracholecystic pressure. If cystic duct patency is not re-established, inflammatory cell infiltration and hemorrhagic necrosis can occur. Acute cholecystitis can either progress to gangrenous cholecystitis (cystic duct remains obstructed) or spontaneous resolution (cystic duct clears). Patients in whom spontaneous clearance of the cystic duct occurs subsequently develop the findings of chronic cholecystitis from repeated acute episodes with subsequent repair processes. Any one of these subsequent episodes can go on to gangrenous cholecystitis, and this may occur in one-fifth of such episodes. This pathophysiologic process explains the

histologic difficulties of diagnosing acute cholecystitis, as there is often the underlying finding of chronic inflammatory fibrosis of the GB wall and the overlap of clinical and pathologic findings of acute and chronic cholecystitis. This is important because the most frequent FP acute cholecystitis scan finding is the scan due to chronic cholecystitis.

*False-Positive Hepatobiliary Scans*

The FP rate for hepatobiliary imaging in acute cholecystitis was initially reported at 2% to 10%, most commonly due to the presence of chronic cholecystitis. Other causes of delayed visualization of the GB include cholelithiasis, recent feeding, prolonged fasting, TPN, and alcoholic liver disease. The introduction of IV morphine resulted in a dramatic reduction in FP cases to 2% (8,12,13).

*False-Negative Hepatobiliary Scans*

Late visualization of the GB, visualization of a nubbin of activity in a dilated proximal cystic duct, perforation of GB (occurs in 10% of acute cholecystitis cases), or dislodgment of an obstructing stone by augmentation have been reported (13,16) as false-negative tests in acute cholecystitis. However, these are infrequent findings.

Various investigators have proposed different times at which nonvisualization of the GB represents an abnormal result. One group combined their data with other published data, which included 10 false-negative cases out of 642 patient studies (17). The false-negative rate of acute cholecystitis is very low (<0.5%) with GB visualization occurring in the first 30 minutes, but it is 40-fold higher if visualization occurs later than 30 minutes after injection (see Fig. 3-7) of tracer (mainly due to chronic cholecystitis).

**Acute Acalculous Cholecystitis**

Acute acalculous cholecystitis was first defined in 1947, and an early large published series was described in post-surgical Vietnam veterans. As much as 10% of acute cholecystitis is acalculous, there is a male predominance, and the age group is generally older than that of calculous cholecystitis patients. A long list of diseases is associated with acalculous cholecystitis, and this type of cholecystitis commonly progresses to a complicated form (perforation, gangrene, or empyema). The mortality is 2 to 20 times that of acute calculous cholecystitis.

Various etiologies have been proposed, including functional obstruction of the cystic duct, periampullary disease, and continuous narcotic administration, which causes stasis of bile in the GB and subsequent inflammation. These pathophysiologic conditions in an arteriosclerotic patient lead to ischemia of the GB. This process is likened to that of stress gastritis and mesenteric ischemia.

Two distinct populations present with acute acalculous cholecystitis. The first includes the patient in the medical or surgical intensive care unit in shock with numerous medical illnesses or the patient recovering from major surgery, burns, or trauma (18). The second group consists of elderly male outpatients with RUQ pain, leukocytosis, and fever together with documented arteriosclerotic vascular disease and hypertension (19). These two populations are either the critically ill or those predisposed to ischemia. Both populations have significantly increased morbidity and mortalities and unfortunately represent diagnostic dilemmas that stress the capabilities of both hepatobiliary imaging and US. In these patients, there is a tendency to proceed with percutaneous cholecystostomy, for both diagnosis and treatment even in the face of normal imaging procedures (20).

### False-Positive Studies

Those most likely to develop acute acalculous cholecystitis include patients who are postoperative, critically ill, have sepsis, have undergone prolonged fasts (>24 hours), or are on TPN. FP scans occur in patients who have no abdominal disease but are on TPN, in alcoholics who have pancreatitis, or in patients with hepatocellular disease. In these instances the GB may contain a gelatinous bile, the result of water resorption from the bile that may be due to bile stasis. Nonvisualization of the GB has been shown to occur in 38% of subjects who had no abdominal symptoms or illness but were on TPN (21). These figures are identical to that of other reports (22,23) and are decreased by pretest CCK-8 administration. The prolonged fast and TPN may have prevented normal bile production and flow because of the absence of intestinal stimulants.

Two studies report on the use of hepatobiliary imaging in patients hospitalized in tertiary care centers rather than the more typical patients being evaluated in the ER or as outpatients (24,25). In one population there were six FP studies on patients on TPN or large narcotic doses or with severe intercurrent illness, and scans were performed using CCK-8 with up to 2.0 mg of morphine. The FP rate was therefore 60% in the 10 critically ill patients but was also 50% in those with hepatocellular disease and even 23% in routine outpatients (24). Delayed imaging reduced these FP rates: four of the 10 FP patients had chronic cholecystitis and five of the six FP patients with severe intercurrent illness were on large doses of morphine, so they might not have responded to the smaller morphine dose (maximum 2 mg) used in the scan protocol. The other study looked at 163 hospitalized patients, of whom 61 were critically ill (25). Here the FP rate of all these inpatients was only 5%, and the sensitivity and specificity of the technique were 99% and 91%, respectively. In the 61 critically ill patients, 38 were true negative, 18 true positive, and five had FP scans, for a sensitivity of 100% and specificity of 88% in this subset. Only one patient was established as FP at surgery, the other four patients were treated with antibiotics and have been called FP for the purposes of analysis. The difference in these two studies (FP rates of 60% and 8%) may be the result of different study inclusion criteria (e.g., chronic cholecystitis), morphine augmentation doses, or time to postaugmentation imaging.

Diagnostic improvements in this distinct population of critically ill patients prone to FP studies could result from the following factors:

- Continuous 15- to 30-minute infusion of prescan CCK-8
- Larger dose of morphine (0.10 vs. 0.04 mg/kg)
- Imaging for 1 hour after morphine instead of the usual 20 to 30 minutes
- Reimaging all patients with GB nonvisualization using US and white blood cell (WBC) scans before surgical intervention (26)

This patient population will be reduced by the recent trend for jejunal tubes to provide oral nutrition in critically ill patients rather than TPN. Although tube feedings have been introduced for cost savings, a secondary benefit is continued GB function, and possibly fewer episodes of cholecystitis and FP hepatobiliary scans in this clinical setting.

### False-Negative Studies

The false-negative rate in acute acalculous cholecystitis is greater than that of calculous disease, but hepatobiliary imaging is still >90% sensitive (27). This figure is greater than the 2% false-negative rate accepted for acute calculous cholecystitis (17).

## Chronic Cholecystitis

Chronic cholecystitis is a common condition without characteristic clinical features. The symptoms range from functional dyspepsia to typical biliary colic. There are no specific radiologic features, and the diagnosis is often made because gallstones are present, although as many as 50% of people in their sixth decade may have gallstones. In chronic cholecystitis the hepatobiliary scan demonstrates delayed GB filling in up to 20% of patients, and GB emptying is reduced with administration of CCK-8. There is considerable overlap of GB ejection fractions (EFs) with the normal population, however, because three-fourths of chronic cholecystitis patients have values that fall into the normal range (28). Hepatobiliary imaging is generally not indicated in chronic calculous cholecystitis. This diagnosis is best left for US evaluation and demonstration of the presence of gallstones.

## Chronic Acalculous Hepatobiliary Disorders

IDA agents have been used in chronic acalculous disorders since 1980 (29), and the GB EF test (see later) was modeled on cholecystokinin-stimulated oral cholecystography and GB sonography. The acalculous conditions in which this scan tech-

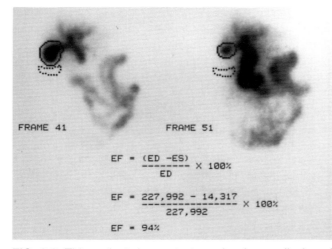

FRAME 41          FRAME 51

$$EF = \frac{(ED - ES)}{ED} \times 100\%$$

$$EF = \frac{227,992 - 14,317}{227,992} \times 100\%$$

$$EF = 94\%$$

**FIG. 3-8.** This patient demonstrates a hard-copy display of GB EF method. In this case, the 10-minute EF is 94%, a normal result. The background region is shown below the GB but should probably be drawn in the liver region.

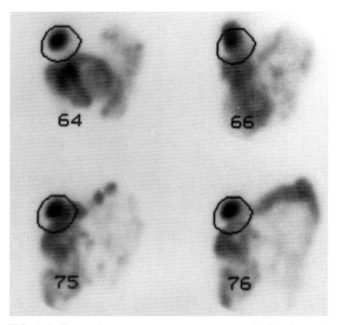

**FIG. 3-9.** These four 1-minute images were obtained at 64, 66, 75, and 76 minutes into the study (4, 6, 15, and 16 minutes after CCK-8 injection), and show the GB moving out of the selected ROI due to patient motion (66-minute image), and large bowel activity moving into the GB ROI (75- and 76-minute images).

nique is used include: chronic acalculous cholecystitis, the cystic duct syndrome, biliary dyskinesia, and evaluation of the sphincter of Oddi. An early review paper of nonradionuclide GB EF tests showed an 88% chance of symptomatic improvement from cholecystectomy if there was an abnormal cholecystographic response to cholecystokinin (30). Some authors showed no significant difference between the various imaging modalities, although others claim US underestimates the true GB EF at the high and low ranges (30,31).

### Biliary Dyskinesia

There is controversy associated with the GB EF test and patients with biliary dyskinesia. These patients were previously labeled *psychosomatic* because they presented with recurrent symptoms suggestive of GB origin yet showed no evidence of any disorder on US or routine hepatobiliary scanning.

There is even greater controversy over the correct dose of CCK-8 in the measurement of GB EF, the duration of infusion, and the expected normal ranges. Using the simplest technique of 3-minute CCK-8 infusions of the package insert dose and a lower limit of normal GB EF at 35%, there have been impressive predictive results in selecting appropriate patients for surgery in this very specific patient population (32). Various other infusion rates have been suggested, and two facts emerge: a rapid IV push of CCK-8 can lead to spasm of the proximal GB, so decreasing the ejection of bile and prolonging administration of the same total dose of CCK-8 results in more uniform and improved GB EFs (33). Because the largest patient populations have used the 3-minute infusion technique, we advocate its routine use but believe that a slower 15- to 30-minute infusion of the same dose results in an improved effect.

The measurement of the GB EF is simple: A region of interest (ROI) is placed about the GB 1 hour after injection of the IDA agent when little further increase in GB filling is expected and background is subtracted. This provides the 100% prestimulated level. The CCK-8 is administered, and 10 and 20 minutes later the residual GB activity is measured and the EF calculated (Fig. 3-8).

Considerable patient movement can occur over the study period, so care must be taken to ensure that GB activity still coincides with the ROI or that bowel activity does not "contaminate" the measurements (Fig. 3-9). If the initial GB EF is low, the procedure is repeated with a double dose of CCK-8. An alternative would be a repeat dose with a more prolonged infusion (e.g., 15 to 30 minutes). The total GB EF measurement is calculated from the initial 60-minute image regardless of whether the first or second CCK-8 injection data are used, and the highest value obtained is the final GB EF reported. Although the largest series of patients has used a lower limit of GB EF of 35% as normal (32), it may be preferable in females to use a lower limit of normal of 20% because it appears that there may be some sex difference in GB EFs (33). We prefer that the patient's symptoms be replicated during CCK-8 infusion as further evidence of GB disease, but using the 3-minute infusion technique, as many as 50% to 65% of all recipients complain of abdominal symptoms, so this clinical sign is nonspecific.

Patients with appropriate symptoms after other likely diagnoses have been ruled out are candidates for the GB EF test. Because of the nonspecific nature of the symptoms, it is important to realize that this test has to date been performed only on highly selected patient populations with nor-

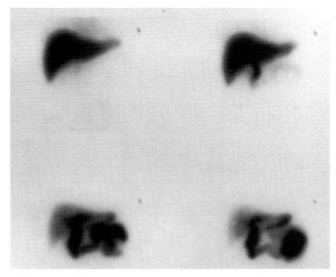

**FIG. 3-10.** This postcholecystectomy patient demonstrates, in these selected 5-minute images, a dilated CBD and minor enterogastric reflux. A similar pattern occurs with narcotic administration and partial CBD obstruction.

mal US and upper GI (UGI) studies. Such patients are likely to get relief with cholecystectomy if the GB EF is low. The same may not apply to larger populations of patients that have not been screened for other diseases.

### Sphincter of Oddi Dysfunction

Hepatobiliary scintigraphy can also diagnose sphincter of Oddi dysfunction (SOD) due to either stenosis or dyskinesia (34) and can be diagnosed by visual prominence of the CBD. In patients with an intact GB, the reservoir function of the GB invalidates the scan criteria of SOD. Other conditions that produce similar images include the postcholecystectomy syndrome, narcotic administration, and partial CBD obstruction (Fig. 3-10). Postcholecystectomy syndrome affects 10% to 40% of patients postoperatively, and although the majority have a nonbiliary etiology, a minority may have a functional biliary tree disorder. SOD may be paradoxically exacerbated by CCK-8 administration (35), and quantitative hepatobiliary scintigraphy with biliary tract and bowel ROIs may be helpful (36). This is a more difficult clinical diagnosis than biliary dyskinesia, and hepatobiliary imaging does not yet have an established role in these conditions, whereas endoscopic retrograde cholangiopancreatography and manometric procedures (basal pressures may be elevated and there may be paradoxic response to CCK-8) are more likely to be helpful in these clinical situations (37).

### Bile Leaks

The majority of bile leaks occur after trauma (e.g., motor vehicle accident, T-tube removal, liver transplantation) and,

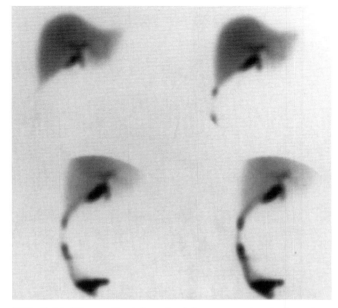

**FIG. 3-11.** The patient has had laparoscopic cholecystectomy. The tracking of tracer down the right paracolic gutter and pooling in the pelvis in these 5-minute images is a typical finding of biliary leak.

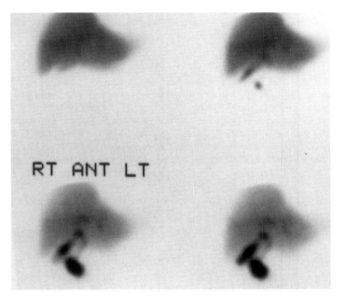

RT ANT LT

**FIG. 3-12.** Five-minute hepatobiliary images of a patient 2 days after laparoscopic appendectomy, at which time the GB was handled with forceps. The GB is unusual, with a "double density" or "target lesion" seen in the lower left image (a central "leaked" nidus of increased activity with a surrounding lesser region of GB activity), a clue of a biliary leak or GB perforation.

more recently, as a complication of laparoscopic cholecystectomy. Many cases are simple to identify (Fig. 3-11). Imaging leaks is difficult by most modalities, but careful inspection of the images is important (Fig. 3-12), and delayed imaging is critical (Fig. 3-13). Overlapping focal

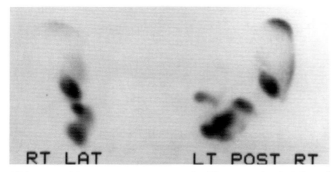

**FIG. 3-13.** The same patient as in Fig. 3-12 had delayed images, which shows an apparent GB with a small focal defect (GB surrounded by leaking bile)—the opposite appearance to the images in Fig. 3-12. No obvious local leakage of tracer but definite tracer is seen about the right lobe of the liver anteriorly and superiorly. Delayed imaging is critical for the detection of bile leaks.

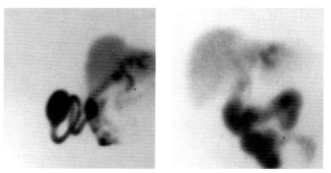

A,B

**FIG. 3-14.** Single 5-minute frames 60 minutes after injection of hepatobiliary agent, obtained 3 days apart. **(A)** The Jackson-Pratt drain and tubing is filled with radioactive bile, some local bile leak is noted in the right paracolic gutter, and minimal GIT activity (<2% total) is present. **(B)** All the tracer is in GIT 3 days later. The difference in size of the liver in these images is due to different formatters used.

bowel activity can cause considerable confusion. The frequency with which the leaked tracer tracks anteriorly over the liver is somewhat surprising (see Fig. 3-13).

A unique application of this test in patients with known bile leaks is the ability to quantify the relative amount of tracer that leaks and the portion that passes normally down the GI tract. When significant amounts of tracer follow the normal route, and in the face of scan evidence of a reducing leak, surgical intervention may be delayed (Fig. 3-14). Such hepatobiliary scans can be repeated at 1- to 2-day intervals if required. Bile leaks in patients with ascites can show free dispersal of the tracer throughout the peritoneal cavity rather than the typical loculated appearance.

### Biliary Obstruction

Extrahepatic biliary obstruction is usually diagnosed by identifying CBD and hepatic duct enlargement on US. This

**FIG. 3-15.** These last two 5-minute frames of 60-minute hepatobiliary scan obtained to rule out acute cholecystitis show a full GB with CBD visualized but nonvisualization of bowel. This is the typical appearance of very early and complete distal CBD obstruction, but in this patient (as in most patients with this pattern) it is due to narcotic (meperidine) administration. Acute cholecystitis was ruled out.

dilatation can take several days to occur, and in the small clinical subset of very acute obstruction, the hepatobiliary scan can be specific. The tracer is rapidly cleared from the blood pool in acute obstruction because secondary cholestasis has not yet occurred. Although hepatocyte excretion is reduced, it may still be sufficient to visualize the intrahepatic system and sometimes the extrahepatic ductal system down to the site of obstruction. The more common scintigraphic pattern of biliary obstruction is nonvisualization of both the intrahepatic and extrahepatic ductal system (including the GB). The passage of tracer to the obstructed site is by diffusion in complete obstruction, so the delineation of the site of obstruction is unusual. An FP scan is possible in postcholecystectomy patients, where the CBD can function as a bile reservoir. In CBD dilatation without obstruction, CCK-8 can cause a rapid washout of GB tracer to rule out CBD obstruction, a maneuver similar to diuretic renography (4). A common cause of apparent obstruction in hospitalized patients is narcotic administration or pancreatitis (Fig. 3-15) or the prior use of CCK-8 that causes delayed visualization of the bowel. Meperidine and fentanyl behave like morphine and can also emulate obstruction.

### Partial Obstruction

Partial obstruction is identified by excellent visualization of the biliary system proximal to the obstruction but with some bowel activity present. Numerous causes of this are possible,

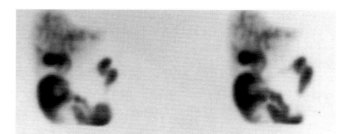

**FIG. 3-16.** The last two 5-minute frames in this scan show visualization of the GB with extrahepatic and dilated intrahepatic ductal system—the hallmark of partial CBD obstruction. This obstruction is due to AIDS-related cholangitis.

including AIDS-related cholangitis due to *Cryptosporidium* (Fig. 3-16). The excellent visualization of the CBD reflects the increased tracer concentration, not the actual ductal dilatation, which is less than the resolution limit of the detector system. One caveat is that, when CCK-8 is used, the bowel may be visualized late because of preferential filling of the GB, which results from the short-term drug effect in GB contraction (minutes) associated with a long-term (hour) effect on the sphincter of Oddi (7). In these patients a repeat dose of CCK-8 can enhance GB emptying and rule out obstruction.

### Postsurgical Indications

Postsurgical indications include bile leaks and postcholecystectomy syndromes (already discussed). In patients who have had Billroth II procedures, complicated gastric surgery, hepatic resections, liver transplantation, or biliary-enteric procedures, the study can help to delineate anatomy. In these studies the tracer can be followed as it is excreted, and evidence of enterogastric reflux, biliary leak, or abnormal tracer passage sought. Delayed views are often very helpful. At times the ingestion of technetium 99m sulfur colloid (Tc-99m SC) in water can outline the stomach and confirm enterogastric reflux or evidence of afferent loop obstruction by localization of tracer to the afferent loop with no passage of tracer beyond the gastric anastomotic site (38).

### Focal Nodular Hyperplasia

Focal nodular hyperplasia and hepatic adenoma are discussed in the section on L/S Imaging. With IDA agents uptake is typically increased in the lesion relative to the adjacent normal liver, especially in delayed imaging.

### Biliary Atresia

Biliary atresia is manifest by delayed blood clearance, increased renal excretion, and hepatocyte uptake without biliary excretion at 24 hours (Fig. 3-17). Urinary activity should not be confused with lower abdominal bowel activity. Although the half-life of Tc-99m is only 6 hours, 24-hour delayed images are obtained, and given the relatively large dose (weight-adjusted 10 mCi [370 MBq]), images are adequate for detection of bowel excretion. The major differential diagnosis is neonatal hepatitis, in which the 24-hour images show some bowel activity. In this clinical situation phenobarbital (5 mg/kg for 5 days in divided doses) helps to separate these conditions by inducing hepatic enzymes and so temporarily increasing hepatobiliary excretion of tracer in hepatitis. The sensitivity is reported as 97%, accuracy is 91%, and specificity is 82% (39). Very severe hepatitis may not be separable from biliary atresia, even with the use of deconvolution analysis (see Quantitation). Hepatobiliary imaging was formerly used frequently to separate these two conditions because the surgical Kasai procedure

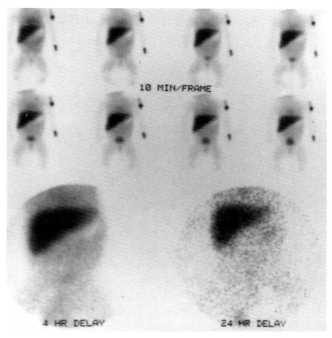

**FIG. 3-17.** Eight 10-minute hepatobiliary images show some urinary bladder but no GIT activity. This is confirmed in 4- and 24-hour delayed views (bottom images). These findings are typical of biliary atresia.

needed to be done early in the patient's clinical course for best results, but now that liver transplantation is an alternative and is performed later in the disease process, this diagnosis does not always have to be made at an early stage, and the demand for this test is declining.

### Choledochal Cysts and Caroli's Disease

Choledochal cysts are a rare phenomenon that can be diagnosed with a sensitivity of 85% by hepatobiliary imaging. They are demonstrated by a defect seen in early images with subsequent filling in on later images, with persistence of the abnormality for up to 24 hours (39). The axis of the cyst is parallel to the CBD. Caroli's disease (congenital dilatation of peripheral intrahepatic ducts) can be manifest by early photon-deficient defects that change to increased uptake due to pooling of the tracer in the dilated ducts.

### Hepatic Trauma

Only blunt trauma is described here because penetrating injuries usually require surgical intervention and rarely necessitate imaging procedures. Trauma to the abdomen introduces the concept of kindred injuries (injury to the liver and kidney or to the spleen and kidney). If left-sided kidney trauma is present, there is nearly always splenic injury. The association of hepatic and right renal injury is not as strong, but the prognosis of hepatic trauma is worse. Twenty percent

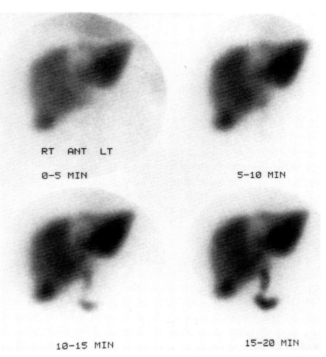

**FIG. 3-18.** The first four 5-minute images of hepatobiliary scan in a patient who had a severe liver laceration, showing persistent defect due to hepatic hematoma.

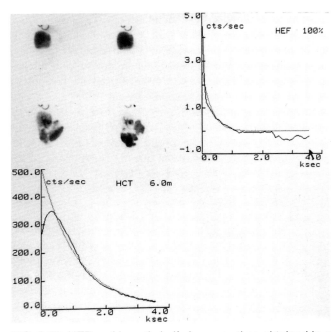

**FIG. 3-19.** HEF and hepatic half-clearance time obtained in a pediatric patient with normal hepatic function.

of patients with viscus damage after blunt trauma are asymptomatic. An L/S Tc-99m SC scan is useful in identifying liver and spleen trauma, but this role has been taken over by computed tomographic (CT) scanning. Severe compressive injuries cause stellate liver fractures, often involving entire lobes, whereas sudden hepatic displacement causes tears that lead to hematomas. Hepatobiliary scans are useful for identifying trauma-associated bile leaks or leaks after partial hepatectomies. During the early parenchymal phase, the liver parenchyma can be evaluated for lacerations (Fig. 3-18).

### Quantitation

The hepatobiliary scan is ideally suited to quantitation. The hepatic tracer uptake cannot be assessed by visual comparison of the cardiac and hepatic tracer concentrations because the hepatic activity represents both hepatocyte and hepatic blood pool tracer content. The measurement of the hepatic extraction fraction (HEF) using time-activity curves generated from hepatic ROIs overcomes this difficulty and provides an assessment of hepatocellular function (4,40). The normal HEF is 90% to 100% and, in acute biliary obstruction, this remains normal in the first few days postobstruction, then within 1 week falls significantly. In contrast, in patients with hepatocellular dysfunction, the mean HEF is reduced directly proportional to the degree of hepatic impairment (41), so this test can be used to separate acute obstruction from hepatocellular disease. The hepatic half-clearance time (HCT) can be measured at the same time. Normal is approximately 25 minutes (range, 5 to 40 minutes) with DISIDA (Fig. 3-19). In general, the HEF and HCT parallel each other, but as the HCT measures clearance of tracer from the hepatocytes it also measures bile flow through the ducts. There is generally an association of HCT and HEF, but in early ductal obstruction there is discordance (42). A definite role for this quantitation has not yet been established, but many are suggested (4).

### GI TRACT HEMORRHAGE

#### Upper GI Bleeding

Common causes of UGI bleeding include peptic ulcer disease, gastritis, esophagitis, and varices. If the bleeding is profuse, then bright red blood per rectum (BRBPR) can occur, although melena is more common. UGI endoscopy and gastric aspiration via nasogastric tube diagnoses UGI bleeding with an accuracy of 90%. In labeled red blood cell (RBC) scans, UGI bleeding is more likely to present with abnormal scans on delayed imaging. The severity of the bleed correlates with the degree of tracer seen in the lumen, and if bowel activity exceeds that of the liver, then significant blood volume replacement and surgery may be necessary.

#### Lower GI Bleeding

Massive lower GI bleeding is usually due to diverticular disease or angiodysplasia and less commonly occurs after polypectomy. Bleeding is usually submassive in other causes, including tumors and inflammatory or ischemic bowel disease. Small intestinal bleeds are less common and are usually due to arteriovenous (AV) malformations, some instances of angiodysplasia, inflammatory bowel disease, various soft-tissue disorders, and occasionally tumors or Meckel's diverticuli. The lesser bleeding episodes are much more difficult to localize.

Massive bleeding is defined as blood loss >30 ml/hr. This is most often due to diverticular disease. Although 80% of all diverticuli are located in the descending colon, 50% of diverticular bleeds arise from the ascending colon. Most (80% to 95%) of these bleeds stop spontaneously, but 25% recur. Although diverticular disease is often present in patients with GI bleeding, the etiology of the bleeding site can only be established by endoscopic or angiographic confirmation that the diverticuli are the cause. Most (80%) instances of angiodysplasia are found in the ascending colon, most stop spontaneously (95%), but most (85%) also recur. Just as in UGI bleeding, the severity of the bleed correlates with the degree of tracer seen in the lumen.

Imaging has several roles:

- To determine whether there is active bleeding
- To localize the bleeding site and guide surgical therapy without requiring angiography
- To identify which patients might benefit from angiography
- To prognosticate by predicting the need for aggressive therapy and transfusion requirements

In general, the nuclear study is more sensitive than angiography for minor bleeding rates, but the angiogram can identify some lesions even when not actively bleeding, such as the vascular tufts of angiodysplasia. The angiogram also provides an opportunity for intra-arterial vasopressin therapy.

Until recently, there was a major controversy over which nuclear imaging technique to use to detect GI bleeding. The competing methods use Tc-99m SC or Tc-99m–labeled RBCs. The Tc-99m SC study in animal experiments shows excellent sensitivity with the ability to detect bleeding rates of only 0.05 to 0.1 ml per minute. The very high target-to-background ratios resulted from sequestration of the nonextravasated tracer into the liver and spleen. Two limitations were present: The hepatic and splenic sequestered activity could obscure bleeding sites in the region, and the blood pool half-disappearance time of 2.5 minutes required that bleeding actually occur while a sufficient concentration of the tracer was still circulating, that is, in the first 10 minutes after injection. The proponents of Tc-99m RBC scans argued that the longer circulating times of that technique increased test sensitivity by detecting intermittent bleeding despite a slightly lower minimal detectable bleeding rate (0.1 to 0.35 ml/min). The minimal detectable bleeding rate of conventional angiography is approximately 1.0 ml per minute.

Our published experience of the two techniques is similar to that of others; for similarly presenting patient populations, there is an increased Tc-99m RBC bleeding detection

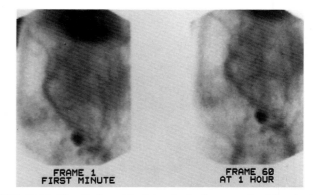

**FIG. 3-20.** The first and last 1-minute frames of a 60-minute GI bleeding study using Tc-99m–labeled RBCs. Multiple collateral vessels are seen throughout the abdomen. A prominent umbilical collection is seen, with a large vessel extending to the liver—the recanalized umbilical vein. The excellent RBC label is demonstrated by the absence of gastric and bladder activity. The persistent intravascular blood pool activity may obscure a GI bleeding site.

rate due to patients identified after the first 10 minutes of radiopharmaceutical injection (43,44). The intermittent nature of GI bleeding explains the nearly 10-fold increase in detection sensitivity with the Tc-99m RBC over the Tc-99m SC method (45). There is, however, one clinical situation in which Tc-99m SC is preferred: patients with collateral abdominal vessels that can obscure bleeding sites in Tc-99m RBC scans (Fig. 3-20). In these patients, the sequestration of the Tc-99m SC radiopharmaceutical in the liver allows the identification of a focal intraluminal collection of tracer otherwise obscured by the plethora of collateral vessels. Dividing a double Tc-99m SC dose into four parts, with repeated injections over 30 minutes or longer, allows for a significant time increase in circulating radiopharmaceutical and so improves test sensitivity (46).

### Radiopharmaceuticals

The preferred radiopharmaceutical is Tc-99m–labeled RBCs. Three labeling methods are used: in vivo, modified in vivo (or "in vivtro"), and in vitro (Table 3-9). The simplest is the in vivo technique, which is accomplished by the IV injection of stannous ion followed 20 minutes later by 20 mCi (740 MBq) of Tc-99m $TcO_4^-$. With this method, the labeling efficiency is approximately 85%, so there is considerable free Tc-99m $TcO_4^-$ excreted by the kidneys

**TABLE 3-9.** *RBC labeling methods*

| Method | In vivo | In "vivtro" | In vitro |
|---|---|---|---|
| Complexity | + | ++ | +++ |
| Infectious risk | None | None | Possible |
| Cost per test | + | + | +++ |
| Label efficiency | 85% | 93% | 98% |
| 24-hr images | Poor | Good | Excellent |

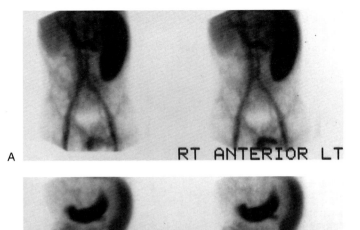

**FIG. 3-21.** Five-minute images obtained after injection of in vitro–labeled Tc-99m RBCs. **(A)** These images, obtained in the first 10 minutes after injection, show the large spleen, bladder void, and penile blood pool. **(B)** These images, obtained 6 hours later, show gastric and small intestine tracer localization indicating UGI bleed. **(C)** At that time, an image of head, neck, and thorax shows excellent blood pool label without thyroid, salivary, or buccal activity to suggest free TcO$_4^-$. This scan indicates UGI bleed originating from the stomach, identified by later images.

**TABLE 3-10.** *Dosimetry for UltraTag*

| Organ | Rads/20 mCi (cGy/740 MBq) |
| --- | --- |
| Total body | 0.30 |
| Spleen* | 2.20 |
| Bladder wall | 0.48 |
| Testes | 0.22 |
| Ovaries | 0.32 |
| Blood | 0.80 |
| Red marrow | 0.30 |
| Heart wall | 2.00 |
| Liver | 0.58 |
| Bone surfaces | 0.48 |

*Critical organ.
Source: Package insert from Mallinckrodt, St. Louis, MO.

need for removal of the patient's blood from the IV lines. Pyrophosphate preparations have the highest stannous ion content of any FDA-approved kit, which explains their continued availability. Mallinckrodt (St. Louis, MO) has the largest stannous content of all kit sets and so is preferred if multiple studies are performed.

The optimal labeling technique is the in vitro method. In this method, blood is drawn from the patient and anticoagulated with anticoagulant citrate dextrose or heparin, and small amounts of stannous ion are added. The mixture is allowed to incubate for 20 minutes while the stannous ion migrates intracellularly. The remaining extracellular stannous ions are then scavenged by additives and Tc-99m TcO$_4^-$ is added. Binding efficiencies >97% are routine, and the tag is very stable, allowing routine imaging at 24 hours without significant secreted free TcO$_4^-$ (see Fig. 3-21). The first Mo-99/Tc-99m generator elution may result in a lower binding efficiency using this technique due to the large number of Tc-99 molecules present (see Chapter 22). Currently, Tc-99m-labeled RBCs (UltraTag) are the only New Drug Application (NDA)-approved radiopharmaceutical available, and additional cost is incurred. Dosimetry is described in Table 3-10. Labeling should be done in a laminar flow hood. If several studies are prepared concurrently, there is the risk of mistakenly reinjecting the patient with another's cells and their potential infectious diseases. For this reason, we label one patient's blood at a time.

and stomach that can complicate delayed images. A poor tag can be confirmed by imaging the thyroid and oral cavity (Fig. 3-21).

The modified in vivo (in vivtro) technique is most often used and has a labeling efficiency of 92% to 95%. In this method the patient's blood is "pretinned" with an IV injection of stannous ion, and 20 minutes later blood is drawn back into an anticoagulated syringe to which 20 mCi (740 MBq) of Tc-99m TcO$_4^-$ is added. This syringe is gently inverted once a minute for 10 minutes, and the contents are reinjected into the patient. This method is simple, has a good label, and can be performed at the bedside or in the imaging room. The technique reduces the possibility of infectious contamination because the system is closed and there is no

### Protocol

Ideally, images should be obtained continuously from radiopharmaceutical injection to identification of bleeding site, but such a procedure is excessively time-consuming and costly. The routine first-time study calls for 1 hour of imaging. Sixty minutes of 10-second images are obtained with the largest field-of-view camera available to image the entire abdomen using a high-resolution collimator. Early protocols included imaging at 5- and 10-minute intervals, but this has been superseded by continuous acquisitions. If the study is done portably, a diverging collimator or separate

**TABLE 3-11.** *Scan interpretation*

Continue until bleeding site is identified
Localize site with 10-sec or 1-min frames
Delayed images help to stratify risk
Penis and uterus often visualized

upper and lower abdominal images will be required. For convenient display purposes, hard-copy images are combined into 5-minute frames. If a bleeding site is seen, 10-second or 1-minute images may better demonstrate the bleeding site (Table 3-11) and identify whether anterograde or retrograde intraluminal passage occurs (Fig. 3-22).

A cine display of the 10-second or 1-minute images, or the subtraction of previous frames, can help highlight the bleeding site (47), and the appropriate shorter-duration (10-second or 1-minute) frames can be selected for hard copy (Fig. 3-23). With older gamma cameras, images may be obtained at 5-minute intervals, but the persistence scope should be constantly monitored because the bleeding site is best identified during the actual bleed. Dramatic changes in scan appearance can occur over 10 seconds, and an alert technologist can document the bleed noted on the persis-

tence scope. If no bleeding site is identified, the patient routinely returns for imaging the next morning to determine if a bleed occurred overnight (see Table 3-11).

If the patient is having a repeat study or if the history suggests an intermittent and relatively mild degree of bleeding that has not been localized by other means, the routine procedure protocol should be modified. A compromise is to image continuously for 1 hour, obtain 10 minutes of images at 2-hour intervals until the end of the work day, and repeat this 10-minute image the next morning. The 2-hour interval compromises localization somewhat, but this may not be a clinical problem because patients who are not bleeding briskly usually have slower tracer transit through their bowel than those with BRBPR. Some clinicians recommend rescanning during the night if bleeding recurs, but if the evidence of bleeding is blood per rectum, the bleeding would have occurred some time earlier. Because nuclear medicine technologists are not available in-house, considerable time delays occur before imaging begins and may result in inaccurate localization. Bleeds of the rectum and anus may occasionally be detected only with the patient's straining on a bedpan.

**Scan Interpretation**

Important points to consider include normal visualization of the male penis during the study; this intensity normally fluctuates over the study duration (Fig. 3-24). In females,

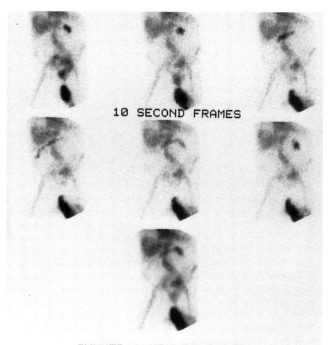

**FIG. 3-22.** The upper two rows of the composite image show 10-second views with intraluminal tracer originating in the splenic flexure and moving retrograde to the hepatic flexure and back in 30 seconds. The images also show dramatic emptying of the rectosigmoid during the same time period. The summed 1-minute image (lower image) does not show this dramatic back-and-forth movement of tracer but rather suggests an elongated collection of blood.

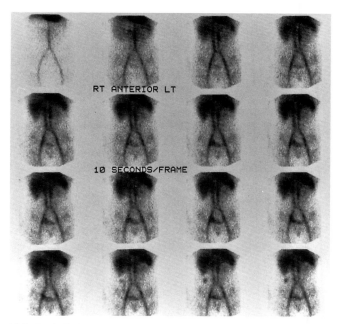

**FIG. 3-23.** This composite image of the first sixteen 10-second frames show a midline suprapubic bleeding site in the terminal ileum that migrates to a focus in the ascending colon in the third minute (bottom row) after injection. The routine 5-minute images incorrectly demonstrated an ascending colon bleeding site. The cine format demonstrated the true bleeding site.

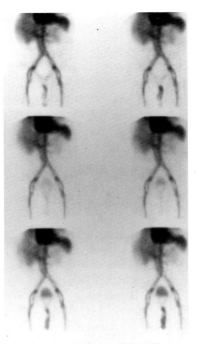

5 MIN/FRAME

**FIG. 3-24.** These 5-minute images of GI bleeding scan at start (upper), 20 minutes (middle), and 40 minutes (lower) into the study. Note the excellent abdominal visualization of both venous and arterial blood pools. These images demonstrate fluctuating penile blood pool intensity. This fluctuating pattern is found in half the male patients studied.

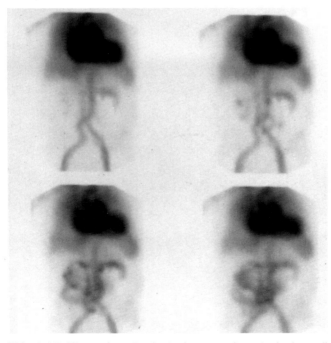

**FIG. 3-25.** These four 5-minute images show typical small bowel bleed. In the initial frame this tracer collection could represent the transverse colon, but subsequent images demonstrate multiple small bowel loops.

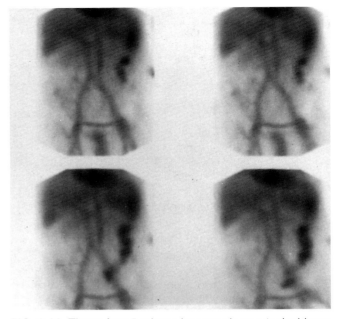

**FIG. 3-26.** These four 5-minute images show a typical large bowel bleed. The descending colon is visualized in the later images, confirming the large bowel site. Incidental note is made of vascular graft between the femoral arteries.

occasionally the region of the uterus may be visualized, which can be related to the menses (48). Care must be taken to recognize these as physiologic findings while not missing a rectosigmoid or anal bleeding site.

When attempting to localize the bleeding site, it is important to recognize the limitations of the technique. In patients with BRBPR there is usually a very rapid transit of tracer through the bowel due to the cathartic nature of blood, so accurate localization of the bleeding site may only be possible with 10-second or 1-minute images (see Figs. 3-22 and 3-23). These images can demonstrate both retrograde and anterograde movement of tracer in the bowel. It is much easier to localize the bleeding site in patients with ileus because of the lack of dispersal of even small amounts of intraluminal tracer. Glucagon has been used to paralyze the bowel and emulate this state (49).

The more intense the luminal tracer, the better the ultimate localization accuracy. One method compares the intraluminal tracer activity with the hepatic blood pool to the accurate localization of bleeding site:

- If the bowel activity is less than the hepatic blood pool, 28% of bleeding sites were accurately localized.
- If luminal activity was equal to the liver, 67% were localized.
- If tracer was greater than that in the liver, 88% were localized (50).

Many physicians terminate the study when identifying the bleed without allowing the study to proceed long enough to enable reliable anatomic localization, for example, small bowel versus large bowel (Figs. 3-25 and 3-26). It is a com-

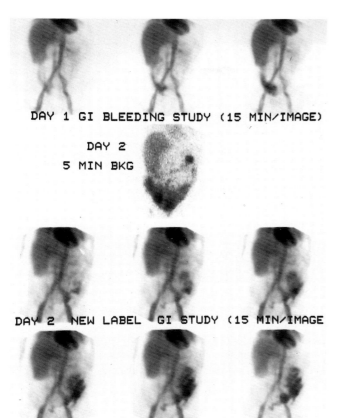

DAY 1 GI BLEEDING STUDY (15 MIN/IMAGE)

DAY 2
5 MIN BKG

DAY 2 NEW LABEL GI STUDY (15 MIN/IMAGE

**FIG. 3-27.** This complicated series of images show the 15-minute composite images of the day 1 study, when a cecal bleed is identified. The patient had a right hemicolectomy and was thought to be bleeding postoperatively (falling hematocrit), so a repeat scan was performed on day 2 after a background image was obtained (second row). The bottom two rows show the second 60-minute study in 15-minute images, and a descending colon bleed is initially suggested (third row), except that the pattern changed to suggest small intestine (bottom row). Given the background image (second row), the interpretation became obvious: a peritoneal bleed surrounding small bowel loops, a complication of surgery the previous day. This extraluminal bleeding site was confirmed surgically.

mon mistake of the less experienced imager to stop the study too early and not be sure whether the site is small or large bowel or even extraluminal (Fig. 3-27).

Recent interpretation schemes include evaluation of the 18- to 24-hour postinjection image when bowel activity is compared to that of the liver. If the luminal activity is greater than hepatic uptake, the likelihood of significant additional transfusion requirements and surgical intervention is increased, and these patients warrant aggressive immediate investigation (45). Bowel tracer that might already have been passed per rectum during that night, however, is not included in this evaluation, and the assessment of these images can underestimate the extent of the bleed, and the bleeding site cannot be identified accurately.

## Clinical Application

Many nuclear medicine departments only perform GI bleeding studies on patients with BRBPR, but others include patients with melena. It is our experience that only patients with BRBPR and significant transfusion requirements (4 U) within 24 hours of imaging have abnormal scans in the first hour (44), but other services have had success in localizing bleeding sites in patients with melena using late 24-hour images (51).

The overall positivity rate of identifying GI bleeding with nuclear medicine studies is approximately 50% (test sensitivity, specificity, and accuracy all in the range of 93% to 95%), of which half (40% to 97%) are accurately localized (47). Localization is most accurate if bleeding is identified early after injection and when considerable intraluminal tracer is present (52,53). The test when positive is abnormal at these times (43,44,52):

- 50% in the first hour
- 25% in the next 4 to 6 hours
- 25% in the next 6 to 24 hours

Sites that are not correctly localized are generally in patients with melena and positive 24-hour images, and although tracer is found in the large bowel, the actual bleeding sites are usually in the stomach, duodenum, and small intestine (45).

The role of nuclear medicine localization imaging should usually be limited to bleeding beyond the ligament of Treitz. Proximal to this, endoscopy is the preferred investigation. Patients who present with hematemesis should go to endoscopy first. If the patient has profuse BRBPR, a Tc-99m RBC scan is done emergently (see algorithm, Fig. 3-28). These patients are not suitable endoscopy subjects because the large amount of blood moving rapidly through the bowel obscures the endoscopic view. If bleeding is mild and melena is present, lower GI endoscopy and proctoscopy are often the initial investigation, with Tc-99m RBC scanning reserved for an all-day procedure starting the next morning with images every 2 hours for 6 to 8 hours and a special emphasis on 24-hour delayed imaging. There is considerable prognostic significance in delayed imaging on these patients: The detection of intraluminal tracer (bleeding) in 24-hour images indicates a clinically more significant bleed than no tracer extravasation into the bowel. This pattern of only 24-hour delayed visualization is seen in approximately half of the population with negative early scans (51) and is usually due to gastric and small bowel bleeding sites. Occasionally, a Meckel's scan is appropriate, but, as in patients with melena, this test can be scheduled electively.

Bleeding from the small intestine is a particularly difficult localization problem given the long length of the small bowel, its mobility, and the distance of the bleeding sites from an orifice suitable for endoscopy. With labeled RBCs, the small bowel can be incriminated as the bleeding bowel by the shape of the bowel lumen tracer localization (see Fig. 3-25). However, exact localization within the 20 feet of

## GASTROINTESTINAL BLEEDING

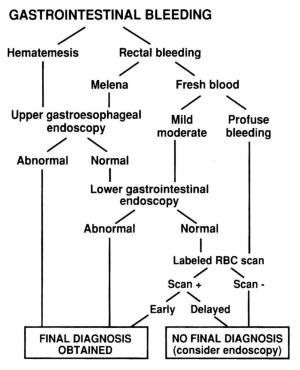

**FIG. 3-28.** An algorithm showing a useful clinical approach to localizing GI bleeding site using nuclear medicine imaging procedures.

small bowel is not possible, and the best we can do is indicate the bleeding site for angiography (superior vs. inferior mesenteric artery distribution). Because of the severity of the consequences of resection of the entire small bowel, the surgeon often attempts to identify the site by intraoperative endoscopic examination. Here the lesion may be located endoscopically while the end of the endoscope is palpated through the bowel wall. More localized resection of small bowel is possible with this technique.

## HEPATIC HEMANGIOMAS

Hepatic hemangiomas represent the most common cause of benign hepatic tumors, with an incidence of 5%, most (85% to 90%) of which are solitary. At least two-thirds are <5 cm, and there is a female preponderance. Hemangiomas can be difficult to diagnose, and most are identified incidentally when abdominal imaging is performed, especially US, for other indications. Considerable time and expense is spent ruling out a malignant etiology. By the time the patient is referred for the nuclear medicine scan, they have often had CT and US images, and the diagnosis may still be uncertain.

### Scan Protocol

The nuclear medicine technique is a labeled Tc-99m RBC scan, and both planar and single photon emission CT (SPECT) images are obtained. The planar image includes a flow study in the view that best displays the potential hemangioma as identified by other imaging modalities, followed by 1-minute images for the next 15 to 20 minutes. SPECT images are then obtained. The dosimetry is as for GI bleeding studies (see Table 3-10).

### Scan Interpretation

The early flow and delayed blood pool scan pattern of a large hepatic hemangioma was first identified serendipitously in 1978, and described as a "perfusion blood pool mismatch" (54). The classic scan pattern ascribed to hemangioma was hypoperfusion during the flow study, with a progressive increase to a hyperperfused lesion on the later images (Fig. 3-29). The delay in the appearance of hyperperfusion results from the virtual absence of arterial flow and the slow mixing of the Tc-99m RBCs with the unlabeled RBC population already present in the confluent loculated

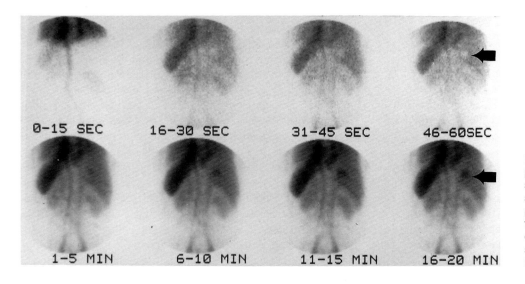

**FIG. 3-29.** The top row shows a posterior flow study (a prior CT scan identified a posterior lesion, so the flow study was performed posteriorly) with hypoperfusion of the lesion (*arrow*). The static delayed images (bottom row) show progressive hypervascularity in the same lesion (*arrow*).

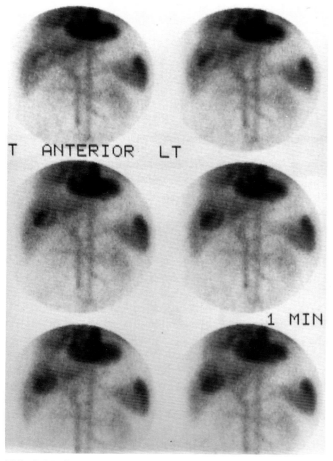

FIG. 3-30. A large hemangioma with progressive filling from the center, as seen in these 1-minute images. The later (lower) images show the lesion beginning to extend superiorly and inferiorly.

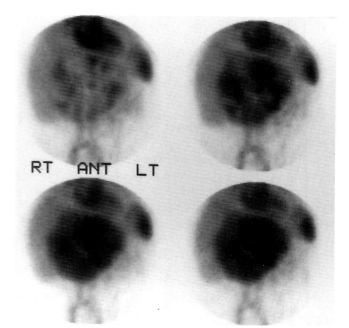

FIG. 3-31. A massive hemangioma with progressive filling in the lesion from the periphery seen in these 5-minute images. The persistent "cold spot" region centrally probably represents a scar.

spaces of the cavernous hemangioma. This pattern is the hallmark of both the nuclear medicine procedure and the dynamic bolus CT technique.

A follow-up report from the initial investigators with 166 patients (55) reported that the perfusion study showed decreased or partial perfusion only in the large or huge (>5 and >10 cm respectively) hemangiomas. The large hemangiomas typically fill in from the center (Fig. 3-30), whereas the huge hemangiomas fill in from the periphery (Fig. 3-31). The overall specificity of the Tc-99m RBC scan for hemangiomas is >95%.

Small hemangiomas may have decreased (20%) or equal perfusion (80%) when compared with the surrounding normal liver, and the classic perfusion blood pool mismatch pattern is not required. These small tumors may or may not be hypovascular, but the imaging modality is not able to discern this, so hypovascularity is not required for their diagnosis. Case reports of hepatocellular carcinomas initially suggested a similar appearance to hemangiomas, but recent large series have shown that hepatocellular car-

cinomas have the opposite scan appearance: hypervascular in the flow study and not hypervascular on delayed imaging (56).

### False-Negative Results

False-negative results usually occur as a result of fibrosis and scarring of the hemangioma, which result in filling defects on Tc-99m RBC scan imaging. Such fibrotic hemangiomas also have atypical bolus CT images. The other causes of false negatives are the size and location of the hemangioma, which may prevent its detection by virtue of the resolution constraints of gamma camera imaging. As many as half of hemangiomas may be <2 cm and therefore difficult to detect by gamma camera imaging, and although the use of SPECT improves the performance considerably, lesions <2 cm are often missed (57). Multihead SPECT devices have higher sensitivities for hepatic hemangiomas: 100% for those ≥1.4 cm, 29% for those ≤1.3 cm (58). Many hemangiomas are peripherally sited and so easier to detect by SPECT, but those deeply located or near portal vessels can be difficult to identify even if >1.4 cm. Because most patients referred for Tc-99m RBC scans have identified hepatic lesions, the decision to perform a Tc-99m RBC or MRI study can be made readily. If the lesion is <1.5 cm or located near a large vessel, MRI is preferred. Otherwise, the lower cost of Tc-99m RBC scanning makes nuclear medicine the preferred imaging modality.

### False-Positive Results

FP results occur in hemangiosarcomas (similar structure to hemangioma) and in some liver tumors (atypical hepatomas or metastases), but these are very rare findings.

## GASTROESOPHAGEAL STUDIES

Some nuclear medicine centers have raised gastroesophageal (GE) studies to an art form and can provide important GI physiologic information about esophageal transit, GE reflux, gastric emptying, enterogastric reflux, and transit times of the small and large bowel. The most common clinically indicated tests are gastric emptying and GE reflux studies. Other studies are requested from motivated gastroenterologists and are already in place where these physicians practice or they bring these protocols with them when they change locations. A very good review is present in the Society of Nuclear Medicine syllabus (59).

### Gastric Emptying

Gastric emptying studies provide a fascinating saga in the history of nuclear medicine radiopharmaceutical development. The study is presently reserved for situations in which endoscopic or radiographic mechanical causes of the patient's symptoms are not identified, or when it is desired to document the effect of pharmacologic agents. Patients who are candidates for drugs that improve gastric emptying, such as metoclopramide, are appropriately studied, and the benefit of drug therapy can be documented objectively. Although most test requests are for symptoms of delayed gastric emptying, some requests are for increased gastric motility as seen after gastrectomy, in duodenal ulcer disease, and the Zollinger-Ellison or malabsorption syndromes. The rate of gastric emptying is related to multiple factors, including gastric pressure gradient from antrum to pylorus, neural and hormonal regulation, and the stomach contents (e.g., volume, solid vs. liquid state, osmolality, pH, fat content, size of solid components). The proximal stomach controls liquid emptying and serves as a gastric reservoir, whereas emptying of solids is largely controlled by the distal stomach, and emptying occurs once the contents have been digested down to small particle sizes (<1 mm). Gastric emptying of liquid test meals is more rapid than that of solid test meals.

### Radiopharmaceuticals

The ideal radiopharmaceutical should behave exactly as the test meal and should not be absorbed onto or through the stomach wall. The classic liquid radiopharmaceutical is

**TABLE 3-12.** *Dosimetry of TC-99m sulfur colloid for oral administration*

| Target organ | Residence time (hrs) | Absorbed dose (mR/0.5 mCi, cGy/18.5 MBq) |
| --- | --- | --- |
| Total body | — | 9.0 |
| Stomach wall | 1.5 | 70.0 |
| Small intestine | 4.0 | 130.0 |
| Upper LI | 13.0 | 240.0* |
| Lower LI | 24.0 | 165.0 |
| Ovaries | — | 48.0 |
| Testes | — | 2.5 |

*Critical organ.
Source: Package insert from CIS-US, Bedford, MA.

indium 111-diethylenetriaminepentaacetic acid (In-111-DTPA), whereas Tc-99m SC is used for solid meals. These can be measured simultaneously with appropriate dual window settings on modern gamma cameras.

Considerable humorous debate has occurred over what is the best solid meal because the tracer should be tightly bound to the solid phase. Initially, in vivo labeling of chicken liver was promoted, but the need to keep a stock of live chickens and a pharmacist able to inject chicken wing veins with Tc-99m SC, willing to slaughter and prepare the bird, and skilled enough to cook the removed liver combined to render this technique impractical. Other foods have been proposed: sautéed store-bought chicken livers, chicken liver paté, oatmeal, egg salads, beef stews, and bran muffins. Tc-99m SC is added during the food preparation. Of all the possible foods, the most stable food-radionuclide complex is in vivo–labeled chicken livers, followed by surface-labeled chicken liver cubes, then Tc-99m SC mixed with eggs before cooking. The scrambled egg breakfast method is most commonly used and is served with toast and orange juice locally, with the radiopharmacist or pharmacy technician assuming the position of *chef de cuisine*. Dosimetry is as described in Table 3-12.

### Protocol

The patient arrives fasted and informed of the test meal. Some patients refuse a meal of scrambled eggs, toast, and orange juice, and then only in exceptional circumstances do we modify the meal type or substitute a liquid test meal because our normal range was obtained using this defined meal. For infants, we add Tc-99m SC to their usual formula and time this with the infant's established feeding routine.

We acquire fifteen 1-minute frames immediately after the test meal is ingested, then we acquire a 1-minute image at 15-minute intervals for up to 2 hours. Some centers insist on obtaining simultaneous anterior and posterior images to be able to calculate the geometric mean, given that the stomach passes from posterior to anterior as the test meal progresses through the stomach from the cardia to fundus. Other cen-

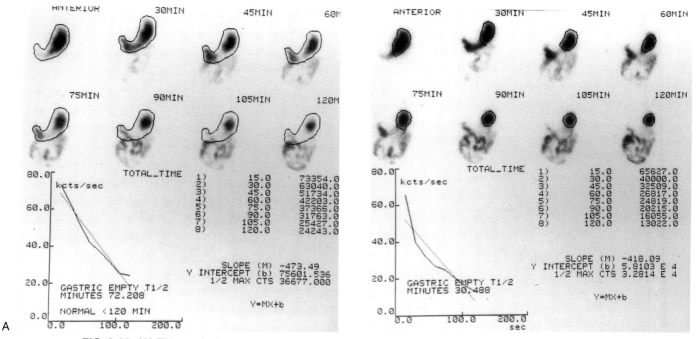

**FIG. 3-32. (A)** This analysis uses a gastric ROI that includes all the stomach and possibly part of the duodenum. In the 45- through 120-minute images, there is some overlap of gastric and small bowel activities. **(B)** In this analysis, the gastric ROI has been fastidiously decreased to include only the body of the stomach activity and to exclude the duodenum. The gastric emptying half-time fell from 72 (large ROI) to 30 (small ROI) minutes, indicating the effect of analysis technique.

ters use left anterior oblique views as a compromise. We use anterior views because this is how we established our normal range.

We use 500 µCi of Tc-99m SC coagulated in the scrambled egg, and this provides sufficient counts in the 1-minute frames to provide good counting statistics (>10,000 counts). The first 15 frames are searched to identify the frame with the greatest counts: the 100% value. This is not necessarily the first frame, even when the geometric mean (summed anterior and posterior images) is used. This lag time to the peak counts has been used as an estimate of disease, but the technique's sophistication is not generally accepted. This composite image is displayed with the next seven 15-minute interval images, and from these eight images the gastric ROI is drawn. The patients lie supine for the first 15 minutes, but between the 15-minute scans thereafter they are encouraged to mobilize. In the later images, there is some superimposition of small bowel and gastric tracer, but this can be reduced by having the patient lie briefly in the left decubitus position before rolling back to the supine imaging position. Nonadherence to a constant gastric ROI can produce striking differences in the gastric emptying half-time, which is calculated from an interpolation of the eight data points. An example is provided where the half-emptying time varied from 30 to 61 and 72 minutes according to ROI selection: a 240% change using the same data set (Fig. 3-32).

### Normal Values

Our normal range extends from 60 to 120 minutes, with a mean of 88 minutes. Studies have shown that gastric half-emptying times vary with the following factors:

- Gender (premenopausal women slower than men)
- Time of day (evening slower than morning)
- Body position (lying down slower than sitting)
- Physical activity (exercise hastens emptying)

These factors can alter gastric emptying by up to 100%. It has been shown that, even in the same patient measured under similar circumstances, significant variations can occur (60).

### Clinical Applications

Despite this intra-individual variability, the test has been clinically useful in therapeutic trials. The most common indication is diabetic gastroparesis, and the efficacy of metoclopramide use can be determined objectively. More recently, IV erythromycin has been shown to have a dramatic effect on increasing gastric emptying, but we have found oral erythromycin to be disappointing in diabetic renal transplant patients. Erythromycin mimics the GI hormone motilin, and if an oral analog is found, this imaging procedure could be quite useful and the demand for the procedure would increase. During these studies evidence of GE reflux can be

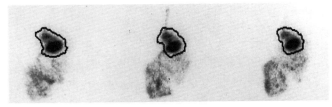

**FIG. 3-33.** This gastric emptying study demonstrates significant reflux in the middle frame (the 105-minute frame). The gastric anatomy is altered by prior surgery.

obtained (Fig. 3-33) but may be missed if frequent sampling is not obtained or sampling periods are too long (61).

## Swallowing Studies

The act of swallowing requires initial relaxation of the upper esophageal sphincter, esophageal muscular peristalsis, gravity, and relaxation of the GE sphincter. These activities must be coordinated for safe and effective swallowing. Once food enters the stomach, the upper and lower esophageal sphincters must contract to prevent pulmonary aspiration and GE reflux—the two conditions nuclear medicine techniques are called on to diagnose. In general, the assessment of oropharyngeal swallowing is better done by dynamic and static radiographic procedures. Quantitative

assessment of bolus clearance by swallowing, however, can be studied by radionuclide techniques.

### Radiopharmaceuticals

Tc-99m SC is again the preferred agent because it is neither absorbed by nor adsorbed to the esophagus or stomach. The radiation dose is an order of magnitude or two less than standard fluoroscopic procedures (see Table 3-12).

### Clinical Applications

#### Esophageal Motility

These techniques can separate patterns of achalasia, diffuse esophageal spasm, and scleroderma (59). In these patients, dysphagia may either be due to the disease itself or mechanical obstruction of an unrelated etiology. These disorders are usually diagnosed radiographically or with manometry, pH reflux studies, and acid perfusion tests. Nevertheless, in half the patients, quantitative nuclear medicine esophageal motility studies may be diagnostic.

The method of Tolin is simple and detects abnormal motility but does not identify the specific etiology (59). A dose of 150 µCi (6 MBq) of Tc-99m SC is ingested by one swallow through a straw with 15 ml of water. The patient is supine to

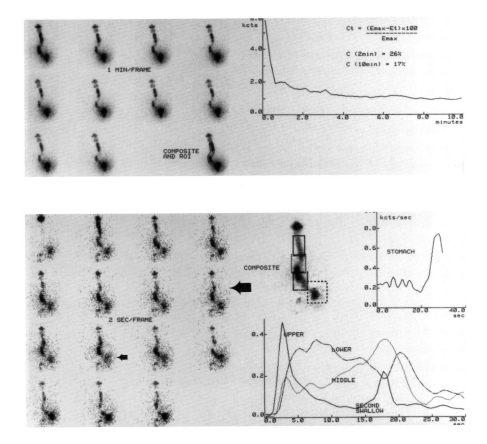

**FIG. 3-34.** First ten 1-minute images of a swallowing study. The lack of esophageal clearance is apparent. At 1 minute, 35% of the tracer remains in the esophagus; at 2 minutes, 26% remains; and at 10 minutes, 17% remains (normal <4%).

**FIG. 3-35.** Fifteen 2-second images on the left side of the panel, with an initial swallow clearing the mouth. Tracer is retained in the lower esophagus until the second swallow (eighth frame, *large arrow*) when there was retrograde passage of tracer back up to the middle esophagus. This patient also has GE reflux, shown by decreasing gastric activity soon after the second swallow (third row, *small arrow*). The upper, lower, and middle esophageal ROI have the tracer content plotted on the lower right, showing the reflux.

prevent the effect of gravity on swallowing. Fifteen seconds later the patient reswallows without additional liquid, and continues these dry swallowing attempts at 15-second intervals for 10 minutes. The initial esophageal tracer content is recorded using a ROI. The normal esophagus empties rapidly and is not readily visualized 10 seconds after the first swallow. By 10 minutes, <4% of the maximal activity should still be in the esophagus, with 90% of the clearance having occurred with the first swallow. This test is 100% sensitive for determining the presence of abnormal motility (Fig. 3-34).

Modifications of this test include dividing the esophagus into the upper and lower esophageal regions, and evaluating the stomach. In normal studies, there is an orderly progression of esophageal transit through these regions, which is documented by higher-frequency data acquisition (2-second frames) during the initial swallow (Fig. 3-35). This method defines regional esophageal dysfunction and can help distinguish, for example, achalasia (marked esophageal retention) from diffuse esophageal spasm (multiple uncoordinated peaks).

### GE Reflux

GE reflux is a very common disease and at times can be confused with cardiac pain. A sensitive noninvasive diagnostic test is very helpful in determining if significant GE reflux is present. The gold standard is acid reflux testing, but this requires intubation and so is both invasive and costly. A simple test is the nuclear GE reflux test, which is performed after an overnight or 4-hour fast.

A quantitative formula is used that is similar to the esophageal motility studies, but the 100% value is the gastric ROI rather than the esophageal ROI. The tracer is generally swallowed but should be instilled by nasogastric tube if the patient has esophageal motility dysfunction. A larger dose of Tc-99m SC (1 mCi [37 MBq]) is used, and the patient flushes the swallowed tracer down with acidified (HCl) orange juice to delay gastric emptying and predispose the individual to reflux.

Fifteen minutes after ingestion of the test dose, the patient is seated or stands in front of the gamma camera, and baseline esophageal ROI is selected for background subtraction. If significant esophageal activity is present, the patient is given more fluid to drink to wash this activity into the stomach. If this cleansing is unsuccessful, the test can be repeated at another time after gastric installation of tracer via nasogastric tube. The patient is then girded with an abdominal binder, and images are obtained as pressure is increased from 0 to 100 mm Hg in 20-mm increments. We use the binder with a Plexiglas block used for IV pyelograms and a blood pressure cuff folded beneath the Plexiglas block. These increments in pressure are intended to induce increased intra-abdominal pressure and reflux. The gastric radioactive contents are measured by gamma camera and the 100% value determined for the quantitation. The counts in the esophagus less the prebinder background are recorded, and expressed as percent of total gastric activity. GE reflux is calculated by measuring:

$$\text{Reflux } \% = \frac{\text{Esophageal counts} - \text{background}}{\text{Initial gastric counts}} \times 100$$

Any value in excess of 4% is abnormal (this figure is the same as for the esophageal retention study), and using this cutoff figure, the test is >90% sensitive.

In the infant population the binder is not used and the tracer is ingested along with the patient's usual formula. Evidence of reflux is sought while the infant is imaged supine, and delayed imaging is performed in an attempt to detect pulmonary aspiration. We suggest that the test be carried out for 60 minutes and that the child return to nuclear medicine after its next nap to determine if any aspiration has occurred. In infants, it is best to time the test with the child's expected feeding and nap times so as to simulate normal conditions and prevent infant restlessness. Rapid clearance of the aspirated upper airway can occur, so sometimes continuous imaging after ingestion is suggested by some services to detect all aspiration with the greatest sensitivity. Another way of documenting aspiration in infants is to squirt a small amount of tracer into the mouth sublingually, using a small volume in a syringe. The baby can be imaged later for evidence of saliva aspiration, which will be demonstrated by bronchial visualization (the "salivagram").

## L/S IMAGING

L/S imaging was the predominant GI study imaging procedure before the introduction of the CT scanner. It has now largely been replaced, except in special clinical circumstances.

### Radiopharmaceuticals and Physiology

Tc-99m SC became the preferred L/S radiopharmaceutical in 1964. It is sequestered in the reticuloendothelial system (RES), and hence the liver, spleen, and bone marrow are normally imaged. Relative tracer uptake is as follows:

- 85% in liver
- 10% in spleen
- 5% in bone marrow

The RES cells of the liver are the Kupffer cells, which comprise approximately 15% of all hepatic cells (62). There is quantitative extraction of tracer by the liver, so the plasma half-disappearance time of Tc-99m SC is 2.5 minutes. Because it is not possible to saturate the Kupffer cells, the relative tracer redistribution away from the liver to the spleen and marrow reflects rerouting of blood flow and identifies decreased portal vein perfusion, that is, portal hypertension. A relative increase in splenic uptake in a patient with no known hepatic disease is seen in hemopoietic disorders, where massive splenomegaly can occur. In septicemia, rheumatoid disease, and melanoma, the spleen can have increased uptake.

**TABLE 3-13.** *Dosimetry* of L/S scan*

| Target organ | Rads/4 mCi (cGy/148 MBq) | | |
| --- | --- | --- | --- |
| | | Diffuse disease | |
| | Normal liver | Early | Advanced |
| Liver | 1.40* | 0.90 | 0.70 |
| Spleen | 0.90 | 1.10* | 1.70 |
| Marrow | 0.11 | 0.19 | 3.20* |
| Testes | 0.01 | 0.08 | 0.13 |
| Ovaries | 0.02 | 0.32 | 0.48 |
| Total body | 0.80 | 0.80 | 0.70 |

*Critical organ in each condition.
Source: Package insert from Squibb Diagnostics, New Brunswick, NJ.

## Scan Protocol

Because the radiopharmaceutical is Tc-99m based and because the tracer is totally sequestered in the RES, only 4 or 5 mCi of Tc-99m SC injected IV is needed for high-quality images. The critical organ is the liver, which receives 1.4 rads (1.4 cGy) per test in patients with normal liver function (Table 3-13). Images are obtained 10 to 20 minutes after injection to allow nearly complete plasma clearance. Multiple planar views, including SPECT images, are obtained.

The GB fossa, cardiac impression, porta hepatis, and falciform ligament can be identified on the normal planar images (Fig. 3-36). In women, the breast can significantly attenuate activity in the superior right lobe on planar imaging, just as in hepatobiliary imaging (see Fig. 3-2). These

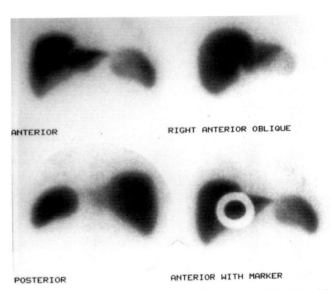

ANTERIOR   RIGHT ANTERIOR OBLIQUE

POSTERIOR   ANTERIOR WITH MARKER

**FIG. 3-36.** Three of the conventional five views of Tc-99m SC scan are shown (right lateral and left lateral views not shown). The falciform ligament defect is shown in the right anterior oblique view. Note that tracer distribution is homogeneous, both organs are of normal size, the splenic uptake does not exceed that of the liver, and bone marrow uptake is absent.

normal variants need to be recognized when looking for focal defects.

## Clinical Applications

### Focal Disease Overview

The hepatic radiopharmaceutical distribution represents Kupffer cell distribution. In focal diseases in which normal liver is replaced (metastases, cysts, abscesses, hemangiomas, hepatic adenomas, hepatomas, hematomas), focal defects are seen. Although the technique is sensitive, it is nonspecific. As is true for all imaging with radiopharmaceuticals, the detection of a photopenic defect in a surrounding volume of normal tracer uptake is difficult and decreases the scan sensitivity for focal disease compared to "hot-spot" imaging, such as bone scanning, in which small lesions are readily visualized. Large lesions and surface lesions are easily identified, and those deep within the right lobe may be missed with planar imaging, even when as large as 6 cm. The imaging principle, however, is very powerful, as the presence or absence of Kupffer cells is a very abrupt signal change when compared to the modest change in CT Hounsfield units between normal and abnormal hepatic tissues. A CT or MRI contrast agent with this amount of signal change would provide a very powerful functional supplement to the excellent anatomic resolution of those modalities.

Despite the image resolution limit of 1 to 2 cm for gamma cameras and the compromise of seeking a "cold" defect in a sea of normal tracer distribution, a review of prospective studies (63) with a short time interval from planar imaging to autopsy (the best correlation possible) show sensitivities of 80% for the detection of metastatic disease and show that the majority of false-negative studies represent lesions <2 cm. With the introduction of SPECT, there has been a significant improvement in test sensitivity compared to conventional planar imaging, and SPECT has now become the accepted method of evaluation of focal disease by nuclear medicine. The recent introduction of multihead SPECT devices has further improved focal disease imaging by allowing the collection of more counts without increasing the likelihood of patient movement. The sensitivity of SPECT liver scanning for detecting focal disease is now approximately 85% to 90%, which is comparable to CT imaging (63).

### Benign Focal Lesions

The common lesions are characterized by their cellular origin.

- Mesenchymal lesions
  Hemangioma (most common)
  Hamartomas, etc.
- Hepatocellular lesions
  Focal nodular hyperplasia (second most common)

Hepatic adenomas (third most common)
Regenerative nodules
• Cholangiocellular lesions
Hepatic cysts
Choledochal cysts and Caroli's disease

All these focal lesions, with the exception of focal nodular hyperplasia, are characterized by absent Kupffer cells and present as cold defects on Tc-99m SC L/S scanning, thus emphasizing the nonspecific nature of the test.

*Focal Nodular Hyperplasia*

Focal nodular hyperplasia (FNH) is a benign tumor with a female preponderance, similar to that seen in hemangiomas. On histology these lesions contain normal hepatocytes and Kupffer cells but have an abnormal hyperplastic arrangement. There is usually a central fibrotic scar, which has a hypervascular arterial supply but no portal venous vessels. Like hemangiomas, these are usually solitary and small (<3 cm). There is normal Tc-99m SC uptake in 50%, increased uptake in 10%, and 40% are represented by either a defect or relative decrease (Fig. 3-37). On IDA imaging there is increased immediate uptake on early images, indicating hypervascularity, and frequently IDA excretion is delayed (45 to 60 minutes), so over time a hot spot may be seen as the rest of the normal liver clears (64,65). Nuclear medicine Tc-99m SC imaging can be reassuring for many patients who present with a mass seen by other imaging modalities because the presence of Kupffer cells implies a benign etiology. In FNH, the triad of hypervascularity on flow study, normal or increased colloid, and increased hepatobiliary uptake and delayed excretion are typical. This demonstration of a hypervascular lesion with an IDA hot spot is very (98%) specific.

*Hepatic Adenoma*

Hepatic adenomas are often estrogen associated, usually due to the oral contraceptive, although occasionally related to anabolic steroids. They are much less common lesions now with the lower estrogen content of oral contraceptives. Histologically, these lesions contain hepatocytes and Kupffer cells but no portal triad. They are usually large, and present with a history of RUQ pain related to lesion ischemia, infarction, and rupture that results from thrombosis of large lesion vessels. These usually present as a defect on the Tc-99m SC scan due to poor vascularity. In distinguishing hepatic adenoma from FNH, the Tc-99m SC scan may be helpful (60% of FNH have uptake vs. 20% adenoma), and there is usually no hepatobiliary uptake.

**Hot Spots on L/S Scan**

Two causes can result in hot spots on L/S scanning: relative regional increase in proportion of Kupffer cells or an increase in perfusion to the Kupffer cells. FNH is associated with a relative increase in numbers of Kupffer cells so it can produce a hot spot.

In cases of reduced flow to the liver there may be a relative sparing of the quadrate lobe (66) as a result of collateral flow via recanalization of the periumbilical vein that empties into the quadrate lobe via the left hepatic vein in patients with collaterals. A dramatic example of this collateral flow is shown in Fig. 3-20. This lobe can appear to be a hot spot. A similar pattern occurs in lung cancer with superior vena cava (SVC) obstruction and the development of abdominal collaterals. When the hepatic vein is thrombosed the caudate lobe may be spared (Budd-Chiari syndrome) because it frequently has its own small venous efferent connections to the inferior vena cava. A Tc-99m SC L/S scan would therefore show a hot spot because there would be a relative increase in perfusion to this lobe due to its maintained venous drainage. Both these conditions cause an increase in relative regional perfusion and result in visualization in the quadrate and caudate lobes, respectively (67).

**Metastatic Lesions**

Liver metastases eventually occur in 30% to 50% of cancer patients and are often the cause of death. Liver metastases occur especially in patients when the primary tumor drains into the portal system, as in colon cancer. Metastases also occur with systemic dissemination via the

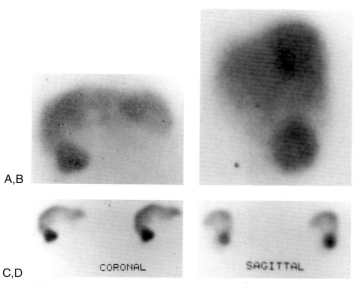

A,B

C,D

CORONAL      SAGITTAL

**FIG. 3-37.** This Tc-99m SC scan shows **(A)** anterior and **(B)** right lateral planar views and **(C)** SPECT coronal and **(D)** sagittal images. This patient has focal nodular hyperplasia with the relatively unusual presentation (10% of patients) of a hot lesion inferiorly in the right hepatic lobe. (Images courtesy of Meriter Hospital, Madison, WI.)

hepatic artery with any primary tumor. Microscopic metastases receive their blood supply by simple nutrient diffusion. In the 1- to 3-mm size, the blood supply is variable, coming from the portal, hepatic arterial, and combined vascular complexes. As the tumor grows, the supply is largely (90%) hepatic arterial, but by the time the tumor is 1.5 to 3.0 cm, the supply again becomes more variable with considerable AV shunting. As the tumor gets even larger it outstrips its vascularity, and central necrosis occurs. This necrotic region can undergo dystrophic calcification (seen in 40% of all liver metastases in patients undergoing bone scanning) (68). There is a significant relationship between size (>8 cm) and the presence of calcification as seen on bone scanning. This is especially common in adenocarcinomas of any etiology.

Metastatic disease presents an image identical to that of any multifocal disease process that causes displacement of Kupffer cells, such as hepatic cysts, abscesses, hemangiomas. Few prospective studies using comparable state-of-the-art imaging equipment have been conducted comparing the different imaging modalities, and in those studies CT had no statistical advantage over Tc-99m SC imaging using receiver operator curve analysis (69). SPECT imaging has improved the detection rate of focal disease, but CT provides the opportunity to evaluate other sites for metastases and is currently the preferred technique.

### Hepatocellular Carcinomas

The most common primary malignant tumor of the liver is hepatoma, and this is most often associated with cirrhosis secondary to alcohol, postnecrotic hepatitis, or hemochromatosis. Sixty-five percent of these appear as solitary defects on L/S scans (Fig. 3-38), 15% are multifocal, and the remainder appear merely as regions of nonhomogeneous tracer uptake or hepatomegaly. Histologically, these tumors appear as groups of abnormal hepatocytes with possible cholangial differentiation but no Kupffer cells. This explains the cold defects seen on Tc-99m SC scans. Many of these tumors take up hepatobiliary agents during delayed imaging (in contrast to FNH, which is hypervascular and has early increased uptake and delayed excretion). Most hepatomas take up gallium 67 (Ga-67) citrate, and the mismatch of cold Tc-99m SC defect with associated normal or increased Ga-67–citrate uptake suggests a hepatoma, abscess, or large metastasis. Although 90% of hepatomas take up Ga-67 citrate, <10% of cirrhotic pseudotumors accumulate gallium.

Patients with hepatoma usually present with a suggestive history. Any suspicious imaging study should warrant the drawing of blood for alpha-fetoprotein estimation, which is elevated in 60% to 70% of hepatoma patients. The fibrolamellar variant, found in younger patients (5 to 35 years of age) with noncirrhotic livers, has only a 10% prevalence of increased alpha-fetoprotein. The latter tumor has a better

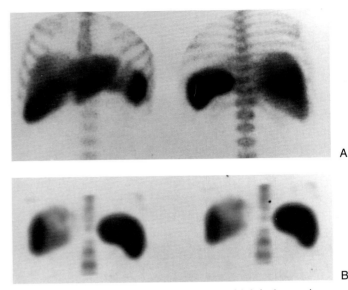

**FIG. 3-38. (A)** Anterior (left) and posterior (right) planar views show the nonhomogeneous tracer distribution, especially of the superior right lobe, colloid shift with increased splenic uptake, and significantly increased bone marrow uptake. The liver is separated from the lateral body wall, suggesting ascites. **(B)** The SPECT coronal views display the superior right lobe focal defect better. The patient had cirrhosis complicated by hepatoma.

prognosis, and these patients often receive a liver transplant. Other primary liver tumors are rare.

### Splenic Indications

The L/S scan can be used to determine whether:

- A spleen is present, absent, or enlarged
- Splenic infarcts or trauma can be identified
- Accessory spleen or splenosis is present
- Situs inversus is present

In all these conditions the Tc-99m SC L/S scan is very useful. One of the most frequent indications for a Tc-99m SC scan is to identify whether a spleen is present or not. In some instances planar and SPECT images will suffice (Fig. 3-39). In other situations a sequential hepatobiliary and Tc-99m SC scan will establish whether a spleen is present: The spleen is visualized by the L/S agent but not the hepatobiliary agent. An example of situs ambiguus is provided to demonstrate this (Fig. 3-40). If SPECT or comparison with a hepatobiliary agent does not convince one that a spleen is present, then a specific spleen scan using heat-denatured RBCs labeled with Tc-99m should be performed. This test heats RBCs for 30 minutes at 49°C to 51°C to damage the RBCs so they are rapidly sequestered by the spleen (Fig. 3-41). Another method is to label the patient's own WBCs with either In-111 or Tc-99m, and the spleen would also be identified by the preferential location of labeled WBCs in the spleen.

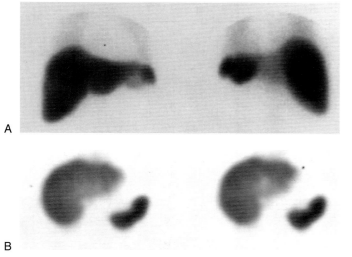

**FIG. 3-39. (A)** Anterior (left) and posterior (right) Tc-99m SC planar images suggest the presence of a small spleen. The posterior view (right) shows the effect due to the displacing and attenuating vertebral column, and a small lateral collection of uptake, possibly splenic, with a more prominent left lobe of liver. **(B)** The SPECT transaxial images unequivocally confirm the presence of a spleen as a separate organ.

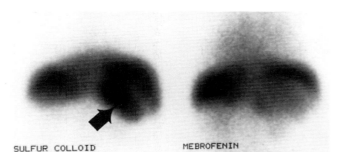

**FIG. 3-40.** Posterior views of Tc-99m SC (left) and hepatobiliary scan (right) show a right-sided spleen that is present on Tc-99m SC scan (*arrow*) but not on the hepatobiliary scan. This patient has situs ambiguus, with spleen and stomach on the right.

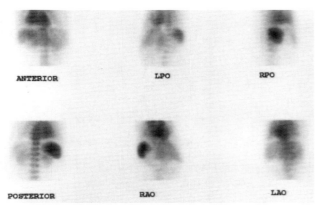

**FIG. 3-41.** SPECT images of heat-denatured Tc-99m RBCs with visualization of the spleen (best seen in posterior view) as well as the blood pool and bone marrow.

**TABLE 3-14.** *Progression of scan changes in diffuse hepatic dysfunction*

Relative increase in size of left lobe
Hepatic tracer diffusely nonhomogeneous
Colloid shift (increased splenic uptake)
Increase in size of spleen
Decreased liver uptake
Increased bone marrow uptake
Separation of ribs from liver and spleen (ascites)
Decrease in size of liver (end-stage disease)
Lung uptake (increased lung RES)

**Diffuse Liver Disease**

The L/S scan is now more frequently ordered for diffuse liver disease than it is for focal disease. The progression in scan findings is listed in Table 3-14, and an example is shown in the planar images of Fig. 3-38. The overall detection sensitivity for diffuse disease is said to be approximately 85%, but the test is nonspecific. The indications include hepatitis, fatty infiltration, and cirrhosis. It appears that alcohol probably has a direct effect on the RE function of the liver (70–72), and the sensitivity of planar imaging using hepatomegaly, splenomegaly, and shift of tracer to the spleen and bone marrow and nonhomogeneous tracer uptake has been reported at 60% to 90%. Using SPECT (71), the sensitivity for steatosis and cirrhosis was greater than CT, US, aminopyrine breath test, or liver function tests. The scan even detects fatty liver, which is the earliest and only reversible stage of alcoholic liver disease (72).

**GASTRIC MUCOSA STUDIES**

Tc-99m $TcO_4^-$ Meckel's scanning was introduced in 1970. Before this, surgical exploration was required to establish the diagnosis of Meckel's diverticulum. This condition results from in utero failure of closure of the omphalomesenteric duct. GI bleeding is the most common presentation of Meckel's diverticulum, but occurs less frequently in patients >40 years in age. Bleeding occurs when gastric mucosa is present in the diverticulum. The bleeding is thought to be due to adjacent ileal ulcers induced by the acid secreted by the ectopic gastric mucosa. Although other radiologic procedures are performed in patients with Meckel's diverticulum, they are usually done to rule out other causes of bleeding.

**Radiopharmaceuticals**

Ten millicuries (370 MBq) of Tc-99m $TcO_4^-$ is used (corrected for patient weight). In the resting patient the stomach is the critical organ (2.5 rads [2.5 cGy]), whereas in the active population the critical organ is either the thyroid or the upper large bowel (Table 3-15).

**TABLE 3-15.** *Dosimetry of Tc-99m TcO$_4^-$*

| Tissue | Dose in rads/10 mCi (cGy/370 MBq) | |
|---|---|---|
| | Rest | Active |
| Stomach wall | 2.50* | 0.5 |
| Thyroid | 1.30 | 1.3* |
| Upper LI wall | 0.70 | 1.2 |
| Lower LI wall | 0.60 | 1.1 |
| Bladder wall | 0.50 | 0.8 |
| Red marrow | 0.20 | 0.2 |
| Testes | 0.10 | 0.1 |
| Ovaries | 0.20 | 0.3 |
| Total body | 0.15 | 0.1 |

*Critical organ.
Source: Package insert from DuPont, Billerica, MA.

**TABLE 3-16.** *Rule of twos for Meckel's diverticulum*

2% of population
½ contain gastric mucosa
Within 2 feet of ileocecal valve
<2 inches long in 80%
2:1 male-to-female ratio
½ are symptomatic by 2 years

ally, posterior views are helpful to differentiate abnormal foci from normal renal collecting system activity. The patient preparation is to be NPO for 4 hours (in infants this is reduced to the usual feeding interval less the 30 minutes of the study to ensure that the infant is not restless during the study).

## Protocol

Pertechnetate is preferentially taken up by the mucus-secreting cells of the gastric mucosa. We image the patient using 1-minute frames for 15 minutes in the anterior view, then obtain two 500,000-count images in the anterior and right lateral views, each at both 15 minutes and 30 minutes. Occasion-

## Scan Interpretation

A positive scan is one in which a site of tracer is seen distinct from the stomach (Fig. 3-42). Generally, this is seen in the right lower quadrant because the Meckel's diverticulum is usually within 2 feet of the ileocecal valve (Table 3-16). It is important to visualize the ectopic gastric mucosa at exactly

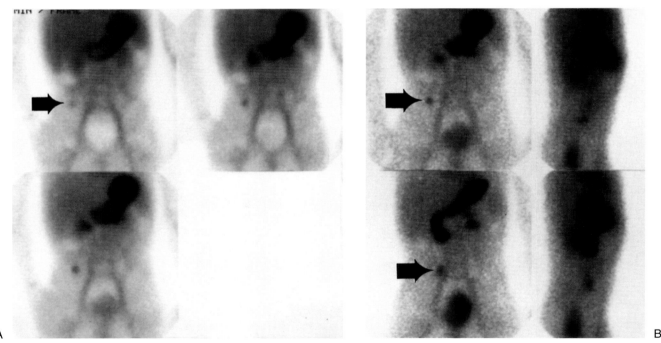

A  B

**FIG. 3-42. (A)** Three 5-minute images of a Meckel's diverticulum scan. As the stomach activity increases, activity in the abnormal focus (*arrow*) in the right lower quadrant increases. This child had a 4-year history of bleeding. Notice that activity in the renal pelves and bladder increases over the study, as tracer is excreted in the urine and fills the bladder. **(B)** The 15- (upper) and 30-minute (lower) images show a slight shift in position (*arrows*) of the abnormal focus between the 15- and 30-minute images as it moves medially closer to the iliac vessels. Over the same period, the duodenum is visualized; note that it lies anterior to (and therefore obscures) the kidney and right renal collecting system. The lateral views (right images) show the Meckel's lesion also. The lower right image shows the duodenal activity anterior to the kidney in the right lateral view.

the same time as normal gastric activity is visualized in the upper abdomen to ensure that a misdiagnosis is not made. In children the sensitivity and specificity is reported as 85% and 95% (73). In adults the sensitivity is only approximately 60%.

### False-Positive Studies

FP studies can result from visualization of the renal pelvis or duodenum (normal routes of excretion of tracer), inflammatory bowel disease, vascular lesions such as AV malformation, intussceptions, and polyps (regions with small bowel inflammation). The visualization of a renal pelvis is the most troublesome FP. The timing of appearance of the renal pelvis with that of the opposite kidney (posterior view helpful), identifying the renal pelvis and calyces, and visualizing the bladder can be very helpful in identifying this FP. Visualization of the duodenum occurs in many patients and is distinguished from the kidney by being anterior on the lateral view (see Fig. 3-42). Recent barium studies and colonoscopy can also cause FP studies due to local trauma and subsequent inflammatory response. Secretion of excess gastric Tc-99m $TcO_4^-$ can mimic a Meckel's diverticulum, and occasionally the test may have to be repeated with nasogastric suction to prevent this.

### False-Negative Studies

The free Tc-99m $TcO_4^-$ in the bladder can obscure pelvic lesions and is the most common cause of false-negative studies.

## Augmented Studies

Pharmacologic intervention has been suggested in Meckel's diverticulum detection. On one hand, pentagastrin has been used to increase the uptake of $TcO_4^-$ in the stomach and presumably the ectopic gastric mucosa. This also increases gastric secretion, so a nasogastric tube with continuous aspiration should be used with pentagastrin to prevent excess tracer passage into the small intestine. Cimetidine has also been used at 300 mg four times a day for 1 day prior to the test, with an additional dose 1 hour before the test. This inhibits release of tracer from the gastric mucus-secreting cells without impairing the uptake and increases the sensitivity of the test to >90% (74). It is equally appropriate to use this drug routinely and when the first study is normal but the diagnosis is still strongly suspected.

## OTHER GI STUDIES

### Hepatic Arterial Perfusion Studies

Hepatic arterial perfusion scintigraphy studies are useful in patients with hepatic arterial catheters inserted for the intra-arterial delivery of chemotherapy for the treatment of liver metastases. This intra-arterial injection of therapeutic agent

allows much higher chemotherapeutic doses without significant systemic effects. The installation of Tc-99m macroaggregated albumin (MAA) has been used to optimize catheter placement in the operating suite using a portable camera, to confirm that appropriate metastatic lesions are being perfused with the therapeutic agent, and to establish that extrahepatic sites (stomach and small bowel) are not perfused. For up to 30% of requests for this test, there is evidence of extrahepatic perfusion, indicating that catheter manipulation or replacement is required. This same technique can be used to routinely check catheter placement in the nuclear medicine department and so prevent the gastric ulceration and infarction sequelae of extrahepatic chemotherapeutic administration. A surprising number of catheters get dislodged, and significant reflux into the celiac axis can occur during chemotherapy infusion, resulting in local or systemic side effects.

The test also evaluates the presence of hepatic tumor AV shunting by obtaining images of the lungs, which are visualized when shunting is present. The degree of shunting can be quantified by comparing the pulmonary to the hepatic distribution of Tc-99m MAA. As many as one-fourth of treated patients demonstrate this shunting.

### Peritoneal Shunts

Evaluation of peritoneal shunts is possible when tracer is instilled into the ascitic fluid of a patient with a possible shunt malfunction. The shunts have either a low-pressure valve (LeVeen shunt) or a pumping device (Denver shunt) inserted into the abdominal wall. The proximal or afferent end of the shunt is placed intraperitoneally, and the distal or

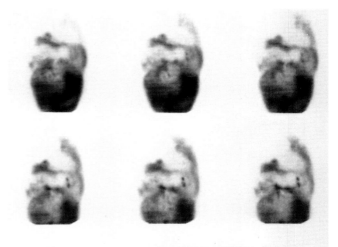

PUMPED EVERY 5 MIN.

**FIG. 3-43.** This study with six 5-minute images shows tracer in the peritoneal fluid after abdominal paracentesis. The later images obtained during intermittent pumping of the Denver valve show gradual accumulation of tracer into the left lung (patient is status post right pneumonectomy). The pump is identified as two dots in the left upper quadrant. This Denver shunt is patent.

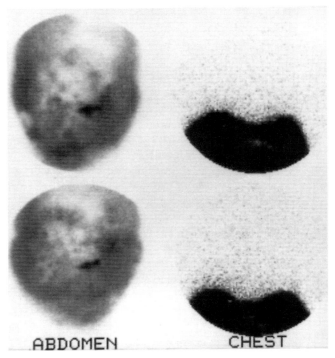

**FIG. 3-44.** Images of abdomen (left) and chest (right; higher image intensity to detect any pulmonary activity) at 15 (upper) and 30 (lower) minutes postinjection. The absence of pulmonary activity indicates a nonfunctioning LeVeen shunt.

efferent end is placed in the SVC. Malfunction most often occurs in the abdominal end. Initial studies used the intraperitoneal instillation of Tc-99m SC, and visualization of the liver indicated the shunt was patent, but this hepatic tracer localization was often obscured by the tracer in the intraperitoneal ascitic fluid. We have switched to using Tc-99m MAA because the presence of pulmonary activity indicated the shunt was not completely obstructed, and the test was easier to interpret. In normal function, the lungs and shunt tubing are visualized within 10 minutes of instillation of tracer intraperitoneally (Fig. 3-43); if not, obstruction is present (Fig. 3-44). Tracer can be injected directly into the Denver pump to check the thoracic end (Fig. 3-45).

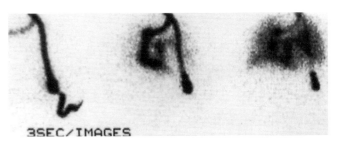

**FIG. 3-45.** Three-second flow images of tracer injected into Denver shunt reservoir showing free flow into the right heart. In this patient with definite obstruction, the site of obstruction was proximal to the reservoir. In the first 3-second image, the injection line is also seen.

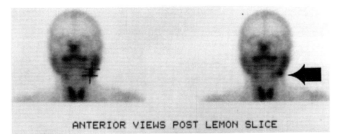

ANTERIOR VIEWS POST LEMON SLICE

**FIG. 3-46.** Delayed anterior images with and without markers about the palpable mass. These images, obtained after lemon juice stimulation, show retention of Tc-99m TcO$_4^-$ in the lesion (*arrow*), a Warthin's tumor. This is a very unusual presentation because the tumor is in a woman, and this lesion is the second Warthin's tumor found.

## Salivary Scanning

Warthin's tumor is one tumor that is uniquely visualized on parotid gland scanning using Tc-99m TcO$_4^-$, which provides an opportunity to make a diagnosis of Warthin's preoperatively. A flow study is first obtained, then 400K count static images are obtained in anterior and both lateral projections. These static images are repeated after administration of citrus juice to induce salivation. Persistent tracer uptake in a region of the parotid gland is correlated with palpation, and if this corresponds with the mass, a Warthin's tumor is likely (Fig. 3-46). These tumors are usually unilateral (90%) and occur predominantly in males (90%).

## Tests Not Available in the United States

Although there are methods of determining GI protein loss, there is no NDA for chromium 51–albumin in this country, so this test is not routinely available. Breath tests can diagnose bacterial overgrowth and test intestinal absorption, but neither has a currently available NDA source. An NDA has just been approved for detecting *Helicobacter pylori* infection (see Chapter 20).

## REFERENCES

1. Winzelberg GG, McKusick KA, Froelich JW, et al. Detection of gastrointestinal bleeding with Tc-99m–labeled red blood cells. Semin Nucl Med 1982;12:139–146.
2. Lull RJ, Morris GL. Scintigraphic detection of gastrointestinal hemorrhage: current status. J Nucl Med Tech 1986;14:79–86.
3. Rubin RA, Liechtenstein GR. Hepatic scintigraphy in the evaluation of solitary solid liver masses. J Nucl Med 1993;34:697–705.
4. Krishnamurthy GR, Turner FE. Pharmacokinetics and clinical application of technetium 99m-labeled hepatobiliary agents. Semin Nucl Med 1990;20:130–149.
5. Datz FL, Christian PE, Hutson WR, et al. Physiological and pharmacological interventions in radionuclide imaging of the tubular gastrointestinal tract. Semin Nucl Med 1991;21:140–152.
6. Firnau G. Why do Tc-99m chelates work for cholescintigraphy? Eur J Nucl Med 1976;1:137–139.
7. Kim CK, Palestro CJ, Solomon RW, et al. Delayed biliary-to-bowel transit in cholescintigraphy after cholecystokinin treatment. Radiology 1990;176:553–556.

8. Choy D, Shi EC, McLean RG, et al. Cholescintigraphy in acute cholecystitis: use of intravenous morphine. Radiology 1984;151:203–207.

9. Brachman MB, Tanasescu DE, Ramanna L, Waxman AD. Acute gangrenous cholecystitis: radionuclide diagnosis. Radiology 1984;151:209–211.

10. Bushnell DL, Perlman SB, Wilson MA, Polcyn RE. The rim sign: association with acute cholecystitis. J Nucl Med 1986;27:353–356.

11. Bohdiewicz PJ. The diagnostic value of grading hyperperfusion and the rim sign in cholescintigraphy. Clin Nucl Med 1993;18:867–871.

12. Kim CK, Tse KKM, Juweid M, et al. Cholescintigraphy in the diagnosis of acute cholecystitis: morphine augmentation is superior to delayed imaging. J Nucl Med 1993;34:1866–1870.

13. Fink-Bennett D, Balon H, Robbins T, Tsai D. Morphine-augmented cholescintigraphy: its efficacy in detecting acute cholecystitis. J Nucl Med 1991;32:1231–1233.

14. Freitas JE, Coleman RE, Nagle CE, et al. Influence of scan and pathologic criteria on the specificity of cholecystitis: concise communication. J Nucl Med 1983;24:876–879.

15. Shea JA, Berlin JA, Escaarce JJ, et al. Revised estimates of diagnostic test sensitivity and specificity in suspected biliary tract disease. Arch Intern Med 1994;154:2573–2581.

16. Achong DM, Newman JS, Oates E. False-negative morphine-augmented cholescintigraphy: a case of subacute gallbladder perforation. J Nucl Med 1992;33:256–257.

17. Hicks RJ, Kelly MJ, Kalff V. Association between false negative hepatobiliary scans and initial gallbladder visualization after 30 minutes. Eur J Nucl Med 1990;16:747–753.

18. Babb RR. Acute acalculous cholecystitis: a review. J Clin Gastroenterol 1992;15:238–241.

19. Savoca PE, Longo WE, Zucker KA, et al. The increasing prevalence of acalculous cholecystitis in outpatients. Ann Surg 1990;211:433–437.

20. Boland GW, Lee MJ, Leung J, Mueller PR. Percutaneous cholecystostomy in critically ill patients: early response and final outcome in 82 patients. AJR Am J Roentgenol 1994;163:339–342.

21. Warner BW, Hamilton FN, Silberstein EB, et al. The value of hepatobiliary scans in fasted patients receiving total parenteral nutrition. Surgery 1987;102:595–601.

22. Shuman WP, Gibbs P, Rudd TG, Mack LA. PIPIDA scintigraphy for cholecystitis: false positives in alcoholism and total parenteral nutrition. AJR Am J Roentgenol 1982;138:1–5.

23. Drane WI, Nelp WB, Rudd TG. The need for routine delayed radionuclide hepatobiliary imaging in patients with intercurrent disease. Radiology 1984;151:763–769.

24. Fig LM, Wahl RL, Stewart RE, Shapiro B. Morphine-augmented hepatobiliary scintigraphy in the severely ill: caution is in order. Radiology 1990;175:467–473.

25. Flancbaum L, Choban PS, Sinha R, Jonasson O. Morphine cholescintigraphy in the evaluation of hospitalized patients with acute cholecystitis. Ann Surg 1994;220:25–31.

26. Fink-Bennett D, Clarke K, Tsai D, et al. Indium-111–leukocyte imaging in acute cholecystitis. J Nucl Med 1991;32:803–804.

27. Swayne LC. Acute acalculous cholecystitis: sensitivity in detection using technetium-99m iminodiacetic acid cholescintigraphy. Radiology 1986;160:33–38.

28. Raymond F, Lepanto L, Rosenthall L, Fried GM. Tc-99m–IDA gallbladder kinetics and response to CCK in chronic cholecystitis. Eur J Nucl Med 1988;14:378–381.

29. Topper TE, Ryerson TW, Nora PF. Quantitative gallbladder imaging following cholecystokinin. J Nucl Med 1980;21:694–696.

30. Davis GB, Berk RN, Scheible FW, et al. Cholecystokinin cholecystography, sonography, and scintigraphy: detection of chronic acalculous cholecystitis. AJR Am J Roentgenol 1982;139:1117–1121.

31. Krishnamurthy S, Krishnamurthy GT. Editorial. Gallbladder ejection fraction: a decade of progress and future promise. J Nucl Med 1992;32:542–544.

32. Fink-Bennett D, DeRidder P, Kolozsi WZ, et al. Cholecystokinin cholescintigraphy: detection of abnormal gallbladder motor function in patients with chronic acalculous gallbladder disease. J Nucl Med 1991;32:1695–1699.

33. Ziessman HA, Fahey FH, Hixson DJ. Calculation of a gallbladder ejection fraction: advantage of continuous sincalide infusion over the three-minute infusion period. J Nucl Med 1992;33:537–541.

34. Pace RF, Chamberlain MJ, Passi RB. Diagnosing papillary stenosis by technetium-99m HIDA scanning. Can J Surg 1983;26:191–193.

35. Fink-Bennett D. Augmented cholescintigraphy: its role in detecting acute and chronic disorders of the hepatobiliary tree. Semin Nucl Med 1991;21:128–139.

36. Sostre S, Kalloo AN, Spiegler EJ, et al. A noninvasive test of sphincter of Oddi dysfunction in postcholecystectomy patients: the scintigraphic score. J Nucl Med 1992;33:1216–1222.

37. Steinberg WM. Sphincter of Oddi dysfunction: a clinical controversy. Gastroenterology 1988;95:1409–1415.

38. Park H, Wellman HN, Madura JA. Hepatobiliary Imaging After Gastrointestinal Surgery. In Biersack HJ, Cox PH (eds), Nuclear Medicine in Gastroenterology: Developments in Nuclear Medicine. Dordrecht, Holland: Kluwer, 1991;47–68.

39. Nadel HR. Hepatobiliary scintigraphy in children. Semin Nucl Med 1996;26:25–42.

40. Chester M, Glowniak J. Hepatobiliary imaging update. J Nucl Med Tech 1992;20:3–7.

41. Doo E, Krishnamurthy GT, Eklem MJ, et al. Quantification of hepatobiliary function as an integral part of imaging with technetium-99m–mebrofenin in health and disease. J Nucl Med 1991;32:48–57.

42. Howman-Giles R, Moase A, Gaskin K, Uren R. Hepatobiliary scintigraphy in a pediatric population: determination of hepatic extraction fraction by deconvolution analysis. J Nucl Med 1993;34:214–221.

43. Bunker SR, Lull RJ, Tanasescu DE, et al. Scintigraphy of gastrointestinal hemorrhage: superiority of Tc-99m red blood cells over Tc-99m sulfur colloid. AJR Am J Roentgenol 1984;143:543–548.

44. Wilson MA, Hellman RS. The detection of gastrointestinal bleeding using nuclear medicine techniques; a local experience and review. Wis Med J 1984;83:15–19.

45. Fink-Bennett D, Eggli DF. Radionuclide imaging in the detection and localization of acute GI bleeding. Imaging Insights 1993;2:1–6.

46. Perlman SB, Wilson MA. The detection of a gastrointestinal bleeding site in patients with liver cirrhosis: which agent to use? J Nucl Med 1986;27:435–436.

47. Maurer AH, Rodman MS, Vitti RA, et al. Gastrointestinal bleeding: improved localization with cine scintigraphy. Radiology 1992;185:187–192.

48. Swayne LC. The uterine doughnut: potential pitfall for technetium-99m gastrointestinal bleeding study. Clin Nucl Med 1989;14:759–761.

49. Froelich JW, Juni J. Glucagon in the scintigraphic diagnosis of small-bowel hemorrhage by Tc-99m–labeled red blood cells. Radiology 1984;151:239–242.

50. Gupta SM, Spencer RP, Chak SP. Significance of intensity of delayed activity during technetium-99m-RBC gastrointestinal bleeding study. J Nucl Med 1991;32:2249–2252.

51. Jacobson AF, Cerqueira MD. Prognostic significance of late imaging results in technetium-99m-labeled red blood cell gastrointestinal bleeding studies with early negative images. J Nucl Med 1992;33:202–207.

52. Winzelberg GG, Froelich JW, McKusick KA, et al. Radionuclide localization of lower gastrointestinal hemorrhage. Radiology 1981;139:465–469.

53. Zuckerman DA, Bocchini TP, Birnbaum EH. Massive hemorrhage in the lower gastrointestinal tract in adults: diagnostic imaging and intervention. AJR Am J Roentgenol 1993;161:703–711.

54. Front D, Hardoff R, Israel O, et al. Perfusion vascularity mismatch in liver hemangiomas. Clin Nucl Med 1978;3:212.

55. Groshar D, Ben-Haim S, Gips S, et al. Spectrum of scintigraphic appearance of liver hemangiomas. Clin Nucl Med 1992;17:294–299.

56. Kudo M, Ikekubo K, Yamamoto K, et al. Distinction between hemangioma of the liver and hepatocellular carcinoma: value of labeled RBC-SPECT scanning. AJR Am J Roentgenol 1989;152:977–983.

57. Birnbaum BA, Weinreb JC, Megibow AJ, et al. Definitive diagnosis of hepatic hemangiomas: MR imaging versus Tc-99m-labeled red blood cell SPECT. Radiology 1990;176:95–101.

58. Ziessman HA, Silverman PM, Patterson J, et al. Improved detection of small cavernous hemangiomas of the liver with high resolution three-headed SPECT. J Nucl Med 1991;32:2086–2091.

59. Maurer AH, Heyman S, Vitti RA, Winzelberg GG. Gastrointestinal Nuclear Medicine. In Siegel R, Kirchner P (eds), Nuclear Medicine: Self-Study Program I. New York: Raven, 1988;59–69.

60. Chatterton BE. Gastric Motility. In Murray IPC, Ell PJ (eds), Nuclear Medicine in Clinical Diagnosis and Treatment. New York: Churchill Livingstone, 1994;393–405.

61. Seymour JC, West JH, Drane WE. Sequential ten-second acquisitions for detection of gastroesophageal reflux. J Nucl Med 1993;34:658–660.

62. Gates GA, Henley KS, Pollard HM, et al. The cell population of human liver. J Lab Clin Med 1961;59:182–184.

63. Wilson MA. Metastatic Disease of the Liver. In Wilson MA, Ruzicka FF (eds), Modern Imaging of the Liver. New York: Dekker, 1989; 631–659.

64. Biersack HJ, Thelen M, Torres JF, et al. Focal nodular hyperplasia of the liver as established by Tc-99m-sulfur colloid and HIDA scintigraphy. Radiology 1980;137:187–190.

65. Boulahdour H, Cherqui D, Charlotte F, et al. The hot spot hepatobiliary scan in focal nodular hyperplasia. J Nucl Med 1993;34:2105–2110.

66. Huang M-J, Liaw Y-F, Tzen K-Y. Radionuclide venography in Budd-Chiari syndrome with intrahepatic vena-caval obstruction. J Nucl Med 1985;26:145–148.

67. Parker FE, Burke TS. Technetium-99m-medronate uptake in hepatic necrosis associated with Budd-Chiari syndrome. J Nucl Med 1992;33:1390–1392.

68. Wilson MA, Liss LF, Studey CL. Uptake of technetium-99m-MDP in hepatic metastases. Noninv Med Imag 1984;1:253–257.

69. Alderson PO, Adams DF, McNeil BJ, et al. Computed tomography, ultrasound and scintigraphy of the liver in patients with colon or breast cancer: a prospective study. Radiology 1983;149:225–230.

70. Rao BK, Weir GJ Jr, Lieberman LM. Dissociation of reticuloendothelial cell and hepatocyte functions in alcoholic liver disease: a clinical study with a new Tc-99m-labeled hepatobiliary agent. Clin Nucl Med 1981;6:289–294.

71. Delcourt E, Vanhaeverbeek M, Binon J-P, et al. Emission tomography for the assessment of diffuse alcoholic liver disease. J Nucl Med 1992;33:1337–1344.

72. Saini S. Editorial: diagnostic imaging of the liver. J Nucl Med 1992; 33:1344–1345.

73. Sfakianakis GN, Conway JJ. Detection of ectopic gastric mucosa in Meckel's diverticulum and in other aberrations by scintigraphy: I. Pathophysiology and 10-year clinical experience. J Nucl Med 1981;22:647–654.

74. Diamond RH, Rothstein RD, Alavi A. Case presentation and discussion: the role of cimetidine-enhanced technetium-99m-pertechnetate imaging for visualizing Meckel's diverticulum. J Nucl Med 1991;32:1422–1424.

*Textbook of Nuclear Medicine,*
edited by Michael A. Wilson.
Lippincott–Raven Publishers, Philadelphia © 1998.

CHAPTER  4

# Pulmonary System

Michael A. Wilson

Lung scans were first performed in the mid-1960s. Since then, there has been a progressive refinement in the lung scan performance and interpretation to the point of its acceptance as a very useful screening modality for pulmonary embolism (PE). There are few other indications for the study (Table 4-1). The doyens on the use of ventilation/perfusion (V/Q) imaging in PE include Wagner, McNeil, Biello, Alderson, Gottschalk, and the groups from the McMaster's and Prospective Investigation of Pulmonary Embolism Diagnosis (PIOPED) studies. There are multiple excellent reviews of this topic, and four that span this era of evolution are suggested (1–4).

V/Q scanning to diagnose PE is a very difficult imaging task, one in which patient management is best served if the radiologist understands the disease process. V/Q scan interpretations span a continuum from the easy, high-probability scans with multiple bilateral segmental mismatches in PE, to the normal scan, which excludes the diagnosis. Most other categories are difficult diagnostic dilemmas for the radiologist and the referring physician.

## HISTORY OF V/Q SCAN

The first perfusion lung scan was performed in 1964 (5). Four years later, the importance of the shape of perfusion defects was reported (6), and the introduction of ventilation scans improved the specificity of lung scanning (7). Eight years after the original report, the segmental nature of V/Q defects in PE was emphasized (8). In 1976, a report by McNeil was prescient, introducing indications for pulmonary arteriograms, many of which are just as relevant today (9). He also discussed both the number and size of anatomic defects and the result when matched and mismatched V/Q abnormalities were present in the same patient (9).

In 1977, Robin described the difficulty in applying V/Q results to the clinical population with his "the emperor may have no clothes" paper (10) that sparked an unprecedented controversy. This resulted in a series of refinements to the V/Q diagnosis of PE, led by Biello, who included the number and size of subsegmental lesions required for a scan to suggest a high probability of PE (11) and descriptions of the "indeterminate" scan, in which each perfusion defect had a corresponding radiographic abnormality. In 1980, McNeil introduced the use of the pretest clinical probability and the effect this has on the scan probability (12). These retrospective papers and others led to the two Northern American prospective series that attempted to define the role of V/Q scanning in the diagnosis of venous thromboembolic disease: the McMaster's and PIOPED series (13,14).

## PULMONARY EMBOLISM

### Pathophysiology of PE

PE can present with a wide range of symptoms—from fatal apoplexy to the mildest symptom complex of fever, tachycardia, and tachypnea that may only be found by the nursing staff who record the patient's vital signs. Many patients with PE are asymptomatic. The symptomatic presentation of PE appears to depend predominantly on two factors: the size of the occlusive phenomenon in the pulmonary arterial tree, and whether pulmonary infarction (or hemorrhage) occurs. The size of the clot reaching the lung determines which size vessel is occluded (main pulmonary, lobar, segmental, or subsegmental arteries). PE can present as massive PE with hypotension, in which symptoms of left ventricular output failure occur because of the extensive pulmonary arterial occlusion. In these presentations, >75% of the pulmonary arterial tree is occluded. These can occur after a single central clot or by a combination of arterial occlusions. It is these patients with massive obstruction who are likely to die acutely from the disease. The role of echocardiography in determining right ventricular dysfunction is likely to become important in risk stratifying PE because of its ability to identify PE patients with massive embolization. Symptoms occur when 30% or more of the

**TABLE 4-1.** *Pulmonary scan frequency*

| | |
|---|---|
| Rule out PE | 95% |
| Quantitative lung perfusion | 3% |
| Lung transplantation | 1% |
| Intracardiac shunts | 1% |

**TABLE 4-2.** *Syndromes of PE in patients with no preexisting cardiac or pulmonary disease*

| Clinical syndrome | PE (n = 117) | No PE (n = 248) |
|---|---|---|
| Pleuritic pain or hemoptysis | 65% | 59% |
| Isolated dyspnea | 22% | 21% |
| Circulatory collapse | 8% | 9% |

Source: Stein PD, Terrin M, Hetes CA, et al. Clinical, laboratory, roentgenographic, and electrocardiographic findings in patients with acute pulmonary embolism and no preexisting cardiac or pulmonary disease. Chest 1991;100:598–603.

**TABLE 4-3.** *Risk factors for DVT*

Age >40 (exponential increase with age)
History of past DVT or PE
Myocardial infarction and heart failure
Immobilization or paralysis (15% <1 week, 80% >1 week)
Peripartum status and large doses of estrogens (but not estrogen replacement therapy)
Multiple trauma or surgery to hips and knees (knee procedures 25% risk, hips 50%)
Prolonged sitting (airplane or automobile travel)
Cancer (increase in coagulability)
Chemotherapy (decreased protein C and S levels)
Tamoxifen (decreased antithrombin III levels)

arterial tree is occluded; these include the sudden onset of dyspnea and tachycardia. PEs, as identified by V/Q scanning, occur in half the patients diagnosed with deep venous thrombosis (DVT) of the calf, yet these small PEs are invariably asymptomatic and clinically unimportant (15).

If pulmonary infarction occurs, patients develop pleuritic chest pain and hemoptysis hours to days later. This clinical presentation is a late development of PE, just as pericarditis is a late development of myocardial infarction. Paradoxically, pulmonary infarction occurs with occlusion of the smaller pulmonary arteries (≤3 mm) that serve subsegmental regions. This is in part explained by the dual blood supply, with the bronchial arteries primarily supplying nutrients in the more proximal bronchopulmonary levels. The dual blood supply also explains why only 10% of embolized regions progress to infarction. The fact that approximately 60% of patients with PE present with pleuritic chest pain and hemoptysis (i.e., pulmonary infarction or hemorrhage) is explained by the multiplicity of emboli in any given patient (16,17). The literature indicates that patients with high-probability lung scans have an average of nine of the 18 bronchopulmonary segments involved (14). This multiplicity is a function of fragmentation in the right ventricle of individual embolized thrombi and repeated embolization of fresh clots from existing distal venous thromboses. Hemoptysis from either pulmonary infarction or pulmonary hemorrhage results from increased bronchial arterial flow that accompanies pulmonary arterial occlusion. This alveolar filling with blood explains many of the chest x-ray (CXR) abnormalities.

### Clinical Presentation of PE

The extent and the rate of occurrence of pulmonary arterial occlusion determines the clinical presentation. The rapid onset of extensive arterial obstruction causes hypotension, tachycardia, nausea, feelings of doom, and diaphoresis. This might result from a Valsalva maneuver, such as that associated with straining at stool, displacing a large iliac vein clot. If a recurrent embolic process gradually leads to significant pulmonary arterial occlusion, it may well be associated with chronic pulmonary hypertension, but this is a rare presentation and occurs in only 2% of PE patients. Dyspnea or tachypnea is present in 90% of patients, and virtually all patients (97%) with PE have one of the triad of dyspnea, tachypnea, or pleuritic chest pain (16).

Dyspnea results from increased dead space and hypoxemia. Hypoxemia results from diversion of blood to nonob-

structed but relatively hypoventilated (the embolized regions have no blood flow but normal ventilation) segments and the shunting that occurs with reflow to atelectatic regions. An increased A-a gradient is found in many patients, but like the lung perfusion scan, this is a very nonspecific indicator of PE. Hypocarbia as a consequence of the tachypnea is a frequent finding and even occurs in patients with chronic obstructive pulmonary disease (COPD). Although local bronchospasm might occur in acute PE, it is unlikely to contribute significantly to hypoxemia and has probably been overemphasized clinically in the past (3).

Many studies have shown that the symptoms of PE are nonspecific. In the PIOPED study, patients who had PE presented the same clinical syndrome (hemoptysis and pleuritic pain, isolated dyspnea or sudden circulatory collapse) as those subsequently found not to have PE (Table 4-2), yet physicians were accurate at predicting which patients had PE (17). This apparent discrepancy is probably explained by the physicians' combining the appropriate symptoms of PE with known risk factors for DVT (Table 4-3). In general, the risk of DVT increases as the number of risk factors increase. Virtually all patients with four or more risk factors have documentable DVT (18).

### Venous Thrombosis and PE

Thrombi causing PE arise from the lower extremities in 90% to 95% of patients. Most lower-extremity thromboses probably begin in the leg veins. With time, these propagate into larger proximal veins. It is the embolization of the

**TABLE 4-4.** *Rules of 50%*

| |
|---|
| 50% of fatal PE is undiagnosed before death. |
| 50% of patients suspected of PE do not have PE. |
| 50% of patients with DVT go on to develop PE. |
| 50% of patients with DVT have a recurrence. |
| 50% of patients with clinical signs of DVT do not have DVT. |

larger vein clots that result in more extensive pulmonary arterial obstruction and symptomatic PE. With the increasing use of central lines, and their moderately common complication of thrombosis of the subclavian veins, there are instances of PE arising from upper limb thrombosis. Iliac vein thrombosis tends to occur in patients undergoing pelvic procedures (postpartum, pelvic fractures, and gynecologic surgery), and thrombi can arise from the right ventricle in right-sided heart disease (myocardial infarction and cor pulmonale).

With venous stasis or endothelial damage there is red blood cell aggregation and clot formation. The clot then propagates by platelet and fibrin accumulation, and the newly formed proximal portion of the clot floats in the venous bloodstream while the distal end becomes organized to the vein wall. As the clot occludes the vein, there can be retrograde and proximal extension of newly formed thrombus. If the clot does not embolize it can recanalize, organize, or lyze. The size of individual thrombi can vary from up to 20 cm in the vena cava to microscopic lesions in the calf. Clots from smaller veins, disruption of large clots in the contracting heart, or fragmentation and lysis of proximal venous thrombi can cause small emboli. The "Rules of 50%" regarding DVT are proposed in Table 4-4.

Prospective studies in the last decade have shown that many patients who develop DVT go on to PE, as diagnosed by V/Q scan:

- 46% of patients with calf thrombi develop PE
- 67% of patients with calf thrombi develop PE if the thrombi extend to the thigh
- 77% of patients with calf thrombi develop PE if the pelvic veins are involved (19)

This study, among other studies, shows a high incidence of PE in DVT, a correlation between the size of the perfusion defects and clinical signs, and importantly, that most PEs are clinically silent (15,17).

### Relevance of Diagnosis and Treatment of PE

The need for treatment in PE was first proposed by Bauer in 1941 (20), when 46% of untreated DVT patients with proximal thromboses had symptomatic PE and 4% had fatal PE. Since the time of this paper, it has been considered unethical not to treat DVT. The efficacy of anticoagulation in the treatment of PE was established in 1960 by a randomized prospective double-blind trial in patients with massive PE

confirmed by right heart failure or x-ray and clinical findings of pulmonary infarction (21). Therapy was 10 days of heparin and 2 weeks with a warfarin-like anticoagulant. The study code was broken after 35 patients, and a significant increase in death and nonfatal recurrent PE occurred in the untreated group (26% each), whereas only one patient died in the treated group (6%), and this from the therapy itself rather than PE. Their conclusions were that anticoagulants

- Reduced mortality
- Treated the actual emboli in the lungs
- Resulted in less heart failure, less death, and less pulmonary infarction
- Obviated the need for the Trendelenburg procedure

Their primary claim was well founded, but their other claims have not stood the test of time.

The greatest risk of death from PE lies in the first hour after the event, and more than half the patients who die of PE do so without the diagnosis being made before death. Most fatal PE occurs in the clinical subset with hypotension with >75% of the pulmonary arterial tree is occluded. In massive PE (defined as >50% arterial occlusion) the death rate is said to be in the range of 25% to 30% (22). In major published series of treated PE in which the patients were classified by symptoms, the death rate was 27% for those with massive hypotensive PE but only 6% for nonhypotensive but symptomatic PE. This combined series included 274 patients and had an overall death rate of approximately 11% (23–25). This suggests that the death rate of patients identified from noninvasive investigations, such as the modern V/Q scan, is lower than those of the earlier studies, when patients were usually identified from their dramatic symptomatic presentation. In the PIOPED data, only 2.5% of treated patients with PE died from the disease, and these had recurrent PE (26).

Treatment of DVT with long-term anticoagulant therapy is not without risk. Few prospective anticoagulant trials are published related to PE, but one such indicates a 30% incidence of hemorrhage and a 3% death rate (27). In the review of anticoagulant use by Levine and Hirsh, four randomized controlled trials involved 159 patients with venous thromboembolism: The average incidence of bleeding was 22.6%, and the major bleeding rate was 8.2% (28).

Clinically apparent recurrent PE occurred in 8.3% of the PIOPED treated population (26), which is similar to another major prospective study (25,29). Recurrence was most likely during the first week of follow-up (26).

Follow-up of low-probability V/Q scans and pulmonary arteriograms without evidence of PE has shown that these patients rarely die from PE or suffer recurrent PE or DVT (30,31). This indicates that most patients with low-probability V/Q scans should not be further investigated if the clinical suspicion is not very high and should be treated with anticoagulants only with great circumspection, given the therapeutic risks. The follow-up of intermediate-probability V/Q scans has been undertaken and, although more studies are required, one abstract indicates that the subgroup of patients with intermediate-probability V/Q scan with large V/Q matches or diffuse lung disease did not have recurrent episodes of PE (32). It is expected that this subgroup will be defined by on-going studies to determine if these patients warrant treatment.

There is, however, another school of thought on this subject. This was presaged by the "emperor has no clothes" article (10), and has been continually fostered by the McMaster's group (13), who believe that V/Q scanning should only be used for ruling out PE when normal scans are found and for identifying PE with high-probability scans. They believe that all other classifications should be considered nondiagnostic. This is discussed further in the sections on Diagnostic Schemes and Alternative Imaging Modalities.

## LUNG SCAN

For the diagnosis of PE both perfusion and ventilation lung scans are required for sensitivity and specificity. Virtually no cases of recent PE in which the perfusion of the lung is normal have been documented; the perfusion scan is 100% sensitive. Most patients with high-probability lung scans for PE have eight or more segmental defects (25,33).

Because multiple possible causes for abnormal perfusion lung scans exist, ventilation scans are required for specificity. In airway or alveolar disease that results in poor alveolar gas exchange, there is a reduction in perfusion due to local reflex vasoconstriction. Although decreased perfusion is expected in alveolar hypoventilation, lowered perfusion in the presence of normal aeration of lung (V/Q mismatch) suggests a primary vascular etiology, the most common being PE.

Baseline V/Q studies in asymptomatic volunteers have demonstrated minor apical abnormalities and changes that "might be indistinguishable" from PE, but this has been thought to occur in no more than 5% of normal subjects. In patients about to undergo elective surgery or radioiodine therapy for thyroid disease, there was a 10% rate of segmental perfusion defects and a 3% rate of V/Q mismatched segmental defects (34).

### Perfusion Scan Protocol

Technetium 99m (Tc-99m) macroaggregated albumin (MAA) is the only commercially available agent although there are several suppliers. Tc-99m microspheres (human albumin microspheres) were previously available and are still New Drug Application (NDA) approved but have been withdrawn from the market by the manufacturer. The MAA is usually supplied in multidose vials for labeling, using the standard "shake-and-bake" stannous ion reduction of the Tc-99m pertechnetate to a suitable binding state for radiopharmaceutical preparation. Adherence to the package insert

**TABLE 4-5.** *Tc-99m MAA dosimetry*

| Organ | Rad/5-mCi dose (cGy/185 MBq) |
|---|---|
| Lung* | 1.02 |
| Whole body | 0.07 |
| Bladder: 2-hr void | 0.15 |
| Bladder: 4-hr void | 0.28 |

*Critical organ.

guarantees that the number of particles contained in the preparation will not be excessive. The particles have a biological half-life of approximately 3 hours and degrade to smaller particles that collect in the kidneys; some free $TcO_4$ is produced.

The lungs contain 200 to 300 billion alveolar capillaries (lumen ~8 μm), 200 million precapillary arterioles (lumen ~35 μm), and millions of terminal pulmonary arterioles (lumen ~100 μm). These represent part of the >20 divisions of the pulmonary arterial tree as it progresses from the main pulmonary artery to the capillary bed. The MAA used in perfusion scanning has a mean size of 40 μm with a range of 10 to 90 μm, so vessels up to the size of a terminal arteriole can be occluded. In patients with chronic pulmonary hypertension (perhaps 2% of all patients with PE), the arterioles are vasoconstricted and so the MAA particles can occlude even more proximal arteries. Several early cases were reported in which massive numbers of labeled particles injected for lung scanning purposes caused the death of the patient. These patients had severe pulmonary hypertension, and the excessive numbers of particles injected resulted in significant additional pulmonary obstruction in seriously compromised patients. Strict adherence to pharmacy protocols using standard package insert instructions ensure that a safe number of particles (100,000 to 700,000) are injected over the entire time the vial is available for use and that adequate statistical images can be obtained. This results in <0.1% occlusion of the peripheral pulmonary arterial tree, even in patients with pulmonary hypertension.

Five millicuries (185 MBq) of the radiopharmaceutical is routinely injected. The patient is injected supine to decrease the hydrostatic gradient between the upper and lower lung lobes that is present in the upright position. This does result in an anterior-posterior gradient that is unimportant.

The MAA is injected after the patient takes several deep breaths to aerate the maximum number of alveoli in the maximum number of pulmonary lobules. The particles should be injected slowly if pulmonary hypertension is present so that the administration can be halted if the patient's condition deteriorates. Withdrawal of blood back into the syringe of MAA can result in multiple hot spots throughout the lungs; this is "clumping" of particles to the blood in the syringe. It has not been a significant problem with the agents currently available. The dosimetry of Tc-99m MAA is provided in Table 4-5.

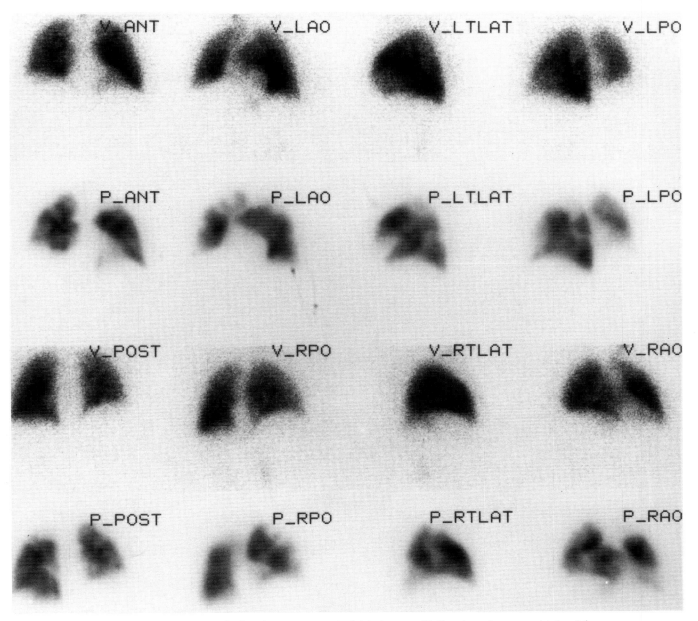

**FIG. 4-1.** An eight-view perfusion lung scan and eight-view ventilation lung images obtained from a dual-headed gamma camera scanner. The ventilation scan is within normal limits, but the perfusion scan shows multiple segmental and subsegmental defects, indicating high probability of PE.

Although some prefer that ventilation and perfusion images be obtained in the sitting position due to decreased diaphragmatic motion in this position, dual-headed imaging devices and ill patients result in the supine position being most commonly used. The ventilation scan should be performed in the same position as the perfusion study, especially when pleural effusions are present, to prevent differences that could result from the positional fluid changes from one study to the other.

We perform eight-view perfusion lung scans (Fig. 4-1), although many nuclear medicine services perform six-view studies. The minimum studies should include anterior, posterior, and both anterior oblique and posterior oblique views. We prefer to add both lateral views as these may help localize specific pulmonary segments. These perfusion lung scans are obtained as planar images, and the use of two-headed and three-headed imaging devices shortens the imaging time required. Most protocols require the anterior and posterior views be collected for 800K counts, the obliques for 700K counts, and the laterals for 600K counts. In doing the lateral views the most perfused lung should be imaged first for 600K counts, and the opposite lung

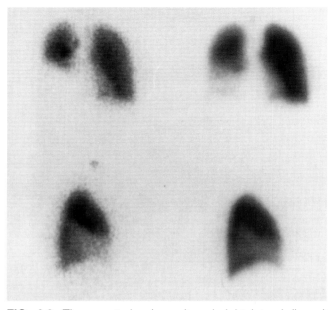

**FIG. 4-2.** These anterior (upper) and right lateral (lower) views demonstrate shine through. The anterior views show virtually no ventilation (left) and minimal perfusion (right) to the right lower and middle lobes. Nearly normal ventilation (left) and perfusion (right) seen in the right middle and lower lobes in the right lateral views (lower) is due to shine through from the opposite left lower lobe.

imaged for the same time period. This latter technique is helpful in instances in which one lung is significantly underperfused and decreases the potential for "shine through" from the opposite normal lung (Fig. 4-2). In all other views the two lungs do not overlap, so shine through is not a problem.

The essence of evaluating the perfusion lung scan is the determination of whether any defect has the distribution of a bronchopulmonary segment and therefore could be the result of pulmonary arterial obstruction. Anatomy texts describe the surface markings of the bronchopulmonary segments, but in a perfusion lung scan the lung surface markings are not visualized. The deeper alveolar capillary bed of the nearest and adjacent segments is visualized, so the individual pattern of segments visible on a perfusion lung scan may be quite different from the surface markings. Aids for correcting this bias to underestimation of segmental perfusion defects include atlases of phantom and patient studies and maps of the surface markings of individual segments (35,36). Unfortunately, these segmental surface markings vary widely in texts, and each individual scan reader or service must decide on its own preference. A gamma camera manufacturer provides a six-view format in the perfusion lung scan format (Fig. 4-3).

The method I prefer to identify individual segments is to compare the defect outlines with charts of bronchopul-

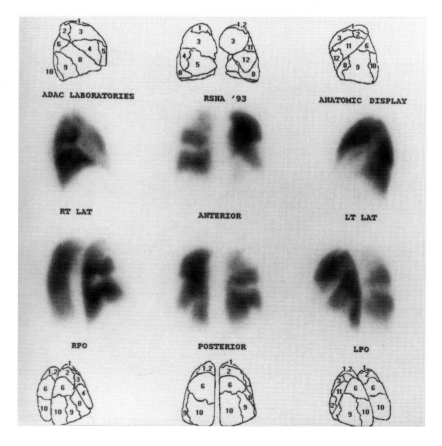

**FIG. 4-3.** An abnormal six-view perfusion lung scan with surface lung segment markings provided. In some views, the actual segmental lesion seen is smaller than the surface markings, for example, the lateral basal defects (#9) on the LPO and RPO views. In the posterior view, the same lesions are overestimated compared to the surface marking. The numbering system for segments is identical to Figs. 4-5 and 4-6. (1, apical; 2, posterior; 3, anterior; 4, lateral; 5, medial; 6, superior; 7, medial basal; 8, anterior basal; 9, lateral basal; 10, posterior basal; 11, lingual superior; 12, lingual inferior.) (Images courtesy of ADAC Laboratories, Milpitas, CA.)

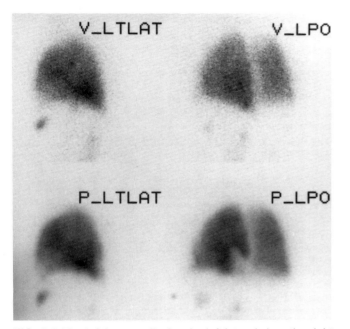

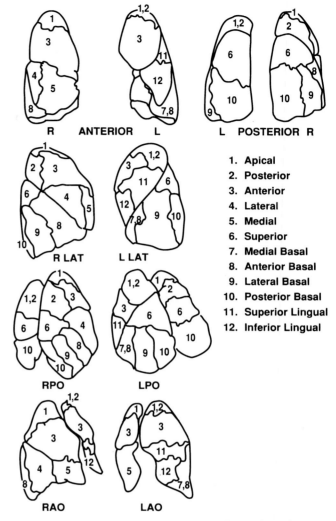

FIG. 4-4. The left images display the left lateral view, the right images the LPO view. The upper images are normal ventilation scans. The lower perfusion images show the posterobasal segment to be nonperfused. This segmental defect is obvious in the LPO view (en face view), and barely discernible in the left lateral view (tangential view). The activity below the lungs is swallowed gastric activity and renal activity from the Tc-99m DTPA aerosol study.

FIG. 4-5. Example of surface markings of bronchopulmonary segments. (Reprinted with permission from McCartney WH. Ventilation-perfusion lung scanning in pulmonary embolus. Clin Nucl Med 1981;6[Suppl]:27–36.)

monary segments. The outlines most useful are tangential views that profile the defect at its surface marking extent and perpendicular views that view the defect "en face" along the axis of the bronchopulmonary segment (Fig. 4-4). In all scan views the defect is heavily influenced by neighboring segments, which makes the individual segments appear much smaller than their surface markings would suggest. In one study, only 44% of full segmental defects deliberately produced in human subjects were recognized as being 75% or more of a segment (large subsegmental); all the others were read as small or moderate-sized subsegmental defects (37). The defects should be viewed in relationship to the surface mapping of bronchopulmonary segments, as given in many articles and texts (Figs. 4-5 and 4-6), and available atlases (35,36) because the use of lung segment reference charts results in significant improvement in observer agreement (38).

It is important when trying to diagnose PE to be familiar with the anatomy and normal lung scan appearance of perfusion scans in which the most emboli are found. In general, the posterior oblique views localize most lower lobe lesions well. Lesions in the midlung zones (superior segment of lower lobes, lingulae, and right middle lobe) are well identified in the lateral, posterior oblique, and anterior oblique views (39,40). Perhaps two-thirds of all acute embolic perfusion defects involve the lower lobes,

with the remainder divided equally between the upper lobes and the middle lobe or lingulae (39). The posterior oblique and anterior oblique perfusion views are said to improve lesion localization in 73% of patients (41). In general, lateral views contribute the least, but they can be particularly effective for separating the anterobasal segments from the right middle lobe and lingulae.

The perfusion lung scan can detect defects due to occlusion of vessels that are 1 mm in diameter, provided the vessel is completely occluded. Only one-fourth of partially occluded vessels are detected with lung perfusion studies (42). The sensitivity of the perfusion lung scan results from the multiple defects typical of PE, so that even if partially occluded vessels are missed there are enough other completely occluded vessels to allow the diagnosis.

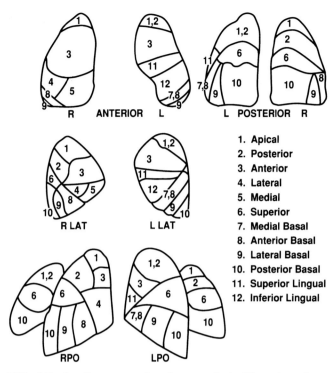

1. Apical
2. Posterior
3. Anterior
4. Lateral
5. Medial
6. Superior
7. Medial Basal
8. Anterior Basal
9. Lateral Basal
10. Posterior Basal
11. Superior Lingual
12. Inferior Lingual

**FIG. 4-6.** Another example of somewhat different surface markings of bronchopulmonary segments. (Reprinted with permission from Morrell NW, Nijran KS, Jones BE, Seed WA. The underestimation of segmental defect size in radionuclide lung scanning. J Nucl Med 1993;34:370–374.)

### Ventilation Scan

Ventilation studies are required to improve the specificity of the diagnosis of PE. Two common radiopharmaceuticals are currently used for these studies (Tc-99m diethylenetriamine pentaacetic acid [DTPA] aerosol and xenon 133 [Xe-133]), and there are four additional tracers that are not readily available (Xe-127, krypton 81m [Kr-81m], Technegas, and Pertechnegas). All have proved satisfactory for imaging, with each having limitations (Tables 4-6 through 4-8).

**TABLE 4-7.** *Physical properties of ventilation radionuclides*

| Ventilation tracer | Physical half-life | Gamma ray keV (abundance) |
|---|---|---|
| Kr-81 | 13.0 secs | 191 (35%) |
| Tc-99m | 6.0 hrs | 140 (89%) |
| Xe-133 | 5.3 days | 81 (36%) |
| Xe-127 | 36.4 days | 172 (25%) |
| | — | 203 (68%) |
| | — | 375 (18%) |

**TABLE 4-8.** *Dosimetry for Xe-133 and Tc-99m DTPA aerosol ventilation studies*

| | Xe-133 (rads/20 mCi [cGy/740 MBq]) | Tc-99m DTPA (rads/20 mCi [cGy/740 MBq])[a] |
|---|---|---|
| Lung | 0.07[b] | 0.10 |
| Red marrow | 0.01 | 0.08 |
| Whole body | 0.01 | 0.01 |
| Kidney | — | 0.03 |
| Bladder | — | 0.18[b] |

[a] Although 20 mCi in nebulizer, ~1 mCi enters bronchopulmonary tree.
[b] Critical organ.

### Xenon 133

Initial investigators used Xe-133, and this has remained the standard because most clinical research studies have used this agent. The inert gas Xe-133 study is performed after first familiarizing the patient with the technique and performing a dry run to demonstrate the sequence and reassure the patient of its simplicity. This is important in COPD patients, who may panic when a face mask is placed over their mouth and nose. The test requires a large inhalation with a 20-second breath-hold that fills the patient's lungs with the inert gas tracer and provides the single-breath "wash-in" image. This good breath-hold image (single-breath wash-in view) is difficult to obtain, especially in patients with COPD. The test is performed in the posterior view because this surveys the largest volume of lung.

**TABLE 4-6.** *Comparison of radiopharmaceuticals (RPs) for ventilation studies*

| | Views possible | Technical difficulty | Pre- or postperfusion | Current availability | RP cost | Equipment cost | Image type | Portable study |
|---|---|---|---|---|---|---|---|---|
| Tc-99m aerosol | All | ++ | Pre (post possible) | Readily available | + | + | Wash-in | Yes |
| Xe-133 | 1–3 | +++ | Pre | Readily available | ++ | ++ | Wash-in/ wash-out | No |
| Xe-127 | 1–3 | +++ | Post | Unreliable supply | +++ | +++ | Wash-in/ wash-out | No |
| Kr-81 | All | + | Post or simultaneous | Daily generator | ++++ | + | Wash-in only | Yes |
| Technegas | All | + | Pre | Not FDA approved | + | ++++ | Wash-in only | Yes |
| Pertechnegas | All | + | Pre | Not FDA approved | + | ++++ | Wash-in only | Yes |

**TABLE 4-9.** *Xenon ventilation scan*

| Phase | Time |
| --- | --- |
| Wash-in (breath-hold) posterior | Single large breath (one posterior 20-sec image) |
| Equilibrium (rebreathing) | 2–3 minutes (four 30-sec posterior images, optional 30-sec LPO and RPO images) |
| Wash-out (clearance) | 2–3 minutes (four 30-sec posterior images, optional 30-sec LPO and RPO image) |

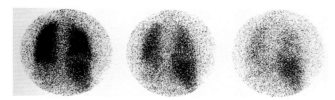

**FIG. 4-8.** This Xe-133 study demonstrates hepatic uptake of tracer, confirming fatty involvement of the liver. The left image is the last equilibrium image while the middle and right images are early wash-out images.

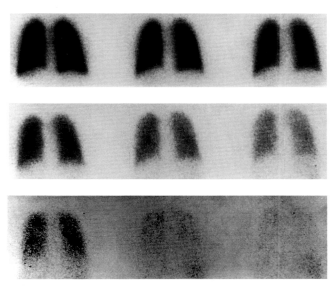

**FIG. 4-7.** Normal Xe-133 ventilation study obtained in the posterior view with initial breath-hold (upper left), followed by four 30-second equilibrium images and four 30-second wash-out images. These images are sequenced from top left to bottom right. The intensity is normalized to the breath-hold image. Note the rapid washout of tracer. (Images courtesy of Dr. Robert Hellman, University of Wisconsin-Milwaukee.)

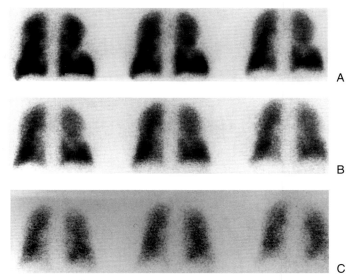

A

B

C

**FIG. 4-9. (A,B)** The initial breath-hold image is not as homogeneous as Fig. 4-7 in this patient's Xe-133 study, with poor air entry into the middle lung zones. **(C)** By the end of the wash-out phase (right) there is considerable tracer still present (abnormal finding), and the pattern is now that of midlung zone retention due to COPD. The intensity of the normalized images shows the degree of retention typical of COPD. (Images courtesy of Dr. Robert Hellman, University of Wisconsin-Milwaukee.)

If the test is stopped at this stage, it is called the single-breath test, but the "wash-out" technique is generally performed. To accomplish this, the single wash-in breath is then exhaled into a closed, shielded container that has been enriched with oxygen, and the tracer oxygen mixture is rebreathed during tidal respiration for 2 to 3 minutes to provide an "equilibrium" image (Table 4-9). For two of these 30-second images the posterior oblique views may be obtained. The patient then continues to breathe from the closed container, and a one-way valve is switched so that with each breath, fresh air is inhaled and the radioactive gas is exhaled into the collection system. During this phase the radiotracer is washed out of the lungs, and areas of abnormal retention are identified. This process continues until the lungs are cleared of Xe-133. The procedure takes approximately 5 minutes to complete (Fig. 4-7). Xe-133 is lipophilic, so fatty liver is readily identified (Fig. 4-8).

This technique is very sensitive for the diagnosis of COPD, which is best identified by regions of increased xenon trapping (retention) and decreased wash-out. These correspond to areas of absent or decreased wash-in seen on the early images, which gradually equilibrate with tracer during the rebreathing or equilibrium phase. The difficulty of air getting into and out of a region of obstructed airway is typical of COPD (Fig. 4-9).

The abnormal retention of tracer in the wash-out images is more sensitive for identifying COPD than the single-breath technique, and the wash-out technique is also more specific for the diagnosis of PE (43). The test can only be done in one view because of the time constraints and the cost of repeated Xe-133 doses. The posterior view is usually selected because it shows the lower lobes, the largest lung volume, and the most common site of emboli. The technique can be expanded by taking left and right posterior oblique views after the first posterior wash-out view, so increasing the number of potential bronchopulmonary segments viewed.

Because of the 80-keV energy of the Xe-133 photon, the ventilation scan is usually performed prior to the perfusion lung scan (Tc-99m MAA, 140 keV). It is possible to do a perfusion lung scan first with a reduced dose (1 mCi [37 MBq] Tc-99m MAA), so that if it is normal, the Xe-133 ventilation study can be omitted. This would typically result in 20% of ventilation scans not being needed. If the perfusion scan is abnormal, the view to best identify regions of potential V/Q mismatch can be profiled using the perfusion scan and the ventilation scan performed in this view. If the patient demonstrates a segmental perfusion defect in the lingulae or middle lobe, a posterior ventilation scan with Xe-133 will not identify mismatch, whereas an anterior or anterior oblique ventilation study might.

### Xenon 127

Another approach has been to use Xe-127, which has 173-, 203-, and 375-keV photons that can be imaged separately from the 140-keV photon of Tc-99m. The ventilation scan can be done in the most suitable view after the perfusion scan, without interference from the Tc-99m photon. This required a medium-energy collimator and better-shielded gas reservoirs than those used in Xe-133 imaging. The supply of this more expensive inert radioactive gas was not reliable, and it is no longer commercially available. The longer half-life of Xe-127 partially overcame its greater cost because less tracer was lost to radioactive decay.

Many hospital radiation safety departments actively discourage the use of radioactive inert gases because they can easily escape from the face mask into the room and so enter the general hospital air circulation. They prefer that nuclear medicine sections use Tc-99m aerosols.

### Krypton 81m

Kr-81m is an alternative inert gas. It is generator-supplied with a parent rubidium 81 half-life of 4.6 hours. The ventilation radiopharmaceutical has a 13-second half-life, and essentially, only wash-in images can be obtained, very similar to single-breath Xe-133 studies. With this radiopharmaceutical, a full eight-view lung scan can be obtained, with 100K to 200K count images that take 1 to 2 minutes per required view. The generator is eluted using oxygen, which is then connected to a face mask. The patient breathes normally via the face mask for image acquisition. The energy of Kr-81 is 191 keV, and so pre-administered Tc-99m MAA and Kr-81 images can be obtained sequentially or simultaneously, if dual window displays are a gamma camera option. Without moving the patient, subtraction techniques can be used to provide parametric images of regional V/Q. The limitation is the parent half-life of 4.6 hours, which requires daily delivery

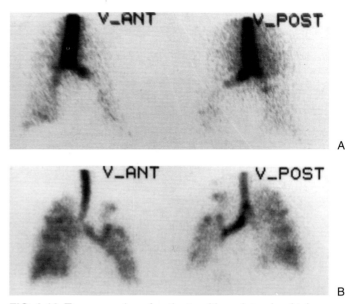

**FIG. 4-10.** Two examples of patients with endotracheal tubes. **(A)** The patient in the upper anterior and posterior ventilation images shows intense aerosol tracer localization in the endotracheal tube with little alveolar activity. **(B)** The patient in the lower images shows tracer predominantly in the left main stem bronchus but, overall, significantly more in the peripheral lung.

of the generator and inadequate availability for emergency after-hours and weekend studies.

### Tc-99m Aerosols

The most commonly used ventilation radiopharmaceutical today is aerosolized Tc-99m DTPA. The tracer is delivered via a commercially supplied nebulizer that received U.S. Food and Drug Administration (FDA) approval in 1983. It is technically difficult to create a uniform aerosol droplet size, and only a small percentage of the tracer reaches the lungs, the majority remaining in the nebulizer, the baffles, and the tubing. A droplet size of 1 to 3 $\mu$m is most likely to be delivered to the alveoli, being deposited by sedimentation. Larger droplets are likely to be deposited by impaction in the oropharynx and at sites of increased turbulence near major airway branching. Uptake in the endotracheal tubes is also increased (Fig. 4-10), but this tracer can be used in ventilated patients.

Despite the technical limitations in some patients, this is a much easier tracer to use in ventilation studies because the patient does not have to learn the breath-hold technique. The patient merely breathes normally with a mask placed over the mouth and nose. If the patient panics, the ventilation procedure can be temporarily halted, then continued when the patient is reassured. Swallowing of the tracer occurs, so the esophagus and stomach are often visualized. The tracer is excreted renally, and the kidneys (critical organ) are usually visualized.

In this technique, eight-view 100K count ventilation image scans are obtained routinely in the supine position for direct comparison with perfusion lung scans. Some prefer the ventilation scan to be acquired in the sitting position for better visualization, but with aerosol agents this results in preferential basal dispersal. The ventilation study is completed first because it is difficult to get large amounts of aerosol into the lungs. Consequently, the perfusion lung scan contains a contribution from the prior ventilation study because Tc-99m is used for both radiopharmaceuticals. We administer the Tc-99m DTPA via the nebulizer to the patient while the patient sits or lies supine in front of a gamma camera, and when the count rate reaches 2,000 cps and appears predominantly in the lungs, we discontinue the administration and start image acquisition. This results in 100K count images that take approximately 60 seconds to acquire.

Although this aerosol agent seems favored over inert gases by radiation safety officers, there appears to be a significant opportunity for local contamination, as reported by some (44). We have not confirmed this with occasional testing for local dispersal of the Tc-99m DTPA aerosol. We have found that if the manufacturer sells a nebulizer said to provide finer droplets, less airway impaction results—for example, the UltraVent kit of Mallinckrodt Nuclear (St. Louis, MO) has resulted in significantly less central impaction in our hands.

The literature on diagnosis of PE using Tc-99m DTPA aerosol studies is not as abundant as that available using Xe-133. The McNeil, Biello, PIOPED, and early McMaster's studies all used Xe-133. Much of the aerosol validation work has come from Alderson's laboratory and shows concordance of Tc-99m DTPA aerosol and Kr-81m studies, as expected, both being primarily wash-in image agents. In the diagnosis of PE, the Tc-99m DTPA aerosol and Xe-133 were quite similar (45,46). Patients with low-probability scans with Tc-99m DTPA who were followed clinically for 1 year showed no PE (47). The second half of the McMaster's prospective trial used Tc-99m DTPA (48), thus establishing the role of Tc-99m DTPA aerosol studies in PE. Indeed, some studies have shown that Tc-99m aerosols were more helpful in diagnosing PE in as many as one-third of the patients (49,50) by reducing the intermediate-probability subset. A large prospective 1,000-patient study using Tc-99m aerosol ventilation scans confirms the utility of this ventilation agent using the modified PIOPED criteria (51). This study also suggests that fewer patients will be classified with intermediate-probability scans.

Care must be taken to calculate the portion of counts seen on the perfusion scan that are attributable to the ventilation study and whether this may obscure a potential V/Q mismatch by simulating a V/Q match (Fig. 4-11). On average, approximately 15% of total "perfusion scan" counts derive from the ventilation scan, but sometimes when inadequate amounts of Tc-99m MAA are administered (e.g., in partial extravasation of Tc-99m MAA dose),

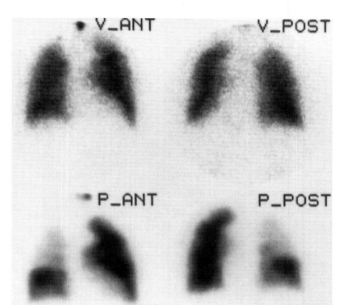

**FIG. 4-11.** The anterior and posterior ventilation views (upper) show normal ventilation. The perfusion views (lower) show reduced tracer in the right middle and upper lung zones compared to the opposite side. A subtraction technique showed this activity in the right upper zones of the perfusion study was due to the prior aerosol study. No perfusion was present.

the aerosol contribution can reach 50% of total Tc-99m counts and identification of mismatches is difficult. We now display on the hard-copy image the maximal pixel count for both ventilation and perfusion scans so that unusual scans can be identified. Subtraction techniques are not very practical with aerosol studies because of potential patient movement between ventilation and perfusion scan images, movement of the centrally impacted aerosol along the major airways by mucociliary clearance, and the physiologic absorption of Tc-99m DTPA across the alveolar membrane.

Some users have performed the perfusion scan first using lower-than-conventional doses of MAA (1 mCi [27 MBq] vs. 5 mCi [185 MBq]), then using dynamic aerosol imaging computer acquisition in the view with the most significant perfusion defect (50). Tc-99m MAA is reduced in the region of the defect, and computer subtraction can be performed to identify mismatch (Fig. 4-12). By this technique, patients with a normal perfusion scan do not require ventilation studies (49).

Other agents have been used for aerosol (see section on Radioaerosol Imaging) studies, such as pyrophosphate, a molecule that produces a finer mist that results in 7% to 15% of the nebulized pharmaceutical reaching the alveoli (50). When mucociliary clearance is to be measured, more central impaction is desired, and a 2- to 5-μm droplet size is preferred for subsequent clearance by ciliary action. Tc-99m sulfur colloid (SC) and Tc-99m human serum albumin (HSA) have been used to perform these types of ventilation studies to investigate ciliary clearance.

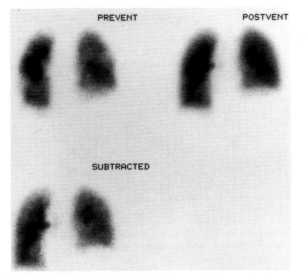

FIG. 4-12. The upper left image is a posterior perfusion scan view obtained prior to the ventilation study. A lateral basal segment defect is profiled on the left. The upper right image is the combined aerosol and perfusion scan images. The lower left image shows a normal ventilation image once the perfusion scan image was subtracted. This patient has a left lateral basal segmental mismatch. (Images courtesy of Dr. Robert Hellman, University of Wisconsin-Milwaukee.)

### New Ventilation Agents

Recent agents, not approved in the United States, include Technegas and Pertechnegas. These agents have been used in Australia. Pertechnegas is available in Canada and is undergoing trials presently in the United States. Here Tc-99m $TcO_4^-$ is vaporized in graphite crucibles heated to 2,500°F in either pure argon (Technegas) or a 20:1 argon-oxygen mixture (Pertechnegas). These minute particles display the alveoli with only one to five breaths compared to Tc-99m DTPA aerosol imaging that requires 3 to 5 minutes of tidal respiration for sufficient alveolar tracer deposition. Although Technegas remains in the lungs, Pertechnegas is absorbed across the alveolar membrane, more quickly than occurs with Tc-99m DTPA aerosol, and so requires top-up breaths of agent every four views. This has the advantage that when the perfusion scans are performed, little background lung ventilation agent is present. FDA approval is eagerly awaited for Pertechnegas and the furnace device. This may represent the most significant nuclear medicine addition to the non-invasive diagnosis of PE.

### Scan Criteria for PE

There are two broad categories of referrals: (1) those in whom PE is to be excluded and (2) those in whom PE is the likely diagnosis.

The three groups of V/Q scans are as follows:

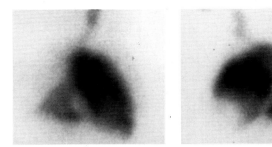

FIG. 4-13. These lateral images show the scan appearance of pleural effusion in two patients. (A) This image shows decreased volume of right lower lobe and increased attenuation due to the moderate amounts of surrounding fluid. (B) This image shows a prominent fissure sign in the left lung, with minimal attenuation due to fluid about the lower lobe

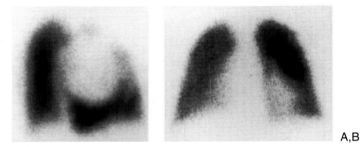

FIG. 4-14. (A) This is an RPO view of a large necrotic tumor with associated nonsegmental perfusion defect. (B) This is a posterior view of a right lower defect with a rim of activity about it (the rim sign). Both patterns indicate a low probability of PE.

- Easy low-probability (normal or very low-probability scan)
- Easy high-probability (multiple V/Q mismatches)
- All other scan combinations

The general hospital distribution of scans is very variable, but in large series this averages

- 55% low-probability or normal scans
- 35% intermediate-probability scans
- 10% high-probability scans

### General Scan Reading

When evaluating scans it is important to identify all V/Q mismatches and to recognize patterns that suggest disease processes other than PE (Figs. 4-13 through 4-15). These scan features include the fissure sign, pleural effusions, pulmonary edema, nonsegmental defects, COPD, the stripe sign, cardiomegaly, and external attenuators.

When reading V/Q scans, I read the perfusion scan first to identify the site, size, and number of perfusion defects. Next, I examine the ventilation scan to see if these nominated perfusion defects are ventilated (i.e., is mismatch

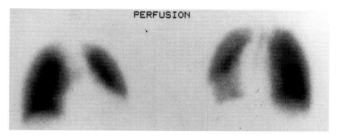

FIG. 4-15. This anterior (left) perfusion image shows cardiomegaly, and the posterior (right) perfusion image shows the associated left-sided pleural effusion.

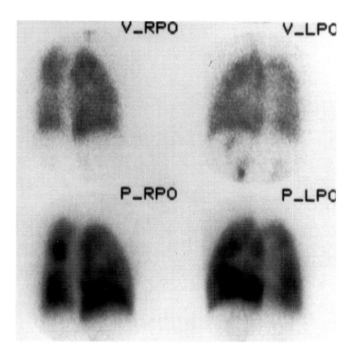

FIG. 4-16. The ventilation scan (upper) shows an abnormal pattern, which the perfusion study (lower) matches exactly. These posterior oblique images are typical of COPD.

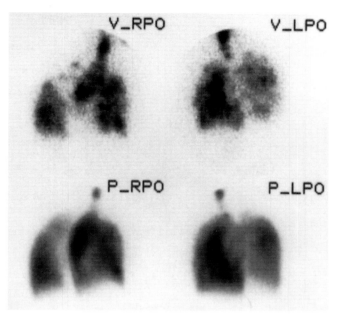

FIG. 4-17. The ventilation (upper) scan shows COPD and the perfusion (lower) scan shows more normal perfusion than ventilation. The right lower lobe posteriorly shows fair perfusion and very reduced ventilation, that is, reverse mismatch, typical of atelectasis. Note the Tc-99m aerosol impaction in the neck region due to the patient's tracheostomy.

present?). The completeness of the perfusion defect (i.e., absent perfusion) is important. When perfusion is merely reduced, the diagnosis of PE is less certain. This scan pattern occurs in 20% to 45% of embolized regions and is explained by partial occlusion of the pulmonary arterial tree by clot (42,52). Partial occlusion is one of the specific pulmonary arteriogram diagnostic features (contrast surrounding an intra-arterial clot), and this difference in features can explain discrepancies in V/Q scanning and arteriography in particular patients.

The degree of V/Q mismatch is important: Those with absent perfusion and normal ventilation are more likely to have PE than those with reduced perfusion and normal ventilation. In a neural network study of the scan features most important in the correct diagnosis of PE, the features of sharpness of outline and completeness of perfusion deficit best established the diagnosis of PE (53). This study demonstrated that of the 20 scan variables input into the network, the best result was obtained by further defining the perfusion component of the two largest mismatches as to sharpness and completeness of the perfusion deficits. Any additional features worsened the network result. Further, the sharpness and completeness of the single largest mismatch was the next best combination. This emphasizes the importance of the completeness of the perfusion deficit to the diagnosis of PE.

Many patients that present to have PE ruled out have matched V/Q abnormalities: In some the matching is exact (Fig. 4-16), and in others the perfusion scan appears much more normal than the ventilation study (Fig. 4-17). These two patterns are typical of COPD and are not due to PE.

### Various Diagnostic Schemes

Over the 30 years since the first abnormal scans associated with PE were described (5,6), there have been significant improvements in the scan criteria for PE. In 1979, Biello published refinements (11) that included both the size of subsegmental defects and the association of CXR abnormalities with perfusion defects (the "indeterminate" scan). In 1987, review articles provided the first detailed schemata of V/Q interpretations, including the numbers of patients studied and the reference sources of their criteria (3,54). The next significant contribution was the PIOPED study (14), their revised criteria (33), and subsequent detailed analyses (16,55). These and other articles (12,56–62) are combined into the author's per-

**TABLE 4-10.** *Probability of PE versus scan patterns*

| Scan category | Scan pattern | Probability of PE (%) |
|---|---|---|
| Very low probability (0–10%) | Normal | 0 |
| | Small SS mismatches | 0 |
| | Q = CXR (due to large effusion) | 5 |
| | Nonsegmental defects | 7 |
| | Stripe sign | 7 |
| | Q << CXR opacities | 8 |
| | Multiple matched V/Q abnormalities (CXR normal) | 9 |
| Low intermediate probability (11–39%) | Single V/Q match (CXR clear)[a] | 14 |
| | Severe COPD, no V/Q mismatch | 19 |
| | Q = CXR | 26 |
| | Small effusion only (CPA blunting) | 27 |
| High intermediate probability (40–84%) | Combined matches and mismatches[b] | 42 |
| | Single moderate SS mismatch | 50 |
| | 1–2 S V/Q mismatches | 72 |
| High probability (85–100%) | Changing V/Q mismatch pattern | 87 |
| | Q >> CXR with mismatch | 89 |
| | > Mismatches in COPD | 95 |
| | ≥2.5 S V/Q mismatches | >95 |

[a] This criteria is controversial; see Single Mismatched Defects (33,61,62,73).
[b] See combined V/Q Matches and Mismatches (12,27,61).
S, segmental; SS, subsegmental; small SS, <25% of segment; match, V and Q abnormal; mismatch, V normal and Q abnormal; Q << (or =, or >>); CXR, size of perfusion defect relative–CXR lesion; CPA, costophrenic angle.
Source: Compiled from references 3, 11, 12, 25, 33, 48, 56–62, and 73.

sonal table of PE probability estimates (Table 4-10). The conversion of the low-probability group to a very low-probability category reflects ongoing PIOPED work, and the division of the scan categories into a low and high intermediate-probability scan reflects a growing feeling that the low-intermediate patients may not warrant aggressive investigation (or therapy [32]), whereas high-intermediate scans do.

This scheme starts with the Biello criteria and adds to it where other papers present additional patients and criteria. Most probability estimates for PE in excess of 40% require the presence of V/Q mismatch. The choice to go with this table using the original Biello criteria as the basis came from these criteria having withstood the test of many challenges. The Biello criteria (11) have been compared to McNeil's, a University of Michigan criteria set based on McNeil's, and to the initial PIOPED criteria (63–65), and in each case the Biello criteria seemed the best diagnostic compromise. Early challenges to the use of any diagnostic criteria other than normal was voiced by Robin (10). Studies that cast doubt on the diagnostic utility of schemata such as Biello's have all been based on small subsets of an institution's total lung scan population who had pulmonary arteriograms because the pretest clinical suspicion of PE did not correspond with the scan result (66,67). This confirms the clinician's role in diagnosis of PE. The doggedness of the pretest clinical suspicion is seen in referring physicians sometimes requiring three low-probability or nearly normal scan interpretations before they abandon their preliminary diagnosis of PE.

Another simpler scheme that classifies the patients with mismatched V/Q defects according to the number of moderate or larger subsegmental V/Q mismatches is excellent for risk

**TABLE 4-11.** *Sensitivity, specificity, and PPV of number of moderate or greater mismatched subsegmental defects*

| Number | Sensitivity | Specificity | PPV (95% CI) |
|---|---|---|---|
| 0 | 100% | 0% | 36% (34–38%) |
| ≥1 | 67% | 86% | 73% (69–77%) |
| ≥2 | 52% | 94% | 82% (78–86%) |
| ≥3 | 44% | 95% | 85% (79–91%) |
| ≥4 | 39% | 97% | 87% (81–93%) |
| ≥5 | 34% | 98% | 90% (84–96%) |
| ≥6 | 30% | 99% | 94% (90–98%) |
| ≥7 | 27% | 99% | 94% (90–98%) |
| ≥8 | 24% | 99% | 93% (87–99%) |

Source: Stein PD, Henry JW, Gottschalk A. Mismatched vascular defects: an easy alternative to mismatched segmental equivalent defects for the interpretation of ventilation/perfusion lung scans in pulmonary embolism. Chest 1993;104:1468–1471.

stratifying patients for PE, and it provides sensitivity, specificity, and positive predictive values (PPV) (Table 4-11) with confidence intervals (68). In Table 4-10, only eight of 18 scan patterns include mismatch as part of the criteria, whereas Table 4-11 requires each scan to have V/Q mismatch. Modifications of these data according to presence of cardiopulmonary disease and prior clinical probability of PE are discussed in detail later. This simpler scheme of counting of V/Q mismatches, derived from the PIOPED study data and described by senior PIOPED authors, provides a means of assessing the PPV for PE, together with confidence intervals for that value.

A study of nuclear medicine physicians' use of diagnostic algorithms for V/Q scan interpretations demonstrated a spectrum of physician interpretive patterns despite a perceived adherence to a uniform institutional diagnostic criteria, and deviations from standard patterns may be associated with diminished diagnostic accuracy (69). The systematic use of a reference chart of bronchopulmonary segments also improves the inter- and intra-observer agreement of V/Q scans (38). When experienced nuclear medicine physicians provided a gestalt or experiential percent probability estimate, it correlated extremely well with the angiography frequency of PE (33) with an almost exact correspondence. When we dictate V/Q reports we include the probability estimate as a percentage. The effect of the scintigraphic diagnosis of PE is evident in a paper that predicted that patient selection bias may exist in studies that correlate the V/Q scan with pulmonary angiography (70). One article in the medical literature highlights the PIOPED study as a worthy study that beneficially affects patient care (71).

## Special Diagnostic Subsets

### Single Defects

Single defects have presented a dilemma. Because the pathophysiology of PE is that of recurrent venous emboli, it seems strange that single defects should provide such a dilemma, especially given that only 7% to 8% of PE presents as single defects (25,29).

### Single Mismatched Defects

Single mismatched V/Q defects have created a perplexing diagnostic dilemma from the introduction of the first diagnostic schemata. Although all agree that multiple V/Q mismatches represent PE, the single V/Q mismatch has been variously placed in the low-, intermediate-, indeterminate-, and high-probability categories (3,11,12,14,27). One review found the overall probability of PE in a single moderate or large subsegmental defect averaged 50%, irrespective of the ventilation scan or CXR findings, although the addition of the ventilation scan and CXR findings resulted in probabilities that ranged from 15% for a matched defect to 90% for mismatched defect with CXR lesion present (62).

### Single Matched Defects

The PIOPED group has reported in their "revised criteria" a higher risk of PE in patients with single matched V/Q defects when compared to multiple matches (33). This finding of increased risk for PE in patients with solitary matched V/Q scan abnormalities is unexplained but may reflect the overall prevalence of PE in the PIOPED study (31%). Another explanation is that the usual diseases that cause multiple V/Q mismatches are COPD and other similar diseases that are generalized processes, making this pattern likely. A subsequent study comparing the revised PIOPED criteria with the original criteria in yet another patient population

**TABLE 4-12.** *Incidence of PE*

| Lung zone | Degree of perfusion defect in triple-matched lesions | | |
|---|---|---|---|
| | Decreased | Absent | Overall |
| Upper and middle | 0% | 25% | 12% |
| Lower | 18% | 61% | 33% |

Sources: Worsley DF, Kim CK, Alavi A, Palevsky HI. Detailed analysis of patients with matched ventilation-perfusion defects and chest radiographic opacities. J Nucl Med 1993;34:1851–1853; and Kim CK, Worsley DF, Alavi A. "Ventilation (V)/perfusion (Q)/chest X-ray" match is less likely to represent pulmonary embolism if Q is only "decreased" rather than "absent" [abstract]. J Nucl Med 1993;34:17.

(72) showed a zero incidence of PE in single matched defect, resulting in a combined probability in PE of 15% in these two series using similar scan interpretation and some common scan readers. This is confirmed in other reviews (62) and in yet a further revision of the PIOPED data (73), so the overall probability of PE with this pattern may be 14%, and it is possible that further studies might lower this pattern into the very low-probability group (<10%).

### Triple Matched Defects

Numerous reports have identified V/Q matches with a clear CXR as low probability of PE, and generally the etiology of these abnormalities is COPD. Published reports indicate that only 4% to 14% of these patients have PE established by pulmonary arteriogram (3,33).

There is a subset of such patients with pulmonary infarction in which radiographic abnormalities are present, the so-called indeterminate scan coined by Biello along with Fischer and McNeil and Alderson (11,74,75). When a radiographic lesion was present of comparable size to the perfusion defect (ventilation scan irrelevant), between one-fourth and one-third of the patients had PE possibly complicated by pulmonary infarction (11,74).

One PIOPED paper, presenting 247 patients with matched ventilation, perfusion, and CXR abnormalities (a "triple match") in at least one lung zone (76), indicated that the overall prevalence of PE was 26%, similar to the reports above. The size of the matching abnormalities did not correlate with PE, but those involving the lower lung zone had a threefold increase in likelihood of PE compared to those in the mid or upper zones (33% vs. 12%). Those with absent rather than reduced perfusion had an even higher likelihood of PE (77) (Table 4-12).

### Combined V/Q Matches and Mismatches

V/Q scan patterns are often seen that do not fit any accepted diagnostic criteria. In the PIOPED study, many combined scan patterns were not reported in the initial analyses. In cases of combinations of matched and mis-

**TABLE 4-13.** *V/Q defects versus probability of PE*

| Type of V/Q defects | Patient numbers | Incidence of PE |
|---|---|---|
| Mismatched | 99 | 88% |
| Mixtures | 33 | 42% |
| Matched | 49 | 4% |

Sources: Spies WG, Burstein SP, Dillehay GL, et al. Ventilation-perfusion scintigraphy in suspected pulmonary embolism: correlation with pulmonary angiogram and refinement of criteria for interpretation. Radiology 1986; 159:383–390; Cheeley R, McCartney WH, Perry JR, et al. The role of noninvasive tests versus pulmonary angiography in the diagnosis of pulmonary embolism. Am J Med 1981; 70:17–22; and McNeil BJ. Ventilation-perfusion studies and the diagnosis of pulmonary embolism: concise communication. J Nucl Med 1980;21:319–323.

matched V/Q defects, the mismatch (the higher-probability pattern) was assigned precedence. In the low-probability studies, there were many exclusions, for example, 137 patients with V/Q matches or triple matches were not included in the initial PIOPED analyses. These, and other scan patterns, represent a very significant proportion of that total patient population. In other studies the abnormal pattern with the highest probability of PE was used (54).

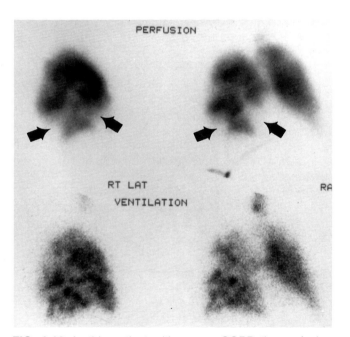

**FIG. 4-18.** In this patient with severe COPD the perfusion (upper) and ventilation (lower) scans show matched and mismatched defects in the right lateral (left) and RAO (right) views. The lateral basal segment of the right lower lobe and the medial segment of the right middle lobe (*arrows*) show mismatched defects. This indicates a high probability of PE despite the coexistent significant COPD (poor ventilation scan and matched defects in middle and upper lung zones).

Early investigators have indicated that the combination of matched and mismatched defects represent a nondiagnostic category for PE. When these publications (12,27,61) are combined, the final probability of PE in patients with a mixture of matched and mismatched defects is half that of patients with only mismatch (Table 4-13). Respected clinician investigators have indicated, over the years, that when both matched and mismatched V/Q defects are present, more mismatches are required for the same probability estimate of PE than if only mismatches are present.

### Severe COPD

In several studies (55,58,75,78), the question of being able to identify PE in the presence of significant COPD is discussed in detail. If perfusion defects are matched with ventilation abnormalities, and if the CXR is clear, then these patients can be placed in the low-probability PE group (see Figs. 4-16 and 4-17). If there are two or more subsegmental or segmental mismatches in a patient with severe COPD (Fig. 4-18) and a normal CXR (58), the probability of PE has been reported as high (95%). This apparent retraction of the discussion on combinations of matches and mismatches above is a consequence of this population with severe COPD, in which there is little well-perfused lung in which V/Q mismatch can be identified. In these patients, only a portion (23%) of emboli are identified as mismatched abnormalities, but most (92%) patients are identified (58).

### Data from PIOPED

The PIOPED data require special mention: This collection of information is impressive in extent, especially because the data are available for future analysis. These data were published as an example of how the clinician can use an article about a diagnostic test and gain sufficient confidence to apply it to his practice (71). To date, at least 30 publications have been released and there are many more to come. The study was a $10 million multicenter prospective randomized trial, and all the clinical, scan, and arteriographic data were put into a computer database to allow future clinical questions to be answered. Already the original PIOPED criteria have been modified and remodified as a result of these analyses (33,73), and these changes have been validated by other studies (72) and even applied to aerosol ventilation imaging (51). It is expected that these data will be able to put V/Q scanning in a clinical context for future generations of referring clinicians. Some of these findings were presented earlier, and others follow.

### Image Interpretation

The overall agreement in reading pulmonary arteriograms and V/Q scans was similar when categorized as to whether PE was very likely (high-probability V/Q scans), very unlikely

**TABLE 4-14.** *Reader agreement in arteriograms and V/Q scans*

| Test result | Reader agreement | |
|---|---|---|
| | Arteriogram | V/Q scan |
| PE likely | 92% | 95% |
| PE uncertain | 83% | 73% |
| PE unlikely | 89% | 93% |

Source: PIOPED investigators. Value of the ventilation/perfusion scan in acute pulmonary embolism. JAMA 1990;263: 2753–2759.

(normal or near normal V/Q scans), or uncertain (low- and intermediate-probability V/Q scans) (14) (Table 4-14).

### Concept of Segmental Equivalence

*Segmental equivalence* is the term developed for determining the total segmental volume involved; for example, four moderate-sized subsegmental defects might be equal to two segments, that is, two-segmental equivalence. The concept of segmental equivalence is now diminished by the simpler alternative of counting all mismatches, provided they are at least of moderate size (16,55,68), as seen in Table 4-11.

### Perfusion Scan Only

Whereas earlier reports indicated that a perfusion scan alone could not identify patients with PE reliably (9,12,27,61), a randomly selected subset of the PIOPED data (79) showed that in patients with multiple segmental perfusion defects the diagnosis of PE using the perfusion scan alone was as good as the V/Q scan. This means full eight-view perfusion studies should be obtained. However, large numbers of patients with an abnormal perfusion scan had intermediate-probability scans, and this increase was at the expense of the low-probability V/Q scan subset. I apply this scan interpretation very carefully to a limited critically ill patient population in whom the scan is being used to rule out massive PE to explain hypotension: If the perfusion scan does not demonstrate typical segmental defects with absent perfusion, PE is unlikely to be the cause of the hypotension.

### Associated Cardiac or Pulmonary Disease

In late 1993, Stein et al. published PIOPED data stratified by the presence or absence of either cardiac or pulmonary disease (68). Patients with cardiac disease were those with a history or evidence of valvular, coronary, or "other" heart disease, and a history of left- or right-sided heart failure. Patients were considered as having pulmonary disease if they had a history of asthma, COPD, interstitial lung disease, prior PE, or other lung disease, or evidence of acute

**TABLE 4-15.** *PPV of PE relative to the number of moderate or larger subsegmental mismatched perfusion defects*

| Cumulative number of defects | PPV (95% CI) | |
|---|---|---|
| | No prior CPD | Any prior CPD |
| ≥0 | 41 (37–45) | 33 (29–37)* |
| ≥1 | 80 (74–86) | 68 (62–74)* |
| ≥2 | 89 (83–95) | 77 (69–85)* |
| ≥3 | 91 (85–97) | 80 (72–88) |
| ≥4 | 89 (81–95) | 84 (76–92) |
| ≥5 | 92 (84–100) | 89 (83–95) |
| ≥6 | 94 (88–100) | 93 (87–99) |
| ≥7 | 96 (90–100) | 92 (86–98) |
| ≥8 | 95 (89–100) | 91 (83–89) |

*$p < 0.05$
CPD, cardiopulmonary disease.
Source: Stein PD, Henry JW, Gottschalk A. Mismatched vascular defects: an easy alternative to mismatched segmental equivalent defects for the interpretation of ventilation/perfusion lung scans in pulmonary embolism. Chest 1993;104:1468–1471.

pneumonia or acute respiratory distress syndrome (ARDS). The study showed that the PPV and specificity of PE based on the V/Q scan could be further stratified according to the presence or absence of prior cardiopulmonary disease (Table 4-15).

### Resolution of Perfusion Defects

The first reported improvement in pulmonary blood flow after a PE was in 1967 (80). Complete resolution occurred as early as 1 week but was exceptional in extensive embolism (Fig. 4-19). Other investigators show that the size of the initial defect was inversely related to complete resolution, as was age, and coexisting heart disease (81). Although young people have all their resolution occur in the first month, older individuals require up to 3 months for resolution to occur (Fig. 4-20). Patients <40 years of age demonstrated some perfusion scan improvement 90% of the time (55% had complete resolution), whereas only 50% of patients >60 years of age showed partial improvement and none had complete resolution (Fig. 4-21).

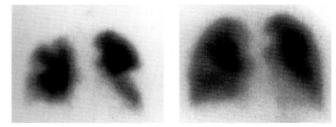

A,B

**FIG. 4-19. (A)** This scan shows multiple segmental and subsegmental defects in the anterior view. **(B)** Two weeks later, there is marked improvement of the defects in the lingulae, right middle, and upper lobes. The different sizes of the images are a consequence of different formatters used.

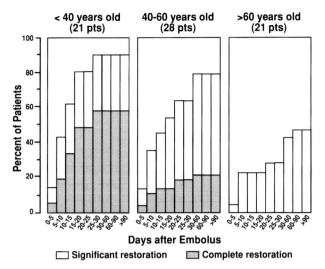

**FIG. 4-20.** Partial and complete resolution rates in three age categories. (Data from Winebright JW, Gerdes AJ, Nelp WB. Restoration of blood flow after PE. Arch Intern Med 1970;125:241–247.)

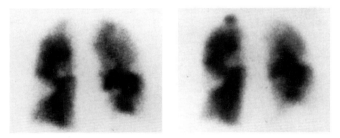

**FIG. 4-21.** Two posterior view scans performed 2 years apart in the same patient. No significant interval changes have occurred in the multiple perfusion defects. A scan performed 5 years later (7 years after first scan) was identical to the two studies shown.

## Underestimation of Disease

Hypoperfusion of entire lung, lobar, or segmental defects associated with mismatch could be due to one of the following:

- Technique—for example, the Tc-99m of the aerosol scan suggests some perfusion (see Fig. 4-11)
- Nonocclusive central vessel (main pulmonary or lobar artery) disease
- Partial reperfusion of defects

Central or lobar saddle emboli can be suggested when relatively unimpressive segmental and subsegmental defects coexist with obvious hypoperfusion of one lung or lobe. This indicates significant and often massive PE with nonocclusive emboli at major arterial bifurcations. These scans may appear to have "hot spots" (82) caused by sparing of some segments in otherwise relatively hypoperfused regions subserved by the partially occluded vessels. It is important to recognize this because the scan pattern suggests less

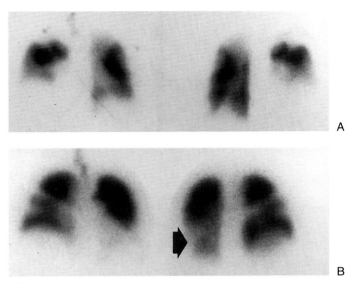

**FIG. 4-22.** Two scans with anterior (left) and posterior (right) images performed 2 days apart. Different gamma cameras account for the change in overall scan size. **(A)** The first scan shows multiple perfusion defects with normal perfusion to only a few segments in the right middle zone and marked hypoperfusion to others, suggesting large proximal (saddle) emboli. **(B)** Two days later, there is considerable overall improvement, but a new segmental defect (*arrow*) has appeared in the left lateral basal segment (posterior view, lower right image). This new defect may reflect either fragmentation of a large central embolus (now with occlusion of the lateral basal segmental artery) or a new embolus.

extensive arterial occlusion than actually exists, and the development of apparent new peripheral defects 3 or 4 days later may only represent fragmentation of the large central PE rather than recurrent emboli (Fig. 4-22). It is important to recognize these patients because of the potential to underestimate the clinical severity of PE. If these patients do throw a new clot, it could become a more hemodynamically significant embolus than otherwise anticipated.

Hot spots can also occur with atelectasis as a result of associated hyperperfusion of the normal adjacent lung (82). In these patients the perfusion lung scan shows regional hyperperfusion without associated V/Q mismatches. Scans like this can demonstrate physiologic shunting (Fig. 4-23) and so explain the patient's dyspnea and hypoxemia. The absence of typical mismatches is the clue to the absence of PE in this hot spot finding, and in these patients there are often reverse mismatch regions of absent or severely reduced ventilation with more normal perfusion (Fig. 4-24).

## False-Positive V/Q Scans

The detection of PE in patients with a past history of DVT or PE can be difficult because mismatched scan patterns may be due to old PE (see Fig. 4-21). Chronic or past PE is the most frequent differential diagnosis for V/Q mismatch. Occasionally, patients that present at emergency rooms with a past

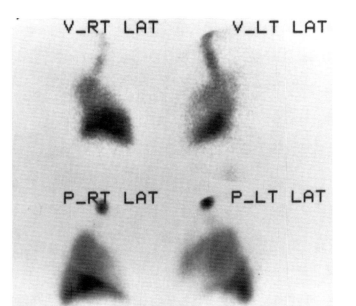

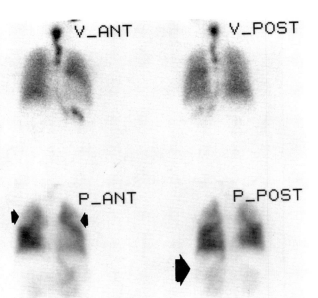

**FIG. 4-23.** This patient had an esophagectomy 2 days prior to this scan and presents with severe hypoxemia with PE to be ruled out. Bilateral symmetric posterior defects in the lateral view ventilation scans (upper row) correspond to pleural effusions in this supine patient. There is hyperperfusion (lower row perfusion scans) of these lower lobes. Most of the pulmonary circulation is to the lower lobes, which are not ventilated, so there is significant scan evidence of shunting to explain this patient's hypoxemia. Similarly, the lingulae and middle lobe have the best ventilation but poor perfusion, further contributing to the shunting process.

**FIG. 4-25.** These ventilation (upper) and perfusion (lower) images (anterior on left, posterior on right) are of a surgically treated tetralogy of Fallot patient with bilateral (*small arrows*) peripheral pulmonary stenoses (regional reduced perfusion and normal ventilation). The renal and faint splenic (*large arrow*) visualization indicates the right-to-left shunt resulting from her shunt procedure.

history of PE have a V/Q scan performed that indicates a high probability of PE. The scan might also have some defects that suggest partial resolution (decreased rather than absent perfusion). In these patients the V/Q mismatch may be due to old disease. Such patients require baseline studies performed 3 months after any clinical presentation, with copies provided to the patient if they seek care at other institutions. Any additional mismatched perfusion deficit at a subsequent clinical presentation would suggest new PE, but the same defects as seen on their baseline studies would not suggest new PE.

A very rare cause of mismatched V/Q abnormalities is seen in the multiple peripheral pulmonary stenoses (Fig. 4-25). More common disease processes that can affect the pulmonary arterial tree and not bronchi include lung tumors and x-ray therapy, which result in extrinsic vessel compression while the presence of bronchial cartilage prevents bronchial obstruction. These processes may result in V/Q mismatch, but such etiology is usually obvious on CXR. Other causes for V/Q mismatch (Table 4-16) include any form of arterial occlusion (Fig. 4-26), primary vascular diseases, and other

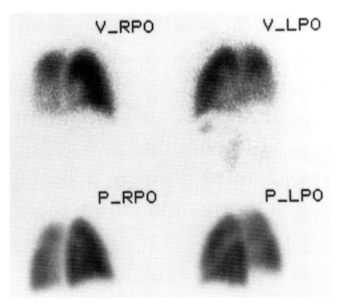

**FIG. 4-24.** An example of reverse mismatch, when perfusion is present uniformly through both lungs but ventilation is virtually absent. This occurs frequently in atelectasis involving the lower lobes.

**TABLE 4-16.** *Causes of FP scans for venous thromboembolism*

| Intravascular | Vessel wall | Extrinsic compression |
|---|---|---|
| Thrombus | Arteritis | Lung cancer |
| Tumor, fat, | Stenosis | XRT |
| parasite, talc | — | Nodal enlargement |

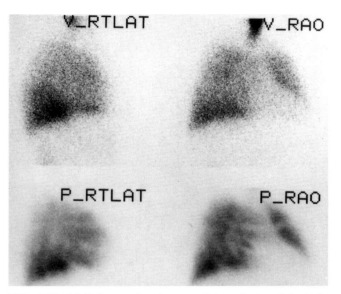

**FIG. 4-26.** Multiple small subsegmental perfusion defects in right lateral and RAO (lower row) mismatched in the ventilation scan (upper row). The probability of thromboembolic PE in this patient is low. We have found these findings in tumor and fat emboli, and this pattern is also said to occur in pulmonary hypertension.

causes of compression of pulmonary arteries without involvement of bronchi (e.g., tuberculous nodal disease, Hodgkin's).

### False-Negative V/Q Scans

False-negative V/Q scans occur when partial occlusion is present. Only 26% of partially occluded vessels demonstrate perfusion defects, whereas 97% of completely occluded vessels >2.0 mm are recognized (42). The perfusion scan does not detect the majority of nonocclusive pulmonary arterial emboli: The very fact that the lesion does not completely occlude the artery allows tracer to pass distally, and although it may produce reduced MAA impaction in the distal arterioles and capillaries, it does not cause absence of tracer (the most important perfusion scan finding of PE). Contrast this with pulmonary arteriography, in which the specific signs of PE include both occlusive and nonocclusive disease: evidence of vessel cutoff (occlusive) or the presence of contrast outlining the clot (nonocclusive). This fact makes segment-by-segment comparisons of V/Q scanning and pulmonary arteriography difficult. Fortunately, patients with clinical symptomatic PE typically have five or more pulmonary segments involved. Although nonocclusive disease is present in 20% to 40% of patient lesions (42,52), other completely occluded vessels usually allow the V/Q diagnosis of PE.

### Practical Diagnostic Strategy

V/Q scanning has a strong influence on patient management because patients with high-probability scans receive

**TABLE 4-17.** Combined clinical and scan probability of PE

| Scan probability (mean) | Pretest clinical probability | | |
|---|---|---|---|
| | High (80–100%) | Medium (20–79%) | Low (0–19%) |
| High (87%) | 96 | 88 | 56* |
| Intermediate (30%) | 66 | 28 | 16 |
| Low (14%) | 40* | 16 | 4 |
| Near normal (4%) | 0 | 6 | 2 |

*Groups reclassified into the intermediate probability group by pretest probability.
Source: PIOPED investigators. Value of the ventilation/perfusion scan in acute pulmonary embolism. JAMA 1990;263: 2753–2759.

anticoagulation, and most with low-probability interpretations are neither treated nor referred for angiography (30). It is important that V/Q scanning correctly classify patients.

In 1980, McNeil looked at the clinical likelihood of PE as obtained from the referring physician and incorporated this with the scan probability of PE (12). This clinical addition increased the chance of the scan interpretation, correctly stratifying the patient status as to having PE or not. This technique has also been used by the McMaster's and PIOPED groups (13,14).

Having a low clinical suspicion and a high-probability scan can downgrade the overall estimate of PE to the intermediate range. Having a high clinical suspicion with a low-probability scan can upgrade the estimate of PE to the intermediate range, according to the PIOPED data (14) (Table 4-17). The utility of this strategy of combining the prior clinical probability with scan probability in deriving a posterior probability for PE cannot be overemphasized. Such clinical information (symptoms, but more important, risk factors for DVT) dramatically recalculates the likelihood of PE in all scan categories (see Table 4-17). The same effect is seen in patients in whom the scan estimate is calculated from adding the number of moderate or larger subsegmental V/Q mismatches, and with this strategy the patients can also be further stratified by the presence or absence of a history (83) of prior cardiopulmonary disease (Table 4-18).

It is generally agreed that pulmonary arteriograms are indicated when one of the following situations is present:

- An intermediate-probability scan
- Strong clinical suspicion of PE with low-probability scan
- Low clinical suspicion of PE with high-probability scan
- Contraindication to anticoagulation in high-probability scan
- To confirm PE before drastic intervention, such as embolectomy

Although arteriograms are frequently performed in these indications the numbers of patients with intermediate-probability scans who are further investigated with an arteriogram is modest. Reports indicate that only half of such patients are studied with angiography (70,84). The use of

**TABLE 4-18.** *PPV of PE: Cumulative number of mismatched defects modified by clinical assessment and presence or absence of cardiopulmonary disease (CPD)*

| Cumulative mismatches | Clinical assessment and CPD | | | | | |
| --- | --- | --- | --- | --- | --- | --- |
| | High clinical | | Intermediate | | Low clinical | |
| | CPD | No CPD | CPD | No CPD | CPD | No CPD |
| ≥0 | 80 | 87 | 36 | 43 | 9 | 38 |
| ≥1 | 89 | 100 | 71 | 78 | 20 | 60 |
| ≥2 | 89 | 100 | 79 | 86 | 29 | 88 |
| ≥3 | 93 | 100 | 83 | 89 | 17 | 80 |
| ≥4 | 93 | 100 | 88 | 88 | 20 | 67 |
| ≥5 | 92 | 100 | 92 | 92 | 25 | 50 |
| ≥6 | 100 | 100 | 95 | 97 | 25 | 60 |

Source: Stein PD, Henry JW, Gottschalk A. The addition of clinical assessment to stratification according to prior cardiopulmonary disease further optimizes the interpretation of V/Q lung scans in PE. Chest 1993;104:1471–1476.

pretest clinical likelihoods can better identify those patients for further study, and several algorithms have been developed to use noninvasive means of identifying venous thrombosis, such as ultrasound (US). Figure 4-27 represents a consensus between the McMaster's and PIOPED groups (85).

The US evaluation for DVT is excellent in patients with leg symptoms and signs (sensitivities and specificities in excess of 90%), but in asymptomatic high-risk patients, the sensitivity is not high (86) and ranges from 38% to 60%. This finding has been confirmed in the radiologic literature, in which the use of Doppler venous US was insensitive (sensitivity, 13%) in identifying patients with DVT with intermediate-probability lung scans who subsequently had angiographically proven PE (87). More recently, physicians have been considering therapeutic decisions concerning the need for fibrinolytics based on the detection of right heart dysfunction (e.g., cardiac echography). The presence of such dysfunction indicates very significant pulmonary arterial occlusion and the potential need of invasive therapy.

Just as Robin voiced dissatisfaction with any PE scan diagnosis other than normal (10), the McMaster's group of Hull has written for a decade that the only good V/Q scan criteria are normal and high-probability scans (13,48) and that all other categories are nondiagnostic. These conclusions have been published in the internal medicine journals, and many medical imagers do not appreciate their existence.

One example (88) found in patients with inadequate cardiopulmonary reserve (pulmonary edema, right ventricular failure, hypotension, syncope, acute tachyarrhythmias, or respiratory failure) a PE death rate of 6% in the group of low, intermediate, and indeterminate category versus 1% without impaired cardiovascular reserve. The authors claim this death rate as evidence of a need for change of nomenclature from low probability to nondiagnostic. The overall death rate (including death

from PE) over the same time period in the impaired cardiovascular reserve group was 41%, the death rate in the unimpaired group was 7% (i.e., a similar sixfold increase in the death rate in the impaired group, in both PE and non–PE-related deaths). This research group has claimed an unacceptable high rate of PE (30%) in low-probability scans in their prospective PE diagnosis study (13,48), but

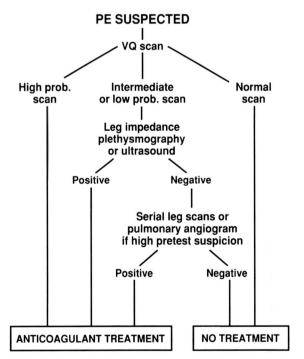

**FIG. 4-27.** This algorithm is the consensus of the McMaster's and PIOPED groups. It combines the results of DVT detection with prior clinical certainty of PE in patients whose V/Q scans are of intermediate probability. (Reprinted with permission from Stein PD, Hull RD, Saltzman HA, Pineo G. Strategy for diagnosis of patients with suspected acute pulmonary embolism. Chest 1993;103:1553–1559.)

their criteria for this category include many intermediate-probability scans because of the simplicity of their scan criteria that does not discriminate between low and intermediate categories as well as other published diagnostic schemes. On the other hand, a publication by the same authors suggests the V/Q scan is cost-effective in the diagnosis of PE (89).

### Diagnosis Synopsis

#### *Relationship of DVT and PE*

- PE and DVT: 50% chance of recurrent PE
- PE but no DVT: recurrent PE unlikely
- One-half of fatal PE patients have both fresh (new) and organized (old) emboli seen at postmortem

#### *Clinical Presentation*

- Tremendous clinical variation occurs in PE.
- 40% to 60% of PE is asymptomatic.
- Hemoptysis and pleurisy indicate infarction.
- Hypotension or syncope indicate massive PE.

#### *V/Q Mismatches*

- 80% are segmental.
- Two-thirds of patients have bilateral emboli.
- Two-thirds of defects are in lower lobes.
- 5% to 7% are solitary.
- Average high-probability scan has eight mismatches.

### Future

The future of V/Q scanning hinges on the possible FDA approval of the new Tc-99m agents Technegas and Pertechnegas, which will vastly improve ventilation imaging. If ventilation images are improved substantially, the current diagnostic criteria may need to be re-evaluated in view of the smaller degree of V/Q mismatch that may be detected. Technegas and the stable alveolar deposition that occurs may make single photon emission computed tomography (SPECT) imaging a possibility, and even with Tc-99m aerosols, SPECT imaging is possible and improves lesion detection. Pertechnegas appears to be the agent that may obtain NDA approval soonest.

There should be a rigorous follow-up of patients with various scan probability estimates to determine whether they are at risk for future death from PE or recurrence of PE. At present it is established that patients with either low-probability V/Q scans (30) or normal pulmonary arteriograms (31) have an excellent clinical outcome. If it is established (as suggested in reference 32) that most patients with low-intermediate probability V/Q scans had an equally benign course, the need to investigate these patients further may be obviated. The PIOPED data may be able to provide this answer because of the clinical follow-up of participants.

## ALTERNATIVE IMAGING MODALITIES

Articles have suggested a role for electron-beam computed tomography (CT), spiral CT, and magnetic resonance imaging (MRI) in PE. In the case of CT, it has been suggested that the modality combines the sensitivity of V/Q scanning and the specificity of angiography (90). Certainly CT is able to identify pulmonary infarcts, but the CT criteria are nonspecific. The CT is superb at identifying large central nonocclusive thrombi that can be missed by perfusion scanning. V/Q scanning can identify these proximal clots if unilateral (see Fig. 4-21), but many scan readers are not aware of these subtle scan findings. Such scans occur several times a year in our practice, when we can indicate the emboli are more massive than the scan might otherwise suggest. Although there are several reports (91), the CT technique has not been thoroughly investigated in patients with few or subsegmental thrombi (92) (the intermediate-probability V/Q scan). Although it is argued that CT has the advantage of evaluating the mediastinum and pulmonary parenchyma, the V/Q scanning combination may have separate advantages in evaluation of COPD patients.

MRI has reliably depicted large and medium sized emboli. A role in the further investigation of intermediate V/Q scans has been suggested (93), especially given that MR angiography can also be used to detect venous thrombi both in the abdomen and the limbs (91). However, sensitivity in detection of PE below the segmental level is a problem for this modality, although many suggest that missing these involved vessels may not be of clinical significance if the thrombi source can be detected (91).

Contrast-enhanced MRI in chronic thromboembolic disease showed greater detection sensitivity, with complete rather than partial vessel occlusion. Forty percent to 45% of lobar and segmental vessels were found to be partially occluded by conventional angiography in this special patient population of chronic disease. The overall detection sensitivity of MRI for segmental vessels was approximately 75%, but this varied according to the occlusion severity; if there was <50% segmental occlusion, detection sensitivity was halved (~40%) (52).

The issue as to whether CT or MRI can replace the V/Q scan will only be resolved when a large study is performed that includes significant numbers of patients with intermediate-probability scans and/or severe COPD. Before such studies are published, alternative diagnostic algorithm proposals to V/Q scanning are premature (94) because these patient populations include the only V/Q scan findings that have been criticized.

## Radioaerosol Imaging

Radioaerosol imaging is described earlier in the section on Ventilation Scan but is reviewed here for other indications. This topic has been well reviewed (95,96).

Radioaerosol studies were first described in 1965 (97), the first use of clear solutions was described in 1973 (98), and before this, viscid (colloidal) solutions of liver and lung perfusion agents were aerosolized. Reliable nebulizers were first available in 1982. For examination of alveolar distribution in patients with COPD, we currently use Mallinckrodt's UltraVent kit set, which appears to provide less central airway impaction.

An aerosol is a mixture of solid or liquid particles or droplets that are stable as a suspension in air. Available radioaerosol systems use jet nebulizers, which pass a stream of oxygen (8 to 10 liters/min) over a small volume (1 to 3 ml) of Tc-99m DTPA or other Tc-99m agent. Sufficiently small submicronic particles form in this mist and can be delivered to the lungs and alveoli, and large particles are removed by baffles built into the device. The particles are deposited in the lungs by sedimentation and gravitational impaction, the site depending on particle size and speed of movement of the aerosol. In regions of turbulence (i.e., COPD, ridged ventilator tubing, tracheostomies, oropharynx [see Fig. 4-10], and regions of excess mucus), impaction of aerosol occurs. Generally, approximately 5% of the tracer enters the peripheral lungs, much settles out in the nebulizer tubing delivery system, and most remains in the nebulizer.

## Clinical Applications

### Bronchial Airways Obstruction

Central impaction occurs in emphysema and asthma, whereas peripheral hot spots typically occur in chronic bronchitis and bronchiectasis.

### Mucociliary Clearance

This testing requires slightly larger particle sizes than are used in the evaluation of alveoli, so that impaction occurs in the airways proximal to the terminal bronchioles. This is achieved by using Tc-99m SC or Tc-99m HSA with aerosol particle sizes of 4 to 5 μm that are cleared by the mucociliary apparatus. These agents are not absorbed, and the critical organs are the lung and major airways.

### Alveolar Capillary Membrane Integrity

The alveolar capillary membrane is composed of the alveolar epithelial surface, the capillary endothelium, and the interstitial space between these two surfaces. In acute

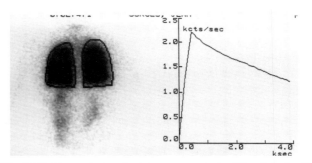

**FIG. 4-28.** Normal alveolar clearance study. (Reprinted with permission from Krasnow AZ, Isitman AT, Collier BD, et al. Diagnostic Application of Radioaerosols in Nuclear Medicine. In Freeman LM (ed), Nuclear Medicine Annual 1993. New York: Raven, 1993;123–193.)

respiratory distress syndrome (ARDS), the solutes that cross the capillary surface pass into the alveoli, causing pulmonary edema as a result of the breakdown of membrane integrity. This differs from pulmonary edema due to congestive heart failure, in which high pressures force fluids across a normal membrane. The rate of disappearance of Tc-99m DTPA aerosol from the lung or the rate of its appearance in the blood can make the distinction between these two causes of pulmonary edema. The normal alveolar clearance has a half-life of 50 to 80 minutes (Fig. 4-28). Accelerated clearances are seen in smokers (this is an acute effect of smoke), ARDS (this effect can be segmental and scattered throughout both lungs), *Pneumocystis carinii* pneumonia, oxygen exposure, interstitial lung disease, bleomycin toxicity, diabetes, sarcoidosis, COPD, and hyaline membrane disease of the newborn.

## OTHER DISEASE PROCESSES

Other disease processes in which lung perfusion imaging can be helpful include congestive heart failure, right-to-left intracardiac shunts, and preoperative evaluation of patients in whom pneumonectomy is being considered.

### Heart Failure

Patients with acute increases in pulmonary perfusion pressures demonstrate increased perfusion to the apical regions compared to normal. Whenever the scan demonstrates better perfusion to the upper lung zones than the lower zones, pulmonary venous pressure is elevated. This occurs in heart failure (Fig. 4-29). The scan finding is not the equivalent of dilated upper lobe veins that occur on the CXR due to chronic pulmonary venous hypertension, rather the scan pattern occurs in acute situations and is a sensitive indicator of heart failure. It can be very reassuring to identify this in patients with unexplained dyspnea when the V/Q scan shows no V/Q mismatch. This can allow the scan

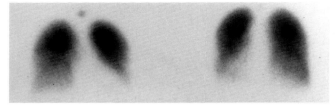

**FIG. 4-29.** Typical scan of patient with raised pulmonary venous pressure. The anterior perfusion scan view is on the left, posterior on the right. The upper lung zones have greater perfusion than the lower lung zones. There is evidence of cardiomegaly. The ventilation scan was normal.

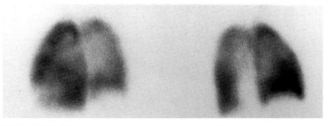

**FIG. 4-30.** These two posterior oblique views show a central and posterior region of decreased perfusion bilaterally. This pattern is symmetric, crosses segmental boundaries, and has reduced rather than absent perfusion. This was associated with the typical CXR findings of pulmonary edema in the same regions. The LPO view (left) also shows a defect due to cardiomegaly.

reader to implicate heart failure as the cause of dyspnea. Many times there is also evidence of pulmonary edema on the CXR (Fig. 4-30).

## Lung Cancer

In the preoperative evaluation of lung cancer patients, the perfusion scan coupled with a forced expiratory volume in 1 second ($FEV_1$) can be helpful in the decision-making process regarding potential pneumonectomy. Many lung cancer patients are smokers and have chronic lung disease with impaired pulmonary function. It can be difficult to wean patients off the ventilator postoperatively if the residual postoperative $FEV_1$ is less than 800 ml. The measurement of the relative perfusion of each lung using the geometric mean of anterior and posterior lung perfusion studies can help prevent this situation (Fig. 4-31). If the estimated residual $FEV_1$ is <800 ml, surgery is contraindicated. In some patients with COPD and cancer, a lobectomy rather than pneumonectomy may be technically possible. By calculating the cancerous lobe's contribution to that lung's total perfusion (using appropriate oblique views without "shine through") and then subtracting this component from the total, one can indicate the result of lobectomy. However, one must also report the potential $FEV_1$ after pneumonectomy, to provide the surgeon with the probability of the patient's

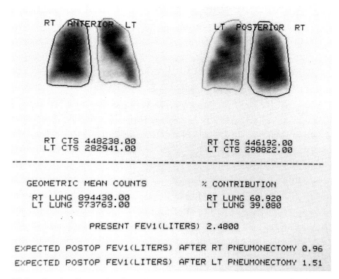

```
        RT  ANTERIOR  LT              LT  POSTERIOR  RT


        RT CTS 448238.00              RT CTS 446192.00
        LT CTS 282941.00              LT CTS 290822.00
-----------------------------------------------------------------
        GEOMETRIC MEAN COUNTS            % CONTRIBUTION
        RT LUNG 894430.00             RT LUNG 60.920
        LT LUNG 573763.00             LT LUNG 39.080

             PRESENT FEV1(LITERS) 2.4800

    EXPECTED POSTOP FEV1(LITERS) AFTER RT PNEUMONECTOMY 0.96
    EXPECTED POSTOP FEV1(LITERS) AFTER LT PNEUMONECTOMY 1.51
```

**FIG. 4-31.** Quantitative lung scan showing the calculated postoperative $FEV_1$.

becoming ventilator dependent if a pneumonectomy is found necessary.

## Lung Transplantation

The role of V/Q scanning in lung transplantation is limited. Preoperative relative perfusion studies can identify the worse lung, and surgeons may prefer to remove this lung first in unilateral transplantation procedures. It is important to remember there is a natural right-left (R:L) difference in perfusion due to the chest volume occupied by the heart: The normal R:L ratio is 55:45. If a single lung transplant is performed, the relative perfusion study may dictate which lung should be transplanted. Other considerations, however, include the surgical technical complexity, which favors removal of the right lung, so the relative perfusion study is just one of the parameters used preoperatively. Single lung transplants have been followed using relative perfusion of the native and donor lungs as measured by the geometric mean of anterior and posterior perfusion lung images. Relative reductions of 5% in perfusion were said to signify rejection, but these results have not been clinically helpful.

## Intracardiac Shunts

Patients with right-to-left intracardiac shunts demonstrate the systemic circulation on lung perfusion scanning, especially vascular organs such as the brain and kidney. This can be an incidental finding during routine V/Q scanning for PE (Fig. 4-32), but the test can also be ordered to establish the degree of right-to-left shunt. If the kidneys are visualized during the routine V/Q scan and Tc-99m DTPA was used as the aerosol ventilation agent, the renal visualization could be attributable to Tc-99m DTPA absorbed across the alveolar

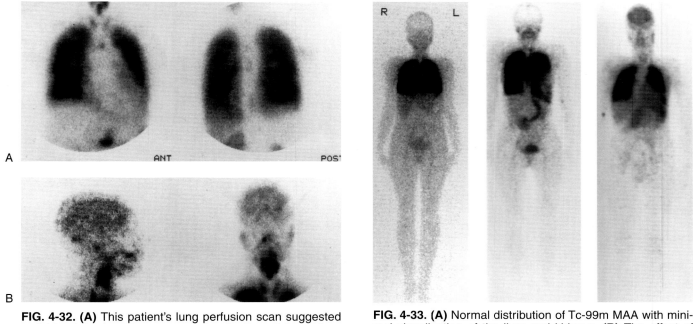

**FIG. 4-32. (A)** This patient's lung perfusion scan suggested a right-to-left shunt because of visualization of the kidney and spleen in the posterior lung view. **(B)** Activity in the cerebral hemispheres confirms a shunt. The activity in the oropharynx is probably explained by impacted Tc-99m DTPA aerosol from the prior ventilation scan.

**FIG. 4-33. (A)** Normal distribution of Tc-99m MAA with minimal visualization of the liver and kidneys. **(B)** The effect of free TcO$_4$ (stomach, bladder, thyroid, and salivary activity). **(C)** A significant (40%) right-to-left shunt with visualization of cerebral cortex.

membrane. However, activity in the cerebral hemispheres establishes a right-to-left shunt. If renal visualization is noted several hours after a Tc-99m MAA perfusion scan, then this activity could also be due to breakdown of the MAA particles and their accumulation in the kidneys as part of the normal MAA biodegradation process.

With a right-to-left shunt quantitative study, whole-body images are acquired, and the relative accumulation of tracer in the pulmonary and systemic circulation is determined by drawing ROIs about the lungs and the entire body. The pulmonary circulation is represented by the lung activity, the systemic is represented by the whole-body activity less that in the lung. Thus, the ratio of activity in the pulmonary and systemic circulation equals the ratio of pulmonary blood flow to shunt flow and the percent of right-to-left shunt can be calculated using this formula:

$$\text{Shunt \%} = \frac{\text{Total body counts} - \text{lung counts}}{\text{Total body counts}} \times 100$$

This calculation should be obtained from data collected immediately after administration of specially prepared and confirmed high-quality Tc-99m MAA to minimize the systemic contribution of counts from loss of Tc-99m from the MAA and biodegradation of the labeled MAA particles. The problems associated with different geometries of tissue distribution may be modified by obtaining the geometric mean of counts with a dual-headed camera. The problem of differential absorption—pulmonary activity being less

attenuated by the air-containing lung compared to the systemic activity being attenuated by tissue equivalent material—cannot be corrected for. Despite these limitations, the technique is valid, but care must be taken to ensure that the shunt is not overestimated by labeled albumin added as a stabilizer to some MAA preparations (demonstrates blood pool of heart, liver, spleen, and kidneys) or septal penetration of the lung activity into the systemic ROI. The test works well with shunts that are significant (>10%; Fig. 4-33), although the number of published reports on this technique is limited (99).

**Intrapulmonary Shunts**

Up to one-fourth of patients with extensive cirrhosis can develop intrapulmonary shunting. The shunting appears to involve the basal pulmonary vasculature, and the patients develop dyspnea when upright, presumably due to redistribution of blood to these basal shunted regions. This shunting can cause hypoxemia and is a relative contraindication to liver transplantation. The perfusion lung scan cannot identify the site of shunting but can identify its presence before it is clinically evident. The scan can quantify the shunt and demonstrate progression. Some shunts have disappeared after liver transplantation (100). Other conditions, such as pulmonary arteriovenous malformation (usually associated with hereditary hemorrhagic telangiectasia), may be diagnosed by this method (99). These conditions differ from

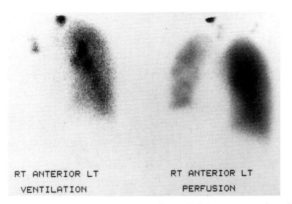

**FIG. 4-34.** This patient had a confirmed right mucus plug that was removed at bronchoscopy after the scan. The ventilation scan (right) shows no ventilation to the right lung. The perfusion scan (left) shows reduced right lung perfusion.

intracardiac shunts in that dynamic images obtained of the pulmonary perfusion study are normal.

### Bronchial Obstruction

There is a reflex pulmonary arterial constriction when ventilation is impaired, such as occurs in bronchial obstruction. Examples include mucus plugging (especially common in paralyzed patients), endotracheal tube placed too low on one side, inhaled foreign bodies, bronchial adenomas, and extrinsic bronchial compression, as from cancer. This vasoconstriction is usually not complete, but typically the blood flow is reduced to 10% of normal if ventilation is absent (Fig. 4-34).

With clearance of the obstruction, perfusion improves immediately: We have encouraged the patient to cough and clear the bronchi and been rewarded with immediate reperfusion of a segmental defect with the administration of an additional dose of Tc-99m MAA.

### REFERENCES

1. Johnson PM. The role of lung scanning in pulmonary embolism. Semin Nucl Med 1971;1:161–184.
2. McCartney WH. Ventilation-perfusion scanning in pulmonary embolus. Clin Nucl Med 1981;6(Suppl):27–36.
3. Alderson PO, Martin EC. Pulmonary embolism: diagnosis with multiple imaging modalities. Radiology 1987;164:297–312.
4. Juni JE, Alavi A. Lung scanning in the diagnosis of PE: the emperor redressed. Semin Nucl Med 1991;21:281–296.
5. Wagner HN, Sagiston DC, McAfee JG, et al. Diagnosis of massive pulmonary embolism in man by radioisotope scanning. N Engl J Med 1964;271:377–384.
6. Poulouse UK, Reba RC, Wagner HN Jr. Characterization of shape and location of perfusion defects in certain pulmonary diseases. N Engl J Med 1968;279:1020–1025.
7. Wagner HN, Lopez-Majano V, Langau JK, et al. Radioactive xenon in the differential diagnosis of pulmonary embolism. Radiology 1968;91:1168–1174.
8. Gilday DK, James AE. Lung scan patterns in pulmonary embolism versus those in congestive heart failure and emphysema. Am J Roentgenol Radium Ther Nucl Med 1972;115:739–750.
9. McNeil BJ. A diagnostic strategy using ventilation perfusion studies in patients suspect for pulmonary embolism. J Nucl Med 1976;17:613–616.
10. Robin ED. Overdiagnosis and overtreatment of PE: the emperor may have no clothes. Ann Intern Med 1977;87:775–787.
11. Biello DR, Mattar AG, McKnight RC, Siegel BA. Ventilation-perfusion studies in suspected pulmonary embolism. AJR Am J Roentgenol 1979;133:1033–1037.
12. McNeil BJ. Ventilation-perfusion studies and the diagnosis of pulmonary embolism: concise communication. J Nucl Med 1980;21:319–323.
13. Hull RD, Hirsh J, Carter CJ, et al. Pulmonary angiography, ventilation lung scanning, and venography for clinically suspected pulmonary embolism with abnormal perfusion lung scan. Ann Intern Med 1983; 98:891–899.
14. PIOPED investigators. Value of the ventilation/perfusion scan in acute pulmonary embolism. JAMA 1990;263:2753–2759.
15. Dorfman GS, Cronan JJ, Tupper TB, et al. Occult pulmonary embolism: a common occurrence in deep venous thrombosis. AJR Am J Roentgenol 1987;148:263–266.
16. Stein PD. Acute pulmonary embolism disease. Disease-a-Month: Masters in Medicine. September 1994;478–523.
17. Stein PD, Terrin M, Hetes CA, et al. Clinical, laboratory, roentgenographic, and electrocardiographic findings in patients with acute pulmonary embolism and no preexisting cardiac or pulmonary disease. Chest 1991;100:598–603.
18. Anderson FA, Wheeler HB. Venous thromboembolism: risk factors and prophylaxis. Clin Chest Med 1995;17:235–251.
19. Kohn H, Konig B, Mostbeck A. Incidence and clinical feature of pulmonary embolism in patients with deep vein thrombosis: a prospective study. Eur J Nucl Med 1987;13:S11–S15.
20. Bauer G. Early diagnosis of venous thrombosis by venography and abortive treatment with heparin. Acta Med Scand 1941;107:136–144.
21. Barritt DW, Jordan SC. Anticoagulant drugs in the treatment of pulmonary embolism. A controlled trial. Lancet 1960;18:1309–1312.
22. Dalen JE, Alpert JS. Natural history of pulmonary embolism. Progress in CV Disease 1975;17:259–270.
23. Alpert JG, et al. Treatment of massive PE: the role of pulmonary embolectomy. Am Heart J 1975;89:413–418.
24. Miller GAH, Hall RJC, Paulth M. Pulmonary embolectomy, heparin and streptokinase: their place in the treatment of acute massive PE. Am Heart J 1977;93:568–574.
25. Urokinase pulmonary embolism trial. Phase I results: a cooperative study. JAMA 1970;214:2163–2172.
26. Carson JL, Kelley MA, Duff A, et al. The clinical course of pulmonary embolism. N Engl J Med 1992;326:1240–1245.
27. Cheeley R, McCartney WH, Perry JR, et al. The role of noninvasive tests versus pulmonary angiography in the diagnosis of pulmonary embolism. Am J Med 1981;70:17–22.
28. Levine MN, Hirsh J. Hemorrhagic complications of anticoagulant therapy. Semin Thromb Hemost 1986;12:39–57.
29. Urokinase-streptokinase embolism trial: a cooperative study. Phase 2 results. JAMA 1974;229:1606–1613.
30. Kahn D, Bushnell DL, Dean R, Perlman SB. Clinical outcome of patients with a "low probability" of pulmonary embolism on ventilation-perfusion lung scan. Arch Intern Med 1989;149:377–379.
31. Novelline RA, Baltarowich OH, Athenasoulis CA, et al. The clinical course of patients with suspected pulmonary embolism and a negative pulmonary arteriogram. Radiology 1978;126:561–567.
32. Jacobson AF, Patel NH. Prevalence of thromboembolic disease in patients with intermediate probability lung scans: association with scan criteria [abstract]. J Nucl Med 1993;34:16.
33. Gottschalk A, Sostman HD, Coleman RE, et al. Ventilation-perfusion scintigraphy in the PIOPED study. Part II. Evaluation of the scintigraphic criteria and interpretations. J Nucl Med 1993;34:1119–1126.
34. Creutzig H, Gonda S, Creutzig A, et al. Frequencies of segmental perfusion and ventilation abnormalities in lung scintigraphy. Eur J Nucl Med 1983;8:401–403.
35. Mandell CH. Scintillation Camera Lung Imaging. New York: Grune & Stratton, 1976.
36. Fogelman I, Maisey M. Lung. In Fogelman I, Maisey M (eds), An Atlas of Clinical Nuclear Medicine. London: Martin Dunitz, 1988; 556–640.
37. Morrell NW, Nijran KS, Jones BE, Seed WA. The underestimation of segmental defect size in radionuclide lung scanning. J Nucl Med 1993;34:370–374.

38. Lensing AWA, Van Beek EJR, Demers C, et al. Ventilation-perfusion scanning and the diagnosis of pulmonary embolism: improvement of observer agreement by the use of a lung segment reference chart. Thromb Haemost 1992;68:245–249.

39. Wilson MA, Pastakia B, Polcyn RE, Gentry L. Re: ventilation-perfusion studies and the diagnosis of pulmonary embolism: concise communication [letter]. J Nucl Med 1980;21:1204–1205.

40. Morrell NW, Roberts CM, Jones BE, et al. The anatomy of radioisotope lung scanning. J Nucl Med 1992;33:676–683.

41. Nielsen PE, Kirchner PT, Gerber FH. Oblique views in lung perfusion scanning: clinical utility and limitations. J Nucl Med 1977;18:967–972.

42. Alderson PO, Doppman JL, Diamond SS, et al. Ventilation-perfusion lung imaging and selective pulmonary angiography in dogs with experimental pulmonary embolism. J Nucl Med 1978;19:164–171.

43. Alderson PO, Biello DR, Khan AR, et al. Comparison of Xe-133 single-breath and washout imaging in the scintigraphic diagnosis of pulmonary embolism. Radiology 1980;137:481–486.

44. Schrave EG, McGray R, Culver RL. Room contamination following Tc-99m-DTPA aerosol ventilation studies. J Nucl Med Tech 1990;18:139.

45. Alderson PO, Biello DR, Gottschalk A, et al. Tc-99m-DTPA aerosol and radioactive gases compared as adjuncts to perfusion scintigraphy in patients with suspected pulmonary embolism. Radiology 1984;153:515–521.

46. Ramanna L, Alderson PO, Waxman AD, et al. Regional comparison of technetium-99m DTPA aerosol and radioactive gas ventilation (xenon and krypton) studies in patients with suspected pulmonary embolism. J Nucl Med 1986;27:1391–1396.

47. Smith R, Maher JM, Miller RI, Alderson PO. Diagnostic utility of Tc-99m DTPA aerosol/Tc-99m MAA lung scintigraphy in patients with suspected PE [abstract]. J Nucl Med 1986;27:923.

48. Hull RD, Hirsh J, Carter CJ, et al. Diagnostic value of ventilation-perfusion lung scanning in patients with suspected pulmonary embolism. Chest 1985;88:819–828.

49. Selby JB, Gardner JJ. Clinical experience with technetium-99m DTPA aerosol with perfusion scintigraphy in suspected pulmonary embolism. Clin Nucl Med 1987;12:1–5.

50. Isitman AT, Collier BD, Krasnow AZ, et al. Impact of postperfusion Tc-99m-PYP aerosol ventilation studies on "moderate probability" Xe-133/Tc-99m MAA lung scans [abstract]. Radiology 1988;169(Suppl):201.

51. Freitas JE, Sarosi MG, Nagle CC, et al. Modified PIOPED criteria used in clinical practice. J Nucl Med 1995;36:1573–1578.

52. Wolf K, Bergin CJ, King MA, et al. Accuracy of contrast enhanced magnetic resonance angiography in chronic thromboembolic disease. Acad Radiol 1996;3:10–17.

53. Fisher RE, Scott JA, Palmer EL. Neural networks in ventilation perfusion imaging. Part I. Effects of interpretive criteria and network architecture. Radiology 1996;198:699–706.

54. Biello DR. Radiological (scintigraphic) evaluation of patients with suspected pulmonary thromboembolism. JAMA 1987;257:3257–3259.

55. Stein PD, Gottschalk A. Critical review of ventilation/perfusion lung scans in acute pulmonary embolism. Prog Cardiovasc Dis 1994;37:13–24.

56. Sostman HD, Gottschalk A. The stripe sign: a new sign for diagnosis of nonembolic defects on pulmonary perfusion scintigraphy. Radiology 1982;142:737–741.

57. Sostman HD, Gottschalk A. Prospective validation of the stripe sign in ventilation-perfusion scintigraphy. Radiology 1992;184:455–459.

58. Alderson PO, Biello DR, Sachariah KG, Siegel BA. Scintigraphic detection of pulmonary embolism in patients with obstructive pulmonary disease. Radiology 1981;138:661–666.

59. Bedont RA, Datz FL. Lung scan perfusion defects limited to matching pleural effusions: low probability of pulmonary embolism. AJR Am J Roentgenol 1985;145:1155–1157.

60. Alderson PO, Dzebolo NN, Biello DR, et al. Serial lung scintigraphy: utility in diagnosis of pulmonary embolism. Radiology 1983;149:792–802.

61. Spies WG, Burstein SP, Dillehay GL, et al. Ventilation-perfusion scintigraphy in suspected pulmonary embolism: correlation with pulmonary angiogram and refinement of criteria for interpretation. Radiology 1986;159:383–390.

62. Catania TA, Caride VJ. Single perfusion defect and pulmonary embolism: angiographic correlation. J Nucl Med 1990;31:296–301.

63. Carter WD, Brady TM, Keyes JW, et al. Relative accuracy of two diagnostic schemes for detection of pulmonary embolism by ventilation-perfusion scintigraphy. Radiology 1982;145:447–451.

64. Sullivan DC, Coleman RE, Mills SR, et al. Lung scan interpretation: effect of different observers and different criteria. Radiology 1983;149:803–807.

65. Webber MM, Gomes AS, Roe D, et al. Comparison of Biello, McNeil and PIOPED criteria for the diagnosis of pulmonary emboli on lung scans. AJR Am J Roentgenol 1990;154:975–981.

66. Braun SD, Newman GE, Ford K, et al. Ventilation-perfusion scanning and pulmonary angiography: correlation in clinical high-probability pulmonary embolism. AJR Am J Roentgenol 1984;143:977–980.

67. Marsh JD, Glynn M, Torman HA. Pulmonary angiography: application in a new spectrum of patients. Am J Med 1983;75:763–770.

68. Stein PD, Henry JW, Gottschalk A. Mismatched vascular defects: an easy alternative to mismatched segmental equivalent defects for the interpretation of ventilation/perfusion lung scans in pulmonary embolism. Chest 1993;104:1468–1471.

69. Scott JA, Palmer EL. Do diagnostic algorithms always produce a uniform lung scan interpretation? J Nucl Med 1993;34:661–665.

70. Sostman HD, Ravin CE, Sullivan DC, et al. Use of pulmonary angiography for suspected pulmonary embolism: influence of scintigraphic diagnosis. AJR Am J Roentgenol 1982;139:673–677.

71. Jaeschke R, Guyatt G, Sackett DL. Users' guide to the medical literature. III. How to use an article about a diagnostic test. A. Are the results of the study valid? JAMA 1994;271:389–391.

72. Sostman HD, Coleman RE, DeLong DM, et al. Evaluation of revised criteria for V/Q scintigraphy in patients with suspected PE. Radiology 1994;193:103–107.

73. Stein PD, Relyea B, Gottschalk A. Evaluation of individual criteria for low probability interpretation of V/Q lung scans. J Nucl Med 1996;37:577–581.

74. Fischer KC, McNeil BJ. The indeterminate lung scan: its characteristics and its association with pulmonary embolism. Eur J Nucl Med 1979;4:49–53.

75. Alderson PO, Rujanavech N, Secker-Walker RH, McKnight RC. The role of $^{133}$Xe ventilation studies in the scintigraphic detection of pulmonary embolism. Radiology 1976;120:633–640.

76. Worsley DF, Kim CK, Alavi A, Palevsky HI. Detailed analysis of patients with matched ventilation-perfusion defects and chest radiographic opacities. J Nucl Med 1993;34:1851–1853.

77. Kim CK, Worsley DF, Alavi A. "Ventilation (V)/perfusion (Q)/chest X-ray" match is less likely to represent pulmonary embolism if Q is only "decreased" rather than "absent" [abstract 58]. J Nucl Med 1993;34:17.

78. Davis RB, Schauwecker DS, Siddiqui AR, et al. Indeterminate lung imaging: can the number be reduced? Clin Nucl Med 1986;11:577–582.

79. Stein PD, Terrin ML, Gottschalk A, et al. Value of ventilation/perfusion scans versus perfusion scans alone in acute pulmonary embolism. Am J Cardiol 1992;69:1239–1241.

80. Tow DE, Wagner HW. Recovery of pulmonary arterial blood flow in patients with PE. N Engl J Med 1967;276:1053–1059.

81. Winebright JW, Gerdes AJ, Nelp WB. Restoration of blood flow after PE. Arch Intern Med 1970;125:241–247.

82. Meignan M, Palmer EL, Waltman AC, Strauss HW. Zones of increased perfusion (hot spots) on perfusion lung scans: correlation with pulmonary arteriograms. Radiology 1989;173:47–52.

83. Stein PD, Henry JW, Gottschalk A. The addition of clinical assessment to stratification according to prior cardiopulmonary disease further optimizes the interpretation of V/Q lung scans in PE. Chest 1993;104:1471–1476.

84. Frankel N, Coleman RE, Pryor DB, et al. Utilization of lung scans by clinicians. J Nucl Med 1986;27:366–369.

85. Stein PD, Hull RD, Saltzman HA, Pineo G. Strategy for diagnosis of patients with suspected acute pulmonary embolism. Chest 1993;103:1553–1559.

86. Davidson BL, Elliot CG, Lensing AWA. Low accuracy of color doppler ultrasound in the detection of proximal leg vein thrombosis in asymptomatic high risk patients. Ann Intern Med 1992;117:735–738.

87. Quinn RJ, Nour R, Butler SP, et al. Pulmonary embolism in patients with intermediate probability lung scans: diagnosis with doppler venous US and D-dimer measurement. Radiology 1994;190:509–511.

88. Hull RD, Raskob GE, Pineo GF, Brant RF. The low probability scan: a need for change of nomenclatures. Ann Intern Med 1995;155:1845–1851.

89. Hull RD, Feldstein W, Stein PD, Rineo GF. Cost-effectiveness of PE diagnosis. Arch Intern Med 1996;156:68–72.
90. Gurney JW. No fooling around: direct visualization of pulmonary embolism. Radiology 1993;188:618–619.
91. Gefter WB, Hatabu H, Holland GA, et al. Pulmonary thromboembolism: recent developments in diagnosis with CT and MR imaging. Radiology 1995;197:561–574.
92. Oser RF, Zuckerman DA, Gutierrez FR. Anatomic distribution of pulmonary emboli at pulmonary angiography: implications for cross-sectional imaging. Radiology 1996;199:31–35.
93. Erdman WA, Peshock RM, Redman HC, et al. Pulmonary embolism: comparison of MR images with radionuclide and angiographic studies. Radiology 1994;190:499–508.
94. Goodman LR, Lipckik RJ. Diagnosis of acute pulmonary embolism: time for a new approach. Radiology 1996;199:25–27.
95. Krasnow AZ, Isitman AT, Collier BD, et al. Diagnostic application of radioaerosols in nuclear medicine. In Freeman LM (ed), Nuclear Medicine Annual 1993. New York: Raven, 1993;123–193.
96. O'Doherty MJ, Miller RF. Aerosols for therapy and diagnosis. Eur J Nucl Med 1993;20:1201–1213.
97. Taplin GV, Poe ND. A dual lung scanning technique for evaluation of pulmonary function. Radiology 1965;85:365–368.
98. Isitman AT, Manoli R, Schmidt DH, et al. An assessment of alveolar deposition and pulmonary clearance of radiopharmaceuticals after nebulization. AJR Am J Roentgenol 1974;120:776–781.
99. Lu G, Shih W-J, Chonc Xu J-Y. Tc-99m MAA total-body imaging to detect intrapulmonary right-to-left shunts and to evaluate the therapeutic effect in pulmonary arteriovenous shunts. Clin Nucl Med 1996;19:197–202.
100. Levin DP, Pison CF, Brandt M, et al. Reversal of intrapulmonary shunting in cirrhosis after liver transplantation demonstrated by perfusion lung scan. J Nucl Med 1991;32:862–864.

*Textbook of Nuclear Medicine,*
edited by Michael A. Wilson.
Lippincott–Raven Publishers, Philadelphia © 1998.

CHAPTER 5

# Genitourinary System

Scott B. Perlman, David L. Bushnell, and W. Earl Barnes

The noninvasive evaluation of renal structure and function has undergone numerous revisions and improvements since the days of the early radiopharmaceuticals, such as ytterbium 169 diethylenetriaminepentaacetic acid (DTPA) and carbon 14 inulin, used to estimate the glomerular filtration rate (GFR), and mercury 203 chlormerodrin, for renal morphology imaging. Current tracer methods used for the evaluation of renal physiology and anatomy represent significant advancements in these areas. These procedures are a significant part of the workload in many nuclear medicine departments and currently represent approximately 20% of the workload at the University of Wisconsin Hospital and Clinics (Table 5-1). This chapter reviews the use of radiopharmaceuticals for the evaluation of renal structure and function. For further information, the reader is referred to several excellent review articles (1–3).

## PHYSIOLOGY OVERVIEW

Renal function is assessed clinically by measurement of blood levels of metabolic products that are excreted renally, such as serum creatinine. This assessment is improved by the actual measurement of the material excreted in the urine, but such prolonged urine sampling (e.g., 24-hour creatinine clearance test) is unreliable because of urine collection difficulties. The tracer method can quantify renal function, and available imaging techniques can determine the relative contribution of each kidney to total function. The quantitative tests are based on two methods: renal clearance, which requires a plasma and urine collection, and plasma clearance, which assumes that tracer is excreted exclusively via the kidneys and therefore requires no urine collection. The most accurate forms of the tracer methods are, in order of accuracy, constant infusion techniques with urine collection, single injection with plasma and urine collection, plasma disappearance techniques with one or more blood samples, and gamma camera techniques.

The plasma clearance of tracer can be measured by two models. The two-compartment model explains the double-exponential plasma disappearance curve, the first compartment representing the volume into which the tracer is immediately distributed (~3 liters in an average adult) and the second representing the closed extravascular extracellular fluid (ECF) space (~11 liters) into which each tracer diffuses to a variable extent. Neither compartment is defined by a particular anatomic space but rather reflect a complex physiologic process. For measurement of GFR using the two-compartment model, multiple blood samples are required early (within minutes) and late (2 to 4 hours) after tracer injection. For effective renal plasma flow (ERPF) or tubular extraction rate (TER) measurements, both early (within minutes) and late (1- to 2-hour) blood samples are required. These highly accurate techniques are somewhat impractical because they require six or more blood samples, and the results are usually falsely elevated in patients with expanded ECF volumes.

Single mono-exponential compartment models (slope-intercept methods) are more practical for clinical use because they require only one or two samples. This method assumes that tracer is distributed in a single compartment and that only renal clearance occurs. The curve is similar to the second slope of the two-compartment model and has the same limitations, but the results obtained are less accurate.

## RADIOPHARMACEUTICALS

Radiopharmaceuticals used for tracer studies should ideally be inert and not metabolized by the kidney, and the kidney should be the only means of excretion of tracer. In practice, when a renal function tracer is injected intravenously (IV), it mixes with the distribution volume (e.g., in blood and ECF volumes): Some may be bound to proteins, some may move into the red blood cells (RBCs), and most should be cleared from the plasma by the kidney. These clearances can be measured by the rate of tracer disappearance from the plasma, tracer renal uptake, or tracer excretion by the kidney. Nuclear medicine techniques can use plasma

**TABLE 5-1.** *Renal examinations performed at University of Wisconsin Hospital and clinics*

| | |
|---|---|
| 56% | Renal transplant examinations |
| 15% | Combined renal and pancreas transplant examinations |
| 6% | Absolute GFR measurements |
| 10% | Diuretic renal examinations |
| 5% | Captopril renal examinations |
| 8% | Miscellaneous other examinations |

**TABLE 5-2.** *Dosimetry for renal cortical imaging agents*

| | Radiation exposure (rads) | |
|---|---|---|
| Tracer dose | Kidneys | Bladder wall |
| DTPA (20 mCi/740 MBq) | 1.80 | 2.30 |
| OIH (300 μCi/11 MBq) | 0.02 | 1.40 |
| MAG3 (10 mCi/370 MBq) | 0.15 | 4.40 |
| GH (20 mCi/740 MBq) | 3.40 | 2.40 |
| DMSA (6 mCi/222 MBq) | 3.78 | 0.42 |

Source: Various package inserts and Eshima D, Taylor A. Technetium-99m mercaptoacetyltriglycine: update on the new 99mTc renal tubular function agent. Semin Nucl Med 1992;22:61–73.

counting, renal uptake, or urine counting methods to provide a variety of ways of measuring renal function.

## Glomerular Function

Glomerular function can be thought of as similar to selective filtration. The GFR can be measured by a substance that is cleared only by glomerular filtration and is not secreted or reabsorbed (4). For the measurement of GFR, the radiopharmaceutical used must be available for glomerular filtration and not be bound to plasma proteins. Inulin is the gold standard of this technique: It is injected by constant infusion, and urinary clearance is measured.

### Technetium 99m DTPA

Technetium 99m (Tc-99m) DTPA, the preeminent glomerular agent, fulfills the first of these GFR requirements but has shown variable degrees of protein binding in certain commercial preparations (5,6), although apparently not in others (7–9). The effect of protein binding can be monitored or avoided by the ultrafiltration of blood samples (5,6). A second caveat is that an abnormal volume of distribution, as found, for example, in patients with edema, leads to inaccurate GFR determination.

### Other Agents

Another approved agent in the United States is iodine 125 iothalamate (Glofil). It is injected subcutaneously and so provides a relatively constant rate of release of tracer into the plasma, in a manner similar to constant infusion. Plasma and urine samples are then collected and measured. An agent used overseas but not approved by the U.S. Food and Drug Administration (FDA) is chromium 51 (Cr-51) ethylenediaminetetraacetic acid (EDTA), which functions similarly to Tc-99m DTPA.

## Renal Tubular Function

The kidneys receive approximately 25% of the cardiac output. The renal plasma flow (RPF) is equal to the renal blood flow multiplied by the proportion of blood that is plasma (i.e., 1 − hematocrit). Therefore, with the normal renal blood flow (RBF) of 1,000 to 1,200 ml per minute, the RPF is 600 to 700 ml per minute (10). Para-aminohippuric acid (PAH) is the gold standard clearance test used to determine RPF. Determining RPF requires a stable plasma level obtained by constant infusion of PAH. For various reasons, PAH is not completely cleared by the kidney, and approximately 10% of the arterial PAH remains in the renal vein. Thus, the estimation of RPF with this technique and other radiopharmaceuticals is referred to as the *effective* RPF (11).

Although the use of labeled PAH would be a sufficiently accurate method of estimating the ERPF, a suitable labeled form is not available. Other radiopharmaceuticals with similar handling by the kidneys are available, such as iodine 131 (I-131) orthoiodohippurate (OIH) and Tc-99m mercaptoacetyltriglycine (MAG3). These two radiopharmaceuticals have proved to be acceptable alternatives to PAH for the estimation of tubular function.

Radiation exposure to the kidneys and bladder wall from Tc-99m MAG3 and I-131 OIH is provided in Table 5-2 (12). It is important to note that these estimates were based on data from normal, healthy volunteers. Exposure levels are significantly greater in cases of renal pathology when renal uptake is spared but clearance is reduced, as occurs with early ureteric obstruction or acute tubular necrosis (ATN). In these instances, renal exposure is much lower using Tc-99m MAG3 rather than I-131 OIH, due to factors that include the longer half-life and the beta particle emission of I-131.

### Orthoiodohippurate

The mechanism of renal clearance of I-131 OIH is by GFR (~20%) and tubular secretion (~80%) (13). Stadalnik et al. have demonstrated the equivalent physiologic handling of both I-123 and I-131 OIH by the kidneys and shown them to be an adequate substitute for PAH (14). In the evaluation of ERPF, I-123 and I-131 OIH have important disadvantages. I-123 OIH is neither FDA approved nor commercially available, and I-131 OIH causes a relatively high radiation exposure to the kidneys and bladder, especially when the clearance is delayed, as in ATN or urinary tract obstruction (see Table 13-1). Image quality suffers

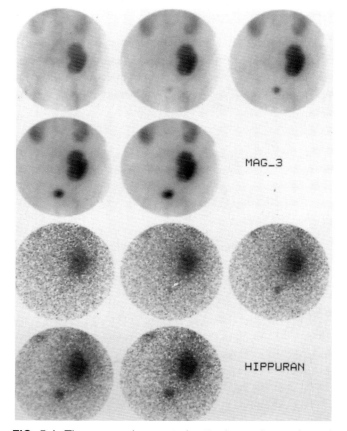

MAG_3

HIPPURAN

**FIG. 5-1.** The scans show anterior 5-minute views of renal transplant study with left pelvic transplant kidney. The MAG3 study shows the renal outline well (including unusual indentation near upper pole), whereas the OIH study (lower two rows) shows the scan appearance with Hippuran. The poorer uptake shows less anatomy, and the unusual shape seen with MAG3 is not apparent. The patient's native kidneys are visualized by the MAG3 study, despite considerable attenuation, and are barely shown on the OIH study.

from the fact that I-131 is not suited to gamma camera crystal thickness (and therefore efficiency) and that relatively small doses of I-131 OIH are administered to keep the patient's exposure to an acceptable level, resulting in inadequate statistics to obtain renal flow data. The administered dose of I-123 OIH is larger than that of I-131 OIH because of its more favorable exposure characteristics, thus resulting in better image quality.

### Tc-99m MAG3

Tc-99m MAG3 is a new radiotracer with similar renal clearance properties to OIH but with the advantages of lower radiation exposure to the patient and significantly improved imaging characteristics (Fig. 5-1) because of the MAG3 (mertiatide) Tc-99m label. This radiotracer is prepared from a kit, thereby making it readily available (although quite expensive) in nuclear medicine departments with an on-site radiopharmacy. The reconstituted kit is stable for up to 6

**TABLE 5-3.** Salient features that contribute to plasma clearance of MAG3 and OIH

| Steady-state studies | MAG3 | OIH |
|---|---|---|
| Tubular extraction efficiency | 50–60% | 90% |
| Glomerular contribution | 11% | 27% |
| Overall clearance | 0.67 | 1.00 |
| Volume of distribution | Smaller | Larger |
| Tracer protein binding | 80–90% | 50–70% |
| Tracer RBC uptake | 5% | 15% |
| Hepatobiliary excretion | | |
|     Normal renal function | 3% | 0% |
|     Renal impairment | 10% | 0% |

Sources: Taylor A, Nally JV. Clinical applications of renal scintigraphy. AJR Am J Roentgenol 1995;164:31–41; Peters AM. Quantification of renal haemodynamics with radionuclides. Eur J Nucl Med 1991;18:274–286; and Eshima D, Taylor A. Technetium-99m mercaptoacetyltriglycine: update on the new 99mTc renal tubular function agent. Semin Nucl Med 1992;22:61–73.

hours (12). Tc-99m MAG3 has an extraction fraction that is approximately 60% to 70% that of OIH, due to lower GFR and lower tubular secretion rate. From their review of the literature, Eshima and Taylor (12) reported a strong linear correlation between the clearance of the kit formulation of MAG3 and of OIH. The specific differences between MAG3 and OIH are listed in Table 5-3, but the renogram curves are comparable (12).

A direct measurement of the ERPF is not obtained with MAG3 because its renal clearance is lower than that of OIH (12). However, the renal clearance of MAG3 can be calculated and appears to provide useful information in the objective assessment of renal function.

### Evaluation of the Renal Cortex

The two radiopharmaceuticals typically used for the functional evaluation of the renal cortex are Tc-99m dimercaptosuccinic acid (DMSA) and Tc-99m glucoheptonate (GH).

DMSA reaches a high concentration in the renal cortex and has a slow urinary excretion rate. Although the renal concentration of GH is not as high as DMSA at 1, 3, or 6 hours, blood clearance and urinary excretion are faster (15). Approximately 50% of the injected dose of DMSA is localized in the kidneys at 1 hour, and >70% eventually accumulates in the kidneys (16), where it is bound to the renal proximal tubular cells (17). It has been estimated that approximately 20% of the injected dose of GH is bound to the renal tubular cells, the majority being cleared by glomerular filtration (17). Both radiopharmaceuticals are useful for imaging the renal parenchyma (Table 5-4). A stable form of DMSA, released in 1995, increases the time the radiotracer can be administered after preparation. The kit shelf life expires approximately 3 months after manufacturing and is therefore expensive to keep in stock if not frequently used. GH, on the other hand, has a longer shelf life,

**TABLE 5-4.** *Radiopharmaceuticals used for renal cortical imaging*

|  | GH | DMSA |
|---|---|---|
| Tubular binding | 10–20% | 40–60% |
| Glomerular excretion | Significant | Minimal |

is stable after kit reconstitution, and, according to the package insert, can be used for up to 6 hours after reconstitution.

## QUANTITATIVE RENAL FUNCTION

### Glomerular Filtration Rate

A variety of nuclear medicine procedures exist for the simple, noninvasive measurement of relative (split) or global (total) GFR. These fall into two broad categories: blood sampling and gamma camera methods. The blood sampling methods measure global GFR accurately, whereas the camera methods measure relative renal function. Because these procedures do not require the continuous infusion of radiotracer or urine collection, they are practical for clinical use, but because actual renal excretion is not measured, these methods do not work if the model constraints are exceeded (e.g., volume expansion or significant renal impairment). Their accuracy exceeds that of creatinine clearance, particularly in patients with mild to moderate renal dysfunction (18,19).

### *Blood Sample Techniques*

Of the methods suitable for general clinical use, blood sample tests are a more accurate way of measuring the GFR than are gamma camera methods. Single- and double-sample single-compartment methods exist, and both have been shown to provide sufficient accuracy for most clinical purposes. A gamma well counter and personnel with the appropriate laboratory skills, including proficiency testing for the purposes of the Clinical Laboratory Improvement Act of 1988, are required.

In the single-sample test, blood is drawn approximately 3 hours after the IV administration of DTPA, and the counts per minute (cpm) per ml are compared to that administered. The error in the single-sample test is approximately 8 ml per minute (8,9,20). At low GFR levels the test is inaccurate, and for these cases the two-sample method or a urine sampling method (21,22) is more appropriate. Two-sample tests require that blood be drawn at approximately 1 and 3 hours after DTPA administration. The advantage of the double-sample method is an error of only 4 ml per minute (6,8,9,20), which approaches the accuracy of two-compartment model tests using multiple samples. Two-sample tests are not as susceptible to error at low GFR levels as are single-sample tests.

### *Gamma Camera Methods*

Because of potential speed and convenience, the gamma camera method of Gates (23–25) is widely used, and many gamma camera manufacturers supply this software. A critical component of this test is the background subtraction, given the low renal clearance associated with purely glomerular filtration. Unfortunately, this method is substantially less accurate than blood sampling methods, although its accuracy compares favorably with that of creatinine clearance. It is recommended that each user validate the method on his or her own system against the commonly accepted clinical tests at her hospital, such as the 24-hour creatinine clearance. The reproducibility of gamma camera GFR measurements, particularly at higher clearances, is good in some laboratories. Serial changes in individual patient measurements can be reliably followed with this technique.

In the Gates method, renal uptake during the second through third minute after injection of DTPA is acquired by drawing regions of interest (ROIs) around the kidneys and applying appropriate background correction. A standard dose must be counted by the gamma camera system to normalize for camera sensitivity. Depth attenuation correction for right and left kidney counts is made on the basis of a formula involving body height and weight, and a regression formula allows the calculation of the GFR. Substantial inaccuracy occurs in this measurement if the correct weight and height are not used in the calculation. The advantage of this renal imaging method is the ability to calculate the differential (relative or split) GFR for each kidney.

### Effective Renal Plasma Flow

RPF can be measured if the tracer is quantitatively (completely) extracted by the kidney on the first passage through the kidney and if no other organ clears the plasma of this tracer. The gold standard for this measurement is PAH, but even with this agent the extraction efficiency is only 90%. OIH is an ERPF agent with an extraction efficiency of approximately 80%, and MAG3 (extraction efficiency of 50% to 60%) can be used to obtain tubular extraction rates. Measuring tubular extraction by ERPF or TER is probably better than by RPF, because tubular injury and certain drugs (e.g., angiotensin-converting enzyme [ACE] inhibitors, cyclosporine) may decrease the tracer clearance without significant alterations in RPF.

### *Blood Sample Techniques*

The clearance of OIH and MAG3 can be measured with a single blood sample drawn at approximately 44 minutes after injection. This shorter delay (compared to Tc-99m DTPA) is due to the more rapid blood clearance of tracer. These tracers are relatively highly protein bound, so they do

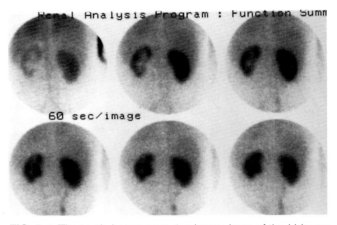

**FIG. 5-7.** These six images are 1-minute views of the kidneys with MAG3. The photopenic defect in the left intrarenal collecting system is obvious in the first 1 to 3 minutes and fills later. Such collecting system activity could imitate renal cortical activity retention.

one of the largest investigations to date, Fommei et al. (37) examined the usefulness the captopril renal scan in a multicenter trial involving 380 patients with hypertension. In patients with normal renal function, a sensitivity of 86% and specificity of 93% were reported for the identification of a RAS ≥70%, and a sensitivity of 93% and specificity of 100% for predicting the blood pressure response to intervention. Kahn et al. used MAG3 captopril renal scintigraphy to separate patients with renovascular hypertension from those with a hemodynamically insignificant RAS (38).

### Summary

In summary, renal scintigraphy using ACE inhibition is a useful method of diagnosing renovascular hypertension, and early data suggest that the test may hold important information about the likelihood of blood pressure control after correction of the stenotic lesion. The classic abnormal scan is prolonged cortical retention with ACE inhibitor, but care must be taken to exclude tracer in the collecting system while including all possible cortical activity. In this respect dilated collecting systems can be a problem, but these are apparent as photopenic defects in the first few images (Fig. 5-7). Thus, the captopril renal scan may represent the physiologic gold standard for the evaluation of patients with possible renovascular hypertension.

## Urinary Tract Obstruction

Urinary tract obstruction can lead to severe impairment in renal function, which may become irreversible. The likelihood of renal damage depends on the severity and duration of the obstruction. Complete urinary tract obstruction may lead to permanent renal damage in less than 1 week, so significant obstruction should be identified promptly for early correction.

Diuretic renal scintigraphy has found widespread use and popularity for the diagnosis of urinary tract obstruction (39). This is largely because it is a relatively simple noninvasive technique that can accurately identify the abnormal urodynamics associated with mechanical obstruction. Other imaging modalities, such as ultrasound (US), commonly used in the assessment of urinary tract obstruction provide anatomic urinary tract information but are incapable of distinguishing obstructed hydronephrotic collecting systems from ones that are merely dilated and not obstructed. These anatomic imaging techniques are unsuccessful in the early stages (approximately within the first 24 hours) of acute urinary tract obstruction, when the collecting system may not have enlarged significantly. In both scenarios, the presence or absence of an obstructing process can often be determined using diuretic renal scintigraphy.

### Radiopharmaceuticals

Although DTPA and I-131 and I-123 OIH have been used extensively over the years for diuretic renal scintigraphy, MAG3 now appears to be the radiopharmaceutical of choice (40,41). This agent combines the advantages of imaging with the favored Tc-99m photon with a relatively high level of radiopharmaceutical uptake by the kidneys due to the combination of glomerular filtration and tubular secretion. The disadvantage is the huge increase in radiopharmaceutical cost over both DTPA and I-131 OIH. The administered activity of MAG3 for diuretic renal scintigraphy should be 50 to 100 μCi/kg for adults and 50 μCi/kg in infants and children, in whom radiation exposure is more of a concern.

### Test Rationale

In the presence of a dilated urinary collecting system, abnormal stasis of urine occurs, even in the absence of obstruction. This is due to a reservoir effect, when urine pools in the dilated collecting system. A renal scintigraphic study performed in such a patient without a diuretic may demonstrate retention of radiopharmaceutical in the hydronephrotic renal pelvis or ureter, even though the urinary tract is patent. The corresponding urinary time-activity curve (renogram) shows a progressive rise and eventual plateau of tracer. However, if urine output from the kidney is sufficient, there should eventually be tracer clearance from the unobstructed dilated system. The images and renogram would then depict a fall in the total radiotracer in the collecting system, signifying that the system is patent.

Initially, abnormal scans with the progressively rising renogram pattern described above were repeated after hydration to produce an adequate urine flow rate. Renograms that normalized after hydration were not considered obstructed. A more reproducible way to ensure an adequate urine output is to administer a diuretic, such as furosemide. The diuretic action of furosemide begins 3 to 5

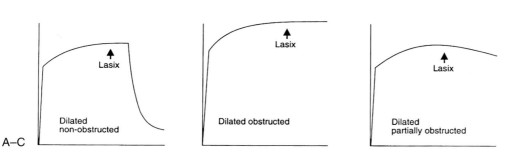

FIG. 5-8. (A) This renogram is a dilated, unobstructed system that shows a gradual rise in activity followed by an abrupt and substantial exponential fall after the diuretic furosemide (Lasix) is given. (B) This renogram is that of an obstructed collecting system showing no decrease in activity after furosemide administration. (C) This renogram is a partially obstructed system, which shows slight fall in activity after furosemide administration.

minutes after injection and is maximal at 20 minutes. In a normally functioning kidney, activity in the urinary tract typically begins to clear within 3 to 5 minutes of intravenous diuretic administration (Fig. 5-8A), although the time depends somewhat on the degree of hydronephrosis and the patient's renal function.

The presence of obstruction alters the effect that a diuretic has on the clearance of urine from the collecting system. In the presence of a true obstructing process, radioactive urine progressively accumulates proximal to the site of obstruction and the renogram progressively rises and then plateaus. This is essentially indistinguishable from the curve obtained in a patient with a hydronephrotic nonobstructed system before furosemide is administered (Fig. 5-8B). The effect of furosemide administration on the renogram is minimal in the presence of complete or high-grade obstruction. If the obstruction is partial, there may be a very modest fall in activity after the diuretic is given (Fig. 5-8C). In long-standing high grade obstruction with renal impairment, the renal concentration of the radiopharmaceutical may be substantially reduced, even to the point that an adequate examination will not be possible.

Many aspects of the methodology for performing diuretic renal scintigraphy have not been well standardized. This may in part explain findings that have been used by some authors to question the reliability of the method for detecting urinary tract obstruction (42). A consortium of experts in this area developed methodologic recommendations that should help to achieve better uniformity in the results obtained with this procedure. Conway published the consensus opinion of this group, and the reader is encouraged to refer to this important discussion of diuretic renal scintigraphy (40).

Adequate hydration is essential for two reasons: (1) to ensure that the results from this procedure are reliable and reproducible and (2) to ensure that the patient does not become hypotensive after the diuresis induced by furosemide. In the presence of significant dehydration, the GFR may be diminished, thus limiting the potential diuretic effect of furosemide. Fluids should be given orally beginning at least 1 hour before the test is begun. For infants and children, it is recommended that a 25-gauge butterfly needle be used to administer 15 ml/kg of normal saline over 30 minutes, beginning 15 minutes before the study (40).

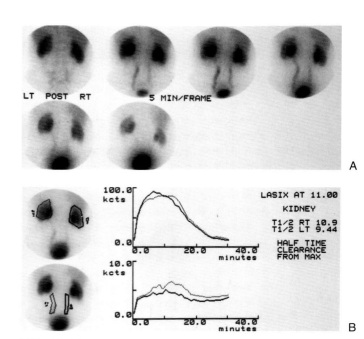

FIG. 5-9. The patient presents with a dilated left renal pelvis and suspected left ureteropelvic junction obstruction. (A) This series consists of six 5-minute images after injection of MAG3. (B) The lower series demonstrates renal and ureteric ROIs identified (left) and the time-activity curve (right) renograms obtained. Furosemide was administered at 11 minutes, and the left renogram promptly falls, thus ruling out obstruction (clearance half-time = 9.44 minutes).

### Scan Protocol

Imaging should be performed using a large–field-of-view gamma camera with a low-energy, high-resolution collimator. This allows simultaneous imaging of the upper and lower urinary tract. Zoom should be applied during image acquisition in children and infants in such a way as to maintain visualization of the entire urinary system (kidneys and bladder). Angiographic phase imaging is performed first. Thereafter, sequential images should be obtained with analog displays formatted based on the local preference of the interpreting physician. We prefer 5-minute images (Fig. 5-9).

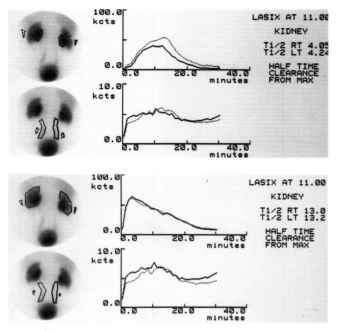

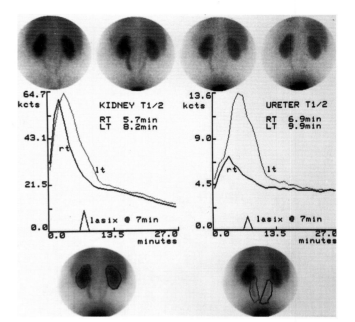

**FIG. 5-10.** These two image series (ROIs on left, renograms on right) of the patient in Fig. 5-9 show dramatically the effect of renal ROI selection. The ureteric renograms and ROIs (lower half of each series) are identical in the two series. The renal ROIs are different in these two series and different from that selected in Fig. 5-9. The lowermost series shows the renal cortical region (often selected for TER calculation) with nearly normal wash-out and no renogram suggestion of obstruction. The upper series shows the renal pelvic ROI only (often used in diuretic scans). It demonstrates a dilated and unobstructed pattern bilaterally, with a progressive rise and plateau until diuretic administration, at which time there is a prompt fall in activity (clearance half-time ~4 minutes). Note that the renogram of Fig. 5-9 is intermediate in pattern between these two renograms.

**FIG. 5-11.** The first four 5-minute MAG3 images are displayed on the top row. The renal pelvis and calyces are not dilated, but the left ureter appears dilated down to the junction of the middle and distal thirds. The renal and ureteric ROIs are displayed in the bottom row. The time-activity curves (renograms) are shown between the images, kidneys on the left and ureters on the right. There was spontaneous drainage of tracer in the renal ROI before furosemide administration (at 7 minutes) so the half-time values (calculated from peak activity) are not influenced by the furosemide. The ureteric ROIs show no abnormality on the right and an obstructive pattern on the left, that promptly clears with furosemide (half-time is normally <10 minutes), confirming a dilated but not obstructed pattern.

When the collecting system activity appears to be maximal on the side and at the site of the suspected obstruction, furosemide should be administered intravenously. Theoretically, the diuretic should not be given until MAG3 has been sufficiently cleared from the blood so that the diuretic response consists of urine that is largely nonradioactive (42). Some have given furosemide at the very beginning of the imaging procedure and found this approach to work well (43). Others routinely give the diuretic exactly 20 minutes after radiopharmaceutical administration, and yet others have administered the diuretic 15 minutes before the administration of tracer. Imaging is generally continued for at least 20 minutes after the diuretic injection (or in the latter protocol, radiopharmaceutical injection).

The consensus report referred to above suggests that the renogram be generated using different ROIs for the pre- and postdiuretic phases of the study (40). Specifically, it is recommended that an ROI encompass the entire kidney and collecting system for the prefurosemide phase to evaluate the relative renal function and that the ROI should probably include only the collecting system for the postdiuretic phase that assesses the dilated collecting system. In practice, most institutions use a single ROI, encompassing both kidney and proximal collecting system, for the entire study period (see Fig. 5-9). For specific assessment of relative renal function in the presence of urinary tract obstruction, it has been suggested that the ROI should be placed around the renal cortex only (Fig. 5-10), excluding the collecting system (44). In Figs. 5-9 and 5-10, the renal ROI selection dramatically affects the renogram shapes.

A separate ROI should be placed over the lower collecting system (ureters) if prior clinical information or images suggest that the obstruction is at the level of ureterovesical junction (42). This is necessary because the time-activity curve for renal pelvis activity alone may show decreasing counts as the urine empties into a dilated distal ureter after administration of the diuretic (Fig. 5-11).

### Normal Scans

A normal scan should show the normal rapid parenchymal uptake and filling of pelvocalyceal system, and the ureters are visualized. There is rapid clearance of the renal

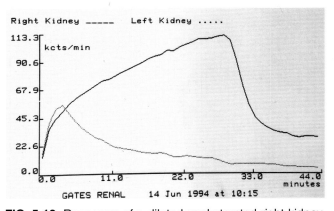

**FIG. 5-12.** Renogram of a dilated unobstructed right kidney. Hydronephrosis is shown on the images (not shown), and the early renogram shows an obstructive pattern. Furosemide was administered at 25 minutes, and there is very prompt wash-out of tracer, indicating a dilated, unobstructed collecting system.

parenchyma and collecting system, so by 20 minutes, using tubular extraction radiopharmaceuticals (e.g., MAG3), more than 70% of the injected dose is in the bladder, and the upper renal tract is only faintly visualized.

### Abnormal Scans

A number of quantitative parameters have been used in addition to the renogram shape in an effort to improve the accuracy of the renogram for detecting urinary tract obstruction. The PTT reflects the interval necessary for tracer to move through the renal cortex to the collecting system, but this is rather involved and requires deconvolution analysis, for which many laboratories do not have software. In an obstructed urinary system the PTT is typically prolonged (45), but because this may also be seen in other renal conditions, it is not specific for obstruction. Another renogram feature sometimes used in assessing urinary tract obstruction is the prolongation of the time at which activity in the kidney is maximal, referred to as $T_{max}$ or *time to peak activity.*

The most frequently used quantitative parameter is the clearance half-time (T-1/2), which represents the time interval after administration of the diuretic necessary for the activity in the dilated renal tract system to decrease by 50%. The interval should probably be measured starting from the point on the renogram at which furosemide is given. A value >20 minutes indicates obstruction, whereas it is generally accepted that a T-1/2 less than 7 to 10 minutes excludes a significant obstruction (42). Values for T-1/2 between 10 and 20 minutes are considered equivocal for obstruction. Although quantitative measures are important, the qualitative appearance of the renogram should also be assessed after diuretic administration. Typically, in the unobstructed system the curve begins to trace downward within 3 to 5 minutes of injection of furosemide (Fig. 5-12), and the appearance tends toward that of an exponential function

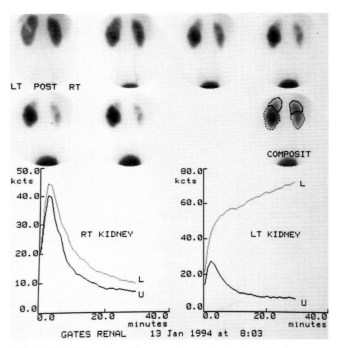

**FIG. 5-13.** This patient has a duplicated left collecting system, which on the images (upper two rows) is suggestive of obstruction of the lower portion. This patient received furosemide at the start of the study (decided from earlier scan). The right kidney (left renogram) is normal. The lower (L) system on the left kidney (right renogram) is obstructed, the upper (U) system drains relatively normally.

(46). In obstruction, the pattern is that of a continual rise or flattening (see Fig. 5-8B,C). The imaging procedure is uniquely suited to evaluation of different parts of the collecting system (e.g., pelvis vs. ureter; see Fig. 5-11) and the different portions of the kidney (e.g., duplicated system; Fig. 5-13).

### False-Positive Studies

In the presence of impaired renal function on the side being evaluated, the results from diuretic renal scintigraphy (especially the T-1/2) may not be reliable due to an inadequate diuretic response (47). We measure the urine output and calculate a urine flow rate, wishing to achieve a urine flow rate of at least 5 to 10 ml per minute after furosemide. Impaired renal function may lead to an interpretation of obstruction, when in fact the collecting system is patent. In cases of severe renal impairment, the collecting system may never visualize at all, making it impossible to ascertain whether obstruction is present. In some cases it is known before the procedure that the patient has impaired renal function, but if impaired function is unilateral, the serum creatinine may be normal. When it becomes apparent that function is abnormal in the potentially obstructed kidney, increased doses of diuretic may be needed, in consultation with the referring physician. If the collecting system shows no wash-out, the patient should be placed upright and if possible ambulated for at least 5 min-

**TABLE 5-5.** *Diuretic renography technique*

| Problems | Possible solutions |
|---|---|
| Poor renal function | Increase diuretic dose. Test may not be possible. |
| Inadequate hydration | Patient safety concerns Ensure adequate hydration. |
| Very dilated collecting system | Delayed images may be helpful. Increase dose. |
| Large noncompliant bladder | Collecting system may not drain. Consider a catheter and upright postvoid images. |
| Ureteric reflux | Consider bladder catheter. |

utes. After this, images of the kidneys are taken to assess the effect of these postural drainage maneuvers on the dilated collecting system and urine drainage (48).

In neonates, renal function may be quite variable as the kidneys slowly mature after birth. Consequently, the diuretic response to furosemide in this group of patients may be unpredictable. Therefore, it has been recommended that hydronephrotic infants (often diagnosed by US prenatally) <1 month in age are not suitable candidates for diuretic renal scintigraphy (40) (see Chapter 11).

In extremely dilated collecting systems, even a good diuretic response to furosemide may be insufficient to clear the dilated (but patent) pelvis or ureter in <20 minutes, resulting in a potentially FP result. A study comparing diuretic renal scintigraphy to the Whitaker test in patients with urinary tract obstruction and varying degrees of hydronephrosis found only a 58% agreement between the two methods when the collecting system volume exceeded 70 ml, compared to an 88% agreement when the collecting system volume was <30 ml (47). Consequently, interpretation of prolonged urinary retention in individuals with very large collecting systems should be done with caution (48).

A noncompliant bladder (usually because it is full of urine) may generate sufficient back pressure in a normal patent urinary system to create the appearance of obstruction on the renogram. In this setting, postvoid images can be used to demonstrate the patency of the urinary tract. For this reason, in infants and children a bladder catheter may be necessary. Significant vesicoureteral reflux (VUR) may make it very difficult to interpret the examination correctly: It may appear obstructed because of the reflux of radioactive urine from the bladder. A bladder catheter can help to eliminate this cause of an FP result.

### Summary

In conclusion, diuretic renal scintigraphy is a valuable tool for the assessment of the patency of the urinary tract. However, it is crucial that careful attention be given to the methodology of the procedure and that the interpreting physician has a good understanding of the potential pitfalls (Table 5-5) associated with this methodology.

### Acute Pyelonephritis

Acute pyelonephritis classically presents with fever, flank pain and tenderness, elevated white blood cell (WBC) count, and pyuria. In many cases (particularly in children) the presentation is not as well defined: Patients with upper urinary tract infection often present with signs and symptoms confined to the lower urinary tract. Consequently, a diagnosis of acute pyelonephritis based on clinical and basic laboratory findings may be unreliable. Sophisticated laboratory methods, such as the antibody-coated bacteria test and detection of serum antibodies directed against the O antigen of the infecting strain, are not sufficiently accurate to be used on a routine basis. A number of imaging modalities have also been used in this setting, and evidence is emerging that renal cortical scintigraphy is probably the gold standard for diagnosis of acute pyelonephritis (49).

Although most cases of treated acute pyelonephritis resolve without any long-term sequelae, improperly treated patients may develop renal scarring, hypertension, and loss of renal function. These adverse sequelae occur most often in children, diabetics, and patients with preexisting renal disease. In these patient categories, it is critical to establish a timely and accurate diagnosis of pyelonephritis because cortical scarring can be avoided with prompt and appropriate therapy (50,51).

### Radiopharmaceuticals

Renal images obtained with either DMSA or GH typically demonstrate focal sites of diminished activity when acute pyelonephritis is present (Fig. 5-14). The cortical

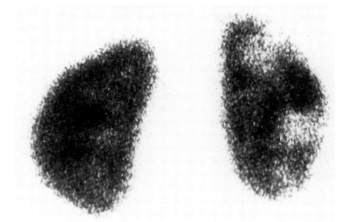

**FIG. 5-14.** Posterior images of Tc-99m DMSA renal activity in a 4-year-old with suspected acute pyelonephritis. Images show three focal regions of decreased DMSA in the right kidney consistent with infection. (Reprinted with permission from Majd M, Rushton HG. Renal cortical scintigraphy in the diagnosis of acute pyelonephritis. Semin Nucl Med 1992; 22:98–111. Copyright 1991, W.B. Saunders.)

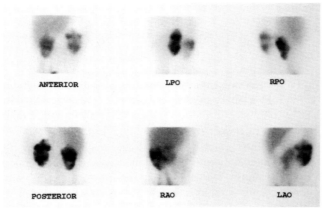

ANTERIOR   LPO   RPO

POSTERIOR   RAO   LAO

**FIG. 5-15.** These images were obtained using a triple-headed camera and show extensive scarring of both kidneys. GH was used, and the liver is visualized.

retention of DMSA is approximately 60% of the injected activity, compared to 20% for GH. Consequently, to achieve similar activity levels in the renal cortex for equivalent imaging, the recommended administered activity for glucoheptonate (150 µCi/kg) is three times that of DMSA (50 µCi/kg).

### Scan Protocol

Imaging commences 90 to 120 minutes after injection and should consist of posterior and posterior oblique planar images using a high-resolution, parallel-hole collimator. In children it is desirable to obtain magnified images with a converging collimator, and for infants a pinhole collimator is appropriate. Single photon emission computed tomography (SPECT) imaging, particularly with the imaging triple detector machines equipped with ultrahigh-resolution collimators, will probably become the method of choice. To date, however, few prospective studies have been performed directly comparing the accuracy of state-of-the-art SPECT to planar imaging for detection of acute upper urinary tract infection.

### Scan Results

#### Normal Scans

The tracer should be evenly distributed through the renal cortical parenchyma. There may be some mild variation in outline, but no definite defects should be apparent.

#### Abnormal Scans

Defects may be single or multiple, unilateral or bilateral, and they are associated with preservation of kidney volume when acute. A regional decrease in kidney size suggests scarring or a chronic process (Fig. 5-15). Less commonly, a generalized decrease in radiopharmaceutical concentration is present in a kidney extensively involved with the acute pyelonephritic process. When a diffuse decrease in renal activity is detected, the kidney should still appear normal in size or even slightly enlarged if acutely infected. The cause of the diminished renal uptake of either DMSA or GH in the presence of pyelonephritis is related primarily to two mechanisms: decreased blood flow to the infected region limiting tracer availability, and direct infectious tubular cell injury impairing tubular tracer uptake.

Studies in animals with experimentally induced acute pyelonephritis show that DMSA has a very high sensitivity (~90%) (52,53). Planar cortical scintigraphy with Tc-99m DMSA has been compared to both intravenous pyelogram (IVP) and US and found to be significantly more accurate than either for detecting acute pyelonephritis (54,55).

Other scintigraphic procedures, such as gallium 67 and WBC imaging, can also be helpful in identifying acute pyelonephritis. Drawbacks of these methods are the extended time required before obtaining results and greater radiation doses (a special concern in children). These procedures may be useful in cases in which the results from cortical scintigraphy are equivocal.

### Other Indications

#### Renal Masses Found by Other Modalities

Renal masses and pseudomasses are often identified by anatomic imaging modalities, such as computed tomography, US, and IVP. The function of the mass is important because normal kidneys may have an unusual anatomic configuration, with unusual-shaped areas of normal tracer uptake, which may represent:

- Pseudotumor
- Dromedary hump (Fig. 5-16)
- Fetal lobulation
- Hypertrophied column of Bertin
- Horseshoe kidney

Other renal masses, such as a renal cell carcinoma, cyst, abscess, metastasis, nephroblastoma, or an area of ischemia, demonstrate absent renal function. Functional renal imaging may help to determine if further investigation, such as a renal biopsy, is necessary.

One of the earliest series examining the usefulness of functional renal imaging to evaluate renal masses used mercury 197 chlormerodrin (56). Subjects are now studied after the IV administration of 15 mCi (550 MBq) of GH followed by planar images of the kidneys, including posterior oblique views. Good sensitivity and specificity are found, but caution must be used in the interpretation of defects in the peripelvic region, where the hilar structures or fat can produce sizable defects (57). DMSA is also an excellent radio-

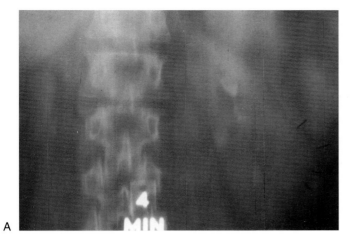

A

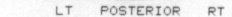

B

**FIG. 5-16. (A)** This anteroposterior IVP image shows a dromedary hump involving the left kidney (*lines*). **(B)** The renal configuration on the GH posterior image corresponds exactly with the IVP and has normal functioning renal tissue in the region of the distorted renal outline. This indicates that the region contains normal kidney tissue.

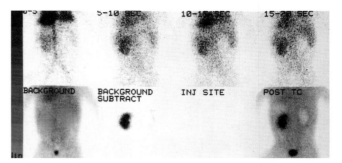

**FIG. 5-17.** This study of an infant shows fair perfusion to the left kidney but a void (photopenic defect) where the right kidney was known to be. The flow study and delayed (post-technetium) images demonstrate absent perfusion and function of the right kidney. This patient's right renal artery was encased by tumor and needed subsequent resection.

pharmaceutical for evaluation of the renal parenchyma, and it can also be used to provide important information about tissue function. SPECT imaging for the evaluation of the renal parenchyma often adds useful information in the evaluation of renal parenchymal function. Examples of when SPECT may be especially useful include the identification of a hypertrophied column of Bertin, better identification of functional renal tissue in a horseshoe kidney, and identification of hematomas or renal infarcts (58).

### Acute Renal Failure

In some patients with acute renal failure (ARF) a perfusion study combined with a TER study using MAG3 can identify potential renal vascular compromise (Fig. 5-17) or urinary tract obstruction and tubular dysfunction. Tubular dysfunction is assessed by stasis of MAG3 in the tubular cells and an abnormal renogram (prolonged tracer stasis with little or no excretion). In patients in whom hypotension was significant and prolonged, this study can separate ATN from acute cortical necrosis. In ATN, perfusion is modestly reduced and cortical uptake is good but there is no excretion, whereas in acute cortical necrosis, flow is severely reduced with virtually no cortical uptake. In patients with ARF, the demonstration of more activity in the kidney than the liver at 1 to 3 minutes using MAG3 indicates that recovery will occur in most, whereas when there is less renal than hepatic uptake of MAG3, dialysis is likely required (59).

### Trauma

At one time, nuclear imaging was important in assessing renal trauma, but the availability of CT has made this redundant. However, the scan can provide an opportunity for following improvement, which is manifest by improving perfusion and function. This can be important when deciding whether a seriously injured and fragmented kidney is worth salvaging. The determination that the fragments are still perfused and have tubular function and that the tracer excretion is occurring without significant extravasation provides an indication for conservative management.

### Ectopic or Dysplastic Kidneys

Sometimes standard imaging procedures cannot localize both kidneys or cannot determine whether some tissue region represents a dysplastic kidney. In these cases, MAG3 imaging may identify the tissue to be a functioning kidney. At times SPECT may be helpful.

### SCROTAL SCINTIGRAPHY

The testicles receive their blood supply from the testicular arteries. These arteries, along with veins, lym-

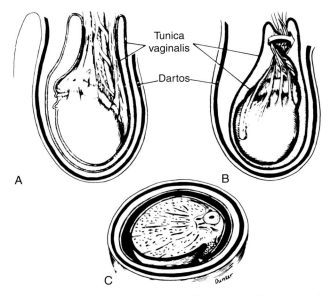

Tunica
vaginalis

Dartos

A

B

C

**FIG. 5-18. (A,B)** The tunica vaginalis completely surrounds the testis and epididymis (bell clapper variation). **(C)** The twist in the spermatic cord leads to testicular torsion. (Reproduced with permission from Holder LE, Melloul M, Chen D. Current status of radionuclide scrotal imaging. Semin Nucl Med 1981;11:232–249.)

phatics, nerves, and the deferent ducts, are located in the spermatic cord (60). In the normal anatomic situation, the epididymis is attached to the testis, and the posterior aspect of the epididymis is attached to the scrotum. The attachment of the epididymis to the scrotum prevents rotation of the testicle within the scrotal sac. The tunica vaginalis covers the testis and the anterolateral aspect of the epididymis. Occasionally, the tunica vaginalis completely surrounds the testis and epididymis, so the testicle and epididymis have no attachment to the scrotum and hang freely in the vaginal sac like a clapper in a bell (Fig. 5-18). This anatomic situation, known as the *bell clapper variation* (61), allows the testis to rotate within the scrotal sac, twisting the spermatic cord and cutting off the testicular blood supply. The early diagnosis and treatment of testicular torsion is important because necrotic changes depend on the duration of ischemia, number of twists in the spermatic cord, and how tightly the arteries within the spermatic cord are compressed (62). Testicular torsion may result in a nonviable testicle if not promptly corrected; hence, it is a surgical emergency. Salvage rates depend on the length of time between onset of symptoms and operation (62). Included in the differential diagnosis of the patient with acute scrotal pain are testicular torsion, epididymitis, orchitis, torsion of the testicular appendix, torsion of the epididymis, and abscess. Thus, it is important that once the diagnosis is considered, the test being used for the confirmation of the torsion must be rapidly available, so that

subsequent surgery will have the best chance of successful revascularization of the testicle.

## Scan Protocol

A rapid, noninvasive technique for evaluation of the blood supply to the testicle is scrotal scintigraphy. The procedure used for testicular scintigraphy has the patient lying supine, with a thin piece of lead placed under the scrotum to attenuate activity from the thighs. Some protocols advocate not using the lead foil under the scrotum for the angiogram phase, because of the importance of evaluating the neighboring major vessels. The penis is taped up to the anterior abdominal wall, away from the scrotum. Tc-99m $TcO_4^-$, 15 to 20 mCi (550 to 740 MBq), is administered as an IV bolus, and dynamic data are acquired for the first minute. Next, a series of static images are acquired for 1 minute each. It is helpful to mark the location of each testicle within the scrotal sac using a radioactive marker, noting the painful side. The converging collimator should be used for adults, and a pinhole collimator is recommended for children.

## Scan Results

### Normal Scans

The findings in scrotal imaging have been described by Holder et al. (61). In the early angiographic phase, the iliac

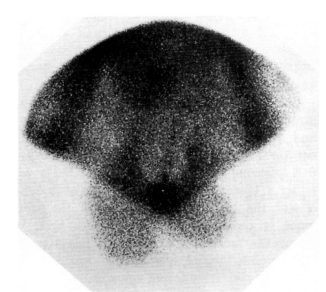

**FIG. 5-19.** Normal scrotal scan. Lead is placed beneath the scrotum in this magnified view. Symmetric activity is present in each scrotum. The mild size asymmetry is within normal limits. (Reproduced with permission from Holder LE, Melloul M, Chen D. Current status of radionuclide scrotal imaging. Semin Nucl Med 1981;11:232–249.)

**TABLE 5-6.** *Scrotal scans*

| Problem | Scan findings |
| --- | --- |
| Acute testicular torsion | Photopenic defect on flow images. Nubbin sign in delays. |
| Late (missed) torsion | Symmetrical halo and central "cold" defect. |
| Epididymitis | Increased flow to painful side. Increased activity laterally in scrotum. |
| Epididymo-orchitis | Increased flow and broad area of increased asymmetric activity. |

and femoral arteries can be clearly defined, but little activity is present in the scrotal area. The normal scrotum and contents have radiotracer activity equal to that in the thigh on the postflow images (Fig. 5-19).

### Abnormal Scans

It is important to know the painful side when interpreting the scan, as unilateral epididymitis or epididymo-orchitis may make the opposite side appear to have decreased flow.

Table 5-6 charts the problems and scintigraphic findings described in the clinical applications below

### Acute Torsion

In acute torsion, a photopenic defect appears in the area of the avascular testicle on the images obtained after the arterial phase (Fig. 5-20), and a "nubbin sign" may be present on the angiogram images. The nubbin is thought to occur in early torsion of the testis, when a nubbin or bump of activity has been noted that extends medially from the iliac artery. This is thought to represent increased flow in the proximal spermatic cord vessels, extending to the site of the twisted spermatic cord (63).

### "Missed" Torsion

In late ("missed") testicular torsion, a symmetric halo of increased activity is present around a "cold" testicle (Fig. 5-21) due to hyperperfusion of the dartos, which has a separate blood supply than that of the testis. Activity around the spermatic cord may also be increased.

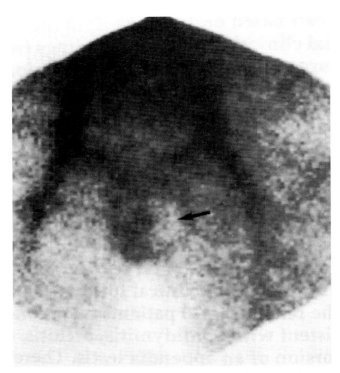

**FIG. 5-20.** An example of acute torsion. The static image shows the photopenic area (*arrow*) representing the torsive left testicle. (Reproduced with permission Middleton WD, Siegel BA, Melson GL, et al. Acute scrotal disorders: prospective comparison of color doppler US and testicular scintigraphy. Radiology 1990;177:177–181.)

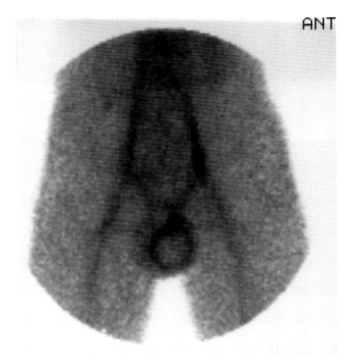

**FIG. 5-21.** An example of missed torsion in a teenager with left testicular pain. Clinical examination demonstrated an enlarged, swollen left testicle. The anterior static image demonstrates a photopenic area surrounded by a hyperperfused rim, consistent with a missed torsion of the left testicle. Surgery later the same day found a gangrenous left testicle. The right testicle was surgically fixated.

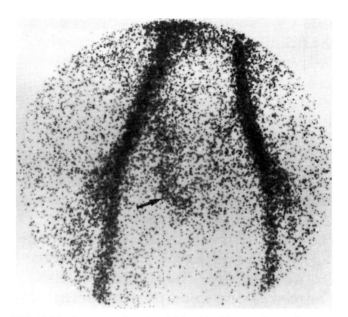

**FIG. 5-22.** An example of epididymitis. The early angiogram phase image shows the area of hyperperfusion in the lateral aspect of the right hemiscrotum (*arrow*). (Reproduced with permission from Middleton WD, Siegel BA, Melson GL, et al. Acute scrotal disorders: prospective comparison of color doppler US and testicular scintigraphy. Radiology 1990;177:177–181.)

### Epididymitis

With epididymitis, flow via the spermatic cord vessels is increased, and a linear area of increased activity (Fig. 5-22) is located asymmetrically in the scrotum (usually laterally). Epididymo-orchitis demonstrates a broader area of increased activity that is asymmetrically located within the scrotum (63).

### False-Negative Scans

A possible problem was described by Holder and coworkers. Normal scans were found in three patients with torsion of the appendix testicle or appendix epididymis, and this is thought to be due to the 2- to 4-mm appendix size being below the resolution limit of the imaging system (61).

### Other Results

Chen and coworkers retrospectively studied 46 patients with various scrotal diseases (64). The radionuclide technique was found to be superior to US, with reported sensitivities for US and scintigraphy in patients with acute scrotal pain (n = 17) of 47% and 94%, respectively, and subacute scrotal pain (n = 6) of 50% and 100%, respectively. Chen et al. concluded that the radionuclide technique should be the first study performed in patients with acute scrotal pain, but scrotal US should be used for patients presenting with a scrotal mass (64). In a more recent series, 28

patients with acute scrotal pain, swelling, or both were studied with both testicular scintigraphy and color Doppler US; seven patients had surgically confirmed testicular torsion. All seven patients had the correct diagnosis made with color Doppler US, and six of seven patients with testicular torsion were correctly diagnosed with testicular scintigraphy. No FP diagnoses were made with either technique (65). Thus, in this series it appears that testicular scintigraphy and color Doppler US are both accurate for the diagnosis of testicular torsion.

## RADIONUCLIDE CYSTOGRAMS

The direct radionuclide cystogram technique is a sensitive method of identifying VUR, as well as determining the residual urine remaining in the bladder after voiding. The technique can also be used to identify urine extravasation (see Chapter 13). The radiation exposure to the patient is very low, because radiotracer is placed in the bladder and then voided. The method results in approximately one-hundredth of the exposure to the bladder and ovaries, and one-two-hundredth of the exposure to the testes compared to the radiographic voiding cystourethrogram (66).

### Technique

A protocol for the procedure in adults is as follows: The patient should have a catheter in place and should lie supine on the table. The gamma camera is below the table with the kidneys, ureters, and bladder in the field of view. Tc-99m DTPA, 1 mCi (37 MBq), should be added to a 500-ml bag of sterile saline that has been warmed to body temperature. (Tc-99m $TcO_4^-$ can be used, but a significant amount may be absorbed through the bladder mucosa and outline the stomach in delayed images.) Dynamic computer acquisition is used at 1 frame per minute. The Tc-99m solution should be instilled into the bladder slowly until the bladder is filled. During filling of the bladder, the persistence scope should be carefully watched for evidence of VUR. If VUR is seen, the volume when VUR first occurred should be recorded. When the patient complains of bladder fullness, and with the catheter in place, the patient should attempt to void. Images should be acquired during voiding, and a postvoid image should be obtained. The volume of urine voided should be measured. The residual urine volume in the bladder is calculated (Fig. 5-23) using the formula below, and pre- and postvoid counts are obtained by selecting ROIs to include the bladder and subtracting the appropriate background from each:

$$\text{Residual volume} = \frac{\text{Voided volume} \times \text{postvoid counts}}{\text{Prevoid counts} - \text{postvoid counts}}$$

A second bladder filling should be performed if the first procedure is normal. To determine the bladder volume in the second fill, the residual volume calculated in the first bladder fill should be added to the volume instilled for the sec-

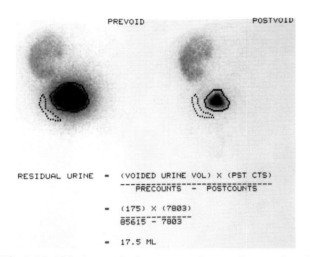

PREVOID                    POSTVOID

RESIDUAL URINE = (VOIDED URINE VOL) X (PST CTS)
                 ------------------------------------
                    PRECOUNTS - POSTCOUNTS

               = (175) X (7803)
                 --------------
                 85615 - 7803

               = 17.5 ML

**FIG. 5-23.** This image is from a renal transplant patient in whom a residual urine was calculated using IV tracer. The residual volume was measured at 17.5 ml.

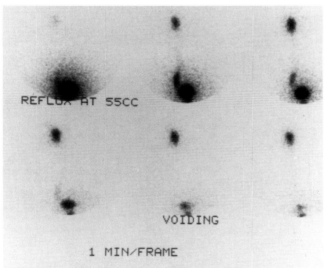

REFLUX AT 55CC

VOIDING

1 MIN/FRAME

TOTAL VOLUME INSTILLED=125CC

**FIG. 5-24.** This radionuclide voiding cystogram was performed on a patient with a spinal cord injury. Left ureteric reflux was noted when 55 ml of the total 125 ml of solution and tracer were instilled.

ond bladder fill. Usually the second fill results in larger instilled volumes (by ~20%).

### Abnormal Scan

An abnormal test occurs when reflux of radiotracer is noted into the ureter or kidneys. A classification of reflux described by Fettich and Kenda (67) is practical:

- Grade I: tracer in ureter
- Grade II: tracer in renal pelvis
- Grade III: tracer in a dilated pelvis

Whether reflux is unilateral or bilateral should also be recorded (Fig. 5-24). The second filling of the bladder has been shown to have improved sensitivity for identifying VUR over earlier protocols that only filled the bladder once. Fettich and Kenda examined 428 children and reported that 161 patients with VUR were identified in the first cycle, 185 in the second cycle, and 231 patients when both bladder fills were combined (67). Therefore, the second fill of the bladder adds important information regarding VUR, with the double-fill technique demonstrating significantly improved sensitivity.

### REFERENCES

1. Blaufox MD. Procedures of choice in renal nuclear medicine. J Nucl Med 1991;32:1301–1309.
2. Taylor A, Nally JV. Clinical applications of renal scintigraphy. AJR Am J Roentgenol 1995;164:31–41.
3. Peters AM. Quantification of renal haemodynamics with radionuclides. Eur J Nucl Med 1991;18:274–286.
4. Investigation of Renal Disease: Glomerular Function. In Sweny P, Farrington K, Moorhead JF (eds), The Kidney and Its Disorders. London: Blackwell, 1989;65.
5. Russell CD, Bischoff PG, Rowell KL, et al. Quality of Tc-99m DTPA for measurement of glomerular filtration: concise communication. J Nucl Med 1983;24:722–727.
6. Goates GG, Morton KA, Whooten WW, et al. Comparison of methods for calculating glomerular filtration rate: Tc-99m-DTPA scintigraphic analysis, protein-free and whole-plasma clearance of Tc-99m-DTPA and I-125-iothalamate clearance. J Nucl Med 1990;31:424–429.
7. Russell CD, Rowell K, Scott JW. Quality control of Tc-99m DTPA: correlation of analytic tests with in vivo protein binding in man. J Nucl Med 1986;27:560–562.
8. Waller DG, Keast CM, Fleming JS, et al. Measurement of glomerular filtration rate with Tc-99m DTPA: comparison of plasma clearance techniques. J Nucl Med 1987;28:372–377.
9. Mulligan JS, Blue PW, Hasbargen JA. Methods for measuring GFR with Tc-99m-DTPA: an analysis of several common methods. J Nucl Med 1990;31:1211–1219.
10. Renal Blood Supply and Its Regulation. In Sweny P, Farrington K, Moorhead JF (eds), The Kidney and Its Disorders. London: Blackwell, 1989;16.
11. Methods for Studying Renal Function. In Hladky SB, Rink TJ (eds), Body Fluid and Kidney Physiology. London: Edward Arnold, 1986;39.
12. Eshima D, Taylor A. Technetium-99m (99mTc) mercaptoacetyltriglycine: update on the new 99mTc renal tubular function agent. Semin Nucl Med 1992;22:61–73.
13. Taylor A, Eshima D, Fritzberg AR, et al. Comparison of iodine-131 OIH and technetium-99m MAG3 renal imaging in volunteers. J Nucl Med 1986;27:795–803.
14. Stadalnik RC, Vogel JM, Jansholt A, et al. Renal clearance and extraction parameters of ortho-iodohippurate (I-123) compared with OIH (I-131) and PAH. J Nucl Med 1980;21:168–170.
15. Arnold RW, Subramanian G, McAfee JG, et al. Comparison of 99mTc complexes for renal imaging. J Nucl Med 1975;16:357–367.
16. Enlander D, Weber PM, dos Remedios LV. Renal cortical imaging in 35 patients: superior quality with 99mTc-DMSA. J Nucl Med 1974;15:743–749.
17. Majd M, Rushton HG. Renal cortical scintigraphy in the diagnosis of acute pyelonephritis. Semin Nucl Med 1992;22:98–111.
18. O'Malley JP, Ziessman HA. Quantitation of renal function using radioisotopic techniques. Clin Lab Med 1993;3:53–68.
19. Russell CD, Dubovsky EV. Measurement of renal function with radionuclides. J Nucl Med 1989;30:2053–2057.
20. Russell CD, Bischoff PG, Kontzen FN, et al. Measurement of glomerular filtration rate: single injection plasma clearance method without urine collection. J Nucl Med 1985;26:1243–1247.
21. Jackson J, Blue PW, Ghaed N. Glomerular filtration rate determined in conjunction with routine renal scanning. Radiology 1985;154:203–205.

22. LaFrance N, Drew H, Walser M. Radioisotopic measurement of glomerular filtration rate in severe chronic renal failure. J Nucl Med 1988;29:1927–1930.

23. Gates GF. Glomerular filtration rate: estimation from fractional renal accumulation of Tc-99m-DTP (stannous). Am J Radiol 1982;138:565–570.

24. Dubovsky EV, Yester MV. Glomerular Filtration Rate, Renal Transit Times, Effective Renal Plasma Flow, and Differential Renal Function. In Gelfant MJ, Thomas SR (eds), Effective Use of Computers in Nuclear Medicine. New York: McGraw-Hill, 1988.

25. Dubovsky EV, Gates GF, Russell CD. Three Approaches to Computer-Assisted Function Studies of the Kidney and Evaluation of Scintigraphic Methods. In Tauxe WN, Dubovsky EV (eds), Nuclear Medicine in Clinical Urology and Nephrology. Norwalk, CT: Appleton-Century-Crofts, 1985.

26. Williams GH. Hypertensive Vascular Disease. In Wilson JD, Braunwald E, Isselbacher KJ, et al. (eds), Harrison's Principles of Internal Medicine. New York: McGraw-Hill, 1991.

27. Nally JV, Black HR. State-of-the-art review: captopril renography—pathophysiological considerations and clinical observations. Semin Nucl Med 1992;22:85–97.

28. Black HJ, Bourgoignie JJ, Pickering T, et al. Report of the working party group for patient selection and preparation. Am J Hypertens 1991;4:745S–746S.

29. Mann SJ, Pickering TG. Detection of renovascular hypertension. State of the art: 1992. Ann Intern Med 1992;117:845–853.

30. Taylor A, Martin LG. The utility of 99mTc-mercaptoacetyltriglycine in captopril renography. Am J Hypertens 1991;4:731S–736S.

31. Geyskes GG, Oei HY, Puylaert CBAJ, Mees EJD. Renovascular hypertension identified by captopril-induced changes in the renogram. Hypertension 1987;9:451–458.

32. Erbsloh-Moller B, Dumas A, Roth D, et al. Furosemide-131I-hippuran renography after angiotensin-converting enzyme inhibition for the diagnosis of renovascular hypertension. Am J Med 1991;90:23–29.

33. Dondi M, Franchi R, Levorato M, et al. Evaluation of hypertensive patients by means of captopril enhanced renal scintigraphy with technetium-99m-DTPA. J Nucl Med 1989;30:615–621.

34. Dondi M, Monetti N, Fanti S, et al. Use of technetium-99m-MAG3 for renal scintigraphy after angiotensin-converting enzyme inhibition. J Nucl Med 1991;32:424–428.

35. Muller FB, Sealey JE, Case DB, et al. The captopril test for identifying renovascular disease. Am J Med 1986;80:633–641.

36. Elliott WJ, Martin WB, Murphy MB. Comparison of two noninvasive screening tests for renovascular hypertension. Arch Intern Med 1993;153:755–764.

37. Fommei E, Ghione S, Hilson AJW, et al. The European Multicentre Study Group. Captopril radionuclide test in renovascular hypertension: a European multicentre study. Eur J Nucl Med 1993;20:617–623.

38. Kahn D, Ben-Haim D, Bushnell DL, et al. Captopril-enhanced 99mTc MAG3 renal scintigraphy in subjects with suspected renovascular hypertension. Nucl Med Comm 1994;15:515–528.

39. Thrall JH, Koff S, Keyes J. Diuretic radionuclide renography and scintigraphy in the differential diagnosis of hydroureteronephrosis. Semin Nucl Med 1981;11:89–104.

40. Conway JJ. "Well-tempered" diuresis renography: its historical development, physiological and technical pitfalls, and standardized technique protocol. Semin Nucl Med 1992;22:74–84.

41. Hvid-Jacobsen K, Thomsen HS, Neilsen SL. Diuresis renography. A simultaneous comparison between I-131 hippuran and Tc-99m MAG3. Acta Radiol 1990;31:83–86.

42. Conway JJ. The principles and technical aspects of diuresis renography. J Nucl Med Tech 1989;17:209–214.

43. O'Reilly PH, Testa HJ, Lawson RS, et al. Diuresis renography in equivocal urinary tract obstruction. Br J Urol 1978;50:76–80.

44. Kalika V, Bard RH, Iloreta A, et al. Prediction of renal functional recovery after relief of upper urinary tract obstruction. J Urol 1981;126:301–305.

45. Verboven M, Achten R, Keuppens F, et al. Radioisotopic transit parameters in obstruction of pelioureteral junction. Urology 1988;32:370–374.

46. Zechmann W. An experimental approach to explain some misinterpretations of diuresis renography. Nucl Med Comm 1988;9:283–294.

47. Kletter K, Nurnberger N. Diagnostic potential of diuresis renography: limitations by the severity of hydronephrosis and by the impairment of renal function. Nucl Med Comm 1989;10:51–61.

48. Shore RM, Uehling DT, Bruskewitz R, Polcyn RE. Evaluation of obstructive uropathy with diuretic renography. Am J Dis Child 1983;137:236–240.

49. Majd M, Rushton HG. Renal cortical scintigraphy in the diagnosis of acute pyelonephritis. Semin Nucl Med 1992;22:98–111.

50. Winberg J, Bollgren I, Kallenius G, et al. Clinical pyelonephritis and focal renal scarring: a selected review of pathogenesis, prevention, and prognosis. Pediatr Clin North Am 1982;29:801–814.

51. Glauser MP, Lyons JM, Braude AI. Prevention of chronic experimental pyelonephritis by suppression of acute suppuration. J Clin Invest 1978;61:403–407.

52. Ruston HG, Majd M, Chaudra R, et al. Evaluation of Tc-99m dimercaptosuccinic acid renal scans in experimental acute pyelonephritis in piglets. J Urol 1988;140:1169–1174.

53. Parkhouse HF, Godley ML, Cooper J, et al. Renal imaging with Tc-99m labeled DMSA in detecting acute pyelonephritis: an experimental study in the pig. Nucl Med Comm 1989;10:63–70.

54. Bjorgvinsson E, Majd M, Eggli KD. Diagnosis of acute pyelonephritis in children: comparison of sonography and 99mTc-DMSA scintigraphy. AJR Am J Roentgenol 1991;157:539–543.

55. Sty JR, Wells RG, Starshak RJ, et al. Imaging in acute renal infection in children. AJR Am J Roentgenol 1987;148:471–477.

56. Pollack HM, Edell S, Morales JO. Radionuclide imaging in renal pseudotumors. Radiology 1974;111:639–644.

57. Older RA, Korobkin M, Workman J, et al. Accuracy of radionuclide imaging in distinguishing renal masses from normal variants. Radiology 1980;136:443–448.

58. Williams ED. Renal single photon emission computed tomography: should we do it? Semin Nucl Med 1992;22:112–121.

59. Lin EC, Gellens ME, Goodgold HM. Prognostic value of renal scintigraphy with Tc-99m MAG3 in patients with acute renal failure. J Nucl Med 1995;36:232P–233P.

60. Splanchnology. In Williams PL, Warwick R, Dyson M, Bannister LH (eds), Gray's Anatomy. Edinburgh: Churchill Livingstone, 1989;1431.

61. Holder LE, Martire JR, Holmes ER, Wagner HN. Testicular radionuclide angiography and stasis imaging: anatomy, scintigraphic interpretation, and clinical indications. Radiology 1977;125:739–752.

62. Haynes BE, Bessen HA, Haynes VE. The diagnosis of testicular torsion. JAMA 1983;249:2522–2527.

63. Holder LE, Melloul M, Chen D. Current status of radionuclide scrotal imaging. Semin Nucl Med 1981;11:232–249.

64. Chen DCP, Holder LE, Kaplan GN. Correlation of radionuclide imaging and diagnostic ultrasound in scrotal diseases. J Nucl Med 1986;27:1774–1781.

65. Middleton WD, Siegel BA, Melson GL, et al. Acute scrotal disorders: prospective comparison of color Doppler US and testicular scintigraphy. Radiology 1990;177:177–181.

66. Lerner GR, Fleischmann LE, Perlmutter AD. Reflux nephropathy. Pediatr Clin North Am 1987;34:747–770.

67. Fettich JJ, Kenda RB. Cyclic direct radionuclide voiding cystography: increasing reliability in detecting vesicoureteral reflux in children. Pediatr Radiol 1992;22:337–338.

*Textbook of Nuclear Medicine,*
edited by Michael A. Wilson.
Lippincott–Raven Publishers, Philadelphia © 1998.

# CHAPTER 6

# Radionuclide Ventriculography

## Jesus A. Bianco and Michael A. Wilson

Radionuclide ventriculography (RVG) is an important but underrated and underused nuclear imaging procedure. Currently, nuclear cardiology represents approximately 25% of a typical large hospital's nuclear medicine workload. The relative distribution of these cardiac tests is approximately:

- Myocardial perfusion imaging (MPI), 84%
- RVG, 15%
- Other cardiac studies, 1%

The major reason for RVG underuse is that MPI provides information related to perfusion and myocardial oxygen consumption (hence cardiac metabolism), whereas RVG provides data only on cardiac function (the result of cardiac metabolism). MPI provides most of the needed practical information because myocardial oxygen consumption is directly related to cardiac function, but there are instances when perfusion and left ventricular (LV) function are dissociated. The clinical significance of this uncoupling of cardiac perfusion and function is not well understood. The recently introduced myocardial perfusion agent technetium 99m (Tc-99m) sestamibi now offers the opportunity of obtaining simultaneous perfusion and ventricular function information (see Chapter 2).

Another reason for RVG underuse is the wide availability of echocardiography, with its recent technological advances of two-dimensional color Doppler and transesophageal echocardiograms. Echocardiograms can measure global and regional LV systolic and diastolic function at rest and at stress and can also offer information on

- Pulmonary artery pressure and valvular stenosis
- Mitral regurgitation and ventricular septal defects
- Myocardial infiltrative disease or scarring
- Pericardial disease, such as thickening or calcification
- Assorted tumor masses and cardiac thrombi
- Potential visualization of left main coronary stenosis

All, or some, of these indications may be present in a patient in whom an RVG is requested, and because echocardiography can provide these answers and also assess ventricular function, echocardiography is often the preferred modality. Currently, twice as many echocardiograms are performed as nuclear medicine MPI and RVG studies combined. Given the wide availability of echocardiography and the newer developments with MRI, the role for RVG will depend on the incremental gains in diagnostic certainty obtained with radionuclide-derived functional assessment.

## GATED RVG

RVG is used for the assessment of LV and right ventricular (RV) function (1) and is performed either by equilibrium gating or as a first-pass procedure. Zaret et al. (2) initially proposed this radionuclide test, and the method as it is known today was developed at the National Institutes of Health (NIH) by Green and Bacharach (3). Burow et al. at the Johns Hopkins Hospital performed RVG by using synchronization of multiple time segments of the cardiac cycle with the electrocardiogram (ECG) (4), calling it multiple gated acquisition (MUGA) cardiac blood pool imaging. *Synchronization* is an appropriate term for these RVG studies because it describes the registration of the radionuclide data acquisition along with the patient's ECG. The RVG may be obtained at rest (rest MUGA) and during exercise (MUGX). The MUGX is particularly relevant because LV function may be normal at rest but abnormal at stress, effectively testing cardiac reserve. With ischemia, valvular dysfunction, and various other mechanical abnormalities, the patient with normal rest MUGA may show decreased function when performing at stress. The concept of cardiac reserve is exemplified in aortic regurgitation, in which the patient has normal LV systolic function for a time, but as the LV dilates the systolic function response to exercise is a fall in LV ejection fraction (EF). This decreased cardiac reserve, evidenced by a fall in LVEF, may be an expression of impending irreversible cardiac damage and is an indication for valve replacement.

## Radiopharmaceutical

Cardiac blood pool imaging is performed with Tc-99m–labeled red blood cells (RBCs) (5), which distribute primarily within the intravascular blood pool. At present, the in vitro labeling method is preferred for its excellent RBC labeling ability (>97% labeling efficiency). In this technique, the pertechnetate ion crosses the intact RBC membrane, but only Tc-99m that has been reduced to a lower oxidation state (e.g., valence [IV]) binds to the beta chain of hemoglobin. Stannous chloride is the preferred reducing agent because it penetrates the erythrocyte membrane. During labeling, the Tc-99m $TcO_4^-$ is brought into contact with erythrocytes pretreated with stannous ions. A nonpenetrating oxidizing agent, sodium hypochlorite, is used to oxidize extracellular stannous ions to prevent extracellular reduction of Tc-99m $TcO_4^-$ and potential labeling of other blood products or tissues. Avoidance of centrifugation lessens the degree of cellular damage that occurs during radiolabeling. We recommend thorough reading of the package insert (UltraTag RBC kit, Mallinckrodt Medical, Inc., St. Louis, MO). The dose of Tc-99m $TcO_4^-$ used is 20 to 30 mCi (740 to 1,110 MBq), according to weight.

Use of fresh Tc-99m $TcO_4^-$ eluate from a molybdenum 99 (Mo-99)/Tc-99m generator that has been eluted within the last 24 hours is recommended to ensure that the proportion of Tc-99 is low (see Chapter 22). Tc-99 would otherwise compete with Tc-99m for the labeling of RBCs. The labeled RBCs have an estimated biological half-life of 29 hours, and 25% of the injected dose is excreted in the urine in the first 24 hours. Table 6-1 lists several of the drugs known to interfere with Tc-99m RBC labeling. The dosimetry is shown in Table 6-2.

## Resting Scan Protocol

Imaging for the MUGA scan is performed by synchronization with the surface ECG and is commenced at least 5 minutes after radionuclide administration to allow complete mixing of the Tc-99m RBCs within the blood pool. The radionuclide concentration is assumed to be constant throughout the blood pool. The LV counts are related to, but are not equal to, the LV volume. The proportionality between LV counts and volume is a complex function of factors that include photon absorption and scattering.

The equilibrium methodology depends on the analysis of a composite sum of 200 to 800 serial cardiac cycles. This requires the recognition of the cardiac cycle initiation, and for this reason, equilibrium studies are computer acquired and synchronized to the R wave of the ECG input. With frame mode acquisition, image data representing preset 30- to 40-millisecond portions of each R-R interval are consecutively collected during the cardiac cycle. The result is a file of two-dimensional (X and Y coordinates) frames, from which parameters such as the LVEF can be derived. The individual frames are grouped with the identical time frames of subsequent beats until, after several hundred beats, a representative cardiac cycle is created. This represents the sum of data from all the time intervals that make up the R-R interval and can be displayed as an endless-loop movie (Fig. 6-1). Frame mode acquisition is used with regular rhythms. Adequate sampling rates use frame durations of 40 milliseconds for studies in patients at rest (MUGA), and of 30 milliseconds' duration for studies in patients performing supine bicycle exercise (MUGX). We specify 24 individual frames of equal duration during the R-R interval because we wish to determine more refined diastolic data.

With the buffered ectopic beat rejection software program, each cardiac cycle is temporarily stored in a buffer. All beats with abnormally long or short R-R cycles relative to that of the predetermined R-R interval can be rejected. The user can preselect a window of acceptance, or the window can be programmed to automatically change with the average of the prior beats. In general, any study with >15% rejected beats should be critically evaluated before use. Buffered ectopic beat algorithms are effective for MUGX scans in which the R-R interval duration changes rapidly and continuously with stress.

In atrial fibrillation, the LVEF derived from an averaged R-R cardiac cycle duration is usually adequate for interpretation, provided not too many beats are rejected due to the varying R-R intervals. In the case of ventricular ectopy, the ectopic and postectopic beats have shorter and longer ventricular filling times, respectively, and result in ventricular volumes that are different from that of normal beats. It is rational to exclude such beats because they degrade the func-

**TABLE 6-1.** *Drugs interfering with Tc-99m RBC labeling*

| Drug | Mechanism |
|------|-----------|
| Heparin | Formation of labeled heparin |
| Methyldopa, hydralazine, preservatives in IV solutions | Oxidation of stannous ion |
| Digoxin, prazosin, propranolol | Unknown mechanism |
| Iodinated contrast media | Competition with anion transport system |

**TABLE 6-2.** *Absorbed dose estimates for labeled RBCs*

| Organ | Rads/20 mCi (cGy/740 MBq) |
|-------|---------------------------|
| Total body | 0.30 |
| Spleen* | 2.20 |
| Bladder wall | 0.48 |
| Testes | 0.22 |
| Ovaries | 0.32 |
| Blood | 0.80 |
| Red marrow | 0.30 |
| Heart wall | 2.00 |
| Liver | 0.58 |
| Bone surfaces | 0.48 |

*Critical organ.
Source: Package insert for Tc-99m labeled RBCs (UltraTag).

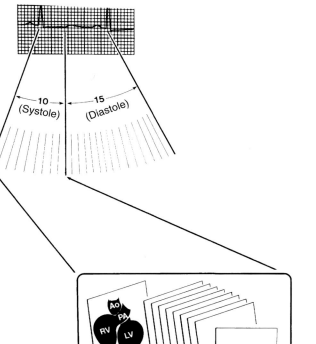

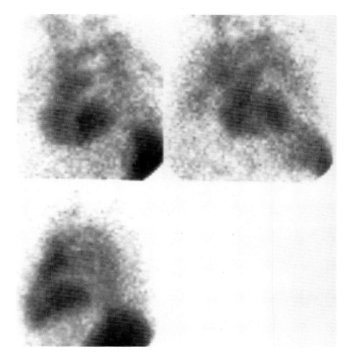

**FIG. 6-2.** Normal three-view MUGA study. The three typical MUGA study projections are 40 to 45 degrees LAO (upper left), anterior (upper right), and 70 degrees LAO (lower left). The ventricles, major vessels, and spleen are clearly identified.

**FIG. 6-1.** The multigated RVG study (MUGA). The ECG's 25 equally divided time intervals and the frames of data collected are synchronized with the ECG into consecutive time intervals during the cardiac cycle. Two frames of the "picture file" are shown. The ED frame represents data acquired from the R wave of the ECG to 30 to 40 milliseconds later. The ES frame represents data when the LV volume (as measured in counts) is lowest. The BKG area of interest is selected at ES.

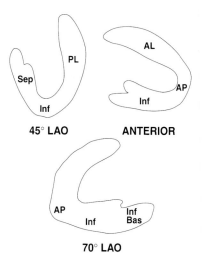

**FIG. 6-3.** One of the conventions for describing the LV myocardial wall segments identified in the typical MUGA views (as shown in Fig. 6-2). (Sep, septal; PL, posterolateral; AL, anterolateral; AP, apical; Inf, inferior; Inf Bas, inferobasal.)

*Wall Motion Interpretation*

tional data obtained. Although drugs (e.g., lidocaine, 100 mg IV) can sometimes abolish the arrhythmia, the computer software is often used to exclude the ectopic and postectopic beats. Each camera manufacturer uses its own method. Resting MUGA studies usually have 200,000 counts in the end-diastolic (ED) frame and should have 6,000 counts in the LV diastolic region of interest (ROI). Lower counts would be expected to decrease the accuracy of the study.

To optimize evaluation of chamber anatomy and wall motion, images are acquired at rest in anterior, the left lateral or 70-degree "steep" left anterior oblique (LAO), and the 40-degree or best septal or "shallow" LAO projections. In a typical MUGA study (Fig. 6-2), the best septal LAO view is acquired first by selecting the orientation that best separates the two ventricles with the interventricular septum positioned vertically. Gating on the R wave of the ECG should be verified, and if necessary, ECG leads should be repositioned to amplify the R wave signal and to minimize other interfering signals such as tall, peaked T waves.

The LV segments are annotated in Fig. 6-3. Inward uniform synchronous contraction of the endocardial boundaries from ED to end-systole (ES) is designated normal contraction

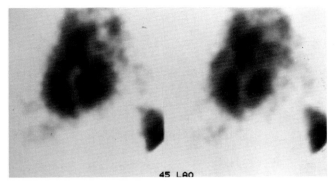

**FIG. 6-4.** This RVG study shows ED (left) and ES (right) frames in a 45-degree LAO view, with normal RV and LV contraction shown by smaller ventricles in the ES frame. The normal spleen is seen in right lower portion of each frame.

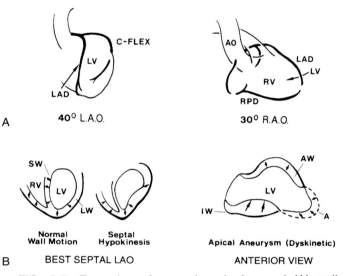

**FIG. 6-5.** Examples of normal and abnormal LV wall motion. **(A)** The coronary arterial distributions in the 40-degree LAO and 30-degree RAO conventional angiographic views. **(B)** Examples of normal LV wall motion, septal hypokinesis, and apical dyskinesis (paradoxic motion typical of an aneurysm). (A, apex; AO, ascending aorta; AW, anterior wall; IW, inferior wall; LW, lateral wall; SW, septal wall; LAD, left anterior descending coronary artery; C-FLEX, left circumflex coronary artery; RPD, right posterior descending coronary artery.)

(Fig. 6-4). Global wall motion abnormalities involve several or all segments of the LV, whereas regional wall motion abnormalities indicate less involvement. Whereas global abnormalities are common in myocardiopathy, regional abnormalities indicate coronary artery disease (CAD). Various abnormal wall motion patterns are defined below (Fig. 6-5):

- Hypokinesis: decreased wall motion
- Akinesis: no wall motion
- Dyskinesis: paradoxic passive expansion (rather than contraction) of a myocardial segment during systole. An LV aneurysm is characterized by localized dyskinesis.

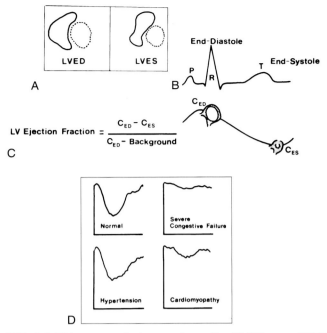

$$LV\ Ejection\ Fraction = \frac{C_{ED} - C_{ES}}{C_{ED} - Background}$$

**FIG. 6-6.** This composite image shows the MUGA scan LVEF calculation method. **(A)** The silhouette of the LV (*dotted boundary*) at ED and ES. **(B)** An ECG cardiac cycle (above) and LV myocardial walls and counts at ED ($C_{ED}$) and ES ($C_{ES}$) superimposed on ventricular TAC (below), to illustrate the basic idea of synchronization of electrical activity and muscle contraction that defines the MUGA technique. **(C)** The method of LVEF calculation with the counts from ED, ES, and BKG ROIs. **(D)** Representative LV count plots for a normal subject and patients with severe congestive failure, hypertension, and cardiomyopathy. (P, P wave; R, R wave; T, T wave.)

### Systolic Function Assessment

Systolic function equates with the determination of the LVEF. The MUGA and MUGX scans allow measurement of the LVEF (Fig. 6-6) in the best septal view. The initial studies determining the correlation between RVG and contrast angiographic LVEF (6) demonstrated a high correlation over a wide range of values; these have now become the gold standard of LVEF methodologies.

To calculate the LVEF, a time-activity curve (TAC) from the LV ROI is generated. An ED frame with the highest number of LV counts and an ES frame with the lowest number of LV counts are chosen for the calculation (see Fig. 6-6). A background (BKG) ROI, frequently crescent shaped, is placed inferolaterally and adjacent to the LV at ES (see Fig. 6-1). The LVEF is calculated as follows (1):

$$LVEF = \frac{ED\ counts - ES\ counts}{ED\ counts - BKG\ counts} \quad (1)$$

The BKG count in MUGA studies traditionally lies between 50% and 70% of the LV activity. The greater the BKG correction, the higher the calculated LVEF. Extracardiac structures (e.g., spleen, descending aorta, left atrium)

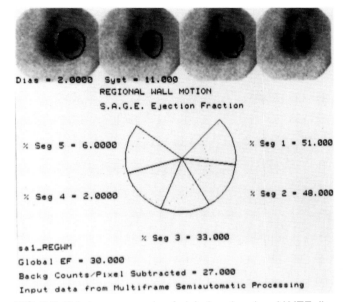

**FIG. 6-7.** This is an example of global and regional LVEF display in a patient with a reduced global LVEF of 30% and scan evidence of septal akinesis. The upper two left images demonstrate diastole (dias, determined to be the second frame), and systole (syst, the eleventh frame) with LV ROIs. The second to right image shows the five segments for which the regional EF was calculated. The regional EFs are shown about the display of segments in the middle of the figure with the systolic edge "dotted" in. The EFs are virtually zero in the septal segments, subnormal in the inferoapex, but near normal in the posterolateral segments.

might falsely elevate the BKG counts and falsely modify the LVEF if included in the BKG region.

The ventricular assessment is usually done in the best septal view and can be done globally or for the major myocardial segments (Fig. 6-7). The global and regional LVEFs are typically as follows:

- Global: >50% (mean 60% ± SD 10%)
- Inferoapical segment: >70%
- Posterolateral segment: 55% to 70%
- Septal segment: 40% to 55%

**Exercise Scan Protocol**

Borer et al. (7) first reported that the LVEF and regional wall motion during exercise was abnormal in many patients with CAD. The protocol for the exercise scan is as follows: After a rest MUGA scan of regional wall motion and LV function is obtained, the patient is asked to perform progressive supine exercise on a bicycle ergometer (8). While the patient exercises, blocks of data are acquired in the best septal projection at each stress level for sufficient duration to obtain reliable information. The workload is expressed in watts at a pedal rate of 50 revolutions per minute. The strategy is to wait for 1 minute at each level for the stabilization of the heart rate after

increasing workloads and to record exercise data at each new workload achieved. The loads can be increased at 25-W or greater increments, to a maximum work load of 100 to 175 W.

Care must be taken to center the heart in the middle of the field of view during acquisition. In most cases, CAD patients can only exercise to 50 to 75 W, but superb athletes can exercise to 150 to 175 W with evidence of lactate production appearing late and resulting in a plateauing of hemodynamic indices. The blood pressure (BP) and pulse are monitored during stress to calculate the double product (systolic pressure times pulse rate), and double products of >24,000 are preferred for optimal peak stress. This peak stress level is more difficult to obtain with supine bicycle stress than with a treadmill, and some centers stress their patients in the sitting position to overcome this limitation.

It is important to achieve sufficient count density (i.e., counts per pixel) in the peak stress stage for analysis, especially because this is to be compared with the rest level. In many studies the exercise data may be suboptimal. If the patient does not appear able to finish a stress level, then judicious lowering of the workload while maintaining the double product ensures satisfactory completion of the study. An early hint of difficulty in completing the stage is a vasoconstriction of the upper limb vessels. Continued encouragement alone or workload decrease may help the patient complete the exercise stage. The ECG is monitored to identify ischemic changes. The minimal load that provides reliable LVEF exercise data is 50 W (8), therefore we like to start patients at the 50-W level. We also prefer to increase stages at 50-W increments if the patients do not have a history of compromised exercise tolerance.

In our laboratory we collect 3,000,000 counts for each stage, and this provides sufficient data to allow diastolic function parameters to be measured. This will require 3 to 5 minutes of data collection per stage of the exercise MUGA scan. The increasing heart rate induced by exercise introduces a technical problem. Although the technologists wait for an apparent stabilization of the heart rate with stress, sometimes the heart rate increases further once data collection has commenced. As a consequence, the later frames in the R-R interval receive less and less data as the R-R interval decreases while the predetermined number of individual time frames (30 to 40 milliseconds) spanning the R-R interval remains constant. This decreases the accuracy of late diastolic data.

*Wall Motion at Stress*

New wall motion abnormalities developing during exercise would suggest significant CAD, but a detailed account of this has not been reported.

*Systolic Function at Stress*

The expected physiologic LV response to exercise is an increase in LVEF, likely mediated by reflex central and humoral catecholamine stimulation. A normal response is either an increase of 5 or more absolute LVEF units or no change whatsoever in the LVEF. When the LV volume is small, the LVEF does not rise with exercise, and when the rest LVEF is high (>70%), significant increments may not occur. This lack of increment may also occur in normal females and all older adults. In patients with CAD, the exercise LVEF drops significantly when the patient exercises to ECG ischemia, but the exercise LVEF may not decline in patients who only exercise to fatigue. The presence of valvular, myopathic, or congenital heart disease may lower the LVEF response to exercise. This may also be the case in patients with hypertension, mitral valve prolapse, or left bundle branch block (LBBB).

### Quality Control Review of MUGA Scans

The time of total acquisition, total counts acquired, percent of rejected beats in each acquisition period (Fig. 6-8) and the stress conditions, duration of stress, workload attained, heart rate, and BP response should be evaluated to ensure the rest and stress studies are adequate.

The two ventricles should be well separated and the septum visualized from the aortic valve plane to the apex (Fig. 6-9; see also Fig. 6-4). The left atrium should lie directly behind the LV. The anterior view should be 45 degrees less oblique than the LAO view, and the steep LAO view 30 degrees more oblique than the LAO view.

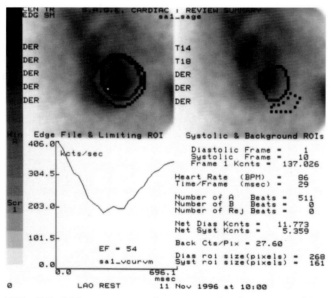

**FIG. 6-8.** This representative composite image provides some data useful for QC. The upper images show the LV diastolic (left) and systolic (right) ROIs, together with BKG ROI (right). The frames used for diastole and systole together with total counts in frame 1 are shown below on the right. The heart rate, time per frame, accepted beats, net diastolic and systolic counts, ROI size, and BKG counts per pixel are shown below. The ventricular TAC is shown on the lower left with the calculated EF.

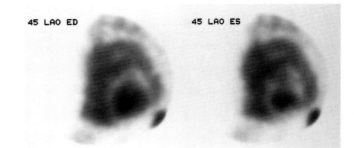

**FIG. 6-9.** This MUGA study shows the 45-degree LAO best septal images at ED and ES with good separation of both ventricles. The LV and the RV contract well, as shown by their smaller size on the ES image. The major vessels are well visualized, and the thoracic aorta is particularly well seen in systole. The BKG ROI should not include the aorta or the spleen.

The ROIs selected for calculation of EF should next be examined to ensure that all are appropriate and do not include activity from adjacent cardiac chambers. The common errors in selection of the LV ROI are inclusion of left atrial counts in the LV ROI with underestimation of LVEF and inclusion of the descending aorta or the spleen (see Fig. 6-9) in the BKG ROI with overestimation of LVEF.

Important considerations in the computation of the LVEF are:

- Shape of the TAC
- Net ventricular diastolic counts >6,000
- Overestimation of ED counts increases LVEF
- Underestimation of ES counts increases LVEF
- A tight ROI around the LV decreases the LVEF
- Inclusion of spleen or aorta in BKG ROI increases LVEF

A systematic count fall-off in the later frames of the cardiac cycle is due to R-R interval variability (e.g., sinus arrhythmia or changing R-R intervals during exercise), with inaccuracies of computation of diastolic events, such as peak filling rate.

Even though the methodologic (4% EF units) and biological (3% EF units) errors in calculation of EF are small, care must be taken in interpreting serial studies in light of the multiple considerations that can affect the measurement. The radionuclide LVEF has become the gold standard for determination of EF because it is noninvasive, it derives from 200 to 800 consecutive normal beats, and it does not require the injection of a volume of contrast, which has the potential to perturb contractions. Below 30%, the LVEF becomes less accurate because the larger ventricular volumes attenuate LV counts, and the relationship between LV counts and volume becomes nonlinear.

For many years (1,4,8), camera manufacturers have used computer programs that track the endocardial edge in the LV chamber to define its border throughout the cardiac cycle by applying threshold criteria, such as the zero intercept of the second derivative. The activity in the chamber

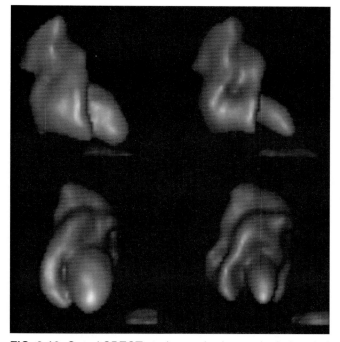

**FIG. 6-10.** Gated SPECT study acquired on a single-headed SPECT system showing the anterior (upper row) and best septal (lower row) views at diastole (left column) and systole (right column ) in a patient with normal RV and LV contraction. The spleen and aorta are seen in the LAO systolic image. (Images courtesy of Dr. James Thomsen, William S. Middleton Memorial Veterans Hospital, Madison, WI.)

at each point of the cardiac cycle is then determined after BKG subtraction using an ROI immediately adjacent to the LV. Automatic determination of the endocardial edge in each frame of the cardiac cycle is known as the variable ROI method, which provides an accurate but less reproducible EF measurement. Workers at NIH have used the fixed ROI method extensively, in which the LV ED ROI endocardial border and adjacent BKG region are used for the LVEF measurement. This fixed ROI method underestimates the LVEF slightly given that ES counts are slightly overestimated because a specific systolic edge and ROI are not used, but LVEFs computed by this method are more reproducible.

## Other Systolic Function Indices

### Right Ventricular EF

The determination of the RVEF by the MUGA method (9,10) is similar to the determination of the LVEF. Because of the difficulty in excluding the right atrium, the RVEF underestimates the true value as assessed by the radionuclide first-pass method (discussed in First-Pass RVG). The RVEF determined by MUGA procedures is reproducible, and typically, the RVEF is 40% ± SD 7%. Occasionally, the cine can identify RV wall motion abnor-

malities because the RV is always well visualized in planar or single photon emission computed tomography studies (Fig. 6-10; see Fig. 6-9).

### Other Indices

#### Stroke Counts Index

The radionuclide ventricular stroke counts are proportional to the volume of blood ejected from the ventricle with each beat. In this calculation, the BKG cancels out (11), and the ventricular stroke count index is the ratio of LV to RV stroke counts:

$$\text{Stroke count index} = \frac{\text{LV (ED counts} - \text{ES counts)}}{\text{RV (ED counts} - \text{ES counts)}} \quad (2)$$

The stroke counts ratio should equal 1.0, but because of the underestimation of the RVEF by MUGA, the normal ventricular stroke counts ratio is mildly overestimated; values between 1.3 and 1.5 are found in normal individuals. Clinically significant aortic or mitral valve (left heart) regurgitation is associated with a stroke counts index >2.0. Combinations of valvular regurgitation and intracardiac shunts invalidate the index. Cardiac failure increases, and right heart valve regurgitation decreases, the stroke counts index. The stroke counts index permits quantitation of the regurgitant fraction:

$$\text{LV regurgitant fraction} = \frac{\text{Stroke counts index} - 1}{\text{Stroke counts index}} \quad (3)$$

#### Stroke Volume Image

The stroke volume and EF images (12) are functional or parametric images extensively investigated at the Boston laboratory of Leonard Holman. To obtain the stroke volume image, the ES frame is subtracted pixel by pixel from the ED frame. Normally, this image shows the pattern of ventricular contraction (the stroke volume or EF "shell") and is used to check endocardial ventricular wall motion and assess the regional EF. Generally, these images are obtained in the best septal projection.

#### Amplitude and Phase Images

The amplitude and phase images (Fig. 6-11) are routinely available in many software packages and are discussed in Chapter 25. The amplitude image is analogous to the stroke volume image and can be used to assess ventricular contraction. The phase image of the ventricles determines the presence of conduction abnormalities  such as right bundle branch block (RBBB) or LBBB (Fig. 6-12) and can be used to identify regions of dyskinesis.

In paradoxic LV motion, a discrete abnormal area of the ventricle is out of phase with the LV (see Fig. 6-11) and can

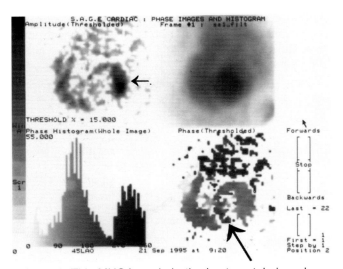

**FIG. 6-11.** This MUGA study in the best septal view shows the raw data (upper right), amplitude image (upper left), phase image (lower right), and phase histogram (lower left). The amplitude image shows good contraction of the posterolateral wall (*small arrow*), with akinesis of inferoapex and some movement of septum (upper left). The phase image shows (*large arrow*) that the septum is out of phase with the remainder of the LV, indicating septal dyskinesis.

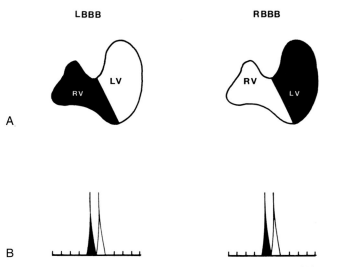

**FIG. 6-12.** Schematic examples of phase images **(A)** and phase histograms **(B)** in cases of LBBB and RBBB. In LBBB, the right ventricle is activated first (*black*) ahead of the LV (*white*), whereas in RBBB the LV is activated first.

indicate an LV aneurysm not appreciated on conventional wall motion analyses. The phase image is abnormal in patients with a ventricular pacemaker, Wolff-Parkinson-White syndrome, bundle branch blocks, and other conduction disorders of the heart. Pavel and colleagues did much of the pioneering work with the phase image (13). Botvinick et al. discuss this topic in more detail in their review (1).

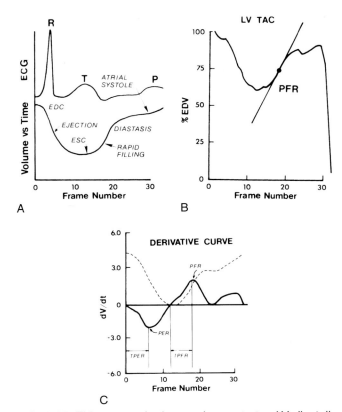

**FIG. 6-13.** This composite image demonstrates LV diastolic events. **(A)** LV TAC during a cardiac cycle in relation to the ECG above it. The diastolic intervals of the TAC are rapid filling, diastasis (slow filling), and atrial systole. **(B)** The derivation of the PFR as the steepest slope of initial rapid diastolic filling of the TAC. **(C)** The typical appearance of the first derivative (*solid line*) of the LV TAC (*dotted line*) showing the location of PER and the PFR. The TPER and the TPFR are also shown. (P, P wave; R, R wave; T, T wave; EDC, end-diastole cycle; ESC, end-systole cycle; EDV, end-diastole volume; PER, peak ejection rate; PFR, peak filling rate; TPER, time to peak ejection rate; TPFR, time to peak filling rate; dV/dt, first derivative of LV volume change.)

## Diastolic Function

For many years, it was thought that LV relaxation was passive, but it is now well established that early ventricular diastole is an active process and that calcium ions play a major role (14). Three distinct phases of LV diastole are described: early rapid diastolic filling, diastasis, and the atrial kick (Fig. 6-13). During the early diastolic filling period, approximately 80% of ventricular filling is accomplished, little occurs in diastasis, and the atrial kick contributes 10% to 15% of total LV filling. The contribution of atrial contraction to cardiac output is critical in some patients with heart failure, and current sequential atrioventricular pacemakers can time the occurrence of atrial and ventricular systole. Increased heart rates, such as those during exercise, result in disappearance of diastasis with little impairment of ventricular filling. When the ventricular TACs of rest and stress are compared, this is obvious (Fig. 6-14). On the other hand, in atrial fibrillation, in which there is no atrial

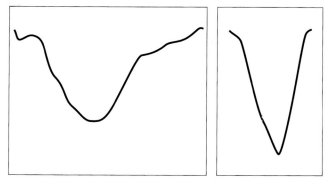

**FIG. 6-14.** Examples of LV TACs as a function of heart rate. **(A)** This image demonstrates expected diastolic events seen well at a physiologic heart rate. **(B)** When the patient is tachycardic, the diastolic phase of the cardiac cycle is shortened.

contraction, there is no discrete atrial kick. This situation contributes to the worsened hemodynamics in patients with atrial fibrillation and heart failure because of the loss of the boost provided by the filling effect of atrial contraction.

Bonow et al. (15) first described diastolic indices with the RVG. They demonstrated that the peak filling rate (PFR) was decreased in many patients with CAD. The PFR is the maximum slope of the early diastolic filling period (see Fig. 6-13) and is obtained by taking the first derivative of the ventricular TAC. Measurement of the PFR requires fast acquisition framing rates of 24 or more frames per heartbeat to ensure sufficiently fine temporal resolution to obtain this measure of diastolic function. The late frames of the ventricular TAC can be count-limited when the heart rate changes over the period of data collection, as occurs during exercise or with marked sinus arrhythmia. The late frames are usually discarded, but, with more dramatic changes in heart rate, critical components of the late ventricular TAC may be lost and the diastolic function analysis compromised. In practice, the user frequently relies on the commercial software provided for PFR analysis. Consultation with other users who routinely use the same software is recommended for better results.

Because the radionuclide PFR is normalized to ED counts, the units are ED volume per second. The normal PFR range in normal individuals is typically 3.3 (±0.6 SD), depending on the laboratory and the software used. PFR values depend on the loading conditions of the heart (aortic pressure and left atrial inflow volume), heart rate, LVEF, and patient age. Bonow et al. showed that the PFR is directly correlated with LVEF (15). Bianco et al. showed that PFR is also directly correlated with heart rate (16) and that, for each increase in rate of 10 beats per minute, the PFR increased 0.4. Stewart et al. have presented age and heart rate normalization data for PFR (17). These kinds of data are important for proper understanding of LV diastolic data. Aging hearts characteristically have a decrease in PFR. The time to peak filling is probably not a useful parameter.

The usual change in diastolic function in disease is a reduction of PFR and an increase in importance of the atrial contri-

bution to LV filling. PFR is subnormal in 90% of patients with myocardial infarction (15) and in 50% to 75% of patients with CAD without evidence of infarction. The atrial (kick) contribution to ventricular filling is increased in aortic stenosis, hypertrophic cardiomyopathy, and other conditions associated with a stiff, noncompliant LV that offers impedance to early diastolic filling. This observation is of importance in ventricular remodeling, which occurs after myocardial infarction, when the LV volume increases over time. Much clinical literature has been written on this topic, and angiotensin-converting enzyme (ACE) inhibitors have been proposed for therapy for these patients because afterload reduction is beneficial. The subject of LV diastole has been thoroughly reviewed (18–20), and these reviews are important because radionuclide PFR assessment of diastolic function remains controversial.

### Clinical Applications of MUGA

#### Chemotherapy Toxicity

The assessment of doxorubicin toxicity effects on LV function (21) is probably the most important application of MUGA scans. With cumulative doses of doxorubicin >500 mg/m$^2$, the resting LVEF frequently declines. This results from a doxorubicin-induced myocyte membrane and mitochondrial cardiomyopathy, which is initially reversible upon discontinuation of the doxorubicin (22). Once established, this cardiomyopathy is irreversible. If after chemotherapy the resting LVEF is 40% or below, the referring physician has to be cautious about further doxorubicin therapy because of this preventable but irreversible cardiotoxicity.

The close surveillance of the resting LVEF in patients on doxorubicin therapy is the best noninvasive diagnostic strategy to prevent doxorubicin toxicity. In doxorubicin toxicity, myocardial perfusion is normal, but abnormalities of glucose and fatty acid metabolism correlate with the myocyte membrane and mitochondrial damage. It has not been found that the exercise LVEF adds new information to the care of patients receiving doxorubicin therapy (10). In patients about to receive doxorubicin therapy, coexistent heart disease requires cardiology consultation before therapy is started.

#### Myocardial Hibernation

The hearts of patients with multivessel CAD, chronic moderate LV systolic dysfunction (LVEF ~30%), and normally perfused or mildly hypoperfused myocardial segments with severe wall motion abnormalities (hypokinesis, resting dyskinesis, or akinesis) are believed to be "hibernating." These LV segments can respond to surgical restoration of coronary flow (23) with improved wall motion. The hibernating segments are considered viable because, despite severe hypocontractility at rest, they improve after coronary revascularization. As a condition for operative revascularization, these segments must demonstrate preoperative inducible ischemia by MPI (24).

### Myocardial Stunning

Another important clinical entity is *myocardial stunning* (25), which refers to regional postischemic depression of LV contractility. Such regions have normal resting cardiac perfusion, altered fatty acid metabolism, abnormal regional wall motion, and abnormal myocardial cell calcium utilization. They normalize after IV catecholamine administration. Postischemic conditions resulting in myocardial stunning include

- Acute myocardial ischemia or infarction
- Recent coronary surgery
- Recent coronary angioplasty

### CAD Prognosis

All cardiac nuclear imaging procedures are useful in CAD prognostication. The exercise LVEF by the first-pass method (see later) has been shown to be very important in identification of severe CAD (26–28). MPI can be used to prognosticate ischemic events in CAD, and the RVG has been shown in several investigations to be a powerful predictor of future cardiac events. In symptomatic patients with CAD, the variables that predict hard ischemic events (myocardial infarction, death, coronary artery bypass graft [CABG] or percutaneous transluminal coronary angioplasty [PTCA] intervention, and recurrent angina) are

- Angiographic severity of CAD
- Presence of ischemia as seen on MPI
- Clinical variables of age and diabetes
- Unstable angina
- Rest and stress MUGA scans

The fall in LVEF with exercise is directly proportional to the angiographic severity of CAD. However, the additional information RVG provides over and above that of MPI needs further investigation. The magnitude of ST depression, the stress LVEF, the exercise double product, and gender are independently predictive of presence of severe CAD (29,30). In fact, inability to continue exercising beyond stage I of the Bruce protocol is predictive of left main or three-vessel CAD. The LVEF is also an important variable for predicting cardiovascular death or myocardial infarction (26,31,32): An exercise LVEF of <0.30 is associated with cardiac events over the next 4 years. These data also apply to patients after acute myocardial infarction (33).

Bonow et al. (34) showed that severe exercise-induced ischemia on MUGA provides independent prognostic information in mildly symptomatic patients with severe CAD without LV dysfunction. Miller et al. (35) demonstrated that patients with one- or two-vessel CAD, impaired LV function, and severe ischemia on exercise MUGA have a higher incidence of future cardiac events.

### Diastolic Function Determination

It is now known that in many CAD patients systolic function may be normal, but the LV may be stiff, with increased impedance to LV filling (18–20). Thus, diastolic heart failure without systolic failure may be present. In these patients, calcium channel blockers, nitroglycerin, or ACE inhibitors rather than digitalis should be given for therapy. After myocardial infarction an LV remodeling process occurs, and it is likely that serial measurements of the LVEF and diastolic parameters may be useful to assess the therapeutic effectiveness of afterload-reducing ACE inhibitors. Typically, the LV is stiff with increased filling impedance in CAD, aortic stenosis, and hypertrophic cardiomyopathy.

### RV Function Assessment

The functional status of the RV (9) is of importance in the assessment and management of patients with

- RV infarction (most patients also have inferior LV infarction)
- Chronic obstructive pulmonary disease (COPD) (with or without cor pulmonale)
- Congenital heart disease (children and adults)
- RV dysplasia or Uhl's syndrome

### Quantitation of Valvular Regurgitation

In patients with single valve dysfunction and no intracardiac shunts, one can assess and quantify aortic insufficiency or mitral insufficiency by the MUGA scan, but this application has not gained popularity.

### LV Aneurysms and Pseudoaneurysms

Aneurysms are common and follow acute myocardial infarction. They are predominantly located at the apex of the LV and frequently contain a luminal clot, but they may also be located at the posterobasal segment. They have scar tissue interspersed with nonischemic tissue. True aneurysms seldom rupture. Pseudoaneurysms (36), on the other hand, are the result of myocardial rupture that becomes contained by the pericardium. Because these can bleed catastrophically, surgical intervention is required. These aneurysms are frequently posterolateral with a "neck" well seen on contrast angiography. On the MUGA scan, these are identified by the visualization of three cardiac chambers: the RV, the LV, and the pseudoaneurysm. They are seen after myocardial infarction, bacterial endocarditis, surgery, and perhaps trauma.

## FIRST-PASS RVG

The injection of tracer into a peripheral vein results in the passage of tracer through the RV then the LV (Fig. 6-15).

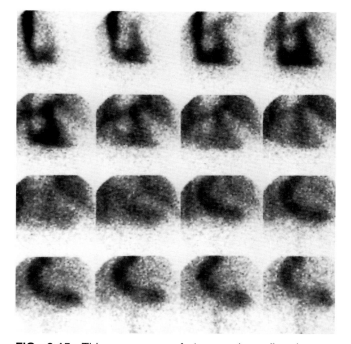

**FIG. 6-15.** This sequence of 1-second cardiac images demonstrates the flow of tracer through the heart, the SVC, and right atrium (upper left images), the RV (upper middle images), and the pulmonary outflow tract and both main pulmonary arteries (upper right images). The lungs are seen in the second row and the LV in the third row. The LV and aorta are visualized in the bottom row.

From these data, the first-pass RVG can be obtained. This has been used since the 1970s to assess global and regional RV and LV performance. The availability of high count rates with the Baird System 77 (now Picker's SIM-400, Picker International, Inc, Cleveland, OH) multicrystal camera enabled investigators to obtain high-quality first-pass studies with high temporal resolution. For many years this was the only means of obtaining useful first-pass data. Much work has been done documenting the usefulness of the first-pass RVG (26,37–42). Multiple studies since 1980 have substantiated the initial observations that both the first-pass and the MUGA scan yield similar data on global and regional left and RV function. Gal et al. have discussed extensively the methodology involved in a first-pass study (42).

## Equipment

### Multicrystal Cameras

A dedicated first-pass multicrystal gamma camera with a 14 × 21 array of crystals and a 6 × 9–inch field-of-view equipped with a 1.5-inch thick parallel-hole collimator are used. The matrix size is 14 × 21 pixels, with a center-to-center crystal spacing of 1.11 cm. The latest version of

this device is a cost-effective means of obtaining first-pass data.

### Single-Crystal Cameras

More recently, single-crystal cameras have been successfully used, particularly the most modern systems that allow high count rate performance, such as the small APEX 215 cardiac system from Elscint (Elscint, Inc, Hackensack, NJ) and the GE ACT (GE Medical Systems, Milwaukee, WI) large field-of-view cameras. The APEX 215 system is a digital, small field-of-view, portable camera equipped with a high-sensitivity, medium-resolution parallel hole collimator. The GE system is a more conventional system with general capabilities but a sufficiently fast count rate (140,000 counts per second with 20% loss in 140-keV window) for first-pass studies, especially if a very high-efficiency collimator is used.

## Scan Protocol

Patients are generally studied at rest in the supine position. Patients have an 18-gauge polytef (Teflon) catheter placed in an antecubital or more proximal vein. The gamma camera detector is placed over the patient's chest in a 20- to 30-degree right anterior oblique projection. A 25-mCi bolus of Tc-99m agent in <1 ml of saline is loaded into an extension tube attached to a catheter. The radionuclide bolus is flushed through this catheter with 20 ml of normal saline. Acquisition is started just before injecting the radionuclide. Using the multicrystal system, stress first-pass studies are performed using a chest point source marker for motion correction. However, motion correction can be undertaken by software control without the need of a marker by using centroid techniques once used for correction of hepatic respiratory motion in liver-spleen scanning.

Counts are accumulated in frame mode for 30 seconds using a rate of 1 frame per 30 milliseconds. A periventricular ROI is chosen as BKG to completely surround, and be contiguous with, the fixed ventricular ROI used. This BKG ROI incorporates the adjacent large vessels and atria. The average counts per pixel in this ring-shaped ROI during ES is used to represent the average BKG per pixel, although some users select the lung region for BKG. The BKG is typically 30% of the LV activity, whereas for the RV measurement the BKG is even less. This low BKG activity is the result of temporal separation of the ventricular activity from the lung in addition to the spatial separation used in MUGA scans. After correcting for BKG, the program searches the TAC and identifies the ED and ES frame numbers for every valid beat, number of beats used, heart rate, total duration of the ventricular phase in seconds, and the first and last frames. The RVEF and LVEF are then calculated using methods similar to MUGA techniques described previously. The ED and ES counts are from a small series (typically

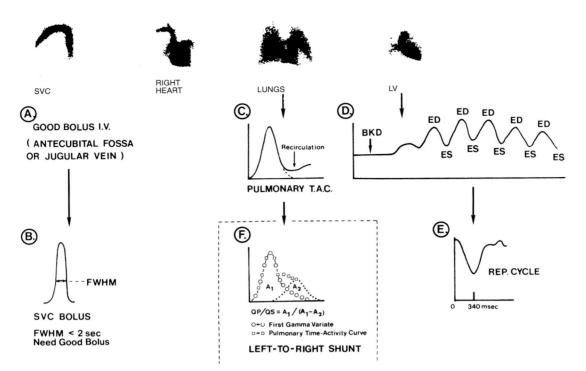

**FIG. 6-16.** This composite illustration shows the typical analysis of first-pass data. **(A)** The upper four panels show the bolus passage through the SVC, right heart, lungs, and LV. It is essential to inject a "compact" bolus with a full-width at half-maximum <2 seconds, as shown in **(B)**. **(C)** Analysis of the TAC in a pulmonary ROI should yield a monotonic curve without "breaks" on the downslope except for normal recirculation. The passage of the bolus through the LV is analyzed in the high temporal resolution mode, and usually 3 to 8 cardiac beats can be resolved. **(D)** Here 5 cardiac cycles are resolved. The BKG is usually 30% of the peak LV activity. **(E)** The individual cardiac beats are summed into a final representative cycle (rep cycle), from which systolic and diastolic parameters are generated. **(F)** When there is a left-to-right shunt, the descending limb of the pulmonary TAC (*squares*) departs from the gamma variate fit (*circles*). The pulmonary/systemic flow (Qp/Qs) seen in a left-to-right shunt is $A_1/A_1 - A_2$. ($A_1$, lung TAC; $A_2$, fraction of blood shunting from left to right.)

three to eight) of frames selected by the operator (Fig. 6-16). Sometimes the individual frames are synchronized with the ECG gate to better select ED and ES, given the statistical fluctuation that results from the relatively low count images. The LVEF using the first-pass technique is calculated in the same way as the gated RVG technique (see Equation 1).

## Quality Control of Technique

The attractiveness of the first-pass method is that it allows the temporal separation of the ventricles in addition to the spatial separation relied on in MUGA and MUGX studies. During a first-pass study, the TAC displays the transit of the bolus through the superior vena cava, right atrium, RV, pulmonary artery, lungs, left atrium, LV, and aorta (see Fig. 6-16). Systemic recirculation of tracer occurs in 10 to 15 seconds. The technical constraints of the first-pass technique are considerable. It is very important that analysis of an ROI placed in the superior vena cava yield a bolus lasting no more than 2 seconds. A poor bolus delivery results in inadequate data for LV and intracardiac shunt studies because the dose is too dispersed. In the case of RV first-pass studies, a bolus that is too compact may have inadequate mixing and so invalidate the model condition of complete mixing within the chamber to be studied.

The TAC data in the RV or LV is inspected and should display the expected diastolic peak and systolic nadir. In general, approximately three to eight cardiac cycles can be found to display the expected LV TAC for subsequent analysis. The decision as to which technique to use (ECG gated or operator-selected ED and ES frames) need not be made before the study is acquired because the rapid frame mode collection allows for recording the physiologic ECG signal.

First-pass studies must have 1,000 to 6,000 counts at ED in the ventricular ROI. They result in a significant statistical uncertainty, especially in patients with low EFs. Green et al. performed a theoretic comparison (43) between the first-pass and gated equilibrium methods in assessing LV function. The data indicated that the MUGA scan tends to possess the greater statistical precision when cardiac output is elevated (such as exercise). The first-pass technique has greater precision when cardiac output is low.

## Clinical Applications of First-Pass RVG

### *Coronary Artery Disease*

The first-pass technique has been used to identify severe CAD (26,31,32) and postsurgical septal abnormalities. Septal function is abnormal postoperatively only in patients who develop a clinical postoperative myocardial infarction (44); otherwise, septal function is maintained in patients who undergo open-heart surgery.

### *Left-to-Right Shunts*

By far the most appropriate indication for the first-pass technique is the detection and quantitation of left-to-right shunts (45,46). With this technique, left-to-right shunts as small as 1.1 to 1.0 (pulmonary-to-systemic flow) can be detected. In 1975, Alderson (47) used the exponential area ratio method to establish left-to-right shunt values. Alderson observed that the downslope of the curve corresponding to the passage of radionuclide through the normal lungs has a monoexponential shape. Its value from the peak activity to the beginning of the early recirculation decreases exponentially to 1% of the maximum. In 1973, Maltz and Treves used a gamma variate method to fit a curve to the TAC (46). In patients with left-to-right shunts, the descending limb of the pulmonary TAC is not exponential and diverges from the purely exponential decay. This is caused by the early recirculation through the shunt. To compute the magnitude of the left-to-right shunt, the pulmonary curve of the first-pass study is first fitted using a gamma variate function and subtracted from the combined normal and recirculation curves (the expected normal pulmonary and the unexpected early pulmonary recirculation) to calculate the shunt.

In practice (see Fig. 6-16F), the points chosen for fitting the gamma variate curve are those approximately 10% before the maximum on the upslope to those just before the start of the recirculation peak, which usually occurs below 70% of the maximum on the downslope. The fitted lung area is represented as $A_1$. The fitted shunt area is presented as $A_2$ and is proportional to the magnitude of the left-to-right shunt.

With these data, and by letting Qp = total pulmonary blood flow and Qs = systemic flow, it follows that:

$$\frac{Qp}{Qs} = \frac{A_1}{A_1 - A_2} \qquad (4)$$

This area ratio method (Qp/Qs) is accurate for shunts between 1 and 3:1. The methodology for computing left-to-right shunts is succinctly shown in Fig. 6-16. This measurement is used for diagnosis or follow-up of patients with intracardiac shunts before or after medical or surgical therapies. Madsen et al. have modified this technique (48). With their algorithm, the gamma variate that is fitted to the first-pass portion of the lung curve is used to generate a curve that simulates the response of a normal lung curve with sys-temic recirculation. The difference between the curve and the observed lung curve is used to yield Qp/Qs.

### *RV Ejection Fraction*

The fact that the right atrium overlaps the ventricle causes artifactual reduction of the MUGA scan measurement of RVEF. The RVEF determined by first-pass angiocardiography is the gold standard measurement of RV function (49). Typically the normal RVEF is 50%, clearly greater than MUGA RVEF. The precise measurement of RV performance by first-pass analysis can be used diagnostically and therapeutically in the assessment of patients with right heart disorders, including

- RV infarction
- COPD
- Intracardiac shunts

### *Right-to-Left Shunts*

Tc-99m macroaggregated albumin (see Chapter 4) can be used to compute right-to-left shunts in the heart and in pulmonary arteriovenous malformations (50,51).

## STRESS ECHOCARDIOGRAPHY

Because the ECG stress test has limited sensitivity, specificity, and predictive power, it is often inadequate as a diagnostic tool. This test is even less helpful in many patient populations, such as nonfasting individuals; some females; those patients with LBBB, previous myocardial infarction, previous PTCA and CABG, rest depolarization abnormalities, inability to exercise, valvular heart disease, or mitral valve prolapse; and those taking drugs such as digoxin, antiarrhythmics, diuretics, and antidepressants.

The echocardiogram can be used to investigate LV function at rest and immediately after exercise for the same purposes as the ECG and as discussed for the gated RVG. Exercise echocardiography can detect regional LV dysfunction immediately after, but not during, exercise. In principle, then, exercise echocardiography should provide similar information to that of the gated exercise RVG (52,53).

Among the advantages of echocardiography are cost, availability, good standardization, absence of ionizing radiation, and the ability to assess valvular or pericardial disease, cardiac tumors, chamber volumes, wall thickness, and pulmonary pressure estimation. The stress echocardiogram can also detect ischemia by identifying a decrease of systolic myocardial thickening.

Among the disadvantages of echocardiography are frequency of suboptimal studies, poor endocardial border definition, observer and operator dependency, regional rather than global LVEF measurements, difficulties in assessing ischemia superimposed on scar tissue, and inability to do treadmill exercise or assess myocardial perfusion.

## DOBUTAMINE ECHOCARDIOGRAPHY

Dobutamine echocardiography is a pharmacologic stress test used as an alternative for patients who cannot achieve maximal exercise (54). Dobutamine is a catecholamine that increases heart rate and decreases BP slightly, and the chronotropic effect may be enhanced by atropine (0.25 to 0.35 mg IV). It causes ischemic regional dysfunction and is the basis for the exercise echocardiographic test. The sensitivity and specificity for detection of CAD are 76% and 89%, respectively, which is very similar to the sensitivity and specificity of MPI (55,56). This intervention can also be used to assess myocardial viability in dysfunctional LV segments (57).

Dobutamine is infused in these tests in 3-minute dose increments of 5, 10, 20, 30, 40, and 50 µg/kg per minute with atropine, if required. End-points of this pharmacologic test are achievement of 85% predicted maximal heart rate, maximum allowable dose, or severe angina. Potential false-positive tests are inadequate endocardial visualization, small vessel disease, or patients with valvular or cardiac muscle abnormalities and LV diastolic dysfunction. The inferior, inferoposterior, and lateral walls may be too deep for good echo signals and so limit its general applicability.

## REFERENCES

1. Botvinick EH, Dae MW, O'Connell JW. Blood pool scintigraphy. Cardiol Clin 1989;7:537–563.
2. Zaret BL, Strauss HW, Hurley PJ, et al. A noninvasive scintiphotographic method for detecting regional ventricular dysfunction in man. N Engl J Med 1971;284:1165–1170.
3. Green MV, Brody WR, Douglas MA, et al. Ejection fraction by count rate from gated images. J Nucl Med 1978;19:880–883.
4. Burow RD, Strauss HW, Singleton R, et al. Analysis of left ventricular function from multiple gated acquisition cardiac blood pool imaging: comparison to contrast angiography. Circulation 1977;56:1024–1028.
5. Chilton HM, Callahan RJ, Thrall JH. Radiopharmaceuticals for Cardiac Imaging. In Swanson DP, Chilton HM, Thrall JH (eds), Pharmaceuticals in Medical Imaging: Radiopaque Contrast Media, Radiopharmaceuticals, Enhancement Agents for Magnetic Resonance Imaging and Ultrasound. New York: Macmillan, 1990;419–460.
6. Folland ED, Hamilton GW, Larson SM, et al. The radionuclide ejection fraction: a comparison of three radionuclide techniques with contrast angiography. J Nucl Med 1977;18:1159–a1166.
7. Borer JS, Bacharach SL, Green MV, et al. Real time radionuclide cineangiography in the noninvasive evaluation of global and regional left ventricular function at rest and during exercise in patients with coronary artery disease. N Engl J Med 1977;296:839–844.
8. Harizi R, Bianco JA, Filiberti AW, et al. Radionuclide ventriculography in normal volunteers performing graded supine bicycle exercise. Am J Noninv Cardiol 1987;1:56–60.
9. Legrand V, Chevigne M, Foulon J, Rigo P. Evaluation of right ventricular function by gated blood pool scintigraphy. J Nucl Med 1983;24:886–893.
10. Zaret BL, Wackers FJ. Nuclear Cardiology II. Evaluation of ventricular function. N Engl J Med 1993;329:855–863.
11. Bough EW, Gandsman EJ, North DL, Shulman RS. Gated radionuclide angiographic evaluation of valve regurgitation. Am J Cardiol 1980;46:423–428.
12. Schad N. Nontraumatic assessment of left ventricular wall motion and regional stroke volume after myocardial infarction. J Nucl Med 1977;18:333–338.
13. Pavel D, Sychra JJ, Olea E. Functional (Parametric) Imaging of Dynamic Cardiac Studies. In Gelfand MJ, Thomas SR (eds), Effective Use of Computers in Nuclear Medicine. New York: McGraw-Hill, 1988;161–205.
14. Barry WH, Bridge JHB. Intracellular calcium homeostasis in cardiac myocytes. Circulation 1993;87:1806–1815.
15. Bonow RO, Bacharach SL, Green MV, et al. Impaired left ventricular diastolic filling in patients with coronary artery disease: assessment with radionuclide angiography. Circulation 1981;64:315–323.
16. Bianco JA, Filiberti AW, Baker SP, et al. Ejection fraction and heart rate correlate with diastolic filling rate at rest and during exercise. Chest 1985;88:107–113.
17. Stewart RAH, Joshi J, Alexander N, et al. Adjustment for the influence of age and heart rate on Doppler measurements of left ventricular filling. Br Heart J 1992;68:608–612.
18. Harizi RC, Bianco JA, Alpert JS. Diastolic function of the heart in clinical cardiology. Arch Intern Med 1988;148:99–109.
19. Lorell BH. Significance of diastolic dysfunction of the heart. Ann Rev Med 1991;42:411–436.
20. Brutsaert DL, Sys SU, Gillebert TC. Diastolic failure: pathophysiology and therapeutic implications. J Am Coll Cardiol 1993;22:318–325.
21. Wagasuki S, Fischman AJ, Babich JW, et al. Myocardial substrate utilization and left ventricular function in Adriamycin cardiomyopathy. J Nucl Med 1993;34:1529–1535.
22. Schwartz RG, McKenzie WB, Alexander J, et al. Congestive heart failure and left ventricular dysfunction complicating doxorubicin therapy: seven-year experience using serial radionuclide angiocardiography. Am J Med 1987;82:1109–1118.
23. Bonow RO, Dilsizian V, Cuocolo A, Bacharach SL. Identification of viable myocardium in patients with chronic coronary artery disease and left ventricular dysfunction: comparison of thallium scintigraphy with reinjection and PET imaging with F-18-fluorodeoxyglucose. Circulation 1991;83:26–37.
24. Baker DW, Jones R, Hodges J, et al. Management of heart failure. III. The role of revascularization in the treatment of patients with moderate or severe left ventricular dysfunction. JAMA 1994;272:1528–1534.
25. Dilsizian V, Bonow RO. Current diagnostic techniques of assessing myocardial viability in patients with hibernating and stunned myocardium. Circulation 1993;87:1–20.
26. Jones RH, McEwan P, Newman GE, et al. Accuracy of diagnosis of coronary artery disease by radionuclide measurement of left ventricular function during rest and exercise. Circulation 1981;64:586–601.
27. DePace NL, Hakki AH, Weinreich DJ, Iskandrian AS. Noninvasive assessment of coronary artery disease. Am J Cardiol 1983;52:714–720.
28. Weintraub WS, Schneider RM, Seelaus PA, et al. Prospective evaluation of the severity of coronary artery disease with exercise radionuclide angiography and electrocardiography. Am Heart J 1986;111:537–542.
29. Gibbons RJ, Fyke FE III, Clements IP, et al. Noninvasive identification of severe coronary artery disease using exercise radionuclide angiography. J Am Coll Cardiol 1988;11:28–34.
30. Taliercio CP, Clements IP, Zinsmeister AR, Gibbons RJ. Prognostic value and limitations of exercise radionuclide angiography in medically treated coronary artery disease. Mayo Clin Proc 1988;63:573–582.
31. Pryor DB, Harrell FE Jr, Lee KL, et al. Prognostic indicators from radionuclide angiography in medically treated patients with coronary artery disease. Am J Cardiol 1984;53:18–22.
32. Lee KL, Pryor DB, Pieper KS, et al. Prognostic value of radionuclide angiography in medically treated patients with coronary artery disease: a comparison with clinical and catheterization variables. Circulation 1990;82:1705–1717.
33. Morris KG, Palmeri ST, Califf RM, et al. Value of radionuclide angiography for predicting specific cardiac events after myocardial infarction. Am J Cardiol 1985;55:318–324.
34. Bonow RO, Kent KM, Rosing DR, et al. Exercise-induced ischemia in mildly symptomatic patients with coronary artery disease and preserved left ventricular function: identification of subgroups at risk of death during medical therapy. N Engl J Med 1984;311:1339–1345.
35. Miller TD, Taliercio CP, Zinsmeister AR, et al. Risk stratification of single or double vessel coronary artery disease and impaired left ventricular function using exercise radionuclide angiography. Am J Cardiol 1990;65:1317–1321.
36. Onik G, Recht L, Edwards JE, et al. False LV aneurysm: diagnosis by noninvasive means. J Nucl Med 1980;21:177–182.
37. Berger HJ, Zaret BL. Radionuclide Assessment of Left Ventricular Performance. In Freeman LM (ed), Clinical Radionuclide Imaging, Vol. 1. New York: Grune & Stratton, 1984;414–436.

38. Ashburn WL, Schelbert HR, Verba JW. Left ventricular ejection fraction—a review of several radionuclide angiographic approaches using the scintillation camera. Prog Cardiovasc Dis 1978;20:267–284.

39. Berger HJ, Mathay RA, Loke J, et al. Assessment of cardiac performance with quantitative radionuclide angiocardiography: right ventricular ejection fraction with reference to findings in chronic obstructive pulmonary disease. Am J Cardiol 1978;41:897–905.

40. Upton MT, Rerych SK, Newman GE, et al. The reproducibility of radionuclide angiographic measurements of left ventricular function in normal subjects at rest and during exercise. Circulation 1980;62:126–132.

41. Jengo JA, Mena I, Blaufuss A, Criley JM. Evaluation of left ventricular function (ejection fraction and segmental wall motion) by single pass radioisotope angiography. Circulation 1978;57:326–332.

42. Gal RA, Grenier RP, Port SC, et al. Left ventricular volume calculation using a count-based ratio method applied to first-pass radionuclide angiography. J Nucl Med 1992;33:2124–2132.

43. Green MV, Bacharach SL, Borer JS, Bonow RO. A theoretical comparison of first-pass and gated equilibrium methods in the measurement of systolic left ventricular function. J Nucl Med 1991;32:1801–1807.

44. Schoolman M, Bianco JA, Khuri SF, et al. The radionuclide evaluation of septal wall function following coronary bypass surgery. Nucl Med Commun 1985;6:159–168.

45. Parker JA, Treves S. Radionuclide detection, localization and quantitation of intracardiac shunts and shunts between the great arteries. Prog Cardiovasc Dis 1977;20:121–150.

46. Maltz DL, Treves S. Quantitative radionuclide angiocardiography. Determination of Qp/Qs in children. Circulation 1973;47:1049–1056.

47. Alderson PO, Jost RG, Strauss AW, et al. Detection and quantitation of left-to-right cardiac shunts in children: a clinical comparison of count ratio and area ratio techniques. J Nucl Med 1975;16:511–516.

48. Madsen MT, Argenyi E, Preslar J, et al. An improved method for the quantitation of left-to-right cardiac shunts. J Nucl Med 1991;32:1808–1812.

49. Iwata K. Alternative method for calculating right ventricular ejection fraction from first-pass time-activity curves. J Nucl Med 1988;29:1990–1997.

50. Gates GF, Goris ML. Suitability of radiopharmaceuticals for determining right-to-left shunting. J Nucl Med 1977;18:255–257.

51. Susuki Y. Quantitation of right-to-left shunt ratio in patients with pulmonary telangiectasis by Tc-99m MAA lung perfusion imaging. Clin Nucl Med 1986;11:84–87.

52. Wann LS, Faris JV, Childress RH, et al. Exercise cross-sectional echocardiography in ischemic heart disease. Circulation 1979;60:1300–1308.

53. Roger VL, Pellika PA, Miller FA, et al. Stress echocardiography. I. Exercise echocardiography: techniques, implementation, clinical applications and correlations. Mayo Clin Proc 1995;70:5–15.

54. Verani MS. Myocardial perfusion imaging versus two-dimensional echocardiography: comparative value in the diagnosis of coronary artery disease. J Nucl Cardiol 1994;1:399–414.

55. Marwick T, Willemart B, D'Hondt AM, et al. Selection of the optimal nonexercise stress for the evaluation of ischemic regional myocardial dysfunction and malperfusion: comparison of dobutamine and adenosine using echocardiography and Tc-99m MIBI single-photon emission computed tomography. Circulation 1993;87:345–354.

56. Marwick T, D'Hondt AM, Baudhuin T, et al. Optimal use of dobutamine stress for the detection and evaluation of coronary artery disease: combination with echocardiography or scintigraphy, or both? J Am Coll Cardiol 1993;22:159–167.

57. Pierard La, DeLandsheere CM, Berthe C, et al. Identification of viable myocardium by echocardiography during dobutamine infusion in patients with myocardial infarction after thrombolytic therapy: comparison with positron emission tomography. J Am Coll Cardiol 1990;15:1021–1031.

*Textbook of Nuclear Medicine,*
edited by Michael A. Wilson.
Lippincott–Raven Publishers, Philadelphia © 1998.

CHAPTER 7

# Thyroid and Thyroid Therapy

Michael A. Wilson

## OVERVIEW

### History

Thyroid studies represent <5% of all nuclear medicine diagnostic studies but the majority (>90%) of nuclear medicine therapies. The role of radionuclides in thyroidology goes back to 1936, when New England endocrinologists heard of Fermi's production of radionuclides in 1934 and asked if radioiodine could be produced. The first radioiodine was produced in 1937, and animal iodine 128 (I-128) tracer studies were published in 1938. In 1939, human studies were performed, and the first attempt to treat hyperthyroidism with radioiodine occurred in 1940. In retrospect, this attempt used diagnostic doses of I-124 rather than therapeutic doses. Later, a battle concerning hyperthyroid therapy raged between surgeons and radioiodine advocates until a thyrotoxic patient was successfully treated with I-130 in 1943. An excellent review of this history and intrigue is provided in a 1983 commentary in the *Journal of the American Medical Association* (JAMA) (1). In 1943, Astwood published on the treatment of hyperthyroidism with thiourea and thiouracil; that remarkable story was published in a 1984 JAMA landmark perspective (2).

Radioiodine was used in the 1950s when I-131 became available, but widespread application of radioiodine treatment was prevented by philosophic concerns about the risk of radiation, which were fueled by the indiscriminate use of irradiation in the treatment of thymus enlargement, acne, tonsillitis, hemangioma, and pertussis. The first mention of the risk of thyroid carcinoma in association with secondary irradiation of the thyroid was made in 1950 (3). This report found that 10 of 28 patients with thyroid carcinoma had had previous irradiation, and the potential relationship was identified. In 1957, follow-up studies recommended abandonment of irradiation because of a tumor rate greater than expected. In 1974, a controlled study showed that as little as 6.5 rads (6.5 cGy) to the thyroid (scalp irradiation given for

tinea capitis) resulted in a severalfold increase in thyroid and brain tumors (4). When confirmation was attempted in similar studies, it was noted that the small dose association applied only to children of Jewish origin. A later large cooperative trial of 26 institutions of tens of thousands of hyperthyroid patients compared treatment by radioiodine, surgery, and drug therapy and found I-131 therapy to be safe (5,6).

In these days of increased awareness of risks of radiation, practicing radiologists giving radionuclide therapies should understand the risks of radioiodine and allow patients to make informed decisions. The radiology therapist must be able to describe the biological risks of radiation rationally and realistically to the patient and the referring physician. Radiologists who are board certified in diagnostic radiology require preceptor statements indicating experience of 10 hyperthyroid and three thyroid cancer therapies for Nuclear Regulatory Commission (NRC) licensure for therapy privileges. They also must be aware of recent NRC regulations concerning the Quality Management Plan (QMP) and rules that require keeping records of dose estimates to individuals exposed to the treated patient, and providing appropriate written instructions.

Nuclear medicine applications to the thyroid continue to evolve. Radioactive iodine uptake (RAIU) was once a mainstay of thyroid diagnosis, but the recent introduction of sensitive, supersensitive, and ultrasensitive thyroid-stimulating hormones (TSHs) (see Chapter 26) have largely replaced the RAIU and the need for suppression and stimulation uptakes and scans (Fig. 7-1). When the TSH radioimmunoassay (RIA) was replaced by the labeled antibody immunoradiometric (IRMA) technique, increased assay sensitivity resulted, and very low TSH levels were measurable. The TSH assay can now separate suppressive, normal, and stimulatory TSH levels and exquisitely define the thyroid's functional status, a role formerly left to RAIU measurements for global assessment and scans for regional assessment.

Following are some important thyroid milestones:

1923: Iodide excess calms patients for surgery

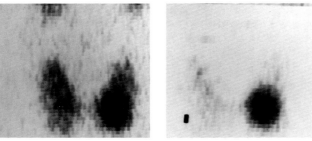

A,B

**FIG. 7-1.** This Tc-99m TcO₄⁻ thyroid scan from 1979 represents images obtained with a rectilinear scanner. **(A)** This scan demonstrates a normal right lobe and increased tracer uptake in the lower pole of the left lobe, where a palpable nodule is present. **(B)** After 7 days of liothyronine (Cytomel) suppression (25 µg tid), this scan shows suppressed normal thyroid (marker shows lateral and lower aspect of palpable right thyroid lobe) and a persistent "hot" autonomously functioning nodule. Both the scanner and the suppression technique are obsolete, replaced by the gamma camera and serum TSH measurements.

1923: External x-ray therapy (XRT) used for hyperthyroidism
1937: Radioiodine first produced
1938: Physiologic I-128 animal studies
1938: I-131 produced at University of California, Berkeley
1943: Bitter dispute regarding the use of radioiodine (1)
1943: Thioureas first used in humans (2)
1946: I-131 available from U.S. Atomic Energy Commission
1948: Geiger-Mueller point-by-point mapping of thyroid
1951: First scanner constructed
1958: First gamma camera built
1964: Gamma camera commercially manufactured

### Thyroid Embryology

The thyroid is one of the largest endocrine organs, with the average mass being 20 g. It develops from the fourth and fifth branchial pouches, is bilobed by 4 weeks in the embryo, and is functional by 10 weeks. The pyramidal lobe (Fig. 7-2) is a remnant of thyroglossal duct tract and is seen in one-third of normal technetium pertechnetate (Tc-99m TcO₄⁻) and I-123 thyroid scans and in two-thirds of scans in patients with Graves' disease. Ectopic tissue can be found anywhere from the site of origin at the base of the tongue (foramen cecum) to the myocardium.

### Iodide Physiology

The thyroid gland clears plasma of iodide, converts it rapidly to iodine, and organifies it into thyroid hormone. Thyroxine ($T_4$) contains four atoms of iodine, which represent 67% of the hormone's molecular weight. The kidneys and thyroid both compete for iodide, the plasma renal clearance (35 ml/min) being approximately twice the normal euthyroid plasma thyroid clearance (20 ml/min). This thy-

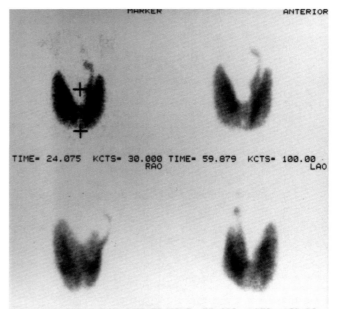

**FIG. 7-2.** A typical thyroid scan format at University of Wisconsin Hospitals. The upper left image shows the thyroid with markers at the hyoid bone (upper) and SSN (lower). The tracer uptake is high (RAIU 60%) because the BKG is low and the thyroid lobes have much more activity than the barely visible salivary glands. The upper right image shows the anterior thyroid image filling much of the field of view because of the pinhole collimator magnification, with a left-sided pyramidal lobe visible. On the RAO (lower left) and LAO (lower right) views, the pyramidal lobe moves away from the pinhole because of its anterior position. Such movement helps distinguish this anterior midline activity from posterior artifacts, such as esophageal tracer. The times and counts recorded help in making decisions about functional status (i.e., crude estimates of uptake).

roidal clearance of plasma is termed *thyroidal trapping*. The thyroid has the ability to vary trapping in excess of 20-fold under TSH control, and in hyperthyroid states the thyroid clearance can approach 200 ml per minute, which explains the very high RAIUs that occur.

The human dietary iodine requirement is about 75 µg daily. The thyroid is the main iodine storage organ (8,000 µg) and contains 100 times the daily dietary requirement, stored in various forms of thyroid hormone and iodotyrosine precursors. The average American diet contains 75 to 700 µg iodide, mostly provided in the form of additives to bread (iodate stabilizer), milk (iodized salt licks used in the dairy industry), and iodized table salt. The gastrointestinal tract absorbs nearly 100% of the ingested iodine, with 90% of the absorption occurring within 1 hour.

Iodide is actively trapped by the thyroid under TSH control, using the adenosine triphosphatase sodium-potassium (ATPase Na⁺/K⁺) pump. There follows very rapid (in seconds) organification of iodide to iodine by peroxidase at the interface of follicular cells and colloid. The iodine is then bound to tyrosine residues on thyroglobulin, a large molecule

**TABLE 7-1.** *Role of TSH*

1. Trapping of iodide
2. Exocytosis of thyroglobulin
3. Organification of tyrosines
4. Coupling of MIT and DIT to $T_3$ and $T_4$
5. Secretion of $T_3$ and $T_4$ (pinocytosis)

**TABLE 7-2.** *Drugs with excess iodine*

| Drug | Utility | Iodine |
|---|---|---|
| Amiodarone | Antiarrhythmic | 75 mg/tab |
| Omnipaque 300 | Contrast agent | 300 mg/ml |
| SSKI | Expectorant | 40 mg/drop |
| Betadine | Topical agent | 12 mg/ml |
| Vitamin with I⁻ | Supplement | 0.15 mg/tab |
| Avadrinal (potassium iodide) | Bronchodilator | 245 mg/tab |

(660,000 molecular weight) that represents 50% to 75% of the thyroid gland by weight. The monoiodotyrosine (MIT) and diiodotyrosine (DIT) are coupled by peroxidase to form triiodothyronine ($T_3$) and $T_4$. Hormone release from the colloid storage is also mediated by TSH. All these processes occur rapidly in response to TSH stimulation (Table 7-1), which is exquisitely sensitive to circulating $T_3$ and $T_4$ levels via the hypothalamic-pituitary feedback mechanism.

In iodine deficiency the thyroid traps iodide very efficiently and converts iodide economically into thyroid hormone. This increased trapping results in increased uptake of iodine (i.e., increased RAIUs) and increased levels of $T_3$ relative to $T_4$ (three rather than four iodine atoms per hormone molecule). When sufficient iodide is provided, the patient becomes euthyroid. As many as 10% of persons in endemic iodine-deficient areas exposed to excess iodine become transiently thyrotoxic (jodbasedow effect). Some patients with multinodular goiter (MNG) may also become thyrotoxic with excess iodine reflecting the autonomous nature of some of their nodules.

With excess iodide (Table 7-2), thyroid hormone production is transiently inhibited (the Wolff-Chaikoff effect) for 10 to 14 days. This iodine excess effect is used before surgical treatment of thyrotoxicosis to decrease the vascularity of the gland and prepare the patient for surgery. Two percent of the American population do not subsequently escape from this transient inhibition, and longer periods of hypothyroidism ensue. Patients with Hashimoto's thyroiditis and partial destruction of the thyroid gland by surgery or radioiodine often do not have this normal escape mechanism from the Wolff-Chaikoff effect, and longer-term hypothyroidism can occur with excess iodide.

Amiodarone, a newer cardiac antiarrhythmic agent, deserves special mention for its effect on thyroid function and circulating $T_4$ levels. Amiodarone is 37% iodine by weight and is usually prescribed in doses of 400 to 600 mg/day. This supplies 150 to 250 mg iodide daily, several hundred times the daily requirement. This excess iodide can produce hypothyroidism or hyperthyroidism in the United States (10% become hypothyroid and 2% become hyperthyroid, with hypothyroidism occurring especially in patients with coexisting Hashimoto's). In iodine-deficient areas, this drug causes the opposite effect (10% hyperthyroidism, 2% hypothyroidism). Amiodarone also consistently alters thyroid hormone levels, increasing total $T_4$, free $T_4$, and the free $T_4$ index in 40% of patients while reducing serum $T_3$ levels. This presumably occurs as a result of inhibition of peripheral deiodination of $T_4$ to $T_3$. The drug is stored in fat tissues and consequently has a biological half-life >100 days. About half the patients on amiodarone have altered thyroid function tests or thyroid status, and these changes persist long after the drug is discontinued.

### Circulating Thyroid Hormones

As described above (see Table 7-1), increased pituitary TSH release results in the formation and release of thyroid hormone. An excess production and release of thyroid hormone is called hyperthyroidism and can be measured by RAIU and circulating hormone levels. The major hormone released is $T_4$, but this acts on peripheral tissues by being converted to the more metabolically active $T_3$. Any $T_4$ not required is converted to reverse $T_3$ ($rT_3$), a metabolically inactive form of $T_3$ providing an exquisitely sensitive peripheral autoregulatory control mechanism in which $T_4$ can be considered a prohormone of $T_3$.

### *Thyroid Feedback Mechanism*

The pituitary produces thyrotropin, or TSH, a large (28,000 d) two-chain molecule that controls the thyroidal uptake of iodide as well as the production and release of thyroid hormones (see Table 7-1). The pituitary gland is exquisitely sensitive to circulating thyroid hormone levels, and this feedback mechanism is the dominant method of adjusting TSH secretion in response to thyroid hormone levels. The hypothalamus, via the tripeptide thyrotropin-releasing hormone, controls the setpoint for thyroid function, resulting in a baseline hormone level that is continuously and exquisitely adjusted by TSH secretion. The effect of thyroid hormone on peripheral organs is therefore dependent on the hypothalamus for the setpoint level, the pituitary via TSH for fine control, the thyroid gland for the maintenance of thyroid hormone blood levels, and the peripheral target site for the conversion of $T_4$ to $T_3$ for cellular action.

### *Hormone Transport*

Thyroid hormones are transported to peripheral tissues by thyroid-binding globulin (TBG), transthyretin, and albumin. Nearly all $T_3$ is bound to TBG, but this binding is of lower affinity than that of $T_4$ to TBG. Seventy percent of $T_4$ is bound to TBG, and the rest is bound to both transthyretin and albu-

**TABLE 7-3.** *Circulating thyroid hormone parameters*

|                    | $T_3$     | $T_4$      |
|--------------------|-----------|------------|
| Serum half-life    | <1 day    | 1 week     |
| Thyroid production | 5 µg/day  | 80 µg/day  |
| Total pool         | 45 µg     | 800 µg     |
| TBG binding        | 100%      | 75%        |
| Free hormone       | 0.3%      | 0.03%      |

min, which have less affinity for $T_4$ than TBG (Table 7-3). Approximately three-fourths of TBG and 99% of transthyretin and albumin are free of hormone, thus demonstrating a huge potential binding capacity for $T_4$ and $T_3$. This results in a small portion (0.03% to 0.3%) of the hormones being free for metabolic effect. The time during which blood bathes the individual cell is only a second or so, insufficient for the dissociation of $T_4$ from the thyroid hormone protein carriers, so the only free forms of thyroid hormone are available to cells.

## Clinical Syndromes

The syndrome that results from the overproduction of thyroid hormone is called *thyrotoxicosis.* Although usually there is an association between hyperthyroidism (increased iodine trapping and production of thyroid hormone) and thyrotoxicosis, there are occasions when these two processes are dissociated. Examples include subacute thyroiditis when stored thyroid hormone is released from the gland but actual thyroid hormone production is inhibited, as manifest by a low RAIU and low levels of $T_3$ relative to $T_4$ ($T_3$ has a shorter serum half-life than $T_4$). In this condition, the excess circulating thyroid is a result of prior release of thyroid hormone rather than excess production of thyroid hormone. Other examples of dissociation of thyroid hormone production and the presence of excess circulating hormone include factitious, accidental (inadvertent ingestion of $T_4$, e.g., "hamburger toxicosis" where thyroid tissue was included in ground beef), and iatrogenic (excess replacement therapy or suppressive therapy for thyroid cancer) thyrotoxicosis. Very rare causes of thyrotoxicosis include extrathyroidal sources of thyroid hormone (functioning thyroid metastases, struma ovarii).

## Diagnosis of Thyroid Disorders

Several blood tests are available for diagnosing thyroid disorders (see Chapter 26). These include the $T_4$ assay, which is elevated in 90% of thyrotoxic patients and depressed in 80% of hypothyroid patients. The best measurement of circulating thyroid hormone is that of the free $T_4$ not bound to TBG and other carrier proteins and therefore available for metabolic function (free $T_4$ by equilibrium dialysis). The measurement of $T_3$ by immunoassay may be the only abnormality in a small number of patients with the unusual form of thyrotoxicosis called $T_3$ *toxicosis* and in other patients with early hyperthyroidism (especially with solitary toxic adeno-

mas). In hypothyroidism the diagnosis hinges on the measurement of an elevated TSH, which indicates thyroid hypofunction and secondary stimulation via the pituitary feedback mechanism. Hypothyroidism due to pituitary disease, with a low TSH, is a very rare clinical condition.

TSH measurement with the labeled antibody technique, especially the later-generation assays, the so-called sensitive, supersensitive, and ultrasensitive assay, have been touted as the single thyroid function test because, besides diagnosing hypothyroidism, it shows suppressed values in thyrotoxicosis. Each new generation of TSH assay has resulted in a 10-fold lower detection limit (see Chapter 26).

## Thyroid Uptake

RAIU was used extensively in the diagnosis of hyperthyroidism and hypothyroidism but has been largely replaced by direct thyroid hormone measurements. In fact, the use of uptakes and scans as routine thyroid test is often inappropriate. The utility of the RAIU test results from the very rapid absorption of iodide from the proximal small bowel, with 90% being absorbed within an hour of oral administration. The RAIU is profoundly influenced by the iodide blood pool, so that contrast media, kelp, health foods, and expectorants rich in iodide can lower the uptake into subnormal ranges (see Table 7-2). The normal 24-hour uptake is 10% to 35%, but for a diagnostic test this must be measured locally and normal ranges constantly checked because of local fluctuations in dietary iodine intake that can result in changes in the normal range. RAIUs have been measured at 6, 24, and 48 hours. The 48-hour RAIU was used to detect hypothyroidism, the delayed measurement enabling a slightly better discrimination from normal than earlier uptake measurements. Six-hour RAIUs were commonly used in thyrotoxicosis and were often combined with I-123 scans, so the study was completed in a day. Twenty-four–hour uptakes were commonly used as a compromise time for these two thyroid conditions and has now become the standard time for uptake measurement. As many as 15% of thyrotoxic patients have a very rapid turnover of radioiodine; therefore, the 24-hour uptake is less than that obtained at 6 hours (7). The RAIUs vary with various etiologies of thyrotoxicosis and can be helpful in confirming the patient's disease process (Table 7-4).

**TABLE 7-4.** *Relative frequency of hyperthyroidism etiologies and their RAIU at the University of Wisconsin Hospital*

| Disease process      | Relative frequency | Local RAIU mean (range) |
|----------------------|--------------------|-------------------------|
| Graves' disease      | 75%                | 63% (32%–96%)           |
| Toxic MNG            | 15%                | 30% (15%–43%)           |
| Toxic adenoma        | 5%                 | 30% (15%–43%)           |
| Thyroiditis          | 5%                 | <2%                     |
| Iodine induced       | Rare               | Low–high                |
| Factitious and other | Very rare          | <2%                     |
| TSH mediated         | Very rare          | Elevated                |

## *Application of Thyroid Uptake*

RAIUs are still used in several conditions, to do the following:

- Identify low-uptake ("nonhyperthyroid") thyrotoxic conditions that do not require ablative therapy (factitious hyperthyroidism, subacute thyroiditis, and thyrotoxicosis of extrathyroidal origin)
- Tailor I-131 therapy to individual thyrotoxic patients (although the actual thyroid residence time is more important than the measured uptake)
- Identify enzyme defects (using the perchlorate discharge test)
- Determine if sufficient uptake occurs to warrant thyroid ablation or thyroid metastatic therapy (done with scans in thyroid cancer)

## *Perchlorate Discharge Test*

The RAIU is measured in the perchlorate discharge test to determine organification defects. The RAIU is usually elevated in patients with enzyme defects, so sufficient uptake occurs within 1 to 2 hours to provide accurate statistical measurement (i.e., 10,000 counts). The patient is then given 1 g oral potassium perchlorate, which, like Tc-99m $TcO_4^-$, is recognized by the thyroid as having a similar charge and size to iodide and, as such, is trapped by the thyroid. Because perchlorate is supplied in gram doses, it is in huge molecular excess (10 to 11 orders of magnitude) over the radioiodine given for the RAIU. The trapped, but not organified, I-131 already taken up by the gland is discharged as the excess perchlorate is trapped; this causes a drop in the thyroid content of I-131 (a positive test is reflected by a 50% relative or 5% absolute decrease in RAIU) and strongly suggests an enzyme defect. This effect is seen in inherited enzyme defect diseases and in 60% of patients with Hashimoto's thyroiditis.

## THYROTOXICOSIS

### Clinical Diagnosis

These are the classic symptoms of thyrotoxicosis:

- Weight loss (despite a good or voracious appetite)
- Increase in number of bowel movements (but not diarrhea)
- Tachycardia at rest (or excess heart rate in response to modest effort)
- Symptoms of heat intolerance, excess perspiration, tremor, nervousness, and sleeplessness (but these symptoms are generally difficult to establish with certainty)

Many patients do not present with classic symptoms, and most symptoms are easily confused with anxiety.

Many patients thrive on the early symptoms of hyperthyroidism, when they need less sleep, achieve more work, and generally feel very alive and well, so that it is often only after successful therapy that these patients finally realize they have been unwell. The most common physical sign of thyrotoxicosis is tachycardia, whereas ophthalmopathy and thyroid bruit are the most specific signs of Graves' hyperthyroidism.

The presence of both classic symptoms and an increased total $T_4$ level is all that is needed for diagnosis and treatment of most thyrotoxic patients (see Chapter 26). This is true despite the fact that only 0.03% of the measured $T_4$ is free and available for metabolic action and that $T_3$ is the more metabolically active thyroid hormone. Although the sTSH test has been advocated as the best single test for screening thyrotoxicosis, it is probably too sensitive to use alone, because many patients have suppressed TSH without evidence of overt thyrotoxicosis (8). Patients often present for treatment with only an elevated $T_4$ done as part of an investigative screen. It is with these patients, who have presumed biochemical proof of hyperthyroidism and a request for I-131 therapy, that the radiologist must exhibit caution before therapy. In some patients, $T_3$ immunoassay, free $T_4$ by equilibrium dialysis, and an sTSH measurement may be required to classify with certainty. Sensitive and, more recently, supersensitive and ultrasensitive TSHs are now the single most powerful tool in assessing thyroid function (8). A normal sTSH level rules out thyroid dysfunction, and a suppressed sTSH without overt signs and symptoms of thyrotoxicosis can diagnose subclinical hyperthyroidism.

### Causes of Thyrotoxicosis

Table 7-4 lists the causative diseases, their frequency, and their RAIU uptakes.

### *Graves' Disease*

Graves' disease is also termed diffuse hyperthyroidism (Fig. 7-3) as a result of the diffusely increased gland size and increased tracer uptake seen on I-123 and Tc-99m $TcO_4^-$ scans. Graves' disease was first described in 1825 by Parry, then by Graves in 1835. Euthyroid Graves' (exophthalmus without evidence of thyrotoxicosis) was described in 1955. Although the immunologic etiology of Graves' is interesting, it does not affect therapy. Several autoantibodies are described, including stimulatory and inhibitory antibodies. The presence of a stimulatory autoantibody to follicular cell receptors causes hyperthyroidism.

Spontaneous remission, a characteristic of Graves', occurs as these antithyroid antibody levels decrease. This spontaneous decrease in circulating stimulatory autoantibody is an important explanation of the onset of hypothyroidism after destructive therapy (both surgery and I-131

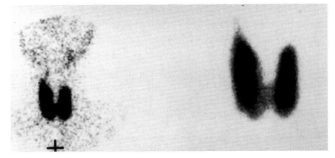

**FIG. 7-3.** The left marker image demonstrates intense localization of thyroidal tracer with minimal background and salivary gland activity, indicating hyperthyroidism. The SSN is marked. The enlarged image on the right demonstrates homogeneous tracer uptake (Graves' disease). Acquisition time was 36 seconds for 100,000 counts. The patient's RAIU was 80% at 24 hours (typical of Graves' disease).

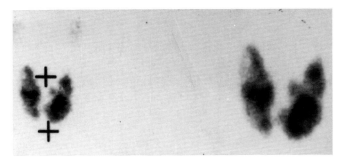

**FIG. 7-4.** The left marker (hyoid and SSN marked) image demonstrates increased and irregular uptake in thyroid with reduced background and salivary gland activity typical of hyperthyroidism. The magnified anterior (right) image demonstrates multiple nodules: some hot, some hot with degenerating portions, and some cold. The RAIU was 43%, at the upper limits for toxic MNGs.

administration). With the destruction of a significant part of the thyroid gland, when the stimulatory autoantibody levels spontaneously decrease, the residual thyroid gland is no longer stimulated to excess production. The production capacity of the remaining thyroid gland is insufficient to produce normal amounts of thyroid hormone, and the patient inevitably becomes hypothyroid.

### Nodular Hyperthyroidism (Toxic MNG)

Nodular hyperthyroidism, or toxic MNG, although a poorly understood condition, is the second most common cause of thyrotoxicosis and occurs especially in older age groups. A goiter may have been present for years, and gland histology shows variable regions of hyperplasia, involution, fibrosis, and calcification. The blood test abnormalities can be subtle, so a single $T_4$ estimation may be insufficient to diagnose toxic MNG. Finding an elevated $T_3$ by immunoassay or free $T_4$ by equilibrium dialysis and evidence of autonomous function (suppressed TSH) is often required for the diagnosis. Patients can present with symptoms referable to a single organ system, which makes the diagnosis easy to overlook. These unusual single-organ presentations include the following:

- Proximal myopathy (difficulty climbing stairs or rising from armchairs)
- Inanition (the apathetic thyrotoxic)
- Unexplained atrial fibrillation

This disease does not spontaneously remit, so antithyroid drugs (ATDs) are not used except as an adjunct to definitive therapy. The thyroid scan demonstrates nodular regions of increased and decreased uptake (Fig. 7-4). The RAIU is not strikingly elevated in this condition and is within the upper half of normal range in as many as 50% of these patients (see Table 7-4).

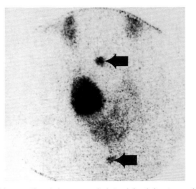

**FIG. 7-5.** This patient has a right-sided hot nodule partially suppressing the remaining palpable left lobe. Radioactive sources (arrows) are located at the SSN (lower) and hyoid bone (upper). Note that the left lobe has less uptake than the salivary glands.

### Solitary Toxic Nodule (Plummer's Disease)

This is a variant of the toxic MNG in which a single adenoma functions autonomously (i.e., is "toxic"). The increased circulating hormone from the nodule suppresses TSH, and consequently the tracer uptake into the adjacent normal thyroid may be less than normal. A solitary palpable nodule, which is often large (>3 cm), suggests this diagnosis in a thyrotoxic patient. A radionuclide thyroid scan is indicated in this group of patients to identify the solitary toxic adenoma and to verify that the rest of the gland is suppressed (Fig. 7-5). If these findings are present, therapy is different than for toxic MNG because the remaining suppressed gland is protected from the I-131 therapy. The scan often demonstrates that a portion of these "hot" nodules are "cold" because of necrosis in part of the hyperfunctioning nodule. The RAIU is in the range of toxic MNG. Patients with solitary hot nodules without thyrotoxicosis have an increased chance of subsequently

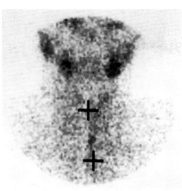

**FIG. 7-6.** The marker (hyoid and SSN) scan shows no uptake of tracer in the region of the thyroid but normal background and salivary gland activity. This patient had classic subacute thyroiditis with 0.4% 24-hour RAIU, ESR of 72, sore throat and tender neck (initially right-sided, "creeping" to include the left side).

developing clinical thyrotoxicosis if one or more of the following is true:

- The nodule exceeds 3 cm in diameter
- The remaining gland tracer uptake is suppressed
- The $T_3$ by immunoassay is at the upper limits of normal (9)

### Thyroiditis

Subacute thyroiditis is an inflammatory disease of the thyroid of presumed viral etiology. The inflammatory process causes the release of much of the stored thyroid hormone, which results in a mild and transient thyrotoxicosis. The transient nature results from the limited amount of thyroid hormone stored in the gland. The erythrocyte sedimentation rate (ESR) is usually elevated. The euthyroid status returns several weeks later, and there is an approximately 10% rate of permanent hypothyroidism. The condition is associated with a tender gland and pain (painful thyroiditis) that is often referred to the ear. The pain can extend from one lobe to another ("creeping" thyroiditis). The pain usually responds to aspirin. Occasionally, steroids are required, in which case there should be a rapid clinical response and fall in ESR if the diagnosis is correct. A painless form of this condition exists (painless thyroiditis) but is difficult to diagnose. Both painful and painless forms may occur more frequently in summer or fall (10). The thyroid scan shows virtually no uptake of tracer into the gland, and the RAIU is <2% (Fig. 7-6).

Another form of thyroiditis can follow pregnancy (postpartum thyroiditis). It can recur, unlike the other forms of thyroiditis. Postpartum thyroiditis and hypothyroidism were first described in 1948, and patients may present with either biochemical hypothyroidism, hyperthyroidism, or hyperthyroidism followed by hypothyroidism. This syndrome can occur for up to 1 year postpartum and occurs in as many as 9% of pregnancies. One-fourth develop permanent hypothy-

roidism, and this may explain the female preponderance of hypothyroidism. It is widely believed that this form of thyroiditis is caused by the immunologic perturbations associated with pregnancy (there is a high incidence of thyroid antibodies in these patients). This condition may be associated with postpartum depression.

### Unusual and Rare Causes of Thyrotoxicosis

- $T_3$ toxicosis: MNGs or iodine deficiency (shift to $T_3$ production)
- Factitious hyperthyroidism (surreptitious thyroid intake)
- Early Hashimoto's thyroiditis (Hashitoxicosis, a rare clinical event that probably results from the combination of Graves' disease and Hashimoto's disease)
- Trophoblastic disease (HCG cross-reacts with TSH)
- TSH-dependent hyperthyroidism (ectopic TSH or abnormal pituitary gland)
- Ectopic $T_4$ source (struma ovarii, hyperfunctioning metastases, inadvertent thyroid hormone ingestion)
- Iodine-induced hyperthyroidism (jodbasedow; occurs with kelp intake or iodination of food products)

## THERAPY FOR HYPERTHYROIDISM

### Antithyroid Drugs

ATDs control symptoms but usually do not provide definitive therapy. They have no long-term role in hyperthyroidism other than Graves', and then only in patients who are young and have a small thyroid gland, mild symptoms, and mild elevations in thyroid hormone levels. Such patients have a higher early spontaneous remission rate than others, but even in this select mild group, only 40% to 70% of patients spontaneously remit in the first year. ATDs are tried for a year, then withdrawn "cold turkey." The patient is then watched for the onset of recurrent symptoms, indicating lack of interval remission. Sometimes patients in whom remission occurs can be predicted by showing decreased thyroid trapping while on $T_3$ (Cytomel) suppression using Tc-99m $TcO_4^-$ scans or early RAIU measurements (11,12). Other Graves' patients, especially older patients with large thyroid glands and significant elevations in thyroid hormone levels and thyroid-stimulating antibodies (TSAbs), have a spontaneous remission rate of only 10% to 20%.

In 1991, Hashizume et al. (13) reported that the routine administration of $T_4$ after starting ATDs and the continuation of $T_4$ after ATD therapy was stopped resulted in a significant decrease in TSH receptor antibodies and Graves' recurrence rates. Follow-up studies by others showed variable results, but most indicate no added remission advantage by the use of $T_4$ (14), so the jury is still out and there is no expectation that the role of radioiodine will be diminished in the future by this therapy technique.

## Mechanism of Action

Propylthiouracil (PTU; 200 mg PO three times per day) and methimazole (MMI; 20 mg PO twice per day) are used in the United States, whereas carbimazole is typically used in Europe. These drugs affect the following:

- Iodide oxidation to iodine
- Thyroglobulin iodination with MIT and DIT
- The coupling of MIT and DIT to form $T_3$ and $T_4$
- Inhibition of thyroglobulin biosynthesis

They have no effect on iodine trapping or thyroid hormone release (compare these actions with TSH as seen in Table 7-1).

Although the organification effect of the drug occurs within 4 hours, and the iodine content of the gland falls by 80% in 4 to 5 days, the large storage capacity for hormone in the gland colloid and the 7- to 10-day biological half-time of $T_4$ means that total symptomatic relief does not occur for several weeks after therapy is initiated. Partial relief can occur in the first week with PTU, probably as a result of inhibition of peripheral $T_4$ to $T_3$ conversion.

## Indications for ATD Therapy

Besides the treatment of Graves' patients with mild hyperthyroidism awaiting the spontaneous remission described above, ATDs can also be used to control symptoms before definitive therapy when the clinician feels the patient cannot continue without symptomatic relief. Alternatively, symptomatic control can be achieved with beta-blockers in patients with lesser symptoms, and an oral propranolol dose of 10 to 20 mg four times per day is effective in nearly all patients. The smaller dose is used in mild symptomatic hyperthyroidism, the larger dose in severe disease. Propranolol takes up to 48 hours to work, and is titrated against the resting pulse, with the desired effect being a heart rate of 70 to 80 beats per minute (bpm). This therapy does not replace primary treatment with ATDs, surgery, or radioiodine but rather ameliorates the tremor, palpitations, stare, anxiety, and amenorrhea that hyperthyroidism produces. Contraindications to beta-blocker use include congestive heart failure and asthma, and in diabetes care must be taken to monitor for hypoglycemia. Some patients develop extreme symptoms of tiredness and lethargy within 48 hours of starting propranolol, precluding its continued use.

## Role of ATD in Pregnancy

Pregnancy is a situation where ATDs are the treatment of choice. The immunosuppressive effect of pregnancy itself causes considerable amelioration of symptoms in the third trimester in patients with Graves' disease. Patients often need their drug treatment sharply reduced or discontinued in late pregnancy. PTU crosses the placental membrane (MMI less so); therefore, fetal hypothyroidism can develop. Unfortunately $T_4$ and $T_3$ do not effectively cross the placental membrane, so hormone supplementation does not correct the induced fetal hypothyroidism. PTU (but not MMI) is secreted in breast milk, so care is required in breast-feeding.

ATD differences are summarized here:

- PTU inhibits peripheral conversion of $T_4$ to $T_3$
- MMI possibly better in pregnancy
  Greater anti-immunogenic effect
  Less crosses the placenta
  Not secreted in breast milk

TSAb crosses the placental membrane, so the patient's baby can develop dramatic thyrotoxicosis postpartum. This is associated with a goiter, and it occurs 1 to 10 days after delivery. Because the half-life of TSAb is months, ATD treatment of these neonates is also necessary for months. High maternal TSAb levels should warn of the possibility of the neonatal thyrotoxicosis.

## ATD Side Effects

The incidence of side effects with ATDs is variable and reports in the literature vary from 4% to 45%. In general, toxicity is related to the dose, and both children and elderly are more susceptible. Major toxic effects are rare and include leukopenia and agranulocytosis (0.5%). However skin rashes, arthralgias, and hepatitis can occur in 5% to 15% of patients. Patients should be warned to promptly discontinue ATDs if they develop a rash, fever, sore throat, joint pains, or jaundice. The hepatitis can be severe and potentially fatal. If the patient reacts to one of these thioamides, another can be administered with only a moderately increased risk of reaction to the new drug.

## Destructive Therapy for Thyrotoxicosis

Definitive therapy of thyrotoxicosis is achieved by destruction of part of the thyroid. Such therapy is usual in toxic MNG and Graves' disease. In these conditions, I like to think of the thyroid gland as a factory that has expanded to fill the entire facility and is working additional shifts, so that thyroid hormone is overproduced. Under conditions of excess hormone production (antibody-stimulated or autonomously functioning nodules), only destruction of part of the physical plant will result in normalization of hormone output. With successful removal of part of the factory, a subsequent spontaneous decrease in TSAb (the delayed spontaneous remission of Graves' disease) will probably result in inadequate thyroid hormone production capacity and hypothyroidism. For this reason, continued lifelong follow-up is a requirement of destructive treatment of Graves' disease. A thyroidectomy scar gives an obvious clue to the physician when the patient presents years later with the vague, depressionlike symptoms of early hypothyroidism, but this obvious stigmata is not present after radioiodine therapy.

### Surgery

Surgery is the oldest therapy, but the risks of anesthesia, recurrent laryngeal damage (~2%), and the possibility of hypoparathyroidism (rare in this subtotal procedure, ~2%) make it less of an option for general application. Even as recently as 1985, radioiodine therapy was frowned on for those <30 years of age, females in the reproductive age, and children, so that surgery was their primary therapy. This is no longer the case. Even in solitary toxic nodules, where surgical extirpation is nearly always effective, radioiodine is now the preferred therapy (15). Where the patient has an excessive fear of radiation that cannot be allayed, or when surgery may otherwise be indicated (e.g., large goiter with compression of trachea), or if definitive therapy is required in pregnancy, then surgery is the preferred therapy. The literature indicates an 85% success rate with the surgeon arbitrarily removing two-thirds to three-fourths of the thyroid. Because few surgeons wish to reoperate on the thyroid because of the increased risk of complications, the 15% of patients with continued thyrotoxicosis due to inadequate resection are usually referred for radioiodine therapy.

### Radioiodine

Radioiodine therapy with I-131 has become the preferred method of treatment for nontransient thyrotoxicosis associated with hyperthyroidism (Graves' disease and nodular hyperthyroidism). The hyperthyroid status can be confirmed by RAIU immediately before the administration of therapeutic radioiodine. An elevated RAIU excludes nonhyperthyroidal causes of thyrotoxicosis, notably factitious thyrotoxicosis and the acute phase of subacute thyrotoxicosis.

### Dose

Radioiodine therapy with I-131 is nearly ideal because it is simple and relatively inexpensive. Patients with allergies to iodine can be heartened by the fact that a therapeutic dose of radioiodine contains trace amounts of iodine (1 ng, or 0.001% of the daily dietary intake). The radioiodine therapy is designed to deliver 5,000 to 10,000 rads (50 to 100 Gy) to the hyperfunctioning thyroid tissue. This could generally be delivered by an empiric dose of 7.5 mCi (278 MBq) of I-131 in patients with Graves' and 15 to 25 mCi (400 to 675 MBq) in patients with nodular hyperthyroidism, but because the RAIU is performed to confirm hyperthyroidism, we use this uptake to help tailor the dose to the individual patient.

### Role of Uptakes

The 24-hour RAIU in Graves' disease is high (mean, 63%; range, 32% to 96%) in our practice over the last 2 years. Toxic MNG disease has lesser uptakes (mean, 30%; range, 15% to 43%), and half of this patient population are within the generally accepted normal range. The uptake is measured after careful evaluation of the patient's medical history and recent medications. The patient should fill out a questionnaire before administration of the uptake test dose (see Chapter 30). Recent local clinical examples of relatively depressed RAIU in Graves' disease include CT scans with contrast, ingestion of seaweed soup, and concurrent treatment of decubitus ulcer with calcium alginate. In all these situations the offending agents were eliminated, and RAIU measurements 2 to 3 weeks later showed threefold increases from an average of 22% with excess iodide into the typical hyperthyroid Graves' range (~65%) (see Table 7-4).

### Regulatory Requirements

When prescribing therapy, the prescription form by the NRC's QMP regulation must contain the following information:

- Radionuclide
- Dose administered
- Chemical and physical form
- Route of administration
- Date (before or that of administration) in NRC-licensed physician's handwriting
- Confirmation that dose given was within 20% of that prescribed
- Confirmation that the correct patient received the dose
- Confirmation that the written directive was followed

The departmental NRC QMP must be in place for all I-131 administrations exceeding 30 μCi, and it must be adhered to. This means there must be appropriate quality assurance follow-up of therapy doses to ensure compliance with NRC regulations. The NRC takes the position that technologists and physicians are equally subject to human error and that procedures, forms, and strict protocols will prevent therapeutic misadministrations. The NRC has enacted further requirements: documentation of the radiation estimate that individuals are likely to receive from the patient and that the patient was provided with adequate written radiation safety instructions.

### Dose Calculation and Administration

The therapeutic doses administered can be calculated as below:

$$\text{Dose} = \frac{\text{Gland size} \times \text{desired dose}}{\text{RAIU at 24 hours}}$$

| Condition | Desired dose |
|---|---|
| Diffuse Graves' | 80 µCi (2.96 MBq)/g |
| Toxic MNG | 150 µCi (5.55 MBq)/g |
| Combined Graves' and nodules | 110 µCi (4.07 MBq)/g |

The severalfold greater average therapy dose for toxic MNG than for Graves' is due to the typically lower RAIU and the relative resistance to therapy (desired toxic MNG dose of 150 µCi [5.55 MBq]/g of gland vs. 80 µCi [2.96 MBq]/g in Graves'). The average dose range of radioiodine administered for nodular hyperthyroidism is 15 to 25 mCi (550 to 775 MBq) of I-131 compared to 5 to 10 mCi (185 to 370 MBq) for Graves' disease.

Although these calculations include gland size and the nature of the tissue (diffuse Graves' disease vs. focal nodular disease), such formulae do not include the most important residence time of I-131 in the gland. The inconvenience of delayed measurements required to determine the residence time outweighs its clinical utility. The determination of the optimal I-131 dose is elusive, and many methods are used. An acceptable practice would be to empirically administer 7.5 mCi (278 MBq) for Graves' patients and 20 mCi (740 MBq) for all nodular disease (the mean doses for such treatments). Alternately, administration of initial doses would ensure successful ablative therapy but high incidences of early hypothyroidism (15 mCi [550 MBq] for Graves', 30 mCi [810 MBq] for toxic MNG) and acceptance of early thyroid hormone replacement therapy. The latter strategy may become important if it becomes generally accepted that early administration of $T_4$ decreases the incidence of worsening or new onset of Graves' ophthalmopathy (15).

A special case of hyperthyroidism is the solitary toxic nodule with hyperthyroidism with suppression of the remainder of the gland. A dose of 15 to 25 mCi is recommended regardless of the uptake because the suppressed normal thyroid tissue will not take up I-131 and is therefore protected from the

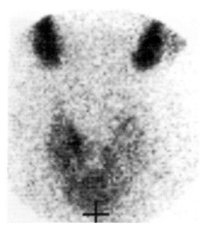

**FIG. 7-7.** The pretreatment scan of this patient is shown in Fig. 7-5. This post-treatment scan shows that the previously hot nodule now has similar uptake to the remainder of the thyroid.

destructive effect (9); post-therapy hypothyroidism is less frequent in these patients (Fig. 7-7). An alternative therapy is surgery, especially if the nodule is large and unsightly.

### Retreatments

In contrast to the use of surgery, where reoperation is not practical for safety purposes, readministration of I-131 is just as practical, safe, and convenient as the initial treatment. It is common to deliver a second dose (~20% of patients in the literature) or even a third or fourth dose (5%). Our current experience of retreatment involves 15% of our therapy population. One should not deliver a subsequent I-131 therapy dose before the previous dose has had its total effect. The factors that play an important role in duration of continuing I-131 effect include the physical half-life (8 days), the residence time (weeks to months), the preformed thyroid hormone storage capacity (months), and the serum half-life of circulating $T_4$ (7 days). All these factors combine to caution therapists not to expect symptomatic relief before 6 to 8 weeks and not to retreat earlier than 6 months after radioiodine therapy unless the patient is overtly clinically and biochemically thyrotoxic. In a typical patient having an early repeat RAIU measurement, as much as half the typical diagnostic uptake dose (several microcuries of I-131) is still present in the thyroid gland from a therapeutic dose administered 2 months earlier. Without the preuptake neck determination (a quality control feature of thyroid uptakes), the RAIU may be overestimated by 50 absolute percentage points.

### ATD Pretreatment

Pretreatment of patients with ATDs before definitive radioiodine therapy results in a decreased intrathyroidal iodine pool and early release of I-131 as thyroid hormone and precursors. This reduces the efficacy of radioiodine treatment by reducing the I-131 thyroid residence time. ATDs need only be administered if the referring clinician feels the patient is at high risk for thyroid storm if the thyrotoxicosis is not alleviated prior to radioiodine therapy. If ATDs are used, they should be discontinued for between 3 and 5 days before the RAIU, and reinstituted, if necessary, 2 days after the therapy dose has been administered. These time intervals are critical to obtaining the appropriate uptake for therapy guidance: Earlier uptakes are low (effect of ATD) and later uptakes too high (due to depletion of the intrathyroidal iodine pool).

### Risk of Thyroid Storm

Patients should be informed of the risk of thyroid storm (very severe thyrotoxicosis endangering life), even though this is extremely rare (more common after surgery). Patients should be warned of resting tachycardia >130 bpm and a fever >103°F. The appearance of these symptoms should bring the patient to the emergency room for evaluation. Most often an intercurrent viral infection is diagnosed rather than thyroid storm. The risk of thyroid storm after I-131 therapy is eliminated by ATD pretreatment, but this advantage is offset by the expected increased radioiodine retreatment rate that occurs with such pretreatment. The radiation to the gland generally exacerbates the patient's symptoms for 2 to 14 days because preformed hormone is released from the irradiated thyroid gland, but this should not be considered abnormal.

When thyroid storm does occur, the objective is to treat symptoms, to prevent peripheral conversion of $T_4$ to $T_3$, to prevent release of more thyroid hormone, and to flood the thyroid with iodine to induce the Wolff-Chaikoff effect. Ipodate (Oragrafin), an oral cholecystographic agent that is 63% iodine by weight, is very useful because it causes a >50% reduction of serum $T_3$ level (an indication of current thyroid hormone production), inhibits thyroid hormone release, and decreases peripheral conversion of $T_4$ to $T_3$ within 24 hours. PTU, but not MMI, decreases the peripheral conversion of $T_4$ to $T_3$, so it is the preferred ATD in this situation. Corticosteroids can be considered because they also divert the peripheral conversion of $T_4$ from $T_3$ to $rT_3$. Propranolol is useful in the treatment of symptoms.

### Radiation Safety

In providing the mandatory radiation safety and protection advice for the family at home (see Chapter 30), two principles apply. First, the I-131 not taken up by the thyroid is excreted renally, so the total remaining will be significantly less 24 hours after administration. A relatively constant amount of I-131 will then be in the thyroid gland and body for the next few days. The NRC guidelines (CFR 20:1301) recommend (in 1997) that family and other individuals receive <0.1 rems (<1 mSv) per year but that doses from medical administrations should not exceed 0.5 rem (5 mSv) (CFR 35:75) and that written instructions should be provided when individuals might receive >0.1 rems (>1 mSv), to comply with as low as reasonably achievable (ALARA) principles, and that records be maintained for 3 years. Those patients who receive >12 mCi (484 MBq) for therapy have dose rates >2 mrem (0.02 mSv) per hour at 1 meter, so precautions are imposed (16). Patients who receive <6 mCi (242 MBq) require no special precautions. Because the thyroid gland of infants and young children is most susceptible to radiation, patients are advised not to carry infants on the shoulder because the thyroid-thyroid distance between patient and infant is shortest in this position. The calculated ovarian dose, assuming a 60% thyroid uptake (i.e., Graves' disease, the common etiology in childbearing age), is approximately 500 mR/mCi (5 mSv/37 MBq) administered, a dose not significantly different than intravenous pyelogram, barium studies, and spine series. Pregnancy is not advised for 3 months after therapy. In general, one should emphasize the following:

**TABLE 7-5.** *Functional status of Graves' disease patients 1 year after therapy*

| Thyroid status | Therapy | |
|---|---|---|
| | Surgery | I-131 |
| Euthyroid | 62% | 59% |
| Hypothyroid | 25% | 35% |
| Hyperthyroid | 14% | 6% |

Source: Data from Becker DV, McConahey W, Dobyns BM, et al. The Results of Radioiodine Treatment of Hypothyroidism: A Preliminary Study. In Fellinger K, Hofer R (eds), Further Advances in Thyroid Research. Vienna: Verlag, 1971;603–609.

- The effect of time and distance on dose
- Flushing the toilet 2 or 3 times after use
- Some restrictions for the first post-treatment day

### Comparison of Destructive Therapies

Comparison of surgery and radioiodine as definitive destructive therapies require looking at immediate specific therapy risks, short-term and long-term hypothyroidism rates, remote risks such as cancer and leukemia, and the genetic effects of radioiodine therapy.

#### Surgery

Surgery is usually a one-time therapy. If the surgeon is unsuccessful at treating the hyperthyroidism at the first operation, the patient is rarely returned for a second attempt because of the disproportionately high surgical complication rate of hypoparathyroidism and recurrent laryngeal nerve injury when operating in a disturbed surgical field. The surgery-specific risk of postoperative bleeding can result in tracheal compression and subsequent anoxia. Thyroid storm is more common after surgery than after radioiodine, but pretreatment with iodide decreases this risk by way of the Wolff-Chaikoff effect. The oft-quoted advantage of surgery over radioiodine is the lower rate of early hypothyroidism. In a large follow-up study of 11,000 patients, however, this merely represents a shift of patients between the hyperthyroid and hypothyroid groups at 1 year (Table 7-5) because the euthyroid cohorts were similar with each treatment modality.

#### Radioiodine

The expected long-term effects of radioiodine therapy include thyroid cancer and leukemia, and the relative risk for these from destructive therapy is shown in Table 7-6. This large multicenter trial dispels any feared consequence of radioiodine (5,6). The rate of leukemia was elevated in all forms of therapy (surgery, radioiodine, and ATDs); this is believed to be an association with the hyperthyroidism itself rather than the therapy. There is no evidence of increased

**TABLE 7-6.** *Long-term leukemia and thyroid cancer follow-up in Graves' disease treatment*

| Mode | Leukemia | | Thyroid cancer | |
| | Number of patients | Rate* | Number of patients | Incidence |
| --- | --- | --- | --- | --- |
| Surgery | 10,731 | 16.0 | 11,732 | 0.5% |
| I-131 | 16,379 | 13.0 | 22,714 | 0.1% |

*Rate per 10,000 patients per year.
Sources: Saenger EL, Thoma GE, Tompkins EA. Incidence of leukemia following treatment of hyperthyroidism. Preliminary report of the cooperative thyrotoxicosis therapy follow-up study. JAMA 1968;205:855–862; and Dobyns BM, Shelline GE, Workman JB, et al. Malignant and benign neoplasm of the thyroid in patients treated for hyperthyroidism: a report of the cooperative thyrotoxicosis therapy follow-up study. J Clin Endocrinol Metab 1974;38:976–998.

fetal defects or cancer in these patients who have received x-ray diagnostic thyroid nuclear medicine tests, nor in the offspring of the Japanese nuclear bomb survivors, who received doses in the 50- to 150-rads (0.5- to 1.5-Gy) range. Although offspring defects were not seen in numerous follow-up studies, no large-scale cooperative study is available to establish this with certainty. The majority of endocrinologists now refer their thyrotoxic patients for radioiodine therapy.

### Hypothyroidism as Complication of Destructive Therapies

Hypothyroidism is both an early and late iatrogenic complication of either form of destructive therapy. Early hypothyroidism can be transient, so replacement therapy should not be considered permanent in the first 6 months after radioiodine therapy. Any replacement undertaken during the first year should also be considered a possible transient condition. The inevitability of hypothyroidism after a destructive treatment of Graves' disease must be emphasized because once the TSAb abates, the capacity of the thyroid gland is insufficient to provide adequate hormone production. The rate of early (first year) hypothyroidism averages 20% but varies with treatment modality (slightly less with surgery than I-131) and administered I-131 dose (greater with higher I-131 doses); it then follows a fairly constant rate of 2% to 3% per annum. This means that within the decade after destructive therapy there is a 50% chance of hypothyroidism, and a 75% within two decades. This inevitability of hypothyroidism has suggested a larger role for empiric rather than calculated therapeutic I-131 dosing (17).

### Destructive Therapy in Nontoxic Goiter

In established goiter-caused obstruction to either the trachea or esophagus, destructive therapy is appropriate. Usually surgery is followed by $T_4$ replacement therapy, especially if the goiter is unsightly. Long-term mean 40% to 60% reductions in volume have been documented after I-131 treatment (18), with most of the reduction occurring in the first 3 months after therapy. This success also occurs in massive thyroid enlargement (19). It had often been argued that I-131 would cause a transient thyroiditis and thyroid gland enlargement and so exacerbate the obstruction, but studies have demonstrated that an occasional 25% volume increase can occur without a mean increase in gland size and with no exacerbation of the clinical presentation (18,19). It should be emphasized that these results apply to functioning nodules in solitary and multinodular glands.

## THYROID IMAGING

The specialty of nuclear medicine developed largely from thyroid imaging departments. I-131 was the major tracer of nuclear medicine for many years. For example, lung scans were performed with macroaggregated albumin labeled with I-131, and rectilinear scanners had 1-inch–thick crystals to stop the high-energy I-131 photons (364 keV [81%], 637 keV [7%], 284 keV [6%]). With the introduction of the gamma camera, Tc-99m became the preferred imaging radionuclide for many reasons, including these:

- Generator production
- No particulate irradiation
- Ideal half-life
- A photon energy sufficient to get out of the body
- A photon readily stopped by the thinner gamma camera crystal

### Indications for Thyroid Imaging

It is my feeling that the indications for thyroid imaging have decreased considerably over the last decade and that thyroid US is rarely indicated. Physical examination (palpation of the thyroid) remains very important in determining whether a patient has a normal, enlarged, or nodular thyroid. Some necks are difficult to palpate (e.g., due to patient size and neck configuration), and some thyroids are difficult to locate and characterize (e.g., low-lying thyroids). In our institution, it is only in these patients that the thyroid scan is approved for investigation of thyroid nodules. The scan can be useful in a small number of patients with thyrotoxicosis, but it is unusual for both a scan and uptake to be needed before treating patients with radioiodine. An example would be a patient with thyrotoxicosis, a 45% uptake (such an uptake could represent either Graves' disease or toxic nodular goiter), and at least one nodule palpable. This clinical situation could be due to a toxic MNG, a solitary hot nodule, or Graves' with associated nodules (Fig. 7-8). The correct therapy dose in a patient with a 45-g gland could vary from 8 to 15 mCi, depending on the etiology.

A smaller subset of patients present the more usual indications for thyroid scans in our institution:

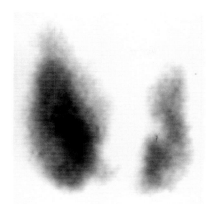

**FIG. 7-8.** This scan is of a patient with goiter and palpable nodules that have intense thyroid uptake with no soft-tissue visualization and RAIU of 67%. The anterior view shows at least two small cold nodules in the left lobe, and at least one small nodule in the lower lateral aspect of the right lobe. The patient should be treated as Graves' with associated MNG disease rather than toxic MNG.

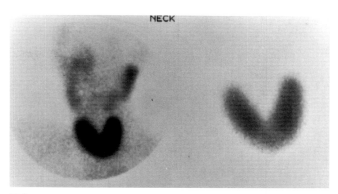

**FIG. 7-9.** This scan was performed bedside in an intensive care unit on a patient with a fractured hip who developed rapid atrial fibrillation. A routine TSH test was zero, and the urgent question was whether this ventilated patient with fever (of 105°F) and tachycardia (130 bpm) had Graves' disease complicated by thyroid storm. The scan looks like an I-123 scan in a subject with Graves' disease but is a Tc-99m $TcO_4^-$ scan. $TcO_4^-$ 20-minute uptake was 30% (normal uptake is 2% to 3%). The diagnosis of early thyroid storm was made immediately, before other thyroid function tests were available.

- Investigation of retrosternal masses (10% are due to substernal thyroids)
- Investigation of neonatal elevations in TSH (athyreotic, ectopic thyroids, or enzyme defects)
- Investigation of anterior neck masses (ectopic thyroid vs. nonthyroidal mass)
- Investigation of ectopic thyroid tissue (no cervical uptake in lingual thyroids)
- Determination of thyroid gland status (confirming subacute thyroiditis [see Fig. 7-6] or thyroid storm [Fig. 7-9]).

**TABLE 7-7.** *Common radionuclides used for thyroid imaging*

| Nuclide | I-131 | I-123 | Tc-99m |
|---|---|---|---|
| Half-life | 8 days | 13 hours | 6 hours |
| Decay process | Beta decay | Electron capture | Isomeric transmission |
| Principle γ | 364 keV | 159 keV | 140 keV |
| Abundance | 81% | 85% | 89% |
| Rads/10 mCi (cGy/370 MBq) | 10,000 | 100 | 1 |
| Rads (cGy)/scan | 100 | 10 | 1 |

## Thyroid Scan Protocol

### *Thyroid Questionnaire*

The thyroid scan patient must fill in the patient thyroid questionnaire (see Chapter 30), including the following information:

- Past and family thyroid history
- Reason for this test and results of previous thyroid tests
- Direct questions about iodine intake, current medications, and recent x-ray contrast agents
- For females, date of last menstrual cycle and whether the patient is currently pregnant, attempting to get pregnant, or breast-feeding

### *Radiopharmaceutical*

The preferred radiopharmaceutical is Tc-99m $TcO_4^-$, which has a much lower thyroid radiation burden than other tracers (Table 7-7). Ten millicuries is injected intravenously, and 20 minutes later, when the thyroidal activity peaks at 2% to 3% of the administered dose, images are taken. A pinhole collimator is used to magnify the images. Views are first taken to demonstrate the relative size and activity of the thyroid gland: The pinhole is moved away from the neck so that the entire thyroid is included in the field of view together with anatomic markers at the suprasternal notch and the hyoid bone or chin (see Fig. 7-2). Such a view includes surrounding soft tissues of the neck and the salivary glands, especially the submandibular glands. It provides an assessment of ratios of thyroid to soft tissue and thyroid to salivary gland, which are an indirect measure of thyroid uptake (see Figs. 7-2 through 7-7, and 7-9). Recording the time and counts provides another indication of thyroid uptake assessment (see Fig. 7-2). Methods of assessing relative size include imaging at a set distance from the pinhole and including a radioactive "ruler." The pinhole is then moved closer to the patient so that the thyroid fills the image, providing improved resolution. Images are obtained in the anterior, left anterior oblique, and right anterior oblique views. The oblique views can identify nodules not apparent on the anterior view alone (Fig. 7-10).

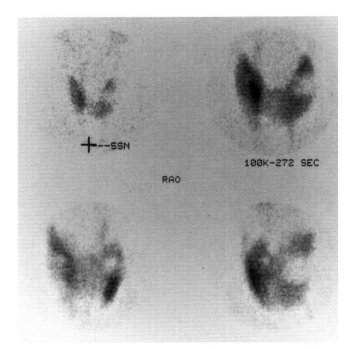

**FIG. 7-10.** This scan demonstrates the power of the oblique views. The upper anterior images with marker (left) and routine magnified view (right) demonstrate a single left lobe nodule. Both oblique views demonstrate an additional smaller right-sided nodule.

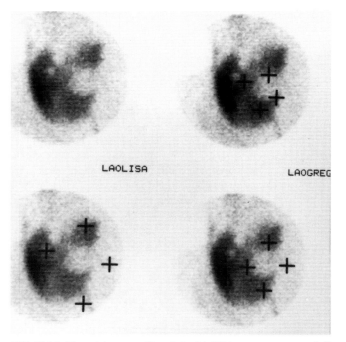

**FIG. 7-11.** Thyroid scan with original LAO image on upper left and thyroid markers around the dominant nodule as marked by staff on the upper right. The markings by Greg and Lisa were made by residents with insufficient skin indentation by the pencil source down to the nodule edge to correctly demarcate the nodule. The pinhole collimator explains the magnification that results.

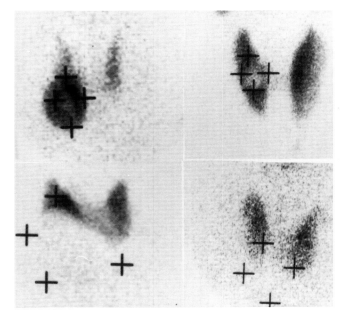

**FIG. 7-12.** All four images represent anterior thyroid scans with markers around palpable nodules. The upper left image demonstrates tracer uptake in the palpable mass—a functional nodule with possible necrotic center. The upper right image shows a small left-sided nodule (1.5-cm diameter) that was hypofunctioning and found to be malignant. The lower left image shows a large left lower pole hypofunctioning nodule distorting the thyroid lobe. The lower right image has a palpable nodule at the medial lower right pole and isthmus region that does not distort the thyroid outline; without palpation, this hypofunctioning thyroid nodule would not be identified.

### Thyroid Palpation

The most common indication for thyroid scanning in the United States is assessing the function of a palpable mass that is considered thyroidal in origin. This can be particularly important in solitary thyroid nodules, where the risk of thyroid malignancy in a solitary functioning (hot) nodule approaches zero compared to a 15% probability in a solitary nonfunctioning (cold) nodule. To make these and similar judgments, it is imperative that the thyroid be palpated at the time of scanning and that the scan abnormality be correlated exactly with the clinical findings.

Any abnormal thyroid palpation findings should be recorded on the scan using markers. Most modern gamma cameras allow for anatomic marking on the images with marks that can be lined up with radioactive source markers: 122-keV cobalt 57 (Co-57) point source for Tc-99m or I-123 and a 356-keV barium 133 point source for I-131. Because of the magnification that occurs with pinhole-to-thyroid distances that are less than the pinhole-to-crystal surface, care must be taken to mark the patient carefully. Small radioactive "pencils" have tips that house the radioactive marker substance (e.g., Co-57). If these radioactive sources are laid at the skin surface without indentation of the soft tissue down to the edges of the nodule being marked, they will be

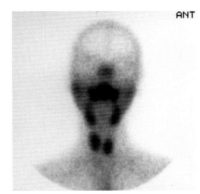

**FIG. 7-13.** The anterior view of this Tc-99m TcO$_4^-$ scan (with parallel hole collimator) demonstrates thyroid, submandibular, and parotid glands as well as a central region of tracer trapped above an upper denture.

significantly closer to the pinhole and the markers will be inappropriately magnified (Fig. 7-11). If the nodule being marked is not directly below the pinhole, then the marks can be both magnified and displaced laterally, and subsequent scan review may suggest an incorrect relationship of the imaged and palpated abnormalities. Without palpation at the time of imaging, the functional nature of the palpable nodule cannot be determined (Fig. 7-12). The procedure is therefore suboptimal, and incorrect interpretations probably represent malpractice.

### Salivary Secretion of Tracer

With Tc-99m TcO$_4^-$ scans, tracer is secreted by the salivary glands, and activity may thus be seen in the hypopharynx, submandibular glands, and parotid glands. If the patient wears a denture or plate, tracer can be trapped behind these devices (Fig. 7-13). This normal salivary secretion of Tc-99m pertechnetate can result in esophageal activity that can emulate ectopic functioning thyroid tissue. Having the patient drink water can be helpful in demonstrating a change in tracer localization, therefore eliminating ectopic functioning tissue as the etiology (Fig. 7-14). Esophageal activity is posterior, so in the oblique views, the activity stays with the lobe being imaged (Fig. 7-15).

### Scan Interpretation

Each time a scan is reviewed, the following steps should be taken:

- Assess ratio of thyroid to background.
- Assess ratio of thyroid to salivary gland.
- Identify all thyroid tissue and nodules.
- Palpate all thyroid tissue and nodules to identify gland suppression.
- Mark and identify cold nodules.
- Mark and identify warm nodules.

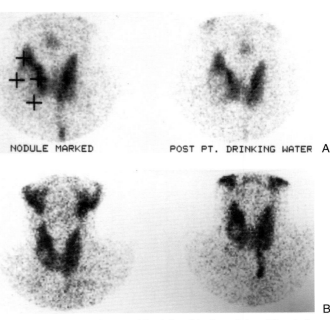

NODULE MARKED          POST PT. DRINKING WATER   A

B

**FIG. 7-14.** Two patients with right-sided nodules. The left-hand images of **(A)** and **(B)** show possible esophageal activity below the left thyroid lobe. The right-hand images were obtained after the patient swallowed water. **(A)** Abnormality clears. **(B)** Abnormality worsens. Both figures confirm non-thyroidal tracer localization because water ingestion will not alter true thyroidal activity: In **(A)**, the esophageal activity was cleared, and in **(B)**, more salivary activity washed into the esophagus.

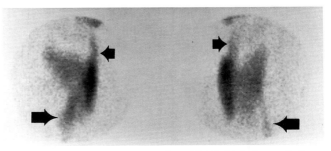

**FIG. 7-15.** The RAO (left image) and LAO (right image) views show an anterior pyramidal lobe (*small arrow*) that moves away from the pinhole direction (to right on LAO view, to left on RAO view) and the posterior esophagus activity (*large arrow*) stays with the lobe to be imaged.

### Exogenous Iodide

For diagnostic imaging purposes, the recent administration of contrast for CT scans is not as much of a problem as generally reported. The role of contrast agents in inhibiting thyroid uptake of Tc-99m TcO$_4^-$ is not well documented. With Tc-99m TcO$_4^-$ imaging, autonomous nodules are visualized even when the thyroid uptake of radioiodine is depressed by exogenous iodide (Fig. 7-16).

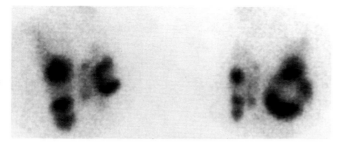

**FIG. 7-16.** This patient received IV and oral contrast with a CT scan 2 days before the thyroid scan. The autonomous nodules are well visualized in the RAO (left) and LAO (right) images. The remaining gland may be suppressed by the contrast or as the result of autonomous function. Note that in the RAO views the right lobe is closer to the pinhole and so is magnified, and in the LAO view the left lobe is magnified; this explains the relative change in nodule sizes between these two images. Incidental note is made of partial necrosis in the left autonomous nodule (a common finding).

Contrast agents administered intravenously, orally, intrathecally, and bronchographically inhibit thyroid iodide uptake, and tables exist that describe the duration of the effect. Intravenous agents that are excreted by glomerular filtration are said to affect RAIU and thyroid scans for 1 to 2 months, oral agents that undergo enterohepatic circulation have an effect for 3 to 6 months, and oil-based agents that are instilled intrathecally or bronchographically can release significant amounts of interfering iodide for years.

The urographic agents are efficiently filtered before significant deiodination of the contrast molecule occurs, so free iodide contaminants present in the initial preparation probably account for the majority of the inhibitory effect. Free iodide is present in ionic and nonionic contrast media at concentrations of only 1 to 20 µg/ml (20), but because 50 to 200 ml may be administered, this represents 50 to 4,000 µg, or 1 to 20 days' requirement of iodine. This is sufficient to transiently suppress RAIU measurements, and it has been calculated that an average radiologic IV contrast dose can cause a 50% reduction in the RAIU at 48 hours. Because iodide is cleared from the plasma twice as quickly by the kidneys as by the thyroid, this effect is short lived. In practice, thyroid scans with Tc-99m $TcO_4^-$ can be performed within days of such procedures, but RAIU values may be significantly reduced, so therapeutic radioiodine applications should be withheld for 2 weeks. When the contrast agent lingers longer (e.g., cholecystographic agents with an enterohepatic circulation and oil-based myelographic agents), there can be continued gradual release of significant amounts of inorganic iodide from the gram doses of contrast agents (20), and significantly higher iodide levels may result that can affect thyroid imaging.

## Clinical Applications

### Thyroid Nodule

Thyroid nodules occur at a 2:1 female-to-male ratio. Palpable nodules are present in 5% to 7% of the population, but US examination, histologic examination of surgical thyroidectomy specimens, and careful routine autopsy examinations reveal a 50% rate of nodular disease. In females, the incidence of nodules is greater and the relationship of age and nodularity is linear, with the percent prevalence indicated by taking the female patient's age in years minus 10 (e.g., a 60-year-old woman has a 50% chance of having a nodular thyroid) (21). The evaluation of thyroid nodules is discussed later under Thyroid Cancer Diagnosis.

### Investigation of Goiter

The development of thyroid enlargement (goiter) occurs worldwide, predominantly as an adaptation to iodine deficiency. This condition has abated in the United States with the introduction of supplemental dietary iodine, such as iodates as a bread stabilizer, iodized salt licks for dairy cattle, and iodized table salt. In the United States, the multinodular colloid goiter is now the most common form of goiter. In this condition, a region of the thyroid becomes more metabolically active, takes up more iodine, and produces thyroid hormone, subsequently undergoing hemorrhage and necrosis. This results in thyroid scans in an initially hot region ultimately becoming cold. This process continues and eventually results in multiple hot and cold nodules present simultaneously. The hot regions can produce thyroid hormone autonomously, so these patients may become thyrotoxic.

### Hashimoto's Thyroiditis

Hashimoto's thyroiditis is the next most common cause of goiter. This disease is known as "the imitator" because thyroid scans in Hashimoto's thyroiditis can be normal or look like solitary cold nodules, MNGs, Graves' disease, or medullary carcinoma of the thyroid (bilateral symmetric defects). These glands can have normal, decreased, and even increased tracer uptake and diffuse or focal defects. Typically, when goiter is present, the gland is firm to palpation, and feels bosselated, like cobblestone paving. The disease is characterized by elevated serum antimicrosomal antibodies. In the early stages, the scan may show a diffuse increase in tracer uptake, and some patients may have RAIUs in the range seen in Graves' disease and present with overt hyperthyroidism. This "Hashitoxicosis" is probably the combination of two separate autoimmune disease processes: Graves' and Hashimoto's thyroiditis. Ultimately, these patients develop hypothyroidism. Sixty percent of them have an abnormal perchlorate discharge test, indicating an organification defect. They develop hypothyroidism with pharmacologic doses of iodide, perhaps due to the inability to escape from the inhibitory (Wolf-Chaikoff) effect of excess iodine.

### Painful Goiter

Painful goiter presents a particular clinical subset. The sudden onset of pain and tenderness associated with a rapidly developing mass is most commonly the result of hemorrhage into a cyst or nodule. In these patients the pain settles in days, the masses regress in weeks, and, although they have the scan appearance of a cold nodule, the lesions are unlikely to be malignant. Pain and tenderness, with referral of pain to the ear or ears, can occur in painful subacute thyroiditis. In these cases, the ESR is elevated, and there is biochemical evidence of mild hyperthyroidism, but the thyroid scan and RAIU show virtually no tracer uptake (see Fig. 7-6). A rapidly growing anaplastic tumor or acute suppurative thyroiditis can be a very rare cause of painful goiter. There is also a painful variant of Hashimoto's thyroiditis.

### Cervical and Substernal Masses

The scan is used to evaluate cervical masses to determine whether they are functioning thyroid tissue. Although many cervical masses can be clinically determined to be thyroidal in origin by palpation alone, some cannot. The thyroid is said to be identified if it moves on swallowing, but any mass attached to the trachea also moves on swallowing. If uptake is present on the thyroid scan in the region of the mass found by palpation, x-ray, CT, or MRI, the mass is normally func-

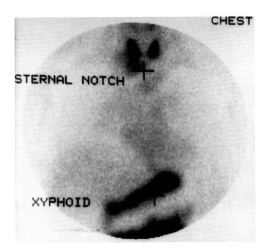

**FIG. 7-17.** The sternal notch and the xiphoid are marked in this large–field-of-view parallel hole collimator image. The thyroid is visualized at the level of the marked sternal notch, and the stomach at the level of the marked xiphoid. There is subtle tracer distribution in the liver and cardiac blood pool. The major blood vessels are seen near the retrosternal portion of the enlarged right thyroid lobe.

tioning thyroid (and therefore benign). In substernal masses, careful correlation of the scan and chest x-ray (CXR) or CT is necessary: The different position used in thyroid scanning (neck extended with a pack beneath shoulders to accentuate extension) versus CXR or CT (neck may be flexed) can account for several centimeters of apparent difference in relative position between cervical lesions identified on the nuclear medicine scan and those detected by other imaging modalities, even when the sternum and clavicle are used in both techniques as anatomic landmarks. The absence of interfering substances such as iodide can be critical to detect poorly functioning thyroid tissue, so the prescan questionnaire is important.

It has been claimed that radioiodine (I-123) scanning is better to identify substernal thyroid extension: This is not due to increased attenuation from the soft tissue and sternum but rather because the Tc-99m $TcO_4^-$ bound to serum proteins can make difficult the visual separation of substernal thyroid from the major thoracic vessels (Fig. 7-17).

### Goiter Compression of Trachea and Esophagus

Radiologists are often asked to review thyroid scans in patients with goiter and symptoms possibly due to tracheal and esophageal compression. Even when tracheal narrowing is shown on a CXR, it is rare that the goiter is causing significant symptomatic compression. No surgical or I-131 destructive therapy should be performed without obtaining respiratory loop volume lung function studies or other procedures to confirm the presence of major proximal airway obstruction. The same caveat applies to presumed esophageal obstruction even when barium swallow studies suggest this. Special swallowing studies should be performed using video x-ray techniques to rule out other, more common causes of dysphagia that may account for the patient's symptoms.

### Ectopic Thyroid

Rests of thyroid cells can be left during development, migrating anywhere from the embryologic origin of the thyroid at the foramen cecum (the base of the tongue) all the way down to the pericardium. These ectopic sites are often midline, the best example being the pyramidal lobe. These thyroid remnants are best differentiated from esophageal activity in thyroid scans by their anterior location and their persistence after water ingestion (see Figs. 7-2, 7-14, and 7-15). In post-thyroidectomy patients, these cell rests are seen more frequently due to TSH stimulation. Upper midline cervical activity, in patients being surveyed for functioning thyroid cancer metastases while maximally TSH stimulated after thyroid remnant ablation, is likely to represent thyroglossal duct tract tissue rather than cancer.

A special case of ectopic thyroid localization is the lingual thyroid. Here the thyroid has not started the normal migra-

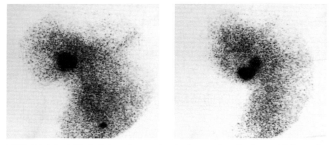

A,B

**FIG. 7-18. (A)** A lateral cervical view of a 9-day-old female with TSH >200 and a lingual thyroid (SSN marked with small radioactive source) with no cervical thyroid. **(B)** An 18-day-old child with TSH of 120 and a sublingual thyroid and residual oral activity noted superior and posterior to the ectopic sublingual tissue. (Courtesy of Dr. Patrick J. Peller, Lutheran General Hospital, Chicago, IL.)

tion, and the thyroid scan shows tracer at the base of the tongue. I-123 has been the stated preferred agent because less background activity from salivary gland secretions is present compared to Tc-99m $TcO_4^-$. Although this is true, most lingual thyroids are readily detected using Tc-99m $TcO_4^-$ scans, and the normal salivary gland and oral biodistribution allows improved localization (Fig. 7-18). Although the thyroid can be found anywhere along the thyroglossal duct tract, most ectopic thyroids are located either in the lingual or sublingual regions, and few cases of completely ectopic thyroids are seen elsewhere. In general, if a lingual thyroid is present, no cervical thyroid can be identified.

### Use of Other Radionuclides

I-131 has a thyroid dose too high for clinical use (1 rad/mCi [1 cGy/37 MBq] of I-131 with 25% uptake) and so is not used for thyroid imaging except in thyroid cancer follow-up. I-123 imaging is performed in many centers, especially smaller hospitals with scheduled patient populations. Iodine radionuclides are theoretically very attractive for thyroid imaging because they assess both trapping and organification processes.

### *Tc-99m $TcO_4^-$ Versus I-123*

Of the five smaller nuclear medicine texts published from 1990 to 1994, four prefer I-123 for thyroid imaging and one suggests that either tracer is equally useful. Of the four major endocrine texts with substantial nuclear imaging sections published in a similar period, one prefers I-123 as the routine radiopharmaceutical, the others prefer Tc-99m $TcO_4^-$. The use of I-123 appears very attractive because it has very favorable physical characteristics: half-life of 13 hours, 159-keV photon, and much less radiation dose per millicurie than I-131. Enthusiasm for its use is tempered by the known contaminants in I-123 production. Using high-energy cyclotrons and the (p, 5n) reaction on tellurium 124

(Te-124), the principal contaminant is I-125. Previous methods of production included large amounts of I-124, which was of high energy and included a positron emission (see Chapter 22). The current suppliers of I-123 delivers the material so that at calibration time (by package insert) there is 97% of I-123, not more than 2.9% of I-125, and 0.1% of all other nuclides (Te-121). Thirty hours later the percentage of contaminants rises to nearly 14%, and therefore the radiation dose increases significantly for the same scanning dose of I-123. This manufacturer makes the tracer 4 days a week, but with the extended expiration time, this provides a 5-day service. If a patient arrives a day late for a thyroid scan, and if the dose ordered for the day before still has sufficient activity to be used, the patient's radiation dose would be considerably increased (i.e., tripled) for comparable scan statistics.

Many articles have been published comparing I-123 and Tc-99m $TcO_4^-$. The consensus is that I-123 produces prettier images, largely as a result of higher thyroid-to-background concentrations. The typical uptake of I-123 at 24 hours is 25%, which is 10 times that of Tc-99m $TcO_4^-$ (2% to 3%) at 20 minutes. Some reports indicate that the image variation detected may be greater among the observers rather than due to the tracer itself (22). When populations with larger numbers of abnormal thyroids were reviewed (23), Tc-99m $TcO_4^-$ appeared more sensitive for the detection of nodular thyroid disease, although the I-123 images were considered of better quality. In an early study (24) comparing I-131 and Tc-99m $TcO_4^-$, there was a marked improvement in Tc-99m $TcO_4^-$ scans in patients with below-normal RAIUs (3% to 15% range), values typical in postcontrast CT patients. Also, Tc-99m $TcO_4^-$ scans are more likely to identify autonomous nodules than are I-123 scans (22,23). For cost, patient and departmental convenience, and for the reasons of better performance after contrast administration and in nodular disease, Tc-99m $TcO_4^-$ may be the preferred agent.

### *Discordant Nodules*

Discordant nodules are those visualized by one tracer as hot and by the other as cold. The 20-minute postinjection Tc-99m $TcO_4^-$ scan demonstrates "trapping," whereas the more delayed, 6-hour I-123 or 24-hour I-131 scan demonstrates "organification" (incorporation of iodine into thyroid hormone). In typical discordant nodules, the nodule traps Tc-99m $TcO_4^-$ but does not organify I-123. These nodules have been described as differentiated enough to trap but not sufficiently differentiated to organify. Approximately 20% of discordant nodules show "reverse discordance"; nodules cold on Tc-99m $TcO_4^-$ while hot on I-123. Discordance occurs in approximately 2% to 8% of random series studying the quality of scans (22), but when patient populations with predominantly abnormal thyroids are studied (solitary nodules, multinodular glands, and history of irradiation) the incidence of discordant nodules increases to 16% to 33% (23,25).

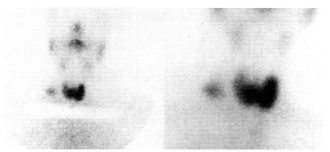

**FIG. 7-19.** This Tc-99m TcO$_4^-$ thyroid scan (left image is a distant view with opaque ruler, right image is a pinhole close-up magnification view) demonstrates decreased uptake in the right thyroid lobe and a region of uptake in the lateral right neck. This was a lymph node metastasis and was also identified on pretherapy I-123 and postsurgical I-131 scanning. The patient was found to have papillary carcinoma with functioning cervical metastases. (Courtesy of St. Clare Hospital, Baraboo, WI.)

There were early reports that discordant nodules had a high incidence of thyroid carcinoma, and many nuclear radiologists and referring physicians still believe that as many as half of these discordant nodules may be cancerous. The available literature on this topic is sparse and poor. The largest number of patients in this literature come from a single atypical case report that refers to 19 patients with either pure follicular cancer (12 of 12 with discordant nodules) or mixed papillary follicular cancer (two of seven with discordant nodules). The single scan provided in this case report is uninterpretable (26). If this series is excluded from the literature, as many reviewers believe it should be, then there is only anecdotal evidence of thyroid cancer in discordant nodules. This anecdotal incidence parallels what we would expect from hot Tc-99m TcO$_4^-$ nodules that have an overall incidence of thyroid cancer variously reported at approximately 1%. Some of the case reports of thyroid cancer associated with hot Tc-99m TcO$_4^-$ discordant nodules had functioning lymph node metastases identified on Tc-99m TcO$_4^-$ scanning. Consequently, they were identified as abnormal and likely to represent thyroid cancer by this scan feature alone (Fig. 7-19), regardless of whether the primary lesion was discordant (27).

### Other Imaging Modalities

Although US is exquisitely sensitive for identifying thyroid nodules, it has no specific features to distinguish malignant from benign nodules, so its utility is greatly diminished. Pure cysts have a minimal chance of associated malignancy, but such pure cysts have a very low incidence, perhaps only one in 500 nodules. The role of US in the workup of thyroid nodules is limited except as an adjunct to fine-needle aspiration (FNA) of thyroid nodules being investigated for thyroid cancer. US and CT may identify incidental cervical lymph nodes that may suggest thyroid cancer, but this is of little clinical benefit, given the additional cost.

Fluorescent scanning is an infrequently used procedure that is able to measure the intrathyroidal content of iodine. The thyroid is irradiated with americium 124, which causes a change in the glandular stable iodine and shows fluorescent iodine x-rays from the thyroid. This has little clinical application.

## THYROID CANCER DIAGNOSIS

Thyroid cancer represents 90% of all endocrine malignancy, but to place thyroid cancer in perspective, it represents <1% of all malignancies. Although its incidence is similar to Hodgkin's disease, the prevalence is much higher because thyroid cancer patients have very long-term survivals. The workup of thyroid cancer is essentially the workup of thyroid nodules. Because 50% of the population have nodules detected by US or at surgery at some time in their lives, there are potentially many patients to investigate, and it is important to identify the appropriate subset for workup. The relationship of age and nodularity is linear, and is reiterated here (21), with the percent female prevalence indicated by taking the patient's age in years less 10; for example, a 60-year-old woman has a 50% chance of having a nodular thyroid.

Thyroid cancer therapy has stirred major controversies and debates in the past 40 years, and, although many publications about advances in thyroid cancer therapy have surfaced, most are flawed. In trials in which a serial change in therapy resulted in better outcomes for thyroid cancer patients, the newer therapy usually occurred when tumors were smaller because of their earlier detection. It is possible that the improved result occurred because the patients were of lower risk because of the smaller tumor size rather than that treatment outcomes were better. For a scientific decision on therapeutic outcome in this low-risk tumor, a study would require a decade to enlist sufficient numbers as well as two to three decades of follow-up. Excellent reviews exist on this topic (28–31).

### Risk Factors

Thyroid cancer experts agree that tumors <1.5 cm should be termed *incidental cancer*. These are frequently found at surgery and autopsy, when up to 35% of the normal population can have such tumors. The prognosis in these individuals is excellent, even in the presence of cervical lymph node metastases (25% of such patients have lymph node involvement). When found at surgery, they do not warrant further surgery or therapy apart from minimal T$_4$ suppressive therapy. Cancers of the 1.5- to 4.0- or 5.0-cm size represent only a moderate risk (28–31). The risk of permanent hypoparathyroidism in bilateral thyroid surgery is approximately 6%, so the surgical risk can outweigh that of the cancer itself in some patients because hypoparathyroidism is an extremely unpleasant iatrogenic disease that is very difficult to manage. Even in the best surgical hands bilateral total thyroidectomy can result in hypoparathyroidism in one-third of the patients.

Factors associated with an increased risk of thyroid nodules being thyroid cancer include

- Solitary thyroid nodule
- Increase in size of thyroid nodule
- Nodule firmness or hardness
- Associated cervical lymph nodes
- Extremes of age (<15 and >40 years old)
- Past history of irradiation

### Thyroid Nodules

Thyroid nodules have a 5% to 10% overall chance of being malignant. It is commonly accepted that solitary nonfunctioning nodules have a risk of approximately 15%, whereas MNGs have a risk of 1% to 5%. European studies suggest the possibility that multiple nodules have a similar risk of thyroid cancer as that of solitary nodules, but this is not substantiated. Any increase in the size of nodule suggests an increased risk of thyroid cancer, except that a rapid increase in nodule size associated with pain suggests hemorrhage into a pre-existing thyroid adenoma or cyst. Firm or hard thyroid nodules are more likely to represent cancer, whereas soft nodules suggest cysts. Cervical lymph nodes, signs of local invasion, and the presence of distant metastases increase the likelihood of thyroid cancer. Nodules at the extremes of age, especially in males, is a further risk factor. The risk of thyroid cancer in a solitary nodule in a child approaches 30%.

### Thyroid Irradiation

There is an increased risk of especially papillary cancers after exposure to 200 to 500 rads (2 to 5 Gy) of external radiation. Cancer induction decreases once the thyroidal dose reaches 1,200 to 1,700 rads (12 to 17 Gy), perhaps as a result of thyroid cell death before malignant transformation (see Chapter 27). Thyroid cancer has been recognized in children irradiated for benign diseases, such as thymus enlargement, acne, hemangiomas, tonsillitis, pertussis, and tinea capitis. This has been described with as little as 6 rads (6 cGy) in children of Jewish origin. The latent period is several years, the incidence peaks at 11 years postirradiation, but tumors have been described as long as 25 years after exposure (32). This does not represent a significant at-risk population now because the indiscriminate use of XRT ceased three decades ago. Large radiation doses delivered internally with radioactive iodine to the thyroid effectively sterilizes the gland. This is established in patients after radioiodine treatment of hyperthyroidism with no significant increase in thyroid cancer. Follow-up studies of diagnostic I-131 use have found no increased risk of thyroid cancer. This is probably a result of

the protracted nature of the irradiation, given the 8-day half-life and ongoing repair of the radiation damage (16).

### Investigation of Thyroid Nodules (Thyroid Cancer)

The investigation of thyroid cancer is essentially that of thyroid nodules (33). The preoperative diagnosis of thyroid cancer is required to prevent unnecessary morbidity associated with either unnecessary operations or unnecessarily extensive operations. Nuclear medicine imaging was the initial and preeminent form of investigation of thyroid nodules a decade ago, but now FNA has replaced it as the primary diagnostic procedure. FNA can establish the diagnosis of papillary carcinoma but cannot distinguish follicular cancers from benign follicular adenomas (as much as 10% to 20% of well differentiated thyroid cancers). Follicular cancers require histologic evidence of tumor capsule breach or vascular invasion to distinguish them from benign follicular adenomas; such determination is not possible with FNA and frequently is not possible at frozen section of a surgical biopsy. This explains the high incidence of reoperation (second operations based on unexpected follicular cancers diagnosed on permanent sections).

### Fine-Needle Aspiration

In FNA, the patient lies supine and a 23- or 25-gauge needle is inserted into the suspicious nodule. The needle is moved within the nodule to aspirate cellular material. The needle is withdrawn and the cells expelled for cytologic preparation and subsequent evaluation (34). In good hands, 85% of specimens are diagnostic (33,34). If not, the procedure can be repeated and the technique improved with US guidance to ensure that solid material in the nodule is aspirated. Although the benign and malignant categories usually represent true negatives and true positives, respectively, 20% of the total suspicious cytology reports turn out to be malignant at surgical biopsy. FNA is somewhat dependent on technique, and sampling errors are higher in small (<1 cm) and large (>5 cm) nodules. Fortunately, these two nodule sizes indicate low- and high-risk parameters, respectively, in and of themselves, and may drive the need for further evaluation and assessment, independent of FNA results. With the use of repeat attempts, 95% of FNA attempts yield sufficient material. The diagnostic categories include the following:

- Benign (75% of all FNAs)
- Suspicious or inadequate sample (20%)
- Malignant (5%)

### Algorithm

The algorithm of clinically solitary nodule investigation presented in Fig. 7-20 would not be universally accepted by

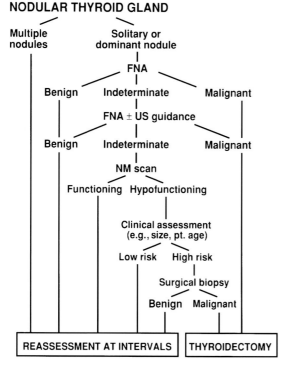

**NODULAR THYROID GLAND**

**FIG. 7-20.** Algorithm for investigating thyroid nodules.

be sent for surgical biopsy (extremes of age, rapid growth, size >4 cm, firmness, fixation, cervical nodes, vocal cord paresis, other evidence of distant metastases, and history of past irradiation) and the other patients can be followed clinically. US evaluation and thyroid suppression with thyroid hormone have virtually no role in thyroid cancer investigation, except that US may be used to follow these patients if the clinician is not comfortable with his thyroid palpation abilities.

### Role of Imaging Modalities

Occasionally, a thyroid scan is helpful because functioning nodules have a very low probability of thyroid malignancy (1%). Fifteen percent of solitary nodules may be functioning and do not warrant further investigation for thyroid cancer. The use of scanning as an initial investigation can be appropriate and does not significantly increase the cost of investigation (35). In patients with extreme fear of cancer, a thyroid scan can quickly be performed and the patient rapidly reassured if the suspicious nodule is functional. The thyroid scan is also appropriate after two failed FNA attempts, as shown in the diagnostic workup algorithm (see Fig. 7-20).

### Discordant Nodules

Discordant nodules were described under Thyroid Imaging. These are nodules visualized by one tracer as hot and by another as cold. Discordance occurs in approximately 2% to 8% of random series studying the quality of scans (22,23), but when patient populations with predominantly abnormal thyroids are studied (e.g., nodular thyroids) the incidence of discordant nodules increases to 16% to 33% (23,25). There were early reports that discordant nodules had a high incidence of thyroid carcinoma, but this probably represents anecdotal evidence of thyroid cancer in discordant nodules, and the true rate is likely to parallel what we would expect from hot Tc-99m $TcO_4$ nodules (i.e., ~1%).

### Concept of the Dominant Nodule

Multinodular glands are not usually further evaluated for thyroid cancer. Some reports have raised the possibility that multinodular glands may house a significant number of cancers. Unfortunately, this would mean that perhaps 40% of normal older women would need workup for thyroid cancer, given their incidence of nodular thyroids. This is where the concept of the dominant nodule is helpful. This term is applied to multinodular glands in which one nodule is significantly larger (twice or more) than the others; this dominant nodule should be investigated like a solitary nodule (Fig. 7-21). The nuclear scan is ideal for this purpose

most imaging departments but is the most cost-effective, rapid, and convenient investigation of clinically suspicious thyroid nodules. Its application, however, reduces nuclear imaging to a secondary role. Arguments can be made for an initial Tc-99m $TcO_4^-$ scan, and thus the elimination of the 15% of patients that have functioning nodules from the need for FNA. The algorithm requires the immediate availability of FNA and cytopathology, which is the case in our institution, where both FNA and scanning can usually be done within an hour or so of the request. This approach using FNA has halved the need of surgery, doubled the yield of carcinoma in surgical specimens, and halved the cost of thyroid cancer investigation and detection (34). Representative costs for several thyroid investigations are provided for comparison (Table 7-8).

Of the small (1% to 5%) subset of patients with no diagnosis after this scheme, the clinically high-risk group can

**TABLE 7-8.** *Thyroid test costs*

| Test | Cost ($) |
| --- | --- |
| $T_4$ RIA | 30 |
| $T_3$ RIA | 40 |
| TSH | 50 |
| Antibodies | 85 |
| Thyroid clinic visit | 200 |
| Thyroid ultrasound | 300 |
| Thyroid nuclear scan | 450 |
| FNA of thyroid | 500 |

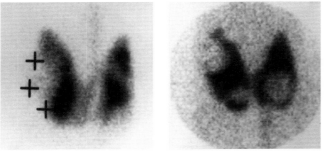

A,B

**FIG. 7-21.** These two MNG thyroid images demonstrate at least three cold nodules in each. **(A)** A dominant nodule (marked) in the left lobe and two smaller nodules in the right lobe. **(B)** Similar-sized nodules in both right and left lobes, that is, no scan evidence of a dominant nodule.

**TABLE 7-9.** *Thyroid cancer variables*

| Histologic type | Age at presentation | 10-year survival |
|---|---|---|
| Familial medullary | 10 years* | 90% |
| Papillary | 45 years | 85% |
| Follicular | 55 years | 70% |
| Sporadic medullary | 40 years | 65% |
| Anaplastic | 65 years | 0% |

*Often diagnosed by screening procedures.

because it identifies only larger nodules (≥1 cm), can adequately compare the sizes of different nodules, and has the added advantage that it may show the clinically dominant nodule as functional and therefore not warranting further investigation. This is especially helpful in patients whose necks are difficult to palpate.

## Tumor Types

### Papillary Carcinoma

Eighty percent of all well-differentiated thyroid cancers are papillary in type. These are commonly multicentric and often spread to regional lymph nodes. The average age of papillary carcinoma patients at presentation is 45 years, and 85% of these patients survive 10 years (Table 7-9). There are two benign variants, the occult or small (<1.5 cm) micropapillary cancer and the encapsulated variant. The rarer tall cell variant in the elderly and the diffuse sclerosing variant in the young are said to have significantly worse prognosis.

### Follicular Carcinoma

In follicular carcinoma, the average age of presentation is slightly older (55 years of age), and the 10-year survival rate is reduced to 70% (see Table 7-9). Follicular cancers spread via the bloodstream to the lung and bone. Although these findings suggest a more aggressive tumor type, most experts agree that the poorer prognosis is related to patient age and tumor size at presentation rather than to an intrinsic difference in tumor aggressiveness. Most follicular carcinomas are encapsulated, and this variety is benign even when minimal tumor capsule or vascular invasion is present. Caution is needed in the workup of follicular carcinomas because FNA cannot separate this cancer from follicular adenomas, and frozen section can be read as nonmalignant in as many as half of the patients at surgical biopsy. These false negative interpretations reflect the need to identify histologic capsular or vascular invasion to diagnose malignancy.

### Other Tumor Types

Other tumor types (~15% of total thyroid carcinomas) include anaplastic carcinoma with a very poor prognosis and medullary carcinoma of the thyroid, often heralded by elevated serum calcitonin levels. Medullary carcinoma presents either as inherited multiple endocrine neoplasia syndromes or a familial form without other endocrine neoplasms. These tumors generally are not referred to the nuclear medicine department, although it is possible that medullary carcinomas will in the future be referred for imaging because of the recent FDA approval of I-131 metaiodobenzylguanidine (MIBG) and indium 111 (In-111) pentetreotide (OctreoScan) and Tc-99m arcitumomab (antiCEA), and possible approval of Tc-99m dimercaptosuccinic acid V (DMSA[V]).

### Prognosis of Tumors

The management of thyroid cancer depends on the expected prognosis. Only patients with potentially aggressive tumors and poor prognosis are treated aggressively with surgery and I-131 therapy. Multiple variables have been shown to be related to prognosis, but multivariate analysis has demonstrated that few are important. Those that are important include

- Age of the patient
- Size of the cancer
- Presence of distant metastases
- Evidence of local invasion
- Completeness of surgical resection
- Occasionally, histologic features
- Possible tumor multicentricity and lymph node involvement

The first three parameters can be assessed before surgery, evidence of local invasion and incomplete resection may be assessed at the time of surgery, and the other features are assessed at histology. Several prognostic scales have been introduced since 1987. The most recent include the acronyms AMES (28), AGES (29), MACIS (30), and that of the U.S. Air Force and Ohio State University (OSU) (31). These and other scales are described in a review article (36).

## Prognostic Scales

Age >40, size >4 to 5 cm, extension of tumor beyond the thyroid capsule into adjacent neck structures, inadequate surgical resection of the tumor, and the presence of metastases in the lung and bone all indicate a worse prognosis and represent the high-risk group. Patients <40 or 50 years of age, tumor size of <4 to 5 cm, and no evidence of local extrathyroidal extension (or distant metastases) indicate a low risk, and in prognostic series 99% of these patients have 20-year survivals (28–31).

### MACIS Scale

The MACIS (Metastases, Age, Completeness of resection, local Invasion, and Size) scoring scale (30), which is similar to other scales, is used as an example. A patient aged 50, with a 4-cm tumor and evidence of extrathyroidal extension, would score 6.2. This prognostic score is defined as such: 3.1 (if aged ≤39 years) or 0.08 times age (if ≥40 years), plus 0.3 times tumor size (in centimeters), plus 1.0 (if incompletely resected), plus 1.0 (if locally invasive histologically), plus 3.0 (if distant metastases are present). As can be seen, age has a significant bearing on the score, and the score has a significant bearing on prognosis. For example, the 20-year cause-specific death rate for each score bracket is as follows:

- Score <6: 1% death rate
- Score 6.00 to 6.99: 11% death rate
- Score 7.00 to 7.99: 44% death rate
- Score ≥8: 76% death rate

### OSU Scale

Some argue that age has an undue effect on the prognostic scores and that Mazzaferri's latest OSU scoring system does not include age but includes tumor multicentricity and presence of nodal disease (31). The addition of more than three lesions or the presence of cervical lymph nodes upgrades a stage I tumor to stage II, as shown in Table 7-10. It is of interest that the occult or microscopic carcinomas have lymph node metastases in as many as one-fourth of patients, with virtually no reported deaths. The OSU stages and 30-year disease-specific death and recurrence rates, are shown in Table 7-10.

### Role of Nodal Metastases

Approximately 40% of adults and 80% of children with papillary carcinoma present with cervical or mediastinal lymph node spread, yet the overall prognosis is still good. Recurrence rates for patients with nodal metastases are established to be slightly higher, but most clinicians believe that the presence of cervical lymph nodes in papillary cancer does not adversely affect the patient's prognosis. This was generally supported, but Mazzaferri's 1994 OSU scale introduces the presence of mediastinal or bilateral cervical metastases and multicentricity as an adverse prognostic factor for papillary carcinoma and the mere presence of cervical nodes as an adverse prognostic factor for follicular carcinoma (31). DeGroot et al. had claimed this in 1990 (37), but corroborating data were not available in North American studies, although generally Europeans agreed with this approach.

## THYROID CANCER THERAPY

### Suppressive and Surgical Therapy

#### Thyroid Hormone Therapy

In all patients with significant thyroid cancer suppressive doses of $T_4$ are important; however, there is a potential risk of osteoporosis in the female population. TSH suppression is important because TSH is believed to play a role in activating tumor growth in well-differentiated thyroid cancer. The degree of TSH suppression should be tailored to the patient's prognosis, and this is possible with the sensitive TSH immunoassays currently available. High-risk patients with distant metastases, extrathyroidal tumor extension, and incomplete surgical excision should be suppressed more completely than patients at lesser risk from thyroid cancer (Table 7-11).

#### Surgery

The extent of surgery remains controversial. All patients do not have total thyroidectomies because even the best surgeons have rates of permanent hypoparathyroidism that vary

**TABLE 7-10.** *Well-differentiated thyroid cancer 30-year death and recurrence rates*

| Tumor grade | Tumor features | Death rate | Recurrence rate |
|---|---|---|---|
| I | Size <1.5 cm | 0% | 8% |
| II | 1.5–4.4 cm or <1.5 cm if >3 lesions or cervical nodes | 6% | 31% |
| III | >4.4 or local invasion | 14% | 36% |
| IV | Any size and distant metastases | 65% | 62% |

Source: Mazzaferri EL, Jhiang SM. Long-term impact of initial surgical and medical therapy on papillary and follicular thyroid cancer. Am J Med 1994;97:418–428.

**TABLE 7-11.** *Suggested TSH suppression for thyroid cancer risk scales*

| Tumor risk scale | | |
|---|---|---|
| MACIS | Ohio State University | TSH level |
| <6 | I | Low normal |
| 6.00–6.99 | II | Below normal |
| >7 | III and IV | Zero |

widely (1% to 32%) in respectable endocrine surgical units (38–41). This iatrogenic condition is very difficult to control, and patients continuously fluctuate between hypocalcemia and hypercalcemia. The risk of permanent hypoparathyroidism in lesser thyroidectomy procedures, such as bilateral subtotal or near total (unilateral total lobectomy, isthmectomy, and subtotal lobectomy on the opposite side) thyroidectomies is much lower, at approximately 6% (31,39). Recurrent laryngeal nerve injury occurs in approximately 2% (31,39) of thyroidectomy procedures and is not as related to the extent of surgery. There is little convincing evidence that total thyroidectomy results in a significant difference in survival when compared to near total procedures. The local recurrence rate and the long-term death rate of unilateral and possibly bilateral subtotal procedures is significantly greater than that of more complete near total or total bilateral procedures in patients with disease of moderate risk (31), so lesser surgical procedures are limited to lower-risk tumors. The removal of enlarged lymph nodes is undertaken at surgery, but radical neck dissections should not be routinely performed. The risk of permanent hypoparathyroidism increases significantly with the extent of lymph node resection (41).

### Radioiodine Therapy

The first demonstration of radioiodine uptake in thyroid cancer occurred in 1940, and the attempted use of therapeutic radioiodine for thyroid cancer dates to 1942. Radioiodine therapy presents an attractive treatment modality because 75% of well differentiated thyroid cancers take up radioiodine. A small number of medullary carcinomas take up radioiodine, but no anaplastic tumors take up I-131. The fact that well differentiated thyroid tumors take up I-131 is somewhat unexpected if one considers that the hallmark of thyroid malignancy is a nonfunctioning nodule as seen on radioiodine or Tc-99m $TcO_4^-$ thyroid scanning.

For functioning thyroid cancer to be visualized by scan, the thyroid remnant should be first destroyed or ablated, confirming that, although thyroid cancers take up I-131, they do not do this as efficiently as normal thyroid. In 1960 (42), it was established that only 10% (Table 7-12) of ultimately proven functioning thyroid cancer metastases were visualized before ablation of the postsurgical thyroid remnant.

**TABLE 7-12.** *Time to visualization of functioning metastases*

|  | Incidence | Cumulative |
|---|---|---|
| Before ablation | 10% | 10% |
| During ablation | 25% | 35% |
| 2 months later | 50% | 85% |
| 4 months later | 15% | 100% |

Source: Pochin EE. Prospects from the treatment of thyroid carcinoma with radioiodine. Clin Radiol 1960;18:113–135.

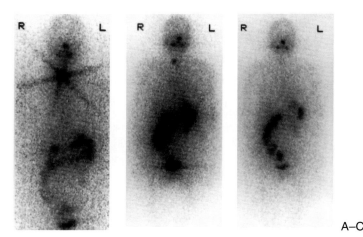

A–C

**FIG. 7-22.** Whole-body anterior images of metastatic survey dose (8 mCi I-131). **(A)** A substantial thyroid remnant is seen, exceeding activity in salivary glands considerably, and representing 0.2% of the administered dose. Note the "star" effect of the collimator due to septal penetration. Repeat surveys after 29.9-mCi ablation doses gave uptakes of 0.02% **(B)** and virtually zero **(C)**. The slight remnant uptake in **(B)**, equal to nose and salivary gland, would not routinely require ablation except in patients with slightly higher-risk tumors.

### *Thyroid Remnant Ablation*

The use of I-131 therapy requires that the thyroid remnant be ablated after surgery. In our establishment, thyroid ablation with radioiodine is only attempted after bilateral near total or total thyroidectomy procedures, that is, in patients with moderate- or high-risk thyroid cancer, in whom we believe it might be desirable to seek functioning metastases for possible treatment. We routinely use outpatient 29.9-mCi (1,110-MBq) doses. Since our change to this dosage schedule in 1984, almost all patients have been successfully ablated (Fig. 7-22), and the average number of doses is not different from the previous higher-dose regimen that was used (Table 7-13). Most centers have not been as successful with low-dose ablations and report only 60% to 80% successful ablation rates. Some studies have shown success with low-dose outpatient ablations in some patients, and that success is probably related to the extent of prior surgical thyroidectomy (43–45).

In our experience, the postoperative thyroid uptake is modest (mean, 0.5% of administered dose; range, zero to 16%), and a 29.9-mCi (1,110-MBq) dose of I-131 as sodium iodide is prescribed on an outpatient basis to ablate the remnant. In patients with high-risk tumors (e.g., local invasion), higher ablation

**TABLE 7-13.** *Low-dose versus high-dose ablation regimen*

|  | Low dose | High dose |
|---|---|---|
| Each dose | 30 mCi | 80+ mCi |
| Mean dose | 38 mCi | 130 mCi |
| Doses needed | 1.35 | 1.4 |

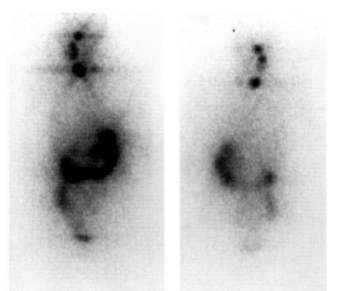

A,B

**FIG. 7-23.** Whole-body anterior **(A)** and posterior **(B)** metastatic survey image using 8.0-mCi (216-MBq) dose of I-131. **(A)** Bilateral remnants (right lobe more than left); two high right cervical lymph nodes; and nasal activity are recognized. The uptake totaled 0.5% of the administered dose. The expected gastric and colonic activity is seen. The patient was admitted to hospital and given 125 mCi (4,625 MBq) of I-131 for remnant ablation and successful treatment of the lymph node metastases (not shown).

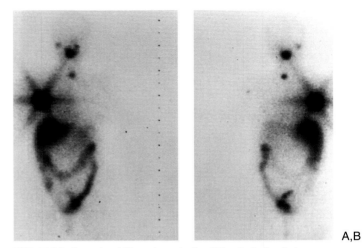

A,B

**FIG. 7-24.** Anterior **(A)** and posterior **(B)** whole-body images after a 94-mCi (3,478-MBq) therapeutic dose of I-131 given 3 days before. There is intense localization in a right rib metastasis (note collimator "star" effect), the thyroid remnant, and the nose. The striking uptake is that in the liver exceeding that of the bowel: This represents labeled thyroid hormones (I-131 PBI) being catabolized in the liver. (Courtesy of Dr. John Weir, Marshfield Clinic, Marshfield, WI.)

doses may be used. If the scan before ablation demonstrates a possible metastasis, such as cervical lymph nodes or pulmonary, skeletal, or other metastases, then the outpatient ablation dose is substituted with the appropriate inpatient therapeutic dose (Table 7-14 and Fig. 7-23), and images can be obtained 4 to 7 days later (Fig. 7-24). We use this simplistic ablation plan because it has been very successful in 10 years of use. Others have introduced approaches that ensure successful ablation with a single dose designed to deliver 30,000 rads (300 Gy) to the thyroid remnant (26 to 246 mCi [962 to 10,000 MBq] were required). Approximately half of these patients can be ablated as outpatients (<30 mCi [1,110 MBq]) with a single treatment (46). Others have demonstrated a relatively uniform remnant ablation rate (63% to 78%), with single I-131 doses ranging between 30 and 150 mCi (1,100 to 5,550 MBq) (47).

Once the thyroid remnant is ablated, any functioning metastases will be more obvious on subsequent metastatic surveys. The ablation process also provides an opportunity for destruction of unrecognized microscopic tumors in the remnant and, with successful remnant ablation serum thyroglobulin

**TABLE 7-14.** *Therapeutic I-131 dose for thyroid metastases*

| Dose (mCi) | Metastatic site |
|---|---|
| 125–150 | Lymph nodes |
| 150–200 | Lung |
| 200+ | Bone |

(sTg) measurements, can assume an important clinical tumor marker follow-up role.

*Controversy About Ablation Dose*

Those who advocate a higher ablation dose suggest possible adjuvant therapy to the thyroid bed region and irradiation of undetected additional tumor sites or small foci of unrecognized extrathyroidal extension.

Those who advocate low-dose ablation argue that significantly higher marrow doses result from the first ablation dose. They believe that the I-131 taken up by the normal remnant thyroid tissue is converted to thyroid hormone and circulates as protein-bound radioiodine (I-131 PBI) with a long serum half-life (weeks). This I-131 PBI is ultimately catabolized in the liver to iodide (see Fig. 7-24). A significant proportion of the total marrow dose in patients treated for metastatic disease can come from the I-131 PBI of the initial thyroid remnant ablation attempt, and in practice approximately 20% of the maximal permissible marrow dose (200 rads [2 Gy]) comes from this I-131 PBI in the high–initial-dose treatment regimen. We advocate outpatient ablation doses to reduce the marrow irradiation of the first ablation attempt. We also use outpatient ablation doses because of the lower cost and greater patient convenience with the same overall ablation efficiency.

*Thyroid Ablation Protocol*

One month after the patient's bilateral surgery, and provided the patient's tumor risk factors indicate the need for

**POST THYROIDECTOMY**

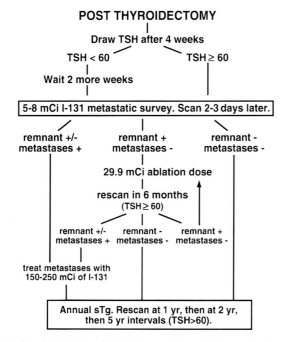

FIG. 7-25. Algorithm of routine post-thyroidectomy follow-up.

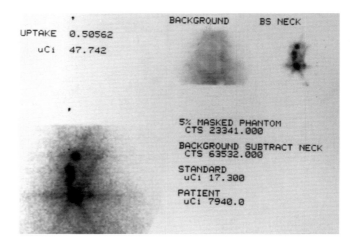

FIG. 7-26. Display of quantitation of patient showing calculation of thyroid remnant and cervical lymph node uptake. This is the same patient as in Fig. 7-22. The uptake was 0.5% (upper left display).

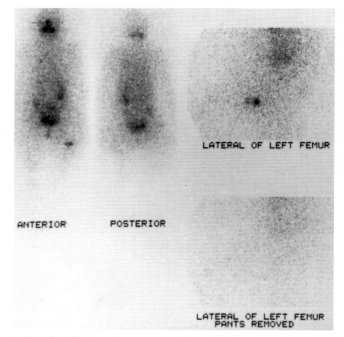

FIG. 7-27. Metastatic survey patient with anterior and posterior whole-body images showing tracer in region of upper left thigh. A spot lateral view of left femur with and without pants removed confirm normal nasal secretions in facial tissues contained in a pants pocket.

aggressive follow-up, a metastatic survey with radioiodine is planned. A TSH is drawn at 4 weeks postsurgery, and if the TSH is >60, the survey is undertaken. If the TSH is <60, a further 2 weeks is allowed before the survey is performed. If a remnant is present, an outpatient ablation dose is administered regardless of TSH (Fig. 7-25). After the initial outpatient ablation dose, repeat metastatic survey scans and ablation doses (if needed) are performed at 6- to 12-month intervals until there is satisfactory ablation of the remnant (mean number of doses, 1.4). When complete remnant ablation is confirmed, scans are repeated 1 and 2 years later, then at 5-year intervals.

### Follow-Up Metastatic Survey Scans

We have used 8 mCi (296 MBq) doses for our follow-up metastatic scans both before ablation and for follow-up studies and followed the required NRC quality management plan. With the introduction of the new NRC requirements regarding doses in excess of 6.5 mCi (240 MBq), and because of the reports of thyroid stunning (see section on Thyroid Stunning) we have recently reduced the metastatic survey dose to 6.0 mCi (222 MBq). The actual uptake of tracer into the cervical region is quantified using the gamma camera and a standard dose using an interpolated background subtraction method (Fig. 7-26). If the remnant is minimal (<0.03%), and if the activity in the remnant as seen on the scan is less than the normal uptake in the nose and the submandibular salivary glands, no ablation is attempted. This is a very rare event in the first postoperative study.

### Technical Artifacts

I-131 is secreted in saliva, so facial tissues, telephones, coffee cups, and drinking glasses can be readily contaminated. Fig. 7-27 demonstrates facial tissues contaminated with nasal secretions in a pants pocket. We have found on several occasions that swallowed saliva in the esophagus can emulate a mediastinal lymph node or pulmonary

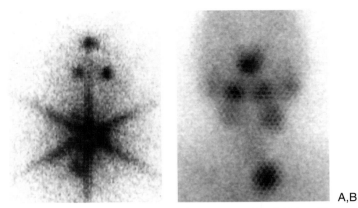

**FIG. 7-29. (A)** This image uses the compromise I-131 collimator (general purpose, high-energy) supplied by the manufacturer. A significant thyroid remnant produces a "star" effect due to the permitted 15% I-131 septal penetration. **(B)** This image, of a different patient, uses the same gamma camera head combined with a high-energy collimator specifically designed for I-131 use. No septal penetration is apparent, but the expected honeycomb pattern of thicker septa is apparent.

**TABLE 7-15.** *Typical distribution of thyroid cancer metastases*

| | |
|---|---|
| Lung | 50% |
| Bone | 20% |
| Lung and bones | 20% |
| Other sites (brain, renal) | 10% |

### Radioiodine Treatment of Thyroid Metastases

Table 7-15 describes the typical sites of thyroid cancer metastases. In our experience, metastatic tumor uptake usually ranges from 0.01% to 22.0% of the administered dose. If the uptake is 0.05% to 0.1% per gram of tissue, one can expect to deliver a therapeutic a dose of 500 to 1,500 rads (50 to 150 Gy) with a 100- to 150-mCi (3,700- to 5,500-MBq) I-131 therapy dose. Typical metastatic lesions take up several percent of the dose, and significant therapeutic results occur. Patients must be admitted to the hospital for such therapies and are now (1997) able to be released when the total body burden of I-131 is <33 mCi or the measured dose rate at 1 m is <7 mR per hour. When these patients are admitted to hospital for I-131 treatment, the nuclear medicine service needs to supply safe yet effective medical care. Time constraints on visitors, medical, and nursing staff should be in effect. Because most patients are well, nursing care is minimal, and the attending nuclear medicine physician can often be the sole caregiver (48). Forms and instructions are provided in Chapter 30.

### Lymph Node Metastases

The metastatic lesions most susceptible to I-131 therapy are lymph node metastases. The majority of these can be success-

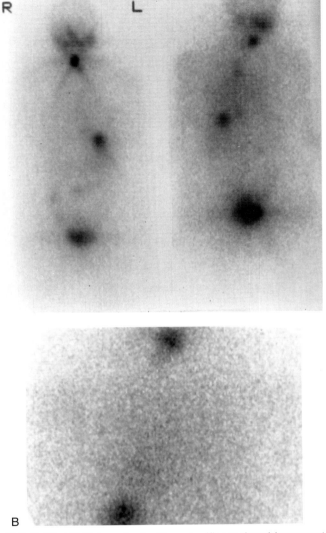

**FIG. 7-28. (A)** This patient with a significant thyroid remnant is being considered for inpatient ablation dose because of the activity seen in the posterior (upper right image) whole-body view centrally. **(B)** After the patient drank 8 oz water, the "lesion" cleared in the posterior spot image, indicating esophageal source.

mass; repeat views after swallowing water can confirm a false-positive scan (Fig. 7-28). Figure 7-29 demonstrates the difference the collimator makes: The medium-energy collimator supplied by most manufacturers for I-131 is really designed for use with In-111 (174- and 243-keV photons) and gallium 67 (98-, 185-, and 300-keV photons), and is a compromise when used with I-131 (364- and 637-keV photons). This is apparent with the septal penetration that occurs when these general purpose, high-energy collimators are used. When using higher-energy tracer, it is essential to use the appropriate "correction" maps (see Fig. 23-19).

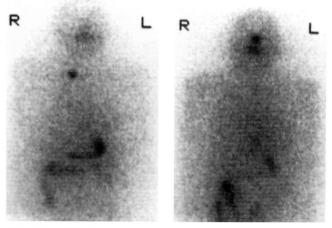

A,B

**FIG. 7-30. (A)** This scan demonstrates a solitary region of I-131 uptake in neck that corresponded to a superficial palpable lymph node. It was resected, and the follow-up scan **(B)** shows no residual lesion activity.

**TABLE 7-16.** *Response of various thyroid metastases to I-131*

|  | Partial resolution | Complete resolution |
|---|---|---|
| Lymph node | 80% | 70% |
| Lung | 75% | 45% |
| Bone | 40% | 5% |

Source: Mazzaferri EL. Thyroid Carcinoma: Papillary and Follicular. In Mazzaferri EL (ed), Endocrine Tumors. Boston: Blackwell, 1993;278–333.

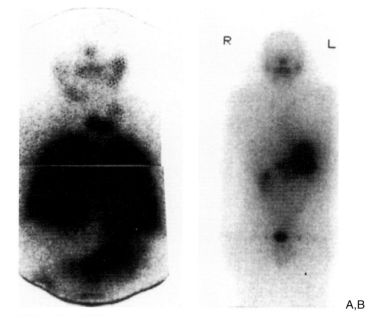

A,B

**FIG. 7-31. (A)** This image is a composite view of two static scans in Polaroid format of head and torso. Functioning thyroid remnant, cervical lymph nodes, and pulmonary metastases are seen, and gastric activity is also present. The patient had a fine reticular infiltrate throughout both lungs on CXR due to metastatic thyroid cancer. Twenty-two percent of the administered dose was calculated to be in the lungs. **(B)** This image is a whole-body scan obtained 8 years later with complete regression on the x-ray and I-131 scan findings. This patient received 600 mCi (22,200 MBq) I-131, with an estimated total pulmonary uptake of 60 mCi (2,200 MBq), and currently has normal pulmonary function tests.

fully treated. If uptake is confined to a cervical lymph node, and if it is clearly palpable and superficial, it is preferable to have it removed surgically rather than ablated with radioiodine. This is true because it can be accomplished simply on an outpatient basis under local anesthetic with complete extirpation of the metastatic disease without irradiation (Fig. 7-30). Metastatic lymph node lesions are effectively treated when doses of 8,000 rads (80 Gy) or greater are delivered to the lesion (Table 7-16). Such doses when calculated for individual patient lesions come close to conventional empiric doses (49,50).

*Pulmonary Metastases*

Lung metastases can take the form of micrometastases seen only on I-131 metastatic surveys, micronodular disease seen occasionally on CXR (Fig. 7-31) or more often on CT, or as macronodules (>1 cm in diameter) readily seen on CXR. These three presentations occur in approximately equal proportions. The microscopic form results in complete resolution in half the patients who receive radioiodine, but the large macronodular lesions rarely take up I-131 or respond to any form of therapy.

*Skeletal Metastases*

Skeletal metastases occur less frequently and rarely respond to I-131, and therefore surgery and XRT should be

contemplated in these patients. Some clinicians believe that screening bone scans are not cost-effective in detecting skeletal metastases (49).

*Therapy Complications*

The complications of radioiodine therapy include the inevitable hypothyroidism of the ablation procedure, short-term risks of sialadenitis and bone marrow depression, and the long-term risks of leukemia and pulmonary fibrosis. Sialadenitis occurs in 10% of patients in the first few days after therapy with 100+ mCi (3,700+ MBq) I-131 and is ameliorated by inducing high salivary flow rates with fluids and acidic hard candy, such as lemon drops. Other transient symptoms include nausea, which may result from fluid overload; thyroid bed pain; change in taste perception; and a dry mouth. Although bone marrow suppression occurs with radioiodine therapy, the effect is mild. Other subacute complications include transient oligospermia in males.

Long-term complications relate to the radiation doses to the marrow and lung and concern leukemia and other solid cancers (49–51) and pulmonary fibrosis (51,52). The risk of leukemia is only significant when the patient receives in excess of 200 rads (2 Gy) to the marrow (possibly 500 to 800 mCi [18,500 to 29,600 MBq] I-131). Patients treated for lung metastases should have pulmonary function tests performed to ensure that significant pulmonary fibrosis does not occur. It has been reported that the lung uptake should not exceed 80 mCi (2,960 MBq) (51,52). Because micrometastases can avidly take up I-131, quantitative uptakes should be performed each time therapy is administered to ensure that excess lung radiation does not occur (see Fig. 7-31).

### Thyroid Stunning

It has been reported that 5-mCi (185-MBq) doses of radioiodine have "stunned" the remnant thyroid (53) and reduced subsequent remnant uptake of I-131 a week later, thus raising the possibility of ineffective subsequent ablation or therapy (Fig. 7-32). Although this does not appear to be a problem given the

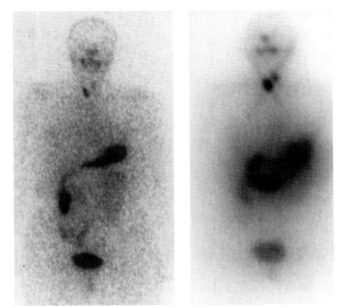

A,B

**FIG. 7-33.** I-123 and I-131 whole-body images. The whole-body images show a slightly different biodistribution of tracer as a result of different timing of the images. **(A)** In the I-123 24-hour image, the bladder is imaged more than bowel. **(B)** In the I-131 48-hour image, the bowel is imaged better than the bladder (because I-131 is in urine already voided). Note the better visualization of the bilateral remnant by the higher dose of I-131.

success of ablations after metastatic I-131 surveys, this finding has been confirmed when significant-sized thyroid remnants are present (54). Suggested approaches to this potential problem of stunning include using I-123 or smaller 2.0-mCi (74-MBq) I-131 doses to detect remnants and then imaging the patient after the ablation dose for improved sensitivity (Fig. 7-33). The reduction of the metastatic survey dose from the conventional 5 to 10 mCi (185 to 370 MBq) to 2 mCi (74 MBq) reduces the sensitivity of detection of metastatic disease fourfold (55). The use of I-123 is also suboptimal because the tracer half-life (one-half day) is not suited to the optimal imaging time (2 to 3 days). Imaging after the ablation dose improves the sensitivity significantly, but images should be obtained later than the routine 2 days used for conventional metastatic survey scans, possibly at 4 or 5 days after ablation (49). This rationale of increasing scan sensitivity by using larger I-131 doses is carried even further in patients who are imaged after empiric therapy doses (see page 185).

### Practical I-131 Applications

#### Patient Selection

Sliding scales of therapeutic intervention have been proposed according to the prognostic indicators before surgery (size, age of patient, presence of metastases), the surgical findings (extrathyroidal extension and incomplete surgical

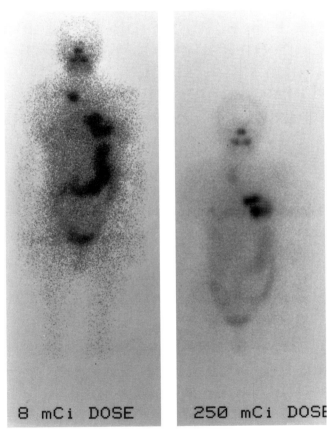

A,B

**FIG. 7-32. (A)** This patient received an 8.0-mCi metastatic survey dose, and the scan showed no remnant, good uptake into a proven medial right clavicular bone metastasis, and uptake into known pulmonary nodules. **(B)** In a scan performed 5 days after a 250-mCi therapeutic dose, the uptake into the pulmonary nodules appears similar, but there is a significant relative reduction in the clavicular lesion when compared to the normal nasal and submandibular activity and the abnormal pulmonary metastases (perhaps stunning of skeletal metastasis).

**TABLE 7-17.** *Treatment and follow-up for patients with various thyroid cancer risks*

| | Thyroid cancer risk | | | |
|---|---|---|---|---|
| | Very low | Low | Moderate | High |
| **Tumor characteristics** | | | | |
| Cancer size (in cm) | <1.5 | 1.5–3.0 | 1.5+ | >4 |
| Patient age | <50 | <50 | — | — |
| Multifocal | No | No | 3+ | — |
| Bilateral nodal involvement | No | No | Yes | — |
| Extrathyroidal extension | None | None | None | Yes |
| Excision margin | Free | Free | Free | Tumor |
| **Treatment** | | | | |
| Surgery type | Lobectomy | Bilateral subtotal[a] | Near total[a] | Total |
| Met survey scan | Not done | Done | Done | Done |
| Scan results | — | No mets | Normal | ± Mets |
| I-131 ablation dose | None | 30 mCi | 30 mCi | 100 mCi+ |
| TSH (T$_4$ suppression) | Replacement | Low normal | Low[b] | Zero |
| Follow-up | Clinical | sTg | Scans + sTg | Scans + sTg |

[a] Sometimes the histologic tumor features are not known at the time of surgery.
[b] Low TSH is up to an order of magnitude below lower limits of normal.

resection), histologic findings (extrathyroidal spread and incomplete resection), and presence of distant metastases (39,56). Table 7-17 is useful in categorizing potential patients for various therapy and follow-up regimens and is similar to the graduated therapy according to the "set of scales" used by Mazzaferri (39) and the "ladder scale" used by the NIH consensus conference (56) on this topic.

### Radioiodine Efficacy

It has been difficult to separate the effect of surgery from I-131 ablation on patient survival, and many respected surgeons still feel that I-131 has little role. However, it is very clear that there is great success in certain individuals treated with radioiodine. This is easily explained when one realizes that 500 to 1,500 rads (50 to 150 Gy) can be delivered to the tumor and that the I-131 beta ray delivers most of its effect within a millimeter of its source, that is, the radiation dose is imparted primarily to the tumor and not the surrounding normal tissue. This is the extremely attractive feature of this therapeutic modality.

Recurrence rates in thyroid cancer after disease-free intervals following initial surgery are higher than one might expect. Both papillary and follicular carcinoma have similar lymph node (8%) and other local site (8%) recurrence rates (39), but distant metastases are more frequent in follicular cancers (12% vs. 4% for papillary cancer). At presentation, significant numbers of patients have metastases: 36% of papillary carcinoma patients have nodal metastases, and 5% have distant metastases versus 17% and 13% (nodal and distant metastases, respectively) for follicular cancer (39). Approximately one-half of all distant metastases (pulmonary, bone, and other) take up I-131, and the death rate in

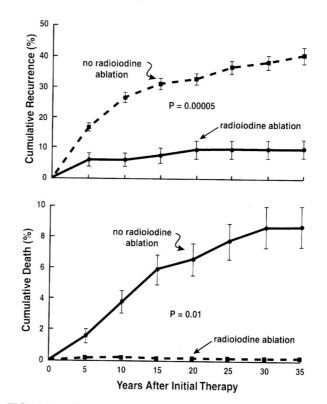

**FIG. 7-34.** These graphs includes stage 2 or 3 tumor patients (OSU scale) treated with (n = 138) and without (n = 802) I-131 to ablate the thyroid remnant. A significant benefit is seen in cumulative recurrence (above) and death (below) rate for those patients treated with I-131. (Reprinted with permission from Mazzaferri EL, Jhiang SM. Long-term impact of initial surgical and medical therapy on papillary and follicular thyroid cancer. Am J Med 1994;97:418–428.)

those patients is halved when compared to patients with distant metastases that do not take up I-131 (39).

Although no prospective randomized and controlled studies unequivocally demonstrate the efficacy of I-131 therapy, there are numerous studies (31,39,50) in which I-131 decreases local recurrence rates and increases life span (Fig. 7-34). Individual metastatic lesions that take up I-131 frequently respond to I-131 therapy.

### Enhancing I-131 Uptake

Methods of enhancing the uptake of I-131 for both diagnostic and therapeutic purposes include low-iodine diet to double the I-131 uptake, ensuring that TSH is >60 at time of I-131 dose administration, and the use of lithium carbonate pretreatment to decrease the release of iodine from the gland and enhance the therapeutic effect without increasing whole-body irradiation. The availability of recombinant human TSH (currently under study) may make thyroid hormone ($T_4$) withdrawal obsolete in the future.

Just as it is wise to check for excess iodine by means of a patient questionnaire (e.g., CT scans), it is wise to suggest restrictions in dietary iodine for a week prior to scans or therapy. Iodine-rich foods to be avoided include the following:

- Iodized salt
- Seafood (including kelp or seaweed)
- Bread
- Milk and dairy products
- Eggs
- Restaurant food
- Foods with red dye number 3

The patient should also be advised to check labels of food prepared from algae derivatives for iodine content.

### Additional Follow-Up Techniques

Additional thyroid cancer follow-up includes sTg measurements, thallium 201 (Tl-201) and Tc-99m sestamibi imaging, CT and whole-body fluorodeoxyglucose (FDG) scanning, and quantitation of I-131 uptake.

### Serum Thyroglobulin

Tg is secreted in small amounts from normal glands at the time of $T_3$ and $T_4$ release. The highest levels of sTg have been seen in patients with skeletal and pulmonary metastases of well-differentiated papillary and follicular carcinomas, provided the tumor has follicular components. Although in the past sTg was not measurable in many patients because of Tg antibodies present in the serum, with improvements in assay systems this problem now affects only 10% of patients. I have found that some laboratories are useful for particular patients when other laboratories using different assay sys-

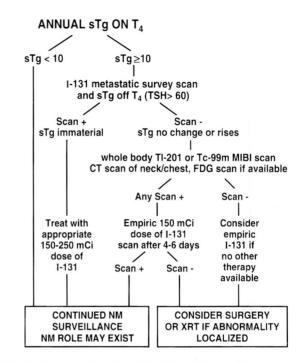

**FIG. 7-35.** Algorithm for high-risk patients after successful ablation of thyroid remnant.

tems demonstrate interfering antibodies. This variability is patient driven rather than assay specific because I have found that all reference laboratories show this variability. Elevations of sTg in thyroid cancer patients is an excellent tumor marker and suggests residual tumor, metastases, or local recurrence of disease. These patients warrant vigorous investigation. The role of sTg in following thyroid cancer patients is one of the major indications for performing remnant ablation to ensure that any detected sTg represents the presence of tumor rather than normal thyroid tissue.

The role of sTg measurement is not yet fully crystallized: Some argue that it can replace the I-131 metastatic survey scan completely as a screening test while the patient remains on $T_4$. Others claim that the sensitivity is maximized only when the patient is off $T_4$ and hypothyroid with an elevated TSH, while yet others claim that both sTg levels off $T_4$ and that metastatic surveys are required for maximal lesion detection (57). There is literature to support all sides of the sTg debate, indicating that sufficient numbers of patients have not yet been studied. Whereas on $T_4$, the sTg <10 ng/ml probably means no further investigation is necessary, elevated values require metastatic surveys (Fig. 7-35). There are patients in whom sTg is elevated, metastatic surveys are normal, and yet the patient has recurrence: This is in part attributed to the fact that only 75% of all tumors take up I-131. We currently perform sTg estimations in all patients undergoing follow-up with I-131 metastatic surveys. We do this with the patient off $T_4$ and while hypothyroid, believing that this is when the sTg is most sensitive (58). I have found a linear relationship between serum TSH and sTg levels in many

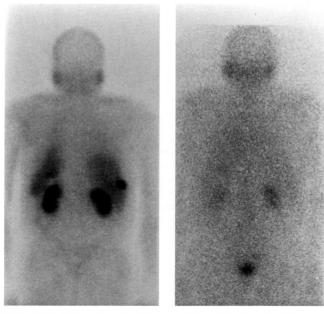

A,B

**FIG. 7-36.** This patient's sTg was 298 off $T_4$. The Tl-201 posterior scan **(A)** shows a rib lesion confirmed on CT, whereas the 8-mCi I-131 scan **(B)** was normal. The rib lesion was surgically removed.

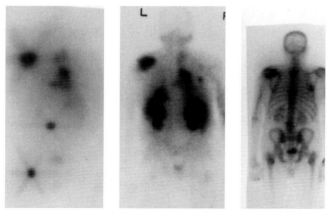

A–C

**FIG. 7-37.** Composite posterior images of I-131 **(A)**, Tl-201 **(B)**, and Tc-99m MDP bone **(C)** scans. Lesions include anterior right cervical soft-tissue local recurrence, left shoulder, right hilar, right rib, thoracic and lumbar vertebrae, and left lesser trochanter metastases. Although all four skeletal lesions were seen on the bone scan, the I-131 scans showed three lesions and the Tl-201 scan just a single rib lesion (not seen on the I-131 scan).

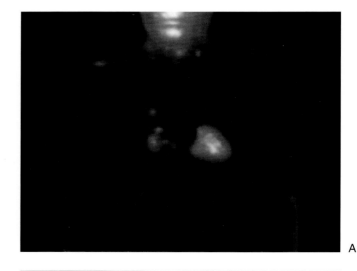

A

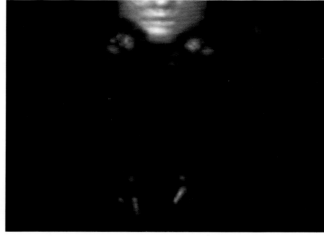

B

**FIG. 7-38.** These anterior upper torso images are three-dimensional reconstructions of two thyroid cancer patient F-18 FDG scans. **(A)** This patient had CT evidence of pulmonary metastases (a 2-cm macronodule and three smaller [4- to 7-mm] satellite lesions). None of these lesions took up I-131 (even with 150-mCi empiric dose) or Tl-201. The FDG scan shows these and many other pulmonary and cervical lesions. **(B)** This patient presented with elevated sTg values, palpable cervical masses, but unimpressive Tl-201 uptake. Bilateral cervical and upper mediastinal lymph nodes are present, but the CT scan showed enlarged right-sided nodes only. Note that the heart is not visualized in this patient, but the renal collecting systems are well visualized.

patients with this tumor marker. Some reports suggest that measurements on $T_4$ are adequate for clinical management (59), and in the years between metastatic surveys we use this test as a means of following the patient (see Fig. 7-35).

### Tl-201 Scans

Some centers have advocated the use of Tl-201 whole-body scans to monitor thyroid cancer, but this has not achieved widespread use in the last 15 years despite the convenience of a 1-day study performed while the patient is on $T_4$ therapy and the relatively good physical imaging characteristics of Tl-201 compared to I-131. In some patients the Tl-201 scan can be abnormal while the I-131 is not (Fig. 7-36). In other patients, both this pattern and the opposite (abnormal on I-131, normal on Tl-201 pattern) can occur (Fig. 7-37). In diagnostic applications, the sensitivity of Tl-201 detection of thyroid cancer in nodular thyroids has been reported since 1977, but unfortunately, Tl-201 uptake also occurs in thyroid adenomas, so this diagnostic technique is not satisfactory. At the same time, the radiopharmaceutical was being tested in thyroid cancer follow-up (60). Here Tl-201 is more successful, and Tl-201 is reported as more sensitive than sTg in the detection of tumor recurrence (61).

### Other Imaging Modalities

In patients with evidence of metastatic disease (abnormal metastatic survey or Tl-201 scans) should be evaluated with CT scans to determine whether surgery or I-131 therapy should be selected for definitive therapy. In addition, if significant lymph node disease is found at initial operation, a neck and upper mediastinal CT with thin-slice acquisition should be undertaken as a baseline assessment to gauge subsequent local nodal recurrence. CT scanning should also be undertaken in isolated sTg elevation when nuclear routine medicine scanning techniques are normal because recurrent cervical nodal disease occurs in both papillary and follicular cancers with about the same overall frequency as distant metastases, so the yield is acceptable and therefore cost-effective.

More recently, FDG positron emission tomography scanning has been used in patients with evidence of elevated tumor markers (Fig. 7-38), although there is some concern that reactive lymph nodes can result in false-positive studies.

### Empiric Therapy Doses

We have been more frequently investigating patients with elevated sTg levels and normal Tl-201 and I-131 metastatic survey scans. In these patients, empiric 150-mCi (5,500-MBq) I-131 therapy doses have been administered, and post-therapy I-131 scans have been abnormal (Fig. 7-39), indicating significant uptake of I-131 and therapeutic potential. In some patients, the sTg has returned to normal. An outpatient compromise is to image after the 32.9-mCi (1,217-MBq) ablation doses, and these can be performed without prior conventional scan doses (5 to 8 mCi [187 to 296 MBq]), which may cause thyroid stunning.

### Quantitative Uptake

Some groups have advocated quantitative uptake and residence time studies to more accurately estimate the delivered

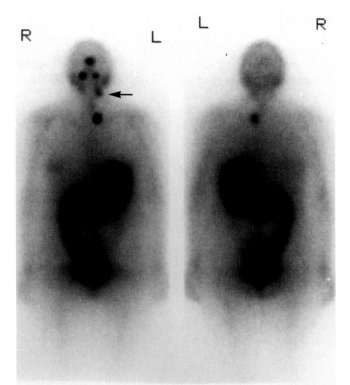

**FIG. 7-39.** This image was obtained after a 150-mCi (5,550-MBq) therapy dose when 15 mCi (555 MBq) of I-131 were calculated to be present in the patient. Prior 8-mCi (296-MBq) metastatic surveys and Tl-201 imaging were normal despite sTg elevation. The anterior and posterior images obtained after the high dose show two lymph nodes: one low left cervical (*arrow*) and one high left cervical, each corresponding with lymph nodes of <1 cm diameter as shown by CT. These were surgically removed, with subsequent fall in sTg.

radiation dose to the thyroid remnant for ablation (50) and to the marrow in therapy of functioning metastasis (52,62). These procedures appear cumbersome, and, given the varying uptakes that can occur with each therapy (Fig. 7-40), the procedures have to be recalculated for each subsequent treatment to prevent inadvertently high patient radiation doses. In some patients with high uptake in metastatic lesions, this or similar quantitative assessments should be considered (see Fig. 7-31).

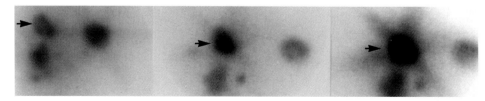

**FIG. 7-40.** These three images (of patient in Fig. 7-37) are anterior views, taken approximately 6 months apart, which show a progressive increase in uptake in the right cervical mass (*arrows*) (note "star" effect on right image) after XRT, with no significant interval change in the uptake to the right hilar mass and left shoulder lesions (*arrows*). Lesion uptake measurements confirmed a progressive increase in cervical tumor mass uptake; before XRT, no I-131 uptake occurred in this mass.

## Long-Term Follow-Up

In patients in whom thyroid cancer is diagnosed but only a hemithyroidectomy has been performed, any suspicion of recurrence should be investigated with sTg and Tl-201 scanning while on $T_4$. An elevated sTg (>30 ng/ml) should be investigated vigorously for local and distant recurrence with CT or US, or both, to identify lesions in the anatomic sites of Tl-201 uptake. It should be remembered that the sTg will be nonspecific and may result from the normal thyroid remnant alone. If I-131 therapy is contemplated, then completion thyroidectomy should be done followed by a metastatic survey and remnant ablation with either the remnant ablation or larger doses (see Table 7-14) if the lesion takes up I-131. Subsequent I-131 whole-body scanning would follow the routine follow-up algorithm (see Fig. 7-25).

In patients in whom the cancer risk was sufficient for total or near total thyroidectomy, the algorithm of Fig. 7-25 is followed. Once thyroid remnant ablation is achieved and no functioning thyroid recurrence or metastasis is identified, follow-up whole-body I-131 metastatic survey scans are repeated at 5-year intervals. With experience of thyroid withdrawal in each individual patient, the time off $T_4$ will be known to ensure that TSH is >60 with the least symptomatic period (3 to 4 weeks in ≥90% patients). Restarting suppressive therapy with both $T_4$ and decreasing doses of $T_3$, if not contraindicated (25 μg three times per day for 3 days, twice per day for 3 days, and once daily for 3 days), results in symptoms of hypothyroidism for the least amount of time. Over the years, I have found that many patients make mistakes with the alternative practice of stopping $T_4$, introducing $T_3$, then withholding all thyroid hormone for the last 2 weeks. Between these 5-year surveys, annual sTg on $T_4$ suppression therapy may be undertaken (see Fig. 7-35).

## Other Thyroid Cancers

The therapy for medullary carcinoma is total thyroidectomy and thyroid hormone replacement. Detection of metastases is difficult in these patients, although recently Tc-99m glucoheptonate, Tc-99m arcitumomab, Tc-99m DMSA(V), I-131 MIBG, and In-111 octreotide have been suggested. The central upper mediastinal lymph node searches are important in this patient population because they are sites of potential local recurrence.

There is no effective therapy for anaplastic carcinoma, and most patients die soon after the diagnosis is made.

## Alternative Therapies

In some patients, XRT is advocated. This group includes

- Patients in whom there is no uptake of I-131, yet CT, US, MRI, Tl-201, or FDG scanning demonstrate metastatic disease
- Patients in whom maximum bone marrow doses are achieved with I-131 and disease persists
- Patients diagnosed with unresectable primary tumor
- Patients with brain metastases (risk of hemorrhage)

The combination of I-131 and XRT can be complementary but is reserved for patients at high risk for local recurrence. Occasionally, patients in whom I-131 lesion uptake was minimal have had increases in I-131 after XRT (see Fig. 7-40). Chemotherapy in the form of doxorubicin has been somewhat effective, with partial response in 20% to 40% of patients. It is commonly used in anaplastic tumors, where a role as a radiosensitizer to complement XRT is also suggested.

## REFERENCES

1. Chapman EM. Commentary: history of the discovery and early use of radioactive iodine. JAMA 1983;250:2042–2044.
2. Landau RL. Treatment of hyperthyroidism. JAMA 1984;251:1747–1748.
3. Duffy BJ, Fitzgerald PT. Cancer of the thyroid in children: a report of 28 cases. J Clin Endocrinol Metab 1950;10:1296–1308.
4. Ron E, Modan B, Preston D, Alfandary E, et al. Thyroid neoplasia following low-dose radiation in childhood. Radiat Res 1989;120:516–531.
5. Saenger EL, Thoma GE, Tompkins EA. Incidence of leukemia following treatment of hyperthyroidism. Preliminary report of the cooperative thyrotoxicosis therapy follow-up study. JAMA 1968;205:855–862.
6. Dobyns BM, Shelline GE, Workman JB, et al. Malignant and benign neoplasm of the thyroid in patients treated for hyperthyroidism: a report of the cooperative thyrotoxicosis therapy follow-up study. J Clin Endocrinol Metab 1974;38:976–998.
7. Aktay R, Rezai K, Kirchner PT, et al. Rapid thyroidal iodine turnover in hyperthyroid patients: incidence and impact on outcome of I-131 therapy [abstract]. J Nucl Med 1995;36:15p.
8. Klee GG, Hay ID. Biochemical thyroid function testing. Mayo Clin Proc 1994;69:469–470.
9. Meier DA, Dworkin HJ. The autonomously functioning thyroid nodule [editorial]. J Nucl Med 1991;32:30–32.
10. Kitchener MI, Chapman IA. Subacute thyroiditis: a review of 105 cases. Clin Nucl Med 1989;14:439–442.
11. Alexander WD, McLarty DG, Horton P, Pharmakiotis AD. Sequential assessment during drug treatment of thyrotoxicosis. Clin Endocrinol (Oxf) 1973;2:43–50.
12. Wilson MA, Hurley PJ. Thyroidal 99m-Tc pertechnetate uptake as a prognostic indicator in hyperthyroidism [abstract]. Aust N Z J Med 1974;4:529.
13. Hashizume K, Ischikawa K, Sakurai A, et al. Administration of thyroxine in treated Graves' disease. N Engl J Med 1991;324:947–990.
14. Hershman JM. Does thyroxine therapy prevent recurrence of Graves' hyperthyroidism? [Editorial] J Clin Endocrinol Metab 1995;80:1479–1480.
15. Tallstedt L, Lundell G, Blomgren H, Bring J. Does early administration of thyroxine reduce the development of Graves' ophthalmopathy after radioiodine treatment? Eur J Endocrinol 1994;130:494–497.
16. Culver CM, Dworkin HJ. Radiation safety considerations for post-iodine-131 hyperthyroid therapy. J Nucl Med 1991;32:169–173.
17. Nordyke RA, Gilbert FI. Optimal iodine-131 dose for eliminating hyperthyroidism in Graves' disease. J Nucl Med 1991;32:411–416.
18. Nygaard B, Faber J, Hegedus L, Hansen JM. [131]I treatment of nodular non-toxic goitre. Eur J Endocrinol 1996;134:15–20.
19. Huysmans DAKS, Hermus ARNM, Corstens FHM, et al. Large compressive goiter treated with radioiodine. Ann Intern Med 1994; 121:757–762.
20. Laurie AJ, Lyon SG, Lasser EC. Contrast material iodides: potential effects on radioactive iodine thyroid uptake. J Nucl Med 1992;33:237–238.
21. Mazzaferri EL. Management of a solitary thyroid nodule. New Engl J Med 1993;328:553–559.
22. Kusic Z, Becker DV, Saenger EL, et al. Comparison of technetium-99m and iodine-123 imaging of thyroid nodules: correlation with pathologic findings. J Nucl Med 1990;31:393–399.

23. Ryo UY, Vaidya PV, Schneider AB, et al. Thyroid imaging agents: a comparison of I-123 and Tc-99m pertechnetate. Radiology 1983;148: 819–822.

24. Strauss HW, Hurley PJ, Wagner HN. Advantages of 99m-Tc pertechnetate for thyroid scanning in patients with decreased radioiodine uptake. Radiology 1970;97:307–310.

25. Dige-Petersen H, Kroon S, Vadstrup S, et al. A comparison of 99m-Tc and 123-I scintigraphy in nodular thyroid disorders. Eur J Nucl Med 1978;3:1–4.

26. Erjavec M, Movrin T, Auersperg M, Golouh R. Comparative accumulation of 99m-Tc and 131-I in thyroid nodules: case report. J Nucl Med 1977;18:346–347.

27. Ryo UY, Stachura ME, Schneider AB, et al. Significance of extrathyroidal uptake of Tc-99m and I-123 in the thyroid scan: concise communication. J Nucl Med 1981;22:1039–1042.

28. Cady B, Rosi R. An expanded view of risk-group definition in differentiated thyroid carcinoma. Surgery 1988;104:947–953.

29. Hay ID. Papillary thyroid carcinoma. Endocrinol Metab Clin North Am 1990;19:545–576.

30. Hay ID, Bergstrath EJ, Goellner JR, et al. Predicting outcome in papillary carcinoma: development of a reliable prognostic scoring system in a cohort of 1779 patients surgically treated at one institution during 1940 through 1989. Surgery 1993;114:1050–1058.

31. Mazzaferri EL, Jhiang SM. Long-term impact of initial surgical and medical therapy on papillary and follicular thyroid cancer. Am J Med 1994;97:418–428.

32. Lindsay S, Chaikoff IL. The effects of irradiation on the thyroid gland with particular reference to the induction of thyroid neoplasms: a review. Cancer Res 1964;24:1099–1107.

33. Robyn J, Mazzaferri EL. Current recommendations for benign and malignant thyroid nodules. Contemp Intern Med 1995;7:44–60.

34. Gharib H. Fine-needle aspiration biopsy of thyroid nodules: advantages, limitations, and effect. Mayo Clin Proc 1994;69:44–49.

35. Van Herle AJ, Rich P, Ljung B-ME, et al. The thyroid nodule. Ann Intern Med 1982;96:221–232.

36. Dalgeroff AJ, Hershman JM. Medical therapy for differentiated thyroid carcinoma. Endocr Rev 1994;15:500–515.

37. DeGroot LJ, Kaplan EL, McCormick M, Straus FH. Natural history, treatment and course of papillary thyroid cancer. J Clin Endocrinol Metab 1990;71:414–424.

38. Grossman RF, Tezelman S, Clark OH. Thyroid Cancer: The Case for Total Thyroidectomy Revisited. In Johnson JT, Didoklar MS (eds), Head and Neck Cancer, Vol. III. Amsterdam: Excerpta Medica International, Elsevier, 1993;879–888.

39. Mazzaferri EL. Thyroid Carcinoma: Papillary and Follicular. In Mazzaferri EL, Samaan NA (eds), Endocrine Tumors. Boston: Blackwell, 1993;278–333.

40. McConahey WM, Hay ID, Wootner LB, et al. Papillary thyroid cancer treated at the Mayo Clinic, 1946 through 1970: initial manifestations, pathologic findings, therapy and outcome. Mayo Clin Proc 1986;61:978–990.

41. Mazzaferri EL, Young RL, Oertel JE, et al. Papillary thyroid carcinoma: impact of therapy in 576 patients. Medicine 1977;56:171–196.

42. Pochin EE. Prospects from the treatment of thyroid carcinoma with radioiodine. Clin Radiol 1960;18:113–135.

43. Johansen K, Woodhouse NJY, Odugbesan O. Comparison of 1073 MBq and 3000 MBq iodine-131 in postoperative ablation of residual thyroid tissue in patients with differentiated thyroid cancer. J Nucl Med 1991;32:252–254.

44. Leung SF, Law MWM, Ho SKW. Efficacy of low-dose iodine-131 ablation of post-operative thyroid remnants: a study of 69 cases. Br J Radiol 1992;65:905–909.

45. Comtois R, Theriault C, Del Vecchio P. Assessment of the efficacy of iodine-131 for thyroid ablation. J Nucl Med 1993;34:1927–1930.

46. Maxon HR, Englaro EE, Thomas SR, et al. Radioiodine-131 therapy for well-differentiated thyroid cancer—a quantitative radiation dosimetric approach: outcome and validation in 85 patients. J Nucl Med 1992;33:1132–1136.

47. Bal CS, Padhy AK, Jana S, et al. Prospective randomized clinical trial to evaluate the optimal dose of I-131 for remnant ablation in differentiated thyroid malignancy [abstract]. J Nucl Med 1995; 36:41P.

48. Castronova FP, Beh RA, Veilleux NM. Dosimetric considerations while attending hospitalized I-131 therapy patients. J Nucl Med Tech 1982;10:157–160.

49. Maxon HR. The role of I-131 in the treatment of thyroid cancer. Thyroid Today 1993;16:1–9.

50. Maxon HR, Smith HS. Radioiodine-131 in the diagnosis and treatment of metastatic well differentiated thyroid cancer. Endocrinol Metab Clin North Am 1990;19:685–718.

51. Leeper RD, Shimaoka K. Treatment of metastatic thyroid cancer. Clin Endocrinol Metab 1980;9:383.

52. Benua RS, Cicale NR, Sonenberg M, Rawson RW. The relation of radioiodine dosimetry to results and complications in the treatment of metastatic thyroid cancer. AJR Am J Roentgenol 1962;87:171–182.

53. Jeevanram RK, Shah DH, Sharma SM, Ganatra RD. Influence of initial large dose on subsequent uptake of therapeutic radioiodine in thyroid cancer patients. Nucl Med Biol 1986;13:277–279.

54. Park H, Park Y, Zhou X. Detection of thyroid remnant/metastasis without stunning: an ongoing dilemma. Thyroid 1997;7:277–280.

55. Waxman A, Ramanna L, Chapman N, et al. The significance of I-131 scan dose in patients with thyroid cancer: determination of ablation. J Nucl Med 1981;22:861–865.

56. Robbins J, Merino MJ, Boice JD Jr., et al. Thyroid cancer: a lethal endocrine neoplasm. Ann Intern Med 1991;115:133–147.

57. Blahd WH. Serum thyroglobulin in the management of thyroid cancer [editorial]. J Nucl Med 1990;31:1771–1773.

58. Ronga G, Fiorentino A, Paserio E, et al. Can iodine-131 whole-body scan be replaced by thyroglobulin measurement in the post-surgical follow-up of differentiated thyroid carcinoma? J Nucl Med 1990;31:1766–1771.

59. Lubin E, Mechlis-Frish S, Zata S, et al. Serum thyroglobulin and iodine-131 whole-body scan in the diagnosis and assessment of treatment for metastatic differentiated thyroid carcinoma. J Nucl Med 1994;35:257–262.

60. Iida Y, Hidaka A, Hatabu H, et al. Follow-up study of postoperative patients with thyroid cancer by thallium-201 scintigraphy and serum thyroglobulin measurement. J Nucl Med 1991;32:2098–2100.

61. Ramanna L, Waxman A, Braunstein G. Thallium-201 scintigraphy in differentiated thyroid cancer: Comparison with radioiodine scintigraphy and serum thyroglobulin determinations. J Nucl Med 1991;32:441–446.

62. Thomas SR, Hertzberg VS, Kereiakes JG, et al. Relation between effective radiation dose and outcome of radioiodine therapy for thyroid cancer. N Engl J Med 1983;309:939–941.

*Textbook of Nuclear Medicine,*
edited by Michael A. Wilson.
Lippincott–Raven Publishers, Philadelphia © 1998.

CHAPTER 8

# Infection

Michael A. Wilson and Rosinda De La Pena

## HISTORY AND PATHOPHYSIOLOGY

For more than two decades, gallium 67 (Ga-67) citrate and indium 111–labeled white blood cell (In-111 WBC) scanning have been used for imaging suspected infection. The role of Ga-67 in inflammatory disease imaging was discovered serendipitously, but the development of In-111 WBC was the result of a conscious search for a WBC labeling procedure (1–4). In the last few years, other infection imaging agents have become available (2,4,5). Infection imaging constitutes approximately 5% of all imaging procedures. Table 8-1 gives the order of indications for infection imaging in a tertiary care hospital.

In the detection of inflammatory disease, these nuclear medicine tests are generally reserved to survey patients without localizing signs or symptoms and patients in whom computed tomography (CT), ultrasonography (US), and magnetic resonance imaging (MRI) have not identified an anatomic lesion. A unique clinical situation is the postoperative patient in whom an ileus makes it difficult to disperse contrast throughout the bowel for CT scanning. In all these presentations, a more general whole-body imaging technique is then indicated (either Ga-67 or In-111 WBC scanning). In specific disease processes, such as a febrile patient with acquired immunodeficiency syndrome (AIDS), a nuclear test may be the preferred screening procedure (6).

A review of the pathophysiology of inflammation helps in the understanding of the role of these radiopharmaceuticals in infection. In acute infection, large quantities of histamine, bradykinin, and serotonin are released by the damaged tissue. This results in an increase in both blood flow and capillary permeability that allows large quantities of fluid and proteins to leak into the locally inflamed tissues, producing edema. This allows many radiopharmaceuticals to localize nonspecifically to the site of infection. The initial cellular phase of the inflammatory response involves phagocytic activity by limited numbers of local macrophages already in the tissue, followed by neutrophil infiltration that begins in 30 minutes and reaches a maximum by 24 hours (this

process helps to explain the success of WBC scans). A slower, longer-lasting monocyte migration to the injured area follows. Chronic inflammation differs from acute inflammation in its less intense hyperemia and vasodilatation, less marked cellular infiltration, and the fact that infiltration involves mainly monocytes.

## RADIOPHARMACEUTICALS

### Ga-67 Citrate

Low–specific activity, reactor-produced Ga-72 was initially evaluated as a potential skeletal imaging agent. Its replacement radionuclide, Ga-67 (a cyclotron-produced, carrier-free agent), demonstrated a significantly different biodistribution from that of Ga-72. In 1968, while under study as a potential bone scanning agent, Ga-67's tumor- and infection-seeking properties were discovered serendipitously. Certain antineoplastics, whole-body irradiation, and iron or gadolinium (for MRI), administered within 24 hours of Ga-67 injection reproduced the bone scan pattern of the low–specific activity Ga-72 tracer. This change in biodistribution is produced by the interference of the binding of Ga-67 to transferrin, the normal blood transport mechanism and perhaps the mode of uptake via transferrin receptors. As a result, soft-tissue retention decreases while skeletal uptake and urinary excretion increases.

### *Physical Characteristics*

Gallium is a member of the group III elements of the periodic table. It is produced in a cyclotron by bombarding a zinc metal target. The physical half-life is 78.2 hours. The principal gamma emissions for Ga-67 are listed in Table 8-2. The predominant measured photons are the 93- and 185-keV gammas, and although their abundance is only 56%, they represent 89% of the measured photons due to improved sodium iodide crystal stopping power of the lower photon energies in the Ga-67 spectrum. Without the use of medium- or high-energy colli-

**TABLE 8-1.** *Indications for infection imaging in tertiary care hospital*

| | |
|---|---|
| Osteomyelitis | 40% |
| Acute cholecystitis | 25% |
| Opportunistic infections | 15% |
| Abscess detection | 10% |
| Others (e.g., infected graft, inflammatory bowel disease) | 10% |

**TABLE 8-2.** *Ga-67 principal radiation emission data*

| Radiation | Mean % of disintegration | Mean energy (keV) |
|---|---|---|
| Gamma-2 | 36* | 93.3 |
| Gamma-3 | 20 | 184.6 |
| Gamma-5 | 16 | 300.2 |
| Gamma-6 | 4 | 393.6 |

*Gamma-1 is a 91-keV photon with 2.9% abundance, and this is included in the gamma-2 (93-keV) window.

mators, the septal penetration contribution from the higher-energy photons is excessive and results in poor images. This is a classic example of the collimator choice being dictated by the radionuclide's total gamma emission spectrum rather than the gamma rays measured (see also Chapter 9).

### Pharmacokinetics

When Ga-67 citrate is injected, the complex dissociates rapidly, and the gallium ion binds to serum proteins, principally transferrin. As much as 80% to 90% of the injected dose may bind immediately to serum transferrin. The non–protein-bound fraction diffuses throughout the extravascular and extracellular space, is excreted by the kidney, and is taken up by the skeleton. At 24, 48, and 72 hours postinjection, approximately 20%, 10%, and 5%, respectively, of the tracer is still bound to plasma proteins.

**TABLE 8-3.** *Dosimetry of Ga-67 injection*

| | Rads/5 mCi (cGy/185 MBq) |
|---|---|
| Whole body | 1.3 |
| Skeleton | 2.2 |
| Liver | 2.3 |
| Bone marrow | 2.9 |
| Spleen | 2.7 |
| Kidney | 2.1 |
| Ovaries | 1.4 |
| Testes | 1.2 |
| GI tract | |
| Stomach | 1.1 |
| Small intestine | 1.8 |
| Upper large intestine | 2.8 |
| Lower large intestine* | 4.5 |

*Critical organ.
Source: Package insert, DuPont Pharmaceutical Division, Billerica, MA.

### Dosimetry

The critical organ is the bowel, despite only 10% excretion occurring by this route. The slow transit through the colon targets it for the highest radiation dose, of approximately 1 rad/mCi (1 cGy/37MBq) (Table 8-3). The liver, spleen, kidneys, bone, and bone marrow receive somewhat lesser doses (approximately 0.5 rad/mCi [0.5 cGy/37 MBq]).

### Mechanisms of Gallium Localization

The similarity in atomic configuration of gallium and the ferric ion helps explain much of the gallium biodistribution. Both transferrin and lactoferrin are metabolized in the liver, and the association of Ga-67 with these proteins explains the significant liver uptake in Ga-67 scanning. Several mechanisms of localization at sites of inflammation are hypothesized. Ga-67 may bind to leukocytes that migrate to, or are present at, the inflammatory lesion, or it may bind to transferrin as it passes into the leukocyte (where it is then bound to intracellular lactoferrin). Leukocytes migrating into a site of infection may degranulate, depositing large amounts of lactoferrin. Ga-67 may also be taken up by pathologic organisms via ferritin (the intracellular iron-storage protein) and siderophores (whose primary function is to trap and incorporate ferric ion).

The relative affinity of Ga-67 for these molecules is as follows, in order of affinity: siderophores, ferritin, lactoferrin, and transferrin. Thus, it seems that gallium may be transported to an abscess bound to plasma transferrin and that translocation of gallium to the abscess is mediated by the higher-binding bacterial siderophores, macrophage ferritin, and polymorphonuclear lactoferrin.

### Altered Biodistribution

Alterations in biodistribution cause scan abnormalities and variants that must be recognized.

Factors that may alter the expected tracer biodistribution of Ga-67 or labeled WBCs and the associated effects are as follows:

- An early In-111 WBC scan (e.g., to identify inflammatory bowel disease [IBD]) will have lung uptake: It should not be confused with diffuse pulmonary inflammatory processes.
- After recent chemotherapy, iron load, or extensive external radiation therapy: A Ga-67 scan may look like a bone scan (see Fig. 9-7).
- After mantle external radiation therapy: Ga-67 scans show increased head and neck glandular uptake (Panda sign) (see Fig. 9-6).
- After chemotherapy (e.g., bleomycin): Increased Ga-67 lung uptake occurs (see Fig. 9-9).
- After external radiation therapy to bone: Decreased regional uptake of labeled WBC and Ga-67 occurs in treated areas.

### Scan Protocol

With modern gamma cameras, at least three of the four photopeaks can be imaged. A medium-energy collimator is used with a large–field-of-view gamma camera. The recommended adult dose is 5 mCi (185 MBq) Ga-67 for infection imaging (10 mCi [370 MBq] is used in tumor imaging; see Chapter 9). After the intravenous (IV) injection, early blood-phase images obtained at 1 to 4 hours may give the first evidence of an inflammatory lesion as a result of the associated hypervascularity and capillary permeability. Routine images are obtained at 24 hours. Whole-body imaging should usually be performed because multiple unsuspected infectious sites can be present (7), and in the referred patient subset, localizing signs are often absent. Single photon emission CT (SPECT) imaging is essential for better delineation of the anatomy of abnormal sites.

Very active sites of infection may accumulate enough Ga-67 within 4 hours to be identified, but detection sensitivity is reduced significantly (to 30% to 70%) of what will be detected at 24 hours. In many cases, lesion identification can be made only on 24-hour images. Images at 72 hours and later can be obtained to follow the progress of Ga-67 in the bowel if it is necessary to differentiate the normal gastrointestinal (GI) route of excretion from abdominal inflammation. Alternatively, over-the-counter laxatives can be prescribed (e.g., bisacodyl or magnesium citrate) for the day before imaging.

Ga-67 scanning disadvantages include the following:

- Delay in imaging needed to allow for adequate blood and soft-tissue clearance
- Poor imaging characteristics of emitted photons
- Normal colonic activity, which can mask areas of abnormal gallium uptake in the abdomen and pelvis (Table 8-4)

Ga-67 scintigraphy has advantages over many anatomic imaging techniques in certain inflammatory conditions, including

- Lesions without well-formed borders, such as those of cellulitis and peritonitis, can be detected as efficiently as abscesses.
- Leukocyte infiltration may not be necessary to detect lesions, so Ga-67 scintigraphy can be used in the neutropenic patient.
- Ga-67 is a good agent for chronic and lymphocyte-mediated inflammation.

**TABLE 8-4.** *Normal Ga-67 visualization*

Liver (uptake greatest in this organ)
Bowel (viscus and bowel wall)
Kidneys and bladder (first 24–48 hrs)
Bone and bone marrow (see scapulae well)
Lacrimal and salivary glands, nasopharynx
Breasts in females (menarche and lactation)

**TABLE 8-5.** *Ga-67 visualization in children*

Thymus (after chemotherapy and radiotherapy)
Lower amounts in bowel lumen
Increased uptake in growth plates

### Normal Studies

When Ga-67 is injected, it is loosely bound to transferrin but readily displaced by other metals that share this transport mechanism (e.g., iron). At 24 hours, 25% of the tracer is excreted renally. At 1 week, 10% is excreted in the bowel, although in children a slightly different biodistribution is seen (Table 8-5). The remaining 65% is distributed through the whole body

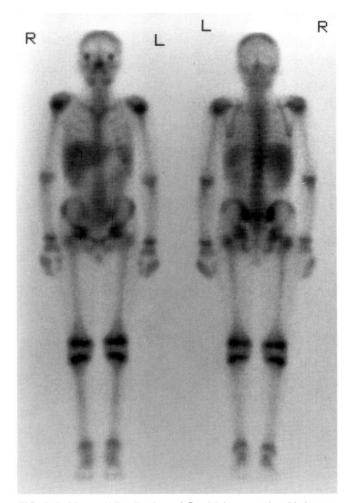

**FIG. 8-1.** Normal distribution of Ga-67 in a youth with immature skeleton. The liver, skeleton, and soft tissues are seen well. Because of his youth, the growth plates are also visualized. The normal route of excretion is the bowel (descending colon visible), but it is less apparent in this patient, a common finding in children. Note that the spleen is less visible than the liver, although the splenic dose rate is similar to that of liver and bone marrow (see Table 8-3).

**TABLE 8-6.** Ga-67 distribution at 1 week

| | |
|---|---|
| Liver | 20% |
| Skeleton | 20% |
| Soft tissues | 25% |

**TABLE 8-7.** In-111 principal radiation emission data

| Radiation | Abundance | Energy (keV) |
|---|---|---|
| Gamma-2 | 90.2 | 171.3 |
| Gamma-3 | 94 | 245.4 |

Source: Package insert, Amersham Corp., Arlington Heights, IL.

**TABLE 8-8.** In-111 WBC dosimetry

| Organ | Dose in rads/500 µCi (cGy/18.5 MBq) | | |
|---|---|---|---|
| | Pure In-111 | Contaminant | Total |
| Spleen* | 13 | 7 | 20 |
| Liver | 1.9 | 0.71 | 2.6 |
| Red marrow | 1.3 | 0.69 | 2 |
| Skeleton | 0.36 | 0.09 | 0.45 |
| Testes | 0.01 | 0.01 | 0.01 |
| Ovaries | 0.19 | 0.01 | 0.2 |
| Total body | 0.31 | 0.06 | 0.37 |

*Critical organ.
Source: Package insert, Amersham Corp., Arlington Heights, IL.

(Fig. 8-1), with a biological half-life of approximately 25 days (Table 8-6). Normal variants include

- Lacrimal (intense), parotid, and submandibular (mild) gland uptake
- Thymic uptake in children <2 years of age
- Thymic hyperplasia in children and teenagers after treatment with either x-ray therapy or chemotherapy
- Hilar node visualization in adult smokers
- Normal breast uptake in females

*Abnormal Studies*

Ga-67 is clinically most useful in chronic inflammatory processes and lymphocyte-mediated causes of inflammation (e.g., sarcoidosis). This tracer is preferred in the following situations:

- Opportunistic infections and nonbacterial infections (especially in immunocompromised patients)
- Patients with fever of unknown origin (FUO) and prolonged history (tumor and chronic infection or inflammation are more likely to be identified)
- Some instances of osteomyelitis (e.g., vertebral osteomyelitis) and discitis

### In-111–Labeled WBC Scanning

Leukocytes are the main cellular component of the inflammatory response. Most neutrophils (90%) reside in the bone marrow, and peripheral sites account for <10% of the total body neutrophil number. Half of all leukocytes are marginated (i.e., attached to endothelial cells). The essential function of the neutrophil is to move rapidly to a site of microbial invasion and to engulf and kill the causative microorganisms. The neutrophils respond to environmental stimuli through a variety of membrane surface receptor molecules that mediate both activation and modulation of phagocytic functions. The neutrophilia seen in acute infection is the result of both increased production and bone marrow release.

In-111 WBC scans were accepted immediately on introduction in 1976. Today, In-111 WBC scanning has largely replaced Ga-67 scanning in infection, except in special circumstances, such as AIDS and some pulmonary diseases (2,3,6). WBC scanning is the technique of choice for abdominal abscess detection and the investigation of secondary osteomyelitis (complicating previous surgery, trauma, etc.). Thirty percent of patients with infection have an unexpected lesion at a second site, and critically ill patients rapidly develop unsuspected new lesions (7).

*Physical Characteristics*

In-111 is produced in a cyclotron and decays by electron capture. The physical half-life is 67.2 hours. Table 8-7 shows the radiation emission data of In-111. There is a significant dose contribution by contaminants (In-114 and In-114m) at the time of expiration, as indicated by the package insert (Table 8-8).

*Dosimetry*

The dosimetry of In-111 WBCs is shown in Table 8-8. The following biodistribution is assumed:

- 30% to spleen
- 30% to liver
- 34% to red marrow
- 6% to remainder of body
- No excretion

In-111 oxine (or In-111 tropolone, an alternative labeling radionuclide) migrates into cells by virtue of cellular lipophilicity; the indium becomes firmly attached to cytoplasm components while the oxine is released. There is concern for the amount of radiation individual leukocytes receive from the conversion and Auger electrons released in the decay process. Multiple In-111 molecules attach themselves to each WBC, so the average radiation dose per cell reaches 1,000 to 2,000 rads (10 to 20 Gy) per day. This is not a problem for leukocytes because they do not replicate and have very short life spans. However, lymphocytes can survive for a long time, and malignant transformation is a concern, but the 15% or so lymphocytes in the total sample labeled probably die from this radiation dose because of their extreme radiation sensitivity (2).

*Preparation*

The only U.S. Food and Drug Administration (FDA)-approved method of preparing In-111 WBC uses In-111 oxine. Because In-111 oxine complexes label both cells and plasma transferrin, the cells must be separated from the plasma to ensure preferential cell labeling. The blood is collected in hetastarch, which helps to settle the red cells, so that after 45 to 60 minutes of standing, the leukocyte-rich plasma (LRP) supernatant can be removed. The LRP contains some red blood cells (RBCs), most of the platelets, and virtually all the WBCs (leukocytes, lymphocytes, and monocytes). The LRP is now centrifuged at 150g for 8 minutes, and the plasma supernatant is removed for later resuspension of the labeled WBCs before reinjection into the patient. This centrifugation step is repeated after resuspending the cell pellet with human serum albumin and saline.

The leukocyte pellet that results from these centrifugations is suspended in normal saline and incubated for up to 30 minutes with In-111 oxine. The normal preferential (90+%) binding of the In-111 oxine to transferrin rather than cells is circumvented by the prior removal of serum. By 15 minutes, labeling is nearly complete, so this incubation time is probably optimal. There are 100 times more platelets and 1,000 times more RBCs than WBCs in the blood to be labeled. The In-111 oxine therefore labels the leukocytes, many platelets, and the few RBCs remaining after the separation process. The labeled WBCs are a mixture of leukocytes and mononuclear cells, but this does not affect their utility in abscess detection and may be a benefit in chronic and lymphocyte-mediated infections. Granulocytes are preferably labeled over RBCs when less than half the cells present are RBCs. When equal numbers of RBCs and WBCs are present, 7% of the label binds to the RBCs. Table 8-9 shows the typical percentage distribution of the label to various blood elements. The labeling efficiency is usually 80% to 90%, and if the efficiency is <40%, the cells should not be reinjected.

Granulocytes and mononuclear cells can only be separated through elaborate density gradient techniques, which require considerable manipulation of cells so that the end result is activated WBCs. WBCs are sensitive to their removal from plasma and become activated, but removal is essential for the labeling process. Excess activation makes In-111 WBC infection-detection technique ineffective because the activated (enlarged) WBCs are sequestered in the pulmonary capillaries and later removed by the liver (normal In-111 WBCs are sequestered by the spleen).

There is concern about the cells' functional capacity once labeled. The labeling should be completed as quickly as practical and the cells then recombined with the patient's plasma. The cells should be injected within 3 hours of removal to ensure optimal viability. Many commercial pharmacies label WBC for nuclear medicine services, and in that case, the time from blood draw to reinjection may be excessive. The In-111 WBCs should be injected as soon as practical, via a large-bore (18- to 20-gauge) needle (not an existing infusion line) using saline (because dextrose can result in cell clumping). Labeling damage can result from the oxine, ethanol, radiation, or physical effects of handling during cell labeling. Among these factors, only oxine was found to exert a significant adverse effect on chemotaxis, but only at concentrations 10 times that typically used. Significant increases in radioactivity per cell do not appear to reduce the functional capacity of the cells (8).

An alternative labeling agent (tropolone) has been used successfully. Its advantage is that labeling efficiency is not reduced by the presence of plasma transferrin. Because separation of the cells from plasma causes most WBC damage, any manipulation of less magnitude should be advantageous. Clinical studies using tropolone in lieu of oxine have not demonstrated a convincing difference, and because this agent is not FDA approved, it is not generally used.

*Scan Protocol*

Both photopeaks should be imaged in routine imaging using a medium-energy collimator. The recommended dose is 500 μCi (18.5 MBq) In-111. Patient images are performed at 24 hours, except if the indication is IBD, in which case early imaging (30 minutes to 1 hour) should be performed to locate site and extent of involvement. Sequential imaging may be used to separate GI bleeding from IBD. In general, studies are performed using the patient's own WBCs, but in patients who need this study and who are extremely leukopenic, ABO-compatible donor cells may be used. We routinely take 50 to 60 ml of patient blood, and the WBC absolute count must exceed 5,000 cells/mm³. If the WBC count is <2,500, either donor cells or Ga-67 is substituted.

*Normal Studies*

Injected In-111 WBCs appear to distribute equally between the marginated pool and the circulating pool. The plasma disappearance half-time is approximately 5 to 9 hours, similar to that of normal unlabeled WBCs. Most marginated cells sequester in the spleen, thus, the spleen is the critical organ. This preference for the spleen does not indicate cellular damage, as it does with some other splenic sequestration agents, such as heat-damaged RBCs. In-111 WBC scans demonstrate the spleen, liver, and bone marrow. Any abnormal focus beyond these normal sites suggests an infection or inflammation (Fig. 8-2).

**TABLE 8-9.** *Cells labeled by In-111 oxine*

| Cell type | % of label used |
|---|---|
| Granulocytes | 60 |
| Mononuclears | 15 |
| RBCs | 7 |
| Platelets | 7 |
| Plasma | 11 |

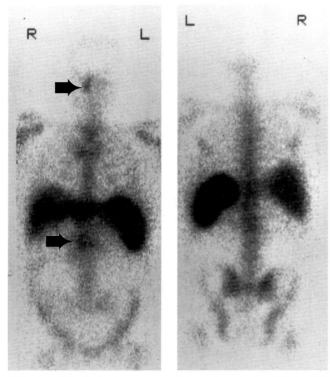

A,B

**FIG. 8-2.** Whole-body anterior **(A)** and posterior **(B)** In-111 WBC scan shows the usual tissue distribution of intense splenic uptake with moderate uptake in liver and bone marrow but no bowel activity. This patient also has mild uptake (*arrows*) in epigastrium (infected pancreatic pseudocyst) and nose (inflammatory reaction to the presence of a nasogastric tube).

*Abnormal Studies*

As many as 10% of injected In-111 WBCs can accumulate in pyogenic abscesses (see advantages of WBC scanning in Table 8-10), and these are clearly visible on a scan with an intensity of uptake equivalent to that of the spleen. Regions of mild and minimal inflammation, such as recent intramuscular injection or early decubitus ulcers, show low degrees of WBC uptake. Sensitivities and specificities are in the 90% to 100% range (see Abscess Detection) for individual diseases, such as abscesses, infected vascular grafts, osteomyelitis, sinusitis, and appendicitis. Early scans (30 minutes to 1 hour) are indicated in IBD, but generally the sensitivity in other In-111 WBC imaging indications (e.g., abscess or osteomyelitis) is only 40% to 70% at 4 hours.

Compared to CT and US, In-111 WBC scans show essentially no statistically significant difference in diag-

**TABLE 8-10.** *In-111 WBC scanning*

| Advantages | Disadvantages |
|---|---|
| 10% of In-111 WBCs accumulate at abscess | 3 hours to label WBCs |
| Whole-body imaging at reasonable cost | Diagnosis takes 24 hours |

**TABLE 8-11.** *False-negative and false-positive In-111 WBC scans*

| False-negative | False-positive |
|---|---|
| Difficulties | Focal localization |
| Small abdominal lesions near the liver and spleen | Central lines, dressings, accessory spleens |
| Disc space infections | Inflammatory response to tumor and foreign body |
| Low-grade infectious processes | Recent hematomas, infarcts, injection sites |
| Chronicity | Healing wounds (7 days) |
| Chronic (>3 wks) processes (e.g., osteomyelitis) | Endometriosis, vaginitis |
| Lymphocyte-mediated inflammation (AFB, viral) | ARDS and transplants |
| Nondelivery | Bowel |
| Skeletal (especially vertebral) | Stomas and drains, infarction, or fistula |
| Encapsulated abscess | Swallowed material (bronchitis and sinusitis), GI bleeding, irritation from enemas |
| Tense pus with microcirculation impairment | Skeletal |
|  | Heterotopic bone formation, trauma, degenerative joint disease, Charcot's joints, rheumatoid arthritis, fracture callus (<2 mos), musculoskeletal tumors |

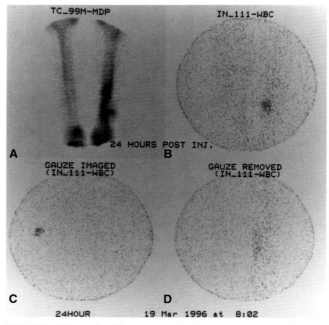

**FIG. 8-3.** This patient had minimal discharge from an ulcer on the left shin; the scan was requested to rule out osteomyelitis. The left anterior tibia bone scan image shows generalized uptake in much of the tibia **(A)**, and the In-111 WBC scan a focal lesion **(B)**. The gauze dressing **(C)** and the wound with dressing removed **(D)** show that In-111 WBC is associated with the minor wound discharge in the dressing, and osteomyelitis is not present.

nostic utility. In-111 WBC scanning is the preferred modality if a whole-body search is indicated because it can be done at less cost than the multiple CT scans, and it has distinct advantages in some clinical situations, such as identification of pseudomembranous colitis even before diarrhea (9). Table 8-11 shows some of the more common false positives and false negatives seen on In-111 WBC scanning (Fig. 8-3).

### Technetium 99m Hexamethylpropyleneamine Oxime WBC Scanning

Technetium 99m hexamethylpropyleneamine oxime (Tc-99m HMPAO) WBC scanning seems to be an ideal imaging candidate because of the marked reduction in radiation exposure ensured by the use of nuclear medicine's favorite radionuclide. Cost, image resolution, and convenience are reasons for the many attempts to replace In-111 with a Tc-99m complex suitable for WBC labeling. This subject is reviewed by Peters (10) and Kipper (11).

Tc-99m HMPAO is a nearly pure granulocyte label with a preference for granulocytes over monocytes and a low tracer elution rate from labeled granulocytes. The lipophilic HMPAO complex readily crosses the WBC membrane and changes into a secondary hydrophilic complex that is trapped in the cell nucleus and mitochondria. The labeling process can occur in the presence of serum plasma, so cellular functional capacity is protected during the labeling process. Animal studies have shown that there is less uptake of Tc-99m WBC than In-111 WBC. In human studies, the clinical results with Tc-99m WBC scans are similar to In-111 WBC studies (12) but can be completed sooner, with 1-hour and 4- to 6-hour imaging times the routine and 24-hour images only occasionally required.

### Normal Studies

The Tc-99m WBC studies look like bone scans, with liver and spleen visualized (Fig. 8-4). The anatomic detail is phenomenal, and many referring physicians prefer these

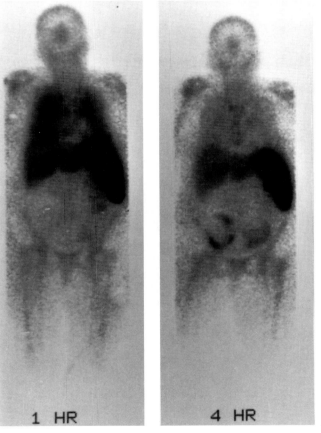

A,B

**FIG. 8-4.** These posterior whole-body images contrast a Tc-99m MDP bone scan **(A)** to a Tc-99m WBC scan **(B)**. The pelvic activity noted on the bone scan corresponds to a urinary ileal drainage conduit (left side) and urine bag (right side). The T7 abnormality, seen as a hot spot on bone scan, is cold on the WBC scan (in this case due to a recent compression fracture). The skeleton is visualized as a result of marrow uptake of labeled WBCs.

**FIG. 8-5.** Anterior whole-body views at 1 **(A)** and 4 **(B)** hours. The delayed 4-hour images show less pulmonary activity (activated cells clear lung) and more GI activity in small bowel loops (hepatobiliary excretion of Tc-99m HMPAO). These are the expected temporal changes. This labeling efficiency was similar to the more normal 40% to 70% reported in the literature, hence the bowel activity. Incidental note is made of tracer in Hickman catheter line (upper right sternum) and splenomegaly.

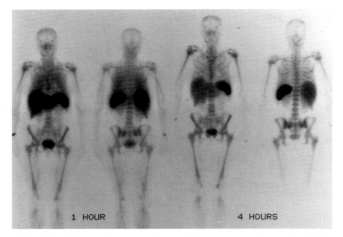

**FIG. 8-6.** These images show 1-hour and 4-hour Tc-99m WBC scans (anterior on the left and posterior on the right in each image pair). The early images show minimal blood pool activity in heart and femoral vessels and modest lung uptake; the 4-hour images show clearance of the blood pool and lung. The bone marrow is very well displayed in this normal individual. This tag was 88%, hence modest bladder and virtually no bowel activity (hepatobiliary excretion of Tc-99m HMPAO) is present in either image.

images to In-111 WBC scans. The 1-hour scans show increased lung uptake but no GI activity (Fig. 8-5) and so can be helpful in ruling out false-positive results of abdominal infection that may result from hepatobiliary tracer excretion. The package insert preparation suggestions give typical labeling efficiencies of 40% to 70%, but by reducing the reconstitution volumes of HMPAO to 1.0 to 2.5 ml, an efficiency averaging 70% can be obtained (Fig. 8-6). Preliminary reports on the use of the newly FDA-approved stabilized HMPAO (with methylene blue) suggest labeling efficiency >90% and prolonged stability and cell viability. Occasionally, 24-hour images are required (especially if 1-hour images are not obtained) because these delayed images establish that GI luminal activity is due to hepatobiliary excretion rather than an intra-abdominal infectious process. Virtually all patients at 24 hours have GI activity (13,14). Some users have found the frequency of bowel visualization at 1 hour in children to be several times that of adults (10).

### Abnormal Studies

In abscess detection, 90% to 100% sensitivities and specificities are regularly obtained.

### Ga-67 Versus Labeled WBC Scans

Compared to Ga-67 images, labeled WBC scans provide important benefits, including higher-resolution images due to better In-111 and Tc-99m imaging characteristics,

higher target-to-background ratio, and absence of abdominal excretion. Advantages of gallium include lower price, immediate availability for IV injection, and no handling of blood products. Strict comparisons between In-111 WBC and Ga-67 scans have been difficult to obtain because of the similarity of the two radionuclide emission spectra and half-lives. This has prevented stringent comparisons of these two radiopharmaceuticals. On the other hand, comparisons of Ga-67 and Tc-99m WBC show improved specificity with the WBC study (15).

### Indications

#### Ga-67 Scan

Indications for gallium imaging include

- Chronic nonpyogenic processes
- FUO
- Granulomatous and lymphocyte-mediated diseases
- Renal infections
- Small children
- Impaired WBC function
- Opportunistic infections

#### WBC Scan

Indications for labeled WBC scanning include

- Acute pyogenic processes
- Nosocomial and neutropenic FUOs
- Postoperative complications
- Abdominal abscess
- Osteomyelitis (especially when complicated)
- Infected prostheses and hardware
- Vascular graft infections

### Identification of Agents

On rare occasions, a scan might be sent for review from an outside hospital without the radionuclide specified. Table 8-12 can help to identify whether Ga-67 or In-111 WBCs were used (Figs. 8-7 and 8-8).

**TABLE 8-12.** *Comparison of normal organ visualization (radiopharmaceutical uptake) in Ga-67 and In-111 WBC scans*

| Organ | Ga-67 | In-111 WBCs |
|---|---|---|
| Bone marrow | + | ++ |
| Skeleton | ++ | — |
| Liver | ++ | + |
| Spleen | + | +++ |

+, mild; ++, moderate; +++, marked.

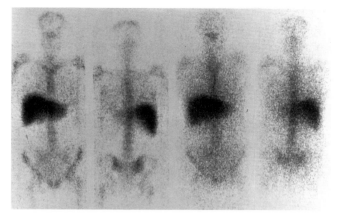

**FIG. 8-7.** This patient received an infection-localizing radiopharmaceutical at an outside hospital, and we were asked to repeat the delayed views on transfer to our hospital. We were told that Ga-67 was administered, but the images on the Ga-67 peaks (two images on right) looked poor, and there was no GI tracer excretion. We rescanned the patient on the In-111 window (two images on left), assuming we were misinformed of the radiopharmaceutical. The spleen is absent because the patient is postsplenectomy. No site of infection was found. The images are amazingly similar, providing a lesson in windowing, peak overlap, and Compton scatter. The clue to the wrong radionuclide was the indistinct organ outlines.

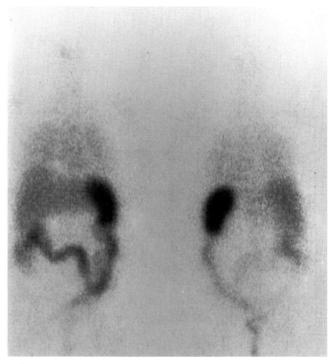

**FIG. 8-8.** Early visualization of bowel and lung in In-111 WBC scan (anterior view on left, posterior on right). The scan could be mistaken for a Ga-67 study, given the bowel activity. The intense visualization of the spleen (In-111 WBC scan likely) and the lung visualization (suggesting early images), suggests the early image protocol for IBD is likely to have been used. This patient had pseudomembranous colitis.

## Other Radiopharmaceuticals

### In-111 Chloride

In-111 chloride has been effectively used by some (16), but image interpretation is difficult. The drug is not FDA approved and so is not available in the United States.

### In-111 Polyclonal Immunoglobulin G

The discovery of nonspecific polyclonal antibodies at sites of active infection led to the testing of an agent already approved for human use by the FDA. This testing also resulted from a serendipitous discovery, when nonspecific immunoglobulin G (IgG) was used as a control for a specific monoclonal antibody (MOAB) being investigated for infection. The nonspecific IgG was unexpectedly found to have similar uptake to the specific MOAB.

Studies to date have shown a sensitivity of 92% and specificity of 95% for infection involving abdominal and pelvic abscesses, infected vascular grafts, and bone and pulmonary infections (17). A wide variety of infections are equally well imaged (gram-positive, gram-negative, and even yeast infections), but there is also accumulation in sterile inflammation (synovitis), recent fractures, and hematomas. The uptake therefore appears to be nonspecific and is presumed to be related to abnormal vascular delivery, increased capillary permeability, and antibody-fragment binding. Treatment with immunosuppressives, antibiotics, and anti-inflammatory agents has not prevented uptake, but uremia decreases the uptake and limits sensitivity. Localization is found in patients with various tumors, including melanoma, gynecologic cancers, lymphoma, prostate cancer, and malignant fibrous histiocytoma.

Most of the studies have used In-111 conjugated to diethylenetriaminepentaacetic acid (DTPA) to label the IgG. No adverse reactions have been reported. The usual dose is 1 mg IgG labeled with 1.5 to 2.0 mCi (55.5 to 74.0 MBq) In-111. The radiation exposure to ovaries, testes, eyes, and marrow is <3 rads (3 cGy). Images are obtained 4, 24, and 48 hours after injection. Human studies demonstrate significant blood pool and liver activity, and significant uptake is also observed in the spleen, kidney, bone marrow, and nasal mucosa. In some patients, faint activity in the large bowel can be observed after 24 hours, and there is some evidence to suggest that this may be more frequent with some but not all manufacturers' products. Disadvantages include a poor target-to-background ratio and imaging that is best delayed to 2 or 3 days. Advantages are its availability in kit form, the absence of need to label WBCs, no human anti-mouse antibody (HAMA) reactions, and the potential for Tc-99m versions or peptide equivalents in the future. These agents are not yet FDA approved.

### Antigranulocyte Antibody

An antigen that cross-reacts with carcinoembryonic antigen (CEA), called the *nonspecific cross-reacting antigen* (NCA), is in abundance on granulocytes, and when anti-NCA antibodies bind to the granulocytes, the WBC function is not impaired. The intact IgG molecule (NCA-95) has been used with I-123 and Tc-99m labels, and an Fab' fragment labeled with Tc-99m has also been used (18).

The Tc-99m–labeled antigranulocyte MOAB shows sensitivity and specificity (95% and 85%) similar to In-111 WBC scanning. This agent is currently going through the FDA New Drug Application (NDA) process, so it is not yet available in the United States. The usual dose is 4.5 mCi (166.5 MBq) I-123 or 15 mCi (555 MBq) Tc-99m. Approximately 10% to 25% of the injected dose is bound to circulating granulocytes, and an equal amount circulates as free Ig. The normal distribution is to bone marrow (55% at 4 hours) and, to a lesser extent, to the liver and spleen. HAMA reactions occur in 40% of patients with the intact IgG but few of the Fab' fragment recipients. The major potential indications appear to be osteomyelitis, soft-tissue infections, abdominal abscesses, and vascular graft infections. It is currently available only in Europe, but clinical trials are published regularly (19,20).

### Nanocolloids

Nanocolloid particles of human serum albumin (<80 nm) developed as marrow and lymphatic agents appear to diffuse into pyogenic and sterile inflammatory lesions and are being investigated for infection imaging. This technique has been used more in Europe and may be a nonspecific plasma marker that diffuses into pyogenic and inflammatory lesions, just like IgG. At present, its role may be limited to the skeleton (5).

### Chemotactic Peptides

Several peptide molecules are being studied, and it is thought that labeled peptide concentration in sites of infection occurs due to increased permeability and labeling of patient WBCs, both at the site of infection and while circulating (21). These agents are years from FDA approval.

## OSTEOMYELITIS APPLICATION

The clinical subtypes of osteomyelitis are categorized as acute, subacute, and chronic. Nuclear imaging with triple-phase bone scans (TPBS) has been used mainly for acute episodes, to diagnose the disease before other radiographic imaging techniques showed abnormality.

Because living organisms can persist in small abscesses or fragments of necrotic bone, resisting all attempts at eradication, months or even years can pass before the residual organisms flare up in recurrent osteomyelitis. This chronic or recurrent osteomyelitis presents a clinical situation that requires different imaging procedures; it is now a common indication for combined bone and WBC scans.

### Presentation

Childhood acute osteomyelitis is associated with the sudden onset of high fever, toxic state, and local signs of inflammation, and it usually involves the metaphysis of tubular bones (see Chapter 11).

In the adult, the acute onset is more insidious, with a relatively longer time between the onset of symptoms or signs and the ultimate diagnosis. It often affects the spine, pelvis, and small bones. When it involves the tubular bones, the epiphysis is more often involved than the metaphysis. *Staphylococcus aureus* is responsible for the vast majority of adult cases, which is in contrast to the multiplicity of organisms in the young.

### History of Nuclear Imaging and Osteomyelitis

The role of nuclear medicine in osteomyelitis was established in 1975, when the bone scan findings of osteomyelitis were recognized before plain-film changes, and effective early treatment precluded the progression to radiographic evidence of bone destruction in 45% of patients (22). In the same year, blood pool imaging was established as part of the nuclear medicine diagnostic criteria, so that osteomyelitis could be distinguished from cellulitis and septic arthritis (23). Also in 1975, Ga-67 was suggested as a useful imaging agent in the diagnosis of chronic osteomyelitis and of infections after open reduction of fractures (i.e., "secondary" osteomyelitis) (24). The cited articles are seminal position statements that established the role of nuclear medicine in osteomyelitis. An excellent review article is that by Schauwecker (25), who helped to establish the role of In-111 WBC and bone scanning in both acute and chronic secondary osteomyelitis (osteomyelitis complicating a fracture site, previous surgery [including prosthesis], past osteomyelitis, or in association with degenerative disease, neuropathic joints, soft-tissue inflammation, or diabetic ulceration).

### TPBS Protocol

The TPBS is very sensitive (94%) for osteomyelitis under all conditions. The scan is very specific (95%) in uncomplicated hematogenous osteomyelitis, especially in children. The TPBS is excellent for ruling out the disease because of

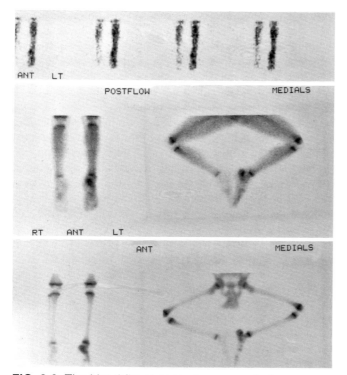

**FIG. 8-9.** The blood flow images (upper row) show generalized hyperemia of the foot, and a focal hot spot in the left os calcis is seen in the blood pool (postflow) image. The straight-leg anterior (left) and frog-leg (right) blood pool (middle row) and delayed (lower row) images of a young child with clinical cellulitis and possible osteomyelitis of the left lower extremity. The delayed images (lower row) confirm the focal spot within the OS calcis of proven osteomyelitis in the midst of slightly increased uptake due to the hyperemia associated with generalized cellulitis.

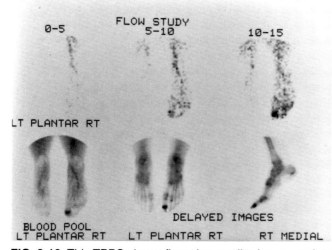

**FIG. 8-10.** This TPBS shows flow abnormality (upper row) to the great toe, and blood pool (left) and delayed (right) images in the lower row. This adult presented with painful toe and had hematogenous osteomyelitis of the base of the distal phalanx of the right great toe.

its very high negative predictive value (NPV), but it is non-specific in secondary osteomyelitis. In the adult population, most patients now present to nuclear medicine with osteomyelitis to be ruled out when secondary bone remodeling is already expected at the same site because of another etiology (e.g., secondary to prosthesis, trauma, previous surgery, past osteomyelitis, local soft-tissue infection, or local ulceration). In these patients, additional tests are required to provide specificity: plain films, MRI, In-111 WBC, Tc-99m WBC, Ga-67, or Tc-99m sulfur colloid marrow scans.

Even the presence of diffuse cellulitis (e.g., from an associated penetrating injury) does not reduce the specificity of the scan for osteomyelitis because the hyperemia of cellulitis is generalized, and there is a more intense focal abnormality at the site of osteomyelitis (Fig. 8-9).

The classic TPBS triad of osteomyelitis is as follows:

- Intense focal lesion in delayed image
- Identical lesion in "blood pool" image
- Increased perfusion in the very early "flow" frames (Fig. 8-10)

### Delayed Imaging

Imaging limbs can be difficult due to modest skeletal uptake of bone tracer. Delayed bone scan images of the feet and hands should be obtained routinely at 6 hours instead of the more common 2 to 3 hours. This results in significantly improved bone-to–soft-tissue uptake ratios. Effectively, it is a compromise between the so-called four-phase bone scan (TPBS plus 24-hour delayed imaging protocol) and the routine TPBS. The patient should be encouraged to ambulate to help decrease the soft-tissue tracer via venous and lymphatic clearance.

### False-Negative Studies

#### False Negatives due to Nondelivery of Tracer

Limitations of this technique occur when blood flow to the lesion is compromised and tracer cannot be delivered. This occurs commonly in arteriosclerosis and especially in diabetics, and it can be partly overcome by delayed 4- to 6-hour imaging. When the bone marrow or subperiosteal compartment is so tense that the bone tracer cannot be delivered by the microcirculation due to intraosseous or subperiosteal pus (26,27), the scan demonstrates a "cold" spot. Although more difficult to identify, this abnormal sign is often present in patients with apparently false-negative studies and occurs in one-third to one-half of adult patients with vertebral osteomyelitis (Fig. 8-11). Such sites often have destructive lesions on the plain film, so the disease process itself is not often missed with routine investigations.

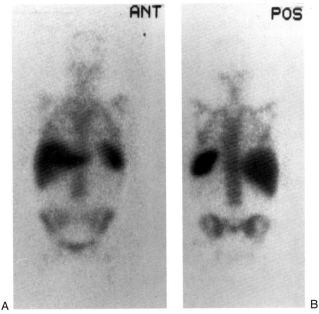

**FIG. 8-11.** This whole-body anterior **(A)** and posterior **(B)** In-111 WBC scan demonstrates a prominent photopenic defect at L5 due to osteomyelitis.

### False Negatives in Neonates

In the infant, osteomyelitis is usually of hematogenous origin, presenting with pain, swelling, and an unwillingness to move the affected region. Involvement of multiple sites is common in this age group. The usual location is the metaphysis with epiphyseal extension, and the infection can extend into the adjacent joint. Many false-negative studies are probably the result of rapid bone destruction.

There is controversy over presentation of osteomyelitis in the first 30 days of life. In these patients, the lesions are often not visualized, or they present as cold spots. This was originally reported in 1980 (28), and the authors assumed that the effect resulted from a destructive form of osteomyelitis that did not allow a bony reaction. Other authors have confirmed the finding, although there is dispute as to how often it occurs (29,30): Its incidence appears to vary between 13% and 100% of neonates. In combined reports, 58% of the infants and 33% of the lesions had normal scans or cold spots (28–31). The pattern is uncommon in older infants. Some believe that the improvement in image resolution that has occurred with modern equipment has reduced these numbers, but all agree that cold spots do occur (31). Great care must be taken when imaging children because most lesions occur in the metaphysis of long bones, so even the slightest asymmetry on the scan (see Chapter 11) can be abnormal and represent a lesion.

### Specificity Improvement

Although the TPBS is exquisitely sensitive, its specificity is poor, so additional imaging tests are required.

### Gallium 67

Initially, Ga-67 was used to improve the specificity of bone scanning after surgery and in chronic osteomyelitis (24). The relative uptake of the bone scan and the gallium radiopharmaceutical in the lesion was compared to either an adjacent bone or to the opposite bone, if paired. The ratio of each tracer was compared qualitatively or semiquantitatively, using computer-derived profiles through the abnormal adjacent bone or opposite normal bone. If infection is a major contributor to the scan lesion, relatively more Ga-67 uptake occurs than would be expected from the methylene diphosphonate (MDP) uptake alone. Despite overall specificity of nearly 70% in these difficult clinical situations, this agent has been replaced by In-111 WBC scanning because of its even greater specificity.

### In-111 WBC

In-111 WBC scanning resulted in excellent specificity in early prospective studies of acute osteomyelitis. Later, larger clinical studies extended this to chronic osteomyelitis. Focal increases in In-111 WBC accumulations are seen in areas of osteomyelitis, but photopenic defects may be seen, especially in spinal osteomyelitis (see Fig. 8-11). In a landmark study, Schauwecker et al. (32) found that the combined bone and In-111 WBC scan diagnostic accuracy (n = 453) was excellent in both acute and chronic osteomyelitis (>88% sensitive and specific), except in central sites containing active bone marrow, where the overall sensitivity fell to 70% (Table 8-13).

The technique of simultaneous bone and WBC imaging has become the gold standard in secondary osteomyelitis. Excellent results occur when bone scans and In-111 WBC scans are obtained and images of each radiopharmaceutical are superimposed (25,32). This reported technique has been modified slightly by acquiring images simultaneously, using the three peaks most modern gamma cameras possess. Bone scans and WBC scans can be acquired simultaneously and regions compared using software localization techniques (Fig. 8-12).

Imaging concerns are that of overlapping peaks (140-keV photon of Tc-99m and 171-keV photon of In-111) and the sum peaks of Tc-99m (photopeaks or Compton scatter) can be detected in the 245-keV In-111 photon window. These

**TABLE 8-13.** *Sensitivity of combined bone and WBC scan for osteomyelitis in proven cases*

| Site | Osteomyelitis | |
| --- | --- | --- |
| | Acute | Chronic |
| Hands and feet | 100% | 96% |
| Middle sites* | 95% | 88% |
| Central marrow sites | 89% | 71% |

*Sites other than hands, feet, and red marrow.
Source: Schauwecker DS. Osteomyelitis: diagnosis with In-111-labeled leukocytes. Radiology 1989;171:141–146.

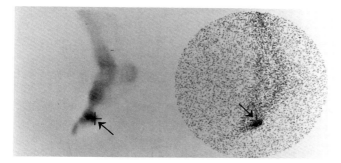

**FIG. 8-12.** These lateral views of the left foot show Tc-99m MDP (left) and In-111 WBC (right) images. Tc-99m and In-111 images are obtained simultaneously and displayed separately, and the cross hair marker is displayed at identical sites in each image. Software localization techniques reveal that the WBC scan is abnormal in the soft tissue of the foot. The cross hair (*arrows*) is posterior to the MDP abnormality but anterior to the WBC lesion.

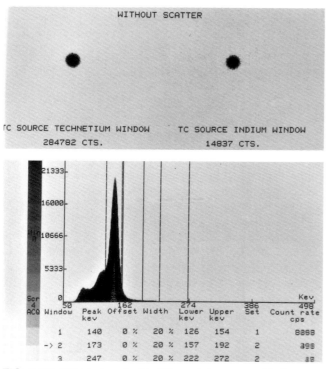

**FIG. 8-13.** This scan of a Tc-99m point source with the routine Tc-99m and In-111 windows used (20% wide Tc-99m centered on 140 keV, and 20% wide In-111 centered on 173 and 247 keV) without scatter material. In the spectrum displayed below, the spread of the Tc-99m photopeak allows >5% of total counts to be imaged in the 173-keV In-111 window and some summed peaks in the 245-keV window.

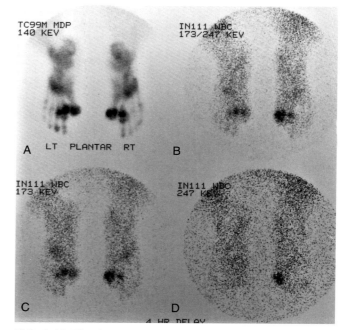

**FIG. 8-14.** The feet of a patient who has had both big toes removed. There is increased uptake in the Tc-99m bone scan **(A)** as a result of the surgery. Osteomyelitis of the stumps is to be ruled out. The 4-hour In-111 WBC images are displayed: both peaks **(B)**, low peak **(C)**, and high peak **(D)**. When the low peak is included, In-111 abnormalities are seen at each of the bone scan lesion sites. When only the upper peak is used **(D)**, there is evidence of increased WBC localization only in the head of the right first metatarsal. At 24 hours, this single abnormal site was confirmed, and the final clinical diagnosis was right-sided first metatarsal osteomyelitis.

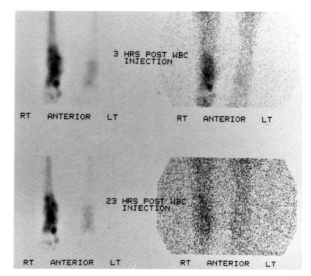

**FIG. 8-15.** The 3-hour images show Tc-99m MDP (upper left) and In-111 WBC (upper right) scans. The In-111 WBC abnormality at the ankle and base of first metatarsal is apparent at 3 hours, but in the 23-hour delayed In-111 WBC images (lower right) there is no scan evidence of osteomyelitis. This 3-hour (early) scan abnormality is due to misregistration of Tc-99m photons in the In-111 photopeak.

peaks result in surprisingly measurable registration in the lower In-111 peak (~5%) (Fig. 8-13). The 40-fold difference in injected tracer activities can make early (3- to 4-hour) images abnormal (Fig. 8-14), but this is unlikely in 24-hour imaging due to the difference in the half-lives of Tc-99m and In-111 (Fig. 8-15). We routinely use this scan combination procedure in all patients suspected of secondary osteomyelitis (e.g., postsurgical, diabetic patients). We routinely obtain 4-hour In-111 WBC scans using only the 245-keV peak for comparison with the 24-hour images. We obtain both peaks at 24 hours (equivalent abundance of 171- and 245-keV peaks improves image resolution), and if there is any difference from the early images, a single 171-keV peak image can be obtained.

### Tc-99m HMPAO WBC

Tc-99m labeled WBCs have largely replaced In-111 in most indications, but we have found infrequent discordant results, with no particular evidence to suggest one technique over the other. Simultaneous Tc-99m MDP bone and Tc-99m WBC scans cannot be obtained because of the identical tracer used, so there has been no wholesale switch to Tc-99m WBC scanning in osteomyelitis, as there has been in other infection imaging sites.

### Troublesome Sites

#### Diabetic Foot

Perhaps the most difficult task in nuclear medicine is the evaluation of osteomyelitis in the diabetic foot. Osteomyelitis is a very common cause of diabetic hospital admissions, and, after trauma, diabetes is the most common indication for lower limb amputation. These patients commonly have progressive Charcot's joints or ulcers, both of which may show WBC uptake and often simulate the scan findings of osteomyelitis. Although in general the sensitivity and specificity of the TPBS is approximately 95% when x-rays are normal, in the feet of diabetics or otherwise compromised patients, meta-analysis has shown that maintaining sensitivities of 80% to 90% by modification of scan criteria would decrease the specificity to 15% to 45% (33). The very high NPV of the TPBS, even in diabetics, makes this a suitable test because some patients with skin ulcers may not have increased bony uptake. With deep ulcers that penetrate deep toward the bone and in patients with Charcot's joints, the bone scan is often abnormal, so the routine use of bone scanning may not be cost effective. Here, tangential views can be of help (Fig. 8-16), but these soft-tissue lesions are often very difficult to separate, especially in the feet (see Fig. 8-12).

The use of In-111 WBC scan with the bone scan as a source of anatomic marker to separate soft tissue from bone allows the diagnosis of osteomyelitis (34) in patients with abnormal bone scans due to neuropathic osteoarthropathy (sensitivity 100%, specificity 83%). Amputations and neuropathic osteoarthropathy can be separated from osteomyelitis using In-111 WBC scans with a sensitivity of 90% and specificity of 90% (35).

Unsuspected osteomyelitis is common in diabetic patients with foot ulcers, of whom two-thirds develop underlying

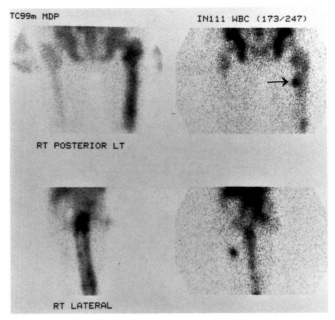

**FIG. 8-16.** Patient is status post prosthetic hip joint surgery and revision. The Tc-99m MDP shows increased tracer uptake in the general region of the prosthesis, with an In-111 WBC focus in the upper medial portion of the bone scan lesion (*arrow*). Tangential right lateral views confirm that the infection site is in the soft tissue.

osteomyelitis. Whereas most cases (~95%) of osteomyelitis have overlying ulcers, only one-third of these patients are clinically suspected of having osteomyelitis (35). One study shows that probing the base of an ulcer and detecting exposed bone is at least as good a detective technique as imaging procedures (sensitivity, 66%; specificity, 85%; and positive predictive value, 89%) (36). The NPV of this clinical procedure is only 56%, which leaves a limited role for nuclear imaging, with its very high NPV.

A recent cost-efficacy study indicates that, given the relatively poor performance of imaging (plain film, bone, In-111 WBC, and MRI scans), a 10-week course of culture-guided oral antibiotic therapy followed by debridement is the most cost-effective management (37) in patients with skin ulcers and suspected osteomyelitis. It is unlikely that this approach will be widely accepted because of physicians' uneasiness with prolonged therapy without a firm diagnosis.

The following points are important:

- A positive bone scan in a patient with a deep ulcer may represent associated synovitis or osteitis rather than septic arthritis or osteomyelitis.
- WBC scans may normalize after as little as 2 weeks of effective antibiotic therapy.
- The value of the bone scan might be in its high NPV in patients with early or shallow ulcers.
- Although In-111 and Tc-99m WBC scans have been compared favorably in osteomyelitis (38), the Tc-99m WBC

scan cannot be used with bone scan to compare radiopharmaceutical uptake because of the common radionuclide.

*Postoperative Sites*

In nonunited fractures, loose prostheses, and other postoperative problems, the abnormal blood pool phase of the TPBS associated with these conditions may cause difficulty in separating hyperemia from osteomyelitis. Combined In-111 WBC and bone scan studies are usually helpful in separating these patients (25,32), but postoperative alterations in bone marrow distribution have resulted in diagnostic errors in the use of bone and In-111 WBC scans after orthopedic surgery. Seabold et al. (39) used radiocolloid bone marrow and In-111 WBC scans to detect osteomyelitis in patients with orthopedic prostheses or fracture nonunion. This combination of tests improved the specificity from 50% (In-111 WBC alone) to 92% (combined marrow and In-111 WBC scan), with only slight decreases in sensitivity (94% to 88%). Soon after joint prosthetic surgery, the adjacent bone might be void of bone marrow, but marrow can develop later and as a consequence this may take up In-111 WBC. The corresponding scan pat-

terns of marrow agent and In-111 WBCs identifies this region as aberrant marrow rather than infection (Fig. 8-17).

*Vertebral Sites*

Central skeletal sites containing active bone marrow may result in reduced detection sensitivity for osteomyelitis because these infected areas may not take up significantly more In-111 WBCs than otherwise normal marrow sites. These sites of osteomyelitis would therefore appear normal or present as cold spots due to impairment in the microcirculation (see Fig. 8-11). In a definitive study of vertebral osteomyelitis, the specificity and sensitivity changed with the diagnostic criteria: With increased In-111 WBC uptake,

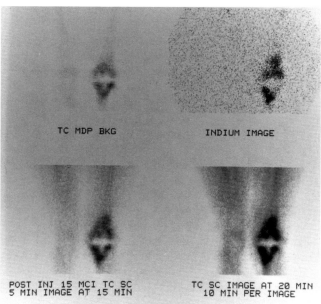

**FIG. 8-17.** This patient is status post left knee prosthesis placement. The TPBS was abnormal, with synovitis (not shown except for delayed anterior image, in upper left). The In-111 WBC scan at 24 hours (upper right) shows increased uptake corresponding to the bone scan abnormality, but with a slightly different configuration (extends higher into femoral shaft and does not involve the lateral tibial plateau region). The bottom row shows Tc-99m SC marrow anterior knee images obtained 24 hours later, the left for 5 minutes, the right for 10 minutes. The Tc-99m SC image extends up into the femoral shaft and has uptake at all the sites seen on the In-111 WBC scan. This indicates expanded marrow spaces around the prosthesis rather than infection.

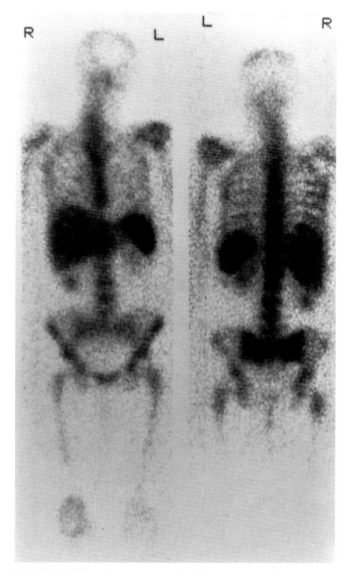

**FIG. 8-18.** This patient presented with streptococcal septicemia and multiple septic joints (e.g., left shoulder, right knee, and possibly left hip). In addition, unsuspected bilateral renal abscesses were identified.

the specificity was 98% (sensitivity, 40%), whereas with either an increase or decrease in In-111 WBC marrow uptake, the specificity fell to 50% (but sensitivity rose to 93%) (40). As many as half these patients with vertebral osteomyelitis have cold defects on In-111 WBC scans. These data also showed that cold defects were rare in the first 2 weeks of symptoms but that cold defects occurred in three-fourths of the patients whose symptoms remained for longer than 2 weeks and in those in whom pus was found. This suggests a progressive osteomyelitis pattern from "hot" to normal to cold. Other causes of a cold defect on In-111 WBC scans include hemangiomas, radiation therapy, avascular necrosis, recent fractures (see Fig. 8-4), metastases, Paget's disease, and degenerative joint disease.

### Septic Arthritis and Disk Infection

The TPBS is very useful in diagnosing septic arthritis by identifying scan abnormalities on both sides of the joint (Fig. 8-18). However, similar patterns occur in inflammatory arthritis. When this process is suspected in a prosthetic joint or after surgical procedures, an In-111 WBC scan can add information, but sometimes a marrow scan is indicated (see Fig. 8-17). Ga-67 scanning has been found to be more helpful in disk space infection, especially when used in conjunction with bone scanning.

### ABSCESS DETECTION AND FUO WORKUP

Abscess detection and FUO workup are considered together for convenience. In 1961, FUO was defined as fever >38.3°C (101°F) present for >3 weeks and failure to reach a diagnosis after 1 week of inpatient investigation. Occult sepsis is described as presumed infection without the Petersdorf criteria. More recently, a new classification was proposed (41).

- Classic FUO: fevers as defined by Petersdorf with no diagnosis in three outpatient visits or 3 inpatient days.
- Nosocomial FUO: fevers in a hospitalized patient in whom infection was not present or incubating on admission. Three days of investigation, including at least 2 days incubation of cultures, is also required for this diagnosis. Possible diagnoses include occult nosocomial infections, infected vascular lines, recurrent pulmonary embolism, transfusion viral infection, and drug fever.
- Neutropenic FUO: fevers in a patient with <500 neutrophils/mm$^3$ (or expected to fall below that level within 1 to 2 days). Three days of investigation, including at least 2 days incubation of cultures, are required. Neutropenic patients are especially susceptible to bacterial and fungal infections.
- Human immunodeficiency virus (HIV)-associated FUO: fevers over a period >4 weeks for outpatients or >3 days' duration in the hospital in a patient with HIV infection.

**TABLE 8-14.** *Causes of FUO*

| |
|---|
| Infection, such as abscesses |
| Tumor, especially lymphoma |
| Collagen disorders |
| Inflammatory diseases |
| Drug reactions, especially antibiotics |

Again, negative investigation after 3 days, including 2 days of culture incubation, is required. Infectious diseases, lymphoproliferative diseases (see Chapter 16), malignancy, and drug fever are possible causes.

Table 8-14 lists some of the more common causes of FUO. Most internal medicine texts do not include nuclear medicine imaging in the workup of FUO in the belief that it is insensitive and nonspecific and suggest CT and US as the only reasonable imaging modalities. If localizing signs are present, then CT and US are indicated because their excellent anatomic resolution allows detailed images of the region, although these techniques require that the inflammatory lesion have well-formed borders. In the absence of localizing signs, when the regional anatomic tests are normal, or in inflammatory lesions without well-formed borders (e.g., peritonitis), whole-body imaging with In-111 WBCs or Ga-67 are excellent diagnostic procedures. In these instances, whole-body nuclear medicine scans are even cheaper than CT scans of several body regions (e.g., of chest, abdomen, and pelvis), and multiple sites of infection, some unexpected, are more likely to be detected with whole-body imaging (7).

Approximately 30% of all classic FUOs are due to infection; another 20% are due to malignancies, including lymphoma; and the remaining 50% go undiagnosed. The longer the fever has been present, the less likely it is to be related to infection. A negative labeled WBC study excludes acute infection. A Ga-67 scan in these circumstances might identify an occult neoplasm, a nonloculated chronic inflammatory process, or a lymphocyte-mediated infection. In these circumstances, a gallium scan would have a higher yield than a labeled WBC scan and should be obtained first. For the nosocomial and neutropenic FUO, the In-111 WBC scan is the study of choice, using donor labeled WBCs if necessary. In the HIV-associated FUO, Ga-67 is the tracer of choice. Even these guidelines are not fixed because there are considerable data to suggest that both agents are indicated in many of these patient populations. Table 8-15 lists typical diseases that might cause occult infection or FUO and their detection sensitivities.

In the role of abscess detection, the Tc-99m WBC scan has excelled (see also Inflammatory Bowel Disease and Graft Infection). Whereas 24-hour imaging is required with In-111 WBC scans to obtain the greatest sensitivity, Tc-99m WBC scans can be performed much earlier in a wide spectrum of abdominal illnesses with excellent results (Table 8-16) (10,42). The bowel activity in the Tc-99m WBC scan,

**TABLE 8-15.** *Typical disease and test sensitivities*

| Disease | Ga-67 scan | WBC scan | Other common diagnostic tests |
|---|---|---|---|
| Abscesses | 85% | 95% | CT, US |
| Colitis | 40% | 80% | Endoscopy |
| Infected graft | 85% | 95% | CT |
| Lymphoma | 95% | — | CT |
| Osteomyelitis | 85% | 95% | MRI |
| PCP | 90% | 40% | CXR, BAL |
| Pneumonia | 40% | 80% | CXR |
| Pyelonephritis | 80% | 80% | GH, DMSA |
| Sarcoidosis | 80% | — | CXR, octreotide |
| Sinusitis | 85% | 95% | X-ray, CT |

**TABLE 8-16.** *Tc-99m WBC scan results at various imaging times*

| Parameter | Time of scan | | |
|---|---|---|---|
| | 0.5 hr | 2 hrs | 4 hrs |
| Sensitivity | 88 | 95 | 96 |
| Specificity | 81 | 85 | 92 |
| PPV | 91 | 93 | 96 |
| NPV | 75 | 88 | 92 |

Source: Lantto EH, Lantto TJ, Vorne M. Fast diagnosis of abdominal infections and inflammations with technetium-99m-HMPAO labeled leukocytes. J Nucl Med 1991;32: 2029–2034.

however, can result in false positives (43) unless serial scanning is performed.

## AIDS AND IMMUNOCOMPROMISED PATIENTS

Ga-67 works well in AIDS and can be used to diagnose the most common clinical presentations: pulmonary and GI infections (1,3,6). Patients with AIDS or who are otherwise immunocompromised are at risk for opportunistic infections and secondary tumor formation. Ga-67 can identify abnormal lymph nodes and associated tumors (except for Kaposi's sarcoma) and has been used to upgrade the AIDS-related complex to AIDS. This topic is discussed in detail in Chapter 16.

### *Pneumocystis Carinii* Pneumonia

The most common presenting symptoms of immunocompromised and AIDS patients are respiratory in nature. The most common opportunistic infection is the protozoan *P. carinii* pneumonia (PCP), which ultimately infects 80% of all AIDS patients. This condition requires invasive testing, such as bronchoalveolar lavage (BAL) or open lung biopsy, for definitive diagnosis. Ga-67 scanning has been recommended as a sensitive but nonspecific test to select symptomatic patients for further invasive investigations. In one

series, Ga-67 imaging was sensitive (94%) but less specific (74%). The sensitivity was 86% and specificity was 85% in patients with abnormal Ga-67 pulmonary uptake and normal or equivocal chest x-rays (CXRs) (44).

The diffuse uptake of Ga-67 into the entire lung is quite specific (80+%) for PCP (45) but may be somewhat difficult to recognize when mild because of the overlying rib activity. If the heart is silhouetted by increased lung uptake, PCP infection is likely. The specificity of the Ga-67 scan abnormality increases with the increase in degree of pulmonary uptake, which has been graded as stages I to IV, according to uptake:

- Stage I: pulmonary uptake equal to that of neighboring soft tissue
- Stage II: pulmonary uptake greater in soft tissue but less in liver
- Stage III: pulmonary uptake equal to that of liver
- Stage IV: pulmonary uptake greater than that of liver

The scan abnormality can be identified 1 to 18 months before CXR findings, but the CXR is abnormal in half the patients at presentation. If the Ga-67 scan is normal, a WBC scan should be obtained (Fig. 8-19) because, although it is less sensitive for PCP, PCP or other extrapulmonary or focal pulmonary causes may be diagnosed (Figs. 8-20 and 8-21) for the fever identified (46). Because prompt treatment improves patient outcome, Ga-67 scanning should be done

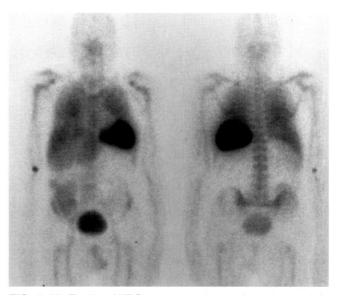

**FIG. 8-19.** Tc-99m WBC scan at 4 hours (anterior on left, posterior on right). The scan shows a renal transplant in right pelvis, effect of XRT in pelvis (lower half of SI joints and sacrum have decreased WBC marrow uptake), injection site in right antecubital fossa, and increased uptake in lungs at 4 hours. This immunocompromised patient was investigated for the lung uptake, and unexpected PCP infection was established. Care must be taken not to overdiagnose pulmonary infection by obtaining delayed (24-hour) images to confirm abnormal lung uptake.

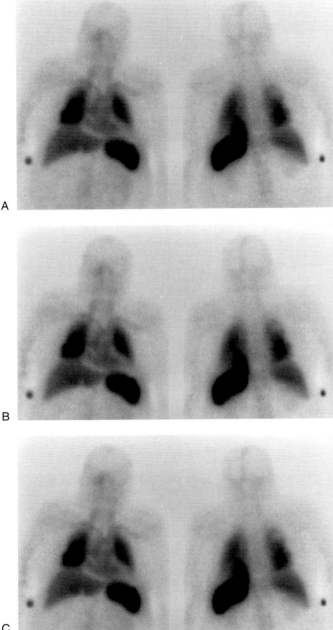

**FIG. 8-20.** This series of images demonstrates anterior (left) and posterior (right) Tc-99m WBC scans obtained at 1 hour **(A)**, 4 hours **(B)**, and 24 hours **(C)**. The injection site (right forearm) is visible in all. The early images show a diffuse increase in lung activity (activated WBCs) with a relative decrease in the right apex. At 4 hours, the lung activity is nearly homogeneous, decreased from earlier but still slightly abnormal, and nasal and esophageal activity is seen (NG tube in place). At 24 hours, the right upper lobe pneumonia has declared itself, and the nasal and esophageal inflammation or infection associated with the NG tube remains apparent.

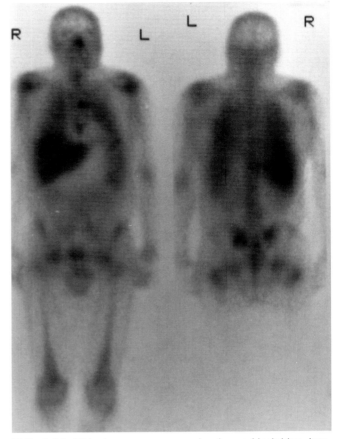

**FIG. 8-21.** This immunocompromised non-Hodgkins lymphoma patient was being investigated for PCP, but the scan also demonstrated generalized pulmonary uptake with parahilar and supraclavicular node involvement. These findings suggest the possibility of PCP plus mycobacterial infection. Note the femoral bone marrow expansion due to lymphoma.

on patients with respiratory symptoms to identify those who require more invasive workup and specific diagnosis.

Other respiratory diseases and organisms detected by Ga-67 imaging include the following:

- Cytomegalovirus
- Bacterial pneumonia
- *Mycobacterium avium-intracellulare* (see Fig. 8-21)
- Toxoplasmosis
- Histoplasmosis
- *Cryptococcus*
- Combinations of these

Thallium 201 (Tl-201) scanning has been suggested in AIDS patients. It serves two purposes in patients with unusual scan patterns. Kaposi's sarcoma is typified by chest lesions with Tl-201 uptake but no Ga-67 uptake, whereas those with focal Ga-67 uptake but no Tl-201 often have mycobacterial infections (47). This subject is discussed in Chapter 16.

## GI Presentations

The second most common site of involvement in AIDS is the GI tract. Just as activity in the lungs greater than that of the liver improves specificity for opportunistic infection, the finding of activity in the abdomen greater than that of the liver is also more specific (60% to 85%) for infection (see Chapter 16).

## INFLAMMATORY BOWEL DISEASE

WBC scanning in IBD has a role in the detection of ulcerative colitis and Crohn's disease. WBC scans are also abnormal in pseudomembranous (see Fig. 8-8) and ischemic colitis but not in irritable bowel syndrome.

Early images are essential in IBD because the WBCs are shed from the abnormal bowel wall regions and migrate through the lumen, thus preventing accurate localization on delayed imaging. The migration might be so rapid in diarrheal patients that shed cells might be passed in the stool by the time of routine 24-hour In-111 WBC imaging, and a normal scan can be obtained. In IBD, 1-hour, 2-hour, and 6-hour images are routine. These early images demonstrate significant pulmonary uptake, which should not be mistaken for additional pulmonary disease (see Fig. 8-8). Delayed images should be obtained routinely because the IBD patient might also present with an abscess, and early In-111 WBC imaging is relatively insensitive (70%) in the detection of abdominal abscesses (43). More recently, Tc-99m WBC has replaced In-111 WBC scans in this patient population (42,43), but early (1- to 4-hour) and late (24-hour) images may be required to differentiate focal abdominal disease from normal hepatobiliary tracer excretion (see Fig. 8-5).

The established role of WBC scanning in IBD is to identify the following:

- Clinical stage of disease
- Extent of bowel involved
- Complicating abscesses (48)

False-positive scans can result from active bleeding causing the passage of labeled WBCs, RBCs, and platelets into the bowel lumen. Ga-67 imaging is not routinely performed in these patients because of the normal bowel excretion of this radiopharmaceutical.

## ACUTE APPENDICITIS

A rare but indicated infection study is the atypical presentation of acute appendicitis. The typical patient who presents with pain that moves to the right lower quadrant, as described by McBurney in 1889, and is associated with point tenderness with or without rebound, provides enough clinical evidence to warrant immediate surgical intervention. Unfortunately, 30% of appendicitis is atypical in presentation and is commonly misdiagnosed in emergency rooms.

In the past, the acceptance of a 15% to 25% incidence of normal histologic appendix in appendectomies was considered good surgical practice. Because the wound infection rate and overall surgical morbidity rate for unrequired laparotomy is similar to that of medically needed appendectomies, the removal of normal appendices is no longer considered good surgery. With suitable radiologic modalities, unnecessary laparotomies are prevented. Studies using WBC and US examinations, alone or in combination, have dramatically reduced the false-positive surgical rate.

Early In-111 WBC scanning at 1.5 to 2.0 hours, with delayed imaging as required, is the routine protocol. A sensitivity of 93%, specificity of 95%, and accuracy of 95% in a trial of 171 patients has been found when the prevalence of disease was 33%, indicating that "easy clinical decisions" were operated on without imaging and that only the atypical presentations were studied (49). In the past, many of these patients would have been admitted and observed for 24 hours and operated on when symptoms and signs became more obvious. As many as 50% of patients with the diagnosis of possible appendicitis are observed for 48 hours, awaiting the typical presentation to emerge. In these patients, early In-111 WBC scanning is excellent (43) at diagnosing acute appendicitis. When the scan was normal, only 5% were false negatives. Perhaps most encouraging is the diagnostic localization of inflammatory disease at other sites in an additional 20% of patients (e.g., colon, pancreas). These are the advantages of WBC scans over US in this population. WBC scanning appears to be an important underused technique, especially if the early imaging advantage of Tc-99m WBC scanning is used (50).

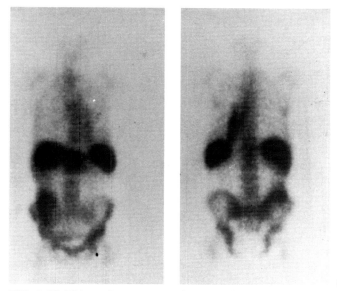

A,B

**FIG. 8-22.** This patient presented with FUO. The anterior **(A)** and posterior **(B)** body images demonstrate increased uptake in the thoracic aortic graft and in the right lower quadrant. An infected vascular thoracic aortic graft was confirmed. The CT of the abdomen showed only thickened bowel loops.

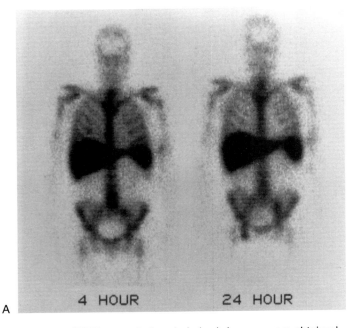

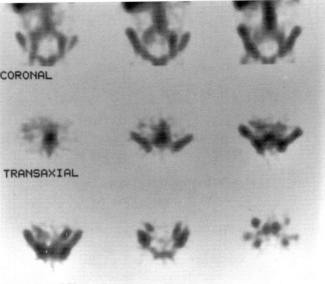

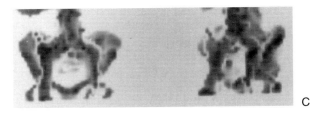

A      4 HOUR      24 HOUR      B

C

**FIG. 8-23. (A)** These anterior whole-body images were obtained 4 hours (left) and 24 hours (right) after injection of In-111 WBCs. The early images show minimal asymmetry in the left iliac region, whereas the 24-hour image shows bilateral abnormalities extending below the groin, especially on the right (only the right-sided infection was suspected clinically). **(B)** SPECT images show abnormalities in the lower aorta, both iliacs, and both femoral grafts. **(C)** Two views of the 3-D reconstruction show these involved vessels quite well. This graft was replaced.

## GRAFT INFECTION

The frequency of synthetic arterial graft infection is relatively low (2% to 6%). The majority involve aortofemoral or iliofemoral grafts, but these infections have a very high morbidity and mortality. In-111 WBC labeling has been shown to be a sensitive (97%) and specific (87%) test in studies that included approximately 200 grafts, and it is useful for the detection of occult vascular graft infections (51). Graft infections are usually manifested by the prompt accumulation of labeled WBCs (Figs. 8-22 and 8-23). Tc-99m WBC scans provide results within 1 to 4 hours of tracer injection; they will largely take over this imaging role. Two weeks after surgery, there should be no WBC localization in an uninfected graft, so the test is valid early in the postoperative period.

## RENAL INFECTION

Accumulation of Ga-67 in the kidneys is normal during the first 24 hours, and patients with normal renal function do not have significant renal accumulation after 48 hours. Renal activity of Ga-67 is considered abnormal in most of these instances:

• It is present beyond 48 or 72 hours.

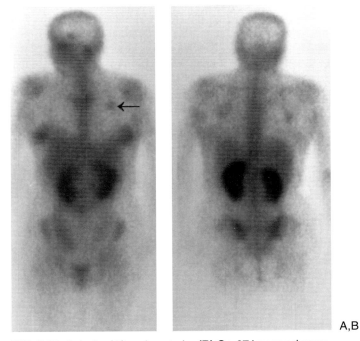

A,B

**FIG. 8-24.** Anterior **(A)** and posterior **(B)** Ga-67 images demonstrating interstitial nephritis due to Goodpasture's syndrome, chronic inflammation at the end of a chest tube drain in left upper chest (*arrow*), and normal breast, lacrimal, and parotid gland visualization.

- It is unilateral.
- It increases with time (e.g., from 24 to 48 hours).

Various intrarenal diseases, such as acute tubular necrosis, pyelonephritis, interstitial nephritis, the nephrotic syndrome, vasculitis, Wegener's granulomatosis, and nephrolithiasis, also produce abnormal uptake (Fig. 8-24). Renal obstruction also shows increased renal uptake of Ga-67 because the excretion route is compromised.

When evaluating children for pyelonephritis, Tc-99m dimercaptosuccinic acid or Tc-99m glucoheptonate are the tracers of choice. Focal abnormalities can be detected before actual distortion of the normal anatomy occurs, thus nuclear scans can detect abnormalities before radiologic changes are present (see Chapters 5 and 11). Labeled WBC scans have also proven useful in the diagnosis of kidney infections, including renal abscesses and perirenal infections (see Fig. 8-18).

## PULMONARY INFLAMMATIONS

Ga-67 scans have been used to determine inflammatory activity in pneumoconioses. These processes have as their earliest pathophysiology an alveolitis, and the process can be identified by BAL. CXR and pulmonary function tests detect old disease, but active inflammatory exacerbations cannot be identified by any of these techniques. Ga-67 scanning is an excellent way of identifying patients with active disease for further investigation.

Debate hinges on whether the best diagnostic means is a semiquantitative scoring system or a quantitative method. All suggested grading systems have in common a scale from low (background activity in the abdomen away from the bowel) to high (hepatic activity). This test applies to sarcoidosis, silicosis, asbestosis, and drug-induced lung changes (e.g., due to bleomycin, busulfan, phenytoin, nitrofurantoin, cyclophosphamide, methotrexate, amiodarone, cephalosporin, and cocaine) (52).

## REFERENCES

1. Alazraki NP. Radionuclide imaging in the evaluation of infections and inflammatory disease. Radiol Clin North Am 1993;31:783–794.
2. Datz FL. Indium-111-labeled leukocytes for the detection of infection: current status. Semin Nucl Med 1994;24:92–109.
3. Palestro CJ. The current role of gallium imaging in infection. Semin Nucl Med 1194;24:128–141.
4. Datz FL, Morton KA. Radionuclide detection of occult infection: current strategies. Cancer Invest 1991;9:691–698.
5. Datz FL, Morton KA. New radiopharmaceuticals for detecting infection. Invest Radiol 1993;28:356–365.
6. Vanarthos WJ, Ganz WI, Vanarthos JC, et al. Diagnostic uses of nuclear medicine in AIDS. Radiographics 1992;12:731–749.
7. Seabold JE, Wilson DG, Lieberman LM, Boyd CM. Unsuspected extra-abdominal sites of infection: scintigraphic detection with indium-111-labeled leukocytes. Radiology 1984;151:213–217.
8. Zakhireh B, Thakur ML, Malech HL, et al. Indium-111-labeled human polymorphonuclear leukocytes: viability, random migration, chemotaxis, bactericidal capacity, and ultrastructure. J Nucl Med 1979;20:741–747.
9. Nathan MA, Seabold JE, Brown BP, Bushnell DL. Colonic localiza-tion of labeled leukocytes in critically ill patients. Scintigraphic detection of pseudomembranous colitis. Clin Nucl Med 1995;20:99–106.
10. Peters AM. The utility of (99mTc)HMPAO-leukocytes for imaging infection. Semin Nucl Med 1994;24:110–127.
11. Kipper SL. Radiolabelled Leukocyte Imaging of the Abdomen. In Freeman LM (ed), Nuclear Medicine Annual. New York: Raven, 1995;81–128.
12. Costa DC, Lui D, Ell PJ. White cells radiolabelled with 111In and 99mTc—study of relative sensitivity and in vivo viability. Nucl Med Commun 1988;9:725–731.
13. Roddie ME, Peters AM, Danpure HJ, et al. Inflammation: imaging with Tc-99m HMPAO-labeled leukocytes. Radiology 1988;166:767–772.
14. Brown ML, Hung JC, Vetter RJ, et al. The radiation dosimetry and normal value study of 99mTc-HMPAO-labeled leukocytes. Invest Radiol 1994;29:443–447.
15. Vorne M, Soini I, Lantto T, Paakkinen S. Technetium-99m HMPAO-labeled leukocytes in detection of inflammatory lesions: comparison with gallium-67 citrate. J Nucl Med 1989;30:1332–1336.
16. Iles SE, Ehrlich LE, Saliken JC, Martin RH. Indium-111 chloride scintigraphy in adult osteomyelitis. J Nucl Med 1987;28:1540–1545.
17. Rubin RH, Fischman AJ. The use of radiolabeled nonspecific immunoglobulin in the detection of focal inflammation. Semin Nucl Med 1994;24:169–179.
18. Becker W, Goldenberg DM, Wolf F. The use of monoclonal antibodies and antibody fragments in the imaging of infectious lesions. Semin Nucl Med 1994;24:142–153.
19. Lind P, Langsteger W, Koltringer P, et al. Immunoscintigraphy of inflammatory processes with a technetium-99m-labeled monoclonal antigranulocyte antibody (MAb BW 250/183). J Nucl Med 1990;31:417–423.
20. Joseph K, Hoffken H, Bosslet K, Schorlemmer HU. In vivo labeling of granulocytes with 99mTc anti-NCA monoclonal antibodies for imaging inflammation. Eur J Nucl Med 1988;14:367–373.
21. Fischman AJ, Babich JW, Rubin RH. Infection imaging with technetium-99m-labeled chemotactic peptide analogs. Semin Nucl Med 1994;24:154–168.
22. Duszynski DO, Kuhn JP, Afshani E, Riddlesberger MM. Early radionuclide diagnosis of acute osteomyelitis. Radiology 1975;117:337–340.
23. Gilday DL, Eng B, Paul DJ, Paterson J. Diagnosis of osteomyelitis in children by combined blood pool and bone imaging. Radiology 1975;117:331–335.
24. Deysine M, Rafkin H, Teicher I, et al. Diagnosis of chronic and post-operative osteomyelitis with gallium-67 citrate scans. Am J Surg 1975;129:632–635.
25. Schauwecker DS. The scintigraphic diagnosis of osteomyelitis. AJR Am J Roentgenol 1992;158:9–18.
26. Russin LD, Staab EV. Unusual bone-scan findings in acute osteomyelitis: case report. J Nucl Med 1976;17:617–619.
27. Trackler RT, Miller KE, Sutherland DH, Chadwick DL. Childhood pelvic osteomyelitis presenting as a "cold" lesion on bone scan: case report. J Nucl Med 1976;17:620–622.
28. Ash JM, Gilday DL. The futility of bone scanning in neonatal osteomyelitis: concise communication. J Nucl Med 1980;21:417–420.
29. Mok PM, Reilly BJ, Ash JM. Osteomyelitis in the neonate. Radiology 1982;145:677–682.
30. Sullivan DC, Rosenfield NS, Ogden J, Gottschalk A. Problems in the scintigraphic detection of osteomyelitis in children. Radiology 1980;135:731–736.
31. Bressler EL, Conway JJ, Weiss SC. Neonatal osteomyelitis examined by bone scintigraphy. Radiology 1984;152:685–688.
32. Schauwecker DS. Osteomyelitis: diagnosis with In-111-labeled leukocytes. Radiology 1989;171:141–146.
33. Littenberg B, Mushlin AI, Diagnostic Technology Assessment Consortium. Technetium bone scanning to detect osteomyelitis: a meta-analysis. J Gen Intern Med 1992;7:158–163.
34. Schauwecker DS, Park HM, Burt RW, et al. Combined bone scintigraphy and indium-111 leukocyte scans in neuropathic foot disease. J Nucl Med 1988;29:1651–1655.
35. Newman LG, Waller J, Palestro CJ, et al. Unsuspected osteomyelitis in diabetic foot ulcers. JAMA 1991;266:1246–1251.
36. Grayson ML, Gibbons GW, Balogh K, et al. Probing to bone in infected pedal ulcers: a clinical sign of underlying osteomyelitis in diabetic patients. JAMA 1995;273:721–723.
37. Eckman MH, Greenfield S, Mackey WC, et al. Foot infections in diabetic patients. Decision and cost-effectiveness analyses. JAMA 1995;273:712–720.

38. Roddie ME, Peters AM, Osman S, et al. Osteomyelitis. Nucl Med Commun 1988;9:713–717.

39. Seabold JE, Nepola JV, Marsh JL, et al. Postoperative bone marrow alterations: potential pitfalls in the diagnosis of osteomyelitis with In-111-labeled leukocyte scintigraphy. Radiology 1991;180:741–747.

40. Palestro CJ, Kim CK, Swyer AJ, et al. Radionuclide diagnosis of vertebral osteomyelitis: indium-111-leukocyte and technetium-99m-methylene diphosphonate bone scintigraphy. J Nucl Med 1991;32:1861–1865.

41. Gelfand JA, Dinarello CA, Wolff SM. Fever, Including Fever of Unknown Origin. In Isselbacher KJ, Braunwald E, Wilson JD, et al. (eds), Harrison's Principles of Internal Medicine (13th ed). New York: McGraw-Hill, 1994;81–90.

42. Lantto EH, Lantto TJ, Vorne M. Fast diagnosis of abdominal infections and inflammations with technetium-99m-HMPAO labeled leukocytes. J Nucl Med 1991;32:2029–2034.

43. Mountford PJ, Kettle AG, O'Doherty MJ, Coakley AJ. Comparison of technetium-99m-HMPAO leukocytes with indium-111-oxine leukocytes for localizing intraabdominal sepsis. J Nucl Med 1990;31:311–315.

44. Barron TF, Birnbaum NS, Shane LB, et al. Pneumocystis carinii pneumonia studied by gallium-67 scanning. Radiology 1985;154:791–793.

45. Kramer EL, Sanger JH, Garay SM, et al. Diagnostic implications of Ga-67 chest-scan patterns in human immunodeficiency virus-seropositive patients. Radiology 1989;170:671–676.

46. Fineman DS, Palestro CJ, Kim CK, et al. Detection of abnormalities in febrile AIDS patients with In-111-labeled leukocyte and Ga-67 scintigraphy. Radiology 1989;170:677–680.

47. Lee VW, Cooley TP, Fuller JD, et al. Pulmonary mycobacterial infections in AIDS: characteristic pattern of thallium and gallium scan mismatch. Radiology 1994;193:389–392.

48. Lantto E, Jarvi K, Krekela I, et al. Technetium-99m hexamethyl propylene amine oxine leucocytes in the assessment of disease activity in inflammatory bowel disease. Eur J Nucl Med 1992;19:14–18.

49. Navarro DA, Weber PM. Indium-111 imaging in appendicitis. Semin Ultrasound CT MR 1989;10:321–325.

50. Rubin RH. In search of the hot appendix—a clinician's view of inflammation imaging [editorial]. J Nucl Med 1990;31:316–318.

51. Brunner MC, Mitchell RS, Baldwin JC, et al. Prosthetic graft infection: limitation of In-WBC scanning. J Vasc Surg 1986;3:42–48.

52. Khan AS, Dadparvar S, Brown SJ, et al. The role of gallium-67-citrate in the detection of phenytoin-induced pneumonitis. J Nucl Med 1994;35:471–473.

*Textbook of Nuclear Medicine,*
edited by Michael A. Wilson.
Lippincott–Raven Publishers, Philadelphia © 1998.

# CHAPTER 9

# Tumor

Michael A. Wilson, Jesus A. Bianco, and Donald J. Stallman

Cancer is the second most common cause of death in the United States. Approximately one million cancers are diagnosed each year in the United States, and 50% of patients with cancer eventually die of their malignancy. Tumor becomes clinically evident when $10^9$ cells are present, which indicates that the lesion may have been present for many years before detection. The patient dies of the tumor mass when this cell number reaches $10^{12}$ cells (approximately 1 kg tumor burden), leaving a therapeutic window between $10^9$ and $10^{12}$ cells. The primary role of tumor imaging is to diagnose and stage cancer accurately, with the ultimate goal of helping in cancer cure and control. If this is not possible, the secondary goal is to provide the optimum quality of life by the appropriate evaluation of patients before intervention, resulting in altered surgical approaches or even cancellation of unnecessary or mutilating surgery if disease is more advanced than expected.

## ROLE OF CONVENTIONAL IMAGING

Tumor spreads locally by direct extension and disseminates widely via blood and lymphatic vessels. This spread is conventionally identified by one or more of the following factors:

- Distortion of local tissue boundaries in the primary organ
- Distortion of adjacent organs by local spread
- Lymph node enlargement in lymphatic spread
- Distorted distant organs in vascular spread

Various imaging techniques are best for determining involvement of the common sites of secondary hematogenous spread: chest x-ray (CXR) and computed tomography (CT) for lung metastases; CT and magnetic resonance imaging (MRI) for liver metastases; and plain film, bone scans, CT, and MRI for skeletal metastases. Imaging is primarily used to stage tumors by defining tumor extent, to assess response to treatment, and to uncover recurrences. Screening for primary tumor is an uncommon indication, the notable exception being mammography.

The rationale of tumor imaging is the need to know the extent of local and distant spread before and during treatment. When tumor size is <1 cm (i.e., <1 billion cells), no imaging method can consistently detect the tumor. MRI and CT as anatomic imaging techniques can identify lesions of 1 to 2 cm with regularity, whereas the nuclear medicine imaging technique often requires slightly larger lesions. The success of the nuclear technique depends more on tracer uptake than tumor size and relies on sufficient activity contrast between tumor and normal tissue. This functional aspect of nuclear medicine imaging explains why it is useful despite an order of magnitude less resolution (centimeters) than conventional radiology (millimeters) under ideal testing conditions.

The distribution of nuclear medicine studies in a typical tertiary care hospital is shown in Table 9-1. Because radiopharmaceuticals are usually administered systemically, whole-body imaging is routinely performed. Thus, nuclear medicine is cost-effective compared to regional CT or MRI scanning, in which body regions are charged separately, so to image equivalent regions (e.g., the torso) a single nuclear charge is made but three separate CT or MRI charges would be required (e.g., CT of chest, abdomen, and pelvis).

Nuclear medicine plays an established role in the staging and therapy of some malignancies. Bone scanning is the most commonly used nuclear medicine procedure in tumor diagnosis (Fig. 9-1), but it is now generally restricted to patients with cancer who present with skeletal pain or who have increasing tumor markers, such as prostate-specific antigen (PSA) or carcinoembryonic antigen (CEA) (see Chapter 1). In the liver, the labeled red blood cell scans can accurately confirm a hepatic hemangioma, and liver-spleen scanning can differentiate benign hepatic lesions with normally functioning Kupffer cells (e.g., focal nodular hyperplasia) from malignant hepatic lesions that do not contain Kupffer cells (e.g., carcinoma). Although there is a veritable explosion of ongoing research to develop unique functional tumor imaging agents, to date, Ga-67 citrate is the most established tumor radiopharmaceutical and is especially useful in the clinical management of lymphoma patients. Tumor imaging of malignancies using

**TABLE 9-1.** *Tumor imaging in a typical referral hospital*

| General availability (FDA approved) | |
| --- | --- |
| Bone scanning for various cancers | 86% |
| Ga-67 tumor scanning (e.g., lymphoma) | 5% |
| I-131 scanning for thyroid cancer | 4% |
| Tl-201 and Tc-99m sestamibi scanning | 3% |
| Labeled MOABs and receptor agents | 2% |
| Limited utilization | |
| Lymphoscintigraphy, hepatic arterial perfusion | |
| F-18 FDG | |
| Limited availability | |
| C-11 amino acids (C-11 methionine) | |
| DNA tracers (C-11 thymidine) | |
| Therapeutic agents (F-18 5-fluorouracil) | |

**TABLE 9-2.** *Tumor-seeking agents*

| Tumor agents | Tracer | Tumor types |
| --- | --- | --- |
| General metabolism | FDG, P-32 | Numerous |
| Specific metabolism | I-131 as NaI | Thyroid |
| Complex compound | MIBG | Neural crest |
| Surface receptors | Pentetreotide | Neural crest |
| Antitumor agents | Bleomycin, 5-FU | Lung, liver |
| Surface antigens | MOABs | Numerous |
| Lymphoscintigraphy | Tc-99m SC | Melanoma, breast |
| Cationic uptake | Ga-67, Tl-201, Tc-99m MIBI | Numerous |

myocardial perfusion agents, such as thallium 201 (Tl-201) and technetium 99m (Tc-99m) sestamibi, hold considerable promise of widespread dissemination through the nuclear imaging community, especially because multicenter trials are under way to determine the utility of some applications in nonacademic centers. Another role that is rapidly becoming the standard of care is lymphoscintigraphy to detect the sentinel lymph node for biopsy (e.g., melanoma) and to aid in subsequent treatment decisions. Advances in monoclonal antibody (MOAB) technology and specific peptide receptor imaging (e.g., pentetreotide [OctreoScan]), along with tumor metabolism (e.g., fluorodeoxyglucose [FDG]) and general metabolic (e.g., labeled amino acids) imaging agents, have contributed to exciting progress in tumor imaging (Table 9-2).

Radiopharmaceutical methods are valuable for their potential to

- Detect occult primary or metastatic disease
- Characterize lesions based on their perfusion, metabolism, or receptor expression
- Determine whether post-therapeutic masses represent scarring or tumor recurrence
- Identify lymphatic drainage beds using the sentinel lymph node concept
- Evaluate actual or potential therapy response using metabolic or neuropeptide agents
- Determine the potential role of therapeutic agents using tracer-radiolabeled analogs
- Treat various diseases

The biological differences between tumor and the normal tissue from which the malignancy arises are minimal, but nuclear medicine can exploit these differences in both diagnosis and treatment. The classic example is that of thyroid cancer, in which three-fourths of well-differentiated tumors can have significant uptake of iodine 131 (I-131), which provides both diagnostic and therapeutic possibilities. I-131 therapy (first successful in 1946) predates conventional cancer chemotherapy and has the unique potential to cure cancer with minimal side effects on adjacent normal tissue. Other successful therapeutic agents include I-131 meta-iodobenzylguanidine (MIBG), which concentrates in neuroblastomas and malignant pheochromocytomas.

## TUMOR PHYSIOLOGY AND MOLECULAR MEDICINE

By the time tumors are detected by imaging methods, they are large, have abnormal neovascularity with increased capillary permeability, and have undergone necrosis as they

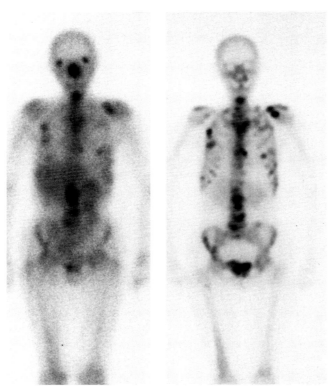

A,B

**FIG. 9-1.** These scans contrast skeletal metastases in the anterior views of a Ga-67 **(A)** and Tc-99m MDP **(B)** bone scan performed on the same patient using the same scanner. The Ga-67 scan shows the normal biodistribution of liver, soft tissue, bowel activity, and lacrimal glands, whereas the bone scan shows the expected skeletal and urinary systems. Every lesion seen in the bone scan is identified in the Ga-67 scan, although the anatomic definition is better with the bone scan due to the higher photon flux and better Tc-99m photon imaging characteristics.

outstrip their blood supply. The nonspecific accumulation of small and large molecules regionally in tumors is a consequence of their easy passage into the local tumor extracellular fluid (ECF) because of the abnormal permeability of the new tumor vessels. Special tumor features can also allow the localization of specific agents; for example, breast tumors can be demonstrated by estrogen and somatostatin receptor agents. These unique biochemical processes can be identified by external imaging with suitable labeling, but the label itself must not interfere with the receptor-ligand binding. When large radioactive labels (e.g., I-131) are used, these must be strategically placed away from the part of the ligand molecule that interacts with the receptor. Smaller-label molecules, on the other hand, can be tolerated at many substituent sites (e.g., fluoride 18 [F-18] as fluoride ion at hydroxyl sites) without affecting receptor binding. Tc-99m and In-111 labels, because of their large size and inability to substitute or attach to existing molecular components (e.g., I-131 binding to tyrosine), require chelator systems that bind the label to the ligand yet displace it at a sufficient distance to prevent receptor-ligand interference (e.g., in-111 diethylenetriamine pentaacetic acid [DTPA] binding to the amino groups of amino acids, either at the terminal amino group or at additional amino groups of phenylalanine and lysine).

Cell surface receptors interact with many atoms of a ligand, and these interactions lead to biochemical changes in the cell. This molecular recognition is a fundamental feature of biological processes, and receptor-ligand and antibody-antigen interactions are examples of it. Currently, the U.S. Food and Drug Administration (FDA)-approved examples of nuclear medicine exploitation of these interactions include several MOABs and the somatostatin receptor, with many agents in various stages of the approval process.

Tumors can have associated specific chromosomal aberrations, and although these findings are particularly prevalent in myeloid neoplasms and soft-tissue sarcomas, to date they have not been exploited by nuclear medicine. With the identification of new tumor-specific abnormalities, greater understanding of tumor growth-promoting and -suppressing factors, and the isolation of oncoproteins, as suggested by the oncogene-antioncogene hypothesis, more specific tumor targets will be developed with better results than those of the present tumor-associated antigens (TAAs). Currently, MOABs have been developed against TAAs only; these TAAs include differentiation antigens (CEAs), tumor-secreting antigens (thyroglobulin), and membrane antigens (tumor-associated glycoprotein 72 [TAG-72]). With the development of more specific tumor markers, the nonspecific normal tissue uptake and the body background that plague the current TAAs will decrease, and tumor contrast will increase. These developments will make imaging simpler, and possibly even practical for screening purposes. The identification of receptor distributions using positron emission tomography (PET), single photon emission CT (SPECT), and planar imaging has been successful to date, but MRI does not seem to have the sensitivity to detect the currently known receptor densities.

**TABLE 9-3.** *Ga-67 tumor avidity*

| Ga-67–avid tumors | Limited Ga-67 avidity |
| --- | --- |
| Hodgkin's lymphoma | Neuroblastoma |
| NHL | Low-grade NHL |
|   High grade | Head and neck tumors |
|   Intermediate grade | Breast |
| Lung cancer | Thyroid |
| Melanoma | Gynecologic |
| Hepatoma | Gastrointestinal |
| Soft-tissue sarcomas | Bladder |
| Brain tumors | Osteosarcoma |
| Testicular tumors | Multiple myeloma |

## GALLIUM

The uptake of Ga-67 citrate into soft-tissue tumors was an unexpected finding of Edwards and Hayes while they were studying Ga-72 as a potential bone scanning tracer (1). They also recognized that tumor uptake decreased following chemotherapy. The Ga-67 scan is clinically useful in lymphomas (2,3), especially Hodgkin's disease (HD), but also in Burkitt's and other aggressive non-Hodgkin's lymphomas (NHL), and virtually all childhood lymphoma. Sensitivity and specificity are as high as 95% in lymphomas, except for low-grade NHL, yet the Ga-67 imaging technique is still not universally embraced by oncologists. This may be because the published results in the 1980s were not ideal. Other Ga-67–avid tumors with possible clinical roles include hepatomas, melanoma, and soft-tissue sarcomas (Table 9-3).

### Radiopharmaceutical

Gallium is a group III element, with multiple valence states, but in biological systems its size and charge are comparable to that of the ferric ion. This similarity to the ferric ion probably explains much of the tracer's biodistribution. Ga-67 is produced in the cyclotron (4) and decays by electron capture to zinc 67, with a half-life of 78.1 hours. In the process of decay, it emits several major gamma emissions in a complex spectrum of 91- to 880-keV photons (Table 9-4) but produces no particulate emission. Two or three of the lower photopeaks are generally used for imaging. We believe that the best photons to image are the 93- and 185-keV photons, which represent 56% of the decay process but account for 81% of the photons detected by gamma camera crystals. This relative detection increase is explained by the lesser stopping power of the relatively thin gamma camera crystals for the higher-energy photons. We typically use three 20% energy windows, including the 93-, 185-, and 300-keV photons, to increase the photon yield. The fourth major photopeak (394 keV) is 4% abundant and is important only for its contribution to image degradation by septal penetration. Some imagers suggest that the 93-keV window should be narrowed to prevent the detection of lead x-rays (73 keV) that result from the septal interaction of high-

**TABLE 9-4.** *Ga-67 spectrum of gamma ray photons*

| keV | Photon abundance |
|---|---|
| 93* | 42 |
| 185 | 24 |
| 300 | 16 |
| 394 | 4 |

*91- and 93-keV gammas combined.
Sources: Compiled from Iturralde MP (ed). CRC Dictionary and Handbook of Nuclear Medicine and Clinical Imaging. Boca Raton, FL: CRC Press, 1990;327; and Leovinger R, Budinger TF, Watson EE (eds). MIRO Primer for Absorbed Dose Calculations. New York: Society of Nuclear Medicine, 1988. It differs slightly from the Ga-67 package insert (Table 8-2).

energy photons (see Fig. 23-4). They also suggest that there is too much septal penetration of the 300-keV photon when medium-energy collimators are used. The Ga-67 gamma ray spectrum represents a difficult technical compromise. Often, the process of trial and error best determines which combination of collimator, scan parameters, and energy windows is best for each particular gamma camera.

Imaging is accomplished after the intravenous (IV) injection of carrier-free Ga-67, which distributes widely throughout the body. More than 99% of circulating Ga-67 is in the plasma, almost all of it bound to transferrin. Ga-67 finally accumulates in the lysosomal fractions of the cell and is thought to enter these cells with transferrin via the CD71 transferrin receptor (5). Other significant protein carriers include ferritin and lactoferrin. Once located intracellularly, the Ga-67 is released from its carrier protein.

Because of this marked protein binding, the plasma Ga-67 residence time is prolonged, with up to 20% persisting in the circulation at 24 hours. During the first 12 to 24 hours the kidneys excrete up to 25% of the injected dose, and renal excretion declines thereafter. Subsequent excretion occurs primarily via the gastrointestinal (GI) mucosa, and this excretion route accounts for 10% to 15% of injected dose, with perhaps one-fifth of the GI activity coming from hepatobiliary secretion. Only one-third of the injected gallium dose is excreted; the remaining two-thirds stay in the body for a long time (Table 9-5). The lower large bowel is the critical organ, due to the prolonged residence time (Fig. 9-2). The estimated absorbed radiation dose to an average adult (70 kg) from an IV injection of 10 mCi (370 MBq) of Ga-67 is shown in Table 9-6.

**TABLE 9-5.** *Biodistribution of Ga-67 citrate*

| Site | Portion | Time |
|---|---|---|
| Body retention | | |
| Soft tissue | 20% | At 1 week |
| Liver, spleen | 25% | At 1 week |
| Bone marrow | 20% | At 1 week |
| Excretion | | |
| Renal | 25% | First day |
| Intestinal | 10% | First week |

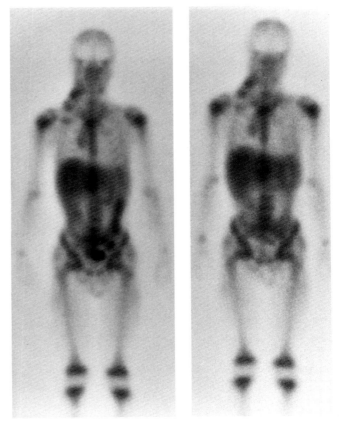

A,B

**FIG. 9-2.** These two Ga-67 scan images were obtained at 48 hours **(A)** and 72 hours **(B)** in a lymphoma patient. The significant epiphyseal activity indicates an immature skeleton. The scan shows abnormal nodal uptake in right cervical, upper right axillary, and right mediastinal regions. Bowel activity changes over the 24 hours shown, with significant clearance from the descending and sigmoid colon. We now routinely perform our first scan at 96 hours rather than 48 hours.

**TABLE 9-6.** *Radiation dosimetry for Ga-67*

| Organ | Rads/10 mCi (cGy/370 MBq) |
|---|---|
| Lower large intestine* | 9 |
| Liver | 4.6 |
| Bone marrow | 5.8 |
| Spleen | 5.3 |
| Ovaries | 2.8 |
| Testes | 2.4 |
| Total body | 2.6 |

*Critical organ
Sources: Compiled from Iturralde MP (ed). CRC Dictionary and Handbook of Nuclear Medicine and Clinical Imaging. Boca Raton, FL: CRC Press, 1990;327; and Leovinger R, Budinger TF, Watson EE (eds). MIRO Primer for Absorbed Dose Calculations. New York: Society of Nuclear Medicine, 1988. It differs slightly from the Ga-67 package insert (Table 8-2).

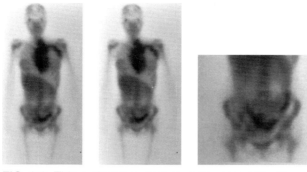

A–C

**FIG. 9-3.** This patient has nodular sclerosing HD with anterior **(A)** and posterior **(B)** whole-body views, and a spot anterior abdomen view **(C)**. Note the normal breast uptake **(A)**, the extensive mediastinal and axillary disease involvement **(A, B)**, and the better bowel definition on the spot view **(C)** due to both increased counts and shorter collimator-to-patient distance.

### Scan Protocol

The recommended Ga-67 dose is 8 to 10 mCi (296 to 370 MBq) in adults, with adjustments for children based on body surface area. Whole-body, spot planar, and SPECT images are often acquired, sometimes at two time points. Tumor imaging may be performed as early as 48 hours postinjection, but because target-to-background ratio increases with time, the best images are obtained 4 or more days postinjection. Scans can be acquired up to 10 days postinjection because of the combination of the relatively long radionuclide half-life and the stable late biodistribution. We now prefer imaging at 96 hours with SPECT of both chest and abdomen, using follow-up studies if bowel activity obscures important regions.

The detection of an abnormality by Ga-67 scintigraphy requires high tumor-to-background ratios, so adequate numbers of photons must be present. Whole-body imaging techniques are typically photon deficient, but they can be used if scanning speeds are slowed (5 to 10 cm per minute) to the equivalent of multiple spot imaging, and adequate numbers of photons are obtained. Spot views of the neck, chest, abdomen, and pelvis can be performed as a function of either time or counts. Typically, 10 minutes per view is adequate, and count-based spot views should contain 1,000,000 to 2,000,000 counts using late-model, large–field-of-view detectors (Fig. 9-3). In spot views of the lung or abdomen, subtle tumor lesions may be missed when the high-activity liver or bowel is in the image; in these cases, displaying at two intensities may be required.

### *Special Views*

Special views are often obtained. Axillary views for lymph node detection can be acquired with a flexed elbow and abducted humerus while the camera is centered over the axilla. These views are acquired for 600,000 counts and should be paired by time. Lateral head and neck views with the head turned (Fig. 9-4) also display the supraclavicular

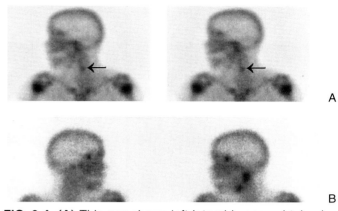

A

B

**FIG. 9-4. (A)** This row shows left lateral images obtained before (left) and after (right) XRT. The patient had Burkitt's lymphoma of a left cervical node (left image, *arrow*); after therapy, the salivary glands are visualized. **(B)** This row shows right lateral (left image) and left lateral (right image, the same as in **A**) spot head views obtained 3 months after therapy. The normal right salivary glands are not seen (left image), but typical post-XRT visualization of the salivary glands is seen on the left (right image). Incidental note is made of the normal bilateral lacrimal gland visualization.

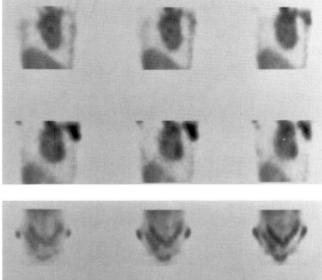

A

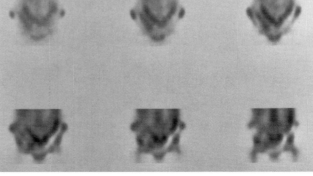

B

**FIG. 9-5.** Coronal SPECT images of the patient in Fig. 9-3. **(A)** These two rows demonstrate extensive mediastinal and axillary disease. **(B)** These two rows show the linear pattern of normal bowel activity. These distributions are better defined in the SPECT images than in the planar images.

fossa well and should be obtained for 600,000 counts. Other areas of considerable interest that might warrant spot views in lymphoma include the groin, antecubital fossa, and popliteal fossa. Enhanced long-bone marrow uptake may be seen in these views due to lymphomatous infiltration, enhanced erythropoietic activity, or cytokine use.

### SPECT Imaging

SPECT imaging is required for high-quality Ga-67 scintigraphy. It has significantly increased the sensitivity and specificity for lymphomas and improved anatomic localization, which is important in radiation therapy planning. SPECT has especially improved sensitivity for mediastinal disease detection due to its ability to detect lesions without obscuration by overlying sternum and underlying spine activity. It has also been helpful in separating abdominal nodal activity from normal bowel, liver, and spleen activity (Fig. 9-5). Impeccable quality control is required for planar imaging and is even more essential for SPECT imaging.

### Normal Scan

The normal Ga-67 scan displays the expected normal Ga-67 biodistribution; any deviation from this pattern indicates disease or treatment effects. Rapid renal excretion occurs during the first 24 hours, resulting in early renal and bladder visualization. Continued renal uptake after 72 hours, however, may indicate inflammation, infection, acute tubular necrosis, acute pyelonephritis, interstitial nephritis, amyloidosis, or impaired renal function (see Chapter 8).

Moderate lung uptake is frequently seen at 6 and 24 hours, but it diminishes with time. Focal pulmonary uptake may be increased by lymphography because the contrast media may cause nodal inflammatory reactions. Mild diffuse homogeneous lung uptake is frequently seen after chemotherapy and may persist for years, and faint hilar activity may be seen in adult smokers but does not indicate active tumor. Asymmetric hilar activity and intense diffuse uptake are not normal.

Soft tissues are prominent at 6 to 24 hours, and normal uptake by the liver, bone marrow, salivary and lacrimal glands, and nasal region occurs at this time. Faint parotid salivary gland uptake should be considered a normal variant, but more intense uptake is frequently seen after adjacent radiation therapy, as a result of radiation sialoadenitis (Fig. 9-6). Diseases affecting salivary gland function, such as Sjögren's syndrome, sarcoidosis (of Panda sign fame: lacrimal, nasal, parotid, and submandibular gland visualization), and systemic lupus erythematosus also show this pattern.

Colonic activity, especially in the ascending and transverse colon, is frequently prominent in delayed images and may persist despite the use of enemas and cathartics. If the patient has two or more bowel movements per day, we do

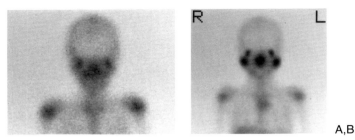

**FIG. 9-6.** These two anterior views of the same patient are taken before **(A)** and immediately after chemotherapy **(B)**. In the space of 2 months this Panda-like appearance (intense nasal, parotid, and lacrimal gland activity) developed, then subsequently regressed. Note also the subtle thymic uptake seen after therapy.

not suggest cathartics. Otherwise, bisacodyl (Dulcolax) and magnesium citrate, purchased over the counter, are suggested the day before the scan. SPECT may be especially helpful in separating abdominal pathology from bowel uptake: The bowel is demonstrated by contiguous activity conforming to an expected bowel configuration (see Fig. 9-5). Delayed imaging is also helpful in discriminating bowel uptake from abnormal abdominal uptake: Lesion uptake is fixed while normal bowel activity progresses along the bowel lumen with time (see Fig. 9-2). Gastric activity has been seen in acquired immunodeficiency syndrome (AIDS) patients.

Liver uptake is typically variable during the first 24 hours and becomes more prominent in 48 to 72 hours as the Ga-67–bound plasma proteins accumulate in the liver. At this time the skeleton is well seen, and in the thorax the sternum, ribs, spine, and scapular tips are prominent. A normal-appearing liver does not exclude a hepatic lesion because the normal liver takes up Ga-67 with an avidity approaching most pathologic lesions. If a liver lesion is suspected, correlation with another imaging modality should be undertaken; for example, Tc-99m sulfur colloid (SC) liver-spleen or CT scans. A lesion identified with these methods should be considered abnormal if any Ga-67 uptake is present, even if it is less than that of adjacent normal liver.

The hepatic uptake may be suppressed by chemotherapeutic agents (Fig. 9-7) for up to 1 week (methotrexate, fluorouracil, actinomycin D, and hydroxyureas), high levels of circulating iron (hemolysis, blood transfusions, and deferoxamine injections), liver failure, azathioprine, and perhaps gadolinium MRI contrast agents. Whenever hepatic uptake decreases, bone uptake usually increases. This pattern occurs frequently in nuclear medicine oncologic practice as clinicians attempt to combine chemotherapy with follow-up Ga-67 scans in cost-saving efforts. Such altered biodistribution occurs universally in the first 24 hours of chemotherapy, but the tumor is often well visualized despite these changes (see Fig. 9-7). This phenomenon is explained by the displacement of Ga-67 from the plasma transferrin by the chemotherapeutic agents and iron, resulting in free ionic

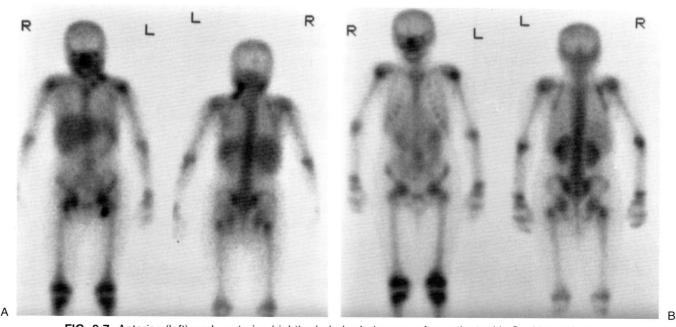

**FIG. 9-7.** Anterior (left) and posterior (right) whole-body images of a patient with Ga-67 uptake into nodes in the posterior cervical, supraclavicular, and bilateral groin regions **(A)**. Four months later, immediately after chemotherapy **(B)**, there is markedly reduced hepatic uptake and resolution of the groin and cervical lesions. This scan shows altered biodistribution (greater renal and skeletal uptake, but reduced hepatic and splenic uptake) because of recent chemotherapy. There is visualization of a new right medial scapular lesion. An intervening 2-month scan performed between therapy cycles showed disappearance of the cervical, but not the groin, lesions.

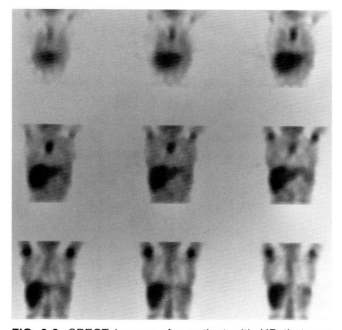

**FIG. 9-8.** SPECT images of a patient with HD that was confined initially to the abdomen. The midline activity (middle row of coronal images) appeared after therapy and is presumed due to thymic hyperplasia. This activity is posterior to the sternum (upper row) and anterior to the spine (lower row). This activity has persisted 2 years after remission induction, with no subsequent clinical relapse (see Fig. 9-11).

Ga-67 that is taken up by the skeleton. This change in biodistribution is to be expected, given that reactor-produced Ga-72, which is of low specific activity, was initially investigated as a bone-scanning radiopharmaceutical.

Splenic uptake is variable, and although the radiation dose to the spleen is similar to that of the liver, the smaller spleen has less absolute uptake and as a consequence is less well visualized. Most causes of splenomegaly therefore result in increased Ga-67 citrate uptake. Breast uptake may be marked when the breasts are stimulated by pregnancy or cyclic estrogens and progesterones, and faint uptake may occur in nonlactating women with no breast abnormalities (see Fig. 9-3).

Thymic activity in children is common, may be extremely variable, and is not necessarily related to the size of the gland as seen radiographically. Thymic uptake should be evaluated cautiously, especially after chemotherapy, when thymic hyperplasia has been reported to occur in 40% of patients. This is first seen 1 to 8 months after chemotherapy induction and can persist for up to 5 years (mean, 1 year) (Fig. 9-8) (6). The increased thymic activity pattern can even appear similar to the configuration of lymph node activity.

**Tumor Uptake of Ga-67 Citrate**

Neoplasms are characterized by neovascularity, increased capillary permeability, necrosis, and delay in new lymphatic

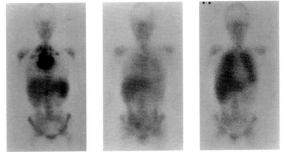

A–C

**FIG. 9-9.** These three images demonstrate bleomycin toxicity. The scans demonstrate pretherapy **(A)**, early post-therapy **(B)**, and late post-therapy **(C)** stages. The normal lung is not seen pretherapy (with prominent mediastinal axillary and supraclavicular nodal disease present), a subtle diffuse lung abnormality is seen early post-therapy, and intense diffuse Ga-67 lung localization is present late post-therapy. Bleomycin is used in common lymphoma therapy regimes. The spleen is seen in **A**, but not in **B** and **C**, as a consequence of splenectomy.

vessel growth. These factors lead to prolonged residence time of macromolecules, such as protein-bound Ga-67 in the interstitial fluid of tumors. The actual mechanism of Ga-67 uptake is complex and not completely elucidated: The initial step involves binding of gallium to transferrin and then transport to the tumor via the blood. This blood supply is essential because necrotic regions show no Ga-67 uptake. The Ga-67 transferrin complex is delivered to the neoplasm via capillaries with increased permeability. In some tumors, Ga-67 citrate is taken up by tumor cells perhaps via transferrin receptors, but some Ga-67 citrate is taken up by associated inflammatory cells (7). Ga-67 uptake scoring has been used to increase the specificity of tumor detection, so the greater the uptake, the more likely the presence of pathology (8). This scoring compares Ga-67 in the tumor to normal sternal and hepatic uptake: 0, no uptake; 1, uptake less than that of sternum; 2, uptake equals that of sternum; 3, uptake greater than that of sternum and less than liver; and 4, uptake equals or exceeds that of liver.

In addition to the normal variants previously described, Ga-67 accumulation may be seen in tumor patients with opportunistic (*Pneumocystis carinii* pneumonia, atypical mycobacteria, tuberculosis, cytomegalovirus, and various mycoses) and other infections (pneumonia), inflammations (sarcoid), interstitial fibrosis, contrast lymphangiography, postirradiation sialoadenitis (see Fig. 9-4), cardiac amyloidosis, and chemotherapy (bleomycin; Fig. 9-9). Diffuse lung uptake can be seen after chemotherapy or irradiation but should only appear after the treatment is started, have less uptake than the known lesions, and be unassociated with anatomic lesion on CT, MRI, or CXR. Focal collections are also seen at injection and Hickman catheter sites.

## Clinical Applications

### Lymphoma

It is estimated that approximately 7,900 cases of HD were diagnosed in 1994 in the United States, compared to 45,000 cases of NHL (9). Fifty percent of these HD cases occur between the ages of 20 and 40 (mean age, ~30 years). In economically developed countries, there is a bimodal incidence of HD, with a major peak occurring in young adulthood (age 30) and a second peak occurring in the later decades of life (age 70). The peak incidence of NHL is later than for HD, with the mean age at presentation being 50 years.

### Hodgkin's Disease

HD is a histologic diagnosis based on the presence of the malignant multinucleated Reed-Sternberg cell. The disease is usually localized and curable, and prognosis is related to disease stage. HD is characterized by an orderly lymphatic spread to contiguous sites and common identification of lymph nodes in the neck and mediastinum (in 60% to 70% of patients); other sites include the spleen (35%), para-aortic nodes (30%), and inguinal and femoral (10%) nodes (10). Spleen involvement in HD cannot usually be detected by Ga-67 imaging. The lung, liver, and bone marrow are involved in 5% to 10% of older patients. There are four types of HD (Table 9-7), but this typing of HD has little prognostic value (11). The nodular sclerosing type is the most common, occurs in young women, and typically involves the mediastinal and cervical lymph nodes.

Clinical staging of HD includes complete history and physical examination to determine the presence or absence of stage B symptoms (e.g., unexplained weight loss, unexplained fever, and night sweats), which occur in one-fourth of all patients. Staging studies should include CT scanning of the chest, abdomen, and pelvis; CXR; bilateral bone marrow aspiration and biopsy; a complete blood count with erythrocyte sedimentation rate; and serum blood tests, including measurement of albumin, lactate dehydrogenate, and liver function tests.

**TABLE 9-7.** *Lymphoma uptake of Ga-67 citrate (relative % distribution in parentheses)*

|  | Ga-67 avidity | Prognosis |
|---|---|---|
| Hodgkin's lymphoma |  |  |
| Nodular sclerosing (60%) | +++ | Good |
| Mixed cellular (30%) | ++/+++ | Poor |
| Lymphocyte depleted (5%) | ++ | Poor |
| Lymphocyte predominant (5%) | +/++ | Poor |
| Non-Hodgkin's lymphoma |  |  |
| High grade (5%) | +++ | Poor |
| Intermediate (60%) | ++/+++ | Moderate |
| Low grade (35%) | + | Good |

+, mild; ++, moderate; +++, marked.

*Non-Hodgkin's Lymphoma*

NHL is more common than HD and is more common in the male. NHL is multicentric, with a nodal distribution similar to HD but more commonly involving regions below the diaphragm. It is characterized by extranodal involvement of bone, kidney, and GI tract. The clinical course varies from indolent to rapidly progressive. The prognosis is related to histology, but this histology is very complex, and no classification is universally accepted. NHL broad classifications use cell type (90% are of B-cell origin); high-, intermediate-, and low-grade tumors; and diffuse or follicular patterns (see Table 9-7). The latest classification, the Revised European American Lymphoma (REAL), requires flow cytometry. In children, the disease is somewhat different in that it is more often extranodal, usually diffuse, high grade, and with lower histologic subtypes (12). Although it is generally agreed that Ga-67 scanning is most sensitive in high- and intermediate-grade lymphomas and poor in low-grade tumors (where Tl-201 is suggested as an alternative), there is evidence of 80% Ga-67 scanning sensitivity even in low-grade types (13).

### Role of Imaging in HD and NHL

The role of Ga-67 imaging in lymphomas is in the assessment of therapy (14), and to accomplish this, a baseline scan is best to establish Ga-67 avidity. With current sensitivities and specificities of between 89% and 100% for both HD and some NHL, it is hard to imagine why this radiopharmaceutical is not used in all lymphoma patients and suggested in textbook management protocols. The only explanation that can be offered is that the radiopharmaceutical development preceded the imaging technology, and the initial clinical experience of individual centers was poor. The addition of SPECT imaging has revolutionized the role of Ga-67 by increasing the sensi-

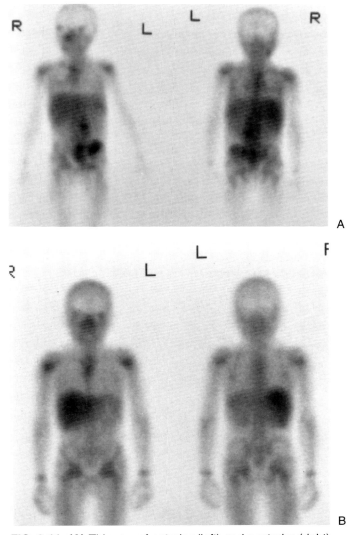

**FIG. 9-11. (A)** This row of anterior (left) and posterior (right) whole-body images show right supraclavicular, mediastinal, abdominal aortic, and massive left iliac adenopathy that displaces the patient's bladder to the right. **(B)** These images, taken 2 years later, demonstrate normalization of Ga-67 uptake while CT and US still demonstrate significant iliac adenopathy. The Ga-67 was correct in indicating no evidence of continuing disease. The later scan shows a slight increase in region of sternum (quite different from the pretreatment mediastinal lesions) that SPECT showed to be probable thymic hyperplasia (see Fig. 9-8). The difference in image size is a result of a different image formatter.

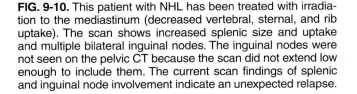

**FIG. 9-10.** This patient with NHL has been treated with irradiation to the mediastinum (decreased vertebral, sternal, and rib uptake). The scan shows increased splenic size and uptake and multiple bilateral inguinal nodes. The inguinal nodes were not seen on the pelvic CT because the scan did not extend low enough to include them. The current scan findings of splenic and inguinal node involvement indicate an unexpected relapse.

tivity and specificity by 50% in chest disease and by approximately 20% at other sites. Today, with the use of larger doses of Ga-67 (10 mCi [370 MBq]) and SPECT technology, along with appropriate quality control to ensure optimal imaging of this multiple-photopeak radionuclide, nuclear imaging is the most cost-effective imaging modality for lymphoma (14). Ga-67 is particularly useful in the detection of disease involving the cervical, mediastinal, hilar, axillary, and inguinal region lymph nodes (Fig. 9-10), but it can also identify disease in the lungs and abdomen. The threshold size for detection of a positive site is approximately 1 cm, but detection depends more on the degree of tracer uptake than lesion size. Ga-67 imaging has several separate and distinct roles in the evaluation of lymphoma, as outlined below.

### Residual Mass After Therapy

A residual mass detected after therapy is a common clinical puzzle (15) because, although the mass may be visible on CT scanning, it may be composed of nonviable lymphoma cells (Fig. 9-11). If the mass is made up of viable cells, the patient must start another chemotherapy regime or radiotherapy (14). Because Ga-67 scintigraphy, CT, and MRI may be discordant at different lymphoma sites before therapy, it is important that baseline gallium scans be obtained before instituting therapy if the scan is to be useful in this role. Optimally, there should be a 3-week interval between the last cycle of treatment and Ga-67 scintigraphy (14) because therapy may decrease the sensitivity of Ga-67 imaging.

### Response to Therapy

Lymphoma (both HD and NHL) patients with abnormal gallium scans after treatment have a significantly worse outcome than those whose scans normalize (Fig. 9-12) (16). The presence or absence of Ga-67 uptake correlates well with patient prognosis after treatment of lymphoma (17,18). The negative predictive value (NPV) of normal gallium scans after lymphoma therapy is 84%; the positive predictive value (PPV) of abnormal scans is 80% for HD and 73% for NHL (14).

The length of time necessary to achieve a response after onset of chemotherapy is also a good predictor of treatment efficacy (19). A complete response is achieved in 70% of lymphoma patients during the first three cycles of treatment (20), and radionuclide imaging with Ga-67 identifies this rapid therapeutic response. It is therefore reasonable to assess the Ga-67 response halfway through treatment as an effective way to measure treatment efficacy (17).

### Diagnosis of Recurrence

The sensitivity and specificity of gallium scans for detection of lymphoma recurrence is very good (21,22), whereas

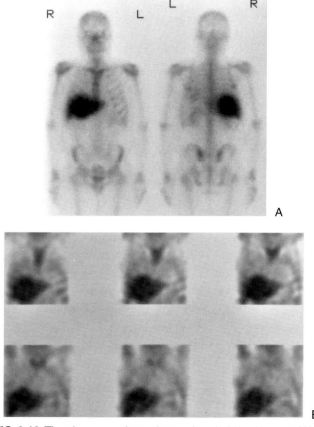

**FIG. 9-13.** The planar anterior and posterior whole body scans **(A)** and coronal SPECT **(B)** images of this adult asymptomatic HD patient are normal 2 years after successful therapy.

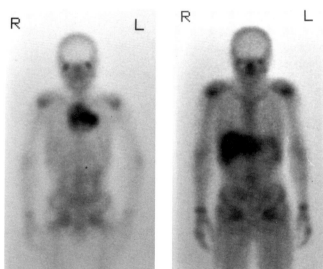

**FIG. 9-12. (A)** This HD patient has a large mediastinal lesion at diagnosis that dramatically disappears with 3 months of therapy **(B)**. The very intense uptake in the mediastinal adenopathy in the early image **(A)** is identical to the classic "lambda sign" of sarcoidosis. Note the absent hepatic uptake due to recent chemotherapy **(A)**. Subsequent images indicated tumor regression **(B)**, and the liver and spleen activity returned to normal (no recent chemotherapy).

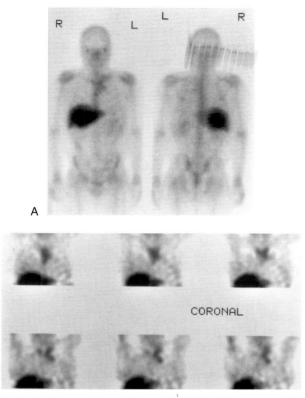

A

B

CORONAL

**FIG. 9-14.** These planar **(A)** and SPECT **(B)** images of the same patient shown in Fig. 9-13 were obtained 3 months later. The scan shows disease recurrence in the mediastinum, a site unaffected at presentation. The time of appearance of this abnormality (2½ years after therapy), the asymmetry of the lesions, and the older age of the patient are not typical of thymic hyperplasia. Tumor recurrence was established.

CT scanning is not as reliable. Given that one-fourth of patients after therapy have recurrences only at new sites (Figs. 9-13 and 9-14), Ga-67 whole-body imaging yields unique additional information (14).

### Other Tumors

Numerous other tumors demonstrate Ga-67 uptake, but this radiopharmaceutical has not found significant usage in these diseases, except perhaps in some hepatoma patients (see Table 9-3). In the majority of those diseases, the role of Ga-67 has been supplanted by newer imaging modes and agents, but several tumors warrant further discussion.

Soft-tissue sarcomas have similar Ga-67 results to lymphoma, with sensitivities of 90% to 95%. Ga-67 uptake is related to tumor grade, and Ga-67 imaging has a possible role in detecting occult disease, restaging tumor, and identifying residual tumor in post-treatment masses. Kaposi's sarcoma is an important exception and is always Ga-67 negative. A positive Ga-67 scan in a patient with known Kaposi's sarcoma would suggest either inflammation or lymphoma (see Chap-

ter 16). Tl-201 and FDG have been used more frequently to image soft-tissue sarcomas.

In lung cancer, the sensitivity of Ga-67 imaging is between 85% and 90% for most cell types, but the current CT investigation of this tumor is satisfactory. F-18 FDG, Tl-201, MOABs, and possibly the somatostatin receptor agent pentetreotide appear more promising as radiopharmaceuticals for lung cancer detection.

The sensitivity and specificity of Ga-67 scanning is reported to be 80% to 99%, but it appears that F-18 FDG will replace this as the best imaging modality to seek distant metastases.

When the diagnosis of hepatoma is not certain, then demonstrated Ga-67 uptake into the lesion, as delineated by another imaging modality, can be useful. Two-thirds of all hepatomas have Ga-67 uptake greater than neighboring liver, one-fourth have uptake equal to the liver, and the remainder have less uptake than normal liver. If there is any Ga-67 uptake at all into a mass lesion suspicious for hepatoma, hepatoma is likely.

## TL-201 AND TC-99M SESTAMIBI FOR TUMOR IMAGING

Tl-201 and Tc-99m sestamibi were initially developed for myocardial perfusion imaging but are gaining increasing acceptance in tumor imaging. They complement conventional CT and MRI anatomic imaging in the clinical problem of separating recurrent viable tumor from surgical or x-ray therapy (XRT) scarring. The role of Tl-201 and Tc-99m sestamibi in benign tumor imaging is exemplified in parathyroid adenoma detection (see Chapter 14).

### Radiopharmaceuticals

The tumor uptake mechanism of these two tracers is not well understood, although several mechanisms are suggested. Neither agent is taken up significantly into inflammatory reactions or necrotic tissue, so these do not explain the mechanism of tumor localization. Both agents gain access to the tumor via the bloodstream and leak into the tumor region through increased capillary permeability associated with the neovascularity, but each agent has other specific uptake mechanisms.

### Thallium 201

Tl-201 occupies two sites on the cellular membrane adenosine triphosphatase pump system (especially in young cells). Intracellular translocation of the tracer results from a cotransport system (especially in older cells). Most Tl-201 remains in the free fluid of the tumor, but significant cellular uptake does occur. The major technical problem with Tl-201 is the decay scheme, which gives off three characteristic x-rays of mercury 201 of low energy over the relatively wide

**TABLE 9-8.** *Decay scheme of Tl-201*

| | Energy | Abundance |
|---|---|---|
| X-ray K$_1$ | 69 keV | 27% |
| X-ray K$_1$ | 71 keV | 47% |
| X-ray K$_2$ | 80 keV | 21% |
| Gamma$_1$ | 135 keV | 3% |
| Gamma$_2$ | 167 keV | 10% |

**TABLE 9-9.** *Radiation absorbed dose estimates of Tl-201 and Tc-99m sestamibi*

| Tissue | Tl-201 (rads/4 mCi [cGy/148 MBq]) | Tc-99m sestamibi[a] (rads/30 mCi [cGy/1,110 MBq]) |
|---|---|---|
| Heart wall | 4 | 0.5 |
| Liver | 1.5 | 0.6 |
| Kidneys | 6.8 | 2 |
| Bladder | 0.8 | 2 |
| Testes | 12[b] | 0.3 |
| Ovaries | 1.5 | 1.5 |
| Thyroid | 9.2 | 0.7 |
| GI tract | | |
|   Stomach wall | 2.8 | 0.6 |
|   Small intestine | 6.8 | 3 |
|   Upper large intestine wall | 4.8 | 5.4[b] |
|   Lower large intestine wall | 4.8 | 3.9 |
| Total body | 5.2 | 0.5 |

[a] Tc-99m sestamibi dosimetry is for radiopharmaceutical injected at rest and uses a 2-hour void.
[b] Critical organ.
Sources: Mallinckrodt, St. Louis, MO (Tl-201); and DuPont Pharma, Billerica, MA, (Cardiolite) package inserts.

energy range of 69 to 80 keV, which is skewed to the 70-keV region (Table 9-8). The patient dose is limited by the radiation dose to normal tissues (Table 9-9).

### Tc-99m Sestamibi

The mechanism of uptake of Tc-99m sestamibi is still under investigation, but appears to be related to the radiopharmaceutical's lipophilicity and negative charge. In addition, the agent enters the cell and is actively transported into the mitochondria, where it is retained. This agent is extruded from this inner space of the tumor cell, apparently facilitated by the permeability glycoprotein (P-gp), which correlates with the degree of expression of the multiple-drug–resistant (MDR) gene. It is hoped that sestamibi may reflect P-gp expression and so become an important prognostic indicator (23). The radiation dose of Tc-99m sestamibi is less than that of Tl-201 (see Table 9-9).

### Scan Protocols

With both tracers, the temporal tracer uptake into tumor is similar to that of the myocardium. Imaging is commenced within 5 minutes after tracer injection (Tl-201, 2 to 5 mCi [75 to 185 MBq]; Tc-99m sestamibi, 20 to 30 mCi [740 to 1,110 MBq]), although many practitioners also obtain delayed imaging at 2 to 4 hours for comparison with the early images. In tumors, wash-out of tracer is generally delayed, so the tumor-to-background tissue ratios rise with time, although the absolute tumor concentration decreases. The imaging protocol depends on the indications: whole-body imaging for metastases (e.g., thyroid cancer) and limited views for specific organs (e.g., brain and parathyroid). SPECT may be helpful at most sites.

### Normal Scans

Normal scans have a remarkably similar biodistribution compatible with the expected uptake into the thyroid, lacrimal, and salivary glands, along with considerable uptake in the myocardial, splanchnic, hepatic, and renal regions (Fig. 9-15). The Tl-201 images can demonstrate prominent muscle uptake, whereas the Tc-99m sestamibi images demonstrate gallbladder and bone marrow uptake not seen with Tl-201. Imaging of the abdomen and the chest is not satisfactory near the heart, liver, and GI and urinary tracts because of the high normal uptake at these sites, especially when patients are injected at rest, when increased liver and GI uptake occurs. If possible, the tracer should be injected when the patient is status NPO to minimize abdom-

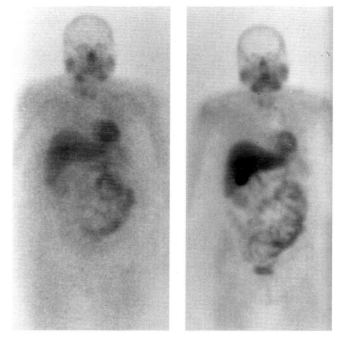

A,B

**FIG. 9-15.** Biodistribution of Tl-201 **(A)** and Tc-99m sestamibi **(B)** in a normal patient. The considerable myocardial, splanchnic, hepatic, and cervical gland uptake limit the diagnostic application in those regions. Twenty minutes after injection, the distribution of both tracers is remarkably similar, except that the Tc-99m sestamibi scan shows prominent gallbladder activity.

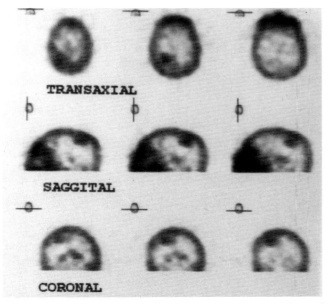

**FIG. 9-16.** These transaxial (upper), sagittal (middle), and coronal (lower) Tc-99m sestamibi images show a recurrent glioma in the right parietal lobe. CT and MRI were not able to differentiate post-therapy scarring from recurrent tumor, whereas the sestamibi scan clearly identifies the mass as containing viable tumor tissue. Activity is also seen in the choroid plexus, especially in the coronal sections.

inal excretion. Tc-99m sestamibi accumulates avidly in the choroid plexus (Fig. 9-16).

### Abnormal Scans

Abnormal Tl-201 or Tc-99m sestamibi uptake occurs in many tumor types (notably low-grade NHL, brain, soft-tissue sarcomas, thyroid and breast tumors). Many roles for these tumor imaging agents have been established that are similar to those of other agents:

- Differentiating benign from malignant disease
- Determining grades of malignancy (especially in brain and soft-tissue tumors)
- Localizing tumor sites for biopsy
- Staging malignant disease
- Evaluating response to therapy
- Differentiating viable tumor from treatment tissue necrosis and scarring
- Determining lymphoproliferative disease in AIDS (especially Kaposi's sarcoma)

### Clinical Applications

#### Brain

Brain imaging is currently the most established role for Tl-201 and Tc-99m sestamibi imaging after parathyroid

adenoma imaging. Tl-201 has been successfully used to diagnose and grade gliomas and to differentiate recurrent or residual viable intracranial tumor (see Fig. 9-16) from postoperative and postradiotherapy scarring (24–27). Sometimes, Tl-201 and brain perfusion imaging can be combined for confirmation of recurrent tumor versus radionecrosis in cases where Tl-201 uptake is not prominent. In contrast to CT and MRI, Tl-201 uptake requires not only breakdown of the blood-brain barrier but also viable tumor cells to demonstrate abnormal uptake (see Chapter 10). It is possible that this tracer may rival F-18 FDG in this role, especially because of the more general availability of the tracers and suitable imaging equipment (i.e., multiheaded scanners). Quantitation of Tl-201 tumor uptake to the mirror-image normal brain tissue region in gliomas and other cerebral tumors is useful, and pretreatment values >1.5 indicate high-grade malignancy. After treatment, a value >1.5 is consistent with residual or recurrent brain tumor (27). Like FDG, the sensitivity of Tl-201 for detection of gliomas depends on the grade of the tumor. Another indication is the differentiation of mass lesions in immunocompromised patients, in whom differentiating lymphoproliferative diseases from infection, such as toxoplasmosis, is difficult (see Chapter 16).

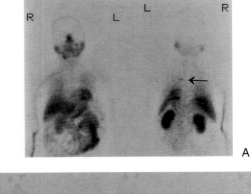

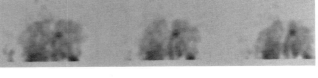

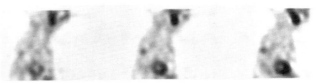

**FIG. 9-17.** This papillary thyroid cancer patient presented with elevated tumor marker (serum thyroglobulin), with a normal I-131 thyroid cancer metastatic survey (using a 30-mCi dose). The planar images **(A)** show a faint abnormality (*arrow*) in the posterior left chest, and coronal **(B)** and sagittal **(C)** SPECT images better demonstrate this lesion. Directed thin-slice CT showed a lesion that had been missed on regular chest CT. This was invading bone and was successfully resected with return of the serum thyroglobulin to normal.

## Bone and Soft-Tissue Tumors

Tl-201 has been more accurate than Ga-67 in detecting primary bone and musculoskeletal tumors, and it is useful in assessing response to therapy in these tumors (28). More recently, Tl-201 uptake has been described in various pediatric tumors, including primary bone tumors and soft-tissue sarcomas as well as lymphoma and brain tumors (29–31).

## Thyroid, Lung, and Lymphoproliferative Tumors

Thyroid, lung, and lymphoproliferative tumors frequently show increased Tl-201 and Tc-99m sestamibi uptake in the primary and secondary lesions, but these tracers are not established as primary imaging procedures. In thyroid cancer, when serum tumor markers (e.g., thyroglobulin) are elevated and there is no I-131 uptake, Tl-201 has a significant role (32), as described in Chapter 7 (Fig. 9-17). Low-grade NHL shows considerable uptake of Tl-201 and Tc-99m sestamibi, and a complementary role to Ga-67 is suggested (13).

## Breast

Tl-201 and Tc-99m sestamibi are taken up into breast adenocarcinoma. Some researchers have found this quality to be very useful in differentiating benign from malignant disease in patients with palpable masses.

### Scan Protocol

Various techniques are proposed, but it appears that prone imaging, with the breasts freely dependent through specially designed imaging tables, is optimal. Lateral and posterior oblique views are obtained 5 minutes after injection. Axillary views are obtained with the patient standing.

### Thallium 201

Benign breast lesions seldom demonstrate abnormal Tl-201 accumulation, whereas palpable breast cancers have an excellent Tl-201 sensitivity (96%) and specificity (88%). The smallest detectable malignancy is approximately 1 cm$^3$ (33), with a 50% to 60% sensitivity for detection of axillary metastases.

### Tc-99m Sestamibi

Tc-99m sestamibi preliminary studies by Khalkhali et al. and Taillefer et al. indicated excellent results, with average lesion sensitivities and specificities of 90% and NPV of 95% (34,35). They used 20 mCi of sestamibi and ultra–high-resolution collimators and 10% photopeaks (Fig. 9-18). The sensitivity and specificity for axillary lymph node detection were approximately 70% and 90%, respectively.

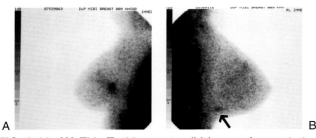

FIG. 9-18. **(A)** This Tc-99m sestamibi image demonstrates uptake into a large palpable breast mass that was an invasive ductal carcinoma by fine-needle aspiration. **(B)** The scan in this image was performed on a patient with a 1.5-cm mass with multiple negative prior biopsies. The lesion was considered of low suspicion and follow-up mammography scheduled for 6 months. The lower central breast Tc-99m sestamibi uptake (*arrow*) was highly suspicious for malignant disease, and excisional biopsy showed infiltrating ductal carcinoma. (Images courtesy of B. David Collier, M.D., Medical College of Wisconsin, and United Regional Medical Services, Milwaukee, WI.)

**TABLE 9-10.** *Adjunctive role of scintiscanning in mammography*

| Mammography grade | Suggested follow-up |
| --- | --- |
| I | None required |
| II | Follow-up mammography in 6 months |
| III and IV | Routine scintimammography, and biopsy if scan is abnormal |
| V | Immediate biopsy |

Source: Khalkhali I, Cutrone JA, Mena IG, et al. Technetium-99m-sestamibi scintimammography of breast lesions: clinical and pathological follow-up. J Nucl Med 1995;36:1784–1789.

### Potential Role of Scintimammography

Because mammography as a screening test has a PPV of only 15% to 40%, Khalkhali and colleagues (36,37) see the role of scintimammography as a means of reducing the number of breast biopsies because of the very high NPV (Table 9-10). A multicenter clinical trial recently completed in the United States and Canada will determine the ultimate clinical usefulness of Tc-99m sestamibi in a general setting. These data are in the preliminary stages of presentation, but NPVs of approximately 90% for fatty and dense breasts and for palpable and nonpalpable lesions are being found.

## DIMERCAPTOSUCCINIC ACID

Tc-99m (V) dimercaptosuccinic acid (DMSA[V]) is a tumor-seeking agent that has been advocated as useful in evaluating medullary thyroid carcinoma (MTC), soft-tissue sarcomas, head and neck tumors, and highly recurrent benign lesions, such as synovial giant cell tumors and aggressive fibromatosis. This tracer is different in structure from the renal agent Tc-99m DMSA(III) but can be prepared in a similar manner from the same commercially supplied vials. Uses of Tc-99m DMSA(V) are similar to those of Ga-67 but with the advantages of 2-hour imaging combined with Tc-99m dosimetry and imaging characteristics. The mechanism of uptake of Tc-99m DMSA(V) is unknown but is likely related to blood flow, phosphate metabolism, or pH. Although DMSA(V) is not currently FDA approved, it can be compounded from the approved DMSA(III) kit set under the practice of pharmacy.

### Scan Protocol

Ten millicuries (370 MBq) of IV Tc-99m DMSA(V) is injected, and whole-body planar images are obtained 2 hours later. Physiologic uptake is present in the nasopharynx, breast, liver, spleen, kidneys, skeletal muscles, and axial skeleton. SPECT investigation has been helpful in separating normal physiologic uptake in the sternocleidomastoid muscles, hypopharynx, cervical spine, sternoclavicular joints, and shoulder joints from head and neck tumors and MTC (38).

### Clinical Applications

#### Medullary Thyroid Carcinoma

MTC, first described as a clinical entity in 1958, arises from the parafollicular cells and secretes calcitonin, which is an excellent tumor marker (39). This histologic subtype represents <10% of all thyroid carcinoma, but it rarely presents to nuclear medicine imaging departments. Three-fourths of cases are sporadic in presentation, the remaining have associated syndromes, including multiple endocrine neoplasia (MEN 2A or 2B) and familial MTC.

In aggressiveness, MTC is intermediate between anaplastic and well-differentiated thyroid cancer. It has a tendency to develop distant metastases and local lymph node involvement, especially in the central upper mediastinum and lateral cervical regions. MTC runs a prolonged course, with patients frequently surviving many years after initial diagnosis, despite the presence of distant metastases. Treatment is total thyroidectomy, with removal of nodes in the primary lymphatic drainage area (40,41). Most patients show diminished calcitonin levels postoperatively, but a significant portion show continued hypercalcitoninemia, indicating residual tumor. Localization of this residual tumor with ultrasound, MRI, or CT has proved difficult, but Tc-99m DMSA(V) is a sensitive, safe, and noninvasive localization method in post-thyroidectomy patients. Significant uptake of DMSA is found in residual tumor and metastatic lesions. Physiologic uptake in central neck structures can limit scan interpretation in that area. SPECT scans have been useful in distinguishing lesions because there should be no significant physiologic uptake immediately lateral to the central neck, the area with the

greatest potential for lymph node spread (38,42). I-131 MIBG, Tl-201, Tc-99m sestamibi, and In-111 pentetreotide have also been shown to accumulate in some patients with MTC. Tc-99m DMSA(V) and In-111 pentetreotide may have comparable sensitivities to detect recurrent MTC (42). Recent literature indicates that the Tc-99m anti-CEA MOAB arcitumomab (released by the FDA in September 1996) has very successfully detected occult MTC secondary disease and may be the imaging procedure of choice (43).

#### Soft-Tissue Tumors

The diagnosis of malignancy in soft-tissue tumors can be difficult, especially in low-grade malignancy, in which diagnosis may be impossible even with needle biopsy due to sampling error. Ga-67 has been used in soft-tissue tumors, but it is not satisfactory in many low-grade malignant tumors or in highly recurrent benign tumors. Tc-99m (V) DMSA accumulates in almost all these tumor types (44,45).

### LYMPHOSCINTIGRAPHY

The lymphatic drainage of tumors provides a common method of tumor spread. MRI and CT routinely measure

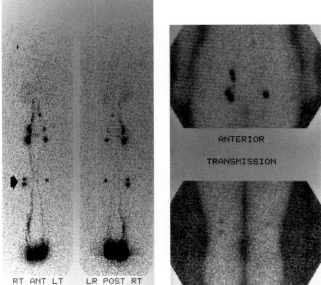

**FIG. 9-19.** Normal lymphoscintigraphy of lower limbs. **(A)** These anterior and posterior whole-body images were obtained soon after injection. Tracer is seen at the injection sites in both legs, along the lymphatics, and in groin and iliac lymph nodes. The arrowhead demonstrates two right knee markers in the anterior whole-body image; the left knee single marker is not arrowed. **(B)** Spot abdomen and knee images were obtained 1 hour later with transmission scans that outline the abdomen and legs. At 1 hour, the lymphatics are no longer seen, and fewer inguinal nodes are visible. The knee markers are faintly seen in the anterior transmission knee images.

lymph node size to predict tumor involvement, and significant increases in node size are suggestive of, but not specific for, tumor. Lymphoscintigraphy is a technique that can demonstrate normal lymphatic drainage patterns well (Fig. 9-19). The preferred radiopharmaceutical (Tc-99m antimony colloid) is a colloid of small size (3 to 30 nm) but is not available because the FDA-approved manufacturer is no longer in business. The next best available agent is Tc-99m SC (particle size 10 to 1,000 nm), which can be filtered to remove the larger particles, creating a nearly ideal particle size (10 to 50 nm). Initially, 220-nm filters were used, but a 100-nm filter is now preferred. With the deposition of these tracers in intradermal and subcutaneous tissue sites, normal lymphatic drainage patterns can be assessed. A long-time routine use of these tracers is to distinguish primary from secondary lymphedema of limbs, an application that is successful and used in many nuclear medicine departments. Lymphoscintigraphy has also been used in the evaluation of lymphangiomas, lymphoceles, chylous ascites, and other chylous leaks. There is a resurgence in the use of lymphoscintigraphy in regions with ambiguous drainage from a known tumor (e.g., melanoma of the trunk or head and neck), as a result of the sentinel node concept (i.e., the first node draining a tumor site is the most reliable indicator of where lymph node metastases might first be found [46]).

## Scan Protocol

Tracer is deposited intradermally (e.g., for melanoma) or subcutaneously (e.g., for breast cancer), and images are obtained immediately and 2 to 4 hours after injection. The immediate scan images (15- or 30-second image sequences) demonstrate the injection site, where approximately 40% of tracer persists; the regional draining lymphatics; and the clos-

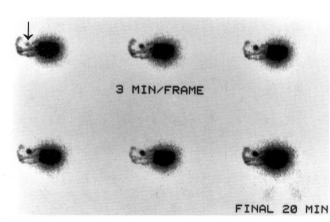

**FIG. 9-20.** This patient was injected about the melanoma excisional biopsy site (midback), and 30-second posterior acquisitions were obtained. These are combined into 3-minute frames, and several draining lymphatic channels are shown, with a sentinel lymph node (*arrow*) identified in the first minute after intradermal injection. In the last image, renal visualization is seen. This sentinel node is axillary, and the lymph channels must course around the posterior axillary fold before moving medially.

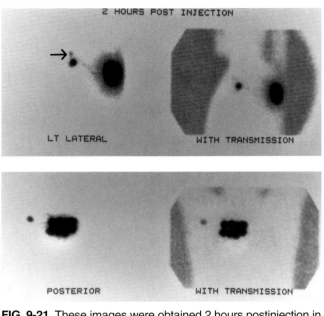

**FIG. 9-21.** These images were obtained 2 hours postinjection in the patient shown in Fig. 9-20. They include the acquired images (left images) and transmission images (right images) outlining the view (**A:** left lateral view with arms raised; **B:** posterior view of upper back with arms raised). **(A)** Two nodes were identified in the axilla with three lymphatic paths (see Fig. 9-20) leading to them (the less clearly visualized node is identified with arrow), and both were well seen 18 hours later in the preoperative images (not shown). Intraoperative probe assessment helped to identify these nodes for histologic evaluation (both were normal).

est lymph node (sentinel node), in the very early images (Fig. 9-20). Dynamic images are important to identify the first node the tracer goes to because unusual patterns can occur (47). The regional lymph node drainage sites are always identified in the delayed images (Fig. 9-21). Once the tracer reaches the thoracic duct, there is drainage into the central venous system, and typically a liver-spleen scan image is obtained. When using the 100-nm filter, we have routinely visualized the kidneys early and not the liver or spleen.

## Clinical Tumor Applications

Because no FDA-approved specific lymphoscintigraphic tracer source is currently available, few nuclear medicine centers in the United States have extensive experience with these procedures. Some centers have experience with internal mammary, vulval, and rectal scintigraphy. In tumor applications, the technique is used to identify lymphatic drainage sites and sentinel lymph nodes. Sometimes the first node visualized is termed an *interval* node, that is, an unexpected lymph node between the primary lesion and the expected regional draining lymph node bed. Abnormal nodes may occasionally be recognized by obstruction to passage of the lymphatic tracer, which may be manifested by a blush about the affected node, as tracer leaks into the adjacent tissue, and the accentuation of unusual collateral pathways.

## Malignant Melanoma

In malignant melanoma, the greatest predictor of prognosis is the presence of lymph node metastases. Most (90%) melanoma patients have clinically localized disease, but approximately 20% of these have undetected regional nodal micrometastases. Lymphoscintigraphy is used to help identify which lymph nodes drain truncal or head and neck melanomas and so to determine which lymph nodes should be sampled for patient staging and therapy planning. There is considerable variation in lymph drainage, so lymphoscintigraphy has the potential to provide an objective means to decide which regional nodes to biopsy in individual patient tumors. The early anatomic descriptions that predict draining lymphatics have been found inaccurate, and there are large areas of head, neck, and trunk where lymphatic drainage is ambiguous. In some centers, this imaging technique is used to identify the most likely sites of spread. To do this, a small sample of colloid is injected intradermally about the tumor site, and the patient is imaged immediately (see Fig. 9-20) and 2 to 4 hours later (see Fig. 9-21). It is important to position the patient as he or she would be placed during the surgical procedure and to obtain orthogonal images for proper three-dimensional localization and improved surgical localization. Intraoperative detection with a gamma ray probe is recommended because some lymph nodes may not be visualized by the conventional dye techniques previously used.

Some studies (48,49) indicate that, in truncal melanoma, 42% to 67% of patients have a single drainage node site (or group) and 30% to 47% have two sites (i.e., 89% to 97% of patients were potential candidates for nodal resection). It has also been shown that the 5-year survival rate improved significantly as a result of lymphoscintigraphy-selected lymphadenectomy (48). One group showed that only 16% of patients had a single lymphatic channel draining the tumor site, many lymphatic channels had indirect paths to the sentinel nodes, and 22% of patients had interval nodes (lymph nodes between the tumor site and the draining nodal bed), which otherwise would not be identified or sampled (49). Some centers use this routinely in stage I and II melanoma; they report 40% to 70% discordance between predicted and actual drainage sites, and changes in surgical management result in 30% to 60% of patients (47).

The value of this test is to identify the first lymph node to drain the tumor because this node invariably contains tumor, if lymphatic spread has occurred. If the histology of these nodes is normal, there is no need to do extensive lymph node dissections, with considerable savings in cost and morbidity (primarily lymphedema in limbs). The identification of the sentinel node also means that more detailed histology, using special techniques, can improve the histologic detection of nodal involvement with tumor. The standard of care is now progressing to the need to stage all melanomas >1 mm thick by this technique.

## Breast Cancer

Breast lymphatics most commonly drain to the axillary region (80% of patients), but internal mammary and supraclavicular drainage also occurs. The rationale of imaging the axilla with Tl-201, Tc-99m sestamibi, and F-18 FDG is to anticipate which patients will require axillary node resection. When tracer is injected immediately adjacent to the tumor, the tumor's lymphatic drainage can be identified. This drainage is unexpected in one-third of patients, with outer quadrant tumors demonstrating internal mammary drainage and inner quadrant tumors demonstrating axillary drainage. One-fifth of patients with upper quadrant tumors show direct drainage to the supraclavicular and infraclavicular nodes (50). Even laterally placed breast tumors can drain primarily via the internal mammary lymphatic system, a system often ignored in treatment planning, and in this region the affected nodes are not seen on routine CT scan. This internal mammary spread explains the solitary sternal metastasis that can be identified on bone scanning (see Fig. 1-19). Internal mammary lymph nodes are multiple and variable, with 10% to 15% of all patients having a unilateral internal mammary lymph chain and approximately 20% demonstrating communication between these parasternal internal mammary lymph chains.

### Internal Mammary Scintigraphy

Internal mammary scintigraphy is carried out by the injection of colloid deep into the posterior rectus sheath, with the needle inserted approximately 3 cm inferior to the xiphoid and 1 to 2 cm medial to the midclavicular line. This is accomplished using a 3-inch, 19-gauge needle held directly cephalad at approximately 45 degrees toward the axilla. The needle is passed deeply through the muscle, and when the posterior rectus sheath is approached, the change in tension is obvious to the operator. If the injection is too forceful, the patient complains of a brief sharp pain as the peritoneum is penetrated. Tracer is injected on the same side as the known breast tumor, and the patient is brought back for imaging 3 hours later. If the internal mammary chain is not seen, this could be the result of inadequate injection technique, a lymphatic chain obstructed by tumor, or a single (and opposite) internal mammary chain. The same side would then be reinjected to decrease the likelihood of technical problems, and the side opposite the tumor would also be injected. In most cases, the diaphragmatic nodes and internal mammary chain are visualized, then the opposite side is injected and the patient brought back for imaging (Fig. 9-22).

Six or seven parasternal nodes are usually visualized extending from the diaphragm to the upper sternum. The upper one or two nodes on the upper sternal chains are visualized universally. Abnormal scan patterns include absent uptake, abnormal collaterals, and partial visualization with crossover to the contralateral chain. The sensitivity for iden-

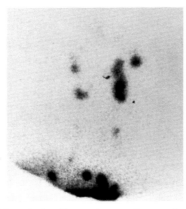

**FIG. 9-22.** This anterior thorax image demonstrates the effect of bilateral injections into the posterior rectus sheath of Tc-99m antimony colloid. Activity is seen in the lowest portion of the image from the injection site and diaphragmatic lymph nodes. Both internal mammary chains are demonstrated. The left is more readily seen because it was injected 3 hours earlier. Normal bilateral internal mammary lymphoscintigraphy. Note that much of the dose remains at the injection site.

tifying tumor presenting as abnormal chains is rather poor. The major indication is to identify patients with unilateral chains or flow crossover to the contralateral chain, so that these patients can have XRT ports extended to include the appropriate internal mammary chain to irradiate the primary lymphatic drainage. It is believed that this lymphatic chain is underestimated in its prognostic importance, but there is evidence that inadequate management of these lymphatic drainage sites is as grave for the patient as the inadequate treatment of axillary spread (51).

### Mammary Lymphoscintigraphy

In this technique, tracer is instilled via a long-bore 23-gauge needle immediately beside the tumor, in the cardinal quadrants, and the lymphatic drainage is mapped. The immediate images demonstrate the tumor's major lymphatic channels and sentinel node(s). An interval node is seen immediately in one-fifth of patients (50). The delayed images at 2 or 4 hours always demonstrate the appropriate drainage nodal bed(s). The identified sentinel node is the one that should be biopsied, and, if positive, that nodal bed should be resected. If the sentinel node is histologically normal, axillary lymph node dissection is not necessary, and cost and morbidity are spared.

### Intraoperative Probes

Intraoperative probe confirmation of the sentinel node localization ensures that the lymph node being sampled is that identified by lymphoscintigraphy (52). Mapping of lymphatic drainage by routine dynamic and static gamma camera imaging is needed to identify unexpected lymph node drainage patterns (e.g., supraclavicular or internal mammary sites in breast cancer, interval nodes in melanoma and breast cancers, and unanticipated lymphatic drainage of melanomas, vulval, or rectal carcinomas). The current standard of surgical care for melanoma now includes lymphoscintigraphy and intraoperative probe use (53). When multicenter trials are complete, it is likely that this imaging technique will also become the standard of care in breast cancer in identification of the appropriate nodes to sample. These individual nodes can be excised, often under local anesthesia with minimal incisions, using the external mapping by nuclear medicine and the intraoperative probe by the surgeon, obviating the diagnostic block dissection and the consequent operative morbidity.

## MONOCLONAL ANTIBODIES

Radioimmunoscintigraphy (RIS) or radioimmunodetection (RAID) is the use of labeled antibodies or antibody fragments against TAAs or tumor-specific antigens to detect primary tumors or their metastases. It may soon become a conventional imaging modality: In December 1992, a TAG-72 MOAB for imaging colorectal and ovarian cancers (satumomab pendetide, OncoScint) was approved by the FDA (see Chapter 15). In mid-1996, a Tc-99m–labeled anti-CEA MOAB (arcitumomab, CEAScan) was approved. In late 1996, an In-111–labeled prostate membrane–specific MOAB (anti-CYT-356 and capromomab pendetide, ProstaScint) and an anti–small cell lung cancer MOAB (nofetumomab mepenten, Verluma) were approved. Various other MOABs are in various stages of approval. Labeled antibodies have been studied in >250 clinical trials since 1978. They have demonstrated clinical usefulness and detection sensitivities of 70% to 85% in colon, rectum, lung, kidney, brain, ovary, breast, and prostate cancers, as well as lymphoma and other hematologic malignancies (54–56).

### History

Pressman was the first to successfully use radiolabeled antibodies, almost 50 years ago. These studies targeted rat osteogenic sarcoma with I-131 labeled anti-rat osteosarcoma antibodies and demonstrated high tumor uptake (57,58). These labeled antibodies were shown to be sequestered with fibrin and fibrinogen within the tumor (59). Subsequently, the use of antibodies against specific tumor-associated markers, such as CEA or human chorionic gonadotropin, was evaluated in mice (60,61). The first clinical study demonstrating successful tumor targeting and imaging in humans used an I-131–labeled goat anti-CEA polyclonal antibody nearly 20 years ago (54).

The injection of an antigen, aided by Freund's adjuvant, into an animal, along with subsequent booster doses, results in antibody production. Multiple lymphocytes, each producing its own clone of antibody, results in the production of polyclonal antibodies. The first large-scale report of successful RIS showed that practical clinical benefits could be achieved and that the following were true:

- Circulating CEA does not block RIS.
- Tumors of 2 cm diameter were consistently detected.
- Tumor uptake was 2.5 times that of adjacent normal tissue.
- Occult tumors could be identified.

Antibodies against TAAs, such as CEA, human chorionic gonadotropin, alpha-fetoprotein, and prostatic acid phosphatase, have all successfully imaged tumors expressing these markers (62–66).

A major advance came in 1975 with the development of MOABs by Kohler and Milstein, for which they received the Nobel Prize in medicine in 1984 (67). Hybridoma technology allowed the development of selected cell lines that produce virtually unlimited quantities of pure, identical (monoclonal) antibody, with a single specificity. MOABs for cancer localization are produced by immunizing a mouse with the specific TAA (ideally, a tumor-specific antigen in the future) to elicit an immune response. A cell suspension is made from the sensitized mouse spleen, and the B-lymphocytes are harvested. These antibody-producing cells are then fused with immortal murine myeloma cells to produce the hybridoma. These hybridoma cells are from a myeloma line that lacks an enzyme essential for DNA synthesis. Only the myeloma cells that successfully fuse with the mouse myeloma cells can survive in a culture media that contains aminopterin, an agent that blocks the alternative pathway of DNA synthesis necessary for the enzyme-deficient immortal cell line. The clone with the best antibody characteristics is subsequently selected, and large-scale antibody production can begin. This process can be carried out in animals or bioreactors, and it results in virtually unlimited supplies of a specific MOAB.

### Problems

The major problem with tumor imaging and therapy with labeled MOABs is the overall poor tumor uptake of MOAB. This is the result of numerous factors, including

- Poor antigen expression and antigen heterogeneity
- Poor tumor perfusion
- Nonspecific uptake by nontumor tissues
- Aggregation with circulating blood pool antigen shed by either the tumor or normal nontumor tissues that also produce the TAA

### Mechanisms to Improve RIS

To overcome these inherent imaging problems, many technical aspects have been addressed, but to date the most

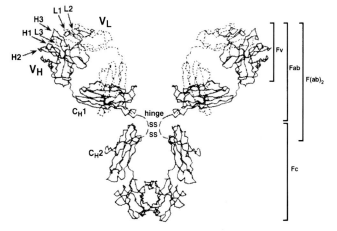

**FIG. 9-23.** This is a diagrammatic representation of an IgG MOAB with the variable fragment (Fv) of heavy and light chain, the constant fragment (Fc) composed of heavy chains only (e.g., $C_H1, C_H2$), and the Fab and $F(ab)_2$ fragments (delineations shown on the right). The six hypervariable regions (H1, H2, H3, L1, L2, L3) within the variable light ($V_L$) and heavy ($V_H$) regions are shown on the left arm. The light chain is dotted, and its complex intertwining with the heavy chain is apparent. The two groups of heavy and light chains are linked by disulphide (SS) bonds at the hinge region. (Modified from Campbell MJ, Niederhuber JH. B-Lymphocyte Responses. In Abeloff MJ, Armitage JO, Lichter AS, Niederhuber JE [eds], Clinical Oncology. Edinburgh: Churchill Livingstone, 1995;103.)

significant refinement of MOAB imaging is based on use of antibody fragments. Whole antibodies are glycoproteins that have a characteristic Y shape and consist of two equal portions, each containing a light (L) and a heavy (H) chain. Each H and L chain has a smaller variable (antigen-specific [Fab]) fragment and a larger constant (complement-fixing [Fc]) fragment, of which the latter determines the antibody class (i.e., immunoglobulin G [IgG] vs. IgM). These antibodies are complex intertwinings of protein chains, with an overall similar shape (the classic and simple Y shape). However, their many infoldings or loops expose various portions of the protein chains to the exterior of the molecule and so make them available for interaction with cell receptors and other ligands (Fig. 9-23). The H chain is divided into four regions—one variable and three constant domains— whereas the smaller L chain has one variable and one constant domain. The constant domains control common features of the antibody (e.g., complement fixation). The uniqueness of the antibody is expressed by the six hypervariable regions (three each on the L and H chains), which are configured so that they are exposed for potential interactions. These hypervariable regions, also termed *complementary determining regions*, are contained in the variable fragment (Fv).

MOAB fragments are produced by enzyme cleavage of the disulphide links that join these equal chains: Papain results in an Fc and two Fab fragments (each approximately 50,000 d), whereas pepsin cleaves the chains at a site closer

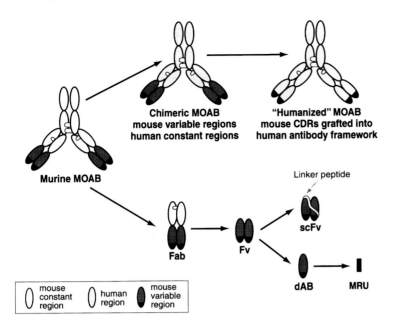

**FIG. 9-24.** Display of the possible modifications of murine MOAB and of the small fragments currently being produced and studied. The Fab antibody fragment contains part of the antibody heavy and light chain. The Fv fragment contains only the variable portion of both heavy and light chain, while the scFv contains the separate Fv fragment heavy and light chains linked as a single chain. The dAB represents variable domain of either the heavy or light chain. The MRU is the molecular recognition unit. (Modified from Campbell MJ, Niederhuber JH. B-Lymphocyte Responses. In Abeloff MJ, Armitage JO, Lichter AS, Niederhuber JE [eds], Clinical Oncology. Edinburgh: Churchill Livingstone, 1995;114.)

to the constant region, resulting in an Fc fragment (50,000 d) and the two Fab molecules still joined by a disulfide bond ([F(ab')$_2$] ≈ 100,000 d). The labeled fragments containing the antigen-specific regions (Fv portion of Fab and F[ab']$_2$) provide high signal-to-background ratios more rapidly than intact IgG (68) because of quicker localization and faster blood clearance and renal elimination rates. The intact MOAB molecule has higher absolute tumor uptake than the smaller fragments, but prolonged biological half-lives (2 to 5 days) require labels with long half-lives (In-111 or I-131). Because of the more rapid metabolism and clearance associated with the use of fragments, earlier tumor imaging can be performed, and shorter half-life radionuclides, such as Tc-99m and I-123, may be used. In general, Fab fragments have biological half-lives of 1.5 hours, and F(ab')$_2$ fragments have half-lives of approximately 10 hours. Low-energy radionuclides with high photon fluxes allow for the use of high-resolution SPECT with significant imaging improvement from increases in lesion detection sensitivity and the ability to fuse SPECT images with MRI or CT images.

The antigen is all important in this imaging modality, and the antibody created can only be as useful as the antigen allows it to be. Although the oncogene-antioncogene theory of cancer suggests that cancer-specific oncoproteins (antigens) will become available, to date, most tumor MOABs use TAAs, which are not specific for the tumor and also exist in normal tissues. These TAAs include dedifferentiation antigens (e.g., CEA and alpha-fetoprotein), cellular secretions (e.g., thyroglobulin), and membrane-stable antigens (e.g., TAG-72). Although MOABs usually have slightly lower antigen-binding affinities than polyclonal antibodies, their potential for massive supply, standardization, and the

probability of future technological advances far outweigh this disadvantage.

Recent technological advances used to improve sensitivity and specificity include the production of second-generation antibodies using purified target antigen rather than the crude tumor cell extract (e.g., CC49 in lieu of TAG-72, with a 10-fold increase in antigen-binding capacity). "Designer" antibodies (69) are another advance, particularly chimeric and humanized antibodies as well as smaller antibody fragments, such as single-chain-binding proteins and molecular recognition units (Fig. 9-24). The chimeric antibodies use manufactured murine Fab fragments attached to human constant regions (Fc fragments), therefore, the murine portion is only one-fourth of the total molecule. In humanized antibodies, the even smaller murine hypervariable region (in the Fv fragment) is incorporated into human IgG, so that only a very small portion of the total molecule is foreign. These modified antibodies have less affinity for the tumor antigen than the murine antibody because the major portion of the IgG molecule derives from humans, and has a different configuration from the original murine antibody. The affinity and avidity characteristics may change as a result of interference with the shape of the murine hypervariable site by the human carrier region.

Various techniques used to improve tumor targeting have included antibody cocktails (combinations of MOABs known to interact with the particular cancer type) and the instillation of the MOAB locoregionally (e.g., intracavitary placement). Other approaches designed to improve the tumor-to-background ratio have included injected unlabeled MOAB to scavenge circulating TAA or a second injected antibody against the MOAB to remove unbound circulating labeled MOAB.

Another method is the injection of a second labeled antigen to identify a specific bifunctional unlabeled antibody after it has distributed in the body and localized at the tumor site. In this instance, the specific tumor MOAB can be allowed to optimally associate with the tumor, a process that can take many days, then the labeled antigen can be injected that localizes the MOAB. The high-affinity streptavidin-biotin system (affinity constant of $10^{15}$ liter/mol, which is several orders of magnitude better than standard MOAB affinity) has been suggested for this role (70). This system is ideal because biotin is a small molecule (244 d) that can be attached to the intact MOAB without interfering with the tumor affinity, and this slightly modified MOAB can then be allowed to slowly accumulate at tumor sites. Streptavidin is a 60-kd molecule that has six exposed tyrosines (excellent for iodination), which rapidly disperse into the tumor ECF by virtue of their small size. In the two-step procedure, the biotinylated antibody or even a cocktail of modified antibodies is injected and allowed to localize for 1 to 4 days. Then, the labeled streptavidin is injected and diagnostic imaging performed. In a refinement using a three-step procedure, the biotinylated antibody is injected, cold streptavidin is injected later in one or two boluses (the first to clear circulating antibody, the second to bind to the antibody located on the tumor), and, finally, labeled biotin is injected for imaging.

Other methods currently being developed for use in MOAB therapy may have application to RIS, including enhancing antigenic expression by alpha-interferon and using interleukin-2 or local XRT to increase tumor vascularity and enhance neovascular permeability to allow better MOAB localization. New approaches include antibodies to tumor necrosis and tumor vessel antigens.

## Scan Protocols

In general terms, the scan protocol and scan findings vary with the following factors:

- Antibody type (e.g., whole or fragment)
- Antibody label (Tc-99m or In-111)
- Amount of antibody injected
- Tumor size
- First or subsequent MOAB injection

Many MOABs react with several tumor types (e.g., OncoScint reacts with colon, prostate, and ovarian cancers). However, not all tumors have these tumor-associated receptors (e.g., only 85% of colon cancers react with satumomab), and not all cells in a patient's particular tumor have the receptor (e.g., 50% of the individual tumor cells in a typical colon cancer have the specific receptors).

The radionuclide used should match the expected or known biological behavior of the MOAB. The radionuclide itself is important: In-111 normally concentrates in the liver, and, consequently, 15% to 25% of the label gets to the liver via transchelation. This often obscures hepatic lesions, which can then only be identified as cold lesions (Fig. 9-25).

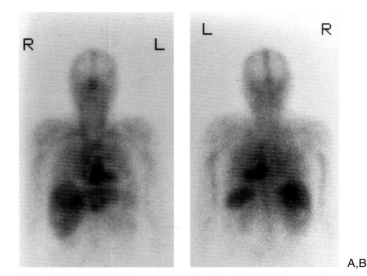

FIG. 9-25. This 24-hour monoclonal antibody image of a patient with known hepatic metastasis shows the inferior right lobe liver lesion as a photopenic defect in both anterior (A) and posterior (B) views. There is considerable blood pool activity, as demonstrated by the heart and major blood vessel visualization. Delayed imaging is preferred to decrease blood pool visualization.

The critical feature that governs imaging success is the amount of labeled MOAB taken up by the tumor, with generally as little as 0.01% of the administered radiopharmaceutical reaching the tumor, and specific activities of only 0.4 to 1.0 µCi/g of tissue being achieved. Some tumors may require large amounts of injected MOAB, even as much as 40 mg of intact MOAB. In general, In-111 is used for intact MOABs because its 68-hour physical half-life matches the biological half-life of the intact MOAB-tumor antigen association (2 to 3 days). Tc-99m is used with antibody fragments because targeting is more rapid (10 hours or less).

The murine MOAB injected is antigenic, so subsequent injections can be affected by the production of human anti-mouse antibodies (HAMA) produced as a result of prior injection. In 10% of patients with HAMA, this results in fever, chills, and rashes, but in 1%, anaphylactic shock can occur. Some MOABs have a low rate of HAMA production, whereas others (e.g., satumomab) have a high rate of HAMA production. In any given murine MOAB, the HAMA rate is proportional to the amount of MOAB injected. The HAMA levels reach a maximum in 1 to 2 weeks after injection and can decrease with time, so sometimes repeat MOAB can be injected after some time, despite a previous HAMA response (see Chapter 15). In the presence of HAMA, the biodistribution is often altered significantly, with rapid hepatic and renal activity and unreliable tumor uptake. This is in part explained by the type of HAMA response (isotypic or idiopathic). HAMAs with an isotypic response react to the Fc fragment, and large 3- to 6-antibody molecule complexes are formed (450 to 900 kd), which are cleared by the reticuloendothelial system (liver, spleen, and marrow). HAMAs with idiotypic response react with the Fv region and interfere directly with the antigen-antibody reaction. The idiotypic response is more likely to occur with chimeric MOABs.

Even when planar images are obtained, impeccable technique is critical. This requirement is especially true in SPECT imaging, and care must be taken to use the appropriate flood correction maps for the particular radionuclide label used. With good technique, SPECT can obtain considerable additional clinical information. This is similar to the lymphoma story, in which poor instrumentation, inadequate Ga-67 doses, and inattention to proper technique resulted in poor reports from many centers, although the Ga-67 technique is now established as invaluable in the management of lymphoma. The package insert of one FDA-approved MOAB (satumomab) recommends images at 48 hours and 72 to 96 hours, but experience suggests that the early images have too much blood pool activity (Fig. 9-25).

### Clinical Applications

The use of satumomab in ovarian and colorectal cancer (Fig. 9-26) is discussed elsewhere (see Chapter 15). Other MOAB agents undergoing active review include those for breast cancer, melanoma, and lymphomas. Numerous worldwide reports, on nearly 4,000 patients with colorectal and

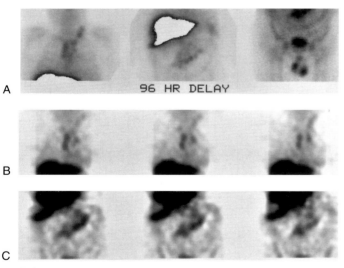

**FIG. 9-26. (A)** The upper row of images displays 96-hour planar views of the chest (left), abdomen (middle), and pelvis (right). The liver has most uptake in this In-111 somatumomab scan, and so it is displayed with a low upper threshold and pixel overflow (white). Incidental note is made of the usual prominent visualization of testes. The lower images are coronal SPECT slices of the mediastinum **(B)** and abdomen **(C)**. The SPECT scan better demonstrates the known hepatic metastasis as a defect and the unknown mediastinal, cervical, and mesenteric nodal metastases. CT scans showed normal-sized (<5 mm) mediastinal lymph nodes. This study precluded partial hepatectomy in this patient, who, prior to the scan, was presumed to have a solitary hepatic metastasis.

ovarian cancers and melanoma, give average figures of sensitivity (75%), specificity (85%), and accuracy (80%). Especially encouraging reports concern prostate cancer, for which the anti-CXT-356 MOAB (arcitumomab, ProstaScint) has been found useful in initial staging and in follow-up situations where increasing levels of prostate-specific antigen occur in previously treated patients. The early reports of a multicenter trial appear very encouraging about diagnosing nodal involvement, although very strict protocols with SPECT and early images are required to allow blood pool identification (71).

General indications for MOABs appear likely to include

- Presurgical staging
- Postsurgical or post-XRT follow-up
- Investigation of rising serum tumor markers
- Checking tumor viability in residual tumor masses seen on CT or MRI
- Determining the potential role of radioimmunotherapy in individual patients

Many of the newer, recently FDA-approved agents use MOAB fragments and are labeled with Tc-99m (anti-CEA MOAB [arcitumomab] and anti–small-cell carcinoma of the lung MOAB [nofetumomab]). Some of these demonstrate excellent sensitivity and PPV; for example, in small-cell lung cancer, preliminary reports suggest that a single MOAB scan is equivalent to the standard battery of imaging tests (PPV of 95%). Now, 20 years after the development of the hybridoma, there is finally an expectation that some of the promise of MOABs is being realized (72).

### Other Peptide Agents

Other peptide agents is a somewhat artificially grouped classification. It includes antibody fragments smaller than the typical Fab molecule (because these smaller molecules are predominantly prepared from recombinant DNA techniques rather than hydridomas), neuropeptide receptor-binding agents (e.g., pentetreotide), or neurotransmitter-like agents (e.g., MIBG). These smaller peptide molecules indicate the true potential of nuclear medicine at the molecular level, and we hope they will revolutionize nuclear medicine in the next century.

#### Smaller Antibody Fragments

MOAB specificity is provided by the variable regions of the H and L chains, and the effector function is performed by the Fc portion. The variable regions are approximately half the size of the smaller fragments, that is, 25,000 d (see Table 9-11), and include three hypervariable subregions (500 to 1,000 d). Several of these hypervariable regions have been prepared and contain only 15 to 30 amino acid residues, compared to >1,300 amino acids of the whole antibody (see Table 9-11). Single-chain-binding proteins (ScFVs), prepared with weights of 25,000 to 30,000 d, consist of only the variable regions of an

**TABLE 9-11.** *MOAB and fragment listed with size and number of amino acids*

| Monoclonal agents | Amino acids | Daltons |
|---|---|---|
| IgG MOAB | 1,500 | 150,000 |
| F(ab¹)₂ fragment | 1,000 | 100,000 |
| Fc fragment | 500 | 50,000 |
| Fab fragment | 500 | 50,000 |
| Fv fragment | 250 | 25,000 |
| ScFV | 250 | 25,000 |
| MRUs | 5–30 | 500–3,000 |
| Peptide analogs | 5–15 | 500–1,500 |

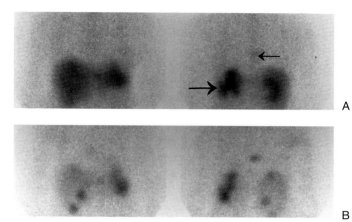

**FIG. 9-27.** This image displays anterior (left) and posterior (right) images of a patient with recurrent metastases in the liver and spine. The pentetreotide scan **(A)** is diagnostically inferior to the MIBG scan **(B)**. In the pentetreotide image, only the local recurrence (*large arrow*) is clearly seen, and the spinal metastasis (*small arrow*) is barely discerned. Several additional lesions are apparent in the MIBG scan.

antibody's H and L chains linked by a 12- to 20-residue peptide. These are folded into a shape that retains antigen-binding capacity. These ScFVs have been shown autoradiographically to gain very rapid tumor access (in hours), to distribute throughout the tumor, and to have low background levels. The total tumor uptake of the ScFV is usually less than that of large intact MOAB molecules, which localize near blood vessels and take 50 to 100 times longer to reach these sites. This reduction in uptake, despite the very rapid access, is due to the lower affinity of these designer MOAB fragments. This decrease in affinity results from the change in configuration of the binding portions of the molecular recognition units (MRUs) in these ScFVs relative to the original MOAB. This change in affinity is even seen in "humanized" MOABs, where the murine Fv fragment is grafted to a human Fc fragment and minor changes result in the murine Fv configuration because the human Fc portion has a slightly different shape from the parent murine intact MOAB. In the case of ScFVs and MRUs, such conformational changes are expected to be more extensive, and, although these small molecules do not produce HAMA, their affinity for the tumor antigen is severely reduced compared to intact murine MOABs. Small peptide analogs of the hypervariable region are undergoing clinical trials as antithrombin agents (see Chapter 19), and it is reasonable to expect antitumor versions in the future.

### Neuropeptide Receptor Agents

Neuropeptides are small molecules formed from amino acids that are secreted by neurons, the gut, and the endocrine system. Neuropeptide examples include thyrotropin-releasing hormone (a tripeptide), somatostatin (14-amino acid chain), and insulin (a large polypeptide chain of 6,000 d). These agents act by binding to specific membrane-associated neuropeptide receptors, and they act predominantly on the gut and endocrine system as either gut and pituitary peptides or hypothalamic releasing hormones.

### Pentetreotide

The recently FDA-approved agent pentetreotide (an eight-amino acid [octreotide] segment of somatostatin) is

90% sensitive in the detection of many neuroendocrine tumors (see Chapter 14), including carcinoids, GI and pancreatic endocrine tumors, pituitary adenomas, and small-cell lung cancer. Pentetreotide also identifies other tumors that express somatostatin receptors, including tumors of the nervous system (e.g., astrocytomas, neuroblastomas, medulloblastomas, and meningiomas), malignant lymphomas, and renal cell carcinomas. Lower incidences of somatostatin receptors occur in breast adenocarcinomas, and even lower incidences occur in ovarian and colonic adenocarcinomas.

### Metaiodobenzylguanidine

MIBG is labeled with I-131 and is available commercially each week. It is labeled with I-123 in some medical centers under institutional investigational new drug rules. MIBG is excellent at identifying pheochromocytomas (Fig. 9-27) and neuroblastomas, and many management protocols routinely use I-131 (I-123 if available) MIBG in the follow-up of such patients. MIBG enters the cell via the reuptake mechanism with other adrenergic precursors (see Chapter 14). This agent has had only limited success in tumor types other than pheochromocytomas and neuroblastomas. In much larger doses, I-131 MIBG has been used therapeutically in neuroblastomas.

## POSITRON EMISSION TOMOGRAPHY

In 1930, Warburg associated high glycolytic rates with malignant transformation (73). This was recently confirmed by cell line studies that demonstrate increased glucose transport and transporter messenger RNA induced by oncogenes (74). In 1972, F-18 5-fluorouracil (5-FU) was labeled, and it was proposed as a determinant of which patients might respond to 5-FU therapy. In 1977, Sokoloff and colleagues developed an autoradiographic technique for quantifying deoxyglucose uptake into tissues (75) that has been applied to PET using FDG (76). For the next decade, PET was confined to the research environment and used very little for clinical research. In 1982, Di Chiro et al. first applied the Sokoloff 2-deoxyglucose autoradiography model to F-18 FDG imaging of cerebral gliomas (77). In the 1990s, whole-body imaging of F-18 FDG in primary and secondary neoplastic disease was introduced, and the role of FDG as the whole-body tumor scan has been suggested (78–80).

PET scanning has the potential to

- Distinguish benign from malignant masses
- Separate treatment effects from tumor recurrence
- Determine tumor grade and proliferation rates
- Predict metabolic response to therapy before measurable changes in tumor size occur

## Radiopharmaceuticals

In general, the tumor PET radiopharmaceuticals can provide qualitative and quantitative information on tumor perfusion and tumor metabolism as well as a means of tracing biodistribution (5-FU) or metabolic effect of cytostatic agents (FDG). Although approximately 200 PET radiopharmaceuticals exist, only 20 are used in oncology. FDG is the most widely used, the most widely available, and best characterized (see Chapter 17). Local distribution centers make FDG available for modern SPECT cameras using 511-keV collimators. The triple-headed camera is especially adaptable to this role, although the sensitivity of lesion detection is not as good as with PET scanners. This new SPECT scanner role has not yet been solidified, and questions remain concerning spatial resolution in noncoincidence systems and attenuation correction in coincidence systems (81,82). Other PET agents used in oncology include amino acids (Carbon 11 [C-11]–labeled methionine, leucine, glutamine, and tyrosine) to measure protein production, DNA tracers (C-11 thymidine) to measure cell proliferation, and estrogen receptors (F-18 estradiol) for breast cancers. There is also the potential to label MOAB, for example, with Ga-68 or I-124. I-124 has a half-life suitable for the intact IgG molecule.

## Protocols

Fasting decreases cardiac uptake (79), and lesions near organs that take up FDG are likely to be missed, such as lymph nodes near the heart or stomach and lesions in or near the brain. Because of this, fasting is recommended when doing whole-body PET imaging. Although quantitation is not generally performed, various simpler qualitative FDG uptake methods used include influx constant $K_1$ and the even simpler dose absorption rate, dose uptake rate, and specific uptake values, which measure the activity in the tumor and relate it to the total injected activity corrected for patient lean body mass (78). At this writing, quantitation of FDG in tumors is controversial (80). Many PET users do transmission scan correction of emission data in the regions of the primary tumor or special interest (e.g., differentiating viable tumor from treatment effect) because of the improved results.

## Clinical Applications

Over the years, populations of oncology patients imaged with FDG were studied, but until 1990, these represented only small pilot studies. More recently, as the desire to establish reimbursement increased, larger patient populations were studied and the technique appeared clinically useful. Relatively small preliminary studies had shown excellent PPVs and NPVs in several clinical situations. Under the guidance of the Institute of Clinical PET (ICP), prospective cost-efficacy studies were commenced, and the results are just now appearing. For a discussion of PET and brain tumors, see Chapter 17.

### FDG Imaging with Gamma Cameras

There is currently considerable discussion (81,82) about the role of conventional gamma camera devices in oncologic, cardiac, and cerebral PET. This development of gamma camera hardware and software reflects the success of FDG PET in several clinical applications and the wider availability of FDG from regional distribution centers that are either established PET centers or commercial nuclear pharmacies. There are two potential imaging methods, and manufacturers are addressing both with special collimators designed for 511-keV photons or electronic upgrades to provide coincidence detection circuitry. This FDG SPECT approach can be applied to existing devices merely by the addition of specially designed collimators (200 to 400 lb apiece), provided the gantry can support this additional weight and the photopeak energy can be increased to include the annihilation photon. The electronic collimation method of the annihilation coincidence detection (ACD) approach requires additional special electronic modifications to increase the count rate capability.

Such modifications to standard gamma cameras add limitations to the already compromised 511-keV detection, such as the poor annihilation photon detected efficiency (18%) by the standard ⅜-inch-thick sodium iodide (NaI) crystal (86% for Tc-99m). Manufacturers sell ¾-

inch crystals for significant increases in efficiency. The SPECT method using 511-keV collimators is compromised by the large amount of lead required for collimation, with the consequent reduction in efficiency. There are some minor improvements in intrinsic resolution with 511-keV photon detection, provided special care is taken to use the appropriate energy maps. The gains include minimal increases in intrinsic resolution (inversely related to square root of energy) and a lower proportion of scattered photons in the photopeak (perhaps 10% compared to the usual 33% in 140-keV photon detection). FDG SPECT works moderately well compared to FDG PET despite 10-fold reductions in counts (300,000 to 3,000,000 vs. 20,000,000 to 30,000,000) and marked reductions in volume sensitivity and image resolution. Despite these significant disadvantages, the technique appears to work satisfactorily.

In ACD, although there are gains in resolution over SPECT imaging, there is a problem in the low percentage of counts that are truly coincidence (approximately 1% of the total counts), especially when FDG-rich organs are located near the region of interest (e.g., brain and heart). Because of this small percentage of true coincidence counts, it is critical to increase the detector's count rate using techniques such as pulse clipping, pulse leading edge detectors, and pulse tail extenders. Initial manufacturer models demonstrated 1% to 2% coincidence rates (1,000 to 2,000 counts per second), but recent models are showing 10-fold increases in these rates. Such ACD technology applies well to the brain, which is close to no other FDG-rich organs, and the coincidence rate can reach 5% of total incident photons. In brain FDG studies, these ACD systems will probably work well.

Unfortunately, in oncologic PET, neither of these compromise gamma camera systems works extremely well with the present technology. The field is developing rapidly, however, and already six manufacturers offer coincidence imaging, and several offer thicker crystals. The initial vendors are offering significant improvements in their high count rate and other technology, and some are contemplating alternative crystals for coincidence detection. These devices will likely be able to do SPECT and FDG imaging well at modest increases ($100,000 to $200,000) in cost over current SPECT-only devices.

Conventional PET struggles for sufficient count rates because of its modest tumor-to-background ratios. Clinical investigators are doing attenuation correction of PET data to better identify subtle lesions. The FDG SPECT technology will not be able to take the PET experience and apply it more generally to the field because of the additional SPECT constraints. With certain lesions, however, such as large solitary pulmonary nodule evaluation, this FDG-SPECT approach appears practical. As a consequence, PET manufacturers are designing smaller three-dimensional PET scanners (e.g., QUESTscanner, Milwaukee, WI) that appear appropriate for clinical use, at prices likely to compete with two- and three-headed coincidence mode SPECT scanners.

### Single Pulmonary Nodules

Early studies using differential uptake rate and standardized uptake value ratios (see Chapter 17) gave sensitivities of 96% to 98% and specificities of 86% to 94% for discriminating between benign and malignant disease in single pulmonary nodules. The potential application is being studied with an ICP-sponsored multicenter trial of indeterminate single pulmonary nodules. Preliminary reports indicate that visual uptake estimates are highly sensitive but less specific and that the techniques work well for lesions >1.5 cm. If the prospective PET studies coordinated by Duke University confirm the early retrospective studies, significant cost savings will be realized in this common disease presentation. There is promise that FDG-SPECT will work with the larger lesions.

### Breast Cancer

Initial axillary lymph node detection studies gave good initial sensitivity and specificity data. Assuming a sensitivity of 90% and specificity of 95%, some 75,000 unnecessary procedures could be saved annually. The ICP prospective study for this evaluation is being coordinated by Case Western Reserve University.

### Colorectal Cancer

Using a multicenter survey with a proposed 96% sensitivity and 88% specificity for the follow-up of colorectal cancer, it is envisioned that PET can replace laparotomy for identifying patients with potential tumor recurrence. This is expected to save 20,900 laparotomies annually. A caveat in abdominal imaging is the significant uptake of FDG in some abdominal organs (e.g., liver), in which mean specific uptake values of 2.2 (a value similar to tumor uptakes) can obscure lesions. Cecal and gastric activity are unexplained findings that also can cause confusion in a significant number of patients. It has been shown, however, that FDG uptake into normal tissues plateaus rapidly after injection, whereas tumor uptakes continue to rise over the course of the scan. This finding may provide a means of discriminating lesions from artifact. Initial small comparisons of FDG with TAA MOABs indicate significant PET superiority in colorectal tumors.

### Other Cancers

A meta-analysis study of FDG in NHL showed a sensitivity of 98%, and there are reports of FDG decrease in responsive tumors as early as 3 days after start of chemotherapy. Small series have demonstrated remarkable FDG uptake in melanoma (see Fig. 17-16), and this has been confirmed by other investigators (83). The tracer has also been usefully applied to lymphomas; head and neck tumors; endocrine neoplasms, such as thyroid cancer (see Fig. 7-39) and parathyroid adenomas; ovarian cancer; renal cancer; bladder cancer; hepatoma; and musculoskeletal tumors. Prostate cancer does not seem to take up FDG as well as other tumors, perhaps as a consequence of its relatively slow growth rate.

## TUMOR THERAPY

The treatment of thyroid cancer with I-131 and treatment of skeletal metastases with strontium 89 (Sr-89) are described in Chapters 7 and 8. The success of radionuclide therapy depends on the degree of tumor localization achieved. Although acceptable levels are achieved with some tracers (I-131 as NaI or MIBG, and Sr-89 as SrCl$_2$) administered systemically, considerable activity remains in normal tissues, circulating in the blood, or in the various elimination routes, resulting in significant radiation doses to normal tissues. If the therapeutic radionuclide can be localized in a site of otherwise limited access, the unwanted irradiation of normal tissues can be significantly reduced or virtually eliminated. Examples include direct implantation into serous cavities and cystic tumors, intra-arterial injection of microspheres into the hepatic artery for liver lesions, and intralymphatic localization for lymph node therapy.

Systemically administered therapies can be divided into three broad categories:

- Simple inorganic compounds (e.g., I-131 as NaI and P-32 as sodium phosphate)
- Complex compounds (e.g., I-131 MIBG)
- Biological ligands (e.g., MOABs and receptor agents)

Nuclear medicine physicians had hoped that MOABs would become the tumor version of Ehrlich's "magic bullet," but most research currently under way is only investigating the limitations of such therapy. Difficulties with MOABs are the relatively low affinities for the tumor and that a very small portion (0.001% to 0.05%) of the administered dose localizes in the tumor, leaving large radiation doses to normal tissues (especially the marrow) unless the tracer is rapidly excreted. Furthermore, it is desirable that human myeloma cell lines be used to prevent HAMA production that would interfere with subsequent therapy, but human hybridoma myeloma lines have been difficult to produce and maintain, and the resultant antibody has generally had lower affinities. Humanized or chimeric antibodies have lesser HAMA rates than purely murine MOABs, but the HAMA response is usually idiotypic and therefore inactivates the Fv fragment affecting the antigen-antibody bond. The most responsive tumors to date in research studies have not been the solid tumors (especially those >2 cm in diameter, with their associated problems of poor vascularity) but rather the lymphoproliferative tumors, such as lymphomas and leukemias, in which dramatic results have occurred (72).

The recent advantages gained for diagnostic imaging MOABs (e.g., antibody fragments) may actually be deleterious in therapy applications. Although fragments labeled with Tc-99m may provide superior images as a result of rapid localization, high photon fluxes, and rapid urinary excretion that clears background activity, the absolute tumor uptake of antibody fragment is less than uptake with the intact antibody, and most MOAB therapy work uses intact IgG molecules. To date, poor tumor penetration, HAMA production, and loss of the tracer (I-131) from the MOAB has hampered the efficacy of MOABs. Methods of increasing the relative tumor uptake of antibody will result from the following:

- Alterations in antibody affinity (e.g., second-generation antibodies)
- Increased tumor neovascularity and permeability (e.g., concomitant XRT, hyperthermia, interleukin 2, and tumor necrosis factors)
- Increased sensitivity of effect (concomitant taxol or hyperthermia therapy)
- Increased antigen expression by alpha-interferon stimulation (upregulation of target antigens)
- Preloading with unlabeled MOAB (to clear nontumor antigen)
- Direct injection into the tumor site (e.g., peritoneal)
- MOABs targeted to epidermal and vascular endothelial growth factors, which are significantly increased in tumors

Approximately 40 therapeutic trials using labeled antibodies are currently under way. With the development of these MOAB uptake enhancers, it is expected that MOAB therapy will ultimately become a reality.

## REFERENCES

1. Hayes RL. The medical use of gallium radionuclides: a brief history with some comments. Semin Nucl Med 1978;8:183–203.
2. McLaughlin AF, Magee MA, Greenough R, et al. Current role of gallium scanning in the management of lymphoma. Eur J Nucl Med 1990;16:771–775.
3. McLaughlin AF, Southee AE. Gallium Scintigraphy in Tumor Diagnosis and Treatment. In Murray IP, Ell PJ (eds), Nuclear Medicine in Clinical Diagnosis and Treatment. Edinburgh: Churchill Livingstone, 1994;711–735.
4. Porter J, Kawana M, Krizek H, et al. $^{67}$Ga production with a compact cyclotron. J Nucl Med 1970;11:352.
5. Podoloff PA. Diffuse lung uptake of Ga-67 citrate in healed lymphoma: another milestone on the road to understanding. Radiology 1996;195:319–320.
6. Peylan-Ramu N, Haddy TB, Jones E, et al. High frequency of benign mediastinal uptake of gallium-67 after completion of chemotherapy in children with high-grade non-Hodgkin's lymphoma. J Clin Oncol 1989;7:1800–1806.
7. Hoffer PB, Bekerman C, Henkin RE. Gallium-67 Imaging. New York: Wiley, 1978;24–38.

8. Chen DCP, Hung GL, Levina A, et al. Correlation of gallium uptake and degree of malignancy in non-Hodgkin's lymphoma [abstract]. J Nucl Med 1986;27:1031.

9. Boring CC, Squires TS, Tong T, Montgomery S. Cancer statistics, 1994. CA Cancer J Clin 1994;44:7–26.

10. Aisenberg AC. Biology, Natural History and Treatment: Malignant Lymphoma. Philadelphia: Lea & Febiger, 1991;16.

11. Schenkein DP. Discussing case records of the Massachusetts General Hospital. N Engl J Med 1995;333:784–791.

12. Hamrick-Turner JE, Saif MF, Powers CI, et al. Imaging of childhood non-Hodgkin lymphoma: assessment by histologic subtype. Radiographics 1994;14:11–28.

13. Ben-Haim S, Bar-Shalom R, Israel O, et al. Utility of gallium-67 scintigraphy in low-grade non-Hodgkin's lymphoma. J Clin Oncol 1996;14:1936–1942.

14. Front D, Israel O. The role of Ga-67 scintigraphy in evaluating the results of therapy of lymphoma patients. Semin Nucl Med 1995;25:60–71.

15. Canellos GP. Residual mass in lymphoma may not be residual disease [editorial]. J Clin Oncol 1988;6:931–932.

16. Front D, Ben-Haim S, Israel O, et al. Lymphoma: predictive value of Ga-67 scintigraphy after treatment. Radiology 1992;182:359–363.

17. Kaplan WD, Jochelson MS, Herman TS, et al. Gallium-67 imaging: a predictor of residual tumor viability and clinical outcome in patients with diffuse large-cell lymphoma. J Clin Oncol 1990;8:1966–1970.

18. King SC, Reiman RJ, Proswitz LR. Prognostic importance of restaging gallium scans following induction chemotherapy for advanced Hodgkin's disease. J Clin Oncol 1994;12:306–311.

19. Hag R, Sowk CA, Franssen E, et al. Significance of a partial or slow response to front-line chemotherapy in the management of intermediate-grade or high-grade non-Hodgkin's lymphoma: a literature review. J Clin Oncol 1994;12:1074–1084.

20. Armitage JO, Weisenberger DD, Hutchins M, et al. Chemotherapy for diffuse large-cell lymphoma—rapidly responding patients have more durable remissions. J Clin Oncol 1986;4:160–164.

21. Weeks JC, Yeap BY, Canellos GP, et al. Value of follow-up procedures in patients with large-cell lymphoma who achieve a complete remission. Clin Oncol 1994;9:1196–1203.

22. Front D, Bar-Shalom R, Epelbaum R, et al. Early detection of lymphoma recurrence with gallium-67 scintigraphy. J Nucl Med 1993;34:2101–2104.

23. Mariani G. Unexpected keys in cell biochemistry imaging: some lessons from Tc-99m sestamibi. J Nucl Med 1996;37:536–538.

24. Black KL, Hawkins RA, Kim TK, et al. Use of thallium-201 SPECT to quantitate malignancy grade of gliomas. J Neurosurg 1989;71:342–346.

25. Loberboym M, Barom J, Feibel M, et al. A prospective evaluation of thallium-201 single photon emission computerized tomography for brain tumor burden. Int J Radiat Oncol Biol Phys 1995;32:249–254.

26. Vertosick FT, Selker RG, Grosman SJ, Joyce JM. Correlation of thallium-201 single photon emission computed tomography and survival after treatment failure in patients with glioblastoma multiforme. Neurosurgery 1994;34:396–401.

27. Slizofski W, Krishna L, Katsetos CD, et al. Thallium imaging for brain tumors with results measured by a semiquantitative index and correlated with histopathology. Cancer 1994;74:3190–3197.

28. Ramanna L, Waxman A, Binney G, et al. Thallium-201 in bone sarcoma: comparison with gallium-67 and technetium-MDP in the evaluation of chemotherapeutic response. J Nucl Med 1990;31:567–572.

29. Nadel HR. Thallium-201 for oncological imaging in children. Semin Nucl Med 1993;3:243–254.

30. O'Tuama L, Treves ST, Larar JN, et al. Thallium-201 versus technetium-99m-MIBI in evaluation of childhood brain tumors: a within-subject comparison. J Nucl Med 1993;34:1045–1051.

31. Howman-Giles R, Uren R, Shaw P. Thallium-201 scintigraphy in pediatric soft tissue tumors. J Nucl Med 1995;36:1372–1376.

32. Ramanna L, Waxman A, Braunstein G. Thallium-201 scintigraphy in differentiated thyroid cancer: comparison with radioiodine scintigraphy and serum thyroglobulin determination. J Nucl Med 1991;32:441–446.

33. Waxman AD, Ramanna L, Memsic LD, et al. Thallium scintigraphy in the evaluation of mass abnormalities of the breast. J Nucl Med 1993;34:18–23.

34. Khalkhali I, Cutrone JA, Mena IG, et al. Technetium-99m-sestamibi scintimammography of breast lesions: clinical and pathological follow-up. J Nucl Med 1995;36:1784–1789.

35. Taillefer R, Robidoux A, Lambert R, et al. Technetium-99m-sestamibi prone scintimammography to detect primary breast cancer and axillary lymph node involvement. J Nucl Med 1995;36:1758–1765.

36. Khalkhali J, Villanueva-Meyer SL, Edell SC, et al. Diagnostic accuracy of Tc-99m sestamibi breast imaging in breast cancer detection [abstract]. J Nucl Med 1996;37:74P.

37. Khalkhali J, Villanueva-Meyer SL, Edell SC, et al. Impact of breast density on the diagnostic accuracy of Tc-99m sestamibi breast imaging in the detection of breast cancer [abstract]. J Nucl Med 1996;37:74P–75P.

38. Udelsman R, Ball D, Baylin S, et al. Preoperative localization of occult medullary carcinoma of the thyroid gland with single-photon emission tomography dimercaptosuccinic acid. Surgery 1993;114:1083–1089.

39. Melvin KEW, Miller HH, Tashjian AH Jr. Early diagnosis of medullary carcinoma of the thyroid by means of calcitonin assay. N Engl J Med 1971;285:1115–1120.

40. Miller HH, Melvin KEW, Gibson JM, Tashjian AH Jr. Surgical approach to early familial medullary carcinoma of the thyroid. Am J Surg 1982;144:420–422.

41. Brunt LM, Wells SA Jr. Advances in the diagnosis and treatment of medullary thyroid carcinoma. Surg Clin North Am 1987;67:263–279.

42. Berna L, Cabezas R, Mora J, et al. 111In-Octreotide and Tc-99m (V) dimercaptosuccinic acid studies in the imaging of recurrent medullary thyroid carcinoma. J Endocrinol 1995;144:339–345.

43. Juweid M, Sharkey RM, Betir LC, et al. Improved detection of medullary thyroid cancer with radiolabeled antibodies to carcinoembryonic antigen [abstract]. J Nucl Med 1996;37:9P.

44. Ohta H, Endo K, Fujita T, et al. Imaging of soft tissue tumors with Tc (V)-99m dimercaptosuccinic acid: a new tumor-seeking agent. Clin Nucl Med 1984;9:568–573.

45. Kobayashi H, Sakahara H, Makoto H, et al. Soft tissue tumors: diagnosis with Tc (V)-99m dimercaptosuccinic acid scintigraphy. Radiology 1994;190:277–280.

46. Morton DL, Wen DR, Cochran AJ. Management of early stage melanoma by intraoperative lymphatic mapping and selective lymphadenectomy. Surg Oncol Clin North Am 1992;1:147–159.

47. Albertini JJ, Cruse CW, Rapaport D, et al. Intraoperative radiolymphoscintigraphy improves sentinel lymph node identification for patients with melanoma. Ann Surg 1996;223:217–224.

48. Aurisch R, Winter H, Buchali K. Scintigraphy of lymphokinetics for removal of lymph paths and nodes in patients with malignant melanoma [abstract]. J Nucl Med 1995;36:194P.

49. Uren RF, Howman Giles RB, Shaw HM, et al. Lymphoscintigraphy in high risk melanoma of the trunk: predicting draining node groups, defining lymphatic channels and locating the sentinel node. J Nucl Med 1993;34:1435–1440.

50. Uren RF, Howman Giles RB, Thomson JF, et al. Mammary lymphoscintigraphy in breast cancer. J Nucl Med 1995;36:1775–1780.

51. Ege G. Lymphoscintigraphy techniques and application in the management of breast cancer. Semin Nucl Med 1983;13:26–34.

52. Alex JC, Krag DN. Gamma-probe-guided localization of lymph nodes. Surg Oncol 1993;2:137–143.

53. Reintgen DS. Editorial: changing standards of surgical care for the melanoma patient. Ann Surg Oncol 1966;3:327–328.

54. Goldenberg DM, DeLand F, Kim E, et al. Use of radiolabeled antibodies to carcinoembryonic antigens for detection and localization of diverse cancers by external photoscanning. N Engl J Med 1978;298:1384–1388.

55. Larson SM. Lymphoma, melanoma, colon cancer: diagnosis and treatment with radiolabeled monoclonal antibodies. Radiology 1987;165:297–304.

56. Goldenberg DM, Goldenberg H, Sharkey RM, et al. Imaging of colorectal carcinoma with radiolabeled antibodies. Semin Nucl Med 1992;33:803–814.

57. Pressman D, Keighly G. The zone of activity of antibodies as determined by the use of radioactive tracers; the zone of activity of nephrotoxic anti-kidney serum. J Immunol 1948;59:141–146.

58. Pressman D, Korngold L. The in vivo localization of anti-Wagner osteogenic sarcoma antibodies. Cancer 1953;6:619–623.

59. Day ED, Planinsek JA, Pressman D. Localization in vivo of radioiodinated anti-rat-fibrin antibodies and radioiodinated rat fibrinogen in the Murphy rat lymphosarcoma and in other transplantable rat tumors. J Natl Cancer Inst 1959;22:413–426.

60. Quinones J, Mizejewski G, Beierwaltes WH. Choriocarcinoma scanning using radiolabeled antibody to chorionic gonadotropin. J Nucl Med 1971;12:69–75.

61. Primus FJ, Wang RH, Goldenberg DM, et al. Localization of human GW-39 tumors in hamsters by radiolabeled heterospecific antibody to carcinoembryonic antigen. Cancer Res 1973;33:2977–2982.

62. Dykes PW, Hine KR, Bradwell AR, et al. Localization of tumor deposits by external scanning after injection of radiolabeled anti-carcinoembryonic antigen. BMJ 1980;280:220–222.

63. Goldenberg DM, Kim EE, DeLand F, et al. Radioimmunodetection of cancer with radioactive antibodies to carcinoembryonic antigen. Cancer Res 1980;40:2984–2992.

64. Goldenberg DM, Kim EE, DeLand F, et al. Clinical radioimmunodetection of cancer with radioactive antibodies to human chorionic gonadotropin. Science 1980;208:1284–1286.

65. Goldenberg DM, Kim EE, DeLand F, et al. Clinical studies on the radioimmunodetection of tumors containing alpha-fetoprotein. Cancer 1980;45:4500–4505.

66. Goldenberg DM, DeLand F, Bennet SJ, et al. Radioimmunodetection of prostatic cancer: in vivo use of radioactive antibodies against prostatic acid phosphatase for diagnosis and detection of prostatic cancer by nuclear imaging. JAMA 1983;250:630-635.

67. Kohler G, Milstein C. Continuous cultures of fused cells secreting antibody of predetermined specificity. Nature 1975;256:495–497.

68. Mach JP, Forni M, Ritschard J, et al. Use and limitations of radiolabeled anti-CEA antibodies and their fragments for photoscanning detection of human colorectal carcinomas. Oncodevel Biol Med 1980;1:49–69.

69. Serafini A. From monoclonal antibodies to peptides and molecular recognition units: an overview. J Nucl Med 1993;34(Suppl):533–536.

70. Mayforth RD, Quintons J. Designer and catalytic antibodies. N Engl J Med 1990;323:173–178.

71. Krynyckyi BR, Li Y, Ganeles A, et al. Patterns of metastatic prostate cancer as determined by In-111 CYT 356 (Prostascint) immunoscintigraphy [abstract]. J Nucl Med 1996;37:10P.

72. Hall S. Monoclonal antibodies at age 20: promise at last? Science 1995;270:915–916.

73. Warburg O. The Metabolism of Tumors. London: Arnold Constable, 1930;75–327.

74. Frier JS, Mueckler MM, Usher P, et al. Elevated levels of glucose transport and transporter messenger RWA are induced by ras or src oncogenes. Science 1987;235:1492–1495.

75. Sokoloff L, Reivich M, Kennedy C, et al. The (14C)deoxyglucose method for the measurement of local cerebral glucose utilization: theory, procedure and normal values in the conscious and anesthetized albino rat. J Neurochem 1977;28:897–916.

76. Phelps ME, Juang SC, Hoffman EJ, et al. Tomographic measurements of local cerebral glucose metabolism in humans with (F-18)-2-fluoro-2-deoxy-D-glucose: validation of method. Ann Neurol 1979;6:371–388.

77. Di Chiro G, DeLaPaz RL, Brooks RA, et al. Glucose utilization of cerebral gliomas measured by F-18 fluorodeoxyglucose and positron emission tomography. Neurology 1982;32:1323–1329.

78. Fischman AJ, Alpert NM. FDG-PET in oncology: there's more to it than looking at pictures [editorial]. J Nucl Med 1993;34:6–11.

79. Glaspy JA, Hawkins R, Hoh CK, Phelps ME. Use of positron emission tomography in oncology. Oncology 1993;7:41–50.

80. Fischman AJ. Positron emission tomography in the clinical evaluation of metastatic cancer [editorial]. J Clin Oncol 1996;14:691–696.

81. Drane WE, Nicole MW, Mastin ST, Kuperus JH. SPECT with 2-(fluorine-18)fluoro-2-deoxy-D-glucose (FDG). Radiology 1995;197:341–343.

82. Macfarlane DJ, Cotton L, Ackermann RJ, et al. Reply [to reference 81]. Radiology 1995;197:343.

83. Steinert HC, Boni RA, Buck A, et al. Malignant melanoma: staging with whole-body positron emission tomography and 2(F-18)-fluoro-2-deoxy-D-glucose. Radiology 1995;195:705–709.

*Textbook of Nuclear Medicine,*
edited by Michael A. Wilson.
Lippincott–Raven Publishers, Philadelphia © 1998.

CHAPTER 10

# Central Nervous System

David L. Bushnell and Scott B. Perlman

Radionuclide central nervous system (CNS) imaging has evolved substantially in the past 15 to 20 years. In the 1960s and 1970s, radionuclide brain imaging was used frequently to assess abnormalities of the blood-brain barrier (BBB) (1) and was the earliest noninvasive imaging technique useful in the detection of tumors, abscesses, stroke, arteriovenous malformations, and hematomas. Technetium 99m (Tc-99m) as pertechnetate and Tc-99m chelated to diethylenetriamine pentaacetic acid (DTPA) have both been used to assess the integrity of the BBB. The preferred BBB agent was glucoheptonate (1,2). With the advent of x-ray computed tomography (CT), this CNS application was quickly replaced. It became clear, however, that to better understand and treat disorders of the brain it would be essential for clinicians to identify abnormalities in regional neurophysiology. Thus, there is an emphasis on developing radiopharmaceuticals and brain imaging techniques that evaluate the functional status of the brain.

Single photon emission CT (SPECT) neuroimaging is a method capable of providing information on the regional perfusion of the brain. This method has been applied to the study of a number of neuropsychiatric disorders (Table 10-1), ranging from cerebrovascular disease to dementia and depression (3). Although we are limited primarily to assessment of neuroperfusion with the current clinically available radiopharmaceuticals, other agents are now being studied that will yield information on many other aspects of brain physiology and pathophysiology, particularly in the realm of neuroreceptor function. Emphasis is also being placed on the ability to fuse the functional SPECT image with corresponding anatomic images of the brain from CT or magnetic resonance imaging (MRI) (4). This image fusion will greatly enhance the ability to localize neurophysiologic abnormalities to specific sites in the brain.

Although SPECT brain imaging continues to carry substantial promise for improving our ability to care for patients with neuropsychiatric disorders, there are currently only a small number of well-established clinical indications for the technique. In large part, this is the result of the limited ther-apeutic options available for most neurologic diseases. Consequently, it has been difficult to demonstrate any positive effect on patient outcome by using SPECT. For example, although SPECT can effectively assist in the diagnosis of Alzheimer's disease, there has been no approved medical treatment for this disorder (until only very recently), so precise diagnosis has had limited effect on patient management. Perhaps with the advent of effective treatments, the method will be applied with greater frequency in the clinical setting. It should be stressed that SPECT neuroimaging has emerged as a valuable and frequently used research tool, and additional applications are likely to be forthcoming as ongoing research studies come to fruition. This chapter deals with the numerous potential clinical applications for this relatively new brain imaging technique. We also briefly discuss several older radionuclide studies of the CNS that are still occasionally used in clinical practice.

## CNS PERFUSION

### Radiopharmaceuticals

Three radiopharmaceuticals have been approved by the U.S. Food and Drug Administration (FDA) for clinical use: Tc-99m d,l-hexamethylpropyleneamine oxime (HMPAO, exametazine), iodine 123 (I-123) *N*-isopropyl *p*-iodoamphetamine (IMP, iofetamine), and Tc-99m ethylcysteinate dimer (ECD, bicisate). Although the future commercial availability of IMP remains uncertain, ECD (FDA approved in 1995) possesses certain advantageous properties relative to IMP and HMPAO. All these radiopharmaceuticals hold in common a high degree of lipid solubility that allows each to readily cross the intact BBB by passive diffusion and distribute in brain tissue. In normal brain tissue, the initial concentration of each agent is directly related to regional cerebral blood flow (rCBF). Table 10-2 summarizes pharmacokinetic data for HMPAO, IMP, and ECD.

**TABLE 10-1.** *Uses of CNS perfusion agents*

Evaluation of regional cerebral perfusion
   Cerebrovascular disease
   Epilepsy
   Dementia
   Psychiatric disorders
   Brain trauma
Evaluation of cerebrovascular reserve

**TABLE 10-2.** *Pharmacokinetic data for HMPAO, IMP, and ECD*

|  | HMPAO | IMP | ECD |
|---|---|---|---|
| First-pass extraction | 70–80% | 90% | 60% |
| Peak brain uptake* | 5% | 6–7% | 6% |
| Time to peak uptake | 1–2 mins | 20 mins | 5 mins |

*As percent of administered activity.

## HMPAO (Exametazine)

After intravenous (IV) injection, the cerebral distribution of HMPAO remains in large part unchanged for several hours, although a significant fraction of the HMPAO diffuses back from brain tissue to blood immediately after initial uptake. As a consequence of this back-diffusion and modest first-pass extraction (see Table 10-2), HMPAO concentration would be expected to underestimate rCBF at higher flow rates. Studies have confirmed that the linear relationship between HMPAO uptake and rCBF is lost at higher levels of perfusion and that HMPAO concentration underestimates rCBF at high flow rates (5). Lassen et al. have proposed a correction for the effect of HMPAO back-diffusion that can be used to preserve linearity between HMPAO cerebral uptake activity and rCBF (6). This issue may be particularly important when SPECT is performed with HMPAO in conjunction with brain-stimulation paradigms that lead to increased rCBF. This loss of linearity between regional brain tracer activity and rCBF at higher flow rates is also observed, at least to some extent, for the other two radiopharmaceuticals discussed here.

Blood clearance is a relatively slow process for HMPAO. The practical consequence of this is the need to delay SPECT acquisition for at least 1 hour after IV injection of HMPAO. Even with delayed imaging, the brain-to-background (primarily blood) ratio is significantly less for HMPAO than for ECD, by a factor of almost 10 (7). It is also crucial that HMPAO be reconstituted with fresh eluate from the technetium generator to ensure adequate labeling.

For HMPAO, the mechanism of retention is still not completely understood. However, in large part it appears related to the formation in the brain of a polar agent, possibly $TcO_4^-$, which cannot back-diffuse across the BBB (8). Interaction of the HMPAO molecule with the glutathione in the brain cells seems to enhance this process (9). There is evidence that HMPAO may bind with certain cytoplasmic proteins in the brain (8).

## IMP (Iofetamine)

Winchel et al. first described the properties of IMP for use as a brain perfusion agent in 1980 (10). IMP was the first radiopharmaceutical released by the FDA for perfusion brain imaging, but it has now been withdrawn by the manufacturer. Although it is similar in several ways to HMPAO, IMP has certain distinct differences (11). Peak IMP brain activity (see Table 10-2) is not reached until roughly 20 minutes after injection. This delay in peak uptake is related, in part, to rapid initial uptake of IMP by lung tissue, which then acts as a reservoir for IMP release after initial blood levels have fallen (12). In the brain, IMP concentration remains reasonably constant for 20 minutes to 1 hour after administration. Thereafter, a process often referred to as *redistribution* takes place, resulting in a shift in IMP concentration away from brain gray matter toward the white matter. The process of redistribution changes the brain concentration of IMP in such a way that the dependence on blood flow is lost and the distribution of IMP becomes determined primarily by the distribution of amine receptor sites. In the presence of an intact BBB, the redistribution phenomenon occurs principally as a result of both wash-in of IMP from other sites in the body (lungs in particular) and regional wash-out of IMP metabolites from the brain (12,13). The mechanism of brain retention of IMP is entirely different from that for the Tc-99m agents and is based on binding of IMP or IMP metabolites to a variety of different amine receptor sites in viable brain synaptosomes (14,15).

## ECD (Bicisate)

In contrast to HMPAO, ECD is characterized by very rapid clearance from the blood after IV injection. A minor degree of wash-out (back-diffusion) of this agent from the brain takes place in a biexponential pattern. However, the degree of initial back-diffusion is substantially less than with HMPAO, and the brain concentration is virtually constant over 1 hour. At 4 hours postinjection, more than two-thirds of the initial activity of ECD remains in the brain (16). Tc-99m ECD is relatively stable and may be injected up to 4 to 6 hours after the agent has been prepared.

The mechanism of brain retention for the two Tc-99m–labeled agents is somewhat similar. In the case of ECD, the brain retention also depends on the formation of a polar technetium complex that cannot cross the intact BBB. This complex is formed, however, after an enzyme-dependent reaction involving ECD occurs when ECD has entered the brain.

Dosimetry data are presented in Table 10-3 for each of these agents.

**TABLE 10-3.** *Dosimetry for approved cerebral perfusion agents*

| | HMPAO (rads/6 mCi [cGy/222 MBq]) | IMP[a] (rads/20 mCi [cGy/740 MBq]) | ECD (rads/6 mCi [cGy/222MBq]) |
|---|---|---|---|
| Brain | 0.46 | 0.35 | 0.40 |
| Whole body | 0.32 | 0.26 | 0.18 |
| Ovaries | 0.84 | 0.26 | 0.44[b] |
| Thyroid | 2.00[b] | 16.20[b] | 0.26 |

[a] Administration of Lugol's solution or saturated solution of potassium iodide before the study reduces thyroid exposure to <1 rad (1 cGy).
[b] Critical organs.

## SPECT Protocols

It is crucial that the environmental conditions at the time of tracer injection be standardized. It is preferable to have the patient in a room with low-level ambient light and sound, but covering the eyes and ears is not recommended because this yields metabolic asymmetries in the cerebral cortex (17,18). Controlled environmental conditions should be maintained for 3 to 5 minutes before injection of any radiopharmaceutical, at least 4 minutes after injection for HMPAO or ECD, and 15 minutes after injection for IMP. The patient's head should be secured to minimize motion during image acquisition.

Correct timing for the initiation of imaging is crucial for each of these radiopharmaceuticals. Imaging should not be initiated for at least 1 hour after injection of HMPAO to allow for blood clearance of the agent. Hayashida et al. have described the "filling out" phenomenon seen on SPECT images in patients with cerebrovascular disease: Lesion contrast becomes significantly greater with time after injection (19). This is presumably due to a continued fall in HMPAO blood pool activity over time. In contrast, imaging with ECD may be initiated 15 to 20 minutes after injection. For both ECD and HMPAO, imaging may be delayed for at least several hours, if necessary, until a time that is suitable for both the patient and the department. In the case of IMP, perfusion imaging should be carried out 20 to 60 minutes after injection. After this time, IMP activity in the brain no longer reflects rCBF due to redistribution of the agent. Numerous attempts have been made to determine whether the redistribution property of IMP has any clinical utility, but to date none has been found, and the routine acquisition of delayed images is therefore not recommended.

## Detector Systems

In contrast to the older, single-detector systems, multidetector rotating gamma camera systems are highly desirable for SPECT neuroperfusion imaging. With ultra–high-resolution parallel-hole or fanbeam collimators, resolution <1 cm full width at half maximum (FWHM) can be achieved.

Because these collimators have very low sensitivity, they can only be used appropriately with the multidetector devices. Although dedicated neuroimaging SPECT systems yield better resolution, their limited flexibility for performing other imaging studies makes them impractical for most nuclear medicine departments until clinical use becomes widespread.

### Acquisition Parameters

A good rule of thumb to follow is that the sampling size (pixel size) during acquisition of a brain SPECT study should be approximately one-third the system resolution. Hence, for system resolution of 1 cm, the pixel size should be approximately 3 mm. The acquisition matrix size and zoom should be adjusted accordingly. Moreover, angular sampling intervals should also be based on system resolution. The number of angular projections through 360 degrees should be equal to the diameter of the brain in pixels times 3.14. Thus, for 3-mm pixels and a brain diameter of 12 cm, the desirable number of projections would be 40 times 3.14, or approximately 120, that is, 3-degree increments.

### Image Reconstruction

Image reconstruction should be performed, if possible, with a filter that has been selected based on the task for which the SPECT images are to be used. For example, if one wishes to identify small, detailed structures in the brain, filtering is desirable because it yields higher-resolution images. Filters can be assessed systematically for specific aspects of performance using SPECT studies of phantoms. Acquisition of phantoms with both simulated lesions and uniform activity distributions is recommended. In this way, important factors, such as image contrast, spatial resolution, and image noise can be reviewed with each filter. Reconstruction filters (e.g., Butterworth, Parzen, Hann) allow the user to select the amount of smoothing by adjusting filter parameters, such as the cutoff frequency. In general, filters that increase image smoothing also reduce resolution. Conversely, those with less smoothing yield a noisier image of the brain but with greater resolution.

Generally, transverse brain images should be oriented parallel to the canthomeatal line because most published results are presented in this fashion. It is advantageous to use laser alignment devices before acquisition to establish this orientation. If such a device is not available, an alternative postacquisition method can be applied to allow display of transverse images in planes approximately parallel to the canthomeatal line. This method consists of drawing a line from the most inferior aspect of the frontal lobe through the midcerebellum and, by the use of software, creating transverse images parallel to this line.

Attenuation correction may be helpful for enhancing the appearance of subcortical gray-matter structures, such as the thalamus and basal ganglia. In general, commercial software

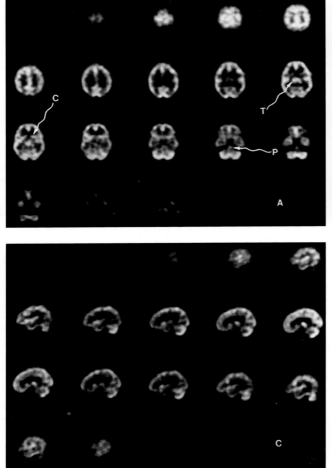

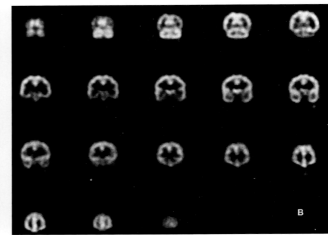

**FIG. 10-1. (A)** Transverse, **(B)** coronal, and **(C)** sagittal SPECT HMPAO images of a normal volunteer. Images were obtained with a triple-detector system using ultra–high-resolution collimators. Structures on transverse images identified by arrows include head of caudate (C), pons (P), and thalamus (T).

allows the user to apply attenuation correction using the Chang method, which assumes a uniform attenuation matrix in the brain, with the user selecting the attenuation coefficient. The efficacy of this type of attenuation correction for improving the diagnostic yield of SPECT has not been established.

### Normal Scan

Normal cerebral distribution is very similar for the three radiopharmaceuticals. The normal HMPAO distribution for the three standard orthogonal planes is shown in Fig. 10-1. If the patient's eyes are open at the time of radiopharmaceutical injection, the most intense region of uptake is seen in the visual cortex in the region of the calcarine fissure. Normal right-left differences in the cerebral cortical activity should be <8% to 10%. This variation depends on the size of the cortical region used in the comparison, larger areas having less side-to-side cortical asymmetry due to pixel averaging. Reconstruction and filtering methods may also influence the degree of asymmetry. The reader is referred to an excellent comparison of normal high-resolution SPECT images with corresponding CT images, including a detailed description of the cross-sectional brain anatomy by Matsuda et al. (20).

### Clinical Applications

#### Acute Cerebrovascular Disease

SPECT neuroimaging is capable of demonstrating abnormalities early in the course of acute cerebral infarction with very high sensitivity that is significantly greater than CT (21,22). Regions of reduced radiopharmaceutical concentration seen on SPECT are often substantially larger than corresponding defects on CT (23). This is probably due to the fact that in patients with infarction, the SPECT defect reflects a combination of infarcted tissue, ischemic tissue beyond the infarct zone, and intrahemispheric diaschisis. In addition, the SPECT defect may appear larger as a result of partial volume effects due to the limited system resolution. Defect contrast in chronic cerebrovascular disease is greatest for IMP, followed by ECD, and then HMPAO (24). The lower reported contrast for HMPAO may be partly due to the fact that HMPAO imaging was often performed at less than the ideal 1 hour postinjection.

In patients with acute neurologic symptoms, SPECT may help to determine in which patients the symptoms will be reversible. SPECT demonstrates perfusion abnormalities in only a fraction of patients who are eventually judged to have a transient ischemic attack (TIA) or reversible ischemic neurologic deficit (RIND). TIAs are defined as clinical events that occur for <24 hours. RINDs are events that occur for 1 to 3 days. Bogousslavsky et al. found that SPECT hypoperfusion that persisted beyond 24 hours after the onset of a TIA indicates a greater risk for developing infarction in the next few days (25).

### Subacute Cerebrovascular Disease

In the subacute period extending from approximately 3 to 15 days postinfarction, SPECT imaging occasionally shows either no decrease in activity or an actual increase in tracer concentration in the region of the infarction (Fig. 10-2). This is the result of luxury perfusion, which represents a regional uncoupling of blood flow and metabolism in which the perfusion exceeds the limited metabolic requirements of the damaged or infarcted tissue. This phenomenon has been described frequently with HMPAO (26) and occasionally with IMP (27); it would theoretically also be seen with ECD. In the subacute phase the concentration of HMPAO in the region of infarction may at times overestimate the degree of actual cerebral perfusion, making the relationship between this increased HMPAO activity and luxury perfusion less clear (28). As a consequence of luxury perfusion, the sensitivity of SPECT

imaging for cerebral infarction, particularly when using HMPAO, may be reduced during the subacute phase.

Diaschisis is a phenomenon in which reduced afferent input (often as a result of infarction) to a region of the brain leads to diminished metabolism in that area and, consequently, reduced perfusion. The specific condition of cerebellar diaschisis is often seen on SPECT images as reduced activity in the cerebellar hemisphere opposite the side of the cortical infarction. Cerebellar diaschisis may be a useful sign to look for in cases where luxury perfusion has rendered the cortical infarct undetectable. Reduced cerebellar activity has also been demonstrated on SPECT images in the setting of vertebral or basilar disease with ischemia or infarction of the cerebellum (29).

### Prognosis in Cerebrovascular Disease

Studies have demonstrated that SPECT imaging is useful for predicting recovery in patients with acute cerebral infarction (30,31); this prognostication is best early in the stroke evolution. There is good evidence that larger or more severe early neuroperfusion SPECT defects predict a poor prognosis (30,31). In patients studied within the first 6 hours, the severity of the defect seen on HMPAO images correlated well with long-term outcome (32). If the HMPAO defect is larger than the hypodense lesion seen on x-ray CT, the potential for recovery appears to be good (33). Lesion location also seems to be important for prognosis (34).

It has been suggested that the late distribution of IMP reflects viable brain tissue and may relate to recovery of neurologic function (35). In chronic infarct, studies have described a central decreased zone of IMP uptake corresponding to a hypodense lesion on CT. A peripheral surrounding zone that is normal on CT has also been described (36). The central zone shows severely reduced IMP activity on both early and delayed images, whereas the peripheral zone shows moderately reduced early IMP activity but normal delayed IMP concentration. This peripheral zone may reflect a penumbra of underperfused or ischemic tissue, which could potentially benefit from interventions designed to improve flow to the jeopardized region. Although redistribution of IMP appears to be an interesting phenomenon, it remains to be determined whether it will be useful for predicting stroke outcome.

### Cerebrovascular Reserve

The degree of anatomic narrowing found in a carotid stenosis does not correlate well with the hemodynamic severity of the lesion (37). The pressure gradient associated with a stenosis in the carotid leads to distal arteriolar dilatation through a process known as *cerebral autoregulation*. Consequently, the magnitude of arteriolar vasodilatation represents an indicator of the hemodynamic severity of carotid stenosis modified by the presence and extent of collateral circulation.

Measurement of the degree of arteriolar vasodilatation may identify patients with carotid stenosis who are at risk

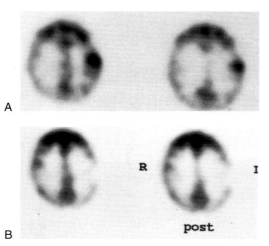

**FIG. 10-2.** Adjacent transverse SPECT/HMPAO image slices from a patient with sudden onset of right hemiparesis and hemianesthesia. **(A)** The initial SPECT images obtained approximately 1 week after onset of symptoms show a large area of intense HMPAO activity in the left parietal region, indicating the presence of luxury perfusion. **(B)** Repeat SPECT images 7 weeks later show a photopenic defect at that site. The initial CT obtained at the time of onset of symptoms was essentially normal.

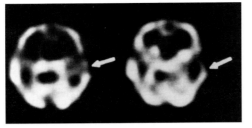

**FIG. 10-3.** SPECT HMPAO images in an elderly male patient, with >75% stenosis of the left carotid artery and a similar degree of narrowing of the right carotid, who was experiencing TIAs in the distribution of the left middle cerebral artery. SPECT images obtained with acetazolamide demonstrate, in two adjacent transverse slices, impairment of perfusion reserve in the left temporoparietal area (*arrows*), suggesting hemodynamically significant stenosis of the left carotid with inadequate collateral supply to this region. The baseline study showed symmetric left and right perfusion (not shown).

for developing hemodynamic or low-flow cerebral ischemic events (38). One method of assessing the degree of regional cerebral vasodilatation is to determine the response of CBF to an exogenously administered cerebral vasodilator. The degree of increase in rCBF in response to such an agent reflects the reserve vasodilating capacity of the distal arterioles and may be used as an indicator of the hemodynamic severity of a large-vessel stenosis.

Both carbon dioxide ($CO_2$) and acetazolamide (Diamox) have been successfully used as vasodilators in conjunction with SPECT for evaluation of brain perfusion (vasodilatation) reserve (39,40). Acetazolamide is somewhat easier to use. Acetazolamide is a carbonic anhydrase inhibitor that causes cerebral vasodilatation, probably by reducing the pH in brain tissue. Increases in rCBF of 30% to 50% approximately 20 minutes after IV injection of acetazolamide are typical in normal subjects (41,42). In many instances, patients with significant carotid stenosis have normal "resting" rCBF patterns, and only after administration of the vasodilator does an asymmetry in perfusion appear (Fig. 10-3) (40).

In clinical practice, Diamox protocol consists of administering 1 g IV Diamox, followed 20 minutes later by the radiopharmaceutical. It is essential that a baseline cerebral perfusion study be performed for purposes of comparison. This is often accomplished by a separate study on a different day, although an alternative method has been proposed that allows the completion of both studies on the same day: A small dose of HMPAO is administered for the first (baseline) study (5 to 15 mCi [185 to 555 MBq]) and a larger dose (20 to 25 mCi [740 to 925 MBq]) for the second (Diamox) study. Image subtraction of the first study from the second yields the distribution of HMPAO associated with Diamox (43).

As an alternative to performing two HMPAO imaging studies on the same day, the dual radioisotope technique pioneered by Devous et al. has been used (44). Tc-99m HMPAO and I-123 IMP are administered sequentially during the baseline and Diamox-stimulation states, respectively, and the distributions of both tracers are then recorded for the two conditions by simultaneous SPECT imaging of the gamma emissions from both agents (44). The protocol consists of administering HMPAO during resting conditions, followed 5 to 10 minutes later by IV injection of the Diamox. Twenty minutes later, IMP is given. The primary advantages of this approach are that it allows completion of the entire procedure in <2 hours and that it yields precise anatomic coregistration of the two SPECT data sets, which is very helpful in the identification of smaller and less obvious asymmetries. For the identification of bilateral symmetric impairment in brain perfusion reserve, quantification of the relative (baseline to Diamox), perfusion change necessitates use of the same radiopharmaceutical (39,45).

The dual isotope technique is most reliable when used in conjunction with the newer SPECT imaging systems with very good energy resolution (<10% FWHM). Using a triple-detector machine (PRISM 3000, Picker International, Cleveland, OH) with a 15% window centered at 140 keV for Tc-99m and a 10% window asymmetric to the high side of 159 keV for I-123, Devous et al. have found that approximately 95% of observed counts came from the gamma emissions for which the window was intended (46). This finding confirms that the technique can be applied successfully without correction for cross-talk between the two radionuclides' photopeaks.

### Cranial Bypass Surgery Assessment

Imaging studies with Diamox performed before and after extracranial or intracranial bypass surgery have demonstrated normalization of perfusion reserve abnormalities after the bypass procedure (47). It has been proposed that carotid stenoses may be classified by the severity of the hemodynamic changes to aid in the selection of patients who might benefit from surgical bypass procedure (48). Studies using HMPAO for both baseline and $CO_2$ inhalation intervention imaging found impaired ipsilateral and sometimes bilateral perfusion reserve in patients with severe unilateral carotid stenosis (45). Another study found good correlation between the degree of perfusion reserve measured by HMPAO with Diamox and the degree of collateral flow, as measured by other techniques (49). Although clarification of the appropriate role of SPECT perfusion reserve imaging in management of patients with occlusive cerebrovascular disease awaits further study, the possibility that this technique will be helpful in predicting low-flow ischemic events appears promising.

### Vasospasm in Subarachnoid Hemorrhage

Ischemia due to cerebral vasospasm represents a major cause of morbidity and mortality following subarachnoid hemorrhage. Identification of reduced cerebral perfusion with SPECT can be used to identify vasospasm, and several studies have indicated the value of SPECT in this setting (50). Soucy et al. found excellent correlation between angiographic evidence for vasospasm and the presence of HMPAO perfusion defects in patients with subarachnoid hemorrhage (51). The ability of SPECT to differentiate early vasospasm from rebleeding as an explanation for the neurologic symptoms can help direct appropriate treatment.

### Carotid Sacrifice Assessment

For patients being considered for surgical ligation of a carotid artery, typically as part of a procedure to remove a locally invasive head and neck tumor, it is important to know the risk of ischemic neurologic sequelae. Preoperative balloon occlusion testing of the carotid artery to be sacrificed has been useful in assessing this risk. Patients who experience neurologic symptoms during the balloon occlusion procedure are not considered acceptable candidates for carotid ligation due to the high risk of ischemic complications. However, the risk may also be high in those who experience no neurologic symptoms during balloon occlusion testing. Studies have demonstrated the efficacy of risk assessment by evaluating perfusion in the territory of the carotid artery with HMPAO injected during carotid test occlusion (52,53).

It is generally accepted that SPECT images that reveal a normal pattern of rCBF distal to the test occlusion site indicate a very low risk of ischemic sequelae after permanent carotid ligation. However, the risk for individuals who demonstrate no neurologic symptoms but show reduced

cerebral perfusion during the occlusion procedure is not as well defined (54). Although some think that the finding indicates increased risk of ischemic neurologic sequelae after ligation, this may not be true for all individuals in this category (55). It may be that the severity of reduced perfusion seen with HMPAO after balloon occlusion, or other indicators of reduced neurologic activity in the affected hemisphere (e.g., crossed cerebellar diaschisis), may be helpful in identifying individuals at greatest risk (Fig. 10-4). It should be stressed that when evaluating results from a balloon occlusion SPECT study, baseline imaging is vital to exclude preexisting abnormalities in the pattern of rCBF. The dual isotope method discussed above may be ideally suited for this purpose.

### Psychiatric Applications

Abnormalities may be present on neuroperfusion SPECT images in various psychiatric disorders. In general, findings with SPECT seem to corroborate earlier results obtained with PET. It is anticipated that these findings will eventually lead to a better understanding of psychiatric disease and improve specific treatments.

### Depression

Psychiatrists often face the problem of distinguishing dementia with secondary depression from depression with pseudodementia. Because abnormalities seen with SPECT in Alzheimer's disease are typically different from the pat-

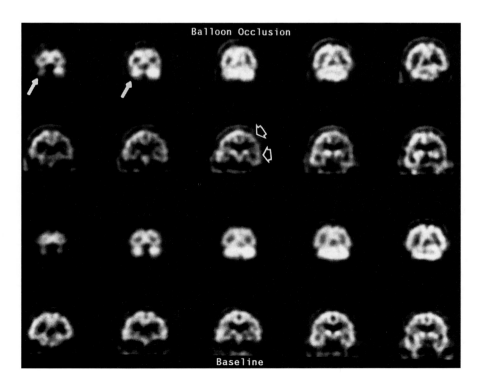

**FIG. 10-4.** These scan images show coronal SPECT HMPAO images (posterior hemisphere and cerebellum upper left, midcerebral hemisphere lower right) obtained during a left carotid artery balloon occlusion test (two upper rows) and again at baseline several days later (two lower rows). The patient was to have a resection of a squamous cell tumor of his neck that would require permanent ligation of the left carotid artery. Because the SPECT images showed a large region of diminished perfusion in the left temporal and parietal regions (*open arrows*), it was felt he would be at increased risk of ischemic neurologic sequelae after ligation. The balloon occlusion images also show cerebellar diaschisis (*solid arrows*) and that the baseline images have a pattern of normal flow distribution in both the cortex and cerebellum. Consequently, the patient underwent a prophylactic bypass procedure before tumor resection and carotid sacrifice. Despite the bypass graft, the patient experienced transient ischemic neurologic symptoms in the distribution of the ligated carotid artery that lasted for several days after the surgery.

tern seen with depression, SPECT can be readily applied to this problem. Individuals with depressive disorders manifest various abnormalities on SPECT perfusion images: Late-onset depression appears to manifest global reductions in cerebral perfusion (56), whereas unipolar depression includes reduced perfusion in the left frontal region and perfusion abnormalities in the temporal lobes (57). These results suggest that there are SPECT perfusion changes in patients with depression distinct from the typical bitemporoparietal defects of Alzheimer's disease.

### Schizophrenia

Perfusion abnormalities have been described in schizophrenic patients in the frontal and temporal lobes and the basal ganglia (58). Some individuals with schizophrenia demonstrate diminished bifrontal perfusion and metabolism (59), and others manifest normal frontal lobe perfusion (60). Actively psychotic schizophrenic patients show increases in perfusion in the prefrontal cortex (61). Certain schizophrenics may lack the ability to activate their frontal lobes in response to cognitive challenges, such as the Wisconsin Card Sort Task (62). Frontal lobe hypoperfusion abnormalities appear to be associated primarily with "negative" symptoms, such as diminution of spontaneity of verbal expression (63). Regions of hyperperfusion in the basal ganglia have been described in schizophrenic patients who manifest primarily "positive" symptomatology, such as delusions or hallucinations (58). Focal hyperperfusion has also been described in the hippocampal region of the left temporal lobe when HMPAO is injected during auditory hallucinations (64).

### Brain Trauma

Although CT remains the standard imaging procedure for assessment of patients with head trauma, many patients have abnormalities on SPECT images in the absence of CT findings (65), especially in minor head trauma. Regions of SPECT hypoperfusion tend to be larger in anatomic extent and appear earlier than corresponding abnormalities on CT. There have been reports of CT lesions in which SPECT results showed that the rCBF was similar to surrounding unaffected brain tissue, a condition not unlike luxury perfusion in cerebral infarction (66). As yet, the clinical importance of this finding has not been determined. There is preliminary evidence that the severity of SPECT defects may predict clinical outcome in patients with head trauma (67), in which case SPECT may play an important role in head trauma management.

### Activation Imaging

Because SPECT measures rCBF and, indirectly, cerebral metabolic activity, it holds potential for evaluating the cere-

bral response to various exogenous stimuli. Using HMPAO, Woods et al. demonstrated a mean increase in cerebral perfusion of 37% in the visual cortex of normal volunteers during a stimulation paradigm consisting of stroboscopic white light (68). Normal subjects imaged during activation and baseline conditions demonstrated a 26% increase in perfusion in the contralateral motor cortex in response to voluntary hand movement (69). Other investigators have used SPECT to demonstrate focal sites of brain activation in normal subjects in response to auditory stimulation (70,71).

Activation studies with SPECT have been successfully performed in patients with cerebral infarction to identify tissue in the region of infarction that retained the ability to respond to appropriate stimuli (72). A study of particular importance in emphasizing the potential clinical utility of activation brain imaging was recently reported by Chollet et al. (73), who measured rCBF using positron emission tomography (PET) in patients with cerebral infarction and hemiparesis. Individuals with good recovery demonstrated activation in the ipsilateral motor cortex during a hand movement paradigm. Studies such as this suggest that the ability to measure brain activation may ultimately be a key that opens the door to future clinical applications for brain SPECT. Although most investigators have performed baseline and activation imaging on different days, the dual radioisotope method with IMP and HMPAO can be used to image activation and baseline states simultaneously. Data suggest that this technique can identify focal cortical activation increases of 10%, providing that the activation focus is of sufficient size.

### Epilepsy

Seizure disorders are a common medical problem. One 1965 study reported the prevalence of epilepsy in Rochester, Minnesota, to be 5.7 per 1,000 people (74). Although the majority of seizures can be controlled with drug therapy, it has been estimated that 10% to 20% of patients who develop epilepsy each year have "medically intractable epilepsy" (75). An important part of the medical workup of these patients is to characterize the seizure type and localize the seizure focus because a significant proportion may benefit from surgical resection of the focus. The workup of these patients includes CT and MRI to identify an anatomic cause for the seizures. Physiologic imaging includes SPECT evaluation of CBF and PET imaging of flow and metabolism.

Most SPECT cerebral perfusion imaging in patients with epilepsy has been performed with patients in the interictal state, when the seizure focus is usually hypoperfused relative to normal brain (Fig. 10-5). Rowe et al. performed both visual and quantitative analysis of SPECT brain perfusion examinations using HMPAO. Using visual analysis, ipsilateral temporal lobe hypoperfusion was identified in the interictal state in 18 of the 46 (39%) patients with a unilateral focus, and contralateral hypoperfusion was seen in three of

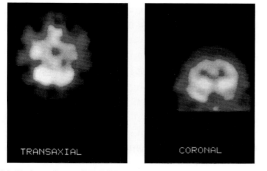

**FIG. 10-5.** Interictal SPECT cerebral perfusion examination using HMPAO in a patient with medically intractable partial complex epilepsy. The selected transaxial and coronal planes demonstrate hypoperfusion of the left temporal lobe.

all 51 (6%) patients with temporal lobe epilepsy. Quantified analysis of temporal lobe asymmetry improved this result by correctly localizing a unilateral seizure focus in 22 (48%) of those patients, but the wrong side was localized in five of all 51 (10%) patients (76). Improved interictal results have been reported using an IMP-like tracer, hydroxymethyliodobenzylproprane diamine (HIPDM). In one such investigation, 24 of 33 patients (73%) had decreased regional cerebral perfusion identified on the same side as the subsequent surgical treatment (77).

In an attempt to improve seizure localization, some investigators have studied patients in the ictal state. During the seizure, perfusion and metabolism of the seizure focus are significantly increased, and SPECT imaging is able to identify the seizure focus as an area of hyperperfusion. Very useful information about the seizure focus, not available from the interictal study alone, may be obtained from ictal studies. Lee and coworkers performed both interictal and ictal SPECT scans on 16 patients with medically intractable complex partial seizures (78). The interictal study correctly localized 56% of the seizure foci, whereas the ictal study localized the seizure focus in 87%, confirming that the ictal procedure was superior.

The addition of the postictal study (when the radiotracer was injected an average of 5 minutes after seizure onset) to the interictal examination has also been shown to improve test accuracy. In a series of 32 patients with intractable complex partial seizures, the interictal scan localized the focus in 53%. The combination of the interictal and postictal scans improved correct seizure focus localization to 72% (79). Adams et al. also reported that the postictal scans added more information than the interictal examinations, and that the best localization occurred when interictal and postictal scans were combined (80).

Ictal studies are technically more difficult to perform than the interictal examinations. The coordination of personnel and radiotracer so that the radiopharmaceutical can be administered at the time of seizure onset is very difficult. Newton and coworkers were able to overcome part of the complexity of the ictal SPECT scan by using a method of rapid radiopharmaceutical preparation and quality control in the preparation of HMPAO, thus establishing the ictal SPECT scan as best (81):

- Ictal scan (n = 51), 97% correct
- Postictal (n = 77), 71% correct
- Interictal (n = 119), 48% correct

It has been suggested that the SPECT perfusion scan may also provide useful information about brain development and maturation in children with idiopathic seizures (82) and about long-term prognosis in patients with intractable seizures and unilateral hemiparesis secondary to hemimegalencephaly (83). This method may also help to explain alternating hemiplegia in which an atypical form of epilepsy is the proposed etiology (84,85).

### Dementia

The differential diagnosis of patients with dementia includes a variety of neurologic diseases:

- Alzheimer's disease
- Pick's disease
- Multi-infarct dementia
- Parkinson's disease
- Progressive supranuclear palsy
- Huntington's disease
- Normal pressure hydrocephalus
- Creutzfeldt-Jakob disease

During life, it may be difficult to accurately diagnose the etiology of the dementia (86) because of the nonspecific clinical presentation of these neurologic disorders, especially early in the disease. The initial workup of these patients includes investigation of a treatable medical cause, such as hypothyroidism, vitamin $B_{12}$ deficiency, thiamine deficiency, progressive multifocal leukoencephalopathy, or neoplasms (87). After possible medical causes of the dementia have been dismissed, a variety of neurodegenerative diseases should be considered. The workup should include anatomic brain imaging (CT or MRI) to exclude a neoplasm or subdural hematoma and to evaluate ventricular size. Although the clinical role of SPECT cerebral perfusion imaging is not yet clearly defined, patterns of abnormal CBF are emerging that are peculiar to specific neurologic disorders. Bonte and coworkers examined the patterns of rCBF in 247 patients with a history of dementia. In 18 patients, the SPECT scan was correlated with clinical and histopathologic diagnosis. Visual interpretation of scans diagnosed 11 of 13 Alzheimer's disease patients and was correct overall in 13 of the 18 patients (88).

### Alzheimer's Disease

Alzheimer's disease is one of the most common causes of dementia and has received the majority of recent attention in

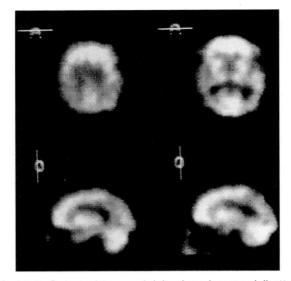

**FIG. 10-6.** Selected transaxial (top) and coronal (bottom) images from a SPECT HMPAO examination in a 73-year-old male with dementia. Note the hypoperfusion of the parietal lobes bilaterally, extending into the temporal lobes. Perfusion is relatively preserved in the occipital and frontal regions of the brain. This scan pattern is consistent with Alzheimer's disease.

the literature. A pattern of decreased CBF in the posterior temporal and parietal region bilaterally is the most common abnormality reported. It is usually bilateral and may be symmetric or asymmetric in its involvement of the brain (89). Many patients also have decreased frontal lobe perfusion.

Various authors have reported similar perfusion deficits in the parietal and temporoparietal regions of the brain in patients with Alzheimer's disease using SPECT (Fig. 10-6), with varying sensitivity and specificity (90). Gemmell et al. (91) reported bilateral temporoparietal perfusion defects in patients with senile dementia of the Alzheimer type (SDAT), but this was the only abnormal feature in 10 of 35 cases (29%). Nearly half (46%) of these patients also had frontal perfusion defects, and 26% did not have bilateral temporoparietal perfusion defects, but these tended to be the least impaired patients. These findings were not specific because similar patterns were also present in multi-infarct dementia (n = 2) and Parkinson's disease (n = 2).

Holman and coworkers (92) prospectively investigated SPECT brain perfusion using HMPAO in 132 consecutive patients with memory or cognitive impairment (52 with Alzheimer's disease). The probability for Alzheimer's disease in various cortical scan patterns was as follows:

- 82% with bilateral posterior temporal or parietal defects only
- 77% with bilateral posterior temporal or parietal defects with additional defects
- 57% with unilateral posterior temporal or parietal cortical defects with or without additional defects

It is important to note that they also reported similar cerebral perfusion deficits in patients with Parkinson's disease associated with dementia (92).

As a more objective way of evaluating the SPECT scans, Hellman et al. (93) developed a semiquantitative method of image analysis. Visual interpretation was compared with manually placed and semiautomatically placed regions of interest. In this small group of SDAT patients, the semiquantitative technique demonstrated temporoparietal decreases in patients in whom the frontal activity was obviously decreased but temporoparietal regions were equivocal on visual analysis (93).

### Other Dementias

Important information about rCBF in other causes of dementia has also been reported. Although results are preliminary at this point, specific patterns are emerging. In patients with multi-infarct dementia, CBF images may demonstrate multiple regions of diminished rCBF (91,94). Reduced CBF has been found in the heads of the caudate nuclei in patients with Huntington's disease (91). Frontal lobe hypoperfusion has been reported in progressive supranuclear palsy and may be especially severe in Pick's disease (89).

### Other Agents in Dementia

Another promising imaging method that may be able to identify patients with dementia involves imaging the cerebral muscarinic receptors using I-123 3-quinuclidinyl-4-iodobenzilate (QNB). Preliminary work has found decreased QNB uptake in the frontal and temporoparietal cortex in patients with the clinical diagnosis of Alzheimer's disease and decreased QNB uptake in the frontal lobes of patients thought to have Pick's disease (95). Others reported similar findings of cortical defects in either frontal or posterior temporal cortex in patients with a diagnosis of Alzheimer's disease, or frontal and anterior temporal defects in patients with the clinical diagnosis of Pick's disease (96).

### Summary

Physiologic imaging of the brain using SPECT techniques will likely play an important role in accurately identifying the cause of dementia. Improvements in hardware and software and introduction of new radiopharmaceuticals will undoubtedly improve the diagnostic accuracy of this method.

## CNS TUMOR IMAGING

Patients being investigated for CNS tumors are usually diagnosed using anatomic imaging. Physiologic imaging is reserved for patients with recurrent symptoms after treatment. Patients with neurologic symptoms due to either recurrent brain tumor or radionecrosis often present with similar signs and symptoms. Anatomic modalities, such as CT and MRI, are often unable to define whether the anatomic changes are due to the prior surgery and radiation therapy or the result of recurrent tumor. Physiologic imaging methods, such as SPECT and PET, have become the most accurate method of identifying recurrent tumor in these patients.

## Thallium 201

One of the best-studied radiotracers for the evaluation of recurrent brain tumors is thallium 201 thallous chloride (Tl-201). Tl-201 is a potassium analog, and its concentration in tumors is related to the CBF, disruption of the BBB, and cell membrane sodium-potassium adenosine triphosphatase activity (97). The technique is relatively simple, and a common protocol is to begin SPECT imaging 5 minutes after the IV administration of 4 mCi (108 MBq) Tl-201.

In an attempt to determine if radionuclides could accurately detect viable tumor in patients with primary brain tumors, Kaplan et al. (98) examined the use of Tl-201, Tc-99m glucoheptonate, and Ga-67 citrate in 29 patients with grade III or IV malignant gliomas. Autopsy correlation was available in seven patients and demonstrated close correlation between Tl-201 activity and the presence of tumor (98). Others have shown that the Tl-201 tumor-cardiac ratio more accurately reflects the clinical status during follow-up than the CT scan (99).

### Tumor Grade

The Tl-201 imaging technique can also be used to determine if a lesion is high or low grade. In a series of 25 patients with gliomas, classified as having low-grade (grade I and II) or high-grade (grade III or IV) malignancy, the Tl-201 index was computed. They reported an accuracy of 89% using a Tl-201 index cutoff of 1.5 (100). In a study relating Tl-201 lesion uptake with the proliferative activity of neoplastic tissue, as evidenced by bromodeoxyuridine, a significant correlation was seen, indicating that Tl-201 uptake was in part related to proliferative activity and determined by tumor grade (101).

### Tumor Recurrence Versus Treatment Necrosis

Increased Tl-201 uptake occurs in viable malignant tumors but not in patients with radiation necrosis (102). High Tl-201 uptake is usually found in recurrent tumor, but low-grade uptake or no significant uptake over background is seen with radiation necrosis (Fig. 10-7). However, the interpretation of moderate uptake of thallium 201 into an area of previous radiation therapy for a brain tumor has yet to be determined.

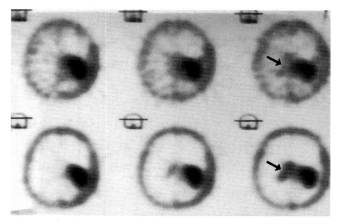

**FIG. 10-7.** Selected transaxial images of a brain SPECT examination using Tl-201 (top) and Tc-99m sestamibi (bottom) in a 12-year-old patient with a glioblastoma multiforme, after surgical resection, chemotherapy, and radiation therapy. High uptake of radiotracer is apparent on both studies, consistent with recurrent tumor. Note the significant uptake of Tc-99m sestamibi in the choroid plexus (*arrows*), which is much less apparent on the Tl-201 images.

## Tc-99m HMPAO and Tl-201 SPECT

In one series of 15 patients with high-grade gliomas and progressively worsening symptoms after radiotherapy, HMPAO and Tl-201 SPECT scans were used to identify tumor recurrence. Eight patients had moderate Tl-201 uptake (compared to contralateral maximal scalp activity), four of these patients had increased or similar HMPAO perfusion when compared to normal brain, and four had decreased perfusion. Those with hypoperfusion showed reactive changes and no evidence of tumor recurrence, and three of four with either normal or increased perfusion had tumor recurrence. These findings suggest that a cerebral perfusion agent may be helpful in evaluating patients with a moderate degree of Tl-201 uptake (103).

## Tc-99m Sestamibi

To improve the accuracy of the identification of viable brain tumor, Tc-99m-methoxyisobutylisonitrile (MIBI; generic name sestamibi) has been advocated in place of Tl-201. Tc-99m sestamibi is readily available in kit form and has the advantages of a Tc-99m radiopharmaceutical: improved availability, larger administered doses, and imaging characteristics that are better suited for a gamma camera. In a series of 19 children with brain tumors, the sensitivity was 67% for both Tl-201 and Tc-99m sestamibi SPECT, with a 91% specificity for Tl-201 and 100% specificity for Tc-99m sestamibi (104). Furthermore, the "growing edge" of the tumor was felt to be more clearly defined with TC-99m sestamibi (104). Both tracers were excluded from normal cerebral tissues, but there was significant Tc-99m sestamibi uptake by the normal choroid plexus (see Fig. 10-7), which persisted despite the administration of 6 mg/kg oral potassium per-

**TABLE 10-4.** *Dosimetry of CSF studies with In-111 DTPA and Tc-99m DTPA*

|  | In-111 DTPA (rads/500 µCi [cGy/18.5 MBq]) | Tc-99m DTPA (rads/mCi [cGy/37 MBq]) |
| --- | --- | --- |
| Spinal cord | 5.00* | 1.333* |
| Brain surface | 4.10 | 0.990 |
| Bladder 2-hr void | 2.10 | 0.047 |
| 4.8-hr void | 5.00* | 0.093 |
| Total body | 0.04 | 0.012 |

*Critical organs (note how void interval affects bladder dosimetry).

chlorate. Choroid plexus uptake of Tl-201 also occurred but was less apparent than Tc-99m sestamibi.

### Summary

Physiologic imaging of brain tumors using either Tl-201 or Tc-99m sestamibi adds clinically useful information regarding tumor viability, patient prognosis, and tumor grading. If a biopsy is needed to determine the presence of viable tumor, these procedures can guide the biopsy to the site most likely to yield important information.

## CEREBROSPINAL FLUID STUDIES

The study of cerebrospinal fluid (CSF) pathways has been accomplished with many radiopharmaceuticals, and this history parallels that of brain scanning in the late 1960s. The first radionuclide test to study CSF flow was used in 1962. In 1964, I-131 human serum albumin (HSA) was first used by Di Chiro. Later, it was extended to shunt evaluations.

### Radiopharmaceuticals

I-131 HSA provided a high–specific activity ligand, and the procedure was safe. When >4 mg HSA was used, there was potential for the development of aseptic meningitis. Various other agents were introduced, but with the availability of indium 111 (In-111) and Tc-99m DTPA, all have been replaced: In-111 DTPA for CSF flow studies over 2 or 3 days and Tc-99m DTPA for studies with shorter time periods (e.g., CSF shunt evaluations and leak studies). Dosimetry is supplied in Table 10-4.

### Scanning Types

#### CSF Shunt Evaluation

Patients with enlarged ventricles may be shunted in an attempt to decrease the symptoms related to the increased CSF pressure and hydrocephalus. Various types of shunts

have been used in the past, including ventriculoatrial and ventriculoperitoneal shunts. Mental status deterioration in a patient with a shunt may indicate shunt malfunction and is not an uncommon event. In a review of the medical records and radiographs of 242 patients with 350 ventriculoperitoneal shunts, 90 complications (25.7%) were found involving the abdominal end of the shunt. The incidence of proximal (ventricular) complications is lower (105).

Obstruction of the shunt may be difficult to diagnose on clinical grounds alone. Imaging procedures, including CT scanning, should be done to establish ventricular enlargement. A physiologic imaging procedure proven to add important information regarding shunt function is the CSF shunt examination. One of the earliest attempts at evaluating function of surgical CSF shunts was reported by Di Chiro and Grove in 1966 (106). Using I-131 HSA and Tc-99m pertechnetate as radiotracers, they were able to successfully evaluate the function of surgical CSF shunts. Over time, changes in the basic method have occurred, although current techniques are still based on the general principle of evaluating the flow of radiotracer from the ventricular

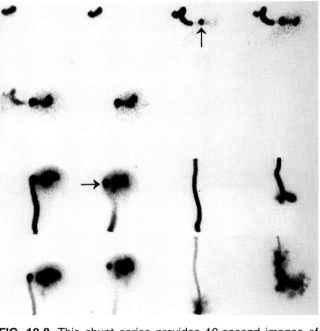

**FIG. 10-8.** This shunt series provides 10-second images of injection of tracer into the reservoir (top two rows). The next row shows 2-minute images obtained immediately after the 1-minute flow study, and these views (lateral head view on left, anterior head view next, shunt tubing in chest next, and shunt tubing in abdomen on right) are repeated 20 minutes later (bottom row). In the flow study, the injection tubing only is seen in the first two frames, the reservoir (*arrow*) is seen in the third frame, and the ventricles in the last three frames. The immediate delayed images show the ventricles, reservoir (*arrow*), and the shunt tubing in the neck, chest (second from right), and abdomen (right image). At 20 minutes the ventricles remain well displayed, the shunt tubing is cleared somewhat, and considerable free spill of tracer is seen in the abdomen.

(proximal) side of the shunt system to the distal (abdominal or cardiac) draining side.

### Scan Protocol

The CSF shunt patency examination involves injecting the proximal portion of the shunt with a small amount of radiotracer (Tc-99m DTPA) while the distal part of the shunt is occluded. Passage of tracer into the ventricle confirms patency of the proximal (ventricular) end. Both ventricles are usually visualized. Descent of radiotracer down the distal shunt, with free entry into the abdomen, confirms patency of the distal (abdominal) part of the shunt (Fig. 10-8). Problems occurring at the distal aspect of the shunt, such as fluid loculation, are seen as a collection of radiotracer that does not spontaneously spread throughout the abdomen nor disperse with changes in patient positioning (107).

The variables that determine the time for clearance from a shunt system include the amount of CSF removed at time of tracer injection, rate of CSF production, CSF circulation through normal pathways, resting ventricular pressure, patient position before test, CSF opening pressure, length of tubing, and changes in ventricular pressure secondary to crying, straining, or coughing.

### Abnormal Scans

When tracer does not flow down the distal limb of the shunt system from the reservoir, and when CSF is obtained and a normal ventricular pressure measured, or tracer flows into the ventricles (Fig. 10-9), then distal obstruction is likely. When this pattern is seen, manipulations to reduce the false-positive rate (approximately half of all abnormal scans) should be undertaken. These include changing the patient position and pumping the reservoir, although there is concern that such manipulations may overcome partial obstructions. *Deceptive patency* describes a patent shunt with inadequate capacity to function properly at all times.

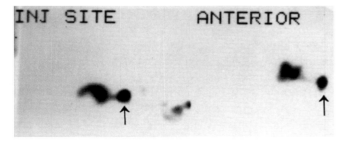

**FIG. 10-9.** In this ventriculoperitoneal shunt patency examination, the radiotracer is present in the reservoir (*arrows*) and lateral ventricles (lateral view on left, anterior view on right) after injection, but it did not enter the distal shunt tubing or the abdomen on the delayed images. The central activity is extracranial and in the injection tubing. This scan pattern is consistent with a distal shunt obstruction.

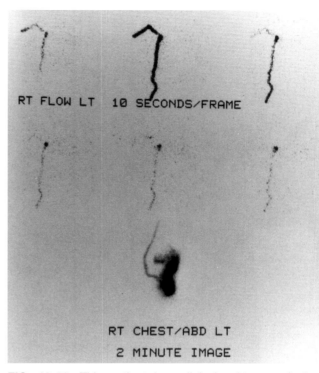

**FIG. 10-10.** This patient has clinical evidence of shunt obstruction. The shunt series shows rapid passage of tracer down the shunt tubing (upper six head and neck injection images) with nearly complete clearance of the reservoir and shunt tubing but no ventricular filling. The lower delayed chest and abdomen image shows free spill of tracer into the abdominal cavity.

Forty percent (23 of 57) of cases shown to be patent by the above means were classified as showing deceptive patency (108). Distal obstruction occurs in approximately two-thirds of all obstructions. Obstruction patterns that should be sought include disconnection of tubing (local extravasation at reservoir or pump mechanism), tubing fracture (local extravasation or delay in tracer passage along tubing), tubing kinking (usually in the patient's neck), tubing migration out of the peritoneal cavity, pseudocyst formation at the peritoneal end of tubing, and obstruction to the tubing at any site.

Obstruction on the ventricular side of the shunt is suggested by inability to aspirate CSF, CSF pressure measurement not possible, and absence of ventricular entry of tracer (Fig. 10-10). If the shunt device has a flap valve, and if the tracer is introduced distal to this valve, tracer does not automatically pass into the ventricles. It is critical to understand the type and mechanism of the implanted shunt to recognize this possibility and to encourage ventricular filling by attempting to occlude the proximal portion of the shunt tubing in the neck during injection. If, on the first attempt, tracer is seen to pass only into the abdomen, the injection needle can be repositioned a little more deeply (through the flap valve if present) and tracer reinjected

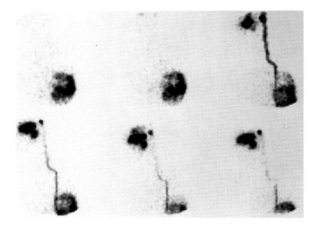

**FIG. 10-11.** This is a six-view reinjection flow study of the head, chest, and abdomen in an infant. Tracer in the abdomen (upper left) is from the prior study, performed minutes earlier, in which ventricular filling was not identified. After repositioning of the butterfly needle, a second dose was injected. The reservoir and tubing are again visualized, reconfirming distal patency, and the ventricles are now visualized during the injection (third frame), thus also establishing ventricular patency.

(Fig. 10-11). Proximal (ventricular) obstruction results from ventricular tubing displacement from the shunt reservoir, obstruction by a fibrin plug, and local encystment. Once tracer reaches the ventricles, it should diffuse into both lateral ventricles normally; if that does not occur, local encystment is a possibility.

In our institution, this test is performed only 10 times per year, but it accounted for most of our peer review interpretive discrepancies until rigorous attention to technical detail was enforced and standardized protocols strictly followed.

*Clinical Applications*

Inaccurate interpretation of the procedure may be due to varying CSF pressure when the shunt study is performed. If the examination is performed only with the patient in the supine position, the CSF pressure may not be high enough to demonstrate flow through the shunt because many patients may have been sitting or standing just before the test; thus, a false positive results. To overcome this problem, CSF flow estimations should be obtained in the supine and erect positions, with the patient being supine for at least 2 hours before the test. A time-activity curve can be generated from the region of the valve chamber if small volumes of tracer are instilled to measure CSF flow rates through the shunt mechanism. In one patient series, flow rates in the supine position were considered normal if >0.1 ml per minute. If flow was slower than this in the supine position, the patient was imaged while sitting up. In a series of 84 examinations performed because of recent deterioration of the patient's

condition, surgical shunt revision resolved the problem in all 59 patients when flow was abnormal in both positions. In the nine cases in which flow became normal in the upright position, four patients spontaneously improved clinically and the CT scan remained unchanged, and five patients continued to deteriorate and required surgical shunt revision. In the 16 examinations showing adequate flow, two patients with continued clinical deterioration demonstrated intermittent obstruction on repeat studies; the other 14 did not require surgical correction (109).

Graham et al. (110) examined 192 shunt patency examinations, of which 140 were ventriculoperitoneal shunts. Patients were placed in the supine position immediately after injection of 1 mCi of Tc-99m DTPA in a small volume of 0.1 ml followed by 0.3 ml CSF. The small volume used was to prevent the visualization of the distal shunt tubing that may be caused by a larger injected volume in an obstructed shunt. If the shunt was not shown to be patent by 45 minutes, the patient was reimaged 15 minutes later, after being allowed to get up and move freely. If radiotracer was still not shown to move down the shunt tubing, the shunt was pumped. In infants, images were obtained every 30 minutes until shunt patency was demonstrated. A test sensitivity of 97%, specificity of 90%, and accuracy of 93% were reported. Functioning ventriculoperitoneal shunts demonstrated passage of radioactivity into the peritoneum within 45 minutes. Infants under 6 months usually demonstrated radiotracer in the peritoneum within 4 hours.

### Radionuclide Cisternography

Although radionuclide cisternography is not commonly performed in most nuclear medicine departments, it can yield useful information about CSF flow patterns and the identification of CSF leaks. Briefly, a lumbar puncture is performed, and approximately 0.5 mCi (18.5 MBq) In-111 DTPA or 10 mCi (370 MBq) Tc-99m DTPA is injected into the lumbar subarachnoid space.

### CSF Leaks

Depending on the suspected area of CSF leak, cotton pledgets are placed in both external auditory canals or two sets of pledgets are placed in the nose, one set high, near the cribriform plate, and a second set lower, near the middle turbinate. A pledget is also placed in the mouth as a control. The patient is imaged, and the pledgets are counted and compared to the counts in the pledget from the mouth and a sample of serum to determine if a leak of CSF has occurred (Fig. 10-12). It should be noted that a small leak of CSF may not be apparent on the images but may be identified by counting the pledgets. This method is a sensitive way of identifying small leaks of CSF not identified by other means.

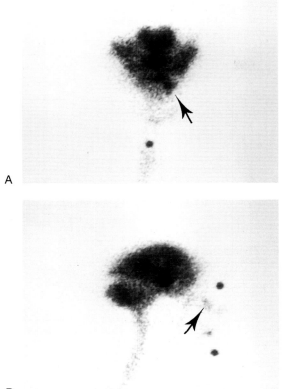

A

B

**FIG. 10-12.** CSF flow study performed on a patient with recent history of head trauma. **(A)** The anterior view shows focal abnormal accumulation of the Tc-99m DTPA (*arrow*). **(B)** The right lateral view also shows the leak (faint accumulation, *arrow*). Markers indicate the level of superior orbital ridge and chin.

*Normal-Pressure Hydrocephalus*

Radionuclide cisternography has also been used in an attempt to identify patients who have normal-pressure hydrocephalus (NPH). In-111 DTPA is injected into the lumbar subarachnoid space, and images of the ventricular system are obtained at 6, 24, 48, and sometimes 72 hours to evaluate CSF flow. Because a specific NPH pattern associated with successful therapeutic intervention has not been identified, this procedure is now rarely performed.

*Demonstrating CSF Flow Patterns*

Occasionally, it is important to determine the exact CSF flow pattern for therapy purposes. This could include the verification of distribution of a chemotherapeutic agent (the very first clinical indication for CSF flow studies in 1962). Here, instillation of the tracer with the therapeutic agent (directly into the subarachnoid space or via whatever administration system is used, e.g., a pump) under identical conditions demonstrates the agent's passage through the CSF pathways.

## EXAMINATIONS FOR THE EVALUATION OF CEREBRAL DEATH

Radionuclide cerebral angiography in the anterior projection using Tc-99m pertechnetate (or other Tc-99m agents) is a technique that can help to determine the diagnosis of brain death. More specifically, this study is used to provide an assessment of cerebral cortical blood flow.

### Radiopharmaceutical

Typically, a 20-mCi (740 MBq) bolus of the Tc-99m radiopharmaceutical is injected intravenously (if possible through a central venous access line), and rapid serial imaging is done of the carotid and intracranial vessels. We routinely use Tc-99m DTPA because of its renal excretion, which allows repeat studies after relatively short time intervals.

### Clinical Application

The findings from radionuclide cerebral angiography have shown excellent correlation in this setting to the results from four-vessel contrast angiography (111). Normal cerebral perfusion as seen on a radionuclide cerebral angiogram is shown in Fig. 10-13. In contrast, cerebral activity is not seen in the presence of brain death, and the absence of intracranial flow is considered a very reliable indicator of brain death (Fig. 10-14).

In approximately 30% of patients who show absent cerebral cortical perfusion, the superior sagittal sinus may be faintly visualized on delayed (1- to 2-minute) images. The normal sagittal sinus activity seen in the early flow images immediately (5 to 10 seconds) after visualization of the anterior and middle cerebral artery territories (see Fig. 10-14) indicates that cerebral perfusion is present. There has been some uncertainty about the significance of delayed visualization of the superior sagittal sinus as it pertains to the diagnosis of brain death. It has been suggested, however, that faint superior sagittal sinus activity does not rule out

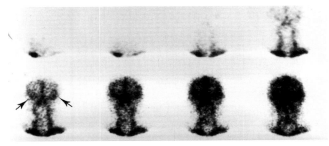

**FIG. 10-13.** Normal cerebral radionuclide angiogram (anterior views) showing the transit of the Tc-99m DTPA through internal carotid arteries, middle cerebral artery territory (*arrows*), and anterior cerebral artery territories. Note that resolution is not adequate for separation of the two anterior cerebral artery territories.

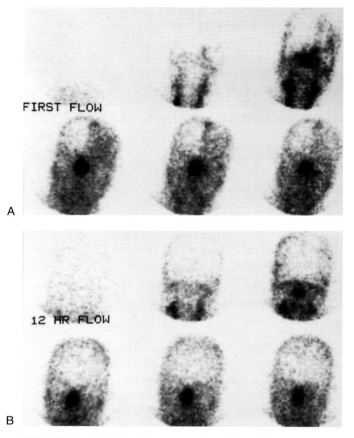

FIRST FLOW

12 HR FLOW

A

B

**FIG. 10-14. (A)** The first cerebral radionuclide angiogram (10-second anterior images) on a patient with recent severe head trauma shows the common carotid artery distribution, absent flow to the right cerebral hemisphere, but flow to the left cerebral hemisphere and prominent sagittal sinus activity in the fourth and fifth frames. **(B)** The flow study was repeated 12 hours later (virtually no background activity seen). Although there is common carotid and external carotid visualization, there is no scan evidence of intracerebral flow nor visualization of the sagittal sinus.

brain death when the angiographic phase shows no intracranial activity (112). In this case, it is assumed the sagittal sinus visualization results from blood draining from the external carotid flow to the skull vault and scalp rather than internal carotid flow.

Tc-99m HMPAO imaging is also useful in the assessment of brain death (113). Standard anterior-view angiographic phase images can be read in the conventional way, and 1-hour delay HMPAO images can be helpful in cases where there is some question about the certainty of the angiographic phase results. Such cases include the presence of slight sagittal sinus activity, compromise of the quality of the bolus during injection, and significant facial, scalp, or skull trauma, which result in hyperperfused regions of the external carotid circulation that obscure the absent intracerebral perfusion. In general, planar HMPAO scans are obtained, including anterior, posterior, and both lateral

views. SPECT images may be helpful to separate overlying external activity and make the diagnosis more certain when significant scalp activity is present.

## REFERENCES

1. McAfee JG, Fueger CF, Stern HS, et al. Tc-99m pertechnetate for brain imaging. J Nucl Med 1964;5:811–827.
2. Hauser W, Atkins HL, Nelson KG, et al. Technetium-99m DTPA: a new radiopharmaceutical for brain and kidney imaging. Radiology 1970;94:679–684.
3. Holman BL, Devous MD Sr. Functional brain SPECT: the emergence of a powerful clinical method. J Nucl Med 1992;33:1888–1904.
4. Holman BL, Zimmerman RE, Johnson KA, et al. Computer-assisted superimposition of magnetic resonance and high-resolution technetium-99m HMPAO and thallium-201 SPECT images of the brain. J Nucl Med 1991;32:1478–1484.
5. Heiss WD, Herholz K, Podreka I, et al. Comparison of Tc-99m HMPAO SPECT with (18F)fluoromethane PET in cerebrovascular disease. J Cereb Blood Flow Metab 1990;10:687–697.
6. Lassen NA, Anderson AR, Friberg L, Paulson OB. The retention of 99m Tc HMPAO in the human brain after intracarotid bolus injection: a kinetic analysis. J Cereb Blood Flow Metab 1988;8(Suppl):13–22.
7. Leveille J, Demonceau G, Walovitch RC. Intrasubject comparison between technetium-99m ECD and technetium-99m HMPAO in healthy human subjects. J Nucl Med 1992;33:480–484.
8. Suess E, Sigismund H, Reither H, et al. Uptake mechanism of technetium-99m-d,-1-HMPAO in cell cultures of the dissociated postnatal rat cerebellum. J Nucl Med 1992;33:108–114.
9. Neirinckx RD, Burke JF, Harrison RC, et al. The retention mechanism of technetium-99m HMPAO: intracellular reaction with glutathione. J Cereb Blood Flow Metab 1988;8(Suppl):4–12.
10. Winchell HS, Horst WD, Braun L, et al. N-isopropyl (I-123) p-iodoamphetamine: single pass brain uptake and washout, binding to brain synaptosomes, and localization in dog and monkey brain. J Nucl Med 1980;21:947–951.
11. Bushnell DL, Eastman G, Barnes WE. Comparison of IMP and HMPAO for SPECT brain imaging. J Nucl Med Tech 1991;19:71–74.
12. Yonekura Y, Fujita T, Nishizawa S, et al. Temporal changes in accumulation of N-isopropyl-p-iodoamphetamine in human brain: relation to lung clearance. J Nucl Med 1989;30:1977–1981.
13. Matsuda H, Tsuji S, Oba H, et al. Autoradiograph analysis of iodoamphetamine redistribution in experimental brain ischemia. J Nucl Med 1990;31:660–667.
14. Kung HF. Neuropharmacology of Iofetamine HCl I-123. In Collier BD, Tikofsky RS (eds), Stroke: A Clinical Update. Milwaukee, WI: Medical College of Wisconsin, 1988;22.
15. Sakai F. Iofetamine SPECT: Metabolism Versus Perfusion. In Collier BD, Tikofsky RS (eds), Stroke: A Clinical Update. Milwaukee, WI: Medical College of Wisconsin, 1988;23.
16. Vallabhajosula S, Zimmerman RE, Picard M, et al. Technetium-99m ECD: a new brain imaging agent: in vivo kinetics and biodistribution studies in normal human subjects. J Nucl Med 1989;30:599–604.
17. Devous MD, Stokely EM, Chehabi HH, Bonte FJ. Normal distribution of regional cerebral blood flow measured by dynamic single photon emission tomography. J Cereb Blood Flow Metab 1986;6:95–104.
18. Mazziotta JC, Phelps ME, Carson RE, Kuhl DE. Tomographic mapping of human cerebral metabolism: sensory deprivation. Ann Neurol 1982;12:435–444.
19. Hayashida K, Nishimura T, Imakita S, Vehara T. Filling out phenomenon with technetium-99m HMPAO brain SPECT at the site of mild cerebral ischemia. J Nucl Med 1989;30:591–598.
20. Matsuda H, Oskoie SD, Kinuya K, et al. Tc-99m HMPAO brain perfusion tomography using a high resolution SPECT system. Clin Nucl Med 1990;15:428–431.
21. De Roo M, Mortelmans L, Devos P, et al. Clinical experience with Tc-99m HMPAO high resolution SPECT of the brain in patients with cerebrovascular accidents. Eur J Nucl Med 1989;15:9–15.
22. Yeh SH, Liu RS, Hu HH, et al. Brain SPECT imaging with 99mTc-hexamethylpropyleneamine oxime in the early detection of cerebral infarction: comparison with transmission computed tomography. Nucl Med Commun 1986;7:873–878.

23. Lee RGL, Hill TC, Holman BL, et al. Predictive value of perfusion defect size using *N*-isopropyl-(I-123)-*p*-iodoamphetamine emission tomography in acute stroke. J Neurosurg 1984;61:449–452.

24. Matsuda H, Li YM, Higashi S, et al. Comparative SPECT study of stroke using Tc-99m ECD, I-123 IMP, and Tc-99m HMPAO. Clin Nucl Med 1993;18:754–758.

25. Bogousslavsky J, Delaloye-Bishof A, Regli F, et al. Prolonged hypoperfusion and early stroke after transient ischemic attack. Stroke 1990;21:40–46.

26. Moretti J-L, Defer G, Cinotti L, et al. "Luxury-perfusion" with Tc-99m-HMPAO and I-123-IMP SPECT imaging during the subacute phase of stroke. Eur J Nucl Med 1990;16:17–22.

27. Bushnell DL, Gupta S, Mlcoch A, et al. Demonstration of focal hyperemia in acute cerebral infarction with iodine-123 iodoamphetamine. J Nucl Med 1987;28:1920–1923.

28. Sperling B, Lassen NA. Hyperfixation of HMPAO in subacute ischemic stroke leading to spuriously high estimates of cerebral blood flow by SPECT. Stroke 1993;24:193–194.

29. Foster NL, Mountz JM, Bluelein LA, et al. Blood flow imaging of a posterior circulation stroke. Use of technetium Tc-99m hexamethylpropyleneamine oxime and single photon emission computed tomography. Arch Neurol 1988;45:687–690.

30. Giubilei F, Lenzi GL, Di Piero V, et al. Predictive value of brain perfusion single photon emission computed tomography in acute ischemic stroke. Stroke 1990;21:895–900.

31. Bushnell DL, Gupta S, Mlcoch A, Barnes WE. Prediction of language and neurologic recovery after cerebral infarction with SPECT imaging using *N*-isopropyl-*p*-(I-123) iodoamphetamine. Arch Neurol 1989;46:665–669.

32. Hanson SK, Grotta JC, Rhoades H, et al. Value of single photon emission computed tomography in acute stroke therapeutic trials. Stroke 1993;24:1322–1329.

33. Mountz JM, Modell JG, Foster NL, et al. Prognostication of recovery following stroke using the comparison of CT and technetium-99m HMPAO SPECT. J Nucl Med 1990;31:61–66.

34. Mlcoch AG, Bushnell DL, Gupta S, Milo TG. Speech fluency in aphasia: regional cerebral blood flow correlates of recovery using single photon emission computed tomography. J Neuroimaging 1994;4:6–10.

35. Gupta SA, Bushnell DL, Mlcoch A, et al. Clinical correlates of late IMP brain distribution in cerebral infarction. Stroke 1991;22:1512–1518.

36. Raynaud C, Rancurel G, Samson Y, et al. Pathophysiologic study of chronic infarcts with I-123 isopropyl iodoamphetamine (IMP): the importance of periinfarct area. Stroke 1987;18:21–29.

37. Powers WJ, Press GA, Grubb RL, et al. The effect of hemodynamically significant carotid artery disease on the hemodynamic status of the cerebral circulation. Ann Intern Med 1987;106:27–35.

38. Levine RL, Sunderland JJ, Rowe B, Nickles RJ. The study of cerebral ischemic reversibility: part II. Preliminary preoperative results of fluoromethane positron emission tomographic determination of perfusion reserve in patients with carotid TIA and stroke. Am J Physiol Imag 1986;1:104–114.

39. Bushnell DL, Gupta S, Barnes WE, et al. Evaluation of cerebral perfusion reserve using 5% $CO_2$ and SPECT neuroperfusion imaging. Clin Nucl Med 1991;16:263–267.

40. Burt RW, Witt RM, Cikrit DF, Reddy RV. Carotid artery disease: evaluation with acetazolamide-enhanced Tc-99m HMPAO SPECT. Radiology 1992;182:461–466.

41. Vorstrup S, Henriksen L, Paulson OB. Effect of acetazolamide on cerebral blood flow and metabolic rate for oxygen. J Clin Invest 1984;74:1634–1639.

42. Cotev S, Lee J, Severinghaus JW. The effects of acetazolamide on cerebral blood flow and cerebral tissue $pO_2$. Anesthesiology 1968;29:471–477.

43. Ebmeier KP, Dougall NJ, Austin MP, et al. The split dose technique for the study of psychological and pharmacological activation with the cerebral blood flow marker 99mTc exametazime and single photon emission computed tomography (SPECT): reproducibility and rater reliability. Int J Methods Psych Res 1991;1:27–38.

44. Devous MD Sr, Gassaway SK. Simultaneous SPECT imaging of Tc-99m and I-123-labeled brain agents in patients using the Prism scanner. J Nucl Med 1990;31(Suppl):877.

45. Oku N, Masayasu M, Hasikawa K, et al. Carbon dioxide reactivity by consecutive technetium-99m HMPAO SPECT in patients with chronically obstructed major cerebral artery. J Nucl Med 1994;35:32–40.

46. Devous MD Sr, Lowe JL, Payne JK. Dual-isotope brain imaging with technetium and iodine-123: validation by phantom studies. J Nucl Med 1992;33:2030–2035.

47. Vorstrup S, Brun B, Lassen N. Evaluation of the cerebral vasodilatory capacity by the acetazolamide test before Ec-Ic bypass surgery in patients with occlusion of the internal carotid artery. Stroke 1986;17:1291–1298.

48. Powers WJ, Tempel LW, Grubb RL Jr. Influence of cerebral hemodynamics on stroke risk: one-year follow-up of 30 medically treated patients. Ann Neurol 1989;25:325–330.

49. Knop J, Thie A, Fuchs C, et al. [99m]Tc HMPAO SPECT with acetazolamide challenge to detect hemodynamic compromise in occlusive cerebrovascular disease. Stroke 1992;23:1733–1742.

50. Davis S, Andrews J, Lichtenstein M, et al. A single photon emission computed tomography study of hypoperfusion after subarachnoid hemorrhage. Stroke 1990;21:252–259.

51. Soucy JP, McNamara D, Mohr G, et al. Evaluation of vasospasm secondary to subarachnoid hemorrhage with technetium-99m HMPAO tomoscintigraphy. J Nucl Med 1990;31:972–977.

52. Mathews D, Walker BS, Purdy PD, et al. Brain blood flow SPECT in temporary balloon occlusion of carotid and intracerebral arteries. J Nucl Med 1993;34:1239–1243.

53. Palestro CJ, Sen C, Muzinic M, et al. Assessing collateral cerebral perfusion with Tc-99m HMPAO SPECT during temporary internal carotid artery occlusion. J Nucl Med 1993;34:1235–1238.

54. Eckard DA, Purdy PD, Bonte FJ. Temporary balloon occlusion of the carotid artery combined with brain blood flow imaging as a test to predict tolerance prior to permanent carotid sacrifice. Am J Neuroradiol 1992;13:1565–1569.

55. Monsein LH, Jeffery PJ, van Heerden BB, et al. Assessing adequacy of collateral circulation during balloon occlusion of the internal carotid artery with Tc-99m HMPAO SPECT. J Neuroradiol 1991;12:1045–1051.

56. Kumar A, Mozley PD, Dunham C, et al. Semiquantitative I-123 IMP SPECT studies in late onset depression before and after treatment. Intl J Ger Psych 1991;6:775–777.

57. Yazici KM, Kapucu O, Erbas B, et al. Assessment of changes in regional cerebral blood flow in patients with major depression using the 99mTc-HMPAO single photon emission tomography method. Eur J Nucl Med 1992;19:1038–1043.

58. Gur RE, Pearlson GD. Neuroimaging in schizophrenia research. Schizophrenia Bull 1993;19:337–353.

59. Cohen RM, Semple WE, Gross M, Nordahl TE. From syndrome to illness: delineating the pathophysiology of schizophrenia with PET. Schizophrenia Bull 1988;14:169–178.

60. Cohen MB, Lake RR, Graham S, et al. Quantitative iodine-123 IMP imaging of brain perfusion in schizophrenia. J Nucl Med 1989;30:1616–1620.

61. Ebmeier KP, Blackwood HR, Murray C, et al. Single photon emission computed tomography with Tc-99m exametazime in unmedicated schizophrenic patients. Biol Psych 1993;33:487–495.

62. Devous MD, Raese JD, Herman JH, et al. SPECT determination of regional cerebral blood flow in schizophrenic patients at rest and during a mental task. J Nucl Med 1986;27:734.

63. Paulman RG, Devous MD, Gregory RR, et al. Hypofrontality and cognitive impairment in schizophrenia: dynamic single-photon tomography and neuropsychological assessment of schizophrenic brain function. Biol Psych 1990;27:337–399.

64. Suzuki M, Yuasa S, Minabe Y, et al. Left superior temporal blood flow increases in schizophrenic and schizophrenia from patients with auditory hallucination: a longitudinal case study using I-123 IMP SPECT. Eur Arch Psychiatry Clin Neurosci 1993;242:257–261.

65. Gray BG, Ichise M, Chung DG, et al. Tc-99m HMPAO SPECT in the evaluation of patients with a remote history of traumatic brain injury: a comparison with x-ray computed tomography. J Nucl Med 1992;33:52–58.

66. Roper SN, Mena I, King WA, et al. An analysis of cerebral blood flow in acute closed head injury using technetium-99m HMPAO SPECT and computed tomography. J Nucl Med 1991;32:684–687.

67. Newton MR, Greenwood RJ, Britton KE, et al. A study comparing SPECT with CT and MRI after closed head trauma. J Neurol Neurosurg Psychiatry 1991;55:92–94.

68. Woods SW, Hegeman IM, Zubal G, et al. Visual stimulation increases Tc-99m HMPAO distribution in the human visual cortex. J Nucl Med 1991;32:210–215.

69. Ebmeier KP, Murray CL, Dougall NJ, et al. Unilateral voluntary hand movement and regional cerebral uptake of Tc-99m exametazime in human control subjects. J Nucl Med 1992;33:1637–1641.

70. Mlcoch T, Bushnell DL, Gupta S. SPECT neuroimaging and language cerebral activation techniques. J Cardiovasc Tech 1990;9:28.

71. Goldenberg G, Podreka I, Steiner M, Willmes K. Patterns of regional cerebral blood flow related to memorizing of high and low imagery words—an emission computer tomography study. Neuropsychologia 1987;25:473–485.

72. Celesia GG, Bushnell D, Toleikis SC, Brigell MG. Cortical blindness and residual vision: is the "second" visual system in humans capable of more than rudimentary visual perception? Neurology 1991;41:862–869.

73. Chollet F, Dipiero V, Wise RJS, et al. The functional anatomy of motor recovery after stroke in humans: a study with positron tomography. Ann Neurol 1991;29:63–71.

74. Hauser WA, Kurland LT. The epidemiology of epilepsy in Rochester, Minnesota, 1935 through 1967. Epilepsia 1975;16:1–66.

75. National Institute of Health Consensus Conference. Surgery for epilepsy. JAMA 1990:264:729–733.

76. Rowe CC, Berkovic SF, Austin MC, et al. Visual and quantitative analysis of interictal SPECT with technetium-99m-HMPAO in temporal lobe epilepsy. J Nucl Med 1991;32:1688–1694.

77. Shen W, Lee BI, Park HM, et al. HIPDM-SPECT brain imaging in the presurgical evaluation of patients with intractable seizures. J Nucl Med 1990;31:1280–1284.

78. Lee BI, Markand OH, Wellman HN, et al. HIPDM-SPECT in patients with medically intractable complex partial seizures. Arch Neurol 1988;45:397–402.

79. Rowe CC, Berkovic SF, Sia STB, et al. Localization of epileptic foci with postictal single photon emission computed tomography. Ann Neurol 1989;26:660–668.

80. Adams C, Hwang PA, Gilday DL, et al. Comparison of SPECT, EEG, CT, MRI, and pathology in partial epilepsy. Pediatr Neurol 1992;8:97–103.

81. Newton MR, Austin MC, Chan JG, et al. Ictal SPECT using technetium-99m-HMPAO: Methods for rapid preparation and optimal deployment of tracer during spontaneous seizures. J Nucl Med 1993;34:666–670.

82. Hara M, Takahaski M, Kojima A, et al. Single photon emission computed tomography in children with idiopathic seizures. Radiat Med 1991;9:185–189.

83. Konkol RJ, Maister BH, Wells RG, Sty JR. Hemimegalencephaly: clinical, EEG, neuroimaging, and IMP-SPECT correlation. Pediatr Neurol 1990;6:414–418.

84. Kanazawa O, Shirasaka Y, Hattori H, et al. Ictal 99m-Tc-HMPAO SPECT in alternating hemiplegia. Pediatr Neurol 1991;7:121–124.

85. Zupanc JL, Dobkin JA, Perlman SB. 123-I-iodoamphetamine SPECT brain imaging in alternating hemiplegia. Pediatr Neurol 1991;7:35–38.

86. Boller F, Lopez OL, Moossy J. Diagnosis of dementia: clinicopathologic correlations. Neurology 1989;39:76–79.

87. Goroll AH, May LA, Mulley AG (eds). Primary Care Medicine. Philadelphia: Lippincott, 1987.

88. Bonte FJ, Tinter R, Weiner MF, et al. Brain blood flow in the dementias: SPECT with histopathologic correlation. Radiology 1993;186:361–365.

89. Bonte FJ, Hom J, Tintner R, Weiner MF. Single photon tomography in Alzheimer's disease and the dementias. Semin Nucl Med 1990;20:342–352.

90. Holman BL, Nagel JS, Johnson KA, Hill TC. Imaging dementia with SPECT. Ann NY Acad Sci 1991;620:165–174.

91. Gemmell G, Sharp PF, Smith FW, et al. Cerebral blood flow measured by SPECT as a diagnostic tool in the study of dementia. Psychiatry Res 1989;29:327–329.

92. Holman BL, Johnson KA, Gerada B, et al. The scintigraphic appearance of Alzheimer's disease: a prospective study using technetium-99m-HMPAO SPECT. J Nucl Med 1992;33:181–185.

93. Hellman RS, Tikofsky RS, Collier BD, et al. Alzheimer disease: quantitative analysis of I-123-iodoamphetamine SPECT brain imaging. Radiology 1989;172:183–188.

94. Komatani A, Yamaguchi K, Sugai Y, et al. Assessment of demented patients by dynamic SPECT of inhaled xenon-133. J Nucl Med 1988;29:1621–1626.

95. Weinberger DR, Mann U, Gibson RE, et al. Cerebral muscarinic receptors in primary degenerative dementia as evaluated by SPECT with iodine-123-labeled QNB. Adv Neurol 1990;51:147–149.

96. Weinberger DR, Jones DW, Sunderland T, et al. In vivo imaging of cerebral muscarinic receptors with I-123 QNB and SPECT: studies in normal subjects and patients with dementia. Clin Neuropharmacol 1992;15:194A.

97. Ueda T, Kaji Y, Wakisaka S, et al. Time sequential single photon emission computed tomography studies in brain tumour using thallium-201. Eur J Nucl Med 1993;20:138–145.

98. Kaplan WD, Takvorian T, Morris JH, et al. Thallium-201 brain tumor imaging: a comparative study with pathologic correlation. J Nucl Med 1987;28:47–52.

99. Mountz JM, Stafford-Schuck K, McKeever PE, et al. Thallium-201 tumor/cardiac ratio estimation of residual astrocytoma. J Neurosurg 1988;68:705–709.

100. Black KL, Hawkins RA, Kim KT, et al. Use of thallium-201 SPECT to quantitate malignancy grade of gliomas. J Neurosurg 1989;71:342–346.

101. Oriuchi N, Tamua M, Shibaszaki T, et al. Clinical evaluation of thallium-201 SPECT in supratentorial gliomas: relationship to histologic grade, prognosis and proliferative activities. J Nucl Med 1993;34:2085–2089.

102. Yoshii Y, Satou M, Yamamoto T, et al. The role of thallium-201 single photon emission tomography in the investigation and characterisation of brain tumours in man and their response to treatment. Eur J Nucl Med 1993;20:39–45.

103. Schwartz RB, Carvalho PA, Alexander E, et al. Radiation necrosis vs high-grade recurrent glioma: differentiation by using dual-isotope SPECT with 201-Tl and 99m-Tc-HMPAO. AJNR Am J Neuroradiol 1991;12:1187–1192.

104. O'Tuama LA, Treves ST, Larar JN, et al. Thallium-201 versus technetium-99m-MIBI SPECT in evaluation of childhood brain tumors: a within-subject comparison. J Nucl Med 1993;34:1045–1051.

105. Agha FP, Amendola MA, Shirazi KK, et al. Unusual abdominal complications of ventriculo-peritoneal shunts. Radiology 1983;146:323–326.

106. Di Chiro GD, Grove AS. Evaluation of surgical and spontaneous cerebrospinal fluid shunts by isotope scanning. J Neurosurg 1966;24:743–748.

107. Mai DT, Vasinrapee P, Cook RE. Diagnosis of abdominal cerebrospinal fluid pseudocyst by scintigraphy. Clin Nucl Med 1993;18:237–238.

108. French BN, Swanson M. Radionuclide-imaging shuntography for the evaluation of shunt patency. Surg Neurol 1981;16:173–182.

109. Brendel AJ, Wynchank S, Castel J-P, et al. Cerebrospinal shunt flow in adults: radionuclide quantitation with emphasis on patient position. Radiology 1983;149:815–818.

110. Graham P, Howman-Giles R, Johnston I, Besser M. Evaluation of CSF shunt patency by means of technetium-99m DTPA. J Neurosurg 1982;57:262–266.

111. Mishkin FS. Determination of brain death by radionuclide angiography. Radiology 1975;115:135–137.

112. Brill DR, Schwartz JA, Baxter JA. Variant flow patterns in radionuclide cerebral imaging performed for brain death. Clin Nucl Med 1985;10:346–352.

113. Wilson K, Gordon L, Selby JB. The diagnosis of brain death with Tc-99m HMPAO. Clin Nucl Med 1993;18:428–434.

# SECTION II

## Specialized Nuclear Medicine

Textbook of Nuclear Medicine,
edited by Michael A. Wilson.
Lippincott–Raven Publishers, Philadelphia © 1998.

CHAPTER 11

# Pediatrics

Richard M. Shore

The application of radionuclide imaging techniques to pediatric patients has similarities and differences compared to adult imaging. The many aspects in which they are similar are covered by other chapters. This chapter considers the differences in technical factors and clinical applications of pediatric radionuclide imaging. The clinical section reflects our case distribution at Children's Memorial Hospital in Chicago (Table 11-1) and emphasizes studies unique to children.

## HISTORIC PERSPECTIVE

In a review of the development of pediatric nuclear medicine, the late historian of nuclear medicine, Dr. William G. Meyers (1), showed one of the earliest pictures of a nuclear medicine procedure, that of a young girl having her thyroid measured by a Geiger-Müller tube. This picture first appeared at a 1941 cyclotron symposium and later in a 1942 issue of *Radiology* (2).

The introduction of radionuclide procedures for children has generally followed initial development in adults. Because the overall volume of nuclear medicine examinations is greater for adults than children, there is more incentive to develop procedures for use in adults. For example, the development of iminodiacetic acid (IDA) derivatives for hepatobiliary imaging was stimulated by their potential use for acute cholecystitis, a prevalent adult disorder. These agents were subsequently shown to be useful in evaluating infants with suspected biliary atresia. Biliary atresia is much less common, however, and there would have been little incentive to develop an agent specifically for it. Radiopharmaceutical development also dictates that pediatric nuclear medicine applications generally follow those for adults because children are usually not studied until adult work has already suggested favorable safety and efficacy.

The development of some specific nuclear medicine procedures of particular interest for pediatrics may be summarized as follows. Radionuclide cystography was first described by Winter in 1959 (3). Subsequent reports by Blaufox et al. (4) and Conway et al. (5) emphasized the use of this technique in children. The potential use of technetium 99m (Tc-99m) pertechnetate for identifying ectopic gastric mucosa was suggested by Harden et al. in 1967 (6), and Jewett and colleagues successfully applied the technique to demonstrate a Meckel's diverticulum in 1970 (7). Cardiac procedures of particular interest for children include the detection and quantification of intracardiac shunts. Left-to-right shunts were first evaluated by the $C_2/C_1$ method of Folse and Braunwald in 1962 (8) and subsequently by gamma variate analysis by Maltz and Treves in 1973 (9). In 1971, Gates and colleagues described the use of perfusion lung scan agents to evaluate right-to-left shunts (10). Evaluation of suspected biliary atresia was initially performed by measuring fecal excretion of I-131 rose bengal, as described by Brent and Geppert (11). Subsequently, I-131 rose bengal was also used for imaging, although this required much larger dosages. When the Tc-99m IDA agents became available, they were quickly used in neonates with suspected biliary atresia, and Majd et al. refined this technique with phenobarbital pretreatment (12).

As with adults, utilization trends in pediatric nuclear medicine have been strongly influenced by the development of radionuclide and alternate techniques. The earliest procedures involved nonimaging applications of radiotracers given in vivo. With the development of Tc-99m pertechnetate and appropriate imaging instrumentation, brain scintigraphy became one of the major imaging procedures in children as well as adults. It provided a noninvasive means of evaluating suspected intracranial mass or inflammatory lesions that otherwise would have required either cerebral arteriography or pneumoencephalography. Then, computed tomography (CT) visualized intracranial anatomy and improved diagnostic specificity, leading to the near elimination of conventional brain scintigraphy. During the time that the use of brain scintigraphy was decreasing, nuclear medicine was experiencing the rapid growth of cardiac procedures. Their use in adults for suspected coronary artery

**TABLE 11-1.** *Case distribution at Children's Memorial Hospital, Chicago*

| Examination | % of imaging procedures |
|---|---|
| Skeletal scintigraphy | 32 |
| Radionuclide cystography | 26 |
| Renal scintigraphy (dynamic and cortical) | 17 |
| Gallium scintigraphy | 2 |
| Meckel's diverticulum | 1 |
| Other | 22 |

disease led to high-volume use. Although there were also many uses for cardiac imaging in children, the indications for these examinations were less frequent and pediatric nuclear cardiology did not experience a similar growth spurt. Rather, pediatric nuclear medicine was experiencing its greatest growth in skeletal and genitourinary procedures, as indicated in Table 11-1.

## TECHNICAL CONSIDERATIONS

Radionuclide examinations must be designed to provide images of sufficient quality to answer the clinical question while minimizing radiation exposure and patient discomfort. The smaller size of pediatric patients argues that the spatial resolution of imaging studies in children should ideally be greater than that for adults. Radiation absorbed doses also need to be minimized in children. Tissues that are still growing and developing are often more radiosensitive than those that are not, and children also have more years ahead of them in which radiation-induced abnormalities may become manifest. Maximizing resolution conflicts with minimizing radiation exposure, however, leading to inevitable compromises in designing radionuclide imaging examinations.

### Radiopharmaceutical Dosage Selection

There are many approaches to determining radiopharmaceutical dosages for children. These generally involve adjusting adult dosages according to patient size along with a minimum dosage, which gives small children dosages larger than the calculated amount. A rational approach to determining radiopharmaceutical dosages and adjusting them for children has been presented elsewhere (13). Radiation absorbed doses for children are slightly smaller than those for adults if dosages are scaled by body weight, and significantly greater than those for adults if scaled by body surface area.

### Imaging Technique

Satisfactory clinical results require optimization of imaging technique for pediatric patients. The importance of basic imaging principles, such as proper patient positioning, reduction of patient-to-collimator distance, and reduction of patient motion, cannot be overemphasized. Proper positioning is particularly important for pediatric skeletal scintigraphy because many abnormalities are located in the metaphyses immediately adjacent to the growth plates. To recognize these lesions, the growth plates must be positioned symmetrically and perpendicular to the camera face so that they are projected as a thin line. Imaging the lower extremities with internal rotation and the toes pointed inward helps to project the tibia and fibula separately from each other. Performing the anterior view with the patient prone and the camera below the table helps to reduce motion and also holds the feet fully extended. The growth plates for the upper extremities are shown in a true frontal projection when the forearms are fully supinated. If arms are imaged posteriorly, sandbags are useful to maintain position. Comparison views of the extremities should be obtained for the same time rather than by counts so that differences in activity can be appreciated.

Spatial resolution depends on intrinsic camera resolution, collimation, and information (count) density. For most pediatric imaging, the need for high spatial resolution requires high-resolution collimation, even though this decreases counting efficiency. Adequate information density must also be obtained, requiring either higher radiopharmaceutical dosages or longer imaging times. To limit radiation exposure, this is usually achieved through longer imaging times. This increases the risk of patient movement, however, which degrades image quality. Accordingly, reduction of movement through a combination of coaching and proper patient handling by the technologist, mechanical immobilization devices, and sedation is essential for obtaining satisfactory radionuclide imaging studies in children.

Optimal patient cooperation may be obtained when the examination is performed in a nonthreatening environment by a technologist who can deal patiently and skillfully with children. In young age groups, immobilization is also often needed, and it is important that immobilization devices not interfere with proper positioning. In some cases, adequate positioning can be obtained with a papoose-type immobilization device. In others, better positioning can be obtained with liberal use of sandbags and imaging performed with the camera beneath the table. Since the 1980s, there has been some shift in emphasis from the use of immobilization to sedation. This is likely related to an overall greater acceptance of sedation in pediatric imaging, which has been needed for CT and magnetic resonance imaging (MRI). Because of potential serious effects, sedation should be used only when proper monitoring is available and only by physicians familiar with the use of these drugs and treatment of complications. The requirements for conscious sedation set by the Joint Commission on Accreditation of Healthcare Organizations are very stringent and must be followed.

## CLINICAL APPLICATIONS

### Skeletal Scintigraphy

Compared to adult nuclear medicine practice, pediatric skeletal scintigraphy is used more often for benign than malignant disorders. The major areas to consider are suspected inflammatory disease, occult skeletal injuries in the limping child, suspected child abuse, and evaluation of avascular necrosis (AVN).

### *Inflammatory Disease*

Acute hematogenous osteomyelitis occurs primarily in otherwise normal children. It is usually due to *Staphylococcus aureus*, and it begins in the metaphyseal regions of major long bones (14). The predominance of metaphyseal localization is believed to be due to slow flow and stasis in the venous sinusoids, which allow bacteria to proliferate. The anatomy of the metaphysis and growth plate may also explain the age-related risk for osteomyelitis to extend from metaphysis into epiphysis. Before 18 months of age, vessels extend across the physeal cartilage and permit the spread of infection. After that time, the physeal cartilage is avascular and forms a relative barrier to the spread of infection (15), although this is not absolute, and transphyseal spread may occasionally be seen, particularly with CT or MRI. With growth plate closure, this barrier no longer exists.

### *Osteomyelitis*

The major clinical utility of skeletal scintigraphy in osteomyelitis is establishing an early diagnosis when the radiographs are normal. The examination typically demonstrates hyperemia on the flow study and increased tracer localization during both early and delayed phases, with the early phase demonstrating not only increased blood pool activity but also specific bone localization. This focally increased localization is typically seen in the metaphysis immediately adjacent to the physis. Distinguishing metaphyseal abnormality from the normally bright physis requires optimal technique. The camera must be positioned perpendicular to the physis. Proper photographic intensity avoids "blooming," which causes the physis to appear rounder and wider than it actually is. With good technique, a metaphyseal abnormality appears as a smudge and obscures the normally sharp linear appearance of the physis (Fig. 11-1).

The pathogenesis of acute hematogenous osteomyelitis helps to explain variant appearances on skeletal scintigraphy. As the inflammatory exudate spreads within the metaphysis, intraosseous pressure increases and may cause vascular compromise, resulting in bone ischemia or infarction. The exudate also spreads into the diaphysis and

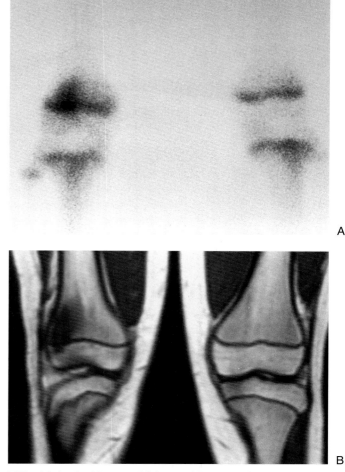

A

B

FIG. 11-1. A 12-year-old boy with acute hematogenous osteomyelitis of the right distal femoral metaphysis. **(A)** The bone scan anterior view shows the typical metaphyseal focal abnormality, which obscures the margin of the adjacent growth plate. Note the slight generalized increase in uptake to the entire knee due to associated mild synovitis. **(B)** The corresponding T1-weighted MRI shows the same metaphyseal location as well as a small amount of extension across physis into epiphysis.

through the cortex to the subperiosteal space (16). This subperiosteal abscess may also interrupt the periosteal vessels, further compromising bone vascular supply. Scintigraphy accurately demonstrates this pathophysiology, and there may be photopenia during this stage of the disease (Fig. 11-2) (17). This is not a false-negative examination but rather a positive finding of severe ischemia or infarction, which must be recognized to establish a diagnosis and identify an increased risk of sequestrum formation.

There are several metaphyseal equivalent regions in flat bones, which are common sites for acute hematogenous osteomyelitis (18), accounting for approximately 25% of all cases. Many of these are located in the pelvis and include sites such as the iliac bone adjacent to the sacroiliac joint, the ischial apophysis, the ischiopubic synchondrosis, and

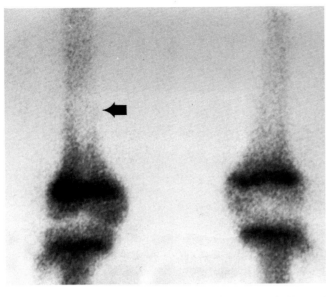

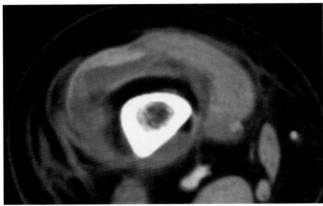

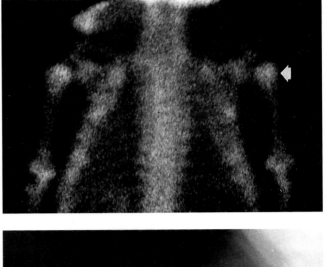

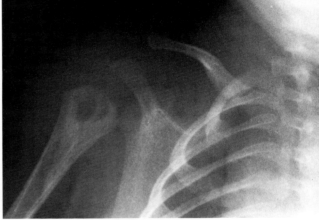

FIG. 11-2. A 10-year-old boy with acute hematogenous osteomyelitis of the right femur associated with knee septic arthritis and soft-tissue abscesses. **(A)** The anterior view of the bone scan shows a photopenic region (*arrow*) at the right distal metadiaphyseal junction together with a generalized increase of the right knee due to associated synovitis. Aspiration of medullary canal at this photopenic site yielded pus. **(B)** Contrast-enhanced CT shows a subperiosteal abscess.

FIG. 11-3. A 1-month-old boy with right shoulder swelling. **(A)** The posterior bone scan view shows only a minimal abnormality with slightly less activity (*arrow*) in that region compared to the normal left side. **(B)** Radiograph shows prominent lytic defect in right proximal humeral metaphysis. Biopsy was compatible with acute and chronic inflammation.

the acetabulum adjacent to the triradiate cartilage. Other metaphyseal equivalent regions are located in the vertebrae, scapula, and calcaneus. These cases are often less obvious clinically than the pelvic sites. Rather than presenting with well-localized pain and tenderness, involvement of the iliac bone may present as back, hip, or even abdominal pain. Recognition of subtle cases depends on knowledge of potential disease sites as well as optimal image quality.

Neonatal osteomyelitis has several features that differ from that seen in older children. There is a wider variety of infectious organisms in neonates, including group B streptococci, enteric coliform organisms, *Candida*, and staphylococcus. Neonatal osteomyelitis also has a greater tendency for multiple sites of involvement, particularly in patients with indwelling vascular catheters. There is controversy about the value of skeletal scintigraphy in neonatal osteomyelitis. For sites of proven osteomyelitis, Ash and Gilday (19) reported that scintigraphy was abnormal in 31.5%, equivocal in 10.5%, and normal in 58%. In contrast, Bressler et al. (20) had no false-negative studies in their series, which they attributed to superior image quality with improved intrinsic resolution, use of magnification, and overall meticulous attention to imaging technique. Recognizing that there is considerable disagreement regarding the sensitivity of scintigraphy for neonatal osteomyelitis, its use in this age group requires optimal technique with greater spatial resolution than that for older subjects. Furthermore, the relatively small bone mass of neonates permits earlier recognition of radiographic bone destruction (Fig. 11-3). Therefore, plain radiographs are often positive at the time of initial evaluation and should be obtained in all cases of suspected neonatal osteomyelitis. Skeletal scintigraphy is also

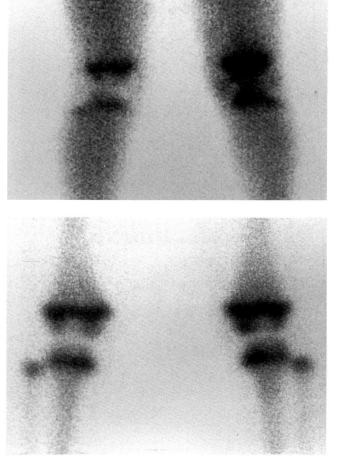

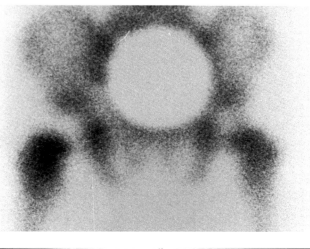

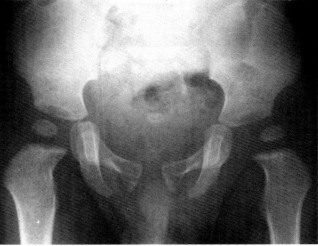

**FIG. 11-4.** A 19-month-old girl with septic knee. **(A)** The early posterior blood pool image shows hyperemia in the region of the right knee, including periarticular tissues. **(B)** The delayed posterior image shows effects of hyperemia with moderately increased localization seen on both sides of knee joint. The physes are well delineated and linear, with no evidence of complicating osteomyelitis.

**FIG. 11-5.** An 11-month-old boy with septic left hip. **(A)** The bone scan posterior view demonstrates absence of tracer localization in the left femoral head, indicating avascularity. Activity in the left proximal femoral metaphysis is increased, suggesting coexistent osteomyelitis. **(B)** The radiograph shows lateral subluxation.

recommended in this age group, not only for evaluation of the suspected site, but also for potential multifocal disease. Scintigraphy is most helpful in regions such as the spine, ribs, scapulae, and pelvis, which are not as easily evaluated by radiographs as are the major long bones.

*Septic Arthritis*

Like acute hematogenous osteomyelitis, septic arthritis is usually a disease of otherwise normal children. Many organisms can be found, and their frequency varies with age group (21):

- Neonates, group B streptococcus
- Between 6 months and 2 years of age, *Haemophilus influenzae* type B

- Older children, *S. aureus*
- Adolescents, gonococcus

Septic arthritis is diagnosed by joint aspiration. Imaging procedures that help to indicate the presence of a joint effusion include ultrasonography (US) (especially for the hip), CT, MRI, and occasionally plain films. Scintigraphy may be used in these patients to survey the skeleton for bone pathology during the initial evaluation of pain or limp. With septic arthritis, hyperemia is centered at the joint rather than at the metaphysis, as in osteomyelitis. This is seen best on the early images, which may show diffuse hyperemia or peripheral hyperemia corresponding to synovitis. The delayed images usually demonstrate mildly increased localization in the bones on both sides of the inflamed joint (Fig. 11-4).

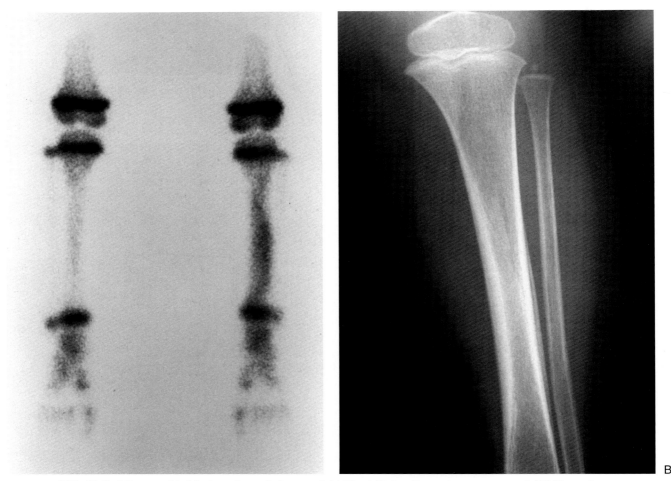

A

B

**FIG. 11-6.** A 2-year-old girl who refuses to bear weight. The initial radiographs were normal. **(A)** The anterior bone scintigraph shows abnormal fusiform tracer localization in left tibial diaphysis. **(B)** The subsequent radiograph shows periosteal new bone formation along the lateral aspect of the tibia. The vertical lucency at the junction of the proximal and mid thirds is a vascular canal. Just medial to it is a faint oblique lucent line corresponding to a portion of the nondisplaced spiral fracture.

After a diagnosis of septic arthritis is established, scintigraphy is useful to determine if there is associated osteomyelitis and to evaluate bone vascularity. Greater activity on one side of the joint than the other suggests specific involvement of that bone. Bone scintigraphy has a major role in evaluating the vascularity of the femoral head in septic arthritis of the hip. Because the hip joint is a tightly confined space, exudate within it can elevate intra-articular pressure and compromise femoral head vascularity, leading to AVN as a major complication (Fig. 11-5).

*Toxic Synovitis*

Toxic synovitis is an inflammatory condition of the hip that generally presents between 5 and 10 years of age (22). Although it may be postviral in etiology, no infectious agents have been isolated. Patients present with unilateral hip pain but do not have the severe limitation of motion that

is usually present with bacterial septic arthritis. US is useful for demonstrating hip effusions, but it cannot distinguish an effusion due to toxic synovitis from one due to septic arthritis. This final determination requires hip aspiration, and the decision to do this must be based on clinical considerations.

Bone scintigraphy may appear normal or show diffusely increased activity in the region of the involved hip. In some cases, the femoral head may be photopenic, reflecting vascular compromise secondary to increased intra-articular pressure. Aspiration of the hip at this stage may relieve this pressure, and tracer uptake into the femoral head can return to normal. Legg-Calvé-Perthes (LCP) disease is a form of AVN of the femoral head that occurs in children and is usually regarded as idiopathic. It is possible that some cases are related to earlier episodes of toxic synovitis. If so, recognition of an ischemic femoral head by scintigraphy and subsequent therapeutic joint aspiration may help to prevent this form of AVN.

### Occult Skeletal Trauma

There are two very different forms of occult skeletal injury in children, and skeletal scintigraphy is useful in both. Occult skeletal injury may apply to toddler fractures, which usually involve the lower extremities and result from relatively minor trauma to the developing skeleton. The term may also refer to fractures in physically abused children in whom the history of injury is withheld.

### Toddler Fractures

Toddler fractures are often thought of as stress fractures occurring in the relatively weak bones of young children. In many instances, they are the result of repetitive stress similar to adult stress fractures, whereas others may be the result of acute compression, such as that which might be sustained in a fall. The key to identifying these injuries scintigraphically and radiographically is awareness of their usual location and clinical presentation. These fractures occur in the lower extremities, which receive the stress of weight bearing and ambulation. The classic toddler fracture is an oblique or spiral fracture of the mid to distal tibia. The initial radiographs are often normal. On follow-up, periosteal new bone is often seen, and demineralization at the fracture site may make the fracture line easier to see. Tibial toddler fractures are usually positive on bone scintigraphy at the time of presentation, typically demonstrating an elongated region of increased localization within the diaphysis (23) (Fig. 11-6). Identification of these fractures allows for symptomatic relief with casting and precludes the need for further testing.

Other common lower extremity occult fractures are the impaction fractures of the tarsal bones, particularly the calcaneus (24) and cuboid (25). At the time of initial symptoms, these are usually not detectable radiographically, and on follow-up they demonstrate a linear band of sclerosis. On scintigraphy, increased localization is usually present (Fig. 11-7). Other processes, such as infection, may also occur in

the calcaneal tuberosity (a metaphyseal equivalent site), and correlation with clinical features is necessary. Other sites to be aware of include the first metatarsal base ("bunk bed" fracture) (26), and the proximal tibia at the metadiaphyseal junction posteriorly.

### Suspected Child Abuse

A problem unique to children is the identification of fractures in suspected child abuse victims. Recognizing that there is controversy surrounding recommendations for imaging (27,28), the following discussion summarizes the considerations useful in optimizing imaging. The occurrence of fractures in abused children is related to age; most are found in infants <2 or 3 years of age, with the highest incidence <1 year (29). Although older children may be abused in many ways, if fractures are present, they are usually accompanied by historical or physical evidence of specific trauma to the fracture site. In the absence of such findings in older children, the yield of both scintigraphy and radiographic skeletal surveys is low.

Many clinical factors determine the need for imaging evaluation of suspected child abuse victims. In some instances the findings on history, physical examination, and social service evaluation may be so convincing that additional evaluation need not be extensive. In most cases, however, the strength of the determination that a child has been abused is aided by the fullest documentation of trauma. For maximum enumeration of fractures, both skeletal scintigraphy and skeletal surveys should be performed because each may find fractures missed by the other method.

Rib fractures in these children are often due to anterior-posterior compression of the chest, which causes the ribs to fracture posteriorly at their articulation with the transverse processes of the vertebrae, laterally, and also anteriorly at the costochondral junctions. These fractures, which are usually multiple and arranged linearly, suggest nonaccidental trauma. Such rib fractures are generally easily demonstrated by scintigraphy (Fig. 11-8), but they are notorious for being missed on radiographs until substantial callus develops (28,30). Scintigraphy is also quite helpful in areas where complex geometry impairs radiographic evaluation, such as the scapula and spine. Scintigraphy can also identify traumatic periosteal injury to the long bone diaphyses that may result from violent grabbing of an extremity (31) (see Fig. 11-8).

Many subtle, nondisplaced "ordinary" fractures may also be more easily shown by scintigraphy than radiography, particularly if examined before callus or demineralization has developed at the fracture site. Conversely, there are also circumstances in which fractures are more easily seen radiographically. Skull fractures are often difficult to document on scintigraphy, and medical centers that rely more on scintigraphy than radiography agree that skull films should always be obtained (28). Healed fractures may return to normal on scintigraphy yet still demonstrate either deformity or cortical thickening indicative of the previous fracture.

A,B

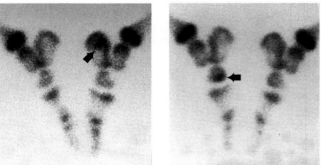

**FIG. 11-7. (A)** Typical stress or impaction fractures of the feet. This image shows lateral views with a linear abnormality in the right calcaneus (*arrow*). **(B)** In a different patient, this image shows lateral views with a fracture of the anterior aspect of the left cuboid (*arrow*).

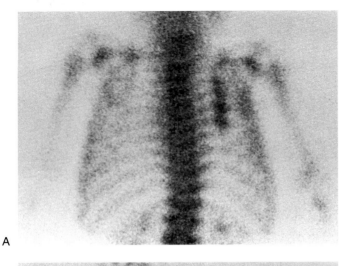

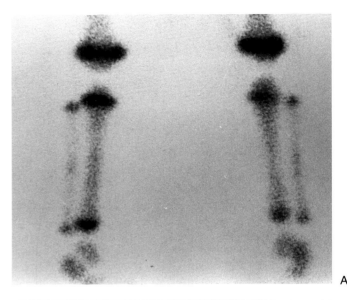

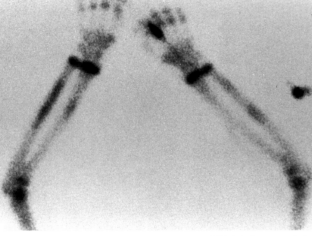

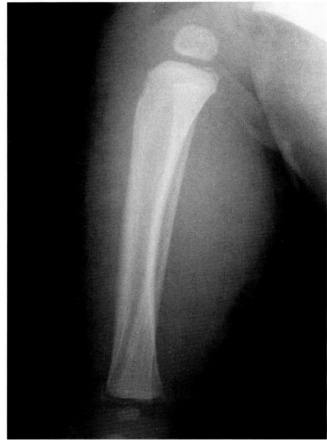

**FIG. 11-8.** Skeletal injury in child abuse. **(A)** This image of the posterior thorax shows posterior rib fractures in a 6-month-old child abuse victim. Note the typical linear distribution of the four consecutive rib fractures. **(B)** This image, with right-side marker source in image, demonstrates several bilateral periosteal injuries to radial, ulnar, and metacarpal diaphyses in a 7-year-old child. The latter injuries were accompanied by bruises.

Metaphyseal fractures may be caused by forcefully grabbing and twisting an extremity or as part of the shaken baby syndrome, which typically occurs as an inappropriate response to prolonged crying by angry adults with poor self-control (29). Such shaking, combined with the relative hypotonicity of infants, leads to severe acceleration and deceleration forces that may have devastating effects, particularly intracranial hemorrhage. In the extremities, these forces are concentrated near the sites of ligamentous insertion at the ends of bones. This often leads to fractures through the metaphysis, usually located just beneath the zone of provisional calcification. This fracture separates the cartilaginous epiphysis along with the metaphyseal zone of provisional calcification from the rest of the metaphysis. The displaced calcific rim, representing the zone of provisional calcification, may appear as a "metaphyseal corner fracture" if it is projected adjacent to the metaphysis. The same fracture may

**FIG. 11-9.** A 2-month-old child abuse victim. **(A)** The anterior bone scan shows increased tibial (and fibular) diaphyseal uptake and asymmetric metaphyseal and epiphyseal activity. **(B)** The left tibial radiograph shows characteristic metaphyseal fractures proximally and distally. The proximal fracture, seen as a corner fracture on this lateral view, was profiled as a bucket handle on the AP view (not shown). A typical bucket-handle fracture is seen distally in the left tibia. Both methods show abnormality, but they demonstrate different aspects of skeletal trauma.

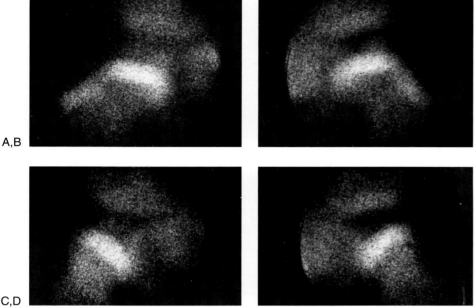

A,B

C,D

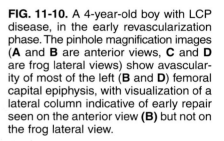

FIG. 11-10. A 4-year-old boy with LCP disease, in the early revascularization phase. The pinhole magnification images (**A** and **B** are anterior views, **C** and **D** are frog lateral views) show avascularity of most of the left (**B** and **D**) femoral capital epiphysis, with visualization of a lateral column indicative of early repair seen on the anterior view (**B**) but not on the frog lateral view.

appear as a "bucket-handle" if it is projected above the metaphysis. These fractures are considered characteristic of child abuse. Whether such fractures can be identified as reliably on scintigraphy as on skeletal surveys is controversial. Activity at the growth plates is normally intense, and we must be able to recognize that region as being irregular or too round or broad in configuration. Asymmetry of growth plate activity certainly helps, but these metaphyseal fractures are often bilateral and symmetric. Performing both a skeletal survey and scintigraphy and interpreting them together maximizes the number of abnormalities that are identified and increases the level of diagnostic confidence (Fig. 11-9). These factors are important in the value of the imaging data for determining whether a child has been physically abused.

### Avascular Necrosis

Skeletal scintigraphy is the most accurate method of demonstrating avascularity of bone. Skeletal localization depends on an intact vascular supply to deliver the radiopharmaceutical to the bone. The greatest usefulness of scintigraphy for AVN is to demonstrate its presence prior to radiographic findings. LCP disease, an idiopathic form of femoral head AVN, affects children between 5 and 10 years of age. In the earliest phases of the disorder, the radiographs are normal even though symptoms are present. During this time, scintigraphy with pinhole magnification views demonstrate complete absence of activity in the proximal femoral epiphysis. This allows a physiologic diagnosis of AVN to be made before radiographic changes.

In patients who already demonstrate radiographic findings of AVN, skeletal scintigraphy may demonstrate the extent of involvement and pattern of revascularization. Con-

way has proposed an extensive classification system for LCP disease based on scintigraphic patterns (32). He observed two distinct patterns of repair in LCP and hypothesized that healing may proceed either by recanalization of existing vasculature or by a slower process of creating new vascular pathways, that is, neovascularization.

For hips that repair via recanalization, by the time radiographs become abnormal, scintigraphy should show a "lateral column" with return of activity to the lateral aspect of the femoral head (Fig. 11-10). With further repair, activity extends from the lateral column anteriorly and medially. Total avascularity of the femoral head in the presence of positive radiographic findings implies that the repair process is delayed and will proceed via neovascularization. These eventually demonstrate base filling, with activity extending progressively from the physis into the head. These scintigraphic patterns may be useful prognostically, with more rapid reconstitution and a better outcome expected from the recanalization pattern.

Besides LCP disease, avascularity of the femoral head may also be caused by septic arthritis, severe cases of toxic synovitis, femoral neck fractures, and other disorders.

Although MRI is also used for evaluating AVN, scintigraphy is directly dependent on blood flow for delivering the tracer to the bone, and so it remains the most accurate means of evaluating the integrity of femoral head vascularity in these disorders.

### Genitourinary Tract Imaging

#### Radionuclide Cystography

Radionuclide cystography is a sensitive and reliable method for demonstrating vesicoureteral reflux, is relatively easy to perform, does not require extensive data processing, and has a very low radiation-absorbed dose. These considerations, along with the prevalence of urinary tract infection (UTI) in children, have made it one of the most frequently performed procedures in pediatric nuclear medicine (see Table 11-1).

A significant advantage of radionuclide cystography compared to the voiding cystourethrogram (VCUG) is the lower radiation dose, which is important because multiple follow-up examinations are often performed. Direct instillation of the radiopharmaceutical into the bladder without systemic distribution keeps whole-body exposure low. Exposure is further limited by emptying the bladder at the conclusion of the examination. This leads to a very low radiation dose to the patient, not only compared to the fluoroscopic VCUG, but also compared to other radionuclide examinations. Ovarian exposure from radionuclide cystography is approximately two orders of magnitude lower than that for a VCUG.

Radionuclide cystography should assess bladder capacity and configuration in addition to vesicoureteral reflux. Reflux may occur during bladder filling, at peak bladder volume, or only during voiding. The pattern of reflux is not simply related to bladder pressure, rather, it is determined by the anatomy of the ureterovesical junction and the effect of bladder contraction on it. In many children, reflux is seen primarily during the filling phase, when bladder volumes and pressures are low. Reflux during this phase may be missed without the continuous monitoring afforded by radionuclide cystography. Serial examinations may show a progressive increase in the bladder volume at which reflux is seen, and this is an encouraging sign of eventual resolution of reflux.

The ability to monitor the patient continuously and to detect smaller amounts of reflux would suggest that radionuclide cystography should be more sensitive for reflux than the VCUG. Several studies have shown that their overall sensitivities are equivalent. Because the VCUG has a higher sensitivity for grade I reflux, it is likely that nuclear cystography is more sensitive for greater degrees of reflux (33). Reflux is an intermittent event, which may not always occur at each bladder filling, and therefore the sensitivity of both examinations can be increased by filling and voiding more than once.

There is widespread agreement that radionuclide cystography is preferable to the fluoroscopic VCUG for follow-up of known vesicoureteral reflux. More controversial is its use as the initial examination. In girls, urethral pathology is extremely rare, and the purpose of the cystogram is to look for reflux. For this, radionuclide cystography suffices, particularly if US is also performed to evaluate for anatomic abnormalities of the urinary tract (34). In boys with suspected lower urinary tract pathology, it is generally considered necessary to exclude posterior urethral valves or other urethral pathology, and a radionuclide cystogram cannot substitute for a carefully performed VCUG.

## Renal Function Analysis

Radionuclide renal function studies include those based on analysis of dynamic imaging data and nonimaging studies with analysis of timed blood samples. Dynamic imaging studies can be analyzed to determine the relative contribution of each kidney toward total renal function (differential function) and to determine the combined function of the kidneys. Most of the work on renal function studies in children has been performed with Tc-99m diethylenetriamine pentaacetic acid (DTPA), which is thought to have a clearance indicative of the glomerular filtration rate (GFR), given that there are some differences between its clearance and that of inulin. It would be desirable to be able to evaluate GFR from the data contained in a dynamic imaging study, and therefore, considerable work has been devoted to this goal in both adults and children.

### Imaging Methods

Piepsz et al. (35) described a theoretically very sound approach in which clearance was determined by the rate of uptake of Tc-99m DTPA into the kidney divided by the plasma concentration. Piepsz used the slope during the accumulation phase (phase II) of the renogram to indicate the rate of tracer accumulation by the kidney. The plasma concentration during that time was determined by a blood pool region of interest calibrated with a single blood sample.

Gates (36) described a much simpler method in an adult population: GFR was estimated by an empiric regression formula with the fractional uptake of Tc-99m DTPA correlated to creatinine clearance. Although the data supporting this method seemed quite good, there are inherent limitations to its use in children. Fractional uptake relates renal uptake to the amount administered rather than the plasma concentration. The implicit assumption that these are equivalent can hold true only if all subjects are the same size, which clearly cannot describe a pediatric population. If a child is given the same amount of tracer as an adult, the child's blood concentration is higher than the adult's. If the same amount is taken up by the kidney, a smaller volume of plasma is cleared in children. Hence, for the same fractional uptake, the child's GFR is lower, although the Gates formula would calculate it as the same.

Combining Piepsz's emphasis on the plasma concentration with the use of an empiric regression, such as that used by Gates, we devised a method for estimating GFR in children (37). The rate of tracer uptake was determined by the slope of the renogram, and the administered dose divided by body weight was used as an index intended to be roughly proportional to plasma concentration. When compared to GFR measured simultaneously by plasma disappearance techniques, this method estimated GFR normalized for body surface area with a mean residual error of 9 ml/min/1.73m². It was also found to be useful in following pediatric patients longitudinally (38).

*Laboratory Methods*

None of these methods for estimating clearance from the renogram is as accurate or reliable as the methods based on analyzing blood samples. The most common methods use plasma clearance kinetics after a single injection of the radiopharmaceutical. Although double-exponential analysis is the most accurate method of evaluating such plasma clearance, the need for at least eight samples has limited its use in children. Single-exponential analysis is more often used, and it requires two or three samples obtained between 2 and 4 hours after injection. Although more convenient, this method often overestimates clearance, particularly in patients with relatively normal renal function. Even more appealing are methods that require a single plasma sample. Although most of this work has been performed in adults, single sample methods have been described in children for several radiopharmaceuticals (39–41). Rather than relying on analyzing plasma clearance kinetics, the single-sample methods are largely empiric, being based on a correlation between the amount of tracer still present in plasma after a specified time and some other measure of clearance. The formulas developed in adults are different from those in children, and they cannot be used interchangeably. It would be desirable if adult formulas could be modified for use in children, which would avoid the need to repeat such work in a pediatric population. Russell et al. (42) used dimensional analysis to demonstrate that adult formulas could be used by adjusting sample collection times by weight divided by area, which is equivalent to the cube root of body weight. Additional verification of such an approach would be useful.

### Diuresis Renography

Evaluation of dilatation of the renal collecting systems and ureters by diuresis renography (43) is the major indication for dynamic renal imaging in children (see Table 11-1). Hydronephrosis is an important sign of obstruction in children, and most of these lesions are congenital. There are also other causes of dilatation of the collecting systems, however, and many systems with significant dilatation are not truly obstructed. The ultimate criterion for obstruction can only be determined retrospectively: Kidneys that are significantly obstructed will demonstrate progression of hydronephrosis or deterioration of function if not corrected. Anatomic studies, such as excretory urography and US, demonstrate the severity of pelvicaliectasis and ureteral dilatation. This dilatation is reflected in a standard renogram by slow transit through the system and prolongation of the drainage phase. This slow drainage does not imply that the dilatation is due to physiologically significant obstruction. Rather, it is a consequence of the dilatation itself. A larger system serves as a "mixing chamber," and the rate of tracer transit through it will be slower. The intent of the diuresis renogram is to minimize the effect of urinary tract dilatation on the rate of drainage by pharmacologically increasing the rate of urine flow through the system. There are clearly limits to this. With massive hydronephrosis, even if the urine flow rate is successfully increased, transit through the system is still slow. The inseparable link between the size of the collecting system and the rate of urinary drainage should warn against relying too much on clearance half-time values. For equivalent urinary flow rates, if a system is twice as large, transit through it takes twice as long. Thus, if drainage half-time values are interpreted dogmatically, obstruction and dilatation will be confused, the very problem that the diuresis renogram was intended to avoid.

In pediatrics, diuresis renography was initially used for children with postnatally recognized hydronephrosis or hydroureteronephrosis. In this population, the diuresis renogram has been helpful in distinguishing obstructed systems from those that are dilated from other causes. This has been demonstrated in many studies in which the diuresis renogram was compared to clinical data, surgical findings, pathologic material, and pressure-perfusion (Whitaker) test results. Although the diuresis renogram is usually accurate in identifying obstruction, false-positive results may be found in the presence of either massive hydronephrosis or substantial impairment of renal function. As long as these conditions are recognized, incorrect conclusions should be avoidable. Experimentally, false-negative studies can also be seen in the presence of acute obstruction (44), but this is rarely a problem with appropriate clinical use of diuresis renography.

More recently, a unique patient population has emerged: infants recognized to have urinary tract dilatation on routine prenatal US screening examinations. Because of its success in older children, diuresis renography has been widely used in these infants. These patients differ from older children, however, in their response to diuresis as well as their underlying disorder, and the role of diuresis renography in neonatal hydronephrosis is not clearly established.

The most widely used diuretic for these studies is furosemide, and its effect is diminished in infants. Furosemide must first be delivered into the lumen of the loop of Henle by either glomerular filtration or tubular secretion, and both of these mechanisms are impaired in infants (45,46). Because of this diminished response to furosemide, an age-dependent dosage schedule has been proposed, with relatively larger doses given to younger children (47), although it is not known if such adjustment produces an equivalent diuretic response. With unilateral hydronephrosis, the contralateral kidney has been used as a control to help determine whether functional immaturity is the cause of insufficient wash-out. If the contralateral kidney had a clearance half-time of <9 minutes, renal function was deemed mature enough to confidently interpret the wash-out phase of the examination (48). Another approach is to simply regard good wash-out as indicative of the absence of obstruction and poor wash-out as an indeterminate finding in this patient population.

Several clinical series have addressed neonatal hydronephrosis (47,49–52). Homsy and colleagues (49) demonstrated that diuresis renograms performed in early infancy correlated poorly with follow-up examination at 3 to 6 months and suggested that the wash-out response on the initial examination should not be used to determine the need for surgery. The findings at 6 months appeared to be more reliable, and thus they recommended initial observation for most patients, with early surgery reserved for those with unequivocal obstruction. Observation during this time appears safe, with no evidence of irreversible functional deterioration (47,49). With surgery, washout often improves, but there is little improvement in function (49–51). Piepsz et al. (50) used functional impairment rather than poor washout as their major criterion for surgery. Most infants with normal function who were followed without surgery showed continued renal growth and functional maturation that was comparable to the nonhydronephrotic kidney. Gordon and coworkers (51) demonstrated that hydronephrotic kidneys with initially good function remained stable, and in some of those with initially diminished function there was spontaneous improvement. Their series had a high incidence of false-positive diuresis renograms in patients who showed no evidence of functional deterioration even though surgery was not performed. They postulated that many cases of in utero hydronephrosis may be due to self-limited obstruction that resolves before birth. In neonates with unilateral hydronephrosis, Koff and Campbell (52) also noted that a poor wash-out response to furosemide did not correspond to any other indication of obstruction, such as further deterioration of function, development of compensatory hypertrophy in the contralateral kidney, or progression of hydronephrosis. Both studies concluded that the tests usually used for identifying obstruction are not useful in this patient population. The diuresis renogram was found to be reliable for excluding obstruction, but failure to demonstrate wash-out was not reliable for positively identifying it. Therapeutically, Koff and Campbell (52) concluded that most infants whose hydronephrosis was discovered by prenatal US could be managed nonoperatively. Similarly, Gordon et al. (51) questioned the role of surgery because many neonatal hydronephrotic kidneys improved spontaneously, and those that did have surgery did not show significant functional improvement.

These clinical series shed some light on the natural history of hydronephrosis discovered in utero, provide no data from controlled studies on the effect of therapeutic interventions, and leave unclarified the role of imaging studies, particularly diuresis renography, in the management of these patients. Although baseline and follow-up diuresis renograms were performed in all these series, their diagnostic role was not defined. It is clear that the response to furosemide diuresis as a test for obstruction was not relied on. Indeed, most investigators have found that positive results for obstruction are likely to be erroneous. Some of these series have relied on the renographic assessment of function as an indicator of the need for surgery, whereas others have shown that many of these kidneys demonstrate functional improvement even without operative intervention. Many investigators appear to have used the diuresis renogram to monitor the functional integrity of these kidneys during the time that the natural history of hydronephrosis discovered in utero was just beginning to be understood. To establish the efficacy of diuresis renography beyond this initial period, however, it will be necessary to demonstrate that the examination contributes to clinical decision making. This will first require a determination of the role of surgery in these patients.

### Renal Cortical Imaging for Infection

Evaluation of children with UTI is another important aspect of radionuclide imaging in pediatric patients. Radionuclides have been used to evaluate UTI since 1964, when abnormal iodine 131 (I-131) hippuran renograms were identified in patients with acute pyelonephritis (53). Much more promising for use in infection are the renal cortical imaging agents Tc-99m glucoheptonate and Tc-99m dimercaptosuccinic acid (DMSA). Both agents demonstrate renal cortical binding, but their renal excretion is quite different. DMSA has minimal excretion, whereas glucoheptonate has considerably more excretion, which provides the opportunity to evaluate the collecting system as well. The cortical localization of these agents reflects regional renal function, and the focal parenchymal defects seen with pyelonephritis may be due to associated cortical ischemia or abnormal tubular transport.

The imaging approach to children with UTI depends on the questions being asked. Vesicoureteral reflux and structural anomalies, particularly those associated with obstruction, must be looked for. Although previously evaluated by the combination of a radiographic VCUG and an excretory urogram, radionuclide cystography may be used to look for reflux and US to evaluate anatomy and evidence of obstruction. Additional information that can be obtained from other imaging studies includes the functional status of the kidneys, whether the kidneys are involved in the acute infection, and whether scars are present from previous episodes of reflux and infection.

The functional status of each kidney is best evaluated with radionuclide imaging. Contrast opacification for excretory urography also depends on glomerular filtration and thus supplies some functional information, but this is not as quantitative as the scintigraphic evaluation.

Knowing whether acute UTI is limited to the bladder or also involves the kidneys is important in patient management. The need for surgical correction of vesicoureteral reflux may depend on whether recurrent infections have included the upper tracts. Fever, the severity of constitutional symptoms, costovertebral angle tenderness, and immunologic features of the infecting bacteria have been correlated with renal involvement, but these are not always reliable.

For the recognition of acute renal infection by imaging, there is considerable variation in the effectiveness of different methods. The excretory urogram is nonspecific and very

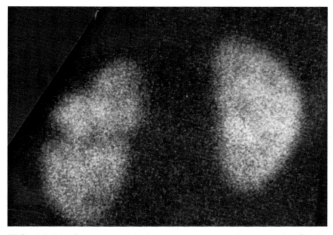

FIG. 11-11. A 4-year-old girl with acute pyelonephritis. Static delayed Tc-99m GH posterior image shows multiple spherical (e.g., lower pole medially) and flare-shaped (mid region laterally) focal defects radiating to the periphery of the left kidney.

insensitive, recognizing acute infection in only 20% to 25% of cases. US is more sensitive and may demonstrate focal renal enlargement and alteration of the normal echo pattern with loss of corticomedullary differentiation. The findings may mimic renal mass lesions. With acute infection, radionuclide cortical scintigraphy typically shows a focal area of diminished tracer localization that may be flare shaped or spherical and often radiates from the pelvicaliceal system to the periphery of the kidney (Fig. 11-11). Acute pyelonephritis should not have renal volume loss, as is seen with scars. Several studies have shown radionuclide cortical scintigraphy to be the most sensitive imaging test for acute pyelonephritis. In some series, cortical scintigraphy was 100% sensitive for identifying acute pyelonephritis (54,55). In others, the sensitivity of cortical scintigraphy was <100% but greater than that of US, which in turn was more sensitive than excretory urography (56,57). Cortical scintigraphy has limitations in evaluation of the extent of infection. US is usually able to identify areas of liquefaction, suggesting a potentially drainable abscess, and CT and US can identify extension of infection into the perinephric soft tissues.

Renal scars may be considered the hallmark of reflux nephropathy. On excretory urography and US, scars have characteristic focal thinning of the renal cortex overlying a dilated and blunted calyx. With cortical scintigraphy, scarring appears as irregularity of the cortical outline and evidence of volume loss. These findings are even more specific for reflux nephropathy if the cortical images are combined with evidence of subjacent caliectasis (Fig. 11-12). This may be seen on the dynamic phase for studies performed with Tc-99m glucoheptonate. With multiple areas of scarring, the kidney is globally small with thinning of the parenchyma; this is recognizable with all imaging methods.

The selection of imaging studies in children with UTI depends on several factors, including age, severity of infection, and results of previous examinations.

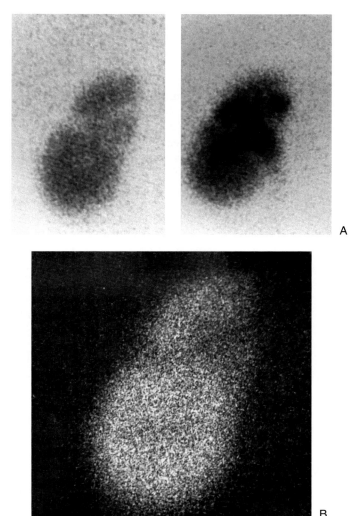

FIG. 11-12. A 4-year-old girl with left reflux nephropathy demonstrated with combined Tc-99m MAG3 and Tc-99m GH imaging, posterior views. (A) The early Tc-99m MAG3 image (left) shows peripheral defects in the left kidney. A subsequent image (right) shows subjacent caliectasis corresponding to the peripheral defects seen in the early images. (B) The Tc-99m GH image shows scarring of the left kidney in the same regions, in a pattern nearly identical to the early Tc-99m MAG3 image. Similar results could have been obtained using dynamic and static imaging performed with Tc-99m GH alone.

There has been a trend toward replacing the VCUG and excretory urogram by radionuclide cystography and US for determining the presence of reflux and abnormalities of the upper tracts. The use of cortical scintigraphy in place of US could also be considered. Clearly this would provide more information regarding function and would have a higher yield in demonstrating focal pyelonephritis. Although anatomic detail is not as well visualized with cortical scintigraphy, it is not certain that significant anatomic lesions would be missed. Most anatomic abnormalities

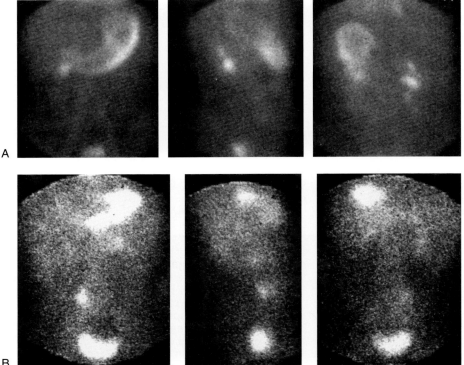

**FIG. 11-13.** Meckel's diverticulum scintigraphy, showing the value of right lateral and posterior views. **(A)** This row of figures shows prominent activity in the right renal collecting system. The anterior view (left) shows the activity in the right side of the abdomen. The right lateral view (center) shows that this activity is posterior, and the posterior view (right) shows the activity even more intensely, along with calyces above and below it, indicating that the major collection is in the renal pelvis. **(B)** This row of images shows a Meckel's diverticulum in the anterior LLQ of the anterior view (left), anteriorly in the lateral view (center), and barely visualized in the posterior view (right).

would be associated with either hydronephrosis and poor drainage or abnormal renal size and configuration. These should be recognized with glucoheptonate, and more complete evaluation could then follow with US, supplemented by excretory urography in some cases. One potential pitfall of such an approach would be the failure to identify duplex systems with a nonfunctioning upper pole associated with hydronephrosis.

### Testicular Scintigraphy

Testicular scintigraphy is useful for torsion of the spermatic cord, which most frequently occurs during adolescence. In most cases, the clinical diagnosis of torsion is quite accurate. Scintigraphy is usually not needed for typical cases, but rather to rule out torsion in patients whose clinical findings suggest that it is unlikely.

### Gastrointestinal Imaging

### Meckel's Diverticulum

The vast majority of examinations looking for a Meckel's diverticulum are performed in children with gastrointestinal bleeding, and scintigraphy is the most sensitive and specific imaging test.

A Meckel's diverticulum is a remnant of the omphalomesenteric duct, which extends from the umbilicus to the antimesenteric aspect of the ileum. The rule of twos (58) indicates the following:

- They occur in 2% of the general population.
- They are located within 2 feet of the ileocecal valve.
- They are symptomatic in 20% of cases.
- They occur in children <2 years of age.

There is considerable variability in the reported frequency of symptoms, with other estimates suggesting that 25% to 40% are symptomatic (59). Approximately 50% of all Meckel's diverticula contain ectopic gastric mucosa. The most common presentation is gastrointestinal bleeding from peptic ulceration of the ileum adjacent to a Meckel's diverticulum that contains gastric mucosa. This bleeding is often painless, may be major, and usually appears to originate from the lower or mid gastrointestinal tract. True melena, such as that seen with gastric or duodenal bleeding, is not characteristically seen with a Meckel's diverticulum. Less frequently, a Meckel's diverticulum may present with obstruction from a fibrous band connecting it to the anterior abdominal wall or from intussusception, with the Meckel's diverticulum serving as a lead point. Some may also become inflamed and present with diverticulitis.

Meckel's diverticulum scintigraphy is based on localization of the pertechnetate anion in ectopic gastric mucosa. Although the acid-producing parietal cells help to define gastric mucosa histologically, it is the gastric mucous cells that trap the pertechnetate anion (60). The alkaline secretion from these cells coats the gastric mucosa and helps to protect it from gastric acidity. Although there are mucous cells throughout the gastrointestinal tract, significant localization of pertechnetate is seen only with gastric mucosa. This may be related to the relative numbers of these cells or to differences in their metabolic activities.

A normal examination demonstrates rapid accumulation in the stomach. This initially conforms to the outline of the stomach, which then fills in as pertechnetate is secreted into the gastric lumen. Subsequent antegrade passage of pertechnetate from the stomach through the duodenum and into jejunum is often seen. There is also some excretion of pertechnetate through the urinary tract. The bladder is always visualized, and the kidneys are often seen, particularly if the collecting system is dilated.

A Meckel's diverticulum demonstrates a focal area of pertechnetate localization, which is usually similar to the stomach in its time of appearance. If the amount of gastric mucosa is relatively small, it may take longer for the Meckel's to be visualized against body background activity. Although a Meckel's diverticulum is usually located in the right lower quadrant of the abdomen (Fig. 11-13), its position is variable, not only between patients, but also over time in the same patient. It is part of the mesenteric small bowel and thus mobile.

Diagnostic difficulties with Meckel's diverticulum scintigraphy include various causes of false-negative and false-positive examinations.

*False-Negative Studies*

Failure to identify a Meckel's diverticulum (i.e., a false negative) may be due to one of the following causes:

- A small amount of gastric mucosa
- Failure to recognize it when present
- Rapid wash-out of activity from a Meckel's diverticulum

Although rapid wash-out has been cited to occur with active bleeding, the bleeding is usually from the adjacent ileum; thus, it is not certain whether this explanation is correct. A Meckel's diverticulum may also be obscured by excessively rapid transit of activity from the stomach through the small bowel. In such cases, pharmacologic augmentation may be useful with cimetidine, which inhibits secretion of pertechnetate from the mucous cells into the lumen (61), or glucagon, which decreases gastrointestinal motility. A Meckel's diverticulum without gastric mucosa cannot be identified by scintigraphy. These do not cause bleeding, and they are generally excluded from consideration in describing the accuracy of scintigraphy.

*False-Positive Studies*

There are many causes for false-positive examinations, including

- Incorrect identification of normal structures, particularly portions of the urinary tract

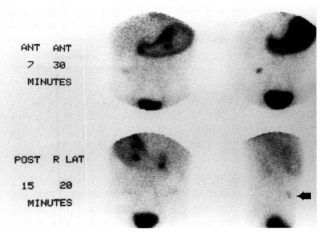

**FIG. 11-14.** Meckel's diverticulum scan, showing the value of time to appearance of lesion. The anterior image obtained at 7 minutes (upper left) shows gastric activity and visualization of both renal pelves. The paired renal pelves are better seen on the posterior 15-minute image (lower left). The 30-minute anterior image (upper right) clearly identifies the Meckel's diverticulum that was in retrospect barely visible at 7 minutes (upper left); note that the increase in gastric activity parallels the increase in the Meckel's diverticulum. The earlier visualization of the pelves suggests a different etiology. The right lateral 20-minute image (lower right) shows the faint Meckel's diverticulum anteriorly (*arrow*).

- Focal areas of hyperemia
- Normal transit of pertechnetate from the stomach
- Ectopic gastric mucosa in structures other than a Meckel's diverticulum

All may be confused with a Meckel's diverticulum.

Focal accumulation in the urinary tract is most likely to be noticed with mild to moderate dilatation of the renal pelvis or ureter. The major features that distinguish this from a Meckel's diverticulum are location and time course of visualization. The kidneys and ureters are retroperitoneal and are more posterior than the intraperitoneal location of a Meckel's diverticulum. This is best demonstrated by a lateral view as well as relative intensity on comparison of anterior and posterior views (Fig. 11-14). Identification of a calyx above or below the renal pelvis additionally confirms that it is urinary tract activity rather than a Meckel's diverticulum. Urinary tract activity often appears earlier (see Fig. 11-14) than a Meckel's diverticulum, and, depending on the size of the collecting system, it may then remain constant or start to diminish while the gastric mucosa is still increasing in activity. A bladder diverticulum may also simulate a Meckel's diverticulum, and determining whether there is complete emptying with voiding may be useful.

Focal areas of hyperemia may be visualized, such as those seen with hemangioma, focal inflammation, and the uterus. In most cases, these should not cause diagnostic difficulty. In the absence of actual concentration of pertechnetate, focal hyperemia should not appear very intense and it should fade in a manner similar to blood pool activity in the spleen and the major abdominal and pelvic vessels. Intussusception has been reported as a cause of false-positive Meckel's diverticulum examinations. This is a potentially significant problem because in some cases the distinction between these entities is not clear clinically, although therapy is quite different (laparotomy for Meckel's diverticulum versus hydrostatic or pneumatic reduction for intussusception). In the absence of ectopic gastric mucosa, visualization of intussusception should simply be due to associated hyperemia, and thus tracer localization should be mild and transient. Alternatively, intussusception may by caused by a Meckel's diverticulum serving as a lead point. Some of these may contain ectopic gastric mucosa and are thus potentially identifiable scintigraphically.

Normal transit of pertechnetate from the stomach through the small bowel is usually recognizable by the time course with which various parts of the gastrointestinal tract are visualized. The final category of false-positive examinations are those that recognize ectopic gastric mucosa in a structure other than a Meckel's diverticulum, usually a gastrointestinal duplication. Such cases may have similar symptoms and generally require surgical excision; their identification on scintigraphy does not constitute a diagnostic failure.

*Diagnostic Accuracy*

Despite these known causes of false-negative and false-positive examinations, scintigraphy is highly effective. In an extensive review of the literature, Sfakianakis and Conway (62) reported that the overall accuracy in 226 surgically proven cases was 90%. In 954 total cases with either clinical or surgical final diagnoses, accuracy was 98%, which is similar to the approximately 95% accuracy suggested by other sources. Although not perfect, the accuracy of Meckel's diverticulum scintigraphy is quite good for abdominal imaging examinations, and it is certainly much better than any other method of diagnosing a Meckel's diverticulum.

### Hepatobiliary Imaging

For the gastrointestinal tract, hepatobiliary scintigraphy is useful for distinguishing biliary atresia from neonatal hepatitis in infants with prolonged jaundice. These studies are aided by therapeutic pretreatment with phenobarbital (12). Interpretation of the scintigraphic findings is also aided by collecting gastric and duodenal samples during the examination.

### Gastroesophageal Reflux

Evaluation of gastroesophageal reflux is a frequent examination in many centers. The major issues regarding this examination are selecting which infants should be studied and how much reflux can be considered within the range of normal. In infants whose clinical problem is spitting up, identification of reflux per se is moot. It is more useful to look for reflux in infants with other clinical problems, such as failure to thrive, wheezing, recurrent atelectasis and pneumonia, and bizarre posturing.

### Thyroid Scintigraphy

In this chapter, only the evaluation of congenital hypothyroidism and thyroglossal duct cyst is considered. Thyroid scintigraphy in infants may be performed with either Tc-99m pertechnetate or I-123 iodide. There are advantages to each of these, and neither is clearly preferable. I-123 iodide delivers a higher radiation dose to the thyroid but a smaller whole-body dose than Tc-99m pertechnetate. I-123 is administered orally, which avoids intravenous injection, but a longer waiting time is needed before imaging. A higher thyroid-to-background ratio is usually considered an advantage of iodide, but visualization of background structures with pertechnetate often helps to define thyroid position in pediatric patients in whom thyroid imaging is warranted.

Congenital hypothyroidism occurs in approximately one in 4,000 newborns (63). It is included in routine screening tests for all newborns because it is relatively common, it can be successfully screened for, it is easily treated, and treatment significantly improves prognosis. In North America, screening programs usually initially measure thyroxine ($T_4$), and for those with low $T_4$ levels, thyroid-stimulating hormone (TSH) is then measured on the initial sample. This procedure recognizes primary hypothyroidism as well as some but not all cases of secondary hypothyroidism due to pituitary insufficiency. In Europe and Japan, screening programs often use TSH elevation as the initial screening test, but this approach does not detect pituitary insufficiency.

Congenital hypothyroidism is most often (90%) due to abnormal morphologic development (thyroid dysgenesis), including complete absence (athyreosis) and more commonly maldevelopment, with thyroid tissue that is small, not bilobate, and usually ectopic. Most ectopic thyroids are midline and located along the path of normal thyroid descent from the region of foramen cecum at the base of the tongue. Less commonly, congenital hypothyroidism may be due to disorders of hormone production.

Congenital hypothyroidism may also be due to fetal exposure to radioiodine, excessive iodide, antithyroid drugs, amiodarone, and other rare causes. Some neonatal hypothyroidism is transient and may be related to developmental immaturity. Transient neonatal hypothyroidism may also occur in infants of mothers with autoimmune thyroid disease and is due to maternal antibodies, particularly TSH-binding inhibitory antibody. Thyroid scintigraphy is useful in distinguishing these causes of congenital hypothyroidism, which is important for prognosis and identifying risk in subsequent pregnancies.

Recognition of thyroid dysgenesis is important because it indicates the need for lifelong thyroid replacement and also because it is sporadic and thus has no increased risk for recurrence in subsequent children. Scintigraphy in thyroid dysgenesis is most definitive when an ectopic thyroid is

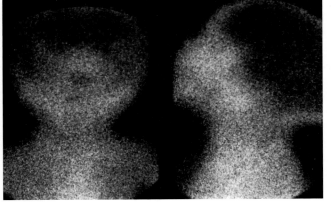

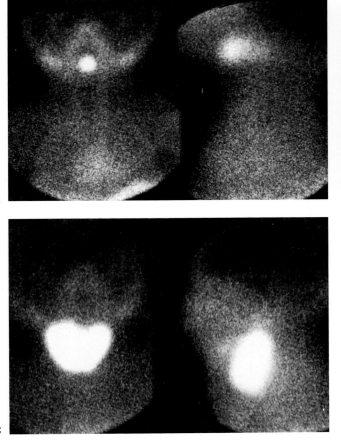

**FIG. 11-15.** Congenital hypothyroidism. Tc-99m pertechnetate provides enough background activity to recognize landmarks and determine thyroid position. **(A)** These images (anterior view on the left, the left lateral view on the right) show thyroid ectopy, with a small round thyroid positioned at the base of the tongue. **(B)** With athyreosis, no thyroid is visualized. **(C)** These images show greatly elevated uptake into an enlarged thyroid gland. In the presence of biochemical hypothyroidism, this finding is compatible with a biosynthetic defect.

identified. These are usually round rather than bilobate and are positioned in the midline and higher than the normal thyroid gland (Fig. 11-15A). With athyreosis, no thyroid tissue is visualized (Fig. 11-15B), but this finding is not as specific because nonvisualization of an anatomically normal thyroid may occur with severe impairment of thyroid function, including that due to TSH-binding inhibitory antibody. A thyroid with normal morphology and normal or decreased uptake may be seen with transient hypothyroidism, and this can be evaluated by discontinuing thyroid replacement. Such a trial is usually not performed until 3 years of age so that the child is not subjected to thyroid insufficiency while the thyroid is needed for neurologic development. A normal-appearing thyroid is also seen with deficiency of thyroxine-binding globulin. In this condition, a low $T_4$ is found by screening programs, even though true hypothyroidism does not exist. TSH measurements should be normal in these children. Patients with disorders of $T_4$ biosynthesis typically have goitrous hypothyroidism. Scintigraphy demonstrates thyromegaly with elevated uptake in most of these patients (Fig. 11-15C), except for those whose defect involves iodide trapping (64). Biosynthetic defects due to enzyme deficiency are usually autosomal recessive in inheritance. In cases where the defect is in iodine organification, the perchlorate discharge test is abnormal.

Thyroid scintigraphy is also useful in the evaluation of suspected thyroglossal duct cyst. These present as midline neck masses located anywhere from the base of the tongue to the level of the thyroid. Because an ectopic thyroid may have a similar position, it is important to be sure that the neck mass does not represent the patient's only thyroid tissue before it is excised. The goal of thyroid scintigraphy is to identify a normal thyroid gland in addition to the midline neck mass. If so, the midline mass may be excised. If it turns out that the mass does represent the patient's only thyroid, it should not be removed. Most patients with thyroid ectopia are either hypothyroid or potentially hypothyroid and are usually given thyroid replacement therapy.

### Other Pediatric Applications

The many other pediatric applications of scintigraphy cannot be reviewed because of space limitations. Oncologic applications include bone scintigraphy for metastatic disease, especially for neuroblastoma, gallium 67 citrate for lymphoma, I-131 meta-iodobenzylguanidine for neuroblastoma, and thallium 201 thallous chloride for brain tumors and soft-tissue neoplasms.

There is considerable variability between centers in the use of pediatric nuclear cardiology. The radionuclide determination of relative pulmonary and systemic blood flow provides accurate quantification of left-to-right intracardiac shunts. In some centers this test is frequently used. In others it is not thought to provide sufficient information above other clinical and echocardiographic evaluation to warrant routine use. Pulmonary perfusion studies with Tc-99m MAA are useful in determining relative pulmonary blood flow in patients who have had systemic-to-pulmonary shunts or repair of pulmonary arterial lesions, such as pulmonary artery sling. In children, thallium myocardial scintigraphy has been used for the coronary lesions associated with Kawasaki syndrome and aberrant origin of the right coronary artery from the pulmonary artery.

As in adult nuclear medicine, functional brain scintigraphy has great potential for evaluating both neurologic deficits and seizure disorders. These studies have been used in the evaluation of perinatal insult, cerebral palsy, infants treated with extracorporeal membrane oxygenation, moyamoya disease, intractable seizures, and psychiatric disorders.

# REFERENCES

1. Meyers WG. Introduction: Historical Perspectives. In Handmaker H, Lowenstein JM (eds), Nuclear Medicine in Clinical Pediatrics. New York: Society of Nuclear Medicine, 1975;1–5.
2. Hamilton JG. The use of radiotracers in biology and medicine. Radiology 1942;39:541–572.
3. Winter CC. A new test for vesicoureteral reflux: an external technique using radioisotopes. J Urol 1959;81:105–111.
4. Blaufox MD, Gruskin A, Sandler P, Goldman H. Radionuclide cystography for detection of vesicoureteral reflux in children. J Pediatr 1971;79:239–246.
5. Conway JJ, King LR, Belman AB, Thorson T. Detection of vesicoureteral reflux with radionuclide cystography. AJR Am J Roentgenol 1972;115:720–727.
6. Harden RMG, Alexander WD, Kennedy I. Isotope uptake and scanning of the stomach in man with Tc-99m pertechnetate. Lancet 1967;1:1305–1307.
7. Jewett TC Jr, Duszynski DO, Allen JE. The visualization of Meckel's diverticulum with Tc-99m-pertechnetate. Surgery 1970;68:567–570.
8. Folse R, Braunwald E. Pulmonary vascular dilution curves recorded by external detection in the diagnosis of left-to-right shunts. Br Heart J 1962;24:166–172.
9. Maltz DL, Treves S. Quantitative radionuclide angiography: determination of $Q_P/Q_S$ in children. Circulation 1973;47:1049–1056.
10. Gates GF, Orme HW, Dore EK. Measurement of cardiac shunting with technetium labeled albumin aggregates. J Nucl Med 1971;12:746–749.
11. Brent RL, Geppert LJ. The use of radioactive rose bengal in the evaluation of infantile jaundice. Am J Dis Child 1959;98:720–730.
12. Majd MM, Reba RC, Altman RP. Effect of phenobarbital on Tc-99m-IDA scintigraphy in the evaluation of neonatal jaundice. Semin Nucl Med 1981;11:194–204.
13. Shore RM, Hendee WR. Radiopharmaceutical dosage selection for pediatric nuclear medicine. J Nucl Med 1986;27:287–298.
14. Dich VQ, Nelson JD, Haltalin KC. Osteomyelitis in infants and children. Am J Dis Child 1975;129:1273–1278.
15. Ogden JA, Lister G. The pathophysiology of neonatal osteomyelitis. Pediatrics 1975;55:474–478.
16. Nixon GW. Acute hematogenous osteomyelitis. Pediatr Ann 1976;5:64–81.
17. Handmaker H. Acute hematogenous osteomyelitis: has the bone scan betrayed us? Radiology 1980;135:787–789.
18. Nixon GW. Hematogenous osteomyelitis of metaphyseal equivalent locations. AJR Am J Roentgenol 1978;130:123–129.
19. Ash JM, Gilday DC. The futility of bone scanning in neonatal osteomyelitis: concise communication. J Nucl Med 1980;21:417–420.
20. Bressler EC, Conway JJ, Weiss SC. Neonatal osteomyelitis examined by bone scintigraphy. Radiology 1984;152:685–688.
21. Welkon CJ, Long SS, Fisher MC, et al. Pyogenic arthritis in infants and children: a review of 95 cases. Pediatr Infect Dis J 1986;5:669–676.
22. Sharwood PF. The irritable hip syndrome in children. Acta Orthop Scand 1981;52:633–638.
23. Miller JH, Sanderson RA. Scintigraphy of toddler's fracture. J Nucl Med 1988;29:2001–2003.
24. Starshak RJ, Simons GW, Sty JR. Occult fracture of the calcaneus: another toddler's fracture. Pediatr Radiol 1984;14:37–40.
25. Englaro EE, Gelfand MJ, Paltiel HJ. Bone scintigraphy in preschool children with lower extremity pain of unknown origin. J Nucl Med 1992;33:351–354.
26. Johnson GF. Pediatric Lisfranc injury: "bunkbed" fracture. AJR Am J Roentgenol 1981;137:1041–1044.
27. Merton DF, Radkowski MA, Leonidas JC. The abused child: a radiological reappraisal. Radiology 1983;146:377–381.
28. Sty JR, Starshak RJ. The role of bone scintigraphy in the evaluation of the suspected abused child. Radiology 1983;146:369–375.
29. Kleinman PK. Diagnostic Imaging of Child Abuse. Baltimore: Williams & Wilkins, 1987;5–28.
30. Smith FW, Gilday DL, Ash JM, Green MD. Unsuspected costo-vertebral fractures demonstrated by bone scanning in the child abuse syndrome. Pediatr Radiol 1980;10:103–106.
31. Conway JJ, Collins M, Tanz RT, et al. The role of bone scintigraphy in detecting child abuse. Semin Nucl Med 1993;23:321–333.
32. Conway JJ. A scintigraphic classification of Legg-Calvé-Perthes disease. Semin Nucl Med 1993;23:274–329.
33. Conway JJ, King LR, Belman AB, et al. Detection of vesicoureteral reflux with radionuclide cystography: a comparison with roentgenographic cystography. AJR Radium Ther Nucl Med 1972;115:720–727.
34. Strife JL, Bisset GS, Kirks DR, et al. Nuclear cystography and renal sonography: findings in girls with urinary tract infection. AJR Am J Roentgenol 1989;153:115–119.
35. Piepsz A, Denis R, Ham HR, et al. A simple method for measuring separate glomerular filtration rate using a single injection of Tc-99m DTPA and the scintillation camera. J Pediatr 1987;93:769–774.
36. Gates GF. Glomerular filtration rate: estimation from fractional renal accumulation of $^{99m}$Tc DTPA (stannous). AJR Am J Roentgenol 1982;138:565–570.
37. Shore RM, Koff SA, Mentser M, et al. Glomerular filtration rate in children: estimation from the Tc-99m-DTPA renogram. Radiology 1984;151:627–633.
38. Shore RM, Koff SA, Hayes JR, et al. Glomerular filtration rate in children: prospective validation and longitudinal utilization of determination from the Tc-99m DTPA renogram. Am J Kidney Dis 1986;8:170–180.
39. Tauxe WN, Hagge W, Stickler GB. Estimation of Effective Renal Plasma Flow in Children by Use of a Single Plasma Sample After Injection of Orthoiodohippurate. In Dynamic Studies with Radioisotopes in Medicine. Vienna: International Atomic Energy Agency, 1974;I:265–275.
40. Tauxe WN, Bagchi A, Tepe PG, Krishnaiah PR. Single-sample method for the estimation of glomerular filtration rate in children. J Nucl Med 1987;28:366–371.
41. Ham HR, Piepsz A. Estimation of glomerular filtration rate in infants and in children using a single-plasma sample method. J Nucl Med 1991;32:1294–1297.
42. Russell CD, Dubovsky EV, Scott JW. Simplified methods for renal clearance in children: scaling for patient size. J Nucl Med 1991;32:1821–1825.
43. Koff SA, Thrall JH, Keyes JW. Assessment of hydroureteronephrosis in children using diuretic radionuclide urography. J Urol 1980;123:531–534.
44. Koff SA, Hayden LJ, Cirulli C, Shore RM. Pathophysiology of ureteropelvic junction obstruction: experimental and clinical observations. J Urol 1986;136:336–338.
45. Mirochnick MH, Miceli JJ, Kramer PA, et al. Furosemide pharmacokinetics in very low birth weight infants. J Pediatr 1988;112:653–657.
46. Stewart CL, Jose PA. Transitional nephrology. Urol Clin North Am 1985;12:143–149.
47. Dejter SW Jr, Eggli DF, Gibbons MD. Delayed management of neonatal hydronephrosis. J Urol 1988;140:1305–1309.
48. Koff SA, McDowell GC, Byard M. Diuretic radionuclide assessment

of obstruction in the infant: guidelines for successful interpretation. J Urol 1988;140:1165–1167.

49. Homsy YL, Williot P, Danais S. Transitional neonatal hydronephrosis: fact or fantasy. J Urol 1986;136:339–341.

50. Piepsz A, Hall M, Ham HR, et al. Prospective management of neonates with pelviureteric junction stenosis: therapeutic strategy based on 99m Tc-DTPA studies. Scand J Urol Nephrol 1989;23:31–36.

51. Gordon I, Dhillon HK, Gatanash H, Peters AM. Antenatal diagnosis of pelvic hydronephrosis: assessment of renal function and drainage as a guide to management. J Nucl Med 1991;32:1649–1654.

52. Koff SA, Campbell K. Nonoperative management of unilateral neonatal hydronephrosis. J Urol 1992;148:525–531.

53. Dodge EA. The use of I-131-labelled "hippuran" renocystogram in the study of acute pyelonephritis. Med J Aust 1964;1:873–881.

54. Handmaker H. Nuclear renal imaging in acute pyelonephritis. Semin Nucl Med 1982;12:246–253.

55. Sty JR, Wells RG, Starshak RJ, et al. Imaging in acute renal infection in children. AJR Am J Roentgenol 1987;148:471–477.

56. Traisman ES, Conway JJ, Traisman HS, et al. The localization of urinary tract infection with $^{99m}$Tc glucoheptonate cortical scintigraphy. Pediatr Radiol 1986;16:403–496.

57. Jakobsson B, Nolstedt L, Svensson L, et al. $^{99m}$Technetium-dimercaptosuccinic acid scan in the diagnosis of acute pyelonephritis in children: relation to clinical and radiological findings. Pediatr Nephrol 1992;6:328–334.

58. Kirks DR, Caron KH. Gastrointestinal Tract. In Kirks DR (ed), Practical Pediatric Imaging: Diagnostic Radiology of Infants and Children (2nd ed). Boston: Little, Brown, 1991;768.

59. Berquist TH, Nolan GN, Stephens DH, et al. Specificity of Tc-99m pertechnetate scintigraphic diagnosis of Meckel's diverticulum: review of 100 cases. J Nucl Med 1976;17:465–469.

60. Chaudhuri TK, Polak JJ. Autoradiographic studies of distribution in the stomach of $^{99m}$Tc-pertechnetate. Radiology 1977;123:223–224.

61. Petrokubi JR, Baum S, Rohrer GV. Cimetidine administration resulting in improved pertechnetate imaging of Meckel's diverticulum. Clin Nucl Med 1978;3:385–388.

62. Sfakianakis GN, Conway JJ. Detection of ectopic gastric mucosa in Meckel's diverticulum and in other aberrations by scintigraphy: I. Pathophysiology and 10-year clinical experience. J Nucl Med 1981;22:647–654.

63. DiGeorge A. Disorders of the Thyroid Gland. In Behrman RE (ed), Nelson Textbook of Pediatrics (14th ed). Philadelphia: Saunders, 1992;1414–1421.

64. Kim EE, Domstad PA, Choy YC, DeLand FH. Avid thyroid uptake of Tc-99m sodium pertechnetate in children with goitrous cretinism. Clin Pediatr (Phila) 1981;20:437–439.

*Textbook of Nuclear Medicine,*
edited by Michael A. Wilson.
Lippincott–Raven Publishers, Philadelphia © 1998.

CHAPTER 12

# Bone Densitometry

Richard B. Mazess

During the 1970s, bone densitometry using the single-photon absorptiometry (SPA) technique developed at the University of Wisconsin was adopted by several hundred researchers. SPA used a low-energy radionuclide source (iodine 125 [I-125] at 28-keV photon) and permitted measurement of the peripheral skeleton (e.g., radius, os calcis). In the 1980s, the SPA approach was supplanted by dual-photon absorptiometry (DPA). This technique, also developed at the University of Wisconsin, used a dual-energy radionuclide (gadolinium 153 [Gd-153] at 44- and 100-keV photons). DPA allowed measurement of the spine, femur, and total body. Approximately 700 nuclear medicine facilities in the United States and approximately 300 international facilities used this approach for research and clinical management of metabolic bone disease. During the same period, several hundred radiology groups adopted quantitative computed tomography (QCT) for assessment of volumetric density of the vertebral body.

Since 1990, these older techniques have been largely displaced by the use of dual-energy x-ray absorptiometry (DEXA). DEXA uses an x-ray source with an increased photon flux to replace the radionuclides used in SPA and DPA. This allows densitometers to provide more reproducible data, better images, and shorter measurement times. In addition, DEXA does not have the sometimes difficult licensing requirements of radionuclide devices or the need for source replacement. As of 1995, there were approximately 5,000 DEXA units worldwide, of which approximately 25% were in the United States. By mid-1997 there were 10,000 DEXA densitometers worldwide.

The explosion in instrumentation for measuring bone density is related to a growing interest in osteoporosis and the recognition that it is an important disease affecting public health. It is estimated that 1,000,000 osteoporotic fractures occur annually in this country. The estimated annual cost of medical treatment and long-term care is approximately $13 billion. Approximately 80% of this is associated with the 200,000 hip fractures that occur each year. Another factor in the clinical acceptance of bone densitometry is that many studies have demonstrated the import of bone densi-

tometry for its two chief clinical applications: (1) to aid in the diagnosis of bone disease and (2) to monitor bone changes during the course of disease or with therapy.

In the past few years, there have been several reviews of bone densitometry that provide a good introduction and give differing perspectives on these developments (1–10).

## PHYSICAL BASIS OF DENSITOMETRY

Bone densitometry using radiation is generally based on the differential attenuation by bone mineral (calcium hydroxyapatite) from the soft tissue in which it is embedded. Single-energy measurements assume that the bone is embedded in a constant thickness of soft tissue. Constant thickness can be achieved by using a water bath, a flexible cuff containing water, or a tissue-equivalent gel molded around a limb. Measurements cannot be done easily on the trunk because of its variable thickness and composition. With dual-energy densitometry, attenuation at the higher energy is used as a measure of overall tissue thickness, so a constant thickness does not need to be artificially maintained. This permits measurement of skeletal areas in the trunk (e.g., spine, femur) as well as measurements over the total body.

## BIOLOGICAL BASIS OF DENSITOMETRY

Bone mineral content (BMC, in grams) and bone mineral density (BMD, in g/cm$^2$) measured by any of the available techniques are of clinical interest because they serve as surrogates for bone strength. Ultimately, BMD also is an indicator of the risk of fracture. Many studies over the past several decades have demonstrated a strong association between measurements of bone mass density and biomechanical tests of bone strength in vitro. The correlations typically are approximately 0.9, indicating that 80% of the variance in strength is associated with BMD. Of great import is the finding that these associations are true for inte-

**TABLE 12-1.** *Comparison of the precision and Z-scores by different available methods at different sites*

| Site | Method | Precision (%) | Difference (%)[a] | Z-score[b] Z[c] | Z-score[b] Z[d] |
|------|--------|---------------|-------------------|------|------|
| Radius | SEXA/DEXA | 1 | 10 | 0.8 | 2.8 |
| Radius | pQCT | 2 | 15 | 0.8 | 2.8 |
| Os calcis | SEXA/DEXA | 2 | 15 | 0.8 | 2.8 |
| Os calcis | US | 2 | 18 | 1.1 | 3.2 |
| Femur | DEXA | 2 | 20 | 1.3 | 3.3 |
| AP spine | DEXA | 1 | 20 | 1.3 | 3.3 |
| Lateral spine | DEXA | 2 | 30 | 1.3 | 3.3 |
| Spine | QCT | 4 | 40 | 1.3 | 3.3 |
| Total body | DEXA | 0.5 | 15 | 1.3 | 3.3 |

[a] Osteoporotics relative to age-matched controls.
[b] The Z-score is the difference between normal and abnormal groups divided by the standard deviation.
[c] Relative to age-matched controls.
[d] Relative to young normal controls.

gral bone strength at sites of osteoporotic fracture, the proximal femur, and the spine, not just for bone sections. Although the correlations typically are 0.9 when the entire adult age range is included, the correlations drop to approximately 0.6 to 0.7 over the narrow range of bone density in the elderly.

Within the population of elderly and osteoporotic individuals, BMD remains a useful predictor of bone strength, accounting for half of the variance, but other factors also relate to the strength of the integral bone. These factors are often referred to as *structure* and include the material properties of bone, such as:

- Microstructure
- Gross anatomic shape of the spine or hip
- Distribution of bone in the area
- Defects in the bone

There is a great deal of debate with regard to structural factors but rather little detailed evidence as to what factors really are important contributors to the increased risk of fracture with aging. Many of the structural changes that occur with aging (i.e., decreased trabecular width, decreased trabecular connectivity, increased trabecular spacing, decreased thickness of the compact wall, and increased cortical porosity) appear to be associated with bone density. Therefore, BMD becomes a surrogate for these structural factors as well as an indicator of bone quantity.

It has been conventional to define osteoporosis in terms of a fracture threshold value, usually the ninetieth centile of patients with clear osteoporotic fracture (spine or femur). Expression of abnormality as Z-scores or centiles is needed because the percentage diminution varies dramatically with the method and site (Table 12-1). This fracture threshold corresponds to a BMD level that is 2.0 to 2.5 SD below the mean level in young normal subjects and approximately 0.5 to 1.5 SD (Z-scores) below the mean level in post-

menopausal women, depending on the site of measurement (see Table 12-1). This criterion provides 90% sensitivity at approximately 70% specificity when spine or femur BMD is used. The World Health Organization recently defined *osteoporosis* operationally as a BMD level 2.5 SD below young normal (11).

Most experts agree that there is little need for concomitant measurement of biochemical markers when bone density is measured. For 20 years, researchers have used urinary calcium and hydroxyproline to indicate elevated bone resorption; serum osteocalcin is increasingly used as a marker of bone turnover. Newer markers of collagen breakdown products in urine are promising but experimental. These markers have very limited diagnostic utility, but they may ultimately prove useful in evaluating short-term changes of bone turnover with therapy, particularly with antiresorptive therapy. However, the high precision error of urinary markers (30% or more), and even serum markers (15%), may preclude their clinical use (Table 12-2). If the precision error is greatly reduced, markers could add to the information provided by densitometry in monitoring, but they are not a substitute.

Epidemiologic data show a strong association in between the risk of fracture, in both retrospective and prospective studies, and bone mass or density (12–14). Typically, the risk of all fractures increases by 50% to 100% (1.5- to 2-fold) for each 10% (1 SD) decrease of BMD at any skeletal site; however, specific risk of spine or hip fracture increases even more (200% to 300%) for each 10% decrease of spine or femur BMD. There also are 20% increases of mortality associated with decreases of BMD, indicating that BMD is an indicator of overall biological state as well as particular skeletal state.

The relationship between BMD and fracture risk is particularly strong for densitometric variables at the sites of osteoporotic fractures. Measurements of BMD in the proximal femur are particularly good indicators of hip fracture,

**TABLE 12-2.** *Biochemical markers compared to spine BMD*

| | Precision error | Postmenopausal (age 55) | | Spinal osteoporosis (age 70) | | Antiresorptive therapy | |
|---|---|---|---|---|---|---|---|
| | 1 SD | Δ | Δ/SD | Δ | Δ/SD | Δ/year | Δ/SD |
| Alkaline phosphatase | 10% | +10% | +1.0 | +20% | +2.0 | −10% | −1.0 |
| Osteocalcin | 25% | +25% | +1.0 | +50% | +2.0 | −25% | −1.0 |
| Urine calcium | 40% | +15% | +1.0 | +40% | +1.0 | −30% | −0.8 |
| Urine hydroxyproline | 30% | +15% | +0.5 | +40% | +1.3 | −30% | −1.0 |
| Urine collagen crosslinks | 30% | +40% | +1.3 | +100% | +3.3 | −60% | −2.0 |
| Spine BMD | 1% | −8.0 | −8.0 | −33.0 | −33.0 | +2% | +2.0 |

Note: Spine changes at menopause or with osteoporosis are much larger relative to precision error. Changes with newer urinary resorption markers with antiresorptive therapy are comparable in sensitivity to spine BMD.

whereas measurements of spine BMD are equally useful predictors of vertebral fractures. Fracture risk for the spine or hip increases by a factor of 2 or 3 for each 1-SD decrease of BMD of the spine or proximal femur, respectively. Measurements at peripheral skeletal sites are far less predictive of spine or hip fracture. The positive predictive accuracy of a future spine or femur fracture is increased by use of spine or femur BMD compared to bone density of the radius, metacarpals, or even the os calcis (which is somewhat superior to the other peripheral sites). As a consequence, the greatest focus of densitometry today is on the measurement of the spine and femur. The femur is considered to be the greatest public health problem, with 90% of the cost of all fracture due to hip fracture, so direct femoral densitometry is increasingly used by experts. To the extent that peripheral measurements are used as a substitute, the os calcis is preferred, because it is far more predictive of hip fracture than other peripheral sites (12).

## MEASUREMENT METHODS

### Single-Energy Densitometry

The SPA technique developed by John Cameron at the University of Wisconsin used a radionuclide source and scintillation detector. A narrow beam of radiation produced by a monoenergetic radionuclide source (I-125 at 28 keV or americium 241 at 60 keV). The beam was detected with a highly collimated scintillation detector coupled to a single-channel analyzer. This allowed the influences of scattered radiation to be minimal. A narrow beam was passed across the area of interest, usually the distal third of the radius or the os calcis. Only peripheral sites could be measured because a constant tissue thickness had to be maintained in the beam path using tissue-equivalent gels or a water bath. Measurements required approximately 10 minutes and had a precision error of approximately 2%. There was not a large cost impediment for this instrumentation (typical cost $20,000 to $25,000), but licensing for use of radionuclides was required, and this entailed minimal training in the United States and elsewhere. In recent years, x-ray sources have been used to replace the radionuclides originally used

for SPA. This new technique has been called single-energy x-ray absorptiometry (SEXA). The new equipment is slightly more expensive than that used for SPA, but it does not require replacement of I-125 at 6-month intervals.

### Dual-Energy Densitometry

Axial densitometry using DEXA is the current standard practice. The technique does not require a constant soft-tissue thickness, as the single-energy method does; this permits scans of the clinically important spine and femur sites. The DPA technique has been largely supplanted by the use of x-ray sources (Fig. 12-1). The most commonly used approach for DEXA closely simulates DPA in that a K-edge filter is interposed in an ultrastable x-ray beam at 80 or 90 kVp to produce a bimodal distribution of energies that approximate the dual-energy radionuclide beam produced by Gd-153 (44 and 100 keV). A samarium K-edge filter gives similar energies (45 and 80 keV). The more common approach with a cerium K-edge filter gives lower energies (40 and 70 keV) but better contrast. Alternatively, the x-ray generator may be rapidly switched between high and low energies (70 and 140 kVp) to achieve the separate energies (approximately 45 and 85 keV effective) required for the dual-energy calculations. The first generation of DEXA instruments provided BMD determinations on the spine and femur in 5 to 8 minutes with a precision error of 1% to 2% in vivo. A second generation of DEXA instruments, with either higher-intensity x-ray sources or linear array detectors, or both, provide these axial scans in approximately 2 minutes (15,16). An even newer generation of DEXA equipment is emerging that provides better imaging capabilities with a spatial resolution approximately three times better (0.5 vs. 2 mm), and acquisition times up to 10 times faster than the first generation. Good contrast resolution is achieved using a fanbeam and slit detector, so the images are of near radiographic quality (Fig. 12-2). This can be important for some clinical applications. These anteroposterior (AP) spine images clearly show extraosseous calcifications (see next paragraph), which can cause artificial BMD calibration by 10% to 20% in the elderly. The femur images show both bone loss from Ward's triangle and cortical thinning, factors that are associated with increased fracture risk.

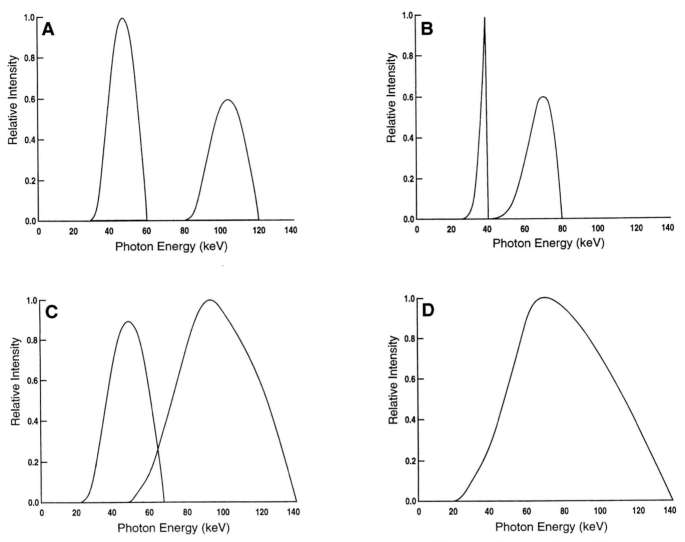

**FIG. 12-1.** The energy spectrum of **(A)** Gd-153 at 44 and 100 keV, **(B)** x-ray with cerium K-edge filter giving peaks at 40 and 70 keV, **(C)** alternating high and low x-rays at 140 and 70 kVp, **(D)** broad-spectrum x-ray source at 140 kVp. (Reproduced with permission from Lunar Corporation, Madison, WI.)

In addition, this third generation of densitometers allows conventional AP spine and femur scans in approximately 10 to 30 seconds (17).

The third-generation densitometers also allow imaging of the lateral spine (L4–T4) in <1 minute. These images are not used for BMD because a series of studies have demonstrated that the diagnostic sensitivity of lateral spine BMD is slightly lower than that of AP spine BMD. The precision error of lateral spine BMD is twice that of AP spine, and the accuracy error of lateral spine BMD is 10% to 15%, which makes it marginal for clinical application. However, the image of the combined lumbar and thoracic spine can be used to measure vertebral heights and deformation. In fact, because BMD need not be measured, a dual-energy scan is not needed, and a higher-resolution single-energy image can be used. Vertebral deformation, which is indicative of wedge and crush fracture, is clinically useful, particularly when considered together with BMD. The presence of a significant deformation at any given level of spine BMD doubles the risk of future fracture. It is thus equivalent to a 10% decrease of spine BMD in terms of fracture risk.

A number of common technical problems are encountered in the routine use of DEXA densitometers. The instruments provided by all manufacturers are extremely reliable and precise, providing long-term precision on phantoms of approximately 0.5%. All instruments provide automated checks on system operation and record quality control data into special databases that provide plots of long-term performance. This allows the user to determine if preventive maintenance, or service, is needed. The most common problems are related to the operator of the instrument rather than the instrument itself. These include the following:

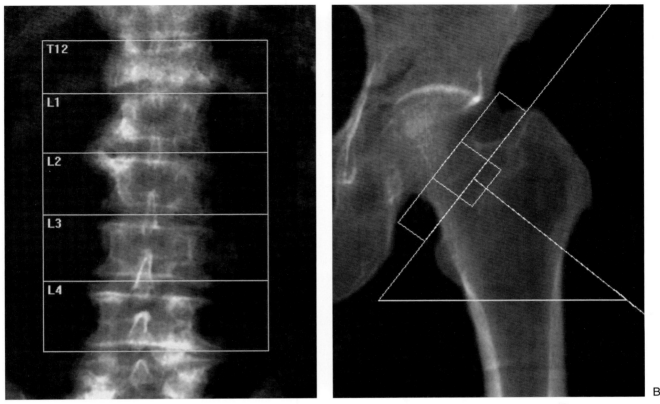

A   B

**FIG. 12-2.** AP spine **(A)** and femur **(B)** images from a third-generation imaging densitometer. (Reproduced with permission from Lunar Corporation, Madison, WI.)

- Misplacement of regions of interest (i.e., misidentification of vertebral level, or angulation of the femur neck)
- Patient positioning errors (starting scans too high or low, or off center)
- Misidentification of patient data files

In some centers, up to 20% of scans are problematic, but with training and experience, only a few percent of all scans present with problems. These problems are largely idiosyncratic and include

- Presence of x-ray contrast agents (barium), buttons, zippers
- Residual dye from myelograms
- Osteophytes and sclerotic facets (>15% prevalence in patients >65)
- Presence of six lumbar vertebrae
- Severe compression fractures

Sclerotic spines are difficult to measure accurately and often have extraosseous calcification combined with osteopenia. A calcified aorta, even when severe, usually does not produce more than a few percent error in densitometry results of the lumbar spine.

Total body scans can be done in approximately 10 to 20 minutes using DEXA. They provide not only BMD of the total body and its subregions but very accurate measurements of soft-tissue composition (fat and lean tissue). Exten-

sive normative databases for all skeletal locations have been derived in many countries to serve as reference data to which abnormal cases may be compared. The DEXA measurement of body composition developed at the University of Wisconsin (18,19) is now considered the gold standard for noninvasive measurement of composition in vivo.

Approximately 90% of determinations today are made on the lumbar spine and femur in AP projection. Approximately 5% are total body determinations. The remaining 5% are used for specialty applications (lateral spine, knees, forearms, lower leg, foot). The DEXA approach has been well accepted in this country and abroad (20); provisional reimbursement has been provided by Medicare in the United States and by national medical insurers in many other countries.

### Quantitative Computed Tomography

QCT provides a volumetric measurement of bone density in the vertebral body but not in the femur. It allows the separation of the cortical and the more metabolically active trabecular bone. QCT is particularly useful in the elderly >65 years of age in whom osteophytes and sclerotic facets complicate conventional AP spine measurements using DEXA. The high radiation dose, even for the more commonly used single-energy QCT approach (typically 1,000 to 2,000 mrem [0.01 to 0.02 Sv] in clinical practice), is as much as 10 times higher than that used in research laboratories. Dual-energy QCT, which is used mostly in Germany, has an even higher radiation dose. The precision error encountered in clinical radiology practices (5% to 10%) is usually several times larger than that achieved in the best laboratories (1% to 2%). Several other problems exist:

- Uncertainties about the accuracy of the measurement due to the large influence of the variable fat content of trabecular bone
- Relatively high cost ($400 per determination)
- Limited accessibility to CT scanners due to heavy use

These problems have led most experts involved with research or clinical management of bone disease to the use of DEXA rather than QCT.

The peripheral skeleton can be measured using QCT, so-called pQCT. A sophisticated but costly ($200,000) special CT scanner is available from Switzerland for very precise monitoring of the peripheral trabecular bone (0.2% precision). Lower-cost equipment (approximately $60,000 or double the price of SEXA instruments) is also available, but this QCT device has a higher precision error (1% to 2%) and provides clinical information comparable to that of SPA or SEXA.

### Quantitative Ultrasound Densitometry

Quantitative ultrasound (QUS) has been used for research on bone for >20 years, but only in the past decade have there been substantial clinical efforts (21). QUS measurements reflect bone structure as well as bone density. In Europe, the focus has been on measurement of broadband QUS attenuation (BUA; measured in dB/MHz), an indication of bone density and bone structure. Measurements are typically done on the highly trabecular bone of the os calcis. BUA is affected by not only the density of trabecular bone but also by the orientation and spacing of the trabecular plates. The speed (or velocity) of sound (SOS in meters per second) also can be measured. The most common approach (developed by researchers at the University of Wisconsin) combines BUA and SOS to give an QUS index, termed *stiffness*, which differs from true biomechanical stiffness. Stiffness provides better precision and diagnostic sensitivity than either BUA or SOS alone. Evidence is accumulating that QUS densitometry provides incremental information beyond that achieved by conventional densitometry. Eventually these devices may be used in conjunction with DEXA to better indicate fracture risk.

Approximately 1,000 QUS densitometers are in use worldwide today. Until recently, many of these were used mostly for clinical research. Clinicians are becoming more familiar with the results obtained in clinical trials, and consequently, these devices are becoming incorporated into clinical use. Their relatively low cost (approximately $25,000), small size, ease of use, and lack of ionizing radiation make them acceptable for the physician in private practice.

## CLINICAL APPLICATIONS

The indications for use of DEXA are diverse. Most experts believe that densitometry is justified in any condition that affects skeletal integrity. The U.S. National Osteoporosis Foundation has outlined four major indications (22):

- Confirm osteopenia in patients presenting with fracture or radiographic abnormality
- Estrogen-deficient women
- Long-term corticosteroid therapy
- Primary hyperparathyroidism

Numerous other conditions, such as renal disease, malabsorption, and immobilization, warrant skeletal examination. In addition, many drug therapies (e.g., heparin, anticonvulsives, methotrexate, thyroid hormone) cause bone loss. Concerned physicians often use densitometry in these conditions. The most common sites for bone densitometry are the AP spine (L2–L4), and the proximal femur but total-body scans are becoming increasingly important.

## CONCLUSION

Bone densitometry is widely used in both clinical research and clinical management today. In the next decade, major improvements will provide better imaging of the key areas: spine and femur. This will allow better assessment of the structure (i.e., distribution of bone) in these areas, as well as identification of potential artifacts. The total-body scans, because they are now achievable in a few minutes, will become more commonly used clinically. Primary physicians (e.g., gynecologists, internal medicine, rheumatologists) may increasingly adopt US densitometry into their practice because of its low cost and wide applicability as a prescreening tool.

## REFERENCES

1. Faulkner KG, Gluer CC, Majumdar S, et al. Noninvasive measurements of bone mass, structure, and strength: current methods and experimental techniques. AJR Am J Roentgenol 1991;157:1229–1237.
2. Grampp S, Jergas M, Gluer CC, et al. Radiologic diagnosis of osteoporosis. Radiol Clin North Am 1993;31:1133–1145.
3. Jergas M, Genant HK. Current methods and recent advances in the diagnosis of osteoporosis. Arthritis Rheum 1993;12:1649–1662.
4. Lang P, Steiger P, Faulkner K, et al. Osteoporosis. Current techniques and recent developments in quantitative bone densitometry. Radiol Clin North Am 1991;29:49–76.
5. Fogelman I, Rodin A, Blake G. Impact of bone mineral measurements on osteoporosis. Eur J Nucl Med 1990;16:39–52.
6. Mazess RB. Bone Densitometry for Clinical Diagnosis and Monitoring. In DeLuca HF, Mazess RB (eds), Osteoporosis: Physiological Basis, Assessment, and Treatment. New York: Elsevier, 1990;63–85.
7. Sartoris DJ, Resnick D. Current and innovative methods for noninvasive bone densitometry. Radiol Clin North Am 1990;28:257–278.
8. Tothill P. Methods of bone mineral measurement. Phys Med Biol 1989;34:543–572.
9. Wahner HW, Fogelman I. The Evaluation of Osteoporosis: Dual Energy X-Ray Absorptiometry in Clinical Practice. London: Martin Dunitz, 1994.

10. Melton LJ, Eddy DM, Johnston CC. Screening for osteoporosis. Ann Int Med 1990;112:516–528.
11. World Health Organization. Assessment of Fracture Risk and Its Application to Screening for Postmenopausal Osteoporosis. Geneva, Switzerland: WHO Technical Report Series, 1994;843.
12. Cummings SR, Black DM, Nevitt MC, et al. Bone density at various sites for prediction of hip fractures. Lancet 1993;341:72–75.
13. Ross PD, Davis JW, Epstein RS, Wasnich RD. Pre-existing fractures and bone mass predict vertebral fracture incidence in women. Ann Intern Med 1991;114:919–923.
14. Melton LJ, Atkinson EJ, O'Fallon WM, et al. Long-term fracture prediction by bone mineral assessed at different skeletal sites. J Bone Miner Res 1993;8:1227–1233.
15. Mazess RB, Chesnut CH III, McClung M, Genant H. Enhanced precision with dual-energy x-ray absorptiometry. Calcif Tiss Int 1992;51:14–17.
16. Blake GM, Parker JC, Buxton FMA, Fogelman I. Dual x-ray absorptiometry: a comparison between fan beam and pencil beam scans. Br J Radiol 1993;66:902–906.
17. Hanson JA, Ergun D, Gauntt D, et al. The EXPERT Imaging Bone Densitometer. In Ring EFJ, Elvins DM, Bhalla AK (eds), Current Research in Osteoporosis and Bone Mineral Measurement III: 1994. Bath, England: British Institute of Radiology, 1994;56.
18. Mazess RB, Peppler WW, Gibbons M. Total body composition by dual-photon (153-Gd) absorptiometry. Am J Clin Nutr 1984;40:834–839.
19. Mazess RB, Barden HS, Bisek JP, Hanson HA. Dual-energy x-ray absorptiometry for total-body and regional bone-mineral and soft-tissue composition. Am J Clin Nutr 1990;51:1106–1112.
20. Kellie SE. Diagnostic and therapeutic technology assessment (DATTA): measurement of bone density with dual-energy x-ray absorptiometry (DEXA). JAMA 1992;267:286–294.
21. Hans D, Schott AM, Meunier PJ. Ultrasonic assessment of bone: a review. Eur J Med 1993;2:157–163.
22. Johnston CC, Melton LJ, Lindsay R, Eddy DM. Clinical indications for bone mass measurements. A report from the Scientific Advisory Board of the National Osteoporosis Foundation. J Bone Miner Res 1989;4(suppl 2):1–28.

*Textbook of Nuclear Medicine,*
edited by Michael A. Wilson.
Lippincott–Raven Publishers, Philadelphia © 1998.

# CHAPTER 13

# Organ Transplants

Scott B. Perlman

Larger medical centers now commonly have active organ transplantation programs. Significant advances in immunosuppression have led to improved graft survival, and this continues to be an important area of investigation. One of the larger problems facing the field of organ transplantation today is the availability of donors. With liver transplantation, for instance, the number of people awaiting transplantation continues to increase (4,095 candidates in 1991, 4,710 in 1992), but the number of donors has remained stable at approximately 3,000 to 3,500 per year (1). The field of organ transplantation will continue to grow as advances are made in several areas, including surgical techniques, immunosuppression, donor organ preservation, and donor organ availability. This chapter reviews the use of radiopharmaceuticals for the evaluation of organ transplant function.

## RENAL TRANSPLANT IMAGING

Kidney transplantation is a frequently performed procedure, and, according to the United Network for Organ Sharing Scientific Registry, 8,161 cadaveric and 2,698 living donor kidney transplants were performed in the United States in 1993 (2). Patients with end-stage renal disease who receive a successful kidney transplant no longer require dialysis and have a better quality of life compared with patients with end-stage renal disease who are on dialysis (3). In children with end-stage renal disease, the kidney transplant is the only therapy that allows normal growth and mental development (4).

After renal transplantation, a number of problems may occur, including acute tubular necrosis (ATN), rejection, arterial or venous thrombosis, urinary extravasation, obstruction, formation of a lymphocele, and cyclosporine toxicity. The three types of rejection typically described are hyperacute, acute, and chronic rejection. Preformed cytotoxic antibodies are responsible for hyperacute rejection. This process is often apparent immediately after transplan-

tation of the kidney. When hyperacute rejection is seen in the operating room, the kidney is removed immediately, before the onset of additional complications, such as disseminated intravascular coagulation. In other cases, hyperacute rejection may not be apparent for 24 to 48 hours. Acute rejection can be caused by cell- or antibody-mediated pathologic processes. Acute rejection usually occurs within 3 months of kidney transplantation. In chronic rejection, the pathologic cause is less clear. This form of rejection may be secondary to several episodes of acute rejection over time (5,6).

Important information about each of these complications may be obtained from radionuclide renal imaging. The technique has undergone numerous revisions and improvements since it was first used in the mid-1960s. Improvements in camera design, software, radiopharmaceuticals, and protocol have all contributed to the technique, so that currently the method has an important role in the evaluation of renal function after transplantation. An active renal transplant program is present at the University of Wisconsin Hospital and clinics, and renal transplant imaging represents a significant portion of the workload in nuclear medicine, estimated at approximately 10%.

### Radiopharmaceuticals

For a more complete discussion of radiopharmaceuticals for renal imaging, see Chapter 5.

The assessment of renal transplant function includes an evaluation of perfusion and function. Tc-99m diethylene-triaminepentaacetic acid (DTPA) is used to evaluate perfusion and function, as reflected by the glomerular filtration rate (GFR) (Fig. 13-1). This radiotracer accurately estimates the GFR because its method of clearance is by glomerular filtration, and it is not secreted or reabsorbed. Tubular function can be evaluated using iodine 131 (I-131) orthoiodohippurate (OIH), which is cleared by GFR (approximately 20%) and tubular secretion (approximately

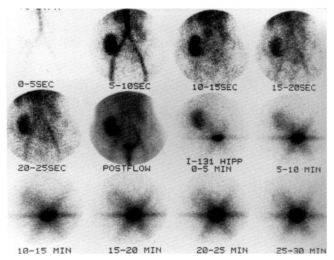

**FIG. 13-1.** Tc-99m DTPA and I-131 OIH images of a living-related renal transplant on the first day after graft implantation. The first five DTPA images represent renal blood flow; the last six OIH images represent renal function. Perfusion of the kidney is excellent (tracer in kidney equal to that in aorta and iliac artery), and extraction and excretion of OIH are prompt, with minimal tracer remaining in the renal transplant at 30 minutes. Note the star effect of septal penetration from using a medium-energy collimator with I-131.

**TABLE 13-1.** Radiation dose to the kidneys from I-131 hippuran under various conditions

|  | Mrads/500 µCi |
| --- | --- |
| Normal | 47 |
| Acute tubular necrosis | 3,000 |
| Total obstruction with: |  |
| 50% uptake | 200,000 |
| 5% uptake | 20,000 |

Source: Adapted from Elliott AT, Britton KE, Brown NJG, et al. Dosimetry of Current Radiopharmaceuticals Used in Renal Investigation. In Cloutier RJ, Coffey JL, Snyder WS, Watson EE (eds), Radiopharmaceutical Dosimetry Symposium. Rockville, MD: HEW Publication (FDA), 1976.

80%). A new radiopharmaceutical that is able to provide important physiologic information is technetium 99m mercaptoacetyltriglycine (Tc-99m MAG3). Although the renal clearance of MAG3 is slower than that of OIH, MAG3 has a number of advantages, including availability in a kit form; favorable dosimetry, especially under pathologic conditions (Table 13-1); superior images because the Tc-99m photon is better suited for gamma camera imaging than the I-131 photons (Fig. 13-2); and a larger dose can be administered while patient exposure remains at an acceptable level.

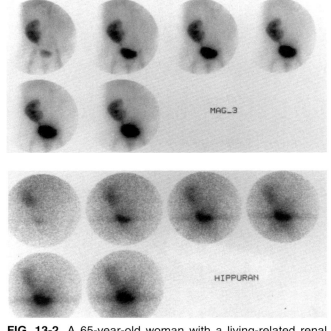

**FIG. 13-2.** A 65-year-old woman with a living-related renal transplant performed more than a year before. Comparison of MAG3 **(A)** and OIH **(B)** images. Overall, there is very good renal graft function present, with prompt radiotracer uptake and excretion. Note that image quality is clearly better with MAG3, but the overall functional information is very similar.

## Imaging Protocol

A common clinical protocol involves the use of 10 mCi (370 MBq) Tc-99m DTPA and 100 µCi (3.7 MBq) I-131 OIH. Before the intravenous (IV) administration of OIH, the patient should be given a few drops of nonradioactive iodine orally, such as saturated solution of potassium iodide or Lugol's solution, to "flood" the iodine pool and minimize the thyroid uptake of free I-131 (according to the package insert, I-131 OIH may contain up to 3% free I-131). The DTPA is administered as an IV bolus in a large vein, and a series of dynamic images (1 frame per second) of the renal graft are obtained over a 1-minute period. After this dynamic data set is acquired, a 400,000-count static image should be acquired. Next, the OIH is administered intravenously, and a series of 1-minute images are obtained over the renal graft and bladder for a total of 30 minutes. If a prior OIH examination has been performed within the last few days, it is important to acquire a background image of the transplant and bladder in the I-131 window to determine how much OIH is present from the previous study. The activity from the prior examination may be substantial if there is significant impairment in function of the renal graft, and this can be subtracted from the activity on the current study for an accurate representation of renal transplant function. Images are reformatted for viewing in a variety of ways, depending on the viewer's and referring physician's preferences.

One common method is to display the perfusion data in a series of images, each representing 5 seconds of summed dynamic data. Functional data may be displayed as a series of images, each summed over a 5-minute period (see Fig. 13-1). Time-activity curves of perfusion, from the early DTPA data, and tubular function, from the OIH data, can be plotted for an objective evaluation of transplant function. The patient should be well hydrated for the examination, so that the effects of hydration status are minimized, allowing more meaningful temporal comparisons. Protocols involving MAG3 are simplified because only one radiopharmaceutical is used to obtain information about both perfusion and tubular function. Objective analysis of renal transplant perfusion and function can be relatively simple, such as review of the renogram curves and images, or more involved and requiring the calculation of objective parameters, such as the ratio of kidney to aorta, renal parenchymal transit time, time-to-peak renal activity, and excretion index. Whatever method is used, the technique should be carefully performed, so that examinations are reproducible and comparable over time.

## Clinical Applications

Radionuclide scintigraphic techniques, using various radiopharmaceuticals, have been shown to add important physiologic information to the assessment of renal transplant function. Soon after the transplant operation, an abrupt decrease in urine output may indicate a vascular problem, such as a renal artery or vein thrombosis, hyperacute rejection, or acute urinary obstruction. In the case of complete renal artery or vein obstruction, the renal scan can quickly identify the total absence of perfusion and function (Fig. 13-3). The renal scan is also very useful in less acute circumstances, such as the evaluation of acute or chronic rejection. One method of evaluating renal perfusion used Tc-99m DTPA to obtain a ratio between the renal and aortic blood flow. A decrease in the kidney-to-aorta ratio of 20% or more from the baseline (usually representing acute rejection) was seen in 26 of 27 patients with complications but was also seen with other clinical problems, such as infection, obstruction, and hypertension. The ≥20% decrease in the ratio of kidney to aorta was seen in 94% of acute rejection episodes. These authors concluded that the ratio of kidney to aorta is a sensitive but nonspecific index for following pathologic changes in the renal allograft (7).

In the early postoperative period, cadaveric transplants and, to a lesser degree, living-related donor transplanted kidneys often have some degree of ATN. In one series of patients with a renal allograft, 2% to 4% of the grafts of patients who had a living-related donor and 18% to 24% of grafts in recipients of cadaveric donors had evidence of ATN (9). Renal scintigraphy performed within a few days of transplantation often demonstrates good graft perfusion and extraction of OIH but with delayed and decreased excretion, usually due to ATN. This pattern is not specific for ATN and

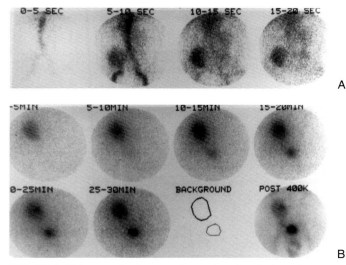

**FIG. 13-3.** An avascular renal transplant in a 40-year-old man with IDDM. This patient had a prior cadaveric renal transplant implanted on the right 9 years earlier, which failed after 7 years. The new cadaveric renal transplant was placed on the left 6 days before this scan. The patient had an acute onset of abdominal pain. **(A)** The perfusion scan demonstrates a good bolus of radiotracer in the aorta and iliac arteries (left image), but the recent renal transplant on the left is avascular. **(B)** The photopenic area, best seen on the right, represents the avascular kidney. A small amount of radiotracer uptake into the older right renal transplant can be seen, especially in the background subtracted image (second from left).

**FIG. 13-4.** This examination, performed on the first postoperative day after a cadaveric renal transplant, demonstrates ATN. **(A)** Perfusion with DTPA is good. **(B)** Extraction of OIH is fair, with decreased and delayed excretion. At 30 minutes, a significant amount of OIH is still present in the renal parenchyma, which is consistent with ATN. The bottom right image is from the DTPA image and demonstrates the ureter visualization not apparent with OIH.

can also be seen with rejection. A baseline renal scan obtained within 2 days after transplantation, when the renal perfusion and function changes due to ATN have usually peaked, establishes an important baseline (Fig. 13-4). On subsequent renal examinations, if the perfusion and function continue to decrease, rejection is the most likely cause,

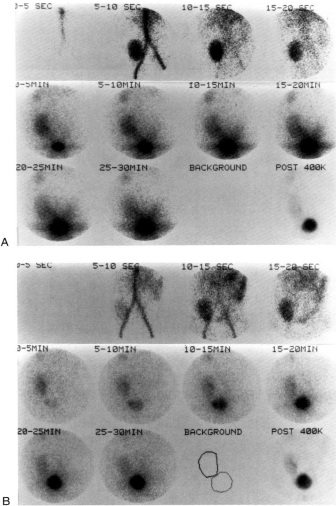

**FIG. 13-5.** Rejection of kidney transplant compared to drug toxicity in a 41-year-old patient with IDDM after receiving a living-related renal transplant. **(A)** This set of scans demonstrates excellent DTPA perfusion images (upper row), together with excellent uptake and prompt excretion of OIH (lower rows). Minimal radiotracer remains in the renal parenchyma at 30 minutes, and the patient's native right kidney is visible, too. **(B)** The examination performed 3 years later, when the serum creatinine level was elevated, shows that the perfusion of the renal transplant has decreased, extraction of OIH has decreased, and excretion is delayed and decreased. These findings can be due to either chronic rejection or cyclosporine toxicity.

although other causes (e.g., cyclosporine toxicity) must also be considered (Fig. 13-5).

In 61 patients who had a cadaveric renal transplant, perfusion (using DTPA) was considered normal if the peak of renal activity occurred within 6 seconds of the radioactivity in the adjacent artery, if the renal radioactivity was greater than or equal to the adjacent artery, and if there was a brief but definite decrease in the renal activity after the peak. DTPA and OIH were used for renal clearance and transit time evaluation. The ratio of renal transplant activity to background at 1 minute was used to evaluate clearance. Normal transit time was defined as a peak in renal parenchymal tracer activity within minutes, followed by a decrease to approximately one-half of the peak in approximately 10 minutes. Two groups of patients were examined, the first within the first 4 days of transplantation (38 studies in 34 patients with abnormal findings likely due to ATN) and the second, 3 weeks after transplantation (62 studies in 27 patients with abnormal findings likely due to rejection). If perfusion was found to be two or more grades better than clearance (on a 5-point scale) in the DTPA study, ATN was considered present. Other parameters were not specific for either ATN or rejection (9).

One series involving cadaveric renal transplant recipients found the combination of Tc-99m pertechnetate and OIH renal scintigraphy to be reliable for the identification of renal transplant rejection. These authors pointed out that a change in a large dose of furosemide therapy made the scan identification of rejection using renal scintigraphy more difficult (10).

The information obtained about tubular function from OIH or MAG3 provides important information about renal graft complications. A comparison of the information obtained from MAG3 and DTPA or OIH renal transplant scintigraphy reported that image quality and time-activity curves were superior with MAG3 and that native kidneys are often visualized with MAG3 despite poor function. There was also a high correlation between the time to peak activity ($T_{max}$) and percentage of peak activity retained at 20 minutes ($T_{20}$) (11). MAG3 has been used to generate a measure of renal parenchymal retention, the $R_{20/3}$, which is the ratio of background-corrected activity in the renal parenchyma in the 1-minute image at 19 to 20 minutes divided by the 1-minute image at 2 to 3 minutes. This parameter was relatively easy to generate and was found to correlate closely with the severity of ATN or acute rejection (12).

The improvement in specificity for determining the cause of the change in tubular function (e.g., using OIH or MAG3) has not been clearly established, in part because of the lack of a satisfactory standard. Renal obstruction, ATN, drug (such as cyclosporin A) toxicity, and rejection can all look similar on the renal scan. Delaney and coworkers compared fine-needle aspiration biopsy, Doppler ultrasound, and radionuclide scintigraphy in 150 episodes of allograft dysfunction in 128 renal transplant patients (13). Although the sensitivity of renal scintigraphy for acute rejection was only 70%, it was still the most sensitive test for the diagnosis of acute rejection. In this investigation, all tests demonstrated a relatively low specificity (13). In one of the largest series to date investigating the usefulness of scintigraphy in the evaluation of the renal allograft, 274 consecutive patients with renal allografts (156 living-related and 136 cadaveric donors) had a total of 1,439 OIH renal scans. Using the effective renal plasma flow determination and an excretion index, the investigators were able to accurately separate acute rejection, chronic rejection, and ATN. Patients with gram-negative sep-

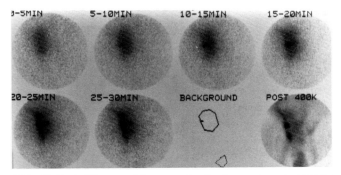

**FIG. 13-6.** A 50-year-old man, who had a cadaveric kidney transplant 2 weeks earlier, presented with right-sided abdominal pain. The DTPA image obtained at the end of this study (bottom right) and the last two OIH images (20 to 30 minutes) show radiotracer outside of the kidney, consistent with a urine leak. The leak was subsequently proved to originate from a renal cyst.

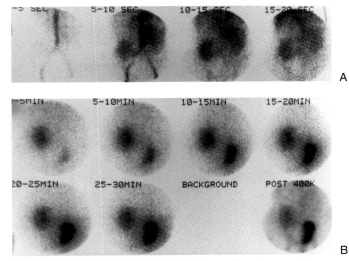

**FIG. 13-7.** A 32-year-old patient with a cadaveric renal transplant. **(A)** The DTPA flow images demonstrate a faint photopenic area inferior and medial to the renal transplant. **(B)** The 5-minute OIH images show extrinsic compression on the right side of the bladder. This is confirmed on the delayed DTPA image (bottom right). The collection was drained, and a lymphocele was confirmed.

ticemia, acute viral illness, and acute glomerulonephritis had changes in renal transplant function that were very similar to acute rejection, whereas the findings in renal artery stenosis were similar to chronic rejection (8).

Extravasation of urine is a postoperative complication established by the demonstration of a fluid collection on an ultrasound or computed tomography (CT) scan, but this finding is nonspecific and may represent a postoperative hematoma or lymphocele. Extravasation can be identified specifically on the renal scan as a collection of radioactive urine outside the renal transplant and bladder. A bladder full of radioactive urine may obscure a leak; therefore, images of the pelvis after voiding are usually necessary. Delayed images are often needed because the kidneys continue to excrete radiotracer into the abdomen, and the leak will become more apparent as the background tissue radioactivity is cleared. The most appropriate length of the delay depends on the renal function and the degree of urine leak. With relatively good function, a delayed image of a few hours should be adequate. With more impaired renal function, or in cases of a small leak, a longer delay is necessary. If renal impairment is considerable and imaging delayed, hepatobiliary excretion of MAG3 may make the diagnosis of leak difficult. On the delayed images, minimal activity should be present in the kidney, ureter, and bladder, especially when the rapidly cleared tubular agent (OIH or MAG3) is used. Thus, a urine leak should be readily identified (Fig. 13-6).

Fluid collections that may be present include urinomas (collections of extravasated urine), lymphoceles, and hematomas. In general, a photopenic defect that remains "cold" over time may represent a lymphocele or hematoma, or even a urinoma, if the defect is long-standing and the urine leak is small. A defect that fills in and becomes "warmer" than the background usually represents a urinoma or urine extravasation. There may even be displacement of the bladder or kidney if the fluid collection is large (Fig. 13-7). In one report, lymphoceles were identified as cold defects that

did not change over time or approached or equaled background activity. If a suspected urinoma shows decreasing activity with voiding, it is unlikely to represent a leak (Fig. 13-8). In one instance, a lymphocele was drained just before a renal scan, and the subsequent activity was greater than background 3 hours later, which may have been due to oozing of radioactivity into the newly forming lymphocele or an inflammatory response, or both (14).

In a postoperative patient in whom the urine output suddenly decreases, obstruction is an important consideration. In early ureteral obstruction, perfusion and tubular extraction remain very good, but excretion beyond the site of obstruction is delayed or absent (Fig. 13-9). The renal scan may demonstrate a dilated intrarenal collecting system and ureter, sometimes up to the point of the ureteral obstruction if the obstruction is acute. With obstruction that has been present for a while, the ureter may not be visualized, being filled with nonradioactive urine that was present before administration of radiopharmaceutical. The renal pelves and calyces may also appear as photopenic defects, thus indicating significantly increased pressure. Delayed images are useful, and urine in the bladder (especially if present in early images) makes high-grade renal obstruction unlikely, although the patient's native kidney may have sufficient function to produce some radioactive urine that enters the bladder. It should be emphasized that proximal renal obstruction, acute rejection, and ATN may have similar appearances on the renal scan, especially in the early postoperative period. Further information about the kidney can be obtained with ultrasonography by demonstration of hydronephrosis, and a diuretic renal scan can evaluate the obstruction physiologically.

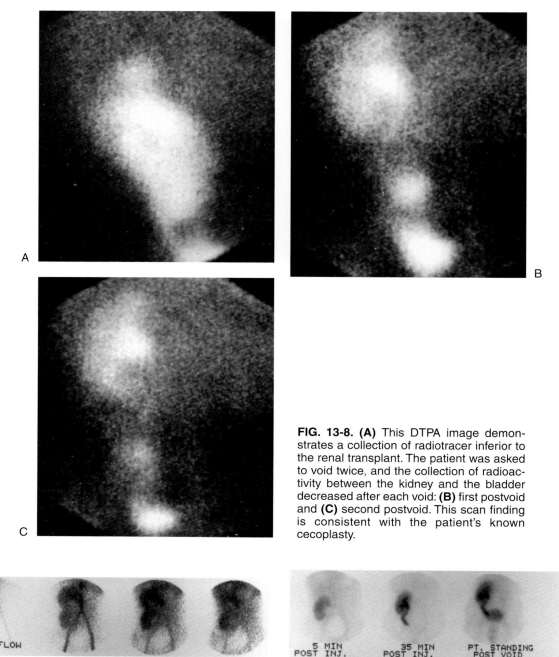

**FIG. 13-8. (A)** This DTPA image demonstrates a collection of radiotracer inferior to the renal transplant. The patient was asked to void twice, and the collection of radioactivity between the kidney and the bladder decreased after each void: **(B)** first postvoid and **(C)** second postvoid. This scan finding is consistent with the patient's known cecoplasty.

**FIG. 13-9.** The renal transplant examination is performed because of an increase in the serum creatinine level approximately 1 month after living-related renal transplantation. **(A)** The DTPA images show good perfusion of the renal transplant. **(B)** Images obtained at 5 minutes show parenchymal activity only; images at 35 minutes show clear visualization of the ureter, but minimal, if any, bladder activity. The postvoid image confirms some tracer drained into the bladder but prominent residual ureteric activity. The patient was found to have a ureteric stricture causing ureteric obstruction.

## Future

Scintigraphic techniques continue to play an important physiologic role in the evaluation of renal transplant function. Methods of objectively estimating the various parameters of renal function, such as GFR determinations or measures of tubular function, continue to undergo refinements. As the accuracy of these methods is established, they will become an important addition to the routine evaluation of renal transplant function because this physiologic information is not available from other imaging methods. Continued improvements in radiotracer methodology, coupled with new developments in radiopharmaceuticals, will continue to improve the accuracy of information provided.

## PANCREAS TRANSPLANT IMAGING

Pancreas transplantation frees diabetic patients from the requirement of exogenous insulin. A major question that remains unanswered is whether an adequately functioning pancreas allograft will prevent the typical long-term diabetic complications that occur in other organs. The donor pancreas is usually from a cadaver, but living-related donor segmental grafts have been used.

Currently, one method of transplantation is to anastomose the pancreas allograft, including a portion of the donor duodenum, to the bladder (Fig. 13-10). This allows the pancreatic exocrine function to be excreted in the urine while protecting the pancreas from urine reflux from the bladder. Serum and urine amylase levels, fasting blood glucose or 2-hour postprandial blood glucoses, and serum C-peptide are often used to monitor the pancreas allograft function. These markers of function become abnormal relatively late in the rejection process, however, when a significant part of the pancreas has irreversibly lost function. In addition to rejection, other postoperative causes of the pancreas graft failure include vascular thrombosis and other vascular complications, infection, and leaks at the anastomotic site. Thus, an accurate method of evaluating pancreatic function would help to improve graft survival.

### Radiopharmaceuticals

One of the earliest radiopharmaceuticals used for the physiologic investigation of pancreatic function was selenium (Se-75) selenomethionine. This radiopharmaceutical was used in the 1960s and 1970s to evaluate the pancreas in patients thought to have a pancreatic carcinoma (15). The radionuclide has a long physical half-life of 120 days and a biological half-life of 70 days. Therefore, to keep patient exposure as low as possible and obtain a useful image, the injected dose used was limited to 250 μCi (9.25 MBq). Early experience with this radiopharmaceutical was encouraging because it was shown to reliably identify abnormal pancreas function in patients with a pancreatitis or pancreatic carcinoma (15). This favorable early experience led investigators to use Se-75 selenomethionine for the investigation of pancreatic allograft function, and the procedure again proved useful (16–18).

Other techniques that have been used to evaluate the pancreas allograft function include thallium-201 (thought to be potentially useful because its uptake depends on cellular viability) (19), indium-111–labeled platelets (20–22), and positron emission tomography using labeled amino acids, such as carbon 11 DL-valine (23), fluorine 18 (F-18) 6-fluorotryptophan (24), and F-18 *p*-fluorophenylalanine

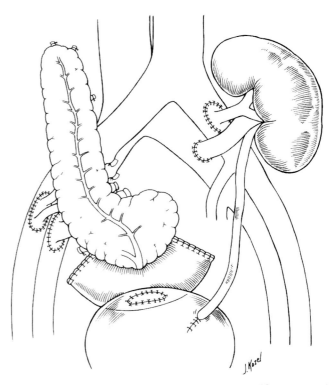

**FIG. 13-10.** Pancreas and renal transplants. (Courtesy of Hans Sollinger, M.D., University of Wisconsin Hospital and Clinics, Madison, WI.)

(25). The labeled platelet and PET imaging methods tend to be expensive, and their complexity precludes their use as a routine clinical tool.

More recently, Tc-99m DTPA has been used to evaluate pancreas transplant rejection. The technique evaluates flow and is relatively simple to perform, and the radiotracer is readily available. Tc-99m DTPA has the added advantage of also providing perfusion information about the renal allograft, which is frequently transplanted along with the pancreas graft.

### Scan Protocol

The imaging procedure is the same as that described for the perfusion part of the radionuclide renal transplant evaluation. Objective semiquantitation of the pancreas allograft perfusion can be performed in a variety of ways. One method uses a Tc-99m index: the percent of the injected Tc-99m DTPA that is present in the pancreas allograft in the third minute of data acquisition after injection. The index decreases during periods of pancreas transplant rejection (26) and provides a relatively objective method of evaluating pancreas graft perfusion. The decreased perfusion may be a sensitive indicator (Fig. 13-11), but it is not specific to the rejection process and may be seen with vascular lesions, rejection, pancreatitis, or infection (27). It should be noted that, although a single pancreas allograft

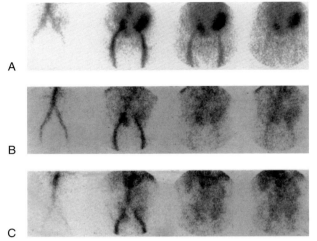

A

B

C

**FIG. 13-11.** A 43-year-old patient with IDDM, who received a combined kidney and pancreas transplant. **(A)** This perfusion scan was performed the first day after transplantation. The 5-second DTPA images demonstrate very good perfusion of both the pancreas (right) and renal (left) transplants in each view. **(B)** The second examination was performed 2 weeks later; perfusion has significantly decreased to both transplanted organs. **(C)** The third examination, 4 days later, shows that perfusion of both organs is even worse. Renal transplant nephrectomy 2 days later demonstrated extensive parenchymal infarction, hemorrhage, neutrophil infiltration, and subendothelial lymphocytes consistent with acute cellular rejection.

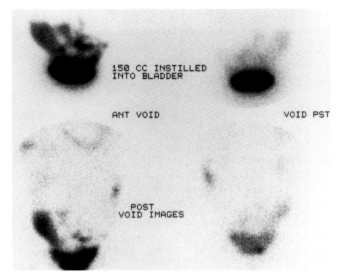

**FIG. 13-12.** This image is from a 32-year-old woman who had had a pancreas and renal transplant performed 18 months earlier. On the evening before this examination, she experienced the acute onset of abdominal pain. After 150 ml saline and radiotracer were instilled into the bladder (upper left, anterior view), extravasation of radiotracer is seen in the peritoneum. After voiding (lower left, anterior view), the amount of activity decreases in the bladder, but extravasated radiotracer is still present outside the bladder. The right-hand images represent posterior views prevoid (upper) and postvoid (lower). A leak was surgically confirmed.

perfusion scan may be difficult to interpret, consecutive studies demonstrating a decrease in perfusion or organ definition are useful for the evaluation of pancreas transplant function (28).

In an attempt to improve technique, other radiopharmaceuticals have recently been used, including Tc-99m hexamethylpropyleneamine oxime (HMPAO), Tc-99m sulfur colloid (SC), and Tc-99m glucoheptonate. Tc-99m HMPAO provides useful information about graft dysfunction, allowing high-quality static images to be obtained (29,30). Scintigraphy using Tc-99m glucoheptonate also provides useful information, although when abnormal, the test is nonspecific (31). George and coworkers (32) used Tc-99m SC to provide a "pancreatic thrombotic index," reflecting vascular injury and thrombosis, and Tc-99m glucoheptonate to evaluate pancreas allograft perfusion and vascular blood pool retention. This method was useful for the evaluation of pancreas allograft function, and when it indicates acute rejection or pancreatitis, the findings may significantly precede hyperglycemia and a decline in the urinary amylase level.

In patients with abdominal pain, extravasation of pancreatic enzymes or urine into the abdomen is an important consideration. Direct radionuclide cystography (technique described in Chapter 5) is a sensitive test for the identification of extravasation, which may occur at the breakdown of an anastomotic site. The technique for these patients should be modified to include anterior images and is a simple, fast, and accurate method of identifying extravasation (Fig. 13-12). The method has been shown to accurately identify urinary extravasation, and it has the advantage of exposing the patient to one-hundredth of the radiation dose of the conventional voiding cystourethrogram (33).

Pancreas allograft evaluation continues to be an important area of investigation. Acceptable sensitivity and specificity have not yet been identified with any technique, in part due to the lack of an accurate standard for pancreas allograft rejection.

## MISCELLANEOUS TRANSPLANT EXAMINATIONS

Radiotracer techniques allow the noninvasive investigation of organ physiology. In general, the methods are very sensitive for the determination of abnormal function, even when high-resolution images obtained from the anatomic imaging modalities are normal.

### Liver Transplantation

A relatively new area of investigation is the evaluation of liver transplant function. Postoperative complications in these patients include vascular complications, rejection, hepatitis, infection, bile leak, and obstruction to the flow of bile. The hepatobiliary examination findings in vascular compromise or ischemia of the liver graft may only be the nonspecific findings of decreased hepatocyte extraction and prolonged blood pool retention of hepatobiliary radiopharmaceuticals (34).

The routine hepatobiliary examination using one of the iminodiacetic acid derivatives, such as mebrofenin, can be a sensitive method of identifying a bile leak or obstruction and evaluating hepatocyte function. CT or ultrasound examination often demonstrates a fluid collection when a bile leak is present. The hepatobiliary examination usually demonstrates an extravasation of radiotracer from the biliary tree in bile leaks, although the exact site of the leak is usually not apparent. Delayed images can be very helpful, allowing the radiopharmaceutical time to clear the liver and adjacent bowel, which may obscure the extravasated activity. Although the small bile leak may not be apparent on the images obtained in the first 1 to 2 hours, these leaks often are easily seen on the delayed images. The length of delay depends on the severity of the extravasation and the degree of parenchymal dysfunction because there is often significant associated cholestasis. Delayed images to 24 hours may be needed. It is important to note, however, that a bile leak may not always present as the more typical focal abnormality; in patients with ascites and bile extravasation the bile leak may be identified as a diffuse increase in activity over the peritoneal region (35). Additional information is provided when there is adequate clearance of radiopharmaceutical into the small bowel, thereby ruling out significant common bile duct (or anastomotic) obstruction (Fig. 13-13). Again, the normal range for the time after radiotracer administration when bowel visualization occurs depends on hepatic function, as demonstrated by the hepatocyte phase of tracer clearance; this information is readily available from the early images. Intrahepatic bilomas can also be identified on the biliary scan as an abnormal collection of radiotracer in the liver (36). Delayed images demonstrate clearance of radiotracer from the normal liver parenchyma and accumulation of radiotracer within the intrahepatic biloma (Fig. 13-14).

To date, there is no proven method of accurately identifying liver transplant rejection. Merion and coworkers (37) have described a promising method of applying a mathematic technique known as deconvolutional analysis to the data obtained from the scintigraphic liver evaluation, including Tc-99m SC, Tc-99m DTPA, and Tc-99m DISIDA (disofenin). Using an estimation of portal blood flow fraction, they were able to identify the presence or absence of rejection in 87% of instances (37). Using a technique that estimated the portal venous-to-arterial hepatic blood flow ratio and the hepatocellular extraction fraction, Knobloch et al. reported a 100% sensitivity and specificity for liver transplant rejection (38). Perfusion indices and uptake parameters derived from quantitative

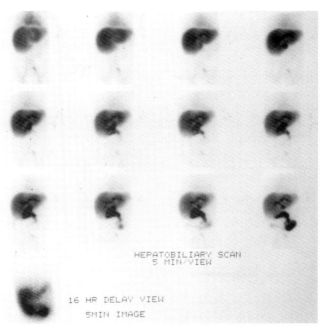

**FIG. 13-13.** A scan of a pediatric hepatic transplant patient, 7 days after the transplant, when a Roux-en-Y obstruction was suspected. The serial 5-minute images show hepatic dysfunction (delayed cardiac blood pool clearance), but while the tracer passes the anastomosis site with some delay, by 16 hours, all activity is in the distal ileum and colon. This study excludes significant anastomotic obstruction.

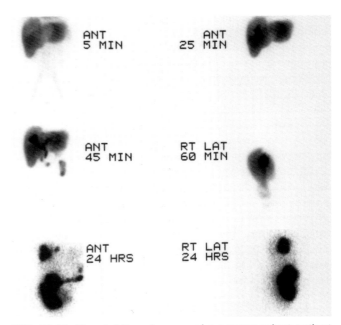

**FIG. 13-14.** Hepatobiliary images of a nontransplant patient who suffered abdominal trauma with hepatic laceration and complicating intrahepatic biloma. Anterior images were obtained at 0 to 5 minutes, 20 to 25 minutes (upper row), and 40 to 45 minutes (middle row, left) together with the right lateral view (middle row, right). At 24 hours (lower row), the anterior and right lateral views confirm the intrahepatic localization of biloma and absence of extrahepatic spread.

hepatobiliary scintigraphy have been found to be useful in the postoperative evaluation of the transplanted liver (39). Useful results from the hepatobiliary examination have also been obtained in liver transplant recipients using the visual interpretation of the hepatobiliary scan to distinguish intrahepatic cholestasis from hepatocyte damage (40). Decreased excretion into the small bowel has been reported with decreased graft survival, although this is not a specific finding for rejection (41).

### Intestinal Transplantation

Intestinal transplantation is a new procedure, and the diagnosis of rejection is a diagnostic challenge. Intestinal permeability may be abnormally increased during rejection, and a technique that can evaluate the permeability of the bowel wall may provide early evidence of rejection. Recently, a promising method was described that used Tc-99m DTPA to evaluate intestinal permeability in two patients who had combined liver-intestinal transplantation. Both patients were administered the Tc-99m DTPA through a jejunostomy tube, and increased Tc-99m DTPA urinary excretion was reported during episodes of rejection (42). Thus, this technique may prove useful in the early identification of rejection.

### Lung Transplantation

Lung transplantation is another area of organ transplantation in which radiopharmaceutical techniques can aid in the post-transplant evaluation. Although most reports are still preliminary, interesting data have been generated on lung ventilation and perfusion in recipients of a single lung transplant. Protocols usually involve baseline or preoperative and follow-up evaluations of lung perfusion and ventilation (43–45) or a comparison of the baseline and exercise data (46). A lung scan demonstrating widespread abnormalities on the ventilation portion of the examination and only mildly abnormal perfusion has been described in a patient who received a heart-lung transplant for primary pulmonary hypertension. Transbronchial biopsies demonstrated obliterative bronchiolitis with no evidence of infection, which is a complication of lung transplantation (47). Lung scintigraphy has provided recent evidence that the hypoxic vasoconstrictive response may be abnormal in the unilaterally transplanted lung (48).

### SUMMARY

Radiotracer techniques have contributed much to understanding the physiology of organ transplantation. Many of these techniques are new, and refinement of current procedures as well as new radiotracer development will continue to increase our understanding of graft func-

tion. Early identification of graft complications will lead to early treatment, resulting in improved graft survival and better patient care.

## REFERENCES

1. Nakazato PZ. Controversial aspects of the current liver donor allocation system for liver transplantation. Acad Radiol 1995;2:244–248.
2. Cadaveric donors recovered between 1988 and 1993. In Unos Update 1994;10:29.
3. Evans RW, Manninen DL, Garrison LP, et al. The quality of life of patients with end-stage renal disease. N Engl J Med 1985;312:553–559.
4. Benedetti E, Hakim NS, Perez EM, Matas AJ. Renal transplantation. Acad Radiol 1995;2:159–166.
5. Nast CC, Cohen AH. Pathology of Kidney Transplantation. In Danovitch GM (ed), Handbook of Kidney Transplantation. Boston: Little, Brown, 1992.
6. Doherty CC. Graft Dysfunction and Its Differential Diagnosis. In McGeown MG (ed), Clinical Management of Renal Transplantation. Boston: Kluwer, 1992.
7. Dunagin P, Alijani M, Atkins F, et al. Application of the kidney to aortic blood flow index to renal transplants. Clin Nucl Med 1983;8:360–364.
8. Diethelm AG, Dubovsky EV, Whelchel JD, et al. Diagnosis of impaired renal function after kidney transplantation using renal scintigraphy, renal plasma flow and urinary excretion of hippurate. Ann Surg 1980;191:604–616.
9. Shanahan WSM, Klingensmith WC, Weil R. 99m-Tc-DTPA renal studies for acute tubular necrosis: specificity of dissociation between perfusion and clearance. AJR Am J Roentgenol 1981;136:249–253.
10. Clorius JH, Kreikorn K, Zelt J, et al. Renal graft evaluation with pertechnetate and I-131 hippuran. A comparative clinical study. J Nucl Med 1979;20:1029–1037.
11. O'Malley JP, Zeissman HA, Chantarapitak N. Tc-99m MAG3 as an alternative to Tc-99m DTPA and I-131 hippuran for renal transplant evaluation. Clin Nucl Med 1993;18:22–29.
12. Li Y, Russell CD, Palmer-Lawrence J, Dubovsky EV. Quantitation of renal parenchyma retention of technetium-99m-MAG3 in renal transplants. J Nucl Med 1994;35:846–850.
13. Delaney V, Ling BN, Campbell WG, et al. Comparison of fine-needle aspiration biopsy, Doppler ultrasound, and radionuclide scintigraphy in the diagnosis of acute allograft dysfunction in renal transplant recipients: sensitivity, specificity, and cost analysis. Nephron 1993;63:263–272.
14. Fortenbery EJ, Blue PW, Van Nostrand D, Anderson JH. Lymphocele: the spectrum of scintigraphic findings in lymphoceles associated with renal transplant. J Nucl Med 1990;31:1627–1631.
15. Miale A, Rodriguez-Antunez A, Gill WM. Pancreas scanning after ten years. Semin Nucl Med 1972;2:201–219.
16. Jamieson NV, McMaster P, Wraight EP, et al. Radionuclide imaging in pancreatic transplantation. Nucl Med Commun 1980;1:291–297.
17. Toledo-Pereyra LH, Kristen KT, Mittal VK. Scintigraphy of pancreatic transplants. AJR Am J Roentgenol 1982;138:621–622.
18. Groth CG, Lundgren G, Arner P, et al. Rejection of isolated pancreatic allografts in patients with diabetes. Surg Gynecol Obstet 1976;143:933–940.
19. Hirsch H, Fernandez-Ulloa M, Munda R, et al. Diagnosis of segmental necrosis in a pancreas transplant by thallium-201 perfusion scintigraphy. J Nucl Med 1991;32:1605–1607.
20. Jurewicz WA, Buckels JAC, Dykes JGA, et al. Indium-111 labeled platelets in monitoring pancreatic transplants in humans. Transplant Proc 1984;16:720–723.
21. Jurewicz WA, Buckels JAC, Dykes JGA, et al. 111-Indium platelets in monitoring pancreatic allografts in man. Br J Surg 1985;72:228–231.
22. Kamps D, Cook K, Lieberman LM, et al. Early detection of pancreatic rejection with indium-labeled platelet scanning. Curr Surg 1984;41:29–32.
23. Washburn LC, Wieland BW, Sun TT, et al. [1-$^{11}$C]DL-valine, a potential pancreas-imaging agent. J Nucl Med 1978;19:77–83.
24. Atkins HL, Christman DR, Fowler JS, et al. Organic radiopharmaceuticals labeled with isotopes of short half-life. V. 18-F-labeled 5- and 6-fluorotryptophan. J Nucl Med 1972;13:713–719.

25. Taylor DM, Cottrall MF. Evaluation of Amino Acids Labelled with 18-F for Pancreas Scanning. In Radiopharmaceuticals and Labelled Compounds. Vienna: International Atomic Energy Agency, 1973;1:433–441.

26. Stratta RJ, Sollinger HW, Perlman SB, et al. Early detection of rejection in pancreas transplantation. Diabetes 1989;38(suppl 1):63–67.

27. Snider JF, Hunter DW, Kuni CC, et al. Pancreatic transplantation: radiologic evaluation of vascular complications. Radiology 1991;178: 749–753.

28. Kuni CC, duCret RP, Boudreau RJ. Pancreas transplants: evaluation using perfusion scintigraphy. AJR Am J Roentgenol 1989;153:57–61.

29. Ford PV, Spieth ME, Vogel JM. The determination of dual pancreatic and renal transplant graft vascular patency with Tc-99m HMPAO. Clin Nucl Med 1993;18:394–399.

30. van der Hem LG, van der Linden CJ, Ticheler CHJM, et al. Early detection of post-transplant pancreatic graft dysfunction with technetium-99m-HMPAO scintigraphy. J Nucl Med 1994;35:1488–1490.

31. Patel B, Markivee CR, Mahanta B, et al. Pancreatic transplantation: scintigraphy, US, and CT. Radiology 1988;167:685–687.

32. George EA, Salimi Z, Carney K, et al. Radionuclide surveillance of the allografted pancreas. AJR Am J Roentgenol 1988;150:811–816.

33. Eckhoff DE, Ploeg RJ, Wilson MA, et al. Efficacy of 99m-Tc voiding cystourethrogram for detection of duodenal leaks after pancreas transplantation. Transplant Proc 1994;26:462–463.

34. Hawkins RA, Hall T, Gambhir SS, et al. Radionuclide evaluation of liver transplants. Semin Nucl Med 1988;18:199–212.

35. Sandler ED, Parisi MT, Shields AT, Hattner RS. Unique scintigraphic findings of bile extravasation in the presence of ascites: a complication of hepatic transplantation. J Nucl Med 1992;33:115–116.

36. Westra SJ, Zaninovic AC, Hall TR, et al. Imaging in pediatric liver transplantation. Radiographics 1993;13:1081–1099.

37. Merion RM, Campbell DA, Dafoe DC, et al. Observations on quantitative scintigraphy with deconvolutional analysis in liver transplantation. Transplant Proc 1988;20:695–697.

38. Knobloch E, Sfakianakis GN, Georgiou M, et al. Improved technique to evaluate liver transplant patients [abstract]. J Nucl Med 1993;34:112P.

39. Brunot B, Petras S, Germain P, et al. Biopsy and quantitative hepatobiliary scintigraphy in the evaluation of liver transplantation. J Nucl Med 1994;35:1321–1327.

40. Kuni CC, Engeler DM, Nakhleh RE, et al. Correlation of technetium-99m-DISIDA hepatobiliary studies with biopsies in liver transplant patients. J Nucl Med 1991;32:1545–1547.

41. Gelfand MJ, Smith HS, Ryckman FC, et al. Hepatobiliary scintigraphy in pediatric liver transplant recipients. Clin Nucl Med 1992;17: 542–549.

42. D'Alessandro AM, Kalayoglu M, Hammes R, et al. Diagnosis of intestinal transplant rejection using 99m-technetium-DTPA (99m-Tc-DTPA). Transplantation 1994;58:112–113.

43. Weissman AF, Greenough R, Deeb M, et al. Quantitative ventilation/perfusion scintigraphy in single lung transplants [abstract]. J Nucl Med 1993;34:43P.

44. Kim E, Kim CK, Palevsky H, Alavi A. Pulmonary perfusion distribution following single lung transplantation is different between the emphysema group and the primary pulmonary hypertension group [abstract]. J Nucl Med 1993;34:43P.

45. Messian O, Selman C, Mal H, et al. Quantitative lung scintigraphy in the follow-up of single lung transplantation [abstract]. J Nucl Med 1992;33:835.

46. Medina LS, Royal HD, Trulock EP, University of Washington University Lung Transplant Team. Quantitative exercise-rest ventilation-perfusion imaging (ex-rest V-P) in patients with single-lung transplants [abstract]. J Nucl Med 1992;33:835.

47. Halvorsen RA, duCret RP, Kuni CC, et al. Obliterative bronchiolitis following lung transplantation diagnostic utility of aerosol ventilation lung scanning and high resolution CT. Clin Nucl Med 1991;16:256–258.

48. Kuni CC, DuCret RP, Nakhleh RE, Boudreau RJ. Reverse mismatch between perfusion and aerosol ventilation in transplanted lungs. Clin Nucl Med 1993;18:313–317.

*Textbook of Nuclear Medicine,*
edited by Michael A. Wilson.
Lippincott–Raven Publishers, Philadelphia © 1998.

CHAPTER 14

# Nonthyroid Endocrine

Michael A. Wilson

In patients with nonthyroid endocrine disease, nuclear imaging can be helpful, but there are two basic premises: All patients should have their endocrine disease already diagnosed by biochemical and clinical evaluation (1), and the imaging procedure should be used to localize the anatomic site (right or left) or classify the process (hyperplasia vs. adenoma). Most referrals come from endocrinologists or surgeons with an established diagnosis. These tests compose <2% of all nuclear medicine procedures, and their use varies according to local available expertise among the competing imaging modalities (Table 14-1).

## PARATHYROID LOCALIZATION

In the past, hyperparathyroidism was diagnosed in symptomatic patients, who were subsequently found to be hypercalcemic, and operative intervention resulted in the removal of a parathyroid adenoma with symptomatic relief. More recently, hyperparathyroid patients are diagnosed as a result of a routine blood screen that demonstrates hypercalcemia (2). Many of these asymptomatic patients have smaller parathyroid adenomas than did the symptomatic patients, reflecting earlier diagnosis. The other common presentation of hyperparathyroidism is that of renal failure, with hypocalcemia leading to hyperplasia of several or all glands (secondary hyperparathyroidism), which occasionally progresses to autonomous growth of one or more of the parathyroid glands (tertiary hyperparathyroidism).

Various parathyroid hormone immunoassays exist, some directed against the N-terminal and others against circulating fragments. In primary and secondary hyperparathyroidism, the N-terminal and intact hormone are elevated. In renal disease, the C-terminal or midmolecule fragment can be elevated because of renal impairment and may not of itself represent increased parathyroid hormone secretion (see Chapter 26).

### Embryology

The parathyroid glands develop from the third and fourth branchial pouches and migrate down to the neck during fetal development. The lower parathyroid glands derive from the third branchial pouch and must migrate further than the upper glands (which arise from the fourth branchial pouch). This longer migration distance is associated with more frequent ectopic locations. The lower parathyroids also migrate with the thymus, which explains their common aberrant location in the thymus. Three-fourths of the upper glands are located behind the thyroid, near the central portion of the gland, and 99% are in close relationship to the thyroid (i.e., juxtathyroidal). Half the inferior glands lie at the inferior pole of the thyroid, and three-fourths are in the region of the lower half of the lobe. The remaining one-fourth of the inferior glands are found extrathyroidally, especially in the thymus and anterior mediastinum.

### Treatment of Primary Hyperparathyroidism

Despite variable sites and numbers of glands (80% of normal subjects have four glands) and the fact that double and triple adenomas are not rare (~5% of all adenomas), the surgeon can localize the parathyroid adenoma or adenomas in 95% of operations (2). Because of this ability, the routine preoperative localization of parathyroid adenomas may seem unnecessary. Certainly, there is little challenge to the role of preoperative localization procedures in patients who have had previous thyroidectomies and parathyroidectomies. Because reoperation is more difficult and hazardous than the original procedure, it is generally agreed that preoperative imaging to localize the adenoma is useful.

In these days of escalating medical costs, the introduction of a presurgical localization technique for an operation that is usually successful appears unnecessary (3), but this localization has proved to be cost effective at the University of Wisconsin Medical School (4). The localization scan has identified both single and double adenomas routinely with excellent sensitivity; therefore, reoperations are rare. With no difference in patient characteristics, the operating time can be reduced by half, with savings in anesthesia and operating room time being sufficient to pay for the localization procedure. This time sav-

**TABLE 14-1.** *Test frequency*

| | |
|---|---|
| Parathyroid localization | 85% |
| Neuroendocrine tumors | 10% |
| Pheochromocytoma localization | 2% |
| Other indications | 3% |

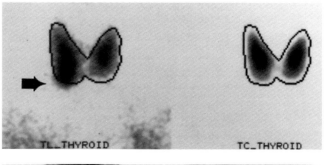

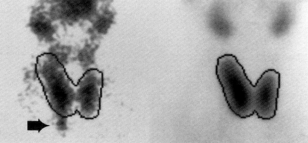

**FIG. 14-1.** The Tl-201 (left) and $TcO_4^-$ thyroid (right) images are displayed for two patients, with the thyroid ROI (as defined by $TcO_4^-$) delineated. **(A)** The discrepancy in tracer uptake in the right lower pole adenoma (*arrow*) of the thyroid is apparent. **(B)** A right thymic parathyroid adenoma (*arrow*) is shown.

ings comes from searching for the scan-localized lesion and its counterpart on the same side rather than all four parathyroid glands. The surgeon can even perform very directed parathyroidectomies under local anesthetic, on an outpatient basis, leaving the opposite side untouched and thus not at higher operative risk if subsequent surgery is required. Although this approach has been deemed controversial, there is evidence that endocrine surgeons are increasingly requesting localization studies in first-time operations.

### Scan Protocols

Multiple protocols have been described for thallium 201 (Tl-201) and technetium 99m pertechnetate (Tc-99m $TcO_4^-$) subtraction scans. More recently, Tc-99m sestamibi (MIBI) was suggested as an improved substitute for Tl-201, and iodine 123 (I-123) was suggested to replace Tc-99m $TcO_4^-$ (abbreviated here as $TcO_4^-$). In 1983, Ferlin and colleagues described the combined $TcO_4^-$ and Tl-201 subtraction imaging technique for adenoma localization in primary hyperparathyroidism (5). This technique required the injection of $TcO_4^-$ to visualize the normal thyroid, then the injection of Tl-201 and the subtraction of the $TcO_4^-$ thyroid image from the combined Tl-201 and $TcO_4^-$ data set. We reversed this order of radiopharmaceutical injection to image the lower-energy Tl-201 photon first, then the higher-energy $TcO_4^-$. Although this modification improves the separation of the two radiopharmaceutical photon energies, the patient must remain immobile longer because $TcO_4^-$ thyroid accumulation is maximal at 20 minutes, so imaging must be carried out for 20 minutes after Tl-201 injection.

The rationale for the test is as follows: Tl-201 is taken up by adenomas and hyperplastic glands in proportion to cellularity and vascularity. The thyroid also takes up Tl-201 and therefore needs to be "subtracted" from the image. This is accomplished by subtracting the $TcO_4^-$ thyroid image.

Each normal parathyroid gland averages 40 mg, whereas the thyroid is normally 25,000 mg. Unfortunately, certain other tissues take up more Tl-201 than normal thyroid and so can mimic parathyroid adenomas. These include thyroid adenomas and carcinomas, and cervical lymph nodes infiltrated with sarcoid, lymphoma, or metastatic cancer.

In this technique, the key element is the subtraction process. In many cases of larger adenomas, the lesion can be identified on the Tl-201 and $TcO_4^-$ image sets (Fig. 14-1). Smaller lesions in general require careful subtraction techniques. Extrathyroidal adenomas are usually detected with-

out subtraction, and early Tl-201 images of the upper chest region may identify these adenomas that lie (in approximate order of frequency) in the thymus (5%), mediastinum (4%), carotid sheath (2%), retroesophageal (2%), lateral cervical (1%), and the suprathyroidal (1%) regions.

Careful subtraction techniques require methods to identify and correct small degrees of patient movement. Constant checks and cross-checks during acquisition, processing, and analysis are required. We acquire the Tl-201 and $TcO_4^-$ data sets in multiple 1-minute frames, then format them into cine mode to detect patient movement and decide on which frames to reject because of movement. If possible, all frames are included, but most studies do not allow this. With the optimal frames combined into composite Tl-201 and $TcO_4^-$ data sets, the thyroid subtraction is performed. It is important that regional variations in Tl-201 and $TcO_4^-$ tracer distribution be identified, but it is never certain which part of the image is normal. The Tl-201 data set is count poor relative to the $TcO_4^-$, so the Tl-201 image is normalized to the $TcO_4^-$ data. The Tl-201 image is slightly overnormalized, so that there are Tl-201 counts present in some pixels in the subtraction image being reviewed. This prevents oversubtraction and obscuration of small adenomas.

The subtraction images must be checked for movement artifact because this can be a powerful source of false-positive images. To do this, we display a composite image with deliberate offset of one data set from the other, with 1 pixel displacement in all directions. This should create a move-

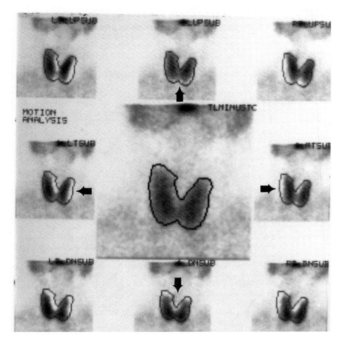

**FIG. 14-2.** This motion analysis display confirms the absence of significant misalignment in the composite $TcO_4^-$ and Tl-201 data sets. Because the $TcO_4^-$ data set is deliberately displaced during the subtraction process, defects are seen opposite to the displacement direction. Viewing the eight directions of pixel shift and the expected defects (*arrows*) confirms the absence of significant movement. If movement is detected, this can be corrected and the analysis repeated to confirm successful realignment.

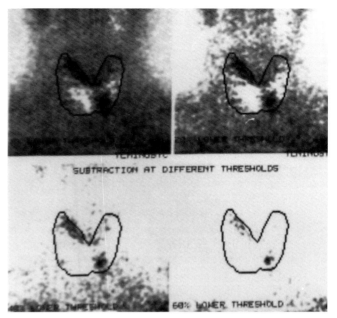

**FIG. 14-3.** Different levels of background subtraction on selected Tl-201 and $TcO_4^-$ subtraction data is shown merely for display purposes. The small left lower adenoma identified was not obvious on the original Tl-201 and $TcO_4^-$ images.

ment artifact on the opposite side from the deliberate displacement direction (Fig. 14-2). If this artifact does not occur, then the data sets are moved to produce the artifact.

The subtraction images are then displayed with various normalization changes and different background subtrac-

tions to check that an optimal procedure has been performed (Fig. 14-3). This technique is described in Table 14-2.

**Clinical Applications**

At the University of Wisconsin Hospital and Clinics (UWHC), parathyroid localization studies are performed on all patients with primary hyperparathyroidism on the day before surgery. Patients with secondary hyperparathyroidism suspected on the basis of renal disease do not usually have preoperative localization procedures because

**TABLE 14-2.** *Acquisition and analysis of subtraction and technique*

| Action | Check |
|---|---|
| 1. Inject 3.0 mCi (111MBq) Tl-201. Image chest and neck for 3 minutes (128 × 128 matrix, 1.33 zoom). | Check for extrathyroidal activity, especially in the thymus. |
| 2. Image neck, zoom 2.67. Acquire 15 1-minute frames. Display as cine. | Check for motion. Clip late images (early images are best). |
| 3. Inject 10 mCi (370 MBq) of $TcO_4^-$. Acquire 15 1-minute frames. Display as cine. | Check for motion. Clip early images (late images are best). |
| 4. Smooth (with 1-2-1 filter) composite $TcO_4^-$ and Tl-201 images. Draw ROI around $TcO_4^-$ image, then superimpose on Tl-201 image. Align using thresholding. | Check superimposition. Move as necessary. (Critical procedure. Check in step 6.) |
| 5. Calculate normalization factor with 10 × 10 ROI over most normal-looking thyroid area. Multiply by 1.2. Subtract composite images. | Check that <10% of all pixels are blank. (This subtraction procedure is critical.) |
| 6. Display 1-pixel shift of $TcO_4^-$ composite from Tl-201 composite image in eight directions (up, down, right, left, and diagonals). | Check for equal edge artifact to verify correct superimposition. (This is a critical review.) |
| 7. Display four extra thresholds (±20, ±40%) to check step 5. Do four more background subtractions. | Check that the threshold and display demonstrate lesion. |

**TABLE 14-3.** *Adenoma size versus test sensitivity*

| Size (mg) | Sensitivity | No. of patients |
|-----------|-------------|-----------------|
| <300 | 58% | 24 |
| 301–600 | 97% | 31 |
| >600 | 100% | 52 |

Source: Wilson MA, Shinners P, Rowe B, et al. Tl-201/Tc-99mO$_4$ subtraction scintigraphy is still the gold standard in parathyroid localization [abstract]. J Nucl Med 1994; 35(suppl):164P.

multiple gland excision is required and all glands must be surgically located.

Given the highly selected patient population with laboratory-proven hyperparathyroidism, specificity is not a problem, and minimal subtraction abnormalities can be reported as probable lesions. Detection sensitivities >90% are possible in primary hyperparathyroidism, and the surgeon should view the images before surgery (Table 14-3). In this era of early detection of asymptomatic primary hyperparathyroidism, the adenoma size has decreased, making localization more difficult. At UWHC, we detect many lesions smaller than the generally reported minimal detection size of 300 mg (2). The smallest so far identified by this method and removed was twice normal (70 mg).

The thyroid gland should be routinely palpated at the time of the study to identify thyroid adenomas that might cause subtraction artifacts, but these patients should not be excluded from the localization procedure. Rather, if two or more lesions are identified by the subtraction technique, all should

be reported. We identify 85% of adenomas correctly in the difficult clinical situations of multiple adenomas, extrathyroidal adenomas, and when thyroid adenomas are present. We have detected lesions outside the thyroid and within the thyroid, and in some patients we have predicted hyperplasia when three or more glands were identified (Fig. 14-4). When the adenoma is medial in the scan images, and especially if an upper gland site is involved, it has often been surgically located in the tracheoesophageal groove.

### New Developments

More recently, investigators have espoused the use of Tc-99m sestamibi as a replacement for Tl-201, and I-123 as a replacement for TcO$_4^-$. Most reports have documented diagnostic advantages of Tc-99m sestamibi over Tl-201, but at UWHC we have not found this advantage in subtraction techniques. The simplest Tc-99m sestamibi protocol has been the comparison of early (20-minute) and late (2- to 4-hour) imaging. Like Tl-201, Tc-99m sestamibi washes out of the normal thyroid with time, and a relative increase in tracer uptake in the parathyroid adenoma is found on

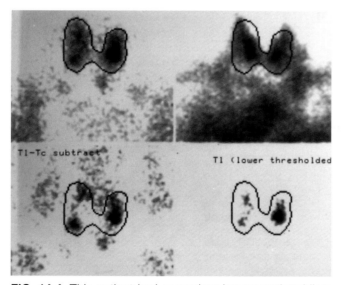

**FIG. 14-4.** This patient had secondary hyperparathyroidism confirmed as hyperplasia of four glands at surgery. The upper left image is Tl-201, the upper right Tc-99m TcO$_4^-$, and the lower images are Tl–Tc subtractions. All images include a thyroid ROI. Four hyperplastic parathyroid glands are visualized: two juxtathyroidal on the right, one upper on the left, and a left thymic. The lower right image is excessively thresholded, and the thymic hyperplastic gland is not visualized.

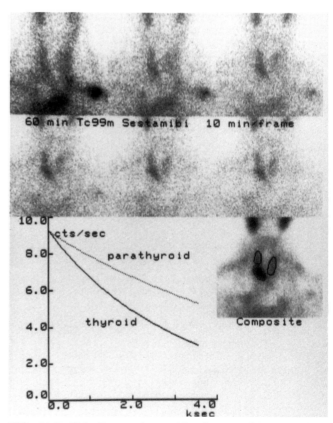

**FIG. 14-5.** This figure shows 60 minutes of imaging (10-minute frames) from time of injection of sestamibi. The washout of sestamibi from both thyroid and a large parathyroid adenoma (ROIs in composite image at lower right) is seen in the lower left graph. Although there are differences in washout rates, the differences are modest.

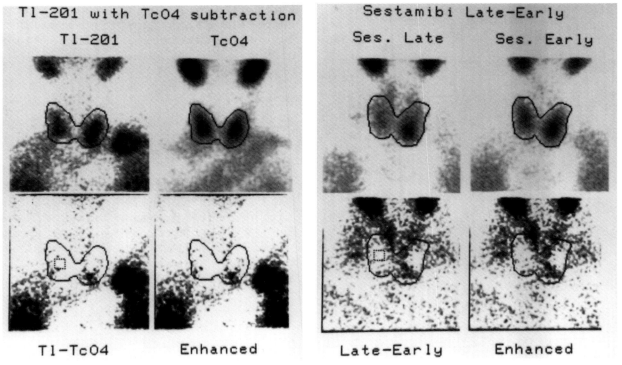

A    TI-TcO4        Enhanced        Late-Early        Enhanced    B

**FIG. 14-6. (A)** TI-201 with $TcO_4^-$ subtraction and **(B)** late Tc-99m sestamibi with early Tc-99m sestamibi subtraction composites show the adenoma relatively well on both sets of images. The small box displayed in the lower left frames is the ROI used for normalization purposes.

delayed imaging (Fig. 14-5). Although Tc-99m sestamibi might be an excellent agent in extrathyroidal adenomas, there have been few rigorous comparisons of the Tl-201/$TcO_4^-$ subtraction technique described here with either the sestamibi/$TcO_4^-$ subtraction or the early and late sestamibi subtraction technique (Fig. 14-6). When we compared these techniques, we found the Tc-99m sestamibi technique (sensitivity, ~75%) was inferior to our more conventional Tl-201 subtraction technique (sensitivity, 100%) in a subset of 20 patients (6).

Some reports have suggested a role for single photon emission computed tomography (SPECT) imaging of Tc-99m sestamibi studies together with the intraoperative measurement of parathyroid hormone to confirm that the adenoma has been removed (7). At UWHC, we have recently begun using the SPECT technique of early and delayed Tc-99m sestamibi imaging and found that excellent localization data are obtained (Fig. 14-7). Stacking transaxial slices and rotating them has produced images of adenomas that look at least as good as our Tl-201/$TcO_4^-$ subtraction scans while adding depth information for the referring surgeon (Fig. 14-8). It appears that the SPECT Tc-99m sestamibi images will be as good as our conventional Tl-201/$TcO_4^-$ subtraction method at locating the side but not the actual site of the adenoma. Because the thyroid is not well visualized by this Tc-99m sestamibi technique, sometimes the SPECT scans may not separate the upper from the lower adenomas. Although Tc-99m

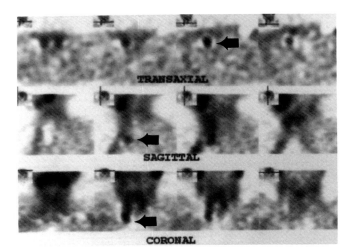

**FIG. 14-7.** Conventional SPECT images of a patient about to undergo adenoma resection. The lesion is detected on delayed Tc-99m sestamibi imaging in the right lower neck, immediately posterior to and below the lower pole of the right thyroid lobe. The adenoma is shown with solid arrows in each slice.

sestamibi appears good for localizing ectopic adenomas, the thyroid subtraction is critical for juxtathyroidal lesions. These are probably best done with simultaneous acquisition of planar or SPECT images (e.g., Tc-99m sestamibi and I-123) with subtraction of the I-123 thyroid image from the sestamibi image (8).

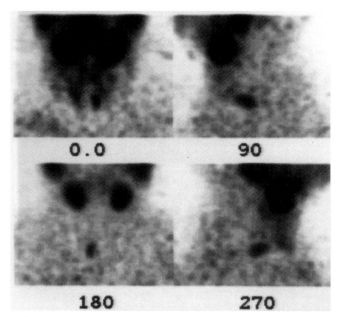

**FIG. 14-8.** Four individual display frames of stacked transverse SPECT Tc-99m sestamibi images at different parts of the rotating format. The images shown are anterior (0-degree), lateral (90-degree), posterior (180-degree), and opposite lateral (270-degree) views of this "rotatogram." The oval shape and the AP orientation of the adenoma is apparent. On the actual rotating image, the size, shape, and position of the adenoma are better displayed than on the individual angle images shown (e.g., 180 or 270 degrees).

From the available experience, there appear to be many ways to localize parathyroid adenomas. Sestamibi's cost will keep it from becoming UWHC's method of choice in locating the site of the adenoma. We currently believe SPECT sestamibi imaging will be reserved for lesions not well seen with our conventional technique and for patients undergoing reoperation.

## ADRENOCORTICAL IMAGING

Adrenal imaging is divided into two types:

1. Adrenocortical imaging with Iodocholesterol
2. Adrenal medullary imaging with meta-iodobenzylguanidine (MIBG)

For a long time, nuclear medicine departments associated with internal medicine departments or strong endocrine sections had a history of frequent use of adrenal imaging (1). These radionuclide studies have largely been overtaken by improved anatomic imaging with computed tomography (CT) and magnetic resonance imaging (MRI), but some roles remain. The indications for NP-59 include endocrine hypertension (e.g., Cushing's and primary aldosteronism), hyperandrogenism, and the evaluation of incidentally detected adrenal masses (incidentalomas) to determine whether or not they are benign "nonhypersecretory" (normal-functioning) adenomas

that do not require further evaluation. The role for MIBG appears to be in following patients with neuroblastoma and the diagnosis of some patients with pheochromocytoma.

### Radiopharmaceutical

The first adrenocortical imaging agent was cholesterol labeled with I-131 (I-131 19-iodocholesterol). Cholesterol, in the form of low-density lipoprotein (LDL) cholesterol, is internalized by specific cell surface LDL receptors and made available as adrenal hormone precursors. The subcapsular zona glomerulosa that produces aldosterone is under the control of the renin-angiotensin system, whereas the zona fasciculata and reticularis are under the control of adrenocorticotropic hormone (ACTH). All three adrenocortical regions can be imaged with the same radionuclide. In 1975, an improved version was produced: I-131 6B-iodomethylnorcholesterol (NP-59). This agent is available from the University of Michigan Nuclear Pharmacy (9) under a physician-sponsored investigational New Drug (IND) Application.

### Adrenocortical Physiology

A portion of the injected NP-59 carried in the LDL fraction is taken up by the adrenocortical cell, esterified, but not further metabolized. The remainder of the NP-59 is excreted in the bile, and there is enterohepatic circulation of this radiopharmaceutical. Uptake is mainly within the zona fasciculata under the control of ACTH. Administration of suppressive doses of dexamethasone suppresses ACTH and therefore suppresses normal adrenocortical uptake of NP-59. In a large proportion of the clinical conditions with normal ACTH secretion (e.g., hyperaldosteronism and hyperandrogenism), suppression of the normal ACTH-dependent adrenal tissue is required to prevent the visualization of normal adrenals.

### Scan Protocol

The tracer is injected by slow intravenous (IV) infusion as the radiopharmaceutical is dissolved in alcohol containing polysorbate 80 (Tween 80); flushing reactions can occur. A dose of 1.0 mCi (37 MBq) per 1.73 m² body surface area is recommended. Before administration, a decision must be made as to whether dexamethasone suppression is to be used. This suppression should be started 1 week before radiopharmaceutical injection and continue over the time of imaging. Because free I-131 may be present in the preparation and liberated in vivo, the thyroid uptake of I-131 is inhibited by the administration of large doses of stable iodine (1 drop saturated solution of potassium iodide (SSKI) three times daily from 2 days before until 2 weeks after radiopharmaceutical administration). Activity in the gut should be reduced by a laxative (e.g., bisacodyl [Dulcolax] 1 mg four times daily). The dosimetry of NP-59 is described in Table 14-4.

**TABLE 14-4.** *Dosimetry of NP-59*

| Organ | Rads/mCi (cGy/187 MBq) |
| --- | --- |
| Whole body | 1.2 |
| Adrenal* | 26.0 |
| Liver | 2.4 |
| Ovary | 8.0 |
| Testis | 2.3 |

*Critical organ.

**TABLE 14-5.** *Altered NP-59 uptake*

| Decreased | Increased |
| --- | --- |
| Glucocorticoids | Excess estrogens |
| Propranolol | Salt depletion |
| Spironolactone | Diuretics |
| High cholesterol | Low cholesterol |

The protocol calls for 50,000-count anterior and posterior images on days 3, 4, and 5, with dexamethasone suppression, and images on day 7, when dexamethasone is not used. If suppression is used, the patient receives 4 mg daily of dexamethasone (1 mg four times daily) for 7 days before and then throughout the imaging study. After 5 days of dexamethasone administration, there is often breakthrough visualization of the normal adrenals. In hyperandrogenism, pelvic images may be required if ovarian tumors are a suspected androgen source.

Agents that affect the adrenal uptake of NP-59 include those that affect the normal hormone secretagogues. Alterations of carrier and uptake mechanism of NP-59 also affect the images (Table 14-5).

**Clinical Applications: Adrenocortical Hypersecretion Syndromes**

The current role of NP-59 imaging is drastically reduced in adrenal hypersecretion syndromes because of its inability to measure hormone status accurately and the exquisite anatomic imaging available with CT and MRI. In most cases, the CT or MRI scan can distinguish adenomas from bilateral hyperplasia, so NP-59 is rarely indicated in these patient populations. When adenomas are small, anatomic imaging modalities may miss them; this patient subset is where NP-59 is used. The radiopharmaceutical cost alone is equivalent to the technical charge of CT and MRI, thus the NP-59 test is not cost-effective in the routine evaluation of adrenal hypersecretion syndromes.

*Cushing's Syndrome*

In Cushing's syndrome, NP-59 was historically very important, but with the exquisite anatomic imaging available with

CT and MRI and the ability to measure excess cortisol production in the plasma and urine, the role of NP-59 has drastically diminished. Comparing the right and left adrenal size with CT or MRI together with the measurement of ACTH can usually differentiate hyperplasia due to excess ACTH from hyperfunctioning autonomous adenoma. The NP-59 scan distinguishes these conditions by demonstrating bilateral visualization of adrenals, in the more common (85%) hyperplastic condition of excess ACTH secretion, from unilateral visualization in the less common adenoma (15%). The current NP-59 role has been reduced to use in patients in whom anatomic imaging is unhelpful and hypersecreting adenoma is still suspected, as with small adrenal tumors. NP-59 is useful in ACTH-independent macronodular hyperplasia causing Cushing's syndrome, where CT may suggest the largest nodule as an adenoma and subtle hyperplasia of the other gland may be missed. Detection rates of 100% are found in clinical use of NP-59 (10). Another indication is diagnosis of recurrence of pituitary Cushing's syndrome (Cushing's disease) after therapeutic pituitary irradiation or bilateral total adrenalectomy. If both adrenals are visualized, pituitary recurrence is suggested, whereas if an adrenal remnant is identified, incomplete total adrenalectomy is established.

*Hyperaldosteronism*

In primary hyperaldosteronism, the role of NP-59 (10) is to separate the more common adenoma (75% of all hyperaldosteronism) from bilateral hyperplastic disease (25%) if CT or MRI have not already established this. In adenomas, surgical treatment is required, whereas in hyperplasia, medical therapy is successful. Normal aldosterone secretion results from renin-angiotensin stimulation, so dexamethasone is used to suppress ACTH and thus much of the normal NP-59 uptake. Bilateral uptake of NP-59 indicates bilateral hyperplasia; unilateral uptake suggests adenoma, provided ACTH is suppressed (Fig. 14-9). The sensitivity and specificity of the dexamethasone suppression NP-59 test is 90% (10). Because most adrenal adenomas are <2 cm, NP-59 imaging can be extremely helpful if anatomic imaging, such as CT, is normal. It is important that the biochemical diag-

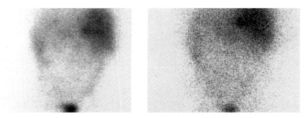

A,B

**FIG. 14-9.** Posterior NP-59 images at 72 **(A)** and 120 **(B)** hours show right adrenal visualization in this patient with hyperaldosteronism due to right-sided adenoma. The normal left adrenal has been suppressed by dexamethasone. Poorer count statistics are seen in the later image.

nosis of primary hyperaldosteronism is made before NP-59 imaging is done because the bilateral uptake scan pattern can be seen in low-renin essential hypertension and secondary hyperaldosteronism.

### Hyperandrogenism and Hirsutism

In adrenal hyperandrogenism and hirsutism, it is also necessary to separate bilateral hyperplasia from unilateral adenoma. Dexamethasone suppression is required. The bilateral increased uptake that occurs in congenital adrenal hyperplasia is suppressed by dexamethasone because the uptake is ACTH mediated. As with hyperaldosteronism, the false impression of bilateral hyperplasia can result from drugs that increase adrenal uptake. This is particularly important because patients who present with menstrual disorders and hirsutism may be prescribed estrogens and oral contraceptives (see Table 14-5). Similar syndromes can result from ovarian hypersecretion, and sometimes images of the abdomen are required to identify ovarian NP-59 uptake as the cause of hyperandrogenism.

### Adrenal Incidentalomas

Adrenal masses are relatively common, with a 1% to 10% autopsy incidence (10–12). Patients with breast and lung cancers that may metastasize to the adrenal have benign adenomas in 9% to 27% of autopsies (11). When should an adrenal mass in patients with cancer be considered a metastasis? In the event that the patient already has metastatic spread elsewhere, the answer may be unimportant, but in other patients, evaluation is required. A common method of evaluation is the size of the lesion: Lesions >5 cm are likely to be cancerous, whereas those <3 cm are likely to be adenoma.

Another way of evaluating adrenal masses is with MRI, where T2 values are higher than normal in malignant tissue. Other MRI sequences and chemical shift imaging have been used to distinguish fatty (benign) from nonfatty (malignant) lesions. Although adenomas in the zona fasciculata are usually fatty, those from other adrenal zones have varying amounts of intracellular fat, which invalidates this generalization. Well-differentiated carcinomas can also contain lipid, as can pheochromocytomas. These histologic variables make diagnosis with MRI unreliable (11).

Patients with incidental adrenal masses should be screened with measurement of urinary free cortisol, serum potassium, and, if indicated, plasma ACTH, renin, aldosterone, and even catecholamines. Patients with hormonal abnormalities should then be managed by endocrinologists.

Nonhypersecretory masses should be investigated. Some have specific CT findings, such as myelolipoma and hemorrhage, but most do not. These "nonhyperfunctioning" masses (adenomas) need to be separated from adrenal carcinoma and metastases. Adenomas tend to be small (<3 cm),

**TABLE 14-6.** *Efficacy of NP-59 adrenal imaging*

| Adrenal diagnosis | Sensitivity | Specificity |
|---|---|---|
| NP-59 | | |
| ACTH independent Cushing's syndrome (adenoma vs. hyperplasia) | 100% | 100% |
| Primary hyperaldosteronism (adenoma vs. hyperplasia)* | 90% | 90% |
| Incidentaloma (adenoma vs. malignancy) | 71% | 100% |
| MIBG | | |
| Pheochromocytoma (n = 1,432) | 88% | 99% |
| Neuroblastoma (n = 137) | 82% | 88% |

*Dexamethasone suppression required.
Sources: Gross MD, Shapiro B. Scintigraphic studies in adrenal hypertension. Semin Nucl Med 1989;19:122–143 and Gross MD, Shapiro B, Francis IR, et al. Scintigraphic evaluation of clinically silent adrenal masses. J Nucl Med 1994;354:1145–1152.

with smooth contours and homogeneous contrast enhancement. Carcinomas tend to be large (>5 cm) and irregularly marginated, with areas of low-attenuation necrosis, calcification, or evidence of direct local invasion or distant spread. Lesions >5 cm are often removed surgically on the presumption that they are malignant.

Masses 1 to 3 cm in size in patients without cancer need no workup except serum biochemical studies to confirm that they are not hypersecreting endocrine tumors. The intermediate-sized masses (3 to 5 cm) require additional workup or can be removed. MRI may help to determine whether the lesion is benign if it looks like the adjacent liver. NP-59 uptake should be concordant with the size of the adrenal mass in a benign adenoma; if discordant, the incidentaloma warrants CT-guided biopsy (12,13). Institutions without NP-59 experience generally proceed directly to fine-needle aspiration (13).

Even in patients with known cancer, benign adenomas are more likely than metastases. This makes discrimination of the etiology of the mass critical because cancer therapy is likely to be different in a patient suspected of metastases. No reliable CT feature exists, so NP-59 and MRI are often used. Although there is some overlap of features in adenomas and metastases on MRI, NP-59 has excellent specificity (Table 14-6), so many lesions need not be biopsied (12,13).

## ADRENAL MEDULLA IMAGING

Functioning paragangliomas are catecholamine-secreting tumors that cause hypertension and paroxysms of headache, perspiration, palpitations, and anxiety. The diagnosis is made by measurement of increased serum free norepinephrine (NE) during paroxysms or, between these episodes, with 24-hour urinary elevations in NE, metanephrine, or the metabolite vanillylmandelic acid. The biochemical diagnosis of pheochromocytoma is not easy (14,15), but when two

**TABLE 14-7.** *Drugs that inhibit MIBG uptake*

| Reuptake mechanism | Depletion of storage vesicle |
|---|---|
| Cocaine | Pseudoephedrine |
| Tricyclic antidepressants | Phenylpropanolamine |
| Phenothiazine | Phenylephrine |
| Labetalol | Labetalol |

**TABLE 14-8.** *Adult I-131 MIBG dosimetry[a]*

| Organ | Rads/0.5 mCi (cGy/18.5 MBq) dose |
|---|---|
| Whole body | 0.11 |
| Adrenals | 0.40 |
| Spleen | 1.10 |
| Heart | 0.70 |
| Ovaries and testes | 0.10 |
| Liver | 1.50[b] |
| Bladder | 1.50[b] |

[a] I-123 MIBG dosimetry is 10% that of I-131 MIBG/mCi, and so a 10-fold increase in tracer can be safely injected.
[b] Critical organ.

or more of these three urine measurements are elevated, the likelihood ratio of disease increases significantly. These paraganglionic cells belong to the amine precursor uptake and decarboxylation (APUD) system, and they store catecholamines in intracellular cytoplasmic vesicles. The World Health Organization divides these rare paraganglionic neuroendocrine tumors according to their site (16):

• Adrenal (pheochromocytomas)
• Aorticosympathetic paragangliomas (e.g., organ of Zuckerkandl)
• Parasympathetic (chemodectomas)
• Unspecified

The level of hormone production in these tumors varies according to type: high in pheochromocytomas, intermediate in aorticosympathetic paragangliomas, and low in parasympathetic paragangliomas. Pheochromocytomas secrete both epinephrine and NE, whereas extra-adrenal paragangliomas secrete only NE.

**Physiology of I-131 MIBG**

NE is synthesized in the adrenergic nerves, adrenal medulla, and neural crest tissues. NE is secreted by these tissues and taken up again into cytoplasmic vesicles by the reuptake mechanism. MIBG is an analog of guanethidine and NE, is taken up like NE by this reuptake mechanism, and is stored in the same vesicles. Unlike NE, MIBG does not bind to the postsynaptic receptors and so does not induce a pharmacologic response. The MIBG not taken up into the neurons is largely (80%) excreted unchanged in the urine over the 4 days after IV administration.

Drugs inhibiting MIBG uptake are listed in Table 14-7. The sympathomimetic group is particularly troublesome because it includes many widely used over-the-counter allergy and diet drugs, such as pseudoephedrine and phenylpropanolamine, that are not considered drugs by many patients. All must be stopped 2 weeks before MIBG scanning to prevent invalidating the scan. Alpha- and beta-adrenergic blocking drugs do not affect MIBG uptake or storage, except for labetalol, which should be discontinued 1 week before scanning.

**Radiopharmaceutical**

The MIBG available to users is labeled with I-131. An NDA in 1994 made MIBG available in the United States

each week. Before the drug is administered, the injecting physician must ensure that the patient is not on medication that will prevent the normal uptake of MIBG and must carefully go over the individual patient's drugs using specific lists of all potentially interfering drugs (see Chapter 30). MIBG labeled with I-123 is probably superior, but because of its 13-hour half-life, is not widely available. MIBG is supplied as a unit dose from Syncor, Inc. (Chatsworth, CA) and can be refrozen and stored for use within 7 days without having to measure free I-131. The dosimetry of MIBG is provided in Table 14-8 from the package insert. The manufacturer's calculation indicates a much lower adrenal dose than previous estimates, and the adrenals are no longer the critical organ.

**Protocol**

Images are obtained at 1, 2, and 3 days after IV administration of 0.5 mCi (18.5 MBq) I-131 MIBG. Thyroid blockade is prescribed 2 days before injection and continued for 6 days. This regimen is less than that required for NP-59 imaging because the tracer does not enter the enterohepatic circulation. If thyroid blockade is forgotten, the planned oral dose administered 1 hour before I-131 MIBG injection provides sufficient initial thyroid blockade. Twenty-minute or 100,000-count images are obtained using high-energy collimators. Many high-energy collimators these days are designed for In-111 and Ga-67, so considerable septal penetration can occur with I-131, producing a "star" effect. If the patient has less than one bowel movement per day, we ask if some foods increase the number of bowel movements. If necessary, we suggest that the patient obtain a mild over-the-counter laxative (bisacodyl and magnesium citrate) to facilitate bowel clearance of tracer. Normal adrenals are seen in 20% of patients imaged, and this is especially so in the later images.

**Clinical Applications**

In 1981, MIBG was introduced to help diagnose adrenal medullary hyperplasia and pheochromocytomas. Neuroblas-

**TABLE 14-9.** *Pheochromocytoma rule of 10%*

| | |
|---|---|
| 10% | Extra-adrenal |
| 10% | Multiple |
| 10% | Malignant |
| 10% | Childhood |
| 10% | Familial |

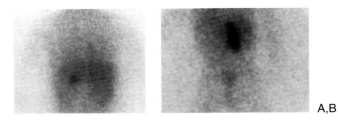
A,B

**FIG. 14-11. (A)** A 24-hour posterior abdominal MIBG scan of a young man with proven familial pheochromocytoma who has had resection of the right adrenal. A new lesion is identified in the left adrenal gland, but no other abnormal sites are detected. **(B)** A 72-hour anterior abdominal MIBG scan of another young man shows increased uptake into a large abdominal neuroblastoma.

tomas were imaged soon after this, and later reports confirmed a role in other tumors.

### Pheochromocytoma

The sensitivity and specificity has been reported as 88% and 99% (see Table 14-6) respectively for MIBG (10) in the detection of pheochromocytoma (Fig. 14-10). Abdominal CT is sensitive for detecting tumors >2 cm in the adrenals, with figures variously reported between 93% and 100% and lesser specificities (14), but small tumors and extra-adrenal tumors are not so readily detected. MRI is reported to have similar sensitivity and specificity because of the tissue characterization: The T1-weighted image intensity of the pheochromocytoma is lower than that of adjacent kidney, liver, or muscle, and the T2-weighted image has high signal intensity (16). The first prospective comparison of the three imaging modes showed that MRI and MIBG had similar detection rates (17). In extra-adrenal tumors and adrenal tumors <1 cm, MIBG has a theoretic advantage because it

* Screens the patient from head to pelvis
* Is highly specific in appropriate populations

* Detects metastases
* Searches for recurrence in postoperative sites

MIBG should be the first test in patients with an increased chance of multiple lesions, extra-adrenal sites (Table 14-9), and prior surgery (Fig. 14-11). Such patients include children who have a 30% risk of extra-adrenal sites, bilateral adrenal disease, multifocal tumors, malignant tumors, and metastases. Conditions associated with multiple tumors (multiple-endocrine neoplasm syndromes, neurofibromatosis, von Hippel–Lindau disease, and familial cases) are also candidates for MIBG.

MIBG labeled with I-123 is superior to I-131 MIBG, but because of the 13-hour half-life, it is only available with a physician-sponsored IND. The role of I-123 MIBG has recently been reported in the detection of pheochromocytoma (18). With I-123 MIBG, incidence of unilateral or bilateral adrenal visualization is increased in approximately one-third of the normal population (i.e., greater than the incidence of pheochromocytoma). Of these patients, one-third had false-positive masses on CT or MRI scans. The degree of tracer uptake was important in improving specificity: Lesions with greater uptake than the liver have a positive predictive value for pheochromocytoma of 100%.

### Neuroblastoma

Neuroblastoma, now the most common indication for I-131 MIBG scanning, is one of the APUD tumors (Table 14-10). MIBG can be used to stage this highly malignant childhood tumor with high sensitivity (90%) and specificity

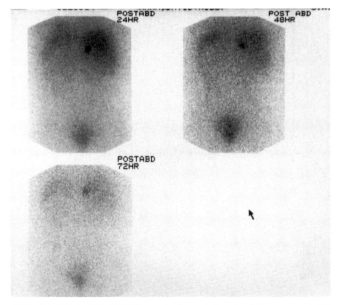

**FIG. 14-10.** I-131 MIBG posterior abdominal images at 24 (upper left), 48 (upper right), and 72 (lower left) hours after injection. The patient is an adult with pheochromocytoma. Note the gradual decrease in lesion intensity with time.

**TABLE 14-10.** *Tumors with MIBG uptake*

Pheochromocytoma
Neuroblastoma
Nonfunctioning paraganglioma
Carcinoid
Medullary carcinoma of thyroid
Pancreatic islet cell tumors

**TABLE 14-11.** *I-131 MIBG therapy*

| Tumor type | Some response | No response |
|---|---|---|
| Pheochromocytoma | 39 | 88 |
| Neuroblastoma | 72 | 186 |

Source: Abstracted from literature (courtesy Brahm Shapiro, M.D.).

(100%) (see Fig. 14-11B and Table 14-6) (10). The extensive list of regions of normal physiologic MIBG uptake (e.g., heart) can lead to false-positive studies if not recognized (19).

### Therapeutic I-131 MIBG

Although diagnostic MIBG scintigraphy is an accepted procedure, the therapeutic use of I-131 MIBG remains experimental. Neuroblastomas are known to be highly radiosensitive, pheochromocytomas less so. Both have been treated with I-131 MIBG. The limiting organ is the bone marrow, and a practical radiation safety problem is the urinary excretion of the MIBG. Urinary catheters can be used in small children with neuroblastoma to decrease contamination. This may necessitate the long-term storage of urine-contaminated materials for hospitalized patients. The same Nuclear Regulatory Commission regulation applied to thyroid therapies applies to MIBG patients on discharge: The patient should emit <7 mR (cGy) per hour at 1 m or a total body burden of <33 mCi (1,221 MBq). Large doses of saturated solution of potassium iodide should be administered before and long after therapy (1 month) to decrease the thyroid burden. Multiple therapeutic MIBG doses are required: at 6- to 8-week intervals for neuroblastomas and at longer intervals for pheochromocytomas. Whole-body irradiation doses of 100 to 200 rads (1 to 2 Gy) may occur with MIBG therapy doses, so thrombocytopenia and neutropenia occur with a similar time course to that of strontium 89 treatment of skeletal metastases. Published response rates are similar to those listed in Table 14-11.

### SOMATOSTATIN RECEPTOR IMAGING

Thirty years ago it was recognized that certain gastrointestinal tract cells were related to neuroendocrine organs (hypothalamus, pituitary, adrenal medulla, etc.). These cells produced peptide hormones and synthesized amines from precursors (the APUD system). This term has been replaced by the neuroendocrine concept because these cells produce peptides and amines that act as both neurotransmitters and hormones.

Somatostatin was discovered in 1978, which led in part to the award of the Nobel Prize to the discoverer. Somatostatin receptors have been identified in many neuroendocrine tumors, and five separate human receptors are described.

These receptors have also been identified in non-neuroendocrine tumors (e.g., breast) and in diseases associated with activated mononuclear white cells (lymphomas and granulomatous diseases, such as sarcoidosis). Activation of these receptors results in the release of inhibitory factors controlling the anterior pituitary, the pancreas, and gastrointestinal functions, including exocrine and gut peptide secretion, gut motility, intestinal transport, and miscellaneous functions, such as splanchnic blood flow and tissue growth and proliferation. Somatostatin roles therefore include paracrine, endocrine, and neurotransmitter modes of action.

### Radiopharmaceutical

Indium 111 (In-111) pentetreotide (OctreoScan) received NDA status in 1994, and approval was granted entirely from data collected overseas. If planar imaging is performed, 3 mCi (111 MBq) is recommended, but if the preferred SPECT imaging is performed, 6 mCi (222 MBq) is required. In >1,000 administrations of this drug, no significant adverse reactions have occurred.

### Scan Protocols

Planar and SPECT images are suggested at 24 and occasionally 48 hours. When abdominal sites are surveyed, early 4-hour images ensure absence of gut activity. Because the abdomen is often imaged in conditions of neuroendocrine tumors, bowel preparation, SPECT, and early images are frequently required. Spot 15-minute images are required, and if SPECT is used, 45- to 60-second acquisition stops are suggested (see Chapter 30).

### Normal Scans

The pituitary, thyroid, spleen, liver (gallbladder in renal failure), kidneys, bladder, and gastrointestinal tract are usually seen in normal individuals. Otherwise, the images are remarkable for the absence of visualization of other sites, so lesions away from those organs are readily identified. Attention to display detail is necessary to ensure that subtle lesions adjacent to the liver, spleen, and thyroid are not missed. False-positive scans can result from recent operative sites, x-ray therapy to the lungs, and bleomycin-induced pulmonary changes. Transient nasal and hilar uptake can be seen in patients with seasonal colds or influenza.

### Clinical Applications

#### Neuroendocrine Tumors

In a large series of neuroendocrine tumors (20) the overall scan detection rate of pentetreotide was 88% (242 of 274). With endocrine pancreatic tumors, the sensitivity was

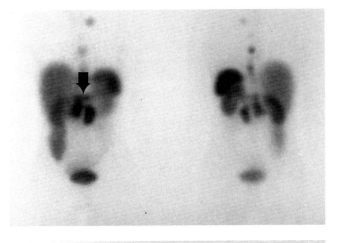

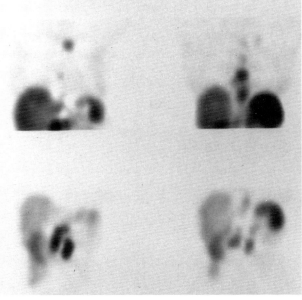

A

B

**FIG. 14-12.** This patient presented with abdominal pain and increased serum gastrin and a past history of Zollinger-Ellison syndrome treated with total gastrectomy 20 years before. **(A)** The planar whole-body anterior (left) and posterior (right) pentetreotide images show multiple abdominal, mediastinal, and supraclavicular nodes. The pancreatic primary tumor (*arrow*) takes up less activity than the metastases. **(B)** The SPECT coronal images show the same lesions better. Prior CT and MRI scans did not identify these lesions, but pentetreotide-directed, thin-cut CT demonstrated some of the lymph node metastases.

100% for gastrinomas (Fig. 14-12 and Table 14-12) and glucagonomas but significantly less than that for insulinomas. In the detection of metastatic gastrinomas, pentetreotide is established as being better than the conventional imaging modalities (ultrasound, CT, MRI, and angiography) and should be the first imaging procedure (21). It appears that some insulinomas have a receptor subtype with which pentetreotide does not interact. In paragangliomas, the sensitivity was 94%, and in one-third of the

**TABLE 14-12.** *Neuroendocrine tumors with somatostatin binding receptors*

| |
|---|
| Pheochromocytoma |
| Carcinoid |
| Pituitary tumors |
| Pancreatic tumors |
| Small cell carcinoma of lung |
| Islet cell tumors |
| Medullary carcinoma of thyroid |

patients, additional sites were identified. In neuroblastomas and pheochromocytomas, the detection rate was 87%, but because of the normal renal route of excretion, occasional nearby tumors may be missed. Sensitivity in small cell carcinoma of the lung was 100%, and in carcinoids it was 96% (pentetreotide has replaced I-131 MIBG as the imaging agent of choice for carcinoid). In medullary carcinoma of the thyroid, sensitivity was 71%, but the normal thyroid and hepatic uptake impaired the detection of residual primary and hepatic metastatic disease.

### Comparison with I-131 MIBG

In the case of pheochromocytomas and neuroblastoma, there is much more experience with I-131 MIBG and I-123 MIBG than with pentetreotide. Early reported sensitivities are nearly identical (90%) for MIBG and pentetreotide (see Fig. 9-27). The dosimetry is similar (Tables 14-13; see Table 14-8), so before switching from MIBG, more experience is probably required, especially because both now have NDA approval and both are expensive. Figure 14-13 shows scans of these two tracers in one patient. The obvious differences in normal distribution influence the choice of imaging agent: The complexity of normal distribution and the sites obscured by this distribution may determine which agent is used in individual patients. In malignant pheochromocytomas, MIBG has been shown to be more sensitive, especially in identifying skeletal, hepatic, and abdominal lesions, whereas In-111 octreotide was able to detect pulmonary metastases better (22). False positives, especially in the lungs, may occur, possibly as a result of inflammatory reaction (20).

**TABLE 14-13.** *Dosimetry of pentetreotide*

| Organ | Rads/6.0 mCi dose |
|---|---|
| Spleen* | 14.8 |
| Kidneys | 10.8 |
| Bladder wall | 6.1 |
| Liver | 2.4 |
| Gonads and red marrow | 0.6 |

*Critical organ.

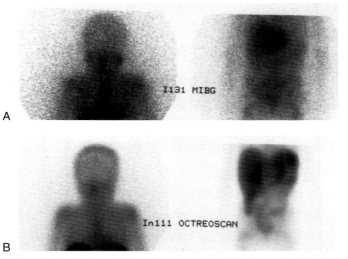

**A**

**B**

**FIG. 14-13.** These 24-hour MIBG **(A)** and In-111 octreotide **(B)** anterior chest (left) and abdominal (right) images were taken of a patient with neuroblastoma in whom no metastases are identified. The differences between I-131 and In-111 are obvious, as are the normal biodistributions of these two tracers. Incidental note is made of the honeycombing of the In-111 image due to use of the high-energy collimator required for I-131 imaging.

### Other Nonendocrine Tumors

Octreotide uptake in non–small cell carcinomas of the lung is 100% sensitive. The uptake is not due to somatostatin receptors in the tumor, however, but probably to cells in the immediate vicinity, possibly immune cells. The metastatic lesions of these tumors do not show uptake, thus confirming that uptake is not due to the tumor itself. These results contrast with neuroendocrine small cell lung carcinomas, which universally demonstrate uptake in the primary site and the metastases. Meningiomas (100%), astrocytomas, and breast tumors (~70%) also demonstrate uptake. In most instances (non–small cell lung cancer being the exception), the octreotide uptake parallels the in vitro receptor presence.

### Granulomatous and Autoimmune Diseases

Pentetreotide uptake is frequently present in sarcoidosis, tuberculosis, and Wegener's granulomatosis. In Hodgkin's disease and, to a slightly lesser extent, non-Hodgkin's lymphoma (mean sensitivity 87%) and in various other lymphomas, uptake is also common (21). Early study results, however, indicate variations in sensitivity according to the individual center and protocols used, so the role of octreotide in lymphomas is not yet defined.

## REFERENCES

1. Beierwaltes WH. Endocrine imaging: parathyroid, adrenal cortex and medulla, and other endocrine tumors. Part II. J Nucl Med 1991;32: 1627–1639.
2. Edis AJ. Asymptomatic primary hyperparathyroidism: a surgeon's perspective. Aust N Z J Med 1992;22:164–166.
3. Goris ML, Basso LV, Keeling C. Parathyroid imaging. J Nucl Med 1991;32:887–889.
4. Wilson MA, Mehta RC, Mack I, et al. Parathyroid localization scans: cost effective and reduced incidence of postoperative hypocalcemia [abstract]. J Nucl Med 1987;28:583.
5. Ferlin G, Borsato N, Camerani M, et al. New perspectives in localizing enlarged parathyroids by technetium-thallium subtraction scan. J Nucl Med 1983;24:439–441.
6. Wilson MA, Shinners P, Rowe B, et al. Tl-201/Tc-99mO₄ subtraction scintigraphy is still the gold standard in parathyroid localization [abstract]. J Nucl Med 1994;35(suppl):164P.
7. Irvin GL III, Prudhomme DL, Deriso GT, et al. A new approach to parathyroidectomy. Ann Surg 1994;219:574–581.
8. Neumann DR. Simultaneous dual isotope SPECT imaging for the detection and characterization of parathyroid pathology. J Nucl Med 1992;37:131–134.
9. Sarkar SD, Beierwaltes WH, Ice RD, et al. A new and superior adrenal scanning agent, NP-59. J Nucl Med 1975;16:1038–1042.
10. Gross MD, Shapiro B. Scintigraphic studies in adrenal hypertension. Semin Nucl Med 1989;19:122–143.
11. Reinig JW. MR imaging differentiation of adrenal masses: has the time finally come? Radiology 1992;85:339–340.
12. Gross MD, Shapiro B, Francis IR, et al. Scintigraphic evaluation of clinically silent adrenal masses. J Nucl Med 1994;354:1145–1152.
13. Falke THM, Sandler MP. Classification of silent adrenal masses: time to get practical. J Nucl Med 1994;35:1152–1154.
14. Bravo EL. Evolving concepts in the physiology, diagnosis and treatment of pheochromocytoma. Endocr Rev 1994;15:356–368.
15. Young MJ, Dmuchowski C, Wallis JW, et al. Biochemical tests for pheochromocytoma: strategies in hypertensive patients. J Gen Intern Med 1989;4:273–276.
16. Van Gils APG, Falke THM, Van Erkel AR, et al. MR imaging and MIBG scintigraphy of pheochromocytomas and extraadrenal functioning paragangliomas. Radiographics 1991;11:37–57.
17. Velchik MG, Alavi A, Kressel HY, Engelman K. Localization of pheochromocytoma: MIBG, CT and MRI correlation. J Nucl Med 1989;30:328–336.
18. Mozley PD, Kim CK, Mohsin J, et al. The efficacy of I-123-MIBG as a screening test for pheochromocytoma. J Nucl Med 1994;35: 1138–1144.
19. Bonnin F, Lumbroso J, Tenenbaum F, et al. Refining interpretation of MIBG scans in children. J Nucl Med 1994;35:803–810.
20. Tenenbaum F, Lumbroso J, Schlumberger M, et al. Comparison of radiolabeled octreotide and meta-iodobenzylguanidine (MIBG) scintigraphy in malignant pheochromocytoma. J Nucl Med 1995;36:1–6.
21. Gibril F, Reynolds JC, Doppman JL, et al. Somatostatin receptor scintigraphy: its sensitivity compared with that of other imaging methods in detecting primary and metastatic gastrinomas. A prospective study. Ann Intern Med 1996;125:26–34.
22. Krenning EP, Kwekkeboom DJ, Bakker WH, et al. Somatostatin receptor scintigraphy with (¹¹¹In-DTPA-D-Phe¹)- and (¹²³I-Tyr³)-octreotide: the Rotterdam experience with more than 1000 patients. Eur J Nucl Med 1993;20:716–731.

*Textbook of Nuclear Medicine,*
edited by Michael A. Wilson.
Lippincott–Raven Publishers, Philadelphia © 1998.

CHAPTER 15

# Labeled Antibodies in Colorectal and Ovarian Carcinoma

Hani Abdel-Nabi

Radiolabeled monoclonal antibodies (MOABs) have gained widespread acceptance as receptor-specific radiopharmaceuticals for clinical applications. Since the hybridoma method was first described by Kohler and Milstein (1), many different MOABs and their fragments have been labeled with a variety of radionuclides for tumor imaging (2). Clinical trials have demonstrated the effectiveness of radiolabeled MOABs in detecting and imaging cancers. The present discussion pertains to the concepts underlying these developments and to recently approved clinical applications in colorectal and ovarian carcinomas, providing more detail than the description in Chapter 9.

## BASIC CONCEPTS

### Antibody Production

Immunoglobulins, or antibody molecules, are produced by plasma cells in higher animals in response to the introduction of foreign substances (antigens) that are generally >1,000 d. As a result, the produced immunoglobulins possess specific binding regions that recognize the shape of particular sites (determinants) on the surface of the antigen. An antigen may have several determinants (epitopes), each of which can stimulate B-lymphocytes. Each B-lymphocyte can differentiate into plasma cells that then secrete a specific immunoglobulin in response to a single antigenic determinant, and this antibody is produced by the family of plasma cells that stems from the single B-lymphocyte. Antigenic challenges evoke a heterogeneous antibody response from a mixture of antibody-producing plasma cells.

If a suitable animal recipient, typically a mouse or rabbit, is immunized with an antigenic agent, serum taken from the sensitized host contains antibodies to several different epitopes of the antigen. Because these antibodies derive from a population of stimulated B-lymphocytes and their daughter plasma cells, the term *polyclonal antibodies* is applied.

### Monoclonal Antibodies

The efficacy of target detection depends on the proportion of specific to nonspecific antibody present in the radiolabeled preparation. Preparations containing a relatively low percentage of specific antibody might not produce an externally detectable level in the target tissue. If individual lymphocytes or plasma cells could be extracted and cloned in tissue culture, however, each clone would have the potential to manufacture a single species (monoclonal) of antibody molecule. Unfortunately, normal antibody-producing cells do not survive in culture media. It was the genius of the two Nobel laureates, George Kohler and Cesar Milstein, to recognize that myeloma cells, which are cancer cells that produce large amounts of identical but nonspecific immunoglobulins and which survive in cultures indefinitely, might be altered by recombinant genetics to construct immortal clones that secrete large amounts of useful single immunoglobulins.

Kohler and Milstein developed a method of producing such monoclonal cell strains by fusing splenic lymphocytes from immunized mice with a mouse myeloma cell, giving rise to clones of hybrid cells called hybridomas (1). Although stimulated lymphocytes do not survive in cell culture and myeloma cells cannot be induced to secrete antigen-specific antibodies, the fusion of these cells using polyethylene glycol results in clones that express both the lymphocyte's property of specific antibody production and the myeloma's immortality (3). Hybridoma cells are selectively grown in hypoxanthine-aminopterin-thymidine medium, which supports neither the unfused lymphocytes nor the myeloma cells alone but does support the fused cells. Hybridomas produced in this manner are then ready for assessment of antibody production and further selective cultivation.

Hybridomas usually generate immunoglobulins of the IgG1 type (or IgG2, a subclass [isotype]), although IgM MOABs have also been produced. IgG molecules comprise two long and two short amino acid chains, referred to as *heavy* (H) and *light* (L) chains, having a total molecular weight of approximately 150,000 d. The chains are linked by disulfide bonds. The IgG isotypes differ structurally in the number of disulfide bonds linking the two H chains, and they differ functionally in their ability to fix complement and to interact with effector cells, such as macrophage and mast cells (4). Immunoglobulins are described as having a single constant portion and two variable regions. The constant region of the antibody molecule includes the Fc fragment, so called because of its tendency to crystallize in vitro. This region is constant for all IgG molecules of the same isotype, is formed of part of the H chains, and can activate components of the immune system. The variable regions, which are unique for each MOAB, are formed from part of the H chain and all of the L chain and contain the two antigen-binding Fab fragments. Antigen specificity resides at these variable sites.

**Antibody Labels**

Antibodies can be labeled with radionuclides using established radioiodination techniques or newer conjugations methods. Chloramine-T, Iodogen, lactoperoxidase, and the Bolton-Hunter reagent can all be used to covalently bond iodine 131 (I-131), I-125, or I-123 to antibodies. One or more iodine atoms can be attached per molecule, depending on the number of tyrosine moieties available for iodination. I-125 is most often used to determine relative tissue distribution in animals. Scintillation camera imaging can be used with I-123, but cost and half-life considerations limit its role. I-131 is more appropriate for imaging patients, but despite its low cost and ready availability, the beta radiation severely limits diagnostic doses. Recently, diethylenetriamine pentaacetic acid (DTPA) has been used to chelate metallic cations, such as indium (In) and technetium (Tc), to antibody molecules. The best results have been achieved with In-111, where the half-life of the label matches the antibody serum half-life. Kits containing antibody-DTPA conjugates designed for in-house labeling with In-111 are currently available.

**MOAB TUMOR IMAGING**

The concept of using radioactive antibodies for tumor localization dates back to the 1940s, when Pressman and Keighley showed that rabbit anti-rat kidney antibodies could be labeled with I-131 and localized in the kidney after intravenous injection (5). A large number of studies have been performed since this initial report. The early studies used radiolabeled polyclonal antibodies and studied animal and human in vitro tumors, in vivo heterotrans-planted human tumors, and patients with a variety of antibodies and malignancies. More recently, radiolabeled MOABs have also been studied with in vitro and in vivo models, and in vivo in cancer patients. These studies confirm that radiolabeled MOABs can be administered safely to patients and that tumor localization is possible. The history of these studies and some of the problems that have arisen is reviewed briefly.

Goldenberg et al. (6) first reported, in 1978, successful tumor detection and localization by scintillation scanning of patients injected with I-131–labeled polyclonal (goat) antibodies to human carcinoembryonic antigen (CEA). Tumor location could be demonstrated 48 hours after I-131–labeled anti-CEA injection in almost all patients. However, scans proved difficult to interpret because of background radioactivity due to the presence of labeled antibody outside the tumor area. To circumvent this problem, Tc-99m albumin and Tc-99m pertechnetate ($TcO_4^-$) were injected before scanning to identify blood pool radioactivity and the nonspecific accumulation of labeled protein in the stomach, bladder, and thyroid. These images were then computer-subtracted from the I-131 antibody images to demonstrate "specific localization" in malignant lesions. Unfortunately, this technique was not easily reproducible and often resulted in the production of artifacts with many false-positive studies (7). Several reports have shown the limited role of polyclonal anti-CEA antibodies in the detection of colorectal tumors (8–11).

Different anti-CEA MOABs and their fragments have been labeled with a variety of radionuclides for imaging colon carcinoma xenografts in animals. Excellent tumor localization was achieved with MOABs compared to polyclonal antibodies (12,13). The first clinical study with I-131 anti-CEA MOABs in patients with colon and pancreatic carcinomas was reported in 1981 by Mach et al. (14). Results of this and other studies showed better sensitivity than similar studies with polyclonal anti-CEA antibodies.

Some of the many problems associated with the low targeting rates are loss of antibody immunoreactivity during labeling with I-131, cross-reactivity with nontarget antigens, interaction of the Fc region with deposition of antigen-antibody complexes in soft tissue, formation of circulating CEA–anti-CEA complexes, and considerable variance in CEA structure (15,16). Many of these problems have been overcome by improved labeling and purification techniques and better tissue screening procedures. Batteries of MOABs are becoming widely available for ready selection and tissue cross-matching. Improved labeling methods that do not affect the antibody's immunoreactivity, combined with the discovery of newer MOABs having minimal cross-reactivity with normal human tissues, have led to a remarkable improvement in patient tumor detection rates.

Precise radiolocalization at the molecular level affords an endless array of applications, and further advances in biotechnology will continue to improve the diagnosis and ultimately the treatment of human disease.

## FIRST APPROVED MOAB

In 1993, the U.S. Food and Drug Administration (FDA) approved the first murine-based In-111–radiolabeled MOAB, satumomab pendetide (OncoScint CR/OV), for the evaluation of patients with newly diagnosed colorectal carcinomas and the detection of recurrences of colorectal and ovarian carcinomas. This new agent was developed to complement and overcome some of the limitations of currently available diagnostic anatomic imaging methods, such as computed tomography (CT) and magnetic resonance imaging (MRI), in staging patients with colorectal and ovarian carcinomas. CT and MRI have only a 65% accuracy for metastatic detection in colorectal carcinoma (17) and have limited value in differentiating postoperative or postradiation changes from recurrent tumor (18,19).

The use of biological molecules reacting with tumor-associated or tumor-specific antigens imparts greater specificity over conventional cross-sectional modalities. Many previously published studies have demonstrated and confirmed the unique ability of radiolabeled MOABs to detect occult recurrent disease in normal-sized lymph nodes, accurately distinguishing local recurrences from postsurgical or postradiation changes (20–22). In ovarian carcinomas, these MOABs have detected diffuse miliary spread (carcinomatosis), which is otherwise undetected by imaging (23,24). Major advantages of radioimmunoscintigraphy (RIS) are that it images the entire body at no additional cost or radiation exposure to the patients and it allows the detection of carcinoma deposits at several sites simultaneously.

Currently, RIS is indicated in the following situations:

- Presurgical staging of extent of disease in patients with primary colorectal cancer (Fig. 15-1)
- Postsurgical evaluation of elevated serum tumor markers in colorectal and ovarian carcinoma patients

As more knowledge and experience are gained, RIS may be a valuable test to confirm the viability of tumors and the tumor targeting of antibodies to be used for chemotherapy or radioimmunotherapy.

### Radiopharmaceutical

The recently approved In-111 satumomab pendetide is a murine monoclonal IgG1 antibody (B72.3) directed against a high–molecular weight, tumor-associated glycoprotein referred to as *tumor-associated glycoprotein 72* (TAG-72) (25). This antibody is expressed by the majority of colorectal and ovarian carcinomas, but it also cross-reacts with other epithelial carcinomas, such as breast, non–small cell lung, pancreatic, gastric, and esophageal cancers. This antibody was initially used in clinical trials with I-131 and more recently with In-111.

In the first study describing their results, Carrasquillo and colleagues demonstrated the ability of this I-131–labeled antibody to target colorectal and ovarian carcinomas (26) and were particularly successful in identifying abdominal carcinomatosis (27). The labeling of indium to the antibody involves oxidation of the carbohydrate moiety found in the constant H chain region and subsequent conjugation of a linker chelator, referred to as *GYK-DTPA* (glycyl-tyrosyl-*N*-E-DTPA), to this oxidized region. This linker technology maintains the antigen affinity and binding characteristics of the antibody because it is far removed from the antigenic recognition sites in the variable region (28). In-111 has been chosen as the isotope to label this antibody because its half-life of 67 hours matches the biological half-life of the antibody (29).

### Clinical Trials

OncoScint CR/OV has been evaluated in a prospective phase III trial involving approximately 20 centers through-

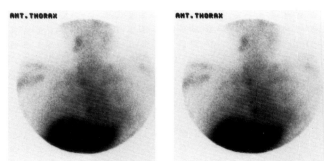

A,B

**FIG. 15-1.** The patient is a 48-year-old white man who had a heme-positive stool on routine examination. Colonoscopy revealed a right colonic lesion. **(A)** A preoperative MOAB scan demonstrated metastatic involvement of several mediastinal lymph nodes. A preoperative CT of the abdomen showed the multiple liver lesions, which are not evident on the MOAB scan. **(B)** The MOAB scan shows normal bowel activity and renal visualization. Palliative surgery was performed, with resection of the primary lesion.

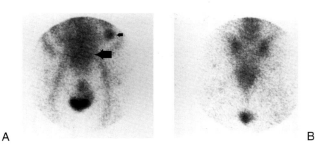

A      B

**FIG. 15-2.** This 70-year-old white man with rectal cancer had an abdominoperineal resection in 1988. The patient presented with pelvic pain and elevation in CEA. A CT scan showed surgical clips in the perineum and a 5 × 4 cm presacral soft tissue mass that had been unchanged for >1.5 years. **(A)** The anterior pelvis scan shows a marked increase in accumulation of the antibody in the presacral area (*large arrow*), later established as tumor recurrence. The site of a left iliac colostomy (*small arrow*) was tumor free. The male gonads are shown (common sites of physiologic MOAB accumulation). **(B)** The posterior scan shows the tumor mass and activity in the gluteal fold.

out the United States. This trial evaluated the ability of OncoScint CR/OV to detect primary or recurrent colorectal cancer (Fig. 15-2) as well as recurrent ovarian cancer. The trial also assessed whether the information from the MOAB scan would affect patient management (30,31).

### Colorectal Cancer

Trial results indicated that the MOAB had a sensitivity of 69% and a specificity of 76% for targeting colorectal carcinomas (either primary or recurrent) with an excellent positive predictive value (PPV) of 97%. The negative predictive value (NPV) is low (19%) because antigenic expression is not present in all tumors. The MOAB scans were superior to CT in the detection of extrahepatic abdominal disease (66% vs. 34%) and pelvic disease (74% vs. 57%), but CT was superior in the liver (84% vs. 41%) (31). The two modalities were found to be complementary when combined, identifying surgically confirmed disease in 88% of patients. In 25% of patients, a potential change in management resulted from the use of the MOAB scan (30).

This study showed that OncoScint imaging was particularly helpful in confirmation of isolated disease in the pelvis or liver, and it was accurate (74%) in eliciting the source of CEA elevation in patients with otherwise negative workup. The sensitivity and specificity of OncoScint was not affected by prior adjuvant therapy or chemotherapy. Increased sensitivity was observed when the TAG-72 expression was found in >50% of the tumor cells (31).

### Ovarian Cancer

In patients with ovarian carcinoma, OncoScint was found to have a sensitivity of 95% in patients with primary disease and a 58% sensitivity in recurrent disease, for an overall sensitivity of 68%. Specificity in recurrent disease was slightly higher (60%) than primary disease (50%), as was the PPV.

False-positive scans were found in 17% and included the following:

- Histologically normal tissue
- Benign ovarian tumors
- Inflammatory tissues
- Adhesions (24)

Because of the rate of false positives, it was felt that OncoScint was more valuable in patients with a diagnosis of recurrent ovarian carcinoma based on either physical findings or rising CA-125, rather than patients with primary disease in whom the potential for false positives was relatively high. Of particular interest was the ability of OncoScint to identify occult disease in 28% of patients, one-third of whom had negative CA-125 and workup. This occurred especially in carcinomatosis and intra-abdominal lymph node metastases, in which MOAB imaging is superior to conventional anatomic imaging modalities.

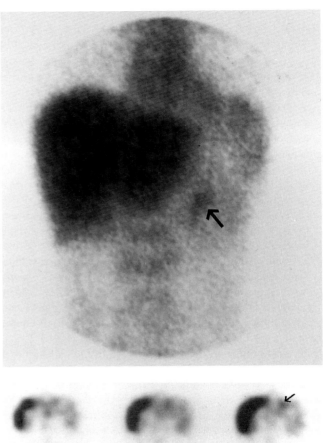

**FIG. 15-3.** OncoScint scan of a female patient after total abdominal hysterectomy and bilateral salpingo-oophorectomy and elevated CA-125 (45 U/ml). Focal accumulation (*arrow*) of the MOAB in the left upper quadrant is seen on **(A)** planar images as well as **(B)** SPECT transaxial views. Disease recurrence was confirmed surgically at that location.

The ovarian study results were similar to those of the colorectal cancer study and showed that OncoScint imaging was far superior to CT (59% vs. 29%) in recurrent tumor and carcinomatosis. In patients with rising CA-125 and otherwise negative workup, a positive OncoScint scan would lead to directed laparoscopy or cytoreduction surgery. In asymptomatic patients with elevated CA-125 levels, a positive OncoScint scan indicates disease recurrence and directs a laparoscopy to this abnormal site instead of "second-look" laparotomy (Fig. 15-3).

### Summary of Phase III Trials

Based on the results of phase III prospective studies in both colorectal and ovarian carcinomas, RIS was shown to have clinical advantages over existing imaging modalities. MOAB imaging is usually disease specific and has a high PPV for adenocarcinoma. In general, the MOAB scan provides pathophysiologic information. It is particularly useful in indicating

- Location of disease
- Extent of disease
- Location of nodal involvement
- Location of distant metastatic spread
- A road map for other diagnostic modalities or procedures

Ideally, RIS should be used in the following situations:

- Initial staging of colorectal cancer patients
- Restaging or reassessing the response to chemotherapy in patients with ovarian carcinomas
- Detecting recurrence in either cancer when an equivocal CT or other findings, such as rising serum markers, are present

Its use would overcome the limitation of standard diagnostic tests in both types of carcinoma.

In ovarian carcinoma, OncoScint imaging is valuable for the following objectives:

- Detecting small tumor deposits (≤1 cm)
- Detecting metastases in normal-sized lymph nodes
- Detecting diffuse miliary disease
- Distinguishing between recurrences from postradiation or postsurgical changes

## PREPARATION AND DOSIMETRY

OncoScint CR/OV is a whole IgG antibody rather than a Fab fragment. This whole IgG is metabolized in the liver, and urinary excretion is only a minor pathway for elimination, thus avoiding the renal tract interference in image interpretation traditionally seen with smaller antibody fragments. The label is cyclotron-produced In-111 and has a half-life of 2.8 days, which closely matches the plasma half-life of the B72.3 MOAB. The two photon peaks (174 and 245 keV) require imaging with a medium-energy collimator. The site-specific In-111 attachment is away from the variable region and preserves the immunoreactivity, thus allowing high tumor targeting.

The OncoScint CR/OV radioimmunoconjugate is supplied as a kit that contains all the nonradioactive components. One vial contains the MOAB, another the sodium acetate buffer and a filter device. The labeling procedure is simple and consists of the addition of the buffering solution to the In-111 chloride, the addition of both to the antibody vial, followed by incubation at room temperature for 30 minutes. At the end of the incubation, the contents of the vial are carefully drawn through a membrane filter (Millipore) to remove any large particles that may have formed during the labeling process. Instant thin-layer chromatography is routinely performed to assess the percent of radioactivity bound to the protein. Because no preservatives are added to the preparation, the kit has an expiration time of approximately 8 hours.

The spleen and liver are the critical organs. The estimated absorbed radiation dose in an average adult patient (70 kg) from a 5.0-mCi (185-MBq) dose of In-111 chloride labeled to OncoScint CR/OV is shown in Table 15-1.

**TABLE 15-1.** *Radiation dose of In-111 chloride labeled to OncoScint CR/OV*

| Organ | Rads/5 mCi (cGy/185 MBq) |
|---|---|
| Whole body | 2.7 |
| Spleen* | 16.0 |
| Liver* | 15.0 |
| Red marrow | 12.0 |
| Kidneys | 9.7 |
| Lungs | 4.9 |
| Adrenal | 4.5 |

*Critical organ.

Very little patient preparation is required, except for a detailed patient history and a history of allergies or previous exposure to murine antibodies. Such exposure would be a relative contraindication because the potential for allergic type reaction could be high in these patients. Allergies to other types of medications or contrast material are irrelevant because they do not lead to an increased risk of adverse reaction.

The most common adverse reactions are hypersensitive allergic-type reactions consisting of fever, transient skin rashes, and rarely transient bronchospasm. These adverse reactions are usually not life threatening and resolve spontaneously. They have been reported in 3.7% of 557 patients who received the antibody intravenously (30).

## SCAN PROTOCOL

Planar images obtained at 72 to 96 hours usually yield high ratios of tumor to nontumor. Although initial studies demonstrated positive localization as early as 48 hours (30,31), the ratio of tumor to nontumor and the vascular and soft-tissue activity tends to decrease the confidence of the interpreter in distinguishing tumors. At the State University of New York (SUNY) at Buffalo, we routinely image the patient first at 96 hours (48 hours is recommended in the package insert) and then at 120 to 144 hours if needed. Single photon emission CT (SPECT) of the anatomic regions most likely to have metastases (i.e., liver, in the case of colorectal cancer, and pelvis, in the case of ovarian carcinomas) is essential for accurate tumor detection. A 35% increase in the detection rate of tumors is achieved by the use of SPECT (32).

For ideal imaging, I recommend performing SPECT of the liver and the lower abdomen separately, either on two separate imaging occasions for patient comfort or on one imaging session if the patient cannot return for the repeat images. Using a single-headed camera, we usually obtain SPECT in a 360-degree rotation with a matrix size of 64 × 64, using a circular orbit and no attenuation correction. Liver SPECT is usually acquired for 20 seconds per stop, whereas SPECT of the lower abdomen or chest is obtained at 45 seconds per stop. Reconstruction is usually performed using a Butterworth filter with cutoff of 0.35, cycle of 5. Images are displayed 2 pixels thick. It is of paramount importance to ensure good quality control of the camera by using an In-111 source and using the two photopeaks (174 and 245 keV) with a 15% window and having appropriate SPECT quality control.

## IMAGE INTERPRETATION

OncoScint CR/OV labeled with In-111 is metabolized primarily through the liver, and 15% to 20% of the injected dose localizes to the liver, which represents the highest concentration in any organ. Other areas of physiologic uptake include the spleen, bone marrow, and genitalia in men, supposedly due to the deposition of transferrin–In-111 complexes in ferritin-rich areas. Early images usually show considerable amounts of blood pool activity in the heart and large vessels, which decreases considerably by 72 to 96 hours and forms the rationale for later imaging times than recommended in the package insert. Activity in the bowel can be seen in up to 15% of patients and is thought to be related to an interaction between the antibody and a weakly antigenic expression of the TAG-72 on normal colonic mucosa. To distinguish bowel from sites of tumor, it is important to recognize the characteristic appearance of the large bowel and to detect changes over time, particularly after the administration of a bowel evacuant (e.g., magnesium citrate and bisacodyl) similar to that used before barium enema and gallium 67 citrate imaging. Nonspecific activity in the large bowel changes over time or with a bowel preparation, whereas activity in a tumor remains fixed or increases with time. Neal and Nabi published a more in-depth description of the practical aspects of immunoscintigraphy with OncoScint CR/OV (33). Occasionally, activity in the urinary bladder may be seen that is related to the metabolism of In-111.

A positive scan compatible with an adenocarcinoma of either the bowel or ovaries is usually based on several features, particularly the location, configuration, and changes in tracer activity over time. Lesion intensity tends to increase over a period of time, and sequential imaging is extremely important in distinguishing true lesions from nonspecific uptake. In our experience at SUNY-Buffalo, confidence in reading these scans increases when it is ascertained that a lesion is seen on two separate occasions, has not shifted in location, and has either the same or increased tracer uptake. We find that lesions that appear at one imaging time only are not true lesions and are usually related to nonspecific uptake.

In-111 chloride–labeled antibodies have been found to localize nonspecifically at colostomy sites (presumably due to the hyperemia [see Fig. 15-2]), sites of degenerative joint disease, organizing abdominal aneurysm, postoperative bowel adhesions, and local inflammatory lesions, including those typically associated with inflammatory bowel disease or secondary to surgery or radiation (34). These can lead to false-positive interpretations, which can be minimized by careful review of the patient's medical history and other diagnostic information.

## HUMAN ANTI-MOUSE ANTIBODY FORMATION

One potential problem arising from the administration of MOABs is the formation of human anti-mouse antibodies (HAMA). This natural phenomenon results from the introduction of foreign protein (the mouse OncoScint MOAB), which triggers the patient's immune response to form antimurine antibodies. These are usually IgG or IgM antibodies; they appear within 2 or 3 weeks and may last 6 months or more. In the phase I, II, and III trials conducted in the United States with OncoScint, HAMA formation was detected in 37% of the patients, half of whom became HAMA negative within 6 months (30). Although it is not a safety issue, the formation and persistence of HAMA in a patient's serum may prevent or limit the application of this technology to one administration. Our experience has demonstrated that the presence of HAMA leads to an alteration in biodistribution with rapid clearance of the antibody, thus reducing the likelihood of tumor detection in subsequent scans to a relatively low level (35). An additional consequence of HAMA formation is the potential for interference with many routinely performed immunoassay laboratory tests, including those not associated with the patient's cancer (see Chapter 26 for a full discussion). There are ways to deal with the HAMA phenomenon and to account for its presence (36), and OncoScint's manufacturer can help in these situations.

Another limitation of HAMA formation is the potential limitation of the number of murine antibody reinjections, which might affect patient follow-up. In one trial, the author and colleagues established the safety of repeated administration of OncoScint in 95 patients who received two to five doses of the MOAB at intervals of at least 4 months in a postoperative surveillance study (35). The study demonstrated the safety of repeated administration of murine antibodies to patients, even those who had developed significant HAMA titers. Only four of 147 repeated administrations developed transient, nonserious adverse reactions (similar incidence to first-time injections). On the other hand, HAMA had a significant effect on the biodistribution of the radiolabeled antibody. In patients with HAMA titers >0.4 µg/ml, rapid clearance of the antibody was evident on both the images and the serial blood samples. These images were characterized by very intense accretion of the antibody in the liver and bone marrow and by reduced and very rapid decrease in the blood pool and soft-tissue levels. It is our belief that this altered biodistribution greatly interferes with the ability of the labeled antibody to detect tumors.

To circumvent HAMA production, investigators have proposed using the Fab or F(ab')$_2$ antibody fragments, which lack the immunogenic Fc portion. Another proposed tactic is the use of antibodies made of the human Fc portion fused to the usual murine antigenic constructs (chimeric or humanized MOABs).

## MOAB Fragments

Although the use of fragments results in low immunogenicity, it is not yet clear whether fragments, particularly those labeled with short-lived isotopes, such as Tc-99m or I-123, will be superior to intact molecules for tumor detection. My department evaluated the efficacy of In-111–labeled intact antibody CYT-372 (an anti-CEA antibody) with its Tc-99m Fab fragment, in 20 presurgical patients with either biopsy-proven carcinoma or high clinical suspicion for colorectal carcinomas (37). Whereas 73% of the tumors were detected with the intact In-111 MOAB, only two of eight adenocarcinomas were detected with the Tc-99m Fab fragment. Excessive persistent radioactivity in the distal bowel, bladder, and kidney contributed to the lower yield. In an extension of this study, we compared the two reagents in the same patients who were injected first with Tc-99m Fab fragment followed by the intact In-111 IgG. The intact antibody identified all lesions in seven patients, whereas the Tc-99m Fab fragment imaged only 53% of the lesions (38).

## Chimeric MOABs

Chimerization of the antibody has been associated with significant clinical problems, particularly low rates of tumor detection and formation of considerable HAMA titers against the antigenic region of the antibody (anti-isotypic) as well as against the Fc portion (anti-idiotypic). Khazaeli et al. have demonstrated that the administration of the chimeric B72.3 was associated with persistently higher HAMA levels and the detection of human antihuman antibodies as well as altered biodistribution (39).

## Humanized MOABs

Human MOABs, being an expression of the immune response of the host, do not elicit an anti-antibody response. Application of human MOABs in clinical trials has lagged considerably behind the application of murine MOABs due to technical factors related to their manufacture, to methods of immortalization and stabilization of clones, and to a good source of sensitized human B-lymphocytes. The development of hollow fiber technology has made possible the large-scale production of human MOABs. We conducted a study with a human MOAB known as 88BV59, which is an IgG3 kappa-class antibody directed against epithelial antigens homologous to cytokeratins 8, 18, and 19. Initial trials of these antibodies in patients with known or suspected recurrent or metastatic colorectal carcinomas demonstrated 75% detection rates for known abdominal and pelvic lesions, particularly when SPECT was used (40). In patients who underwent surgery, the sensitivity of the antibody imaging was slightly greater than CT, with a detection rate of 68% of tumors within the abdomen and pelvis (CT rate was 40%). In a subgroup of patients presenting with rising serum CEA levels and no evidence of recurrent disease by conventional diagnostic imaging (41), we could identify lesions in 50% of patients with a specificity of 75% (PPV of 50% and NPV of 75%). Occult, previously unsuspected lesions were detected and surgically confirmed in six patients. Of importance is the fact that patients who had previously been subjected to murine antibodies and had detectable HAMA levels in their sera could be imaged safely with 88BV59 with no cross-reactivity.

## CONCLUSION

RIS is a clinically important diagnostic tool that has been developed to overcome the limitations of currently existing anatomic imaging modalities. This is readily demonstrated by OncoScint. The current use of these biological molecules against tumor-associated or tumor-specific antigens imparts both theoretically and practically greater specificity than conventional cross-sectional imaging modalities. A major advantage of RIS is that the entire body is screened at no additional radiation dose to the patient, allowing the detection of carcinoma deposits at several sites simultaneously. OncoScint has been found to be particularly helpful in the following situations:

- Presurgical staging of disease extent in patients with primary colorectal carcinoma and elevated CEA
- Postsurgical evaluation of elevated serum tumor markers in patients with colorectal and ovarian cancer
- Patients with equivocal or suspicious recurrences, particularly in the pelvis
- Patients with presumed isolated resectable liver metastases

In the future, RIS may be a valuable test to confirm the viability of tumors and provide prognostic information by confirming tumor targeting before chemotherapy or radioimmunotherapy.

Although clinical trials of these molecules, and smaller molecules, continue at a relatively slow pace, approval by the FDA for clinical implementation hinges on the ability of these agents to affect patient management, change outcomes, and provide cost-effective ways to stage patients with carcinomas and to screen postoperative patients at high risk of developing recurrences.

# REFERENCES

1. Kohler G, Milstein C. Continuous culture of fused cells secreting antibody of predefined specificity. Nature 1975;256:495–496.
2. Goldenberg DM, Larson SM. Radioimmunodetection in cancer identification. J Nucl Med 1992;33:803–814.
3. Milstein C. Monoclonal antibodies. Sci Am 1980;243(4):66–74.
4. Weir DM. Experimental Immunology. Philadelphia: Davis, 1967; 258–272.
5. Pressman D, Keighley G. The zone of activity of antibodies as determined by the use of radioactive tracers; the zone of activity of nephistoxic anti-kidney serum. J Immunol 1948;59:141–156.
6. Goldenberg DM, Deland F, Kim EE, et al. Use of radiolabeled antibodies to carcinoembryonic antigen for the detection and localization of diverse cancers by external photoscanning. N Engl J Med 1978;298:1384–1388.
7. Ott RJ, Grey LG, Zievonic NA, et al. The limitations of the dual radionuclide subtraction technique for the external detection of tumors by radioiodine-labeled antibodies. Br J Radiol 1983;56:101–108.
8. Sullivan DC, Silva JS, Cox CE, et al. Localization of I-131 labeled goat and primate anti-carcinoembryonic antigen (CEA) antibodies in patients with cancer. Invest Radiol 1982;17:350–355.
9. Dykes PW, Bradwell AR. Carcinoembryonic antigen radioimmunodetection. Gastroenterology 1983;84:651–653.
10. Mach J, Carrel S, Forni M, et al. Tumor localization of radiolabeled antibodies against carcinoembryonic antigen in patients with carcinoma. N Engl J Med 1980;303:5–10.
11. Nabi HA, Hinkle GH, Olsen JO, et al. Iodine-131 labeled anti-CEA polyclonal antibody detection of gastrointestinal cancer. J Nucl Med 1984;25:P113.
12. Hedin A, Wahren B, Hammarstrom S. Tumor localization of CEA containing human tumors in nude mice by means of monoclonal anti-CEA antibodies. Int J Cancer 1978;30:547–552.
13. Wahl RL, Parker CW, Philpott GW. Improved radioimaging and tumor localization with monoclonal F(ab')$_2$. J Nucl Med 1983;24:217–225.
14. Mach J, Buchegger F, Forni M. Use of radiolabeled monoclonal anti-CEA antibodies for the detection of human carcinomas by external photoscanning and tomoscintigraphy. Immunol Today 1981;2:239–249.
15. Mauligit GM, Struckey S. Colorectal carcinoma. Evidence for circulating CEA-anti-CEA complexes. Cancer 1983;52:146–149.
16. Banjo C, Shuster J, Gold P. Intermolecular heterogeneity of the carcinoembryonic antigen. Cancer Res 1974;34:2114–2121.
17. Zerhouni EA. RDOG (Radiology Diagnostic Oncology Group) Update. Part 2. Radiology 1992;185(suppl):64P.
18. Freeny PC, Machs WM, Ryan JA, Bolen JW. Colorectal carcinoma evaluation with CT: preoperative staging and detection of post-operative recurrence. Radiology 1986;158:347–359.
19. Thompson WM, Halvorsen RA. Computed tomographic staging of gastrointestinal malignancies, II. Invest Radiol 1987;22:96–105.
20. Nabi HA. Radiolabeled Antibodies in Clinical Nuclear Medicine: A Technology Coming of Age. In LM Freeman (ed), Nuclear Medicine Annual. New York: Raven, 1993;1–27.
21. Doerr RJ, Abdel-Nabi H, Merchant B. Indium-111 ZCE 025 immunoscintigraphy in occult recurrent colorectal cancer with elevated carcinoembryonic antigen level. Arch Surg 1990;125:226–229.
22. Haseman MK, Brown DW, Keeling CA, Reed NL. Radioimmunodetection of occult carcinoembryonic antigen-producing cancer. J Nucl Med 1992;33:1750–1757.
23. Surwit EA. Impact of $^{111}$In-CYT-103 on the Surgical Management of Patients with Ovarian Cancer. In Maguire RT, Van Nostrand D (eds), Diagnosis of Colorectal and Ovarian Carcinoma. Application of Immunoscintigraphic Technology. New York: Dekker, 1991;125–140.
24. Surwit EA, Krag DN, Katterhagen JG, et al. Clinical assessment of $^{111}$In-CYT-103 immunoscintigraphy in ovarian cancer. Gynecol Oncol 1993;48:285–292.
25. Colcher D, Hand PH, Nuti M, Schlom J. A spectrum of monoclonal antibodies reactive with human mammary tumor cells. Proc Natl Acad Sci U S A 1981;78:3199–3203.
26. Carrasquillo JA, Sugarbaker P, Colcher D, et al. Radioimmunoscintigraphy of colon cancer with iodine-131 labeled B72.3 monoclonal antibody. J Nucl Med 1988;29:1022–1030.
27. Carrasquillo JA, Sugarbaker P, Colcher D, et al. Peritoneal carcinomatosis: imaging with intraperitoneal injection of I-131 labeled B72.3 monoclonal antibody. Radiology 1988;167:35–40.
28. Rodwell JD, Alvares VL, Lee C, et al. Site specific covalent modification of monoclonal antibodies: in-vivo and in-vitro evaluations. Proc Natl Acad Sci U S A 1986;83:2632–2636.
29. Maguire RT, Schmelter RJ, Pascucci VL, Conklin JJ. Immunoscintigraphy of colorectal adenocarcinoma: results with site-specific radiolabeled B72.3 ($^{111}$In-CYT-103). Antibody Immunocong Radiopharm 1989;2:257–269.
30. Doerr RJ, Abdel-Nabi H, Krag D, Mitchell E. Radiolabeled antibody imaging in the management of colorectal cancer: results of a multicenter clinical study. Ann Surg 1991;214:118–124.
31. Collier BD, Abdel-Nabi H, Doerr RJ, Harwood SJ. Immunoscintigraphy performed with In-111 CYT-103 in the management of colorectal cancer: comparison with CT. Radiology 1992;185:179–186.
32. Nabi HA, Erb DA, Cronin VR. Superiority of SPECT to planar imaging in the detection of colorectal carcinoma with $^{111}$In monoclonal antibodies. Nucl Med Commun 1995;16:631–639.
33. Neal CE, Abdel-Nabi H. Clinical immunoscintigraphy of recurrent colorectal carcinoma. Appl Radiol 1994;25:32–39.
34. Abdel-Nabi H, Chan HW, Doerr RJ. Indium-labeled anti-colorectal carcinoma monoclonal antibody accumulation in non-tumored tissue in patients with colorectal carcinoma. J Nucl Med 1990;31:1975–1979.
35. Abdel-Nabi H, Harwood SJ, Collier BD, et al. Repeated administration of OncoScint (In-111-CYT-103) in colorectal carcinoma patients. Interim report of safety, efficacy and HAMA development. J Nucl Med 1993;34:213P.
36. Hansen HJ, LaFontaine G, Newman ES, et al. Solving the problem of antibody interference in commercial "sandwich" type immunoassay of carcinoembryonic antigen. Clin Chem 1989;35:146–151.
37. Nabi HA, Doerr RJ. Colorectal carcinoma imaging with In-111 labeled intact anti-CEA MAb CYT-372 and its Tc-99m Fab' fragment CYT-380 [abstract]. Antibody Immuno Radiopharm 1993;6:50.
38. Abdel-Nabi H, Doerr RJ, Maroli AN, et al. Localization of colorectal carcinomas with In-111 intact anti-CEA MoAb CYT-372 and its Fab' fragment (CYT-380) labeled with technetium: comparative results within the same patients [abstract]. J Nucl Med 1994;35:219.
39. Khazaeli MB, Saleh MN, Liu TP, et al. Pharmacokinetics and immune response of 131I-chimeric mouse/human B72.3 (human gamma 4) monoclonal antibody in humans. Cancer Res 1991;51:5461–5466.
40. DeJager RL, Abdel-Nabi H, Serafini A, et al. Current status of cancer immunodetection with radiolabeled human monoclonal antibodies. Semin Nucl Med 1993;23:165–179.
41. Abdel-Nabi H, DeJager R, Evans N, et al. Detection of occult colorectal carcinoma with Tc-99m labeled human monoclonal antibody 88BV59 [abstract]. J Nucl Med 1994;35:86.

*Textbook of Nuclear Medicine,*
edited by Michael A. Wilson.
Lippincott–Raven Publishers, Philadelphia © 1998.

CHAPTER **16**

# Acquired Immunodeficiency Syndrome

Hussein M. Abdel-Dayem

## EPIDEMIOLOGY

Acquired immunodeficiency syndrome (AIDS) is a serious epidemic and a major health concern in the United States. In St. Vincent's Hospital and Medical Center in New York, this population represents approximately 20% of the nuclear medicine workload, but at most other centers the proportion is much lower. To date, >1.2 million Americans have been infected by the human immunodeficiency virus (HIV), with >400,000 having clinical manifestations of AIDS. There have been more than 270,000 reported deaths in this country since the onset of the disease in 1981 (1–3). AIDS is induced by integration of the HIV into the cellular immune system (4). The initial event appears to require exposure to a body fluid containing HIV by an individual with macrophage immune stimulation (5,6). According to the Centers for Disease Control (CDC) records through December 1990, there are five high-risk groups for AIDS infection (4):

* Homosexuals, 59%
* Intravenous (IV) drug abusers, 29%
* Blood product recipients, 5%
* Those having sexual contact with AIDS patients, 4%
* Children with in utero contact, 3%

The epidemic of AIDS is changing in mode of transmission as the number of homosexual and pediatric cases (typically hemophiliacs) decreases and heterosexual transmission increases.

HIV-infected individuals may proceed through three pre-AIDS classification groups before developing classic AIDS (Table 16-1). The acutely HIV-infected individual may have a viral syndrome (group I), which may be forgotten. For a period of up to 36 months, the standard HIV antibody test is negative in HIV-exposed individuals (group II), but extensive HIV nucleic acid replication methods are positive during this latent period (7). If lymphadenopathy persists, but the AIDS criteria of dementia, wasting, opportunistic infections, or tumor involvement is not present, the patient is categorized as having AIDS-related complex (ARC) (pre-AIDS group III). The patient finally develops AIDS.

Health problems in patients with AIDS are complicated by other medical and social problems. Many patients with AIDS in both homosexual and heterosexual groups may be drug or alcohol abusers, may be infected with other venereal diseases, or may have more than one disease process. As the ability to prolong the life of patients with AIDS improves and as the number of heterosexual patients with AIDS increases, new patterns of disease will be seen.

Preferential involvement of the T-helper lymphocyte CD4 by HIV accounts for most of the complications. As the number of T-lymphocytes decreases, and as a result of the lack of immune response, the pattern of opportunistic, neoplastic, and lymphoproliferative diseases in these patients with AIDS increases and the biology of disease is different from that seen in non–HIV-infected patients. Neoplastic and infectious diseases are more aggressive in patients with AIDS (8), resulting in wider dissemination and more central necrosis in the lesions.

## CLINICAL PRESENTATION AND INVESTIGATION

Fever, weight loss, and gastrointestinal (GI) symptoms are usually the presenting symptoms of AIDS. The accurate and rapid localization of the site of infection is necessary to start appropriate treatment. Verification of the diagnosis of opportunistic infections, especially in the respiratory and GI tract, is sometimes difficult, exhausting to the patient, and very costly. Anatomic imaging modalities, such as planar radiography and computed tomography (CT), are not sensitive in the early stages of infections and, if abnormal, are frequently nonspecific.

Nuclear medicine has the advantage of being sensitive in detecting specific image patterns early in the presentations of opportunistic infections, neoplastic involvement, and HIV-specific diseases, such as encephalopathy. Gallium 67 citrate (Ga-67) whole-body scans are the most commonly used nuclear technique in AIDS (9,10). Ga-67

**TABLE 16-1.** *HIV infection status*

| Group | HIV status | Clinical status |
| --- | --- | --- |
| Pre-AIDS group I | Acutely HIV infected | May or may not develop viral infection symptoms |
| Pre-AIDS group II | Asymptomatic HIV carrier | Standard serology negative for 3 years |
| Pre-AIDS group III | AIDS-related complex | Persistent lymph node enlargement but no AIDS criteria |
| AIDS group IV | AIDS | AIDS criteria: HIV dementia, wasting syndrome, opportunistic infections, specific tumors |

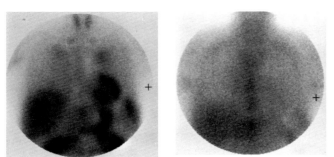

A,B

**FIG. 16-1.** An example of KS with **(A)** Tl-201–positive and **(B)** Ga-67–negative scans. (The cross hair indicates the patient's left side.) The patient's CXR was normal. This scan pattern suggests KS.

uptake is seen in both opportunistic infections and tumors. Thallium 201 chloride (Tl-201) has been widely used recently for imaging viable tumor tissues, and increased uptake is not found in acute infectious processes (11,12). Kaposi's sarcoma (KS) is Tl-201 positive, whereas Ga-67 citrate uptake is negative in KS (13,14). Tl-201 uptake in tuberculous, granulomatous, or inflammatory lesions is reported to decrease when 2-hour images are compared to early 30-minute images, which is the opposite of what occurs in neoplastic tissues (15). Sequential Tl-201 and Ga-67 scans have been used successfully (16) to differentiate opportunistic infections such as KS and lymphoreticular neoplasia (Fig. 16-1).

## RADIOPHARMACEUTICALS

The following radionuclides have been used for diagnostic purposes in patients with AIDS:

- Ga-67
- Tl-201
- Indium 111 (In-111) or technetium 99m (Tc-99m) white blood cells (WBCs)

Other organ-specific radionuclides include

- Tc-99m hexamethylpropyleneamine oxime (HMPAO) for central nervous system (CNS) dementia
- Tc-99m diethylenetriamine pentaacetic acid (DTPA) or Tc-99m mercaptoacetyltriglycine (MAG3) for acute tubular necrosis (ATN), nephritis, and drug toxicity

- Tc-99m iminodiacetic acid (IDA) for hepatitis and cholangitis
- Tc-99m aerosols for pulmonary diseases

In this chapter, a new approach for nuclear medicine studies in patients with AIDS is described. It developed from our experience at St. Vincent's Hospital and Medical Center of New York, which is one of the nationally recognized centers for the treatment of AIDS.

## Gallium Scanning in AIDS Patients

In patients with AIDS, a Ga-67 dose of 5 to 8 mCi (185 to 296 MBq) meets the requirement of good image quality for both planar and single photon emission CT (SPECT) acquisition. Because of the physiologic excretion of Ga in the bowel, abdominal imaging at 48 hours makes the differentiation of abnormal Ga-67 uptake due to AIDS-related colitis or enteritis difficult to separate from normal physiologic excretion. We find that images obtained 4 hours after injection are the best compromise. Because time is important in patients with AIDS and early diagnosis is necessary, we compared 24- and 48-hour planar and SPECT imaging of the lungs and found that SPECT is essential in all Ga studies, and that planar and SPECT 24-hour images of the chest did not miss any lesions when compared with 48-hour images. Accordingly, we recommend this Ga-67 protocol and have found it to be satisfactory in >90% of these patients:

- 4 hours planar whole body (option of SPECT for the abdomen)
- 24 hours planar whole body (SPECT required for the chest)

Occasionally there is high background activity that requires 48-hour imaging of the chest.

Any bowel activity in the 4-hour Ga-67 scan is significant in an AIDS patient who has fever. Figure 16-2 shows abnormal bowel gallium activity at 4 and 24 hours with no abnormal chest activity, suggesting that AIDS-related colitis is the cause of the patient's symptoms and fever. The cecum, ascending colon, and transverse colon are the sites most commonly involved. Activity equal to or greater than that of the liver indicates involvement of the bowel by either opportunistic infection or neoplastic process. However, we found that there is no relationship between the grade of Ga-67 uptake and the incidence of diarrhea.

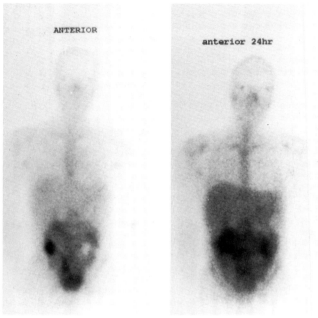

**A,B**

**FIG. 16-2. (A)** The 4-hour Ga-67 anterior view shows increased bowel activity without abnormal lung uptake. **(B)** The 24-hour image shows that Ga-67 uptake in the bowel has become more intense. Without the 4-hour image it might be difficult to determine whether the 24-hour bowel activity is physiologic or pathologic, but the increase in bowel uptake confirms AIDS-related colitis in this feverish patient.

**TABLE 16-2.** *Differentiating pulmonary KS from acute infectious and other neoplastic processes*

|  | Tl-201 | Ga-67 |
|---|---|---|
| Opportunistic infections | Negative | Positive |
| KS | Positive | Negative |
| Neoplastic lesions | Positive | Positive |

**TABLE 16-3.** *Sequential Ga-67 and Tl-201 scans in AIDS*

|  | Ga-67 | | Tl-201 | |
|---|---|---|---|---|
|  | Ga+ | Ga− | Tl+ | Tl− |
| KS (n = 23) | 1 | 22 | 21 | 2 |
| KS and opportunistic infection (n = 15) | 9 | 6 | 12 | 3 |
| Opportunistic infection (n = 21) | 13 | 8 | 11 | 10 |
| Neither (n = 12) | 0 | 12 | 0 | 12 |

**TABLE 16-4.** *Sensitivity, specificity, and accuracy of sequential Tl-201 and Ga-67 scans in AIDS patients*

|  | Sensitivity | Specificity | Accuracy |
|---|---|---|---|
| KS alone | 91% | 80% | 86% |
| KS plus infection | 40% | 80% | 66% |
| Overall | 71% | 80% | 78% |

## Tl-201 Scanning and KS

KS affects approximately 15% of patients with AIDS. Almost all cases occur in homosexual or bisexual males, with a sex ratio (M:F) of 50:1. The disease appears to be a result of sexual rather than parenteral transmission because it is seen rarely in hemophiliacs, and women with KS are more likely to be partners of bisexual males than of IV drug abusers. These observations might suggest that KS is caused by an unidentified agent that is transmitted sexually, and the disease has been linked to cytomegalovirus (CMV).

Pulmonary involvement occurs in 20% of patients with KS and is nearly always preceded by the more commonly documented cutaneous or visceral disease. Diagnosis of skin lesions is usually confirmed by clinical examination and excisional biopsy. KS involvement of the trachea and bronchi is usually confirmed visually by bronchoscopy without biopsy because of the fear of excessive bleeding. The diagnosis of KS involvement of the lung parenchyma is difficult because the radiograph and CT findings are nonspecific.

In 1988, Lee and coworkers reported that KS is Tl-201 avid and Ga-67 nonavid (13,14). Sequential Tl-201 and Ga-67 scans differentiate pulmonary KS from acute infectious or other neoplastic processes using the simple scheme shown in Table 16-2.

Planar and SPECT Tl-201 images are acquired 20 minutes after the IV injection of 4 mCi (148 MBq) Tl-201 chlo-

ride. When Tl-201 is abnormally increased, the images are repeated 2 hours later, and Ga-67 scans are obtained at 4 and 24 hours, either injected on the same day or the next day (see Fig. 16-2). We evaluated sequential Tl-201 and Ga-67 scans (Table 16-3) to determine the sensitivity, specificity, and accuracy (Table 16-4) in correctly diagnosing KS involve-

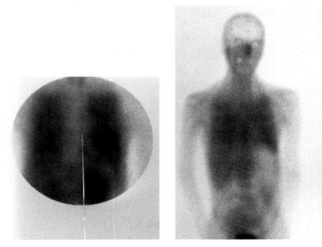

**A,B**

**FIG. 16-3.** Diffuse increased uptake in the lungs of both **(A)** Tl-201 and **(B)** Ga-67 images in an AIDS patient with PCP. (Reprinted with permission from Abdel-Dayem HM, DiFabrizio L, Kowalsky, et al. Diffuse thallium uptake in the lungs in PCP. Clin Nucl Med 1994;19:287–291.)

ment of the lungs in patients with AIDS (16). The accuracy of sequential Tl-201 and Ga-67 scans in diagnosing pulmonary KS decreases in the presence of opportunistic infections (see Table 16-4).

Diffusely increased Tl-201 pulmonary uptake is seen in the early images (which correlates with increased Ga-67 uptake) (18). Figure 16-3 shows examples of diffusely abnormal Tl-201 and Ga-67 scans for *Pneumocystis carinii* pneumonia (PCP) involvement. Focal abnormalities of increased Tl-201 and Ga-67 uptake can also be seen in tuberculosis. Patients with AIDS can suffer KS and opportunistic infection simultaneously.

### In-111 WBC Scans

Labeled WBCs (with In-111 or Tc-99m HMPAO) can be used to diagnose opportunistic pulmonary infections, such as PCP and CMV pneumonias, and GI conditions, such as esophagitis and inflammatory bowel disease. In these conditions, the labeled WBC is reserved for situations when Ga-67 and other anatomic imaging or investigations are not helpful. Labeled WBC scans have a particular application in bone and joint infections and in CNS infections, for which the detection rate exceeds that of Ga-67 or other imaging procedures.

## PATHOLOGIC CONDITIONS

### Infections

#### Pneumocystis Carinii *Pneumonia*

PCP is usually the first pulmonary manifestation in two-thirds of patients with AIDS, and eventually, >80% of patients with AIDS develop PCP (19). Ga-67 scintigraphy is abnormal in >85% of PCP cases and detects PCP in asymptomatic patients with normal chest x-rays (CXRs) (20). Due to reports of In-111 WBC scans being abnormal in only 39% of active PCP cases, whereas Ga-67 scans are abnormal in 93%, and because of the risks of handling HIV-infected blood during the labeling procedure, Ga-67 is the preferred radiopharmaceutical for pulmonary imaging (21). Because Ga-67 scans result in early detection, and thus early therapy and a better prognosis, the scan should be used more often for patients presenting with fever and cough and normal CXR. The specificity of intense Ga uptake in HIV-infected individuals when the concurrent CXR is normal approaches 100%.

Unfortunately, up to 50% of positive Ga-67 scans can represent conditions other than PCP, but the etiology of the positive Ga-67 scan can be suggested by the uptake pattern. The characteristic pattern of diffusely increased bilateral Ga-67 lung uptake with an intensity greater than liver (without nodal or parotid uptake) has a specificity of 90%

for PCP (9,21). The presence of heterogeneous diffuse lung uptake may have a higher predictive value than homogeneous uptake (22,23). Due to increasing use of therapy with aerosol pentamidine, Ga-67 uptake in PCP may be limited to the upper lobes due to less effective therapeutic access of the aerosol treatment to this region. Follow-up Ga-67 scans can be helpful in determining cure or etiology of new pulmonary symptoms. Once the plain chest film becomes clearly abnormal, Ga-67 avidity decreases and may become nearly normal. This state likely reflects a decrease in the number of immune functioning lymphocytes and is associated with a high fatality rate. Pulmonary pathology is virtually ruled out if both Ga-67 lung uptake and CXR are normal.

Because of rapid aerosol clearance from the lungs, Tc-99m DTPA aerosol imaging may detect PCP in patients with AIDS who have had negative Ga-67 images (24). Aerosol imaging is nonspecific, however, because it is frequently abnormal due to other etiologies, such as smoking and chronic obstructive pulmonary disease; thus, it is not recommended.

#### Lymphocytic Interstitial Pneumonitis

Lymphocytic interstitial pneumonitis (LIP) is common in pediatric AIDS patients. LIP is a noninfectious process characterized by diffuse lymphocytic infiltration of the lung parenchyma and parotid gland. The CXR may be normal, resemble PCP, mimic other viral infections (e.g., CMV), or be radiographically indistinguishable from miliary TB. Fortunately, Ga-67 scintigraphy appears to have a diagnostic pattern for LIP, with symmetric parotid uptake and low-grade diffuse lung uptake without nodal uptake (25) (Fig. 16-4A).

#### Cytomegalovirus

Although CMV is a frequently detected pathogen in patients with AIDS, its significance is controversial. Low-grade pulmonary Ga-67 uptake with perihilar prominence associated with eye uptake (retinitis is the most frequent clinical presentation), adrenal uptake (adrenalitis is the most frequent autopsy finding), renal uptake beyond 48 hours, and persistent colon uptake (Fig. 16-4B) in patients with diarrheal symptoms is a pattern suggestive of CMV (25). If high-grade pulmonary uptake is seen, superimposed PCP must be considered. When CMV is present with PCP, the patient's prognosis is worse.

#### Bacterial Infection

Intense Ga-67 uptake in a lobar configuration in the absence of nodal and parotid uptake suggests bacterial pneumonia (Fig. 16-4C). This is usually apparent on CXR, and the

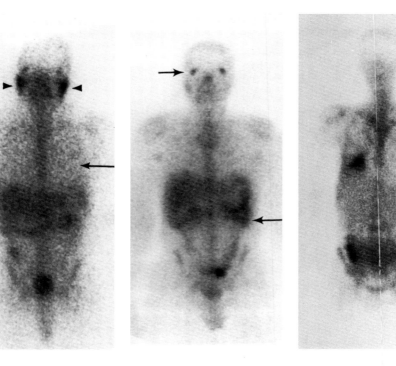

**FIG. 16-4.** Anterior whole-body gallium scans in **(A)** lymphocytic interstitial pneumonitis, showing bilateral increased gallium uptake in both parotids (*arrowheads*) and minimal diffusely increased uptake in both lung fields (*arrow*); **(B)** CMV, with increased uptake in both orbits (*arrow* to right orbit) and the colon (*arrow* in abdomen); and **(C)** bacterial pneumonia involving right lower and left midlung zones. (Contributed by Dr. William Ganz, Associate Professor of Radiology, University of Miami, Miami, FL.)

A–C

patient has a positive sputum culture. However, Ga-67 scans are only 65% sensitive in bacterial pneumonia in AIDS.

### Other Infections

Unusual aggressive infections, such as actinomycosis or nocardiosis, may be suggested when both pulmonary and local bone uptake are noted in a patient with AIDS. Needle biopsy can be negative in these aggressive bacterial infections.

### Mycobacterial Infections

*Mycobacterium avium-intracellulare* (MAI) causes widespread disease in 25% to 50% of patients with AIDS. Many who are treated for the tubercule bacillus (TB) have atypical mycobacterial infections, such as MAI, and do not respond to therapy. Patchy lung uptake and extrahilar nodal Ga-67 uptake patterns suggest atypical mycobacterial infection and require a more aggressive therapy than is used for TB. Because delays in diagnosing atypical mycobacterial infections contribute to the high morbidity associated with these infections, routine evaluation of nonhilar (particularly axillary and inguinal) nodes on Ga-67 scans may prompt earlier and possibly more effective therapy. The more usual TB is suggested when Ga-67 uptake is present only in the hilar nodes, involves pulmonary lobes, or is associated with effusions.

TB or infection reactivation in patients with AIDS is a serious problem. In New York City there are >200,000 IV drug abusers, 20% (40,000) of whom may be positive for tuberculin purified protein derivative (PPD), 55% (110,000) HIV infected, and 11% (22,000) are coinfected (26,27). It is expected that 15% of the 22,000 coinfected (PPD positive and HIV infected) will have TB activation within 2 years, which means 3,300 new cases of TB in New York City alone. In the United States, 10 million people have latent TB infection and 1 million are HIV infected. The overlap of the two populations will be a significant factor in the next decade.

The diagnosis of TB usually coincides with or precedes the diagnosis of AIDS. In Florida, the diagnosis of TB preceded that of AIDS by 1 month in 50% of cases and was made within 1 month in 30% (28). Given these findings, it seems that a lower degree of immune suppression may be required for mycobacterial TB activation than for opportunistic infections. The clinical presentation of active TB among HIV-infected individuals differs from that seen in persons with normal immunity, especially in the later stages of AIDS, when the symptoms may be subtle with atypical presentations. Early cavitating lesions in the upper lobes of the lungs and late extrapulmonary disease are commonly due to lymphatic or hematogenous dissemination that occurs in 40% to 70% of patients (27). Extrapulmonary TB involves the mediastinum, lymph nodes, visceral abscesses, bone, and brain.

Extrapulmonary TB is more common in patients with AIDS, blacks, IV drug users, heterosexuals, and those with lower CD4 counts and is associated with poor prognosis. Verification of the diagnosis is by microscopic examination and cultures of the sputum. PPD testing should be performed on all HIV patients, and all TB patients should be tested for HIV, as recommended by the CDC. Anergy may be present in >50% of patients with advanced AIDS. In all patients with

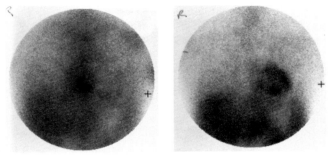

**A,B**

**FIG. 16-5. MAI infection. (A)** The Ga-67 scan shows increased uptake in lower mediastinum, but **(B)** the Tl-201 scan shows no mediastinal uptake.

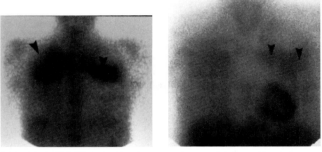

**A,B**

**FIG. 16-6. (A)** TB infection in upper lung, which on Ga-67 scan, shows increased uptake (left more than right) and **(B)** similar increased uptake on Tl-201 scan taken within 24 hours of each other.

AIDS with a negative PPD test, a CXR should be obtained, and individuals should be examined for extrapulmonary TB. Prophylactic treatment for TB with 300 mg isoniazid daily for at least 12 months should be administered to all PPD-positive individuals who are HIV positive, drug abusers, or have close contact with active TB pulmonary disease.

MAI TB lesions are usually Ga-67 avid, but Tl-201 uptake depends on the host cellular reaction. The lesions could behave like an acute inflammatory abscess (i.e., Tl-201 negative; Fig. 16-5) or like a granulomatous lesion (i.e., Tl-201 positive; Fig. 16-6).

### Neoplasms

KS and lymphocellular neoplasia are the most common forms of neoplastic disease encountered in AIDS. Nodal Ga-67 uptake is usually due to lymphoma or mycobacterial infection. AIDS-related lymphomas (ARLs) are primarily of the B-cell type and include Burkitt's, non-Burkitt's, and immunoblastic sarcomas. ARLs occur in 2% to 5% of patients with AIDS and tend to be highly aggressive with poor prognosis. In general, ARL occurs late in the course of the disease and is primarily extranodal, involving the CNS, the GI tract, and the bone marrow. Thoracic involvement has been reported in 9% to 31% of ARL patients and presents as either solitary or multiple pulmonary masses. Associated features include pleural effusions, alveolar or interstitial infiltrates, and paraspinal masses. Asymmetric adenopathy involving the axilla, supraclavicular regions, neck, or pulmonary hila may be the early manifestations of ARL.

Lymphadenopathy is common in HIV-positive patients and patients with AIDS. Causes include reactive follicular hyperplasia (50%), ARL (20%), mycobacterial infections (17%), KS (10%), and, more rarely, metastatic tumor, multiple-organism opportunistic infection, and drug reaction. When mediastinal or hilar adenopathy is seen, it indicates serious pulmonary infection or neoplasms (e.g., mycobacterial infection, lymphoma, or KS).

## CLINICAL MANIFESTATIONS

### GI Manifestations

As the largest lymphoid organ in the body, the GI tract is a potential reservoir for HIV. Defects in cellular and humoral defense mechanisms predispose the GI tract to a wide spectrum of viral, fungal, bacterial, and protozoan pathogens, which cause relentless morbidity and in some cases death (29). GI symptoms, particularly diarrhea, occur in 30% to 50% of North American and European patients with AIDS and in nearly 90% of patients in developing countries. Diarrhea may be associated with nausea, anorexia, malaise, and other mononucleosis-like symptoms at the time of seroconversion. Later, diarrhea is often the presenting symptom of full-blown AIDS and is characterized by large-volume stools, the presence of blood, and abdominal pain, depending on which pathogen is present.

Esophagitis is a common complication in AIDS. If eye, adrenal, or major colonic uptake is seen on Ga-67 scans, CMV is likely (30). Oral and esophageal candidiasis is the most probable cause of dysphagia in AIDS. Unless oblique or lateral chest images are obtained, Ga-67 or In-111 WBC scans may not detect this esophagitis. If Ga-67 or In-111 WBC uptake is seen outside the esophagus, CMV esophagitis or other opportunistic infections should be considered because candidiasis is rarely systemic. In 60% of candidiasis cases, other opportunistic infections are present.

Etiologies to be considered in the presence of abnormal bowel uptake on Ga-67 or In-111 WBC scans include the following:

- Delayed physiologic excretion (sigmoid and cecum)
- *Cryptosporidium* (proximal small bowel)
- *Isosporidium* (immigrants with proximal small bowel)
- CMV (diffuse colon with eye, adrenal, low-grade lung, and ileal or esophageal uptake)
- Giardiasis (travel history in endemic area)
- GI tumors (obstructive hold-up proximal to location of tumor and associated typical CNS and marrow sites for ARL)
- Bacterial infections such as *Salmonella* or *Shigella* (diffuse intense colonic uptake)

- Herpetic or gonococcal proctitis (intense rectal uptake in homosexuals)
- TB (ileal with pulmonary and hilar nodes)
- Antibiotic-induced colitis (patient on antibiotic with diffuse colonic uptake)

## CNS Manifestations

Opportunistic infections, CNS ARL, and AIDS encephalopathy are the main etiologies of CNS involvement in patients with AIDS. The most common cause of focal encephalitis in HIV-positive individuals is *Toxoplasma gondii*, which is best diagnosed with CT. Other conditions, including lymphoma, abscesses, fungal infections, progressive multifocal leukodystrophy, TB, CMV, KS, and hemorrhage, can all mimic the CT pattern of toxoplasmosis. Ga-67 scans are often negative, and AIDS CNS infection appears to be better diagnosed by In-111 WBC scans (18,19). Magnetic resonance imaging (MRI) and In-111 WBC scans show improvement after toxoplasmosis therapy much earlier than with CT, and they are useful for patient follow-up.

Tl-201 and F-18 fluorodeoxyglucose (FDG) scans have been recommended to differentiate toxoplasmosis from CNS lymphoma (12,31). Toxoplasma lesions are usually hypometabolic on FDG and have low Tl-201 uptake (with lesion-to-brain ratio of 1.6:1). On the other hand, lymphoma lesions are characteristically hypermetabolic on FDG images, and Tl-201 lesion-to-brain ratios average 2:1.

A large percentage of patients with AIDS may develop HIV-induced dementia. Initial manifestations of AIDS dementia complex or HIV encephalopathy are usually subtle, such as mental fatigue and difficulty reading. Increasing apathy along with mental slowing may be mistaken for depression and paranoid psychosis. The differentiation

between a functional depression or psychosis and an early manifestation of HIV encephalopathy is not easy to make clinically and yet has important implications for treatment. Neuroleptics used for treatment of psychosis are more likely to cause serious extrapyramidal symptoms in patients with AIDS. Early documentation of HIV encephalopathy is important because zidovudine (AZT) has been shown to ameliorate cognitive dysfunction, albeit often temporarily (32). It is important to differentiate HIV encephalopathy from other psychiatric disorders because treatment is different. Both CT and MRI are typically normal in early disease and show nonspecific findings in the late stages (33).

FDG positron emission tomography and Tc-99m HMPAO SPECT brain perfusion imaging are more sensitive than x-ray CT or MRI. In a report from St. Vincent's Hospital, 94% of HIV patients showed multifocal cortical and subcortical areas of hypoperfusion, some of whom improved with AZT therapy (33). Figure 16-7 shows an example of advanced HIV encephalopathy.

## Musculoskeletal Manifestations

Although the musculoskeletal changes in patients with AIDS are not as common as GI, pulmonary, or CNS manifestations, a wide range of soft-tissue and bony changes have been described (30,34). Bone Ga-67 and WBC scans have been used to diagnose septic arthritis and osteomyelitis in patients with HIV. Joint pain is a common symptom in HIV-positive individuals. When bilateral joint uptake is seen, it is more likely to be due to the HIV-related Reiter's syndrome, psoriatic arthritis, or AIDS rheumatoid arthritis rather than septic arthritis (35).

A wide range of opportunistic and nonopportunistic organisms may cause infection of the skin, subcutaneous tissue, muscles, bones, and joints, resulting in cellulitis, skin ulcers, soft-tissue phlegmon and abscesses, osteomyelitis, and septic arthritis. Infection of the hands is relatively common, and in some cases osteomyelitis may follow. When needed, Ga-67 or WBC scan correlative studies can confirm osteomyelitis. In one center, WBC scans appear to detect 91% of bone infections, compared to 60% by Ga-67 (20). Twenty percent of acute infections are "cold" on WBC scanning; the clinician should consider these cold spots potential infections and suggest Ga-67 or MRI imaging to confirm the diagnosis. CT or MRI muscle masses or muscle uptake of bone scanning agents may represent AIDS-related myositis or KS. Myositis takes up Ga-67, whereas KS takes up only Tl-201. KS is the primary consideration in patients with AIDS with cutaneous vascular lesions and muscle or skeletal changes.

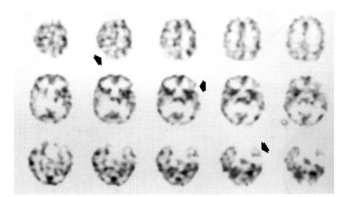

**FIG. 16-7.** HIV encephalopathy. SPECT brain perfusion study showing multiple subcortical areas of perfusion defects affecting almost every part of the brain: the cerebral cortex (*arrows*), basal ganglia, and cerebellum. (Reprinted with permission from Abdel-Dayem HM, Scott AM, Macapinlac HA, et al. Role of Thallium 201 Chloride and Tc-99m Sestamibi in Tumor Imaging. In Freeman LM [ed], Nuclear Medicine Annual 1994. New York: Raven, 1994;181–234.)

## Cardiac Manifestations

HIV commonly involves the heart and may be manifest as ventricular dilatation with reduced ejection fraction in HIV-

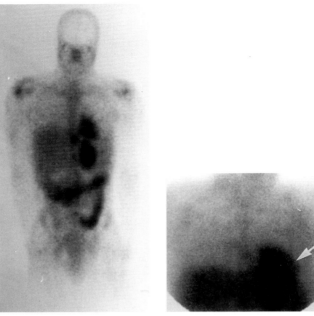

A,B

**FIG. 16-8. (A)** Whole-body image showing that Ga-67 scan is better than **(B)** Tl-201 scan in identifying cardiac lymphoma. The Ga-67 scan at 48 hours shows intense uptake involving the whole heart, epigastric region, and hepatic focus. The Tl-201 scan shows barely discernible perfusion defect in the anterior wall (*arrow*) of the left ventricle.

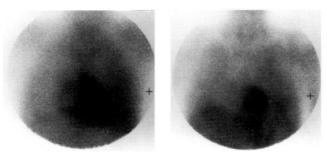

A,B

**FIG. 16-9.** Anterior thorax views of **(A)** Ga-67 and **(B)** Tl-201 scans. The Ga-67 scan shows evidence of acute pericarditis with increased uptake around the heart; the Tl-201 scan shows normal myocardial uptake.

related myocarditis in the pre-AIDS state. The congestive failure may be detected only with depressed diastolic function in more than one-third of cases (36,37). Ga-67 uptake is seen in the pre-AIDS and pericardial effusions, pericarditis, endocarditis, and neoplasms, such as cardiac lymphoma (usually the aggressive Burkitt's lymphoma). Tl-201 uptake in cardiac lymphoma is not helpful because of the normal Tl-201 uptake and is rather identified by decreased myocardial uptake (Fig. 16-8). The Ga-67 scan is more helpful than other imaging modalities in locating the extent of the disease. Figure 16-9 is an example of Ga-67 and Tl-201 in acute pericarditis.

## Renal Manifestations

Abnormal localization of Ga-67 in the kidneys has been correlated with impairment of renal function in the patients with AIDS (38). The degree of proteinuria correlates to the degree of renal Ga-67 uptake. Increased Ga-67 uptake and renal size raises the suspicion of AIDS nephropathy. The differential diagnosis includes infiltrative lymphoma or leukemia, drug toxicity, CMV nephritis, and recent transfusions. Abnormal cortical Tc-99m MAG3 uptake is usually seen in ATN, drug toxicity, and nephritis. Focal defects on Tc-99m renal scans suggest either tumor or infection, and if the defect takes up Tl-201, tumors such as KS or lymphoma are likely.

## PRECAUTIONS FOR HEALTH CARE WORKERS

In health care workers caring for the AIDS patient, the risk of HIV conversion is low unless they themselves are in one of the high-risk categories. Health care workers exposed to HIV-containing fluids are not known to have a higher incidence of AIDS than others. There is no study to show that there is any risk associated with either airborne exposure or casual contact (5,39). Avoiding health care–related work when ill, and the routine use of precautions, such as disposable gloves, minimizing contact with body fluids, appropriate gown and mask infection control, sterile technique, and needle precautions, is suggested to avoid the rare HIV conversion in health personnel. Unless a health care worker is immune stimulated, hepatitis is a greater danger than AIDS from needle-stick exposures. To protect oneself, hepatitis vaccine and needle-stick precautions are suggested. Also, the standard use of dilute chlorine bleach, which kills HIV on surfaces, instruments, and needle-injured skin, is recommended as part of all hospital procedures. If a worker is exposed to HIV, prophylactic AZT administration may be more risky than no treatment because the risk of drug side effects is higher than the risk of HIV conversion.

## REFERENCES

1. Mertens TE, Belsey E, Stoneburner RL, et al. Global estimates of HIV infection and AIDS: further heterogenicity in spread and impact. AIDS 1995;9:S251.
2. Mertens TE, Burton A. Estimates and trends of the HIV/AIDS epidemic. AIDS 1996;10:S221.
3. Konki P. Epidemiology and Natural History of Human Immunodeficiency Virus Type 2. In DeVita VT Jr, Hellman S, Rosenberg SA (eds), AIDS: Biology, Diagnosis, Treatment and Prevention (4th ed). Philadelphia: Lippincott–Raven, 1997;127–145.
4. Gallo RC, Salahuddin SL, Popovic M, et al. Frequent detection and isolation of cytopathic retrovirus (HTLV-III) from patients with AIDS and at risk for AIDS. Science 1984;224:500–503.
5. Wachter H, Fuchs D, Hausen A, et al. Who will get AIDS? Lancet 1986;2:1216–1217.
6. Fuchs D, Hausen A, Hengster P, et al. In-vivo activation of CD4+ cells in AIDS. Science 1987;235:356.

7. Imagawa DT, Lee MH, Wolinsky SM, et al. Human immunodeficiency virus type I infection in homosexual men who remain seronegative for prolonged periods. N Engl J Med 1989;320:1458–1462.
8. Revision of the case definition of acquired immune deficiency syndrome. MMWR Morb Mortal Wkly Rep 1987;36(suppl): 1S–15S.
9. Woolfenden JM, Carrasquillo JA, Larson SM, et al. Acquired immunodeficiency syndrome: Ga-67 citrate imaging. Radiology 1987;162: 383–387.
10. Kramer EL, Sanger JJ, Garay SM, et al. Gallium-67 scans of the chest in patients with acquired immunodeficiency syndrome. J Nucl Med 1987;28:1107–1114.
11. Sehweil A, Abdel-Dayem HM, McKillop J. Thallium Kinetics in Malignant Tumors [doctoral thesis]. Glasgow, Scotland: Glasgow University 1988.
12. Abdel-Dayem HM, Scott A, Macapinlac H, et al. Role of Thallium 201 Chloride and Tc-99m Sestamibi in Tumor Imaging. In Freeman LM (ed), Nuclear Medicine Annual 1994. New York: Raven, 1994;181–234.
13. Lee UW, Rosen MP, Baum A, et al. AIDS related Kaposi's sarcoma: finding in thallium-201 scintigraphy. AJR Am J Roentgenol 1988; 151:1233–1235.
14. Lee UW, Fuller JD, O'Brien MJ, et al. Preliminary Kaposi sarcoma in patients with AIDS: scintigraphic diagnosis with sequential thallium and gallium scanning. Radiology 1991;180:409–412.
15. Ganz WI, Nguyen TQ, Mnaymneh W, et al. Use of early, late and SPECT thallium imaging in evaluating activity of soft tissue and bone tumors [abstract]. J Nucl Med 1993;34:33P.
16. Abdel-Dayem HM, DiFabrizo L, Aras T, et al. Prospective evaluation of sequential Tl-201 and Ga-67 scans in AIDS patients [abstract]. J Nucl Med 1993;34:172P.
17. Abdel-Dayem HM, DiFabrizo L, Aras T, et al. Accuracy of sequential Tl-201 and Ga-67 scans in the diagnosis of pulmonary Kaposi's sarcoma in AIDS patients [abstract]. Eur J Nucl Med 1993;20:837.
18. Abdel-Dayem HM, DiFabrizio L, Kempf J, et al. Diffuse thallium uptake in the lungs in PCP. Clin Nucl Med 1994;19:287–291.
19. Padhani A, Kuklman JE. Pulmonary manifestations of AIDS. Appl Radiol 1993;22:13–19.
20. Bitran J, Bekerman C, Weinstein R, et al. Patterns of gallium-67 scintigraphy in patients with acquired immunodeficiency syndrome and AIDS related complex. J Nucl Med 1987;28:1103–1106.
21. Palestro GS, Swyer AL, Aim CR, et al. Relative efficiency of In-111-leukocytes and Ga-67 imaging in AIDS patients [abstract]. J Nucl Med 1991;32:1003.
22. Barron JP, Birnbaum NS, Sharel B, et al. Pneumocystis carinii pneumonia studied by Ga-67 scanning. Radiology 1985;154:791–793.
23. Kramer EL, Sanger JH, Garay SM, et al. Diagnostic implications of Ga-67 chest scan patterns in human immunodeficiency virus-seropositive patients. Radiology 1989;170:671–676.
24. Rosso J, Guillon JM, Parrot A, et al. Technetium-99m-DTPA aerosol and gallium-67 scanning in pulmonary complications of human immunodeficiency virus infection [abstract]. J Nucl Med 1992;33:81–87.
25. Smith RC, Ganz WI, Cohen D, et al. Characteristic pattern of lymphocytic interstitial penumonitis on Ga-67 citrate scans [abstract]. Radiology 1993;20:228.
26. Pitchenik A, Burr J, Fertel D. Tuberculosis in HIV infected patients: epidemiology, infectivity, clinical features, response to treatment, prognostic factors and long-term outcome [abstract]. International Congress for Infectious Disease, Montreal, Canada. July 15–19, 1990;152.
27. Pitchenik AE, Fertel D. Mycobacterial Disease in Patients with HIV Infection. In Wormser GP (ed), AIDS and Other Manifestations of HIV Patients. New York: Raven, 1992;277–313.
28. Rieder HL, Cauthen GM, Bloch AB, et al. Tuberculosis and acquired immunodeficiency syndrome. Arch Intern Med 1989;149:1268–1273.
29. Smith PD, Quinn TC, Strober W, et al. NIH conference.Gastrointestinal infections in AIDS. Ann Intern Med 1992;116:63–77.
30. Ganz WI, Serafini DM. The diagnostic role of Ga-67 in the acquired immunodeficiency syndrome. J Nucl Med 1989;30:1935–1945.
31. Macapinlac HA, Scott AM, Yeh SDJ, et al. The role of Tl-201 SPECT and F-18 FDG PET in the diagnosis of CNS lymphoma vs. toxoplasmosis in patients with AIDS [abstract]. Radiology 1993;189:114.
32. Brunetti A, Berg G, DiChiro G, et al. Reversal of brain metabolite abnormalities following treatment of AIDS dementia complex with 3'-azido-2',3'-dideoxythymidine (AZT, zidovudine): a PET FDG study. J Nucl Med 1989;30:581–590.
33. Masdeu JC, Yudd A, Van Heertum RL, et al. Single-photon emission computed tomography in human immunodeficiency virus encephalopathy: a preliminary report. J Nucl Med 1991;32:1471–1475.
34. Scott JA, Palmer EL, Fischman AJ. HIV associated myositis detected by radionuclide bone scanning. J Nucl Med 1989;30:556–558.
35. Calabrese LH. The rheumatic manifestations of infection with the human immunodeficiency virus. Semin Arth Rheum 1989;18:225–239.
36. Acierno LI. Cardiac complications in acquired immunodeficiency syndrome (AIDS). A review. J Am Coll Cardiol 1989;13:1144–1154.
37. Holladay AO, Siegel RJ, Schwartz DA. Cardiac malignant lymphoma in acquired immunodeficiency syndrome. Cancer 1992;70:2203–2207.
38. Sfakianakis GN, Fayad F, Fernandez JA, et al. Ga-67 renal hyperactivity in AIDS patients and its relationship to laboratory renal data [abstract]. J Nucl Med 1988;29:909.
39. Weiss SH. Occupational Issues Related to the HIV Epidemic. In Warsiver GP (ed), AIDS and Other Manifestations of HIV Infection. New York: Raven, 1992;559–608.

Textbook of Nuclear Medicine,
edited by Michael A. Wilson.
Lippincott–Raven Publishers, Philadelphia © 1998.

CHAPTER 17

# Clinical Positron Emission Tomography

Scott B. Perlman and Charles K. Stone

Positron emission tomography (PET) represents a major advance in clinical imaging because it improved on previous imaging modes in both spatial resolution and the ability to correct for attenuation. The quantitative nature of PET has led to its inclusion in standard diagnostic paradigms used in research and clinical imaging. Although PET imaging was first used clinically in neurology and cardiology, the development of whole-body protocols is providing exciting new information and will likely play a central role in the management of cancer patients, where PET can be used to evaluate the extent of disease and to monitor the response to therapy.

## POSITRON EMISSION TOMOGRAPHY

A review of instrumentation and a comparison with single photon emission computed tomography (SPECT) is provided in Chapter 24.

Briefly, PET imaging is based on the detection of the two 511-keV gamma rays that originate from the annihilation of a positron. Although the energy of the positron depends on the particular nuclide, the energy of each of the resulting divergent annihilation photons is constant at 511 keV, representing half of the mass energy equivalent of the positron at the time of annihilation. With the emission of photons at 180 degrees with respect to each other, 360-degree data acquisition is generally performed. Scintillation events recorded without a corresponding event in the opposing detector are termed *random* or *single* events and are discarded.

### Advantages

Coincidence detection results in improved sensitivity over high-energy collimation, lessens the effect of photon scatter on image quality, and allows the use of an extrinsic pin source to determine the photon attenuation in each subject. The principal advantage of PET is its capacity to perform measured attenuation correction and so to yield quantitative data with biologically active tracers. Other advantages over standard gamma camera imaging include greater temporal and spatial resolution, decreased attenuation with higher-energy gamma emission (Table 17-1), and the capacity to administer greater activity levels due to the shorter isotope half-life of positron emitters.

### Disadvantages

One limitation of PET is that spatial resolution is related to the energy of positron emission, which differs for each agent. Positrons with higher energy travel farther in tissue before annihilation, thus limiting the ability to resolve discrete structures and decreasing image resolution (Table 17-2). The identical energy of the PET annihilation gamma emission prevents simultaneous imaging of two different PET tracers or the imaging of a second tracer before the decay of the first. Although dual isotope techniques (e.g., technetium 99m bone and indium 111–labeled white blood cell scans in complicated osteomyelitis) are not feasible with PET, rapid sequential studies are possible because of the rapid decay of positron emitters.

A few limitations to the widespread use of clinical PET imaging are worth noting. PET scanning requires either an on-site cyclotron, proximity to a regional distribution positron radiopharmaceutical source, or the use of a positron generator (e.g., strontium 82[Sr-82]/rubidium 82 [Rb-82]). A cyclotron requires a substantial capital investment. The lack of reimbursement for many clinical indications remains a major limitation to widespread clinical use, although progress has been made. Two agents, Rb-82 and F-18 fluorodeoxyglucose (FDG), have U.S. Food and Drug Administration approval for New Drug Applications. Furthermore, Medicare determined in March 1995 that the technology is "reasonable and necessary" in the case of Rb-82 and myocardial perfusion imaging (MPI), so this indication is reimbursable in the Medicare outpatient population. It is almost certain that the technology will be

**TABLE 17-1.** Attenuation of gamma emissions

| Photon (keV) | HVL (cm) | |
|---|---|---|
| | Lead | Water |
| Positron (511) | 0.40 | 8.0 |
| Tc-99m (140) | 0.03 | 4.6 |

**TABLE 17-2.** Physical characteristics of more common PET isotopes

| Isotope | Source | Half-life (mins) | Energy (MeV) | Range (mm) |
|---|---|---|---|---|
| C-11 | Cyclotron | 20.00 | 0.96 | 4.1 |
| N-13 | Cyclotron | 10.00 | 1.19 | 5.4 |
| O-15 | Cyclotron | 2.00 | 1.72 | 8.2 |
| F-18 | Cyclotron | 110.00 | 0.64 | 2.4 |
| Rb-82 | Generator | 1.25 | 3.35 | 15.9 |

**TABLE 17-3.** PET perfusion tracer characteristics

Isotope production
    Cyclotron (on-site or regional)
    Generator
Isotopic half-life
Myocardial kinetics
    First-pass extraction fraction
    Myocardial uptake of tracer
    Freely diffusible
    Membrane transport
    Cytosolic binding
Biological activity
    Labeled endogenous substance
    Cation
    Coordination complex

**TABLE 17-4.** PET perfusion tracers

| PET tracer | Biological activity | First-pass extraction |
|---|---|---|
| N-13 NH$_3$ | Transanimation | 75% |
| O-15 water | Diffusible tracer | 95% |
| Rb-82 | K$^+$ analog | 35% |

widely used in the near future because research continues to demonstrate the important and unique information available from PET imaging.

## PHYSIOLOGIC IMAGING WITH PET

Radiotracers have been developed to assess three major areas of organ physiology: perfusion, metabolism, and neuronal innervational activity. The underlying physiology, available radiopharmaceuticals, imaging technique, and image data analysis are reviewed here.

### Perfusion Imaging

#### Perfusion Tracers

One of the earliest clinical applications of PET was in MPI. Since the 1980s, a number of PET perfusion tracers have been developed with various attributes. PET perfusion tracers in general can be classified according to the physical characteristics of the radionuclide and the biological activity of the tracer (Table 17-3).

The physiologic characteristics of the tracer are related to the first-pass extraction of the tracer by an organ, the cellular uptake mechanism, and intracellular metabolism (Table 17-4). These agents have used the imaging advantages of PET to derive improved qualitative and quantitative assessment of organ perfusion.

The choice of which tracer to use at a particular PET center is highly dependent on the local logistics of tracer production and delivery, the sensitivity of the PET scanner, and the clinical question. The short half-life of oxygen 15 (O-15) water requires the delivery of tracer by a pneumatic tube system or juxtaposition of the cyclotron or linear accelerator and a high-sensitivity PET scanner able to handle the rapid

dynamic data acquisition. The use of Rb-82, obtained from an Sr-82/Rb-82 generator, allows for cardiac imaging without a cyclotron, but a steady clinical demand is needed to justify the cost of the generator system. Nitrogen 13 (N-13) NH$_3$ is a perfusion tracer with a half-life of 10 minutes that lies between the extremes of availability of O-15 and Sr-82. Newer tracers are being developed, such as copper 62 pyruvaldehyde thiosemicarbazone (Cu-62 PTSM), specifically to overcome some of the limitations of the current tracers.

#### Quantitation of Perfusion

The quantitative nature of PET has allowed investigators to describe myocardial, brain, or tumor blood flow in absolute terms of milliliters per minute per gram of tissue. In general, two means of quantitation of organ perfusion have been validated, but their application is somewhat organ and tracer specific. One method of quantitation is the normalization of tissue uptake to the amount of tracer injected. This approach is analogous to the laboratory method of measuring perfusion with radiolabeled microspheres. The microsphere arterial reference method is considered the standard for measuring perfusion when the spheres are of sufficient size that all are trapped at the capillary level (i.e., 100% extraction of the tracer by the tissue). Microsphere blood flow ($F$) in milliliters per minute per gram is calculated as follows:

$$F = \frac{T_{act} \times R_{rate}}{T_{wt} \times R_{act}} \qquad (1)$$

where $T_{act}$ = the tissue activity for the tracer, $T_{wt}$ = the tissue sample weight in grams, $R_{act}$ = the activity in an arterial ref-

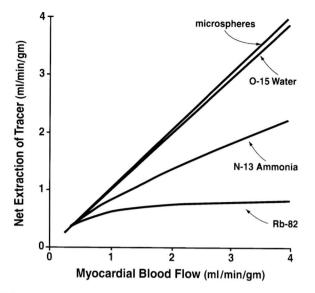

**FIG. 17-1.** A plot of the net PET radiopharmaceutical extraction against myocardial blood flow demonstrates the differences in extraction fraction of O-15 water, N-13 ammonia, and Rb-82 compared to microspheres. (Reprinted with permission from Schelbert HR. Principles of Positron Emission Tomography. In Marcus ML, Schelbert HR, Skorton DJ, Wolf GL [eds], Cardiac Imaging: A Companion to Braunwald's Heart Disease. Philadelphia: Saunders, 1991;1142.)

erence sample, and $R_{rate}$ = withdrawal rate for reference sample in milliliters per minute.

For partially extracted tracers, in contrast to microspheres, only a fraction of the tracer is extracted with each circulation through the organ (Fig. 17-1). The first-pass extraction fraction declines with increasing flow, as defined by the Renkin-Crone model (1,2):

$$E = (1 - e^{-PS/F}) \qquad (2)$$

where $E$ = the first-pass extraction fraction, $PS$ = the permeability-surface area product in milliliters per minute per gram, and $F$ = blood flow to organ.

Thus, for partially extracted tracers, the uptake of a tracer in an organ is not only related to the blood flow ($F$) to the organ but also to the first-pass extraction ($E$) of the tracer such that

$$FE = U_T \left( \int_0^T c_a \, dt \right)^{-1} \qquad (3)$$

where $U_T$ is tissue uptake at time $T$, $c_a$ is arterial blood radioactivity concentration, $\int c_a \, dt$ is the sum of arterial activity up to the time point $T$ (arterial input function). This relationship can be derived from dynamic PET scans because of the quantitative nature of the imaging modality. For cardiac and some other chest studies (e.g., evaluation of single pulmonary nodules), the input function may be

obtained directly from the scan by placing a region of interest (ROI) over the left ventricle (LV) blood pool cavity and integrating the ventricular activity over time (3). For cerebral and other organ studies away from the chest, the input function may be obtained from rapid arterial sampling, although this can be modified by using arterialized venous sampling (venous sampling of a heated distal vein). Tissue activity is obtained from an ROI placed over the organ on the final frame of a dynamic study or from a static emission study. Obtaining the input function from the dynamic scan obviates the conversion of tissue activity to millicuries per milliliter. The tissue activity is corrected for the partial volume effect, the size of the ROI, the resolution of the scanner, and the spillover effect (tracer from adjacent organs and structures).

This method of quantitation of flow has been applied most frequently to the partially extracted tracer N-13 NH₃. A major limitation for all the partially extracted tracers is the nonlinearity in tissue uptake activity at higher flow rates, due to the shorter transcapillary transit time and less time available for extraction. This is corrected for by using a PS product, which is obtained from the analysis of changes in extraction fraction at different flow states in laboratory preparations or derived from in vivo animal PET data using microsphere blood flow determinations.

A second and more complicated method of quantitation has been the application of parametric modeling to dynamic studies to determine organ perfusion. This approach was first applied to the diffusible tracer O-15 water (4,5), but it has also been applied to the less highly extracted tracers Rb-82 (6) and N-13 NH₃ (7). With this approach, distribution rates of tracer in different cellular and extracellular compartments is estimated by fitting the dynamic data.

**Metabolic Imaging**

A brief review of cellular metabolism is necessary to highlight the variety of biochemical pathways that can be analyzed by PET metabolic tracers. Cerebral metabolism is largely dependent on plasma glucose levels and glucose metabolism and relatively independent of fatty-acid and ketone levels or hormonal changes. In contrast, the heart is omnivorous and metabolizes several substrates, principally plasma free fatty acids, but it also uses glucose and ketones. The rate of use of substrates depends on the myocardial energy needs, circulating levels of these substrates, oxygen levels, and hormone concentrations. Many tumors have glycolysis rates as well as protein and amino acid use rates that are significantly greater than those of normal tissues. These increased metabolic rates can be used clinically for diagnosis and monitoring therapeutic interventions.

Glucose was the first substrate studied with PET, and the PET glucose tracer FDG is the most commonly used PET

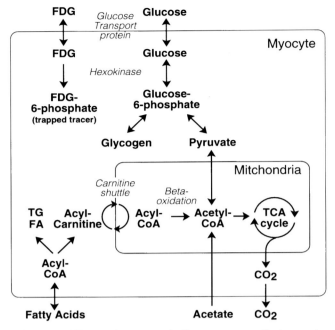

**FIG. 17-2.** The various metabolic processes that can be measured using PET are demonstrated with a schematic diagram of a cell with mitochondrion. FDG uptake results from glucose transporter proteins, and FDG is handled similarly to the substrate glucose. Hexokinase acts on glucose and FDG to produce the appropriate 6-phosphate version. Although glucose-6-phosphate is metabolized further, FDG-6-phosphate is trapped. Fatty acids (FA), the preferred cardiac metabolite substrate, can be converted into triglycerides (TGs), remain as FA stores, or be shunted to the mitochondria via the carnitine shuttle to beta-oxidation. (Adapted with permission from Schwaiger M, Hutchins GD. Evaluation of coronary artery disease with positron emission tomography. Semin Nucl Med 1992;22:210–223.)

radiopharmaceutical (Fig. 17-2). Glucose transport across the cellular membrane is an example of facilitated transport, and it occurs via glucose transporter proteins. The rate of transport is affected by, but not dependent on, circulating plasma levels of insulin. The rate-limiting step in glucose uptake is the phosphorylation by hexokinase of glucose to glucose-6-phosphate in the intracellular cytoplasm. Glucose-6-phosphate is either incorporated into glycogen for storage purposes or metabolized to pyruvate for energy production. After the formation of pyruvate, a second major branch point occurs, in which pyruvate either undergoes anaerobic metabolism to lactate or aerobic metabolism in the Krebs cycle.

Although fatty acids represent a major metabolic substrate for the heart, the study of this substrate occurred later than glucose study due to the complexity of fatty acid metabolism (see Fig. 17-2). This complexity is related to the variety of circulating fatty acids, extensive metabolic steps within the cytoplasm, exchange with cytoplasmic lipid pools, and the transport of fatty acids across the mitochondrial membrane by the carnitine shuttle. The final metabolic

pathway is the cleavage of terminal portions of fatty acid chain into acetyl coenzyme A units (beta-oxidation) for incorporation into the Krebs cycle.

In stark contrast to the more complex glucose and fatty acid metabolic pathways, ketone metabolism is simple (see Fig. 17-2). The incorporation of ketones into the Krebs cycle is rapid, with few mitochondrial intermediary steps.

Two major types of PET metabolic tracers have been developed. The trapped tracers are designed to be metabolized along a specific metabolic pathway until a structural modification prevents further metabolism and the tracer is retained in that organ. The rate of tracer uptake depends on the reaction and transfer rates before the step that halts further metabolism, with reaction rates beyond this step not directly assessed. The classic PET agent of this type is FDG. The second type of metabolic tracer is metabolized completely in the organ, with the tracer label lost from the organ as a labeled metabolite. The rate of loss of signal from the organ is proportional to the rate of metabolism of the substrate, assuming that there is no loss of intact tracer from the organ of interest. Classic PET tracers of this type include carbon 11 (C-11) glucose for glucose metabolism, C-11 acetate for ketone metabolism and oxidative phosphorylation rates, and C-11 palmitate for fatty acid metabolism.

### Trapped Tracer Method

FDG is transported into the cytoplasm and phosphorylated by hexokinase to FDG-6-phosphate but is thereafter essentially trapped because it cannot undergo isomerization (see Fig. 17-2). The dependence of FDG uptake and trapping on these few metabolic steps simplifies the kinetic modeling of FDG. Although the rate of organ uptake is proportional to the phosphorylation rate of exogenous glucose, subsequent metabolic steps for glucose can only be inferred. Thus, the relative fraction of glucose being incorporated into glycogen stores or metabolized immediately (either aerobically or anaerobically) is unknown. To lessen the glycogen deposition rate, patients are studied in a controlled state rather than during or after stress, when glycogen repletion rates are high.

The rate of glucose metabolism by the heart is very dependent on circulating levels of the more preferred metabolic substrates (fatty acids, lactate, and ketone bodies) as well as circulating hormones (catecholamine and insulin). For FDG image acquisition, the heart and metabolic milieu must be manipulated to favor glucose metabolism. Three methods optimize FDG uptake: oral glucose bolus (8), the insulin clamp (9), and fatty acid suppression (10,11). The most common approach has been to stimulate insulin secretion by the administration of an oral glucose bolus 40 to 50 minutes before tracer injection.

In clinical protocols, the low first-pass extraction for FDG means that a significant delay of 30 to 50 minutes after injection is necessary to allow organ uptake for imaging. The standard cardiac clinical protocol for imaging is ingestion of 50 to 75 g of glucose, waiting 45 to 60 minutes to allow absorption, injection of 8 to 10 mCi FDG, and obtaining 10- to 20-minute static images 40 minutes after injection. In diabetic patients, scans are performed with the administration of insulin to maintain the blood sugar in the 110- to 130-mg/dl range. For cardiac imaging, attenuation correction of emission data is performed by obtaining a transmission image before injection of FDG (measured attenuation correction). New software algorithms allow for the simultaneous acquisition of transmission and emission data using rotating external source pin technology. Clinical sites with this capability can acquire the emission data before the transmission data. Studies then can be done more efficiently and with fewer patient movement artifacts because of the close temporal proximity of the transmission and emission acquisitions. Because of the glucose dependency of the brain, cerebral FDG studies are performed without glucose loading. The symmetric anatomy of the brain allows the use of calculated attenuation correction with assumed attenuation coefficients.

### Dynamic Tracers

#### Fatty Acid Metabolism

Fatty acid metabolism has been measured using C-11 palmitate. The conventional C-14 constant infusion laboratory technique has been applied to in vivo PET imaging by obtaining dynamic scans of the organ of interest with a C-11–labeled fatty acid (most commonly palmitate). ROI analysis determines the rate of loss of tracer from the organ, which is equated with the beta-oxidation rate of exogenous fatty acids. This approach assumes that the fatty acid tracer has adequately filled the cytoplasmic lipid pools and that all ROI signal loss is the result of C-11 carbon dioxide production. In some physiologic conditions (e.g., cardiac ischemia), significant back-diffusion of intact tracer may occur, leading to an overestimation of circulating fatty acid oxidation rates (12).

#### Ketone Metabolism

Another dynamic tracer used for assessment of cellular metabolism is C-11 acetate. Because some organs prefer ketones as an exogenous substrate, dynamic studies of labeled acetate have been very useful in the determination of rates of the Krebs cycle and, indirectly, oxidative phosphorylation. Studies are performed in a similar manner to C-11 palmitate, with wash-out rates determined from ROI analysis of the organ of interest (13).

#### Methionine Metabolism

Methionine is an essential amino acid that can be labeled with C-11. This radiotracer allows the study of amino acid metabolism and is especially useful in patients with primary brain tumors, which have increased demand for methionine. The technique has been especially helpful in delineating tumor extent.

### Quantitation of Metabolism

Just as in perfusion studies, metabolic data may be reviewed qualitatively or quantitatively. For most clinical studies, qualitative reading of the data is performed with static images displayed with a color scale set to maximum activity.

#### Graphical Analysis

The most common means of quantitating organ glucose uptake rates (GURs) is to use the graphical analysis of Patlak and colleagues (14). For this procedure, a dynamic image protocol with 5-minute images is performed throughout the period of FDG uptake. Arterial or arterialized venous blood samples are obtained at frequent intervals for F-18 activity and plasma glucose levels. The glucose uptake rate ($K_i$) is estimated from the following relationship:

$$\frac{C_t}{C_p} = K_i \left( \int_0^T C_p \, dt \right) (C_p)^{-1} + b \qquad (4)$$

where at time $T$, $C_t$ is the tissue radioactivity concentration and $C_p$ is the plasma F-18 radioactivity concentration.

The model assumes that activity comes into equilibrium quickly between plasma and cell and that there is a unidirectional tracer flow into the cell. Plots of $C_t/C_p$ versus the integral of $C_p$ from 0 to time $T$ divided by $C_p$ at time $T$ (the "stretch time") are fitted as straight lines by conventional least-squares methods, and the slopes of the best-fit lines are taken as estimates of $K_i$.

Organ GURs are then calculated as follows:

$$\text{GUR} = \frac{K_i \times \text{Gluc}}{\text{LC}} \qquad (5)$$

where LC is the lumped constant and Gluc is the plasma glucose level.

The LC is a ratio of tracer uptake to substrate use, and it refers to the relative preference of the organ for the tracer rather than the substrate being examined. For the study of FDG and glucose in the heart, the LC often used is 0.67, as determined by Ratib et al. in isolated heart preparations (15).

#### Standardized Uptake Ratio

The SUR is defined as the mean ROI activity (mCi/ml) divided by the total injected activity per kilogram of body weight (16). Alternative names include differential uptake ratio (DUR) and differential absorption ratio (DAR) (16). This technique is often used in oncology applications, especially in separating benign from malignant disease and in following up treatment effects. If uptake is uniform throughout the body, the SUR is unity. This simple technique works for FDG and adds a level of objectivity to the image analysis to distinguish malignancy from normal tissue or radiation necrosis when visual assessment is not obvious. Reported important factors to control in this measurement include determination of tissue activity at the same time after injection in patients and correcting for plasma glucose and lean body mass. Furthermore, if the SUR is applied to a small ROI, an inaccurate ratio may result.

### Compartment Modeling

Compartment modeling is the most complex form of quantitation and is now routinely performed only for research purposes. In this method, a model is created for the tracer studied, and several compartmental pools (e.g., plasma and brain FDG) and metabolic products (FDG or FDG-6-phosphate) are defined for measurement and calculation of time-activity curves (TAC). The models for FDG require the following:

- Input function (plasma TAC from arterial blood)
- Model of FDG behavior
- Initial estimate of model parameters
- Tissue TAC (from scanner)
- Best fit of data to the model

Fitting functions are then performed with parameters determined as the best fit to the TAC.

## Neuronal Imaging

The third area of clinical PET studies is centered on neurotransmitter synthesis for presynaptic and postsynaptic binding studies. The central biosynthetic steps for catecholamine neurotransmitter synthesis is the hydroxylation of tyrosine to dopa and subsequent decarboxylation to dopamine. Dopamine is transported to storage vesicles in nerve terminals, where norepinephrine is formed by dopamine β-hydroxylase, then stored and released by exocytosis on nerve stimulation. Multiple hormonal factors modulate the exocytic process, including negative feedback by norepinephrine and the postsynaptic response via specific $\alpha_1$- or $\beta_1$-adrenergic membrane receptors. Adrenally released epinephrine also interacts with $\beta_1$ receptors and $\beta_2$ receptors. The major physiologic response to adrenergic stimulation occurs via the $\alpha_1$ receptors, which account for peripheral vasoconstriction; the $\beta_1$ receptors, which cause the cardiac inotropic response; and the $\beta_2$ receptors, which are responsible for the cardiac chronotropic response and peripheral vasodilatation.

Several tracers have been developed for imaging different aspects of the nervous system with PET. Cerebral studies to assess the rate of catecholamine synthesis have been conducted with the labeled catecholamine precursor F-18 DOPA. Cardiac studies have been performed with labeled precursors, labeled neurotransmitters, norepinephrine analogs for study of presynaptic uptake, and postsynaptic adrenergic receptor antagonists. Adrenergic receptor studies have been performed in vivo by adapting the in vitro laboratory method of receptor-binding assays.

## CLINICAL PET APPLICATIONS

PET imaging using the tracer technique provides unique information about in vivo biochemistry and physiology. In clinical cardiac imaging, PET has proved very useful for the evaluation of myocardial ischemia and viability. Clinical indications for PET imaging in neurology include the evaluation of primary central nervous system (CNS) tumors, epilepsy, and dementia. PET whole-body imaging uses include staging cancer and providing information on tumor response to therapy. FDG has been the most common radiopharmaceutical used, with perfusion agents the next most common (N-13 $NH_3$ and Rb-82), although other radiotracers, such as C-11 methionine, F-18 fluorodopa, and C-11 HED (the neuroreceptor analog meta-hydroxyephedrine) may gain in prominence.

FDG is a glucose analog that, under steady-state serum glucose conditions, accurately allows the estimation of rate of use of exogenous glucose (3,14). At 30 to 40 minutes after the intravenous administration of FDG, the static image obtained is in direct proportion to the glucose metabolism that has occurred over the previous 30 to 40 minutes. To quantitate these images, the input function can be obtained with serial arterial or arterialized venous samples obtained during the FDG uptake period; or the dynamic LV activity curve can be used for the input function. From the curve generated from the input function and the rate constants, quantitated data can be obtained. Thus, with this relatively simple and noninvasive procedure, glucose metabolic rates in vivo can be measured. Although this quantitated method is available in most PET centers, most clinical PET applications do not use the quantitative technique, and the simpler visual interpretation is preferred.

## Brain PET

### FDG Protocol

In general, patients should fast for a minimum of 4 hours before the injection of FDG to prevent hyperglycemia and to achieve good brain uptake of radiotracer. In cases in which hyperglycemia is possible, the patient's blood sugar is checked before FDG is injected. This may be done quickly

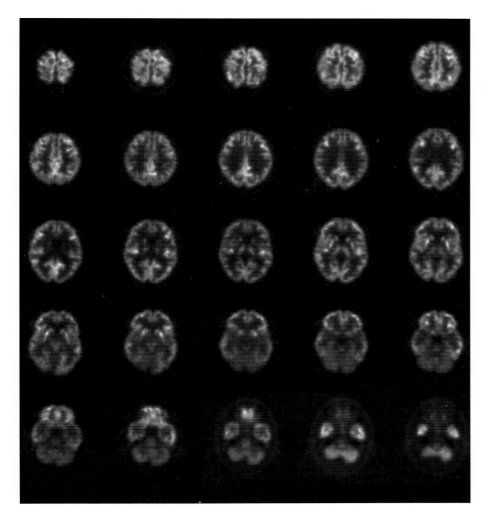

**FIG. 17-3.** Normal PET FDG scan of the brain showing 25 of the 35 routinely obtained transaxial images acquired using the General Electric Advantage PET scanner (Waukesha, WI).

and inexpensively using a finger stick and a small glucose meter. If hyperglycemia is present, one may wish to postpone the examination until the blood glucose level is controlled or administer a small amount of insulin to maintain blood glucose within the normal range. If FDG is injected during hyperglycemia, relatively poor brain uptake of FDG usually results. For quantitation, it is critical to have a stable blood glucose level, and some centers recommend a significantly longer period of fasting.

The patient should be injected in a quiet, dimly lit room and remain there for the 40-minute FDG uptake period. The patient should be encouraged to void to reduce the radiation exposure dose to the bladder and surrounding organs. The patient then enters the PET scanner for image acquisition. The imaging parameters used vary from scanner to scanner, depending on system sensitivity, axial field of view (FOV), and whether a measured or calculated attenuation correction method is used.

The emission scan varies according to injected dose, organ uptake, and scanner sensitivity. FDG brain emission scans are acquired for approximately 30 minutes (Fig. 17-3). In scanners with a small axial FOV, one must be sure that the entire area of interest is included; if not, multiple axial FOVs may be necessary.

Modern PET scanners can acquire a transmission scan after the emission scan; therefore the patient does not need to lie in the scanner during the FDG uptake period. This is a great improvement over earlier scanners, in which the transmission scan was acquired first, and then the patient had to lie perfectly still during the 40-minute FDG uptake period before the emission scan was started. Motion during this uptake period caused a misregistration of the transmission and emission data sets, leading to misregistration of the attenuation images. For nonquantitated clinical brain imaging, the calculated attenuation correction works well, and it is applied to the emission scan after the images are acquired. The calculated program is satisfactory in most situations, but it should not be used if attenuation might be unusual, such as when the skull thickness is significantly different from one side to the other.

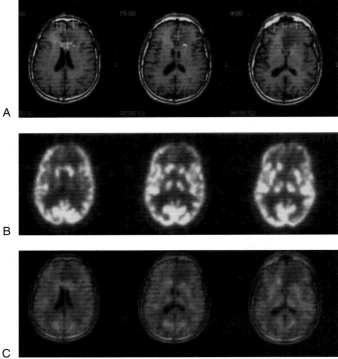

**FIG. 17-4.** PET and MRI fusion in a young man with recurrent left frontal anaplastic astrocytoma who had prior radiation and chemotherapy. **(A)** Three contiguous transaxial MRIs. **(B)** This row shows similar slices of a PET FDG scan. **(C)** This row displays the fused MRI FDG images. The PET FDG scan demonstrates evidence of recurrent tumor anterior to the head of the left and right caudate and crossing the midline. Decreased FDG uptake in the left frontal lobe is consistent with changes secondary to prior radiation therapy. The far left fusion image shows the lesion crossing the midline, with anatomic "bearings" provided by the MRI scan and metabolic activity from the PET scan.

## Image Fusion

The information supplied by anatomic (computed tomography [CT], magnetic resonance [MR]) imaging can be combined with PET physiologic imaging for anatomic and physiologic correlation. This comparison is often difficult, in part because of the different way the image planes are acquired for the MR, CT, and PET images. An important software advance in this area is image coregistration or fusion that reorients one data set to the other. The final image represents the combination of metabolic and structural information (Fig. 17-4) and helps to localize regions of FDG uptake with greater accuracy. The fusion image may help to determine, for example, whether the metabolic area represents recurrent tumor or normal displaced gray matter.

One method of image fusion allows the retrospective combination of data from CT, MR, and PET images. This method also allows registration of sequential studies performed on the same subject, allowing one to closely follow the change in lesion size or shape. A major advantage of this method is that

it does not require special landmarking of the patient and can be applied to images that have already been obtained (17).

## CNS PET

### Primary Brain Tumors

The degree of PET FDG uptake can provide important information about the metabolic characteristics of a tumor. Early work in patients with primary cerebral gliomas at the National Institutes of Health showed a correlation between PET FDG scan glucose use and tumor or malignancy grade (18). Further work performed by this group and others found PET FDG imaging to be accurate in identifying recurrent tumor.

Primary brain tumor treatment often includes radiation therapy and surgery. When the patient presents after therapy with new symptoms, these may be due either to radionecrosis or recurrent tumor, and the symptoms can be indistinguishable. If recurrent brain tumor is present, the patient may then undergo radiation therapy, chemotherapy, or surgery, but if the clinical symptoms are due to radionecrosis, then further radiation therapy is not necessary and may worsen the patient's condition. With MR and CT, there may be difficulty in differentiating radiation necrosis from recurrent tumor because both may have associated edema, contrast enhancement, and the appearance of a recurrent mass. Radionecrosis shows minimal or no FDG uptake (Fig. 17-5),

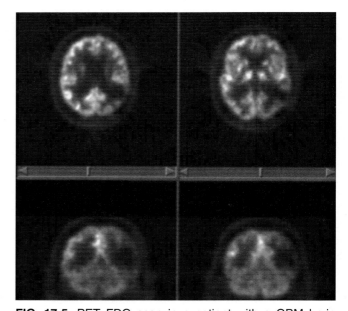

**FIG. 17-5.** PET FDG scan in a patient with a GBM brain tumor, with prior surgical and radiation therapy. The scan (transverse images above, coronal slices below) demonstrates a small area of severely reduced glucose use in the left posterior parietal hemisphere, with surrounding regions of mildly reduced FDG uptake. The PET FDG scan is consistent with a combination of prior surgery and radiation therapy. There is no evidence of recurrent tumor.

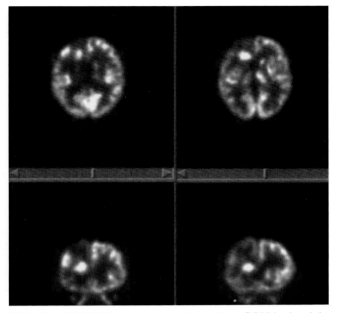

**FIG. 17-6.** PET FDG scan in a patient with a GBM in the right frontal lobe, with previous surgical resection. The scan (transverse slices above, coronal slices below) demonstrates significantly increased areas of FDG uptake centrally and peripherally, consistent with a recurrent GBM (confirmed surgically). Adjacent areas of decreased FDG uptake are secondary to a combination of prior surgical and radiation therapy.

whereas recurrent tumor shows elevated FDG uptake (Fig. 17-6). This PET technique is frequently the only way to make this subtle but critical clinical distinction.

The scan may also be useful in evaluating the biological behavior of low-grade gliomas because biopsy results are very dependent on the site the sample is taken from. Although anatomic imaging methods can define the anatomic characteristics of the suspected neoplasm, it is often difficult to direct the biopsy site with these methods. In such cases, PET imaging of the brain can direct the biopsy to the most metabolically active area, thus significantly improving biopsy accuracy (19).

PET FDG imaging may also provide prognostic information. Patients with malignant gliomas and prior brain irradiation were imaged before chemotherapy, then 1, 7, and 30 days after chemotherapy. Those with increased FDG uptake on the first postchemotherapy day had shorter survival times. The authors speculated this was consistent with tumor re-energization, which may imply that the tumor can repair prior damage and continue to grow (20). Patients with a high-grade hypermetabolic tumor on PET scanning have a significantly shorter median survival compared to patients with hypometabolic lesions (21). Fourfold lesser survivals occurred when FDG uptake in the area of the tumor was higher than the normal contralateral brain region (22).

In clinical PET, accurate data can often be obtained without quantitation. A relatively simple ratio of tumor to whole brain or contralateral normal brain regions, and simple visual analysis can be very valuable. For most clinical examinations, semiquantitative image analysis methods (SUV, DUR, DAR) or even simple visual analysis is adequate for image interpretation and can perform significantly better than the quantitative glucose metabolic rates, which involve more invasive arterial blood sampling (23).

A second radiotracer that appears very promising for the evaluation of recurrent brain tumor is C-11 methionine, an amino acid that accumulates avidly in malignant tissue because of increased tumor metabolic demands. This tracer can also document recurrent tumor. C-11 methionine has been found useful for defining the extent of the tumor, whereas FDG better determines the grade of malignancy and the separation of recurrent brain tumor from radiation necrosis (24). PET imaging with C-11 methionine has also been reported to be useful in the evaluation of pediatric brain tumors (25).

### Epilepsy

Approximately 150,000 people in the United States develop epilepsy each year, and approximately 10% to 20% have medically intractable epilepsy. A thorough investigation of the patient's seizure disorder includes characterization of the seizure type by diagnostic testing, to identify a structural or metabolic cause, and an adequate trial of the appropriate antiepileptic drugs (26). After this workup, if the patient's seizures are not adequately controlled (medically intractable epilepsy), surgical intervention should be considered.

Various types of electroencephalographic (EEG) recordings are performed in these patients, often in association with video monitoring: sphenoidal leads, subdural and epidural electrodes and grids, and depth electrodes (26). CT and MR are used for structural imaging, and physiologic information about blood flow or metabolism is obtained from SPECT and PET. Much of the work performed on medically intractable epilepsy has been done in patients with partial complex seizure disorders of temporal lobe origin. FDG imaging is very useful for identifying the seizure focus (Fig. 17-7). The accuracy of identifying a hypometabolic temporal lobe on interictal PET scanning has increased to 85% as PET scanner resolution has improved (27). The use of surface EEG recordings and PET imaging has significantly decreased the need for costly and invasive depth electrode recordings. A paper reported that, at the University of California, Los Angeles (UCLA), 77 of 84 children (92%) with a seizure disorder who were operated on did not require chronic invasive monitoring because of the FDG scan (28). This is an important consideration because a separate surgical procedure and considerable expense is required for the placement of subdural or epidural grid electrodes for chronic intracranial monitoring (29).

The PET examination is usually performed with the subject in the interictal state. Some recommend postponing the PET scan if the patient has had a seizure within the last 12

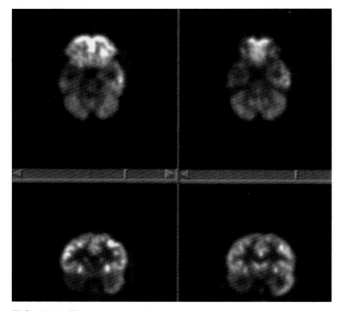

**FIG. 17-7.** This young patient with medically intractable partial complex seizures was being considered for surgical resection of the seizure focus. The scan (transverse slices above, coronal slices below) is performed with the subject in the interictal state and demonstrates a severe reduction of FDG uptake in the right temporal lobe, especially in the lateral aspect. This is consistent with a seizure focus in the right temporal lobe. A right anterior temporal lobectomy, including amygdalohippocampectomy, was performed, and the patient became seizure-free.

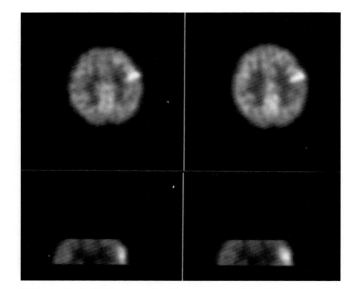

**FIG. 17-8.** A PET scan of a 7-year-old child with continuous partial seizures secondary to Rasmussen encephalitis. The FDG was injected during a seizure and shows a hypermetabolic seizure focus in the left parietal region seen in both the transverse (upper) and the displayed portion of the coronal (lower) slices. A left partial hemispherectomy was performed, which temporarily ended the seizures. (Images courtesy of Dr. Ross Levine, University of Wisconsin Hospital and Clinics, Madison, WI.)

hours, thereby ensuring that the brain metabolic rate is in the basal state. FDG scans show a "hot" seizure focus during an ictus (Fig. 17-8), but because of the unpredictable onset of epilepsy and the prolonged period of FDG uptake, the ictal PET scan is difficult to accomplish. To obtain optimal scan results, one needs to know the seizure state of the person before and during the FDG uptake period. EEG monitoring during this period may be necessary.

Although the temporal lobe histopathologic abnormality may be confined to the mesial temporal lobe (e.g., mesial temporal sclerosis) the metabolic changes seen on the PET scan often involve both the mesial and lateral aspect of the temporal lobe, and in some cases the lateral temporal lobe region may be more hypometabolized. Even though the pathologic changes are usually limited, the metabolic PET scan derangements can be very impressive (30).

In patients with medically intractable partial complex epilepsy, the FDG scan can be an important predictor of postoperative seizure control in subjects who had a temporal lobectomy on the same side as the temporal lobe hypometabolism (31). Patients with temporal lobe epilepsy and extratemporal FDG hypometabolism may have a worse surgical outcome (27). In patients with bilateral temporal lobe seizure foci, both lobes may be hypometabolic, but visual interpretation of temporal lobe activity may, in some cases, identify only the more severely affected lobe. Temporal

lobectomy on the side where PET imaging demonstrated the more significant abnormality has correlated with significant improvement in postoperative seizure frequency. Sometimes, a seizure-free recovery occurs, despite known bilateral seizure foci. FDG imaging has also proved useful in identifying the seizure focus in patients with infantile spasms, Lennox-Gastaut syndrome, and Sturge-Weber syndrome (32).

### Dementia

As life expectancy increases, so does the incidence of dementia. The differential diagnosis for the cause of the decline in a patient's cerebral function is described in Chapter 10. Although the cause is sometimes revealed by careful history, physical examination, laboratory testing, and anatomic imaging, the cause of the dementia remains unknown in a significant number of patients. In these patients, functional imaging plays an increasingly important role. Although adequate therapies are not yet available, the accurate classification of the dementia is an important and necessary first step in patient management.

The most common cause of dementia in the elderly is Alzheimer's disease (AD), and anatomic imaging is neither sensitive nor specific. PET imaging of blood flow and metabolism has demonstrated a typical pattern for AD (Fig. 17-9). Clinical PET imaging is usually performed using FDG. Simple visual interpretation of the images, or ROI analysis, enables identification of alterations in cerebral

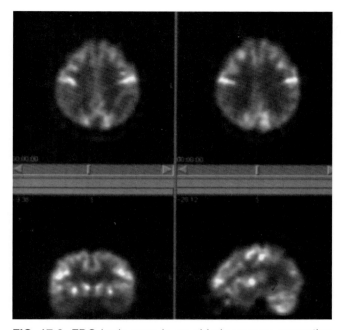

**FIG. 17-9.** FDG brain scan in an elderly woman presenting with dementia. The FDG PET scan with transverse (upper), coronal (left lower), and sagittal (right lower) images shows significantly reduced FDG uptake into both parietal and temporal cerebral cortices. Sparing of metabolism in the primary sensory and motor cortex is seen well in the transverse and coronal images. This scan is typical of Alzheimer's disease.

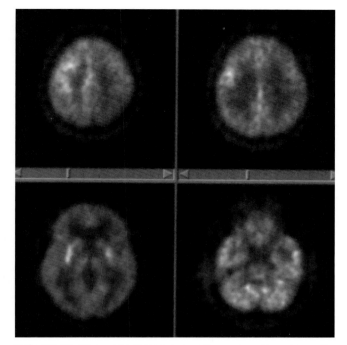

**FIG. 17-10.** The patient has a rapidly progressive dementia of unknown etiology. The EEG showed generalized slowing, whereas the MRI was normal for the patient's age. The PET scan shown here (various transverse images) reveals generalized poor uptake of FDG throughout much of the cerebral cortex bilaterally and slightly worse uptake in the left hemisphere. The patient expired a few months later, and Creutzfeldt-Jakob disease was found at autopsy.

metabolism. Patients with AD have decreased blood flow, decreased oxygen metabolic rate, and decreased glucose metabolic rate in the parietal, temporal, and frontal cortical regions of the brain, with sparing of the sensorimotor and visual cortex. These PET imaging features are evidence of synaptic dysfunction in the associated cortices in the early stages of AD (33).

In one of the larger series to date, Salmon and coworkers studied 129 patients with dementia, 65 of whom were thought to have AD (34). In patients with probable AD, 97% of PET scans were abnormal, although a variety of scan patterns were identified. Most had either bilateral or unilateral temporoparietal hypometabolism, or frontal greater than the temporoparietal hypometabolism (34).

Many patients with dementia have significant cortical atrophy, and correction of the cerebral metabolic rate estimation for this atrophy is necessary to estimate the cerebral glucose metabolic rate (35). The absolute quantity of glucose used by the whole brain may be the more important measurement in patients with AD than the metabolic rate per unit of brain weight (36). The group who made that finding reported that atrophy-weighted total brain metabolism (a combination of metabolic and volumetric measurements) appeared to be better than absolute whole-brain or mean cerebral metabolic rate measurements in the identification of abnormal brain metabolism in patients with AD compared with controls.

Patients with multi-infarct dementia have multiple focal regions of FDG hypometabolism scattered throughout the brain (37,38). Various patterns of abnormal brain metabolism have been reported that correlate with less common forms of dementia. Although few cases of FDG scanning in patients with Pick's disease have been reported, hypometabolism in the frontal lobes, which may extend into the anterior temporal lobes, has been found (34,39). In Huntington's disease, hypometabolism of the caudate and putamen may precede significant atrophy. There is evidence that the caudate nucleus may be hypometabolic in asymptomatic subjects who carry the autosomal dominant gene (40). A form of dementia can be seen in patients with Parkinson's disease, and in one small series, the FDG hypometabolism involved the frontal, temporal, parietal, occipital, sensorimotor, and striatal regions (41). Hypometabolism has been reported throughout the entire brain in patients with Creutzfeldt-Jakob disease (Fig. 17-10) (41,42). Interesting patterns of glucose hypometabolism have been reported with other forms of dementia, such as progressive supranuclear palsy, Wilson's disease, and normal-pressure hydrocephalus. Mazziotta and colleagues present a detailed discussion of PET imaging of dementia in their review article on PET imaging in dementia (43).

## Cardiac PET

### Image Format

Traditionally, cardiac PET images have been displayed as transaxial images in the conventional CT orientation of the observer looking up from the patient's feet, with the anterior aspect at the top of the image and the right side of the body on the left side of the image, with planes displayed superior to inferior. Recently, investigators have reoriented the transaxial views into the standard cardiac axial views of horizontal and vertical long-axis and short-axis views, as seen in SPECT cardiac imaging. For clinical image review, a late emission image or summed late dynamic frames are used. Some investigators have also used the bull's-eye format for their final image display. Gated imaging is also possible, with display of systolic and diastolic images.

### Quantitative MPI Methods

#### Rb-82 Flow Reserve

In Rb-82 imaging, the most common quantitation has been the semiquantitative relative uptake method. This method calculates the ratio of uptake of Rb-82 in a myocardial segment at rest and after pharmacologic stress with adenosine or dipyridamole (44).

#### Correction of Extraction Fraction

A more quantitative method of determining myocardial blood flow was proposed by Schelbert and coworkers. Using various flows above baseline, the investigators were able to calculate the PS product in animals for N-13 $NH_3$ (45), verify it in the PET scanner, and then apply it to humans (46,47). In humans, they demonstrated the expected two- to threefold increase in myocardial blood flow with pharmacologic stress.

#### Kinetic Modeling

Dynamic imaging of the heart during administration of a PET tracer allows myocardial uptake and clearance measurements. Parametric modeling of these data allows one to derive kinetic rates. This approach was first applied to O-15 water imaging by the Hammersmith and Washington University groups (4,5). The major advantages of O-15 water are the ability to give large doses of O-15, because of its short half-life, and the high first-pass extraction fraction. However, the short myocardial residence time and rapid tracer diffusion limits the data acquisition interval. This and the spillover of ventricular chamber blood pool activity into the myocardial ROIs have limited the technique. Parametric modeling has also been applied to N-13 $NH_3$ by Hutchins and coworkers (7) and to Rb-82 by Bergmann and colleagues (6). A three-compartment model was used by Hutchins to estimate the $K_1$

of ammonia (7), and a two-compartment model has been used with Rb-82 to quantitate perfusion (6,48).

### Myocardial Perfusion Imaging

#### Pathophysiology

Several investigators have used PET MPI to elucidate the pathophysiology of coronary artery disease (CAD) in humans. PET imaging was used because of its noninvasive nature and its quantitative capability to measure changes in perfusion. Gould and coworkers demonstrated that coronary blood flow limitations with CAD occur at critical stenoses of >85% diameter stenosis (49–51). With coronary vasodilatation, however, less critical forms of disease are apparent with a decrease in coronary blood flow distal to the stenosis, secondary to the impairment of vascular reserve in the diseased coronary segment. These changes in flow were measured directly or by assessment of perfusion with PET.

These studies were important clinically in demonstrating that one of the first manifestations of CAD is a decrease in coronary flow reserve. Coronary vasodilatation due to exercise increases flow to two to three times resting level. Direct coronary vasodilatation by exogenous adenosine or dipyridamole increases coronary blood flow fourfold. CAD atherosclerotic plaque first interferes in the vasodilatory response, and it is only with marked luminal narrowing by the plaque that resting blood flow is diminished. Pharmacologic vasodilatation with dipyridamole or adenosine tests the coronary reserve by vasodilating the coronary arterial bed. With the decrease in vasodilatation at the site of an atheromatous plaque, the increase in resistance in the bed leads to a relative decrease in flow with stress (coronary steal). In more severe forms of impaired coronary vascular reserve, myocardial ischemia is precipitated when distal flow decreases to a level below that of resting blood flow.

Later studies by Gould and coworkers have demonstrated the effects of coronary anatomy and risk factor reduction on coronary vascular tone. These investigators have been able to show that the decrease in coronary reserve with CAD is reversed with coronary angioplasty (52) or a 90-day intensive cholesterol-lowering trial (53).

Investigators at the Hammersmith Hospital in London have demonstrated changes in coronary vasomotor tone with mental stress and smoking by Rb-82 PET. They were able to demonstrate transient perfusion abnormalities after arithmetic computations (54) or cigarette smoking (55). These studies were seminal in the description of the impact of coronary vasomotor tone on luminal diameter.

#### Clinical Studies

The conventional hallmark of the noninvasive diagnosis of CAD is the assessment of coronary vascular reserve using a tracer injected at stress, which redistributes at rest (e.g.,

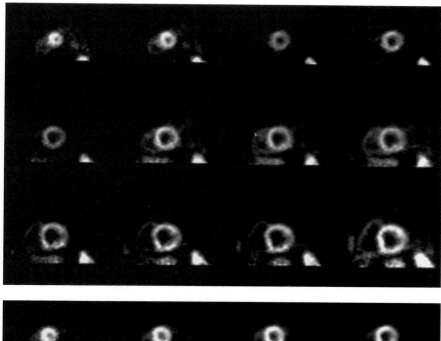

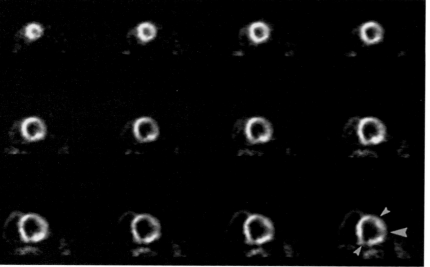

**FIG. 17-11.** The PET MPI scan shows 12 short-axis slices (of 25 total cardiac slices) at rest **(A)** and the same 12 at stress **(B)**. The dipyridamole stress images **(B)** show a moderate-sized lateral defect (*large arrowhead*) and smaller anterolateral and inferoseptal defects (*small arrowheads*). At rest **(A)**, the lateral wall defect persists, but the smaller anterolateral and inferoseptal defects normalize. This patient demonstrates both impaired coronary vascular reserve in the inferolateral and anterolateral segments and infarction in the lateral segment.

thallium 201 [Tl-201] chloride), or separate injections at stress and rest of tracers that are retained or washed out without redistribution (e.g., technetium 99m sestamibi). MPI with PET has also been applied clinically for the detection of CAD (Fig. 17-11).

The three common MPI tracers, Rb-82, N-13 NH$_3$, and O-15 water, have been compared to coronary angiography as the gold standard. Sensitivity for the detection of CAD has ranged from 87% to 97%, with specificities of 78% to 100% (Table 17-5) (56). Direct comparisons with Tl-201 planar and SPECT imaging show an improvement in sensitivity or specificity, or both, for PET, suggesting a role as the primary noninvasive imaging study for detecting CAD for PET. In a direct comparison of PET and SPECT MPI, Stewart and coworkers found an increase in specificity (84% PET, 53% Tl-201 SPECT) and predictive accuracy (85% PET, 79% Tl-201 SPECT) (59). Go

**TABLE 17-5.** *PET dipyridamole stress MPI*

| PET tracer (reference) | Number of patients | Sensitivity (%) | Specificity (%) | Accuracy (%) |
|---|---|---|---|---|
| N-13 NH$_3$ (57) | 35 | 97 | 100 | 98 |
| NH$_3$ + Rb-82 (58) | 193 | 82 | 95 | 88 |
| Rb-82 (59) | 81 | 85 | 84 | 85 |
| Rb-82 (60) | 135 | 95 | 82 | 92 |
| Rb-82 (61) | 225 | 83 | 91 | 89 |
| Rb-82 (62) | 287 | 87 | 88 | 88 |
| Mean PET (56) | — | 88 | 90 | 90 |
| Mean SPECT (59,60) | — | 82 | 64 | 78 |

Source: Adapted with permission from Schwaiger M. Myocardial perfusion imaging with PET. J Nucl Med 1994;35:693–698.

and colleagues also demonstrated an advantage for PET over SPECT in sensitivity (95% vs. 79%) and specificity (82% vs. 76%), leading to an increase in predictive accuracy (92% vs. 78%) of Rb PET over Tl-201 SPECT (60). Of particular clinical utility might be the higher specificity of PET imaging due to attenuation correction. This has prompted the use of PET imaging in patients with potential false-positive perfusion planar or SPECT scans, particularly in individuals with angiographically normal vessels but continued symptoms.

MPI PET has also been applied to other selective instances, as when the results of myocardial gamma camera imaging, coronary arteriography, and clinical symptomatology are discrepant. One clinical scenario is a patient with typical symptoms of angina pectoris, negative conventional MPI scan, and negative or equivocal coronary artery angiography; in this case, the higher sensitivity of PET is used to determine if abnormalities in coronary vascular reserve do exist. MacIntyre and coworkers (63) reviewed patient outcome after a true positive PET scan and false-negative Tl SPECT and found a 63% successful revascularization rate. If SPECT data were used alone, the predictive capability was inferior (63). Another scenario is a patient with no symptoms or atypical symptoms but a positive MPI scan; in this case, the higher specificity of PET is used to verify the gamma camera results as a true positive rather than a false positive. Gould et al. (64) used MPI PET imaging as a primary imaging step, justifying the increased cost of PET by the cost savings of fewer coronary angiograms. Use of MPI PET as a primary imaging tool of CAD is limited because only Rb-82 is approved for reimbursement by the Health Care Financing Agency and because the generator carries a high monthly cost.

A clinical concern of PET MPI has been the lack of prognostic data derived from the maximal functional aerobic capacity on the treadmill stress test that accompanies standard SPECT imaging. The standard PET imaging procedure is best adapted to pharmacologic stress, where the drug may be infused after transmission imaging without moving the patient. In these patients a separate treadmill study must be performed to assess functional aerobic capacity. The development of simultaneous transmission and emission imaging may allow the use of treadmill exercise directly in conjunction with MPI PET and so provide simultaneous functional capacity and electrocardiographic data.

### Myocardial Metabolism

Similar to MPI studies with PET, myocardial metabolic studies have an important role in the study of CAD pathophysiology and have been applied in clinical diagnostic and therapeutic decision making.

### Pathophysiology

The classic dictum in cardiology before the 1980s was that chronic resting myocardial wall motion abnormalities indicated previous myocardial infarction and irreversible damage. The second tenet was that the dysfunction associated with acute myocardial ischemia was transient and immediately reversible. Later, Rahmitoola (65) described clinical studies from the catheterization laboratory in which chronic wall motion abnormalities improved on ventriculography after nitroglycerin administration in the setting of decreased myocardial perfusion due to CAD. This *hibernating myocardium*, or dysfunctional myocardial segments, were shown to improve in function after revascularization (65,66). In animal preparations, Braunwald and Kloner also described the delay in recovery of systolic function (myocardial stunning) after myocardial ischemia despite restoration of flow (67). Hibernating myocardium and myocardial stunning are two examples of reversible myocardial mechanical dysfunction related to decreased perfusion from CAD.

Tillisch and coworkers at UCLA were the first investigators to demonstrate the perfusion metabolic derangements of regional myocardial wall motion abnormalities with PET (68). They identified two patterns of perfusion and FDG uptake in patients with chronic heart disease. In a study of 17 patients with CAD and resting wall motion abnormalities, PET imaging with N-13 ammonia and FDG was obtained before bypass surgery. The effect of revascularization on wall motion was determined after surgery with a repeat assessment of wall motion. They defined segments having an ammonia defect but FDG uptake (the "mismatch" pattern) as having a reversible wall motion abnormality while those segments having both an ammonia and FDG defect (the "matched" pattern) as being scarred. Examples are shown in Fig. 17-12. Complex combinations can occur in one patient (Fig. 17-13). The investigators found that the mismatch pattern had a positive predictive accuracy of 85% for the return of function after revascularization, whereas the matched pattern had a negative predictive accuracy of 92% for the lack of return of function.

PET has also been used as a surrogate viability end point in Tl-201 scintigraphy studies. In one study, stress, redistribution, and reinjection Tl-201 imaging were compared to rest and redistribution imaging. On a segmental basis, the investigators determined a concordance rate of 79% on the stress, redistribution, and reinjection protocol for viability (defined as reversible Tl-201 defects) with the rest-redistribution protocol (69). In 20 of the 41 patients studied, FDG and O-15 water PET were used to determine the presence of myocardial viability. In this subgroup, the discordant segments with irreversible Tl-201 defects on the stress, redistribution, reinjection protocol were analyzed for the severity of count depression. The discordant segments that had only mild to moderate count depression (15% to 50% decreases) on the stress-reinjection protocol were found on the rest-redistribution Tl-201 protocol to be viable in 89% of patients and on the PET study to be viable in 98% of patients. PET in this study was used to confirm the presence of viability rather than the assessment of changes in regional wall motion after revascularization.

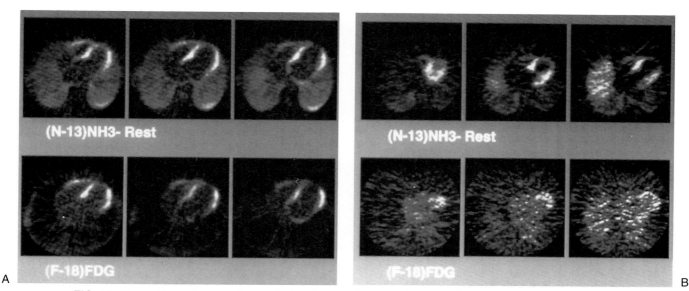

**FIG. 17-12. (A)** These images demonstrate a large apical "matched" rest flow (N-13 NH$_3$) and metabolic (F-18 FDG) apical defect. **(B)** These images demonstrate a "mismatched" flow and metabolic apical defect, where the only FDG uptake occurs in the unperfused region.

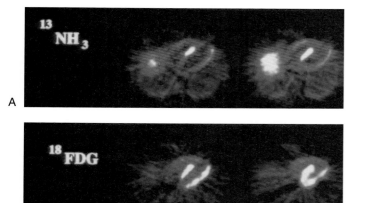

**FIG. 17-13.** Flow **(A)** and metabolic **(B)** images show a matched apicoseptal defect and a mismatched lateral wall defect.

**TABLE 17-6.** *PET viability scan patterns*

| Blood flow | Glucose use | PET scan description | Pathophysiologic interpretation |
|---|---|---|---|
| Normal | Intact | No defect | Normal myo-cardium |
| Reduced | Intact | Mismatch | Viable myo-cardium |
| Reduced | Reduced | Matched defect | Scar or infarct |

*Cardiac Applications*

The concept of hibernating myocardium has generated intense clinical interest. Several clinical trials have demonstrated the efficacy of coronary revascularization, as measured by decreased mortality in patients with CAD and impaired LV function. However, revascularization by coronary artery bypass graft (CABG) surgery carries increased risk in patients with LV dysfunction and reduced benefit in individuals with dysfunction secondary to scar. Thus, a major area of interest has been the graft determination of whether dysfunctional myocardium is scar or viable.

A variety of metabolic tracers have been used to assess myocardial metabolism in infarction, ischemia, and cardiomyopathy. The largest role for metabolic tracers has been to identify metabolic activity (i.e., viability) in a myocardial segment that is hypoperfused and dysfunctional so as to determine the likelihood of functional recovery after revascularization. Three tracers have been used for viability (FDG, C-11 acetate, and Rb-82), but the majority of studies have been performed with FDG. The common protocol used for myocardial viability assessment is a resting NH$_3$ scan for perfusion assessment and an FDG scan for determining glucose use. The majority of readings are done on a qualitative basis, comparing glucose use to blood flow. Three scan patterns have been proposed (Table 17-6). Within the mismatch group, three patterns of glucose use relative to segmental blood flow have emerged. Perfusion defects have been associated with enhancement of FDG uptake greater than the normal perfused segments (see Fig. 17-12B), uptake equal to normally perfused segments, and mild reduction in FDG compared to the normally perfused segment. A generally accepted criterion of viability is FDG uptake at a level of at least 70% of FDG uptake in the normally perfused segment.

Three reviews summarize the PET viability data (70–72). The first prospective data using N-13 NH$_3$ and FDG resting PET imaging are from UCLA, where prognosis in heart fail-

## Match

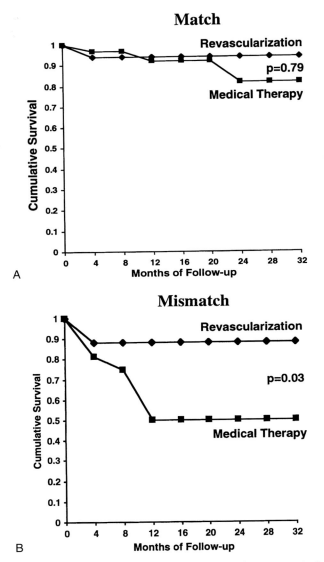

**A**

## Mismatch

**FIG. 17-14.** The cumulative survival rates for revascularization (*diamonds*) and medical therapy (*squares*) for matched defects **(A)** and mismatched defects **(B)** using N-13 ammonia and F-18 FDG scanning performed at rest. (Modified with permission from Di Carli MF, Davidson M, Little R, et al. Value of metabolic imaging with positron emission tomography for evaluating prognosis in patients with coronary artery disease and left ventricular dysfunction. Am J Cardiol 1994;73:527–533.)

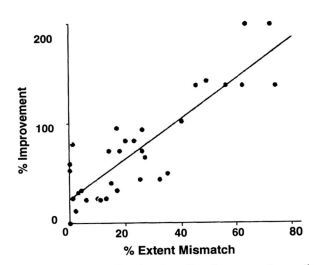

**FIG. 17-15.** A graph showing the linear postoperative improvement in functional capacity against percent mismatch. (Modified with permission from Di Carli MF, Asgarzadie BA, Schelbert HR, et al. Quantitative relation between myocardial viability and improvement in heart failure symptoms after revascularization in patients with ischemic cardiomyopathy. Circulation 1995;92:3436–3444. Copyright 1995, American Heart Association.)

ure patients was compared for medical therapy and revascularization (73). A PET mismatch pattern (i.e., reduced perfusion and increased glucose metabolism) predicted a lower annual survival rate with medical therapy than a matched defect (50% vs. 82%), and revascularization in the PET mismatch patient group significantly prolonged survival (88% vs. 50%) (Fig. 17-14).

A second study from the UCLA group looked at the predictive capability of PET perfusion and FDG imaging for determining the recovery of function after CABG (74). In patients with ischemic cardiomyopathy, they demonstrated a significant correlation of the extent of PET perfusion-metabolism mismatch (Fig. 17-15) with improvement in functional status after CABG. The authors showed that patients with a large mismatch preoperatively had a greater improvement in functional capacity after CABG. These data highlight the prognostic importance of PET perfusion-metabolism mismatch for the medical and surgical therapy of ischemic cardiomyopathy. Further larger-scale, multi-center, randomized trials should confirm these single-center studies.

The other tracers that have been used for assessment of myocardial viability are acetate and Rb-82. The Washington University group has advocated the use of acetate to demonstrate myocardial viability (75). Such an approach is in contrast to FDG imaging, in which, instead of assessing the early rates of glucose metabolism, the more terminal metabolic step of oxidative phosphorylation is measured. Gropler et al. (76) compared the predictive capability of acetate to FDG in the recovery of regional function after revascularization. In a series of 34 patients, they demonstrated that the metabolic rate by acetate had better positive and negative predictive capability in determining the recovery of function than FDG (positive predictive capability of 67% vs. 52%, and negative capability of 89% vs. 81%). Recently, Gould and coworkers proposed the use of Rb-82 kinetics for the determination of viability (77). Because Rb-82 is a potassium analog, the cellular uptake requires the presence of intact membrane function. Infarcted or scarred myocardium does not retain rubidium because of a lack of cellular membrane transport. Gould et al. found a correlation ($r = 0.93$) in rubidium wash-out kinetics with infarct size by FDG (77). Vom Dahl et al. (78) also measured the changes in wash-out kinetics in normal, viable, and infarcted myocardium and found that the clearance half-time of rubidium was significantly shortened in infarcted myocardium, with viable myocardium having lesser decreases in clearance half-time.

Thus, three PET tracers have been used clinically for the determination of viability. Although the greatest work has been done with FDG, more extensive trials are needed to compare the three tracers. The choice of tracer at a local site will probably depend on the logistics of production of the tracer.

### Receptor Studies

Although some cardiac PET studies have been done with labeled precursors to determine neurotransmitter synthesis, more interest has focused on postsynaptic adrenergic receptor densities and presynaptic catecholamine uptake rates. This interest comes about because of the disruption of myocardial innervation that occurs with myocardial infarction and the down-regulation of beta-adrenergic receptors that results from congestive heart failure. Delforge et al. (79) have demonstrated in vivo measurement of beta-adrenergic receptors with the receptor ligand C-11 CGP 12177 (a labeled beta-blocker). The same group has also studied muscarinic receptors in the heart (80). Another approach has been to study presynaptic function with labeled neurotransmitter analogs. Schwaiger and colleagues (81) have extensively studied the *N*-methyl sympathomimetic meta-hydroxyephedrine labeled with C-11 (C-11 HED). Using dynamic PET, they have shown decreased retention of C-11 HED in patients with cardiomyopathy and after cardiac transplantation, two physiologic states of cardiac denervation. Further studies are needed to determine the prognostic value of presynaptic and postsynaptic receptor studies in the outcome of myocardial infarction or cardiomyopathy. The current hypothesis is that patients with myocardial denervation, as measured by synaptic receptor density, are at higher risk for sudden cardiac death.

## Oncologic PET

Many tumors have an elevated rate of glucose use due to an increased rate of glycolysis. For this reason, FDG is a very useful radiotracer for the evaluation of the primary tumor and sites of metastatic disease. Advances in scanner technology have led to high-quality, rapid whole-body images that allow whole-body evaluations for metastatic disease. Follow-up scan examinations after chemotherapy or radiotherapy may provide early information about tumor response, before lesion size decreases. A major indication for the FDG whole-body scan is the evaluation of lymph node involvement for improved staging of disease. The technique is also useful at the end of conventional chemotherapy or radiotherapy courses, to determine if viable tumor remains.

Most of the preliminary work performed to date has used FDG, although other radiopharmaceuticals, such as C-11 methionine, are under investigation. To improve the subjective visual assessment of FDG images, investigators have applied various semiquantitative methods to add a level of objectivity (e.g., SUR and DUR).

### Scan Protocol

The typical protocol is performed with the patient in the fasting state (minimum of 4 to 6 hours after a light meal) after the injection of 10 mCi (370 MBq) F-18 FDG. Whole-body images are acquired 40 to 60 minutes later. Improved image quality and accuracy are obtained with measured attenuation correction of the whole body, although this is currently not practical in the clinical setting. The primary tumor region should be imaged for a longer period (approximately 20 minutes) for improved statistics and resolution, and the routine use of measured attenuation correction is recommended for this limited acquisition region. Variations in measured attenuation correction techniques applicable to whole-body imaging are under development and may soon be available. Quantitation to obtain the absolute metabolic rate is usually not necessary. Visual interpretation is often aided by ROI comparison of one area to the contralateral or adjacent areas, and this is usually adequate for clinical purposes.

### Image Fusion

In a further attempt to improve the diagnostic utility of PET imaging in oncology, investigators at the University of Michigan have developed a method of coregistering the physiologic FDG data with the higher-resolution anatomic images of the CT or MR scan (see Fig. 17-4). This method uses external fiducial markers during each examination to obtain accurate alignment of the scans. The resulting data, referred to as *anatometabolic fusion images* will undoubtedly represent an improvement over the independent interpretation of the individual modalities (82).

### Tumor Types

#### Melanoma

PET scanning using FDG has been investigated in malignant melanoma (Fig. 17-16) (83). The scan has been

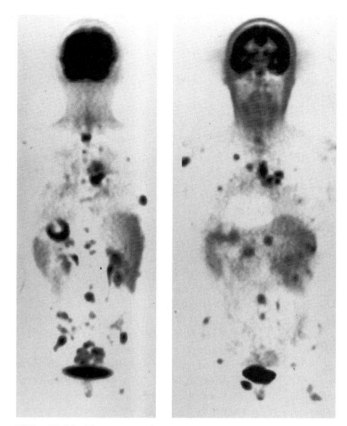

**FIG. 17-16.** Two coronal planes of the whole-body FDG image show normal brain uptake and multiple regions of melanoma metastases. (The left side of the images represents the left side of the patient.)

compared to the physical examination, biopsy results, and other imaging procedures. Most visceral and lymph node metastases in the abdomen, head, and neck were seen, but the technique was not as successful in identifying pulmonary metastases.

### Breast

Adler and coworkers studied FDG uptake in patients with breast masses to evaluate uptake of radiotracer in benign and malignant breast lesions and the role of FDG in evaluating the axillary lymph nodes (84). Reduced FDG uptake was noted in benign breast masses, whereas malignant masses had significantly elevated FDG accumulation. They reported a sensitivity of 96% and specificity of 100% for the detection of benign versus malignant disease. Sensitivity was 90% and specificity was 100% for detection of axillary lymph node metastases (Fig. 17-17).

### Focal Pulmonary Abnormalities

Patients with focal pulmonary abnormalities were prospectively studied with FDG to determine if benign and malignant disease could be correctly identified using the degree of FDG uptake. SURs were ≥2.5 in all patients with bronchogenic carcinoma, whereas lesions with <2.5 SUR were benign. Using this threshold value for detection of a benign lesion, the sensitivity was 89% and specificity was 100% (85). Other investigators have also reported significant FDG uptake in lung cancer (86).

### Bronchogenic Cancer

An SUR ≥2.5 was used to evaluate residual chest x-ray lesions in bronchogenic carcinoma in 43 patients; sensitivity of 97% and specificity of 100% was found for persistent or recurrent tumors (87). FDG PET imaging is important in staging the extent of mediastinal disease (Fig. 17-18) and was found to be more accurate than CT in patients with suspected non–small cell lung cancer (88). Using FDG scanning, with measured attenuation correction and correction for the regional blood volume using C-11 CO, Nolop and coworkers reported that the tumor uptake of FDG was significantly greater than normal lung tissue, but there was no

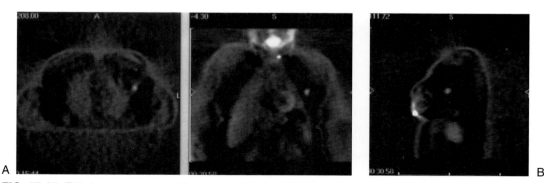

A                                                                                           B

**FIG. 17-17.** This breast cancer patient demonstrates FDG uptake in an axillary lymph node (confirmed to be tumor) and probable supraclavicular lymph node (as yet unconfirmed) in these transaxial (left) and coronal (right) images **(A)** and sagittal image **(B)**.

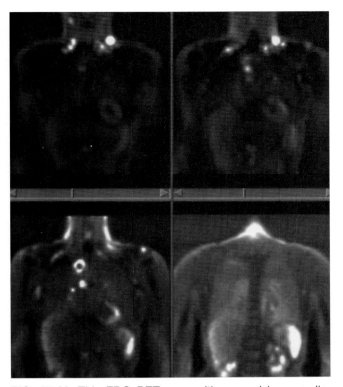

**FIG. 17-18.** This FDG PET scan with coronal images displayed was performed in a patient with small cell lung cancer. The scan demonstrates a large hypermetabolic primary tumor with a central area of decreased uptake, consistent with viable tumor and central necrosis, as well as numerous areas of metastatic disease in the supraclavicular and hilar regions. Normal cardiac, hepatic, splenic, and renal collecting system activity is apparent.

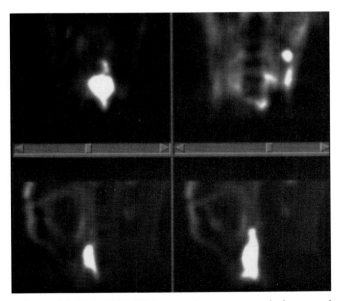

**FIG. 17-19.** This PET FDG scan (upper coronal views and lower sagittal views) of the neck in a patient with a squamous cell carcinoma of the left piriform sinus. The scan demonstrates intense FDG uptake into the primary tumor in all views and a metastatic left cervical lymph node in the right-side coronal and sagittal views.

relationship between the type of tumor and the degree of FDG uptake (89).

*Soft-Tissue Tumors*

Using a slightly different form of semiquantitative analysis (DUR) to interpret FDG uptake in various soft-tissue masses, Griffeth et al. (90) were able to differentiate benign from malignant tissue (Fig. 17-19). In this series, simple visual assessment was inferior to the DUR method. The DUR for malignant lesions was 6.4 times greater than DUR for benign lesions, and there was no overlap between groups. This semiquantitative technique may add important information as to whether a lesion is malignant.

*Other Tumors*

The literature in the area of PET imaging in various areas of oncology is growing rapidly. Investigators have imaged patients with lymphoma (91,92) and head and neck tumors (93). Although the majority of the investigations to date in the area of PET imaging in oncology have been performed using FDG, other radiopharmaceuticals will likely contribute a great deal to our knowledge of the functioning of these neoplasms. A few examples are the evaluation of C-11 methionine use (94) and the evaluation of glioma hypoxia using F-18 fluoromisonidazole (95).

## REFERENCES

1. Crone C. Permeability of capillaries in various organs, determined by use of the indicator diffusion method. Acta Physiol Scand 1963;58:292–305.
2. Renkin EM. Transport of potassium-42 from blood tissue in isolated mammalian skeletal muscles. Am J Physiol 1959;197:1205–1210.
3. Gambhir SS, Schwaiger M, Huang S-C, et al. Simple noninvasive quantification method for measuring myocardial glucose utilization in humans employing positron emission tomography and fluorine-18 deoxyglucose. J Nucl Med 1989;30:359–366.
4. Bergmann SR, Fox KAA, Rand AL, et al. Quantification of regional myocardial blood flow in vivo with H$_2$$^{15}$O. Circulation 1981;63:1248–1257.
5. Bergmann SR. Quantification of Myocardial Perfusion with Positron Emission Tomography. In Bergmann SR, Sobel BE (eds), Positron Emission Tomography of the Heart. Mount Kisco, NY: Futura, 1992;97–127.
6. Herrero P, Markham J, Shelton ME, et al. Implementation and evaluation of a two-compartment model for quantification of myocardial perfusion with rubidium-82 and positron emission tomography. Circ Res 1992;70:496–507.
7. Hutchins GD, Schwaiger M, Rosenspire KC, et al. Noninvasive quantification of regional blood flow in the human heart using N-13 ammonia and dynamic positron emission tomographic imaging. J Am Coll Cardiol 1990;15:1031–1042.
8. Berry JJ, Baker JA, Pieper KS, et al. The effect of metabolic milieu on cardiac PET imaging using fluorine-18-deoxyglucose and nitrogen-13-ammonia in normal volunteers. J Nucl Med 1991;32:1518–1525.
9. Knuuti MJ, Nuutila P, Ruotsalainen U, et al. Euglycemic hyperinsulinemic clamp and oral glucose load in stimulating myocardial glucose utilization during positron emission tomography. J Nucl Med 1992;33:1255–1262.
10. Knuuti MJ, Yki-Jarvinen H, Voipio-Pulkki LM, et al. Enhancement of

myocardial (fluorine-18) fluorodeoxyglucose uptake by a nicotinic acid derivative. J Nucl Med 1994;35:989–998.

11. Stone CK, Holden J, Stanley W, Perlman SB. Effect of nicotinic acid on exogenous myocardial glucose uptake. J Nucl Med 1995;36:996–1002.

12. Rosamond TL, Abendschein DR, Sobel BE, et al. Metabolic fate of radiolabeled palmitate in ischemic canine myocardium: implications for positron emission tomography. J Nucl Med 1987;28:1322–1329.

13. Armbrecht JJ, Buxton CB, Schelbert HR. Validation of (1-$^{11}$C) acetate as a tracer for noninvasive assessment of oxidative metabolism in positron emission tomography in normal, ischemic, postischemic and hyperemic canine myocardium. Circulation 1990;81:1594–1605.

14. Patlak CS, Blasberg RG, Fenstermacher JD. Graphical evaluation of blood-to-brain transfer constants from multiple-time uptake data. J Cereb Blood Flow Metab 1983;3:1–7.

15. Ratib O, Phelps ME, Huang SC, et al. Positron tomography with deoxyglucose for estimating local myocardial glucose metabolism. J Nucl Med 1982;23:577–586.

16. Fischman AJ, Alpert NM. FDG-PET in oncology: there's more to it than looking at pictures [editorial]. J Nucl Med 1993;34:6–11.

17. Levin DN, Pelizzari CA, Chen GTY, et al. Retrospective geometric correlation of MR, CT, and PET images. Radiology 1988;169:817–823.

18. Di Chiro G, DeLaPaz RL, Brooks RA, et al. Glucose utilization of cerebral gliomas measured by (F-18) fluorodeoxyglucose and positron emission tomography. Neurology 1982;32:1323–1329.

19. Hanson MW, Glantz MJ, Hoffman JM, et al. FDG-PET in selection of brain lesions for biopsy. J Comput Assist Tomogr 1991;15:796–801.

20. Rozental JM, Levine R, Nickles RJ. Changes in glucose uptake by malignant gliomas: preliminary study of prognostic significance. J Neurooncol 1991;10:75–83.

21. Alavi JB, Alavi A, Chawluk J, et al. Positron emission tomography in patients with glioma. Cancer 1988;62:1074–1078.

22. Patronas NJ, Di Chiro G, Kufta C, et al. Prediction of survival in glioma patients by means of positron emission tomography. J Neurosurg 1985;62:816–822.

23. Kim CK, Alavi A, Reivich M. New grading system of cerebral gliomas using positron emission tomography with F-18 fluorodeoxyglucose. J Neurooncol 1991;10:85–91.

24. Ogawa T, Kanno I, Shishido F, et al. Clinical value of PET with F-18-fluorodeoxyglucose and L-methyl-C-11-methionine for diagnosis of recurrent brain tumor and radiation injury. Acta Radiologica 1991;32:197–202.

25. O'Tuama LA, Phillips PC, Strauss LC, et al. Two-phase (C-11) L-methionine PET in childhood brain tumors. Pediatr Neurol 1990;6:163–170.

26. NIH Consensus Conference. Surgery for epilepsy. JAMA 1990;264:729–733.

27. Swartz BE, Tomiyasu U, Delgado-Escueta AV, et al. Neuroimaging in temporal lobe epilepsy: test sensitivity and relationships to pathology and postoperative outcome. Epilepsia 1992;33:624–634.

28. Chugani HT, Shewmon DA, Shields WD, et al. Positron emission tomographic scanning in pediatric epilepsy operation: UCLA experience in 84 patients. Ann Neurol 1991;30:483.

29. Chugani HT. The use of positron emission tomography in the clinical assessment of epilepsy. Semin Nucl Med 1992;22:247–253.

30. De La Pena R, Perlman SB, Levine R, et al. PET scan findings in patients with temporal lobe epilepsy of mesial temporal origin [abstract]. J Nucl Med 1992;33:1014.

31. De La Pena RC, Perlman SB, Ramirez LF, et al. PET/FDG imaging and post-surgical outcome in subjects with complex partial epilepsy [abstract]. J Nucl Med 1993;34:22P.

32. Chugani HT. The use of positron emission tomography in the clinical assessment of epilepsy. Semin Nucl Med 1992;22:247–253.

33. Fukuyama H, Ogawa M, Yamaguchi S, et al. Altered cerebral energy metabolism in Alzheimer's disease: a PET study. J Nucl Med 1994;35:1–6.

34. Salmon E, Sadzot B, Maquet P, et al. Differential diagnosis of Alzheimer's disease with PET. J Nucl Med 1994;35:391–398.

35. Chawluk JB, Dann R, Alavi A, et al. The effect of focal atrophy in positron emission tomographic studies of aging and dementia. Nucl Med Biol 1990;17:797–804.

36. Alavi A, Newberg AB, Souder E, Berlin JA. Quantitative analysis of PET and MRI data in normal aging and Alzheimer's disease: atrophy weighted total brain metabolism and absolute whole brain metabolism as reliable discriminators. J Nucl Med 1993;34:1681–1687.

37. Benson DF, Kuhl DE, Hawkins RA, et al. The fluorodeoxyglucose F-18 scan in Alzheimer's disease and multi-infarct dementia. Arch Neurol 1983;40:711–714.

38. Kuhl DE, Metter J, Riege WH, et al. Local cerebral glucose utilization in elderly patients with depression, multiple infarct dementia, and Alzheimer's disease. J Cereb Blood Flow Metab 1983;3:S494–S495.

39. Goto I, Taniwaki T, Hosokawa S, et al. Positron emission tomographic (PET) studies in dementia. J Neurol Sci 1993;114:1–6.

40. Kuhl DE, Phelps ME, Markham CH, et al. Cerebral metabolism and atrophy in Huntington's disease determined by F-18-FDG and computed tomographic scan. Ann Neurol 1982;12:425–434.

41. Goto I, Taniwaki T, Hosokawa S, et al. Positron emission tomographic (PET) studies in dementia. J Neurol Sci 1993;114:1–6.

42. Holthoff VA, Sandmann J, Pawlik G, et al. Positron emission tomography in Creutzfeldt-Jakob disease. Arch Neurol 1990;47:1035–1038.

43. Mazziotta JC, Frackowiak RSJ, Phelps ME. The use of positron emission tomography in the clinical assessment of dementia. Semin Nucl Med 1992;22:233–246.

44. Hicks K, Ganti G, Mullani N, Gould KL. Automated quantitation of 3D cardiac PET for routine clinical use. J Nucl Med 1989;30:1787–1797.

45. Shah A, Schelbert HR, Schwaiger M, et al. Measurement of regional myocardial blood flow with N-13 ammonia and positron-emission tomography in intact dogs. J Am Coll Cardiol 1985;5:92–100.

46. Schelbert HR, Phelps ME, Huang S-C, et al. N-13 ammonia as an indicator of myocardial blood flow. Circulation 1981;63:1259.

47. Krivokapich J, Smith G, Huang S, et al. $^{13}$N-ammonia myocardial imaging at rest and with exercise in normal volunteers. Circulation 1989;80:1328–1337.

48. Goldstein RA, Mullani NA, Marani SK, et al. Myocardial perfusion with rubidium-82. II. Effects of metabolic and pharmacologic interventions. J Nucl Med 1983;24:907–915.

49. Gould KL, Lipscomb K, Hamilton GW. Physiologic basis for assessing critical coronary stenosis. Am J Cardiol 1974;33:87–94.

50. Gould KL, Schelbert HR, Phelps ME, Hoffman EJ. Noninvasive assessment of coronary stenoses with myocardial perfusion imaging during pharmacologic coronary vasodilation. V. Detection of 47% diameter coronary stenosis with intravenous N-13 ammonia and positron emission tomography in intact dogs. Am J Cardiol 1979;43:200–208.

51. Gould KL. Identifying and measuring severity of coronary artery stenosis: quantitative coronary arteriography and positron emission tomography. Circulation 1988;78:237–245.

52. Goldstein RA, Kirkeeide RL, Smalling RW, et al. Changes in myocardial perfusion reserve after PTCA. Noninvasive assessment with positron tomography. J Nucl Med 1987;28:1262–1267.

53. Gould KL, Martucci JP, Goldberg DI, et al. Short-term cholesterol lowering decreases size and severity of perfusion abnormalities by positron emission tomography after dipyridamole in patients with coronary artery disease. A potential noninvasive marker of healing coronary endothelium. Circulation 1994;89:1530–1538.

54. Deanfield JE, Shea M, Kensett M, et al. Silent myocardial ischaemia due to mental stress. Lancet 1984;2:1001–1005.

55. Deanfield JE, Shea MJ, Wilson RA, et al. Direct effects of smoking on the heart: silent ischemic disturbances of coronary flow. Am J Cardiol 1986;57:1005–1009.

56. Schwaiger M. Myocardial perfusion imaging with PET. J Nucl Med 1994;35:693–698.

57. Schelbert HR, Wisenberg G, Phelps ME, et al. Noninvasive assessment of coronary stenoses by MPI during pharmacologic coronary vasodilation. VI. Detection of CAD in man with IV N-13 NH$_3$ and PET. Am J Cardiol 1982;49:1197–1207.

58. Demer L, Gould K, Goldstein R, et al. Assessment of coronary artery disease severity by positron emission tomography: comparison with quantitative arteriography in 193 patients. Circulation 1989;79:825–835.

59. Stewart R, Schwaiger M, Molina E, et al. Comparison of Rb-82 PET and Tl-201 SPECT imaging for detection of CAD. Am J Cardiol 1991;67:1303–1310.

60. Go RT, Mararde TH, McIntyre WJ, et al. A prospective comparison of Rb-82 PET and Tl-201 SPECT myocardial perfusion imaging utilizing a single stress in the diagnosis of CAD. J Nucl Med 1990;31:1899–1905.

61. Simone GL, Mullani NA, Page DA, Anderson BA Sr. Utilization statistics and diagnostic accuracy of a nonhospital-based positron emission tomographic center for the detection of coronary artery disease using rubidium-82. Am J Phys Imag 1992;7:203–209.

62. Williams BR, Mullani NA, Jansen DE, Anderson BA. A retrospective

study of the diagnostic accuracy of a community hospital-based PET center for the detection of coronary artery disease using rubidium-82. J Nucl Med 1994;35:1586–1592.

63. MacIntyre WJ, Go RT, King JL, et al. Clinical outcome of cardiac patients with negative thallium-201 SPECT and positive rubidium-82 PET myocardial perfusion imaging. J Nucl Med 1993;34:400–404.

64. Gould KL, Goldstein RA, Mullani NA. Economic analysis of clinical positron emission tomography of the heart with rubidium-82. J Nucl Med 1989;30:707–717.

65. Rahimtoola SH. A perspective on the three large multicenter randomized clinical trials of coronary bypass surgery for chronic stable angina. Circulation 1985;72(suppl V):123–135.

66. Braunwald E, Rutherford JD. Reversible ischemic left ventricular dysfunction: evidence for the "hibernating myocardium." J Am Coll Cardiol 1986;8:1467–1470.

67. Braunwald E, Kloner RA. The stunned myocardium: prolonged, postischemic ventricular dysfunction. Circulation 1992;66:1146–1149.

68. Tillisch J, Brunken R, Marshall R, et al. Reversibility of cardiac wall-motion abnormalities predicted by positron emission tomography. N Engl J Med 1986;314:884–888.

69. Dilsizian V, Perrone-Filardi P, Arrighi JA, et al. Concordance and discordance between stress-redistribution-reinjection and rest-redistribution thallium imaging for assessing viable myocardium. Comparison with metabolic activity by positron emission tomography. Circulation 1993;88:941–952.

70. Schelbert HR. Metabolic imaging to assess myocardial viability. J Nucl Med 1994;35(suppl):8S–14S.

71. Schelbert HR. Merits and limitations of radionuclide approaches to viability and future developments. J Nucl Cardiol 1994;1:S86–S96.

72. Maddahi J, Schelbert H, Brunken R, De Carli M. Role of thallium-201 and PET imaging in evaluation of myocardial viability and management of patients with coronary artery disease and left ventricular dysfunction. J Nucl Med 1994;35:707–715.

73. Di Carli MF, Davidson M, Little R, etc. Value of metabolic imaging with positron emission tomography for evaluating prognosis in patients with coronary artery disease and left ventricular dysfunction. Am J Cardiol 1994;73:527–533.

74. Di Carli MF, Asgarzadie BA, Schelbert HR, et al. Quantitative relation between myocardial viability and improvement in heart failure symptoms after revascularization in patients with ischemic cardiomyopathy. Circulation 1995;92:3436–3444.

75. Gropler R, Siegel B, Sampathkumaran K. Dependence of recovery of contractile function on maintenance of oxidative metabolism after myocardial infarction. J Am Coll Cardiol 1992;19:989–997.

76. Gropler R, Geltman E, Sampathkumaran K, et al. Comparison of carbon-11-acetate with fluorine-18-fluorodeoxyglucose for delineating viable myocardium by positron emission tomography. J Am Coll Cardiol 1993;22:1587–1597.

77. Gould KL, Yoshida K, Hess MJ, et al. Myocardial metabolism of fluorodeoxyglucose compared to cell membrane integrity for the potassium analogue rubidium-82 for assessing infarct size in man by PET. J Nucl Med 1991;32:1–9.

78. Vom Dahl J, Muzik O, Wolfe ER Jr, et al. Myocardial rubidium-82 tissue kinetics assessed by dynamic positron emission tomography as a marker of myocardial cell membrane integrity and viability. Circulation 1996;93:238–245.

79. Delforge J, Syrota A, Lancon J-P, etc. Cardiac beta-adrenergic receptor density measured in vivo using PET, CGP 12177 and a new graphical method. J Nucl Med 1991;32:739–748.

80. Syrota A, Comar D, Paillotin G, et al. Muscarinic cholinergic receptor in the human heart evidenced under physiological conditions by positron emission tomography. Proc Natl Acad Sci U S A 1985;82:584–588.

81. Schwaiger M, Hutchins GD, Wieland DM. Noninvasive Evaluation of the Cardiac Sympathetic Nervous System with Positron Emission Tomography. In Bergmann SR, Sobel BE (eds), Positron Emission Tomography of the Heart. Mount Kisco, NY: Futura, 1992;231–254.

82. Wahl RL, Quint LE, Cieslak RD, et al. "Anatometabolic" tumor imaging: fusion of FDG PET with CT or MRI to localize foci of increased activity. J Nucl Med 1993;34:1190–1197.

83. Gritters LS, Francis IR, Zasadny KR, Wahl RL. Initial assessment of positron emission tomography using 2-fluorine-18-2-deoxy-D-glucose in the imaging of malignant melanoma. J Nucl Med 1993;34:1420–1427.

84. Adler LP, Crowe JP, Al-Kaisi NK, Sunshine JL. Evaluation of breast masses and axillary lymph nodes with (F-18) 2-deoxy-2-fluoro-D-glucose PET. Radiology 1993;187:743–750.

85. Patz EF, Lowe VJ, Hoffman JM, et al. Focal pulmonary abnormalities: evaluation with F-18 fluorodeoxyglucose PET scanning. Radiology 1993;188:487–490.

86. Abe Y, Matsuzawa T, Fujiwara T, et al. Clinical assessment of therapeutic effects on cancer using F-18-2-fluoro-2-deoxy-D-glucose and positron emission tomography: preliminary study of lung cancer. Int J Radiat Oncol Biol Phys 1990;19:1005–1010.

87. Patz EF, Lowe VJ, Hoffman JM, et al. Persistent or recurrent bronchogenic carcinoma: detection with PET and 2-(F-18)-2-deoxy-D-glucose. Radiology 1994;191:379–382.

88. Wahl RL, Quint LE, Greenough RL, et al. Staging of mediastinal non–small cell lung cancer with FDG PET, CT, and fusion images: preliminary prospective evaluation. Radiology 1994;191:371–377.

89. Nolop KB, Rhodes CG, Brudin LH, et al. Glucose utilization in vivo by human pulmonary neoplasms. Cancer 1987;60:2682–2689.

90. Griffeth LK, Dehdashti F, McGuire AH, et al. PET evaluation of soft-tissue masses with fluoro-2-deoxy-D-glucose. Radiology 1992;182:185–194.

91. Newman JS, Francis IR, Kaminski MS, Wahl RL. Imaging of lymphoma with PET with 2-(F-18)-fluoro-2-deoxy-D-glucose: correlation with CT. Radiology 1994;190:111–116.

92. Hoffman JM, Waskin HA, Schifter T, et al. FDG-PET in differentiating lymphoma from nonmalignant central nervous system lesions in patients with AIDS. J Nucl Med 1993;34:567–575.

93. Jabour BA, Choi Y, Hoh CK, et al. Extracranial head and neck: PET with 2(F-18)fluoro-2-deoxy-D-glucose and MR imaging correlation. Radiology 1993;186:27–35.

94. Leskinen-Kallio S, Huovinen R, Nagren K, et al. (C-11) methionine quantitation in cancer PET studies. J Comput Assist Tomogr 1992;16:468–474.

95. Valk PE, Mathis CA, Prados MD, et al. Hypoxia in human gliomas: demonstration by PET with fluorine-18-fluoromisonidazole. J Nucl Med 1992;33:2133–2137.

*Textbook of Nuclear Medicine,*
edited by Michael A. Wilson.
Lippincott–Raven Publishers, Philadelphia © 1998.

CHAPTER 18

# Nonendocrine Therapy

G. John Weir

## TREATMENT OF SKELETAL METASTATIC DISEASE

### Historical Overview

Radionuclide treatment of malignancies involving the bone marrow is one of the first recorded medical uses of radioactivity. Marshall Brucer has told the story of early investigations and uses of phosphorus 32 (P-32) and strontium 89 (Sr-89) in polycythemia, leukemias, and metastatic bone disease (1,2). The first patient treatment with Sr-89 took place in 1940. The first article published in the *Journal of Nuclear Medicine* (1960) was devoted to treatment of prostate carcinoma metastatic to bone with a P-32 phosphate complex (3).

Interest in treatment of metastatic bone disease lagged over a number of years. The untimely death of Charles Pecher and the intervention of World War II (1,2) impeded further work with Sr-89. P-32–labeled phosphate continued to be used for polycythemia and some platelet disorders. Toxicity to the bone marrow probably militated against its continued use for skeletal metastatic disease. Many believe that P-32 phosphonate complexes have greater bone marrow toxicity than Sr-89, but this is not well established (4,5). Work with Sr-89 was renewed in 1976 in Europe (6) and in 1977 in the United States (7). The U.S. Food and Drug Administration (FDA) released Sr-89 for use in painful skeletal metastatic disease in 1993.

### Physiology

The agents used for treating skeletal metastatic disease are incorporated into skeletal tissue, into either the bone matrix or bone marrow. They all decay primarily or exclusively by beta emission, and the energy of emission is deposited locally, minimizing whole-body exposure. Sr-89 is a calcium analog and is incorporated into newly forming bone mineral, just like older bone scanning agents. Phos-

phonate complexes are laid down in bone mineral as part of the hydroxyapatite crystal, like the current imaging agents. P-32 has been used both as a phosphonate complex and as P-32 sodium phosphate. The latter formulation preferentially concentrates in reproducing cells and therefore is found especially in bone marrow. All the agents accumulate in bone proportional to bone turnover and are preferentially concentrated at sites of increased deposition of new bone. Metastases commonly stimulate new bone deposition and so concentrate more activity than adjacent normal bone. These agents are usually reserved for use only in metastases that demonstrate bone formation by bone scan. Even metastases that appear lytic by x-ray evaluation show active deposition of bone by scintigraphy; therefore they are appropriate candidates for therapy.

## STRONTIUM 89

### Dosimetry Considerations

Sr-89 has a maximum beta energy of 1.4 meV and a maximum penetration of approximately 5 mm at water density. The half-life is 50.5 days. The amount of administered activity incorporated into bone is quite variable, depending largely on the amount of metastatic disease (8). Excretion of the remainder is primarily renal, with some fecal excretion possible, and retention is greater in patients with extensive metastases. Retention at metastatic sites is greater than that of normal bone. Estimation of the dose delivered to the lesion is difficult because of the short distances involved in absorption of energy, but it has been calculated at approximately 800 to 8,000 rads/mCi (21 to 231 cGy/MBq) (9). The absence of gamma emission simplifies handling of the patient and excreta after administration of the dose. Urinary incontinence presents some inconvenience, but this can be handled in most patients with catheterization for a few days. Toxicity resulting from use of Sr-89 is essentially limited to bone marrow toxicity, discussed in the next section. The material is mildly caus-

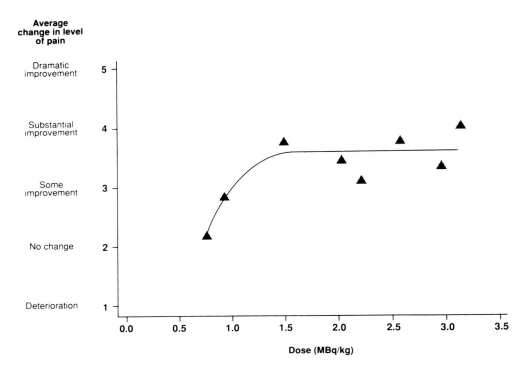

**FIG. 18-1.** Dose-response curve for Sr-89 taken from data on file at Amersham International. Data are combined from U.S. and U.K. trials. Curve is fitted, points are means. (Reprinted with permission from Ackery D, Yardley J. Radionuclide-targeted therapy for the management of metastatic bone pain. Semin Oncol 1993;20[suppl 2]:27–31.)

tic, and administration via a free-flowing intravenous line to prevent soft-tissue damage is appropriate.

**Efficacy**

Not all studies with Sr-89 have shown a clear dose-response relationship. However, the threshold of effectiveness is approximately 20 µCi/kg of body weight (0.7 MBq/kg) (10), and although doses of up to 20 mCi per patient have been used (11,12), it appears that response plateaus at about 40 µCi/kg (1.5 MBq/kg). The dose-response curve (Fig. 18-1) indicates that 40 to 50 µCi/kg is the best dose for most patients. Bone marrow toxicity is definitely observed with the higher doses but is difficult to document at the lower doses. Many patients have depressed blood elements because of previous therapy or bone marrow replacement by metastases.

Unit doses of 4 mCi are readily available and economical, and they fit the dose-response curve quite well. Published reports (6,7,11,13) show that 70% to 80% of patients treated achieve some pain relief; approximately 20% are able to stop all analgesic use and return to activity levels similar to those they enjoyed before the onset of the pain syndrome. Some results are indeed spectacular: Patients who were bedridden with pain have returned to full activity, including work. Results other than pain relief are difficult to document. Some patients respond with evidence of sclerosis of lesions, as seen by x-ray or computed tomographic examination, and with improvement in tumor markers. One placebo-controlled, double-blinded study showed statistically significant reduction in tumor markers (11). This study used a higher dose than most but obtained significant bone marrow depression. Response was measured in a different manner than most other studies, making comparisons difficult, but there was no greater pain control with the higher dose.

Prediction of response in individual patients is elusive. Response has not been related to extent of disease, type of malignancy, location of disease, analgesic dose used, or other discernible parameters. I have treated >100 patients, and the response rate in evaluable patients has been similar to that reported in the literature. My clinical impression is that most patients who did not respond had pain related to soft-tissue or spinal cord involvement in addition to, or instead of, pain due to skeletal metastases.

Response to treatment occurs over days to a week or two, not immediately. A number of patients respond with exacerbation of pain beginning 2 to 14 days after treatment, before relief is noted. Additional, unnecessary radiation therapy may be started if this is forgotten by the patient and referring physician. This "flare" of pain has been noted as a predictor of a good response (13). Responses may last up to 1 year but average 4 to 6 months. Those who respond to the first treatment usually respond to subsequent administrations, but in most cases later responses are not as long-lasting as the first. We have treated patients up to five times, and others relate even more repeat treatments.

The phase III trials of Sr-89 were difficult to quantify because of a large number of unevaluable patients. Response was measured at 3 months, but a number of patients in our series responded well, although pain recurred within 3 months. We wanted to judge these as responders but could not do so on the protocol, so the actual response rates may be slightly higher than those reported from these trials.

Optimal treatment protocols in conjunction with other agents remain to be worked out. It seems reasonable to use local radiation therapy and Sr-89 together when a patient presents with diffuse disease and an area of impending pathologic fracture. Use much earlier in the disease process, in conjunction with other therapy, may be efficacious and may protect from the bone marrow toxicity that is seen with multiple areas of radiation therapy or extensive use of chemotherapy. It is hoped that protocols will be developed to assess these therapeutic questions.

All malignancies when metastatic to bone seem to respond uniformly to treatment. On the other hand, Sr-89 has not been found useful in the treatment of primary bone malignancy.

### Protocol for Treatment with Sr-89

The patient should have documented skeletal metastatic disease by recent bone scan. They should be experiencing pain, and, by clinical judgment, the pain should be due to the metastatic disease. A recent blood count should be available. Although patients with low blood counts have been treated, generally a white blood cell count $\geq 2,500$ and a platelet count $\geq 60,000$ is desirable. The patient, or the patient's agent, should give informed consent for treatment; whether consent is oral or written depends on local practice. The pharmaceutical manufacturer provides educational materials that are convenient and well written. No patient preparation is necessary.

A unit dose of 4 mCi is easy and economical to use. If the patient weighs <45 kg or >90 kg, adjustment for weight is indicated. The dose should be documented in the dose calibrator. Although dose calibrator measurements of beta emitters have poor accuracy, they are sufficient to ensure against major mistakes. Even though the decay is beta, use of a syringe shield during injection protects the administrator from auger radiation.

To ensure against extravasation, a free-flowing intravenous line should be started. Use of a three-way stopcock allows rinsing of the dose syringe and checking during infusion to ensure that the intravenous line is still infusing correctly. If extravasation inadvertently occurs, only mild irritation is expected, and tissue destruction is unlikely. The extravasated portion of the dose is absorbed faster if the area is treated with warm compresses. The area of infusion can be checked with a survey meter to document the absence of extravasation. The syringe and infusion apparatus can again be checked in the dose calibrator after infusion to document administered dose. These materials become radioactive waste and must be handled as such.

Appropriate follow-up of the patient should include blood counts at periodic intervals to document any change in counts. This can be arranged by the referring physician or by the nuclear medicine unit, depending on local custom, but these patients require that their primary or oncology physician be in overall control of their care.

## OTHER AGENTS

Phosphonate complexes concentrate in bone mineral. Metallic ions can be chelated with phosphonate complexes and the resulting compound utilized to deliver metallic radioactive ions to bone mineral. This mechanism has been exploited with two agents currently under evaluation for use in treatment of metastatic bone disease.

Samarium 153 (Sm-153) ethylenediaminetetramethylene phosphonate (EDTMP) has been used at the University of Missouri and at Fremantle Hospital, Western Australia (14,15). Sm-153 decays with emission of two beta particles with an average penetration of 0.83 mm in water. Twenty-eight percent of decays result in a 103-keV gamma, which allows imaging. The half-life of 46.3 hours is significantly shorter than Sr-89. This may have advantages for handling of patients and excreta.

Diphosphonate chelated to rhenium 186 with hydroxyethylidene diphosphonate (Re-186[Sn]HEDP) has been developed and evaluated at the University of Cincinnati (16,17). It emits a beta particle with penetration of 1.0 mm in soft tissue and 0.5 mm in dense bone. A 137-keV gamma ray with 9% abundance allows imaging. The half-life of 3.8 days minimizes patient and handler exposures but allows more time for processing and shipping than the shorter half-life of Sm-153.

Published reports for both of these phosphonate complexes indicate that toxicity and response profiles are very similar to Sr-89. These two agents remain under investigation and review by the FDA. (Note: Sm-153 ethylenediaminetetramethylene phosphonate has now been released by the FDA and is commercially available.) Nonradioactive pharmaceuticals with a direct action on bone have been assessed for use in treating metastatic bone pain, but results have been disappointing (18).

## OTHER NONENDOCRINE THERAPY

These topics are well summarized in *Nuclear Medicine Therapy*, a textbook by John Harbart (19). P-32 administered as sodium phosphate has been used extensively in the treatment of polycythemia rubra vera and various thrombocythemias. It is used less now than before because newer nonradioactive agents have been developed. It is still the agent of choice for patients with thrombocytosis as the primary problem.

Colloidal chromic phosphate P-32 is occasionally used for treatment of omental disease especially due to ovarian carcinoma. Gold 198 and colloidal yttrium 90 have been used in the past but are no longer available. Colloidal P-32 chromic phosphate is also used in the treatment of malignant ascites and pleural effusions, which develop as a result of peritoneal or pleural seeding with tumor and are resistant to conventional therapies, such as sclerosing agents in pleural effusions. The suitability of this treatment can be determined by instillation of a conventional unabsorbable radionuclide (technetium 99m sulfur colloid), which would emulate the therapeutic distribution. Imaging the patient would determine if there would be a suitable distribution of therapeutic tracer and what volume of carrier fluid and what maneuvers should be used to ensure this distribution.

Beta-emitting isotopes, especially yttrium 90, have been used with applicators to deliver localized superficial radiation therapy, primarily in the treatment of pterygia.

Various nuclides and preparations have been used for intra-articular therapy, especially in rheumatoid arthritis. Interest in this area continues, but no agent is currently approved for use.

A variety of antibodies and chelating agents have been used in experimental procedures for delivering radiation to malignancies, and some of these may be approved for routine use in the future. The special cases of endocrine and neuroendocrine therapies are described in Chapters 9 and 14.

## REFERENCES

1. Brucer M. Vignettes in Nuclear Medicine. Nos. 7, 81. St. Louis: Mallinckrodt Nuclear, 1966–1983.
2. Brucer MA. Chronology of Nuclear Medicine. St. Louis: Heritage, 1990.
3. Kaplan E, Fels IG, Kotlowski BR, et al. Therapy of carcinoma of the prostate metastatic to bone with P-32 labeled condensed phosphate. J Nucl Med 1960;1:1–13.
4. Silberstein EB, Elgazzar AH, Kapilivsky A. Phosphorus-32 radiopharmaceuticals for the treatment of painful osseous metastases. Semin Nucl Med 1992;22:17–27.
5. Silberstein EB, Williams C. Strontium-89 therapy for the pain of osseous metastases. J Nucl Med 1985;26:345–348.
6. Firusian N, Mellin P, Schmidt GC. Results of 89-strontium therapy in patients with carcinoma of the prostate and incurable pain from bone metastases: a preliminary report. J Urol 1976;116:764–768.
7. Robinson RG. Radionuclides for the alleviation of bone pain in advanced malignancy. Clin Oncol (R Coll Radiol) 1986;5:39–49.
8. Blake GM, Zivanovic MA, McEwan AJ, Ackery DM. Sr-89 therapy: strontium kinetics in disseminated carcinoma of the prostate. Eur J Nucl Med 1986;12:447–454.
9. Breen SL, Powe JE, Porter AT. Dose estimation in strontium-89 radiotherapy of metastatic prostate carcinoma. J Nucl Med 1992;33:1316–1323.
10. Ackery D, Yardley J. Radionuclide-targeted therapy for the management of metastatic bone pain. Semin Oncol 1993;20(suppl 2):27–31.
11. Porter AT, McEwan AJB, Powe JE, et al. Results of a randomized phase-III trial to evaluate the efficacy of strontium-89 adjuvant to local field external beam irradiation in the management of endocrine resistant metastatic prostate cancer. Int J Radiat Oncol Biol Phys 1993;25:805–813.
12. Kloiber R, Molnar CP, Barnes M. Sr-89 therapy for metastatic bone disease: scintigraphic and radiographic follow-up. Radiology 1987;163:719–723.
13. Robinson RG, Preston DF, Spicer JA, Baxter, KG. Radionuclide therapy of intractable bone pain: emphasis on strontium-89. Semin Nucl Med 1992;22:28–32.
14. Farhanghi M, Holmes RA, Volkert WA, et al. Samarium-153-EDTMP: pharmacokinetics, toxicity and pain response using an escalating dose schedule in treatment of metastatic bone cancer. J Nucl Med 1992;33:1451–1458.
15. Turner JH, Claringbold PG, Hetherington EL, et al. A phase 1 study of samarium-153 ethylenediaminetetramethylene phosphonate therapy for disseminated skeletal metastases. J Clin Oncol 1989;7:1926–1931.
16. Maxon III HR, Schroeder LE, Thomas SR, et al. Re-186(Sn)HEDP for treatment of painful osseous metastases: initial clinical experience in 20 patients with hormone-resistant prostate cancer. Radiology 1990;176:155–159.
17. Maxon III HR, Thomas SR, Hertzberg VS, et al. Rhenium-186 hydroxyethylidene diphosphonate for the treatment of painful osseous metastases. Semin Nucl Med 1992;22:33–40.
18. Campa III JA, Payne R. The management of intractable bone pain: a clinician's perspective. Semin Nucl Med 1992;22:3–10.
19. Harbart J. Nuclear Medicine Therapy. New York: Thieme, 1987.

*Textbook of Nuclear Medicine,*
edited by Michael A. Wilson.
Lippincott–Raven Publishers, Philadelphia © 1998.

CHAPTER 19

# Deep Venous Thrombosis

James E. Seabold

Acute deep venous thrombosis (DVT) is the most common disease of the vascular system. There are approximately 5 million cases of DVT per year in the United States, and approximately 10% of these patients have pulmonary embolus as a dynamic complication (1,2). More than 90% of pulmonary emboli originate in the lower limbs, and up to 70% of patients with DVT have a positive lower limb contrast venogram (1–4). Moreover, 50% to 67% of patients with DVT eventually develop post-thrombotic syndrome and have a high incidence of recurrent DVT (5,6).

## CLINICAL DIAGNOSIS OF DVT

Unfortunately, a clinical diagnosis of DVT is not very reliable and is incorrect approximately 50% of the time. In serial follow-up studies, 40% to 60% of patients with positive lower limb contrast venograms are asymptomatic (1–4,7–9). In patients with symptoms thought to be due to DVT, normal venogram rates range from 46% to 70%. Thus, in patients with an increased risk for DVT, a high index of clinical suspicion is needed to initiate the appropriate diagnostic study. Venous stasis, endothelial injury, and altered coagulability in various combinations are the major factors that initiate DVT (1,2,8).

A significant step in establishing the diagnosis of DVT is the clinical recognition of which patients should undergo diagnostic testing (1,2,8). Anyone with sudden swelling of a lower limb, especially if accompanied by pain or tenderness, is a candidate. A high index of suspicion for DVT is needed in patients with predisposing factors, such as recent hip, knee, or abdominal surgery; trauma; pregnancy; stasis secondary to congestive heart failure; prior DVT; varicose veins or inactivity from illness; obesity; hypercoagulable states secondary to birth control medications; polycythemia or dysproteinemia; and accelerated clotting factors, either familial or associated with various malignancies. Noninvasive imaging should be considered in these patients even if there are only minimal signs or symptoms, particularly in the postoperative period (1,7–9).

## CLINICAL SEQUELAE OF DVT

All lower limb thrombi do not pose the same risk of embolization. Most thrombi arise in the calf in the soleal sinuses or near a venous valve, and 20% to 45% of thrombi propagate to the iliofemoral veins, which greatly increase the likelihood of pulmonary emboli (1–4,7). In one prospective study of 101 consecutive patients who had symptoms of DVT, 88% had proximal deep vein thrombi detected by contrast venography. Fifty-one percent of these patients had high-probability ventilation-perfusion lung scans, even though they did not have symptoms of pulmonary embolism (4). Furthermore, even in the absence of clinical suspicion for pulmonary emboli, 35% to 51% of patients with clots detected above the knee have evidence of pulmonary emboli (1–4).

Although most pulmonary emboli originate above the knee, there is a high correlation between distal vein (popliteal and below-the-knee) DVT and postphlebitic syndrome, skin pigmentation, and leg ulcers. Approximately two of every three patients who have an acute lower limb DVT develop signs of postphlebitic syndrome within 3 years (5,6). In addition, one in every five patients has symptoms severe enough to interfere with daily life, and approximately one in seven is incapacitated to the extent of not being able to work. Controversy continues over the effectiveness of thrombolytic agents in preventing postphlebitic syndrome and whether sufficient emboli arise from below the knee to warrant anticoagulation. Nevertheless, early diagnosis and anticoagulant therapy of lower limb DVT, including thrombi below the knee, would appear to be indicated in the majority of patients.

## DVT DETECTION

The non–nuclear medicine methods of detection of DVT rely primarily on the indirect recognition of altered vascular pathways of venous return that result from partial or total venous occlusion. There is considerable interest in the role of magnetic resonance imaging (MRI) for DVT. MR angiography provides the potential for imaging all important venous channels, even proximal upper limb veins. To date, however, the cost and limited availability of MRI have restricted the general acceptance of this modality. Computed tomography (CT) can detect DVT in the abdomen, pelvis, and limbs (2). CT is superior to conventional contrast venography for proximal disease and should be considered for use in complicated cases involving the abdomen or pelvis.

### Contrast Venography

The standard for the detection of DVT has been contrast venography, and all other techniques are usually compared with its results. With the use of a saline flush and nonionic contrast media, side effects are few, and the incidence of postvenographic thrombophlebitis is 1% to 3% (2,8,10). The diagnostic criteria for a positive venogram are intraluminal filling defect or abrupt vessel cut-off with signs of collateral circulation (7,8).

Contrast venography, however, is an invasive procedure and has certain limitations. In 20% to 25% of patients, either the procedure cannot be performed or there is inadequate visualization of the deep system to permit detection of thrombi (2,8). An inadequate study is often due to intraluminal changes from prior venous thrombosis or dilution of contrast material in the upper venous system. Difficult venous access due to obesity, severe edema, or cellulitis of a limb can make this procedure time consuming and an adequate study hard to obtain. Contrast media allergy, congestive heart failure, and renal insufficiency all increase the incidence of side effects or complications. In addition, a portable study technique is often needed for patients who are too unstable to be transported to an angiography suite.

### Labeled Fibrinogen Test

Other methods have been used for several years, both to supplement contrast venography and to improve DVT detection. Iodine 125 (I-125)–labeled fibrinogen scanning was one of the early noninvasive techniques (7–9). The sensitivity of this technique was poor above the midthigh due to increased background activity from the bladder and the larger adjacent blood vessels. There was also a 24- to 48-hour time delay to obtain results. Because of the high cost of production and concern about transmission of infectious agents via a labeled blood product, this radiopharmaceutical has been withdrawn from the market.

### Plethysmography

Plethysmography, which measures the capacity of the venous system to fill and empty, is another noninvasive screening technique (2,7–9). It is most useful in symptomatic

patients who have had no prior episodes of DVT; however, it does not identify the specific cause of decreased venous flow or distinguish between acute or old DVT. This technique is not reliable in patients with cord injuries, strokes, arterial vascular insufficiency, impaired venous return from right heart failure, external compression of veins, or prior DVT. The sensitivity of this method below the knee is only 30%, so it was often performed in conjunction with labeled fibrinogen (8,9). Further, the sensitivity of plethysmography varies greatly, depending on the patient population. A prospective study of postoperative orthopedic patients found the sensitivity of plethysmography to be <50% for detecting early proximal leg DVT, compared with contrast venography results (9).

### Radionuclide Venography

#### Technetium 99m Macroaggregated Albumin Venography

Technetium 99m–labeled macroaggregated albumin (Tc-99m MAA) is a noninvasive procedure that is used as a screening technique and has an accuracy for DVT in the thigh of 80% to 90% (7,11,12). Tc-99m MAA venography (Fig. 19-1) can be performed before and in conjunction with a lung scan by

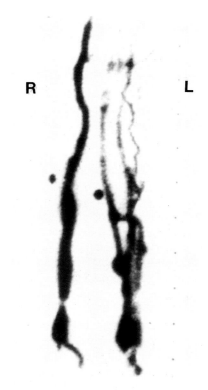

**FIG. 19-1.** This 36-year-old patient presented with left lower limb swelling and pain of 2 days' duration. Tc-99m MAA venogram shows a normal pattern of radioactivity in the deep venous system of the right leg and abrupt cut-off of activity in the deep system of the left calf, with evidence of collaterals in the left thigh. This confirms a left DVT.

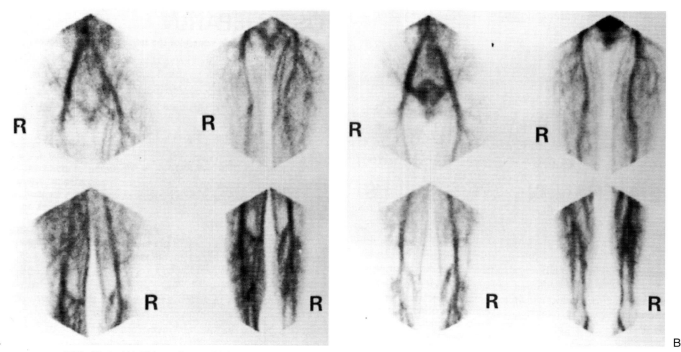

A                                                                         B

**FIG. 19-2. (A)** This collage of labeled RBC scans shows the venous system of the anterior abdomen and thighs (upper) and the posterior thighs (left lower) and legs (right lower). There is asymmetry of venous channels with collateralization from an extensive left-sided DVT (right side indicated, *R*). **(B)** This collage of the same patient shows views obtained 10 days after heparin therapy, when the Tc-99m RBC venography has reverted to normal. (Reprinted with permission from Lisbona R, Derbekyan V, Novales-Diaz JA, Rush CL. Tc-99m red blood cell venography in deep venous thrombosis of the lower limb. An overview. Clin Nucl Med 1985;10:208–224.)

injecting the radiotracer in the dorsal pedal vein. Tourniquets are applied just above the ankle to evaluate the dynamic flow and patency of the deep venous system. It is most useful in acute-onset symptomatic patients who have had no prior DVT because it does not reveal the cause of the venous obstruction (intrinsic vs. extrinsic or acute vs. old DVT).

Some Tc-99m MAA scans may show a "hot spot" on delayed images because the tagged aggregate adheres to the thrombus. This can also occur when radiotracer is trapped behind a venous valve, however, and by itself it is not a reliable sign of DVT (11). Tc-99m MAA venograms require nearly complete venous obstruction for a positive test and are unreliable in the calf because of the numerous vessels. Many venographic studies are performed with a single set of tourniquets placed at the ankles. Using standard diagnostic criteria in 20 consecutive patients, a 20% false-positive interpretation rate was observed when tourniquets were placed only above the ankle rather than above both the knee and ankle (12). Additional tourniquets placed above the knee decreased the false-positive studies by enhancing the preferential blood flow through the deep venous system.

### Tc-99m–Labeled Red Blood Cell Venography

Tc-99m–labeled red blood cell (RBC) or Tc-99m human serum albumin (HSA) blood pool venography is a simple noninvasive test that affords a direct image of the venous system (Fig. 19-2), from which abnormal morphology can be inferred (13,14). In the limbs, blood pool images preferentially show the deep venous system because this is a low-pressure compartment that holds a large fraction of the total blood volume compared with the smaller arterial channels or the superficial veins. In DVT, clotted veins become ill defined or interrupted on the scintigraph because of the reduced blood content of the affected channels. Venous congestion and visualization of collateral channels that serve as alternative pathways of drainage are also seen in some DVT cases. The combined results of six clinical studies yielded a mean sensitivity of 89% and a mean specificity of 84% for lower-limb DVT (14).

Tc-99m RBC venography relies on alterations in the normal venous anatomy, but it does not determine the cause of the venous obstruction or the likely age of the obstruction. In addition, femoral vein anatomy is variable, conforming to the conventional single popliteal-femoral vein anatomy only 65% of the time (7). Approximately 5% of patients have complete duplication of the femoral and popliteal veins, and approximately 20% to 25% have duplication of the femoral vein. These additional vessels can mimic collateral vessels and lead to a false-positive interpretation of the radionuclide venogram. Finally, the specificity of an abnormal radionuclide venogram decreases markedly in patients who have had prior episodes of DVT (11,14).

## Ultrasonography

Duplex and triplex or color Doppler ultrasonography are currently used extensively in many centers as the initial screening procedure for DVT (2,15–20). In symptomatic patients, pooled results of duplex Doppler studies yielded a sensitivity of 92% to 95% with a specificity of 97% to 100% from the popliteal vein to the groin (15,16). Equivocal studies are obtained in 1% to 6% of patients because of gross obesity, severe wound edema, or poor compliance, but Doppler also reveals other causes of leg swelling in 5% to 15% of patients.

The enhancement of real-time ultrasound with color Doppler permits real-time encoding of Doppler flow signals as a color map, allowing direct visualization of flow within vessels. Color Doppler is less demanding and less time-consuming than conventional duplex imaging. It also has been reported to have a sensitivity equal to that of duplex Doppler imaging and to be more accurate in the symptomatic outpatient population (16,17).

"Compressibility" of a deep vein is considered one of the most sensitive and specific criteria for Doppler detection of DVT (15,16). In one series of 36 patients with intermediate-probability lung scans, however, Doppler compression detected lower-limb DVT in only two of 15 (13%) patients who had pulmonary emboli detected by angiography (18). Even with the addition of color Doppler, the sensitivity of this method is poor for the detection of calf DVT (17,19). In addition, the significance of abnormal findings is uncertain in patients with prior episodes of DVT, unless a normal study is obtained in the interim (16,20). Approximately 50% of patients show venous compression abnormalities indistinguishable from the original findings 6 to 31 months after an acute episode of DVT. A test that indicates if there is acute or active DVT is often needed to improve diagnostic accuracy in patients who have had prior episodes of DVT or postphlebitic syndrome.

Color Doppler has been shown to have a poor sensitivity for the detection of proximal DVT in asymptomatic high-risk patients (2,17,19). The pooled results of six color Doppler studies yielded an overall sensitivity of 59% for the detection of proximal DVT in asymptomatic high-risk patients. A multicenter prospective study of prophylactic antithrombotic therapy in 319 patients undergoing elective hip or knee replacement revealed a sensitivity of only 38% for proximal DVT and 20% for the entire limb, when color Doppler was compared with contrast venography (19). Thus, the type of patient to be evaluated is an important factor in determining which imaging study should be performed. Although Doppler imaging can be repeated in 3 to 7 days, there are many patients at risk for proximal DVT or pulmonary embolus in which a rapid and sensitive diagnostic test that detects the presence of active DVT would complement the results of color Doppler.

## ACTIVE THROMBUS DETECTION

Nuclear medicine provides the potential for detection of the ongoing thrombus formation, hence the means of discriminating between old and active new clot formation. This would be especially valuable in determining the clinical significance of venous thrombosis in patients who return for the diagnosis of pulmonary embolism when there is a past history of embolic disease. Labeled fibrinogen scanning (described earlier) is the earliest agent used for the purpose of detecting active clot formation.

### Labeled Platelets

Indium 111 (In-111)–labeled platelet scintigraphy (Fig. 19-3) is a sensitive and specific test for the detection of active DVT (21,22). Approximately 15% to 30% of patients, however, require 18- to 24-hour delayed imaging for "diagnostic results," particularly patients with venous stasis or low-grade thrombosis. Another limitation is the high number of false-negative scans in patients receiving concurrent heparin or warfarin therapy (Fig. 19-4). Heparin therapy should be withheld for 4 to 8 hours before platelet labeling and should not be restarted until positive images for DVT are obtained. This technique also requires 1.5 to 2.0 hours for labeling and rein-

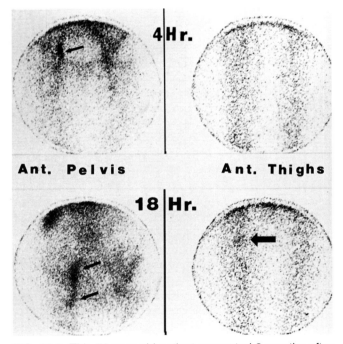

**FIG. 19-3.** This 72-year-old patient presented 3 months after a hip fracture with progressive right leg pain and swelling of 5 days' duration. The In-111 platelet scan shows increased tracer localization along the course of the right common iliac vein (*arrow* in upper left image) at 4 hours, with progression by 18 hours (*arrows* in lower left image). A new focus was also identified in the right thigh (*large arrow* in right lower image).

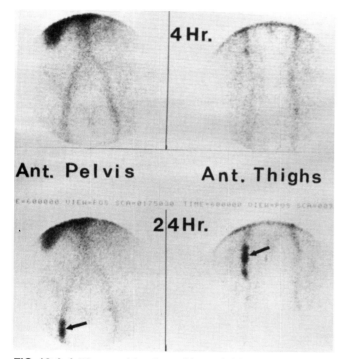

**FIG. 19-4.** A 50-year-old patient with a painful swollen right calf. In-111 platelet images show asymmetric blood pool pattern in the thighs at 4 hours, evolving over 24 hours into a discrete linear pattern (*arrow*) in the right thigh. This is an example of an equivocal 4-hour scan in a patient who was receiving intravenously administered heparin up to 4 hours before imaging.

jection of the patient's platelets. Venous trauma, venipuncture, or persistent asymmetric increased blood pool activity in the popliteal or inguinal regions can cause false-positive studies (22). The availability and cost of In-111 oxine and the time required to obtain a diagnostic study have limited the use of this procedure in many centers. Tc-99m hexamethylpropyleneamine oxime–labeled platelet scintigraphy has been reported to be a useful alternative method for diagnosing active DVT and avoids the need to use In-111 oxine (23).

## Labeled Antibodies

New radiopharmaceuticals are evolving for the detection of acute DVT (24). The small molecular size of Fab' and (Fab')$_2$ fragments of monoclonal antibodies allows renal filtration that results in a more rapid clearance of blood-background activity and earlier diagnostic imaging. Radiolabeled antiplatelet antibodies and Tc-99m–labeled T2G1s antifibrin antibody have undergone clinical trials. Monoclonal antibodies specific for plasmin-digested fibrin, including GC4, 15C5, 3B6/22, and radiolabeled thrombus-binding peptides have also shown promise as thrombus imaging agents.

Tc-99m T2G1 antifibrin has undergone fairly extensive human clinical trials. Immediate blood pool images are obtained, as well as 1.5- to 2.0-hour and 4- to 6-hour

images after intravenous radiopharmaceutical injection. Tc-99m labeling allows 2- to 4-minute planar images to be acquired, compared to 10- to 15-minute images for In-111–labeled agents. Another advantage is that this agent localizes at the site of active thrombus formation in patients receiving anticoagulants. Limitations include dissociation of labeled Tc-99m and lysis of the labeled antibody from the clot, poor binding to "chronic" thrombi, a delay of 2 to 6 hours before diagnostic results can be obtained in many patients, and a study cost that is likely to be greater than Doppler imaging.

## Future Agents

Radiolabeled thrombus-binding peptides that have very rapid renal clearance appear to be the most promising new radiopharmaceuticals for the detection of DVT (24). Small synthetic peptides that bind to platelets have been designed to mimic the binding of larger proteins involved in the clotting process and are not likely to initiate a human immune response. In humans, Tc-99m–labeled synthetic peptide (P-280) has shown good localization in acute DVT by 1 to 4 hours, and this agent is currently completing phase III trials (Fig. 19-5). Early studies of P-748 have shown that this peptide may afford a more rapid test for the detection of active arterial and venous thrombi, even at 1 hour (Fig. 19-6). Not

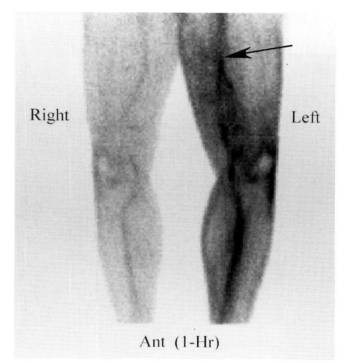

**FIG. 19-5.** This 23-year-old patient presented with a 4-day history of left leg pain and swelling. The 1-hour P-280 anterior view scan shows abnormal uptake starting in the thigh (*arrow*) and continuing distally along the active DVT at 1 hour. On Doppler ultrasound, a femoropopliteal clot was identified.

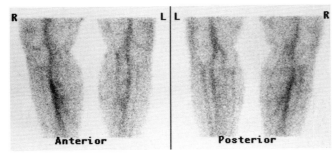

**FIG. 19-6.** This 46-year-old man with left hemiplegia and prior myocardial infarction presented with 1 to 2 weeks of intermittent left-sided chest pain, dyspnea, and bilateral pitting edema of the lower limbs. A Tc-99m P-748 peptide scan shows abnormal localization along the course of a deep vein in both popliteal regions and calves (right greater than left), indicating bilateral active venous thrombosis. Pulmonary embolism was found on ventilation-perfusion lung scanning.

only do they have clinical utility in patients with postphlebitic syndrome and suspected DVT, they also hold promise for the detection of the arterial or venous emboli.

Radiolabeled peptides can be used in patients with a high suspicion for DVT and a negative Doppler examination, rather than waiting 3 to 10 days for a repeat ultrasound examination. It can add specificity for acute DVT in patients with prior episodes of DVT and abnormal Doppler findings to help differentiate between postphlebitic syndrome and acute DVT. In addition, active thrombosis in accessory or duplicated deep veins may be missed by ultrasound techniques but detected with these agents.

## REFERENCES

1. Moser KM. Venous thromboembolism. Am Rev Resp 1990;141:235–249.
2. Weinmann EE, Salzman EW. Deep-vein thrombosis. N Engl J Med 1994;331:1630–1641.
3. Kruit WHJ, De Boer AC, Sing AK, Van Roon F. The significance of venography in the management of patients with clinically suspected pulmonary embolism. J Intern Med 1991;230:333–339.
4. Huisman MV, Buller HR, ten Cate JW, et al. Unexpected high prevalence of silent pulmonary embolism in patients with deep venous thrombosis. Chest 1989;95:498–502.
5. Strandness DE Jr, Langlois Y, Cramer M, et al. Long-term sequelae of acute venous thrombosis. JAMA 1983;250:1289–1292.
6. Monnreal M, Martorell A, Callejas JM, et al. Venographic assessment of deep vein thrombosis and risk of developing post-thrombotic syndrome: a prospective study. J Intern Med 1993;233:233–238.
7. Ferris EJ. Deep venous thrombosis and pulmonary embolism: correlative evaluation and therapeutic implications. AJR Am J Roentgenol 1992;159:1149–1155.
8. Kramer FL, Teitelbaum G, Merli GJ. Panvenography and pulmonary angiography in the diagnosis of deep venous thrombosis and pulmonary thromboembolism. Radiol Clin North Am 1986;24:397–418.
9. Hull RD, Raskob GE, Gent M, et al. Effectiveness of intermittent pneumatic leg compression for preventing deep vein thrombosis after total hip replacement. JAMA 1990;263:2313–2317.
10. Morris TW. X-ray contrast media: where are we now, and where are we going? Radiology 1993;188:11–16.
11. Hayt DB, Blatt CJ, Freeman LM. Radionuclide venography: its place as a modality for the investigation of thromboembolic phenomena. Semin Nucl Med 1977;7:263–281.
12. Vansant JP, Habibian RM, Melton RE. The effect of varying tourniquet applications on the flow pattern of lower extremity radionuclide venography. Clin Nucl Med 1990;15:783–786.
13. Leclerc JR, Wolfson C, Arzoumanian A, et al. Technetium-99m red blood cell venography in patients with clinically suspected deep vein thrombosis: a prospective study. J Nucl Med 1988;29:1498–1506.
14. Pinson AG, Becker DM, Philbrick JT, Parekh JS. Tc-99m-RBC venography in the diagnosis of deep venous thrombosis of the lower extremity: a systematic review of the literature. J Nucl Med 1991;32:2324–2338.
15. White RH, McGahan JP, Daschbach MM, Hartling RP. Diagnosis of deep-vein thrombosis using duplex ultrasound. Ann Intern Med 1989;111:297–304.
16. Cronan JJ. Venous thromboembolic disease: the role of US. Radiology 1993;186:619–630.
17. Mattos MA, Londrey GL, Leutz DW, et al. Color-flow duplex scanning for the surveillance and diagnosis of acute deep venous thrombosis. J Vasc Surg 1992;15:366–376.
18. Quinn RJ, Nour R, Butler SP, et al. Pulmonary embolism in patients with intermediate probability lung scans: diagnosis with Doppler venous US and D-dimer measurement. Radiology 1994;190:509–511.
19. Davidson BL, Elliott CG, Lensing AWA. Low accuracy of color Doppler ultrasound in the detection of proximal leg vein thrombosis in asymptomatic high-risk patients. Ann Intern Med 1992;117:735–738.
20. Baxter GM, Duffy P, MacKechnie S. Color Doppler ultrasound of the post-phlebitic limb: sounding a cautionary note. Clin Radiol 1991;43:301–304.
21. Ezekowitz MD, Pope CF, Sostman HD, et al. Indium-111 platelet scintigraphy for the diagnosis of acute venous thrombosis. Circulation 1986;73:668–674.
22. Seabold JE, Conrad GR, Kimball DA, et al. Pitfalls in establishing the diagnosis of deep venous thrombophlebitis by indium-111 platelet scintigraphy. J Nucl Med 1988;29:1169–1180.
23. Honkanen T, Jauhola S, Karppinen K, et al. Venous thrombosis: a controlled study on the performance of scintigraphy with Tc-99m-HMPAO-labeled platelets versus venography. Nucl Med Commun 1992;13:88–94.
24. Seabold JE, Rosebrough SF. Will a radiolabeled antibody replace indium-111-platelets to detect active thrombus? J Nucl Med 1994;35:1738–1740.

*Textbook of Nuclear Medicine,*
edited by Michael A. Wilson.
Lippincott–Raven Publishers, Philadelphia © 1998.

CHAPTER 20

# Nonimmunoassay Laboratory Tests

G. John Weir

Laboratory tests, including blood volumes, Schilling tests, and urea breath tests, are usually only a small portion of the work load in nuclear medicine practices. However, these and other laboratory-like tests have been quite important in the development of our specialty (1). Some of these tests have been widely used in the past, as is attested by the majority of references being >20 years old. The paucity of use today is not the result of inaccuracy or difficulty in performance; rather, the lessons learned from prior use have developed the referring physician's knowledge to the point that we no longer need to use these tests as frequently. This may account for the less frequent use of blood volumes recently. When blood volume determination was popular in the 1950s, clinicians were not able to estimate blood volume and surgical blood losses with precision. The use of blood volumes taught them to estimate losses more accurately, and continued use of the test became less necessary. Other tests are less commonly used today because of improvements in technology and understanding of physiology. Unfortunately, the radiation hysteria gripping many people and the political problems associated with disposal of radioactive waste have also contributed to the declining use of these tests.

These tests are all a form of tracer chemistry. In their simplest form, a known quantity of tracer is added to an unknown volume, mixing occurs, and a known quantity of the mixture in question is removed and quantitated. The ratio of the quantity measured after mixing to the quantity added is multiplied by the volume removed to obtain the unknown volume. In the case of a radioactive tracer:

$$\frac{\text{Activity added} \times \text{sample volume}}{\text{Activity in sample}} = \text{Unknown volume}$$

The prerequisites for such a test are presented in Table 20-1. In addition to the absolute requirements listed, it is helpful if the tracer can be easily detected with high accuracy and if the tracer is inexpensive and readily available. Radioactive tracers meet the absolute requirements very well, and, although they are readily available, their infrequent use makes them relatively expensive compared to the more routinely used imaging tracers. The unique utility of radiotracers is their lack of biological toxicity. We can detect radioactivity in minute amounts (parts per trillion or greater). Therefore, nearly any chemical entity, if made radioactive, can be administered to living organisms, including human, in such small amounts that toxic reactions are nonexistent but the desired metabolic pathways can be traced accurately.

## BLOOD VOLUMES

In principle, blood volume determination is a straightforward tracer problem. Complications arise because of the following factors:

- The blood is not a single system but has two components: plasma and red blood cell (RBC) mass.
- Uniform mixing is not readily achieved, so labeled RBCs must be allowed to circulate for 30 to 60 minutes to ensure uniform mixing, especially in patients with splenomegaly.
- Plasma tracers exhibit leakage into extravascular fluids.

The volume of white cells and platelets is negligible and does not affect the measurement. Many patients in whom we wish to do these studies have splenomegaly, and sampling must be done early enough that plasma leakage is minimal but late enough to ensure uniform mixing.

### History

The measurement of plasma volume was stimulated by studies of hemorrhagic shock (2). The early dyes used were unable to trace the loss of plasma during shock, whereas radioactive labels allowed plasma loss to be traced. RBC volume had been measured with phosphorus 32 (P-32) (3) and radioiron (4), but P-32 was eluted from the cells and radioiron was difficult to acquire. Also, radioiron is later reused by the bone marrow, which complicates the measurement. Sterling and Gray (5) discovered that chromium

**TABLE 20-1.** *Absolute requirements for tracer measurements*

The tracer must not change (or be toxic to) the system to be measured.

The volume added to the system must be so small as to be negligible (or is known and therefore can be taken into account in the calculations).

The system to be measured must not alter the tracer to preclude its measurement.

The tracer must mix uniformly with the system to be measured.

The tracer must remain within the system to be measured.

51 (Cr-51) could label RBCs with fewer problems, and it has become the accepted agent.

## Pathophysiology

The RBC mass is pathologically elevated in polycythemia. Secondary polycythemia arises from conditions that impair oxygen delivery to the tissues, including pulmonary diseases, abnormal hemoglobinopathies, sleep apnea, and cardiac disorders. Primary polycythemia occurs in polycythemia rubra vera, which is probably a relative of the leukemias. Measurement of the RBC mass alone does not distinguish between primary and secondary forms of polycythemia because a relative increase in the concentration of hemoglobin occurs in stress erythrocytosis, often referred to as Gaisböck's syndrome. The problem in this condition is a contracted plasma volume rather than an increase in absolute RBC mass. It tends to occur in hypertensive, middle-aged males and can only be distinguished with certainty by the measurement of the RBC mass. Plasma volume alterations also occur in congestive heart failure, low serum protein conditions, and debilitating illnesses. Complex situations with multiple organ disease can be difficult to sort out, and plasma volume determinations can help to guide therapy.

## Radiopharmaceutical

RBC mass is determined with Cr-51, which is commercially available as sodium chromate. When incubated with whole blood or RBCs, the radioactive chromate ion freely diffuses into the RBCs. Once inside the cell, the chromate is reduced to chromic ion ($Cr+3$), which is retained in the cell, bound to proteins. The chromate ions remaining in the mixture can be reduced to chromic ion with ascorbic acid, and no further labeling will occur. The spleen is the critical organ and receives a dose of 3.9 mrad (0.039 mGy)/µCi (0.037 MBq) administered dose. A common dose for RBC mass determination is 50 µCi (1.85 MBq), resulting in a dose of approximately 200 mrad (0.2 cGy) (6). The whole-body dose from 50 µCi (1.85 MBq) of Cr-51 approximates 14 mrad (0.14 mGy) (7).

The plasma volume is determined using human serum albumin labeled with iodine 125 (I-125), and the critical organ is the blood, receiving 26 mrad (0.26 mGy) from a dose of 10 µCi (0.37 MBq) (6).

## Procedure

### Plasma Volume

I-125–labeled albumin is usually obtained as unit-dose syringes. One syringe can be used to prepare a standard for all syringes in a shipment lot. If this is done, the syringes should be checked to ensure consistent activity content through the lot. One syringe is injected intravenously via an indwelling intravenous catheter, and the injection should be flushed with saline. We have found that we can draw the sample for counting from the same catheter if we withdraw and discard 5 to 10 ml of blood immediately before drawing the sample. For most purposes, a single sample drawn at 15 minutes after injection provides satisfactory accuracy. The blood sample is centrifuged and plasma pipetted for counting purposes. Alternatively, samples can be obtained at 10, 20, and 30 minutes for greater accuracy, with the activity plotted against time from injection, and the resulting line traced backward to zero time.

### RBC Volume

A blood sample of approximately 25 ml is incubated with acid-citrate-dextrose (ACD) anticoagulant solution. Cr-51 as the chromate ion is added, and the sample is incubated at room temperature for 10 minutes. The cells are then washed, or ascorbic acid is added to reduce the chromate to chromic ion, to stop the labeling process. This mixture is divided, with part to be used for a standard and a known amount reinjected into the patient. After 30 minutes (longer if the patient has splenomegaly), a blood sample is drawn for counting and RBC mass determination.

RBC mass and plasma volume can be determined simultaneously, using the difference in energies of the emissions to determine activity of Cr-51 and I-125 simultaneously. Chapter 30 presents the procedure in detail.

## Normals

One of the biggest controversies in blood volume determination is the method of expressing the results and comparing them to normals. Results can be compared to normals as milliliters per kilogram of body weight or can be related to body surface area (8,9).

## Future Developments

We have long believed that RBC mass cannot be reliably estimated by determining plasma volume and calculating the RBC mass from the hematocrit. The problem is that measured hematocrit varies, depending on the source of the blood sample, and differs with samples obtained from arteries, large veins, or capillaries. None of the samples equals "whole-body hematocrit," which is the value needed. Recent work challenges this assumption (10): Fairbanks and associates have shown that RBC mass determined from plasma volume and a correction for venous hematocrit to whole-body hematocrit is nearly identical to values obtained by direct measurement of RBC mass. The correction value they use is 0.864. When one critically compares their results to earlier statements that a simple, uniform correction was not possible, a difference in patient population is obvious. The earlier studies included many patients with disease, often advanced disease. The later studies are mostly of normal subjects or patients with early polycythemia rubra vera. Indeed, the patients who deviated from the correction factor most in the Fairbanks study were primarily those with more severe disease.

Most laboratories have long held the belief that because we use Cr-51 we are directly determining the RBC mass. Because of the difficulty in obtaining a pure sample of RBCs for counting, we routinely count whole blood and calculate the RBC mass from the hematocrit. This hematocrit value is the value of the sample counted and does not bring in the difficulties inherent in whole-body hematocrit, as discussed above. Nevertheless, we are in fact using Cr-51 to determine the whole blood volume and obtaining RBC mass from a calculation. Any whole blood label would work just as well as Cr-51, and because Cr-51 has become expensive, it is an expensive laboratory procedure.

## RBC SURVIVAL AND SEQUESTRATION STUDIES

RBC survival and sequestration studies have been used to confirm anemias that result from either hemolysis or abnormal sequestration of RBCs in the spleen. The indications are relatively rare, but in some therapeutic decisions concerning the value of splenectomy, the studies are valid.

### Radiopharmaceutical

The radiopharmaceutical is Cr-51 as $Na_2CrO_4$, and the RBCs are labeled in a fashion similar to blood volume determination, except that a larger dose is used (120 µCi [4.44 MBq] vs. 40 to 60 µCi [1.5 to 2.2 MBq]). Unfortunately, the cost is high: approximately $260 per 250 µCi (9.25 MBq). The price hinders the routine use of this test unless several patients can be scheduled simultaneously so as to efficiently use the radionuclide. As described above, the Cr-51 chromate rapidly enters the RBC in the presence of ACD anticoagulant, is reduced to the chromic ion, and is bound to the beta chain of hemoglobin, becoming an effective RBC label. The Cr-51 has a half-life of 27.8 days and emits a gamma ray of 320 keV, with an abundance of only 9%.

When Cr-51 is incorporated into RBC, the spontaneous elution rate is approximately 1% per day. In addition, the cohort of cells labeled have an average life span ranging from senescent (life expectancy, ~0 days) to that of immature RBCs (life expectancy, ~120 days). The combination of this average RBC age and elution rate results in an effective

Cr-51 RBC half-life of approximately 25 to 35 days (the average RBC life is 60 days) (11).

### Cr-51 RBC Half-Life

Blood samples are obtained 24, 48, and 72 hours after injection, then on Mondays, Wednesdays, and Fridays of each week for 2 to 4 weeks. The hematocrit is determined for each sample, and each sample is centrifuged so that the plasma can be discarded. The volume is restored using water (effectively eliminating plasma Cr-51), and the samples finally are counted together at the end of the study (eliminating the need for decay correction). The Cr-51 RBC survival can then be plotted on semilog paper to linearize the curve. Then the patient's effective half-life is calculated, with the normal being 25 to 35 days.

False positives (abnormally reduced half-life) can occur from various problems, including careless handling of cells while labeling and nonhemolytic loss of RBCs (gastrointestinal or genitourinary blood loss).

Prolonged normal survival times—that is, false-negative results—exist when the patient is transfused during the procedure, effectively eliminating the basis of the tracer method (i.e., addition to the volume measured).

### Cr-51 RBC Sequestration

If the Cr-51 RBC half-life is reduced below normal, the procedure can be used to determine if there is significant splenic sequestration of RBCs and, therefore, the potential for a therapeutic response to splenectomy. For this possibility, there must be a significant and progressive increase in splenic uptake relative to the other expected site of RBCs, for example, blood pool or liver (normal deposition site of Cr-51 from senescent labeled RBCs).

### Methodology

This test is prolonged because it requires regular monitoring of RBC uptake into the spleen and liver and comparison of this uptake to the background vascular activity (cardiac blood pool). This is achieved by using the thyroid uptake probe and positioning it over the liver (anteriorly over the ninth and tenth right ribs, between the midclavicular and anterior axillary line, angled 15 degrees cephalad), the spleen (posteriorly over the left ninth and tenth ribs, at the posterior axillary line), and the precordium (over the fourth left interspace, 4 cm to the left of the sternum, angled 15 degrees medially). These organ counts are obtained at 1, 2, and 3 days after injection, then 3 times a week for another 2 weeks or until the RBC Cr-51 half-time study is completed. The uptake ratios of spleen to heart, liver to heart, and spleen to liver are obtained for each time interval. The spleen-to-liver ratio is normally 1:1, and active sequestration results in a 2:1

to 4:1 uptake. Because the liver can also sequester RBCs, the spleen-to-heart ratio may be a better discriminator of splenic sequestration, the abnormal being >2:1. The therapeutic implication of increased splenic uptake is splenectomy. This test is described in Chapter 30.

## SCHILLING TEST

### Overview

Vitamin $B_{12}$ is not synthesized by plants or animals but rather by microorganisms in the gastrointestinal tract of animals. The major sources of human vitamin $B_{12}$ are meat and dairy products. For absorption, vitamin $B_{12}$ must first be complexed with intrinsic factor (IF), which is secreted by the gastric fundus. The IF-$B_{12}$ complex is then absorbed in the terminal ileum. Vitamin $B_{12}$ deficiency is a serious illness causing both hematologic and neurologic complications. Although the megaloblastic anemia and white blood cell and platelet decreases are readily reversible, the subacute combined degeneration of the spinal cord needs early treatment to reverse. The deficiency is readily treated by the systemic replacement of the vitamin. Vitamin $B_{12}$ levels in blood can be determined by a radioligand assay, but the assay does not give information about the cause of the deficiency. Deficiencies can result from the following:

- Malabsorption due to absence of the necessary IF in the stomach (gastrectomy or pernicious anemia)
- Dietary lack of the vitamin may also cause deficiency
- Certain bacterial overgrowths within the bowel (microorganisms consume vitamin $B_{12}$ and prevent absorption)
- Inability to absorb the IF-$B_{12}$ complex in the terminal ileum (terminal ileal resection or disease states, e.g., Crohn's disease).

Many methods of measuring vitamin $B_{12}$ absorption have been devised, including timed serum whole-body uptakes and fecal estimates of orally administered samples of labeled vitamin $B_{12}$. All clinical measurements currently performed make use of a modification of the urinary excretion method developed by Schilling (12). Radioactive vitamin $B_{12}$ is given orally, and the blood transport proteins are saturated by giving an excess of nonradioactive $B_{12}$ intramuscularly. Absorption is not affected, but much of the absorbed material is excreted in the urine because of the saturation of the transport proteins. Measuring radioactivity in the urine then indirectly indicates the amount of absorbed vitamin $B_{12}$.

### Procedure

#### Patient Preparation

The patient should not have had other procedures with administration of radioactivity recently because these can interfere with urine counting. Contrast agents can interfere with absorption, so orally administered barium and CT contrast should not be performed in conjunction with the procedure. To ensure absorption, the patient should fast for 8 hours before the study and continue fasting until the nonradioactive vitamin $B_{12}$ injection is administered 2 hours after the start of the test. If the patient has been taking vitamin $B_{12}$, it should be stopped 3 to 4 days before the test.

#### Administration of Isotope

A capsule of vitamin $B_{12}$ labeled with radioactivity is given orally with a small amount of water. Capsules can be labeled with various isotopes of cobalt (Co), a normal component of vitamin $B_{12}$, the most commonly used isotopes being Co-57 and Co-58.

#### Administration of Flushing Dose

Two hours after ingesting the labeled vitamin $B_{12}$, nonradioactive $B_{12}$ is injected. Usually, 1 mg is given intramuscularly.

#### Urine Collection

A small sample of urine can be collected before the study to evaluate for radioactivity; this ensures that there is no confounding activity from previous tests. The patient should void just before injection of the flushing dose. Starting from that time, a 24-hour specimen is obtained. The specimen can be evaluated for creatinine excretion as a check on adequacy of collection.

#### Evaluation

The urine specimen is measured for volume, and a specimen is prepared for counting. A standard of the administered dose is prepared (this is usually part of the materials received from the test vendor). The standard and dose given to the patient should be checked to be certain they are the same lot number. Standard and specimen are counted and the percentage of urinary excretion of the administered dose calculated.

$$\% \text{ Excretion} = \frac{(\text{Urine counts/ml} - \text{BKG}) \times \text{urine volume} \times 100}{\text{Standard counts/ml} \times \text{dilution factor}}$$

#### Normal Results

A normal result is usually considered >10% excretion of the administered dose within 24 hours. Excretion of 5% to 9.9% is considered borderline, and <5% is abnormal, indicating failure to absorb vitamin $B_{12}$.

#### Confounding Factors

The most common cause of problem is incomplete urine collection. Normal values assume near-normal renal function;

severe renal failure makes the test inappropriate. Collecting an additional 24-hour urine sample can help, especially in the male population, in which benign prostatic hypertrophy (resulting in urinary retention) and mild renal failure can result in significant tracer excretion in the second 24-hour sample (in the elderly male population, 10% to 30% of excreted tracer is routinely found in the second urine collection).

### Further Evaluation

An abnormal test indicates failure of absorption but does not indicate the etiology. Absorption can fail because of a lack of IF in the stomach, because of a problem in the ileum, or because the administered dose is used by bacteria or parasites in the intestine. To evaluate these possibilities, a second part can be performed using vitamin $B_{12}$ already bound to IF. Such capsules are available from vendors. If the first part is abnormal, but the second part (with IF) is normal, then the problem is absence of IF (i.e., pernicious anemia). Severe lack of vitamin $B_{12}$ can affect reproducing cells in the intestinal mucosa and cause or exacerbate malabsorption of the vitamin. This deficiency can be reversed within a few days, and the administered intramuscular $B_{12}$ can be enough to reverse malabsorption due to intestinal mucosal problems. In this situation, one would assume IF deficiency, but the real problem might be dietary deficiency. A three-stage test is sometimes performed after a course of antibiotic therapy to reverse potential bacterial overgrowth.

### Alternative Methods

At least one vendor supplies a product (Dicopac, Mediphysics, Inc., Arlington Heights, IL) that performs the first and second parts of the Schilling test simultaneously. The product includes vitamin $B_{12}$ bound to IF and labeled with Co-58 and vitamin $B_{12}$ without IF and labeled with Co-57. The two can be differentiated by energy window counting, and the absorption of both can be determined at one time. This test is a very simple and convenient method that overcomes many of the technical and patient problems associated with the 24-hour urine collection. This test is described in Chapter 30.

### Radiation Exposure

The administered dose is commonly on the order of 0.63 μCi (23 KBq) Co-57. This results in a dose of approximately 0.003 rads (0.03 mGy) to the whole body and 0.08 rads (0.8 mGy) to the liver, which is the critical organ.

## UREA BREATH TEST

*Helicobacter pylori* bacteria is established as an etiologic factor in gastritis. Nearly all patients with duodenal ulcer and most with gastric ulcer are infected with this organism, and eradication significantly reduces the recurrence rates of these diseases. This infection is also related to gastric adenocarcinoma and lymphoma.

### Pathophysiology

The urea breath test (UBT) is based on the presence of urease-producing *H. pylori* organisms in the stomach of afflicted individuals (13). Other urease-producing organisms do not normally colonize the stomach. The presence of urease in breath samples while urea is present in the stomach indirectly establishes the presence of *H. pylori*. If patients are administered carbon 14 (C-14)–labeled urea, urease present in the stomach of those with *H. pylori* infection results in the production of C-14 $CO_2$, which is absorbed into the circulation, exhaled, and counted in the breath: the UBT.

### Procedure

C-14 urea is administered orally to the patient, breath samples are obtained periodically by the patient exhaling through a straw, and the exhaled breath is passed through a solution of hyamine in methanol that traps an exact amount of $CO_2$. An indicator is added to establish saturation of hyamine with $CO_2$. These samples are then added to a liquid scintillation cocktail and the patient sample (obtained at 10 or 20 minutes) counted, along with a background (i.e., 0 minute) sample and a calibrated standard, if percent dose exhaled is to be measured.

### Normal Results

The normal cut-off value depends on the activity of C-14 urea administered and the C-14 $CO_2$ trapped (i.e., amount of hyaline trapping solution). For 5 μCi (0.185 MBq) of C-14 urea and 1 mmol of $CO_2$ trapped, a positive test is defined as >1,000 counts per minute in the 20-minute sample (14). The UBT is both sensitive (90% to 100%) and specific (78% to 100%) compared to biopsy-based tests (13).

### False-Positive Results

False-positive results occur if urease-producing bacteria are in the stomach. This can result from oral flora with urease activity (patients are instructed to brush their teeth carefully) or when gastric pH rises and the stomach becomes colonized (e.g., achlorhydria, antacid use, $H_2$-receptor antagonist use [discontinued for 24 hours], and uremia).

### False-Negative Results

The most common causes of false negatives are performing the UBT too soon after a course of antibiotics, bismuth (30 days), sucralfate, or omeprazole (7 days); in conditions of rapid gastric emptying (e.g., surgery); or in a nonfasting state (patient must fast for 6 hours before the test).

## Clinical Application

The diagnosis of the presence of *H. pylori* can be done with the UBT (using either stable C-13 and mass spectroscopy, or radioactive C-14 methodologies) and by serology, which works well in most patient populations except the elderly and those that do not have a systemic antibody response to *H. pylori*. Clearing of the *H. pylori* infection results in healing of the gastritis. Serology remains positive for some time after treatment, however, so it is unreliable in treatment follow-up before 6 months. Because the UBT can be used 1 month after therapy, it has significant advantages over other testing methods.

A simple, single, timed breath test using an encapsulated C-14 urea (obviates oral flora false positives) was just released by the FDA for New Drug Application. The dosimetry using 1 to 10 µCi (0.037 to 0.37 MBq) is <1 mrad (0.01 mGy) to the critical organ (bladder wall).

## REFERENCES

1. Silver S. Radioactive Nuclides in Medicine and Biology. Philadelphia: Lea & Febiger, 1968.
2. Fine J, Seligman AM. Traumatic shock IV. J Clin Invest 1943;22:285–303.
3. Hevesy G, Koster KH, Sorensen G, et al. The red corpuscle content of the circulating blood determined by labeling the erythrocytes with radiophosphorus. Acta Med Scand 1944;116:561.
4. Hahn PF, Balfour WM, Ross JF, et al. Red cell volume circulating and total as determined by radioiron. Science 1941;93:87.
5. Sterling K, Gray SJ. Determination of the circulating red cell volume in man by radioactive chromium. J Clin Invest 1950;29:1604–1613.
6. International Committee for Standardization in Hematology. Recommended methods for measurement of red-cell and plasma volume. J Nucl Med 1980;21:793–800.
7. Cloutier RJ, Watson EE. Radiation Dose from Radioisotopes in the Blood. In Cloutier RJ, Edwards CL, Snyder WS (eds), Medical Radionuclides: Radiation Dose and Effects. Springfield, VA: U.S. Atomic Energy Commission, 1970.
8. Nadler SB, Hidalgo JU, Block T. In Surgery. 1962;51:224–232.
9. Hurley PJ. Red cell and plasma volumes in normal adults. J Nucl Med 1975;16:46–52.
10. Fairbanks VF, Klee GG, Wiseman GA, et al. Measurement of blood volume and red cell mass: re-examination of $^{51}Cr$ and $^{125}I$ methods. Blood Cells Mol Dis 1996;22:169–186.
11. International Committee for Standardization in Haematology. Recommended method for radioisotope red cell survival studies. Br J Haematol 1980;45:659–666.
12. Schilling RF. Intrinsic factor studies. II. The effect of gastric juice on the urinary excretion of radioactivity after the oral administration of radioactive vitamin $B_{12}$. J Lab Clin Med 1953;42:860–866.
13. Atherton JC, Spiller RC. The urea breath test for *Helicobacter pylori*. Gut 1994;35:723–725.
14. Marshall BJ, Plankey MW, Hoffman SR, et al. A 20-minute breath test for *H. pylori*. Am J Gastroenterol 1991;86:438–445.

# Fundamentals of Nuclear Medicine

*Textbook of Nuclear Medicine,*
edited by Michael A. Wilson.
Lippincott–Raven Publishers, Philadelphia © 1998.

# CHAPTER 21

# Physics of Radioactive Decay

Onofre T. DeJesus

## HISTORICAL PERSPECTIVE

Nuclear medicine is a subspecialty of radiology aimed at the diagnosis and therapy of disease. Undoubtedly, nuclear medicine is a major beneficial application of the advances made in this century in understanding the atomic nucleus. Other radiologic imaging modalities, such as x-ray computed tomography (CT), magnetic resonance, and ultrasound imaging, wherein external sources of radiation are used, detect altered anatomy due to pathologic variations in some local physical property of tissues and organs (e.g., attenuation of x-rays in CT scanning). In contrast, nuclear medicine procedures involve administration of small amounts of radiotracers, whose distribution provides images related to biochemical and physiologic properties of tissues or organs. Specific radiotracer distribution is achieved by the proper choice of labeled compounds based on molecular or cellular characteristics of the target tissue or organ. Altered localization or kinetics of radiotracer signify pathophysiologic function.

As a therapeutic modality, nuclear medicine similarly involves administration of internal radioactive sources, which target pathologic tissues or organs based on biochemical and physiologic mechanisms of localization. In contrast, conventional radiotherapy involves external sealed sources of intense radiation focused on the diseased organ or tissue. Besides its clinical applications, nuclear medicine has also made fundamental contributions to our understanding of human biochemistry and physiology with the application of in vitro and in vivo radiotracer techniques. This chapter describes the basic physics of nuclear medicine and introduces topics described in more detail in subsequent chapters.

The beginnings of nuclear medicine and the whole field of radiology can be traced to the Wilhelm Roentgen's discovery in 1895 that invisible and very penetrating radiations, which he called *x-rays,* were being emitted by electrodes in an evacuated glass tube maintained at high voltage. A year later, Henri Becquerel reported that similar unknown rays coming from uranium salts were, like Roentgen's x-rays, exposing photographic plates in the absence of any external stimulus. This particular property of uranium salts was called *radioactivity* by Marie Curie, who with her husband, Pierre, later isolated other elements (e.g., radium and polonium) that were more radioactive than uranium. The subatomic origin of radioactivity was first suggested in 1903 by the New Zealander Ernest Rutherford, who speculated that the radiations were the result of the transmutation of one element into another. Rutherford identified two uranium radiations: alpha particles, which could be stopped by 0.02-mm-thick lead foil, and beta particles, which were more penetrating but could be stopped by thicker (1-mm) lead foil. Alpha particles were found to be doubly positively charged ions with four times the mass of hydrogen and were subsequently identified as helium nuclei. Beta particles were found to have mass approximately $\frac{1}{2000}$ of the hydrogen atom and unit negative charge, similar to the cathode ray or electron, which was discovered earlier by J.J. Thomson in 1897. A third, more penetrating radiation called *gamma rays* (continuing the use of the Greek alphabet), which were not bent by electric or magnetic fields, were then detected. Gamma rays were found to be electromagnetic, similar to light, but with higher energies (shorter wavelengths).

It is interesting that a conceptual picture of the atom was still not clear when these particles were identified. Various descriptions of the atom were proposed during this period. Thomson speculated that the atom was made up of electrons embedded in a positively charged mass that was uniformly distributed over the volume of the atom, like raisins in a plum pudding. Bragg, on the other hand, described alpha particles as flying clusters of thousands of electrons. In 1911, using simple laws of mechanics, Rutherford proposed a nuclear or planetary model of the atom to explain the results of experiments wherein alpha particles were observed to be scattered as much as 180 degrees as they traversed targets made of different materials. This model of the atom involves a massive positively charged nucleus surrounded by orbiting negatively charged electrons. The mass of the atom is concentrated in the nucleus, with dimensions in the range of $10^{-15}$ m (femtometer, fm, also called *fermi*) and densities of approximately $10^{14}$ g/cm$^3$. This nuclear model of the atom was dismissed by others when it was first proposed because, it was argued, if this were the case, the negatively charged electron would gradually lose energy as it orbits the nucleus and eventually spiral toward the positively charged nucleus, leading to atomic collapse. This atomic model did not find favor until the quantized nature of the electronic shells was proposed by Bohr in 1913. Bohr's quantum theory described electronic levels, wherein electrons are confined in discrete energy levels, and specified that energy in the form of x-rays is absorbed or emitted as electrons move between these energy levels. This description of electronic states satisfactorily explained atomic spectra of the elements and supported Rutherford's nuclear model.

In addition to the proton, a second nuclear constituent, the neutron, earlier predicted by Rutherford to exist as a "close combination of proton and electron," was detected by Chadwick in 1932. A neutron is slightly bigger than a proton but carries no charge, which made it difficult to detect. The discovery of the neutron completed our current simple picture of the atom. Neutrons also explained why atoms of some elements have similar chemical properties but different masses. For example, the presence of a neutron in the hydrogen atom describes deuterium, which has the same chemical properties as hydrogen but with double its mass. Elements are currently organized in the periodic table by their atomic number, Z, which is the number of protons and, in a neutral atom, also the number of electrons. Atoms with the same atomic number Z but with different mass number, A (the sum of the number of protons and neutrons), are called *isotopes*. Isotopes of an element have identical chemical properties and thus are not separable by chemical means. Isotopes may be stable or radioactive. Although *nuclide* refers to the nucleus without consideration of extranuclear electrons, this distinction should be kept in mind when using the terms *radioisotope* and *radionuclide*. Atoms with the same A but different Z are called *isobars*, whereas nuclei with the same N (the number of neutrons or the difference between the mass number A and atomic number Z) but different A are called *isotones*. Nuclei with the same A, Z, and N but in different energy states are *isomers*. Isomers are radionuclides that are in some nuclear-excited or metastable state and that de-excite to the ground state by the emission of a gamma ray, via a process called *isomeric transition* (IT).

## ELEMENTARY PARTICLE PHYSICS

Spurred by the knowledge of the nucleus and the mathematics developed to explain its physics, scientists in the second half of this century elucidated elementary particles and forces in nature from astrophysics to particle physics. Three fundamental natural forces were recognized: gravitational, strong, and electroweak forces. The more familiar gravitational forces describe interactions of bodies in the galactic

**TABLE 21-1.** *Fundamental forces and elementary particles in the Standard Model*

| Fundamental forces | Exchange particles |
|---|---|
| Gravitational | "Gravitons" |
| Strong | "Gluons" |
| Electroweak | Photons, $W^+$, $W^-$, $Z^o$ |

| Elementary particles | Examples |
|---|---|
| Leptons | Electrons, $\beta^+$, $\beta^-$, $\mu$, $\tau$ |
| Quarks | Up, down, strange, charm, top, bottom |
| Quark composites: Hadrons | |
| Baryons | Nucleons (protons and neutrons) Hyperons |
| Mesons | Pions and kaons |
| Elementary vector bosons | Exchange particles (listed above) |

space. Strong forces that bind nuclear particles, such as nucleons (protons and neutrons), are $10^{38}$ times stronger than gravitational forces (at ~2 fm). Electroweak forces are those involved in electric fields and magnetic fields, as described by Maxwell's equations, and those in weak forces, which are involved in lepton (e.g., electron) interactions and beta decay. Glashow and Weinberg and Salaam laid the groundwork for unifying electromagnetic theory with the theory on weak interactions and shared the Nobel Prize in physics for this work.

There are three classes of elementary particles: leptons, quarks, and elementary vector bosons. Each of these elementary particles has a corresponding antiparticle (some particles, such as photons, are antiparticles of themselves). The leptons, which interact via weak forces, comprise the following:

- Electrons ($e^-$, $\beta^-$, $\beta^+$)
- Muons, whose masses are approximately 200 times that of electrons
- Tauons, whose masses are approximately 3,500 electron masses

Each lepton is associated with a neutrino, an almost massless particle that carries energy and momentum.

Quarks, on the other hand, are subnuclear particles that interact via weak and strong forces and have charges of either $-\frac{1}{3}$ or $+\frac{2}{3}$. The smallest stable free particle under ordinary conditions is made up of three quarks. There are six basic quarks: up and down, strange and charm, and top and bottom. With experimental evidence supporting the existence of the top quark, first reported by an international group of collaborators at Fermilab (1), all six quarks have now been observed. Hadrons, which are composite particles of quarks, can be subdivided into baryons and mesons. Baryons are either nucleons or hyperons. Nucleons are stable particles composed of three-quark combinations of up (*u*) and down (*d*) quarks; for example, protons are *uud* composites, and neutrons are *udd* combinations. Hyperons, on the other hand, are unstable particles containing at least one strange (*s*) quark, such as Σ, which is a *uds* composite. Mesons are unstable combinations of quark-antiquark pairs; for example, pi mesons or pions and k mesons or kaons, which are observed only in high-energy reactions. The elementary vector bosons are exchange particles mediating the fundamental interactions. This third class of elementary particles, called *vector bosons* or *exchange particles,* comprise the following:

- Photons, the exchange particles for electromagnetic interactions, and weak-force bosons (W+, W−, and Zo), which are massive exchange particles with masses approaching 90 to 100 times the nucleon mass, mediate lepton interactions
- Strong-force bosons or gluons, of which there are eight, mediate quark interactions
- Gravitons, postulated to be the long-distance exchange forces mediating gravitational forces

The current organization of fundamental forces and elementary particles is summarized in Table 21-1.

## NUCLEAR FORCES AND STABILITY

The repulsion of positively charged protons in nuclei is dominated by strong forces at short distances. These forces, supplied by protons and neutrons, prevent the composites of nucleons from flying apart. As the distance between protons in larger nuclei increases as atomic number Z increases, the same strong forces become less able to overcome repulsive coulomb forces. More uncharged neutrons are therefore required to provide strong forces to maintain the stability of the nucleus. Thus, nuclear diameter is a major factor in nuclear stability. The stability of a nucleus can be deduced from the binding energy of the nucleons. The actual measured mass of a stable nucleus is smaller than the sum of the masses of the constituent nucleons in a nucleus. This mass difference, or mass defect, represents the binding energy of the nucleus. Because mass is related to energy ($E = mc^2$), where one atomic mass unit, *u*, is equivalent to 931.5 MeV, the mass defect in units of u can be converted to binding energy in megaelectron volts. As an example, our current atomic mass unit is based on the most common isotope of carbon, C-12, whose mass is taken to be exactly 12.0 u. Thus, the mass defect for C-12 atom is 0.09906 u (combined masses of six electrons, six neutrons, and six protons is 12.09906 − 12.00000), and therefore its nuclear binding energy is 92.22 MeV (0.09906 u × 931.5 MeV/u). This gives a binding energy per nucleon of 92.22/12 or 7.685 MeV. A plot of binding energy per nucleon against mass number A (Fig. 21-1) shows that maximum binding energy per nucleon values is approximately 8.8 MeV per nucleon, centering around mass number 60 (iron and nickel). Beyond A = 60, the binding energy per nucleon decreases monotonically to approximately 7.45 MeV at A of 255. The relative stability of a nucleus with respect to other nuclei can be deduced from this plot. From the point of view of energet-

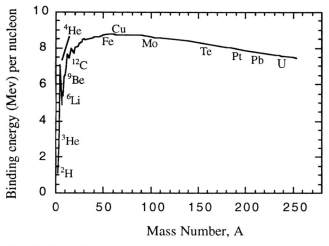

**FIG. 21-1.** Binding energy, in megaelectron volts, per nucleon versus mass number A.

ics, alpha decay or fission can occur in high-Z nuclei because the decay daughters formed have lower Z and thus higher binding energy per nucleon. A semi-empiric mass equation, which contains contributions of mass or volume, surface area, coulomb energy, and nucleon pairing, has been found to fit the plot shown in Fig. 21-1. This convergence of theory and experiment has brought about a better understanding of the factors contributing to nuclear stability.

The notion that nucleon pairing contributes to nuclear stability was suggested by the finding of unusual stability exhibited by nuclei with certain proton or neutron numbers: 2, 8, 20, 28, 50, 82, and 126. Nuclear stability of nuclei with these "magic numbers" were explained by closed nuclear shell structures, analogous to completely filled electronic shells associated with chemical unreactivity (or stability) of noble elements.

## RADIOACTIVE DECAY

The driving force for any nucleus to disintegrate spontaneously is the formation of more stable product nuclei, wherein the binding energy per nucleon of the product nuclei is higher than that of the parent nucleus. Thus, nuclear transformations, which give off energy (exothermic reactions), are more likely to occur spontaneously than are those that require energy (endothermic reactions). Other forces, however, such as coulomb barriers in alpha decay and fission, have to be overcome for these spontaneous nuclear transformations to occur. Coulomb barriers, which prevent external charged particles from penetrating the nucleus, as observed in the early alpha-scattering experiments performed in Rutherford's laboratory, also prevent alpha particles or any other charged fragment from leaving the nucleus. Quantum mechanical treatment of the nucleus, which allows alpha particle to "tunnel" through the potential barrier, successfully explained alpha decay and predicted the half-life of alpha-emitting radionuclides.

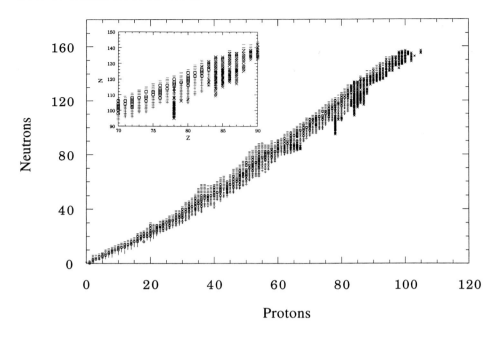

**FIG. 21-2.** Neutron number versus proton number of stable and radioactive nuclei. The stable nuclei are represented by open circle (o). Those that decay by negatron, positron, electron capture, and alpha emission are represented by −, +, bar, and x.

## Alpha Decay and Fission

As mentioned earlier, an alpha particle is a helium 4 (He-4)$^{+2}$ ion, which is a relatively stable nucleus by virtue of having paired neutrons and paired protons. An example of alpha decay is the decay of uranium 238 (U-238): U-238 → Pu-234 (plutonium 234) + (He-4)$^{+2}$. This is the first of 14 transformations in this naturally occurring decay series, which end in the formation of stable lead 206 (Pb-206).

Due to its mass, an alpha particle has a short range and thus deposits most of its energy along its short track, which causes highly localized ionization. Thus, alpha particles are useless in radionuclide imaging because the internally administered source must have radiations able to penetrate the body and reach the external imaging camera. However, the short-range, high–linear energy transfer (LET) of alpha particles causes highly localized ionizations, which lead to significant radiation damage to biological systems. This localized destructive property of alpha particles may be useful in internal radiotherapy for malignant diseases. (Further discussion of radiation dosimetry and its radiobiological consequences is found in other chapters.)

Fission is the splitting of a large nucleus into two smaller nuclei, accompanied by the release of tremendous amounts of energy and one or more neutrons. Spontaneous fission is not as prevalent as alpha decay, again because the coulomb barrier keeps large composites of nucleons inside the nucleus. However, neutron-induced fission is highly probable in some fissionable nuclei, such as U-235 and Pu-239. Each fission process produces one or more neutrons, which can induce another nucleus to fission and so on, leading to a chain reaction. This chain reaction can be uncontrolled, as in the atom bomb, or controlled, as in reactors used for power generation, research on nuclear structure, or radioisotope production. In nuclear medicine, fission is an important process in the production of radioisotopes either in the reactor, as a source of neutrons, or in the recovery of useful fission products, such as molybdenum 99 (Mo-99) or iodine 131 (I-131). The advantage of fission-produced radioisotopes is the very high–specific activity radionuclides obtained.

## Beta Decay

A plot of proton number Z versus neutron number N for all the known nuclides (Fig. 21-2) shows that low-Z materials stable nuclides have a proton-to-neutron ratio of 1:1. As the size of the nucleus increases (increasing Z and N), the proton-to-neutron ratio increases to approximately 1.0:1.5; thus the need for strong forces of the uncharged neutrons to overcome the repulsive charges of the protons as the size of the nucleus increases. Figure 21-2 also shows that the naturally stable nuclei (represented by o) lie along a so-called line of stability. A nucleus above this line (−) decays by β$^-$ emission, whereas nuclei below the line (x or !) decay by β$^+$ and electron capture (EC), respectively, to a daughter nucleus that would likewise lie on this line of stability. Thus, beta decay is the decay process that returns neutron- or proton-rich nuclides back to the line of stability.

When beta particles were first identified as electrons, no distinction was made between those that originate from the nucleus and those that are extranuclear. The electron was thought to exist in the nucleus as an entity before Fermi developed a beta decay theory, which does not propose that electrons reside in the nucleus. Fermi proposed that beta particles are created in the nucleus as gamma particles are created in the nucleus. Fermi's theory of beta decay therefore differentiated beta particles from extranuclear electrons.

## Negatron Decay

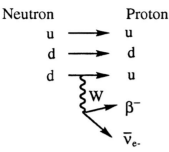

Neutron          Proton

**FIG. 21-3.** A neutron transforms to a proton with the accompanying emission of β⁻ particle and neutrino.

## Positron Decay

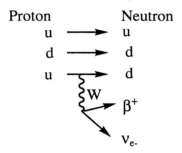

Proton          Neutron

**FIG. 21-4.** A proton transforms to a neutron with the accompanying emission of β⁺ particle and neutrino, $v_{e-}$.

There are three types of beta decay: negatron (β⁻), positron (β⁺), and EC. The energy requirements for these decays to occur in a nuclide, $A_Z$, of atomic number Z and atomic mass $M_Z$ decaying into daughter $A_{Z \pm 1}$ with mass $M_{Z \pm 1}$, are as follows:

Negatron decay: $A_Z \rightarrow A_{Z+1} + \beta^- + v_{e-}$    $M_Z > M_{Z+1}$

Electron capture: $A_Z \rightarrow A_{Z-1} + \beta^+ + v_{e-}$    $M_Z > M_{Z-1}$

Positron decay: $A_Z \rightarrow A_{Z-1} + v_{e-}$    $M_Z > M_{Z-1} + 2m_e$

where $m_e$ is electron mass or 0.511 MeV. These energy requirements follow the previously mentioned observation that exothermic reactions involving loss of energy (mass) can occur spontaneously.

The three beta decays, which involve, in the simplest terms, the transformation of a neutron to a proton or vice versa can be satisfactorily described using the quark model. In negatron decay, a neutron (*udd*) transforms to a proton (*uud*) with the accompanying emission of β⁻ particle and neutrino (actually the antineutrino, $v_{e-}$, by convention) (Fig. 21-3).

In positron decay, a proton (*uud*) transforms to a neutron (*udd*), with the accompanying emission of β⁺ particle and neutrino, $v_{e-}$ (Fig. 21-4). The third type of beta decay involves the capture of an orbital electron and the emission of monoenergetic neutrino (Fig. 21-5).

## Electron Capture Decay

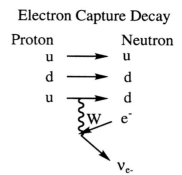

Proton          Neutron

**FIG. 21-5.** Capture of an orbital electron and the emission of a monoenergetic neutrino.

### Negatron Decay

Negatron (β⁻) decay occurs when a nuclide is neutron-rich (see Fig. 21-2). Most radioisotopes are produced via neutron absorption in a reactor, wherein a nucleus captures a neutron and increases its mass number by 1, and the nucleus decays by β⁻ decay. In the early days, beta decay was thought to violate the energy conservation law because β⁻ decaying nuclides emitted beta particles with a spectrum of energies, from almost zero to a maximum energy characteristic of the radionuclide corresponding to the Q value (energy) for the decay. To explain this seeming violation, Pauli proposed that an unobserved particle called a neutrino, which carried the unaccounted energy, was also emitted in beta decay. In 1953, Reines and Cowan reported the first observation of neutrinos via inverse beta reaction in a nuclear reactor. This conclusively demonstrated the existence of these almost massless and difficult-to-detect particles. Reines received the Nobel Prize for physics in 1995 for this work.

By convention, in the examples of decay schemes shown below, the direction of the arrow follows the relative positions of the nuclides in the periodic table of elements; that is, the decay of a Z nuclide to a Z + 1 daughter is represented by an arrow pointed to the right, the decay to a Z – 1 daughter has the arrow pointed to the left, and decay without a change in Z is represented by an arrow pointed down. An example of β⁻ decay is that of phosphorus 32 (P-32) to sulfur 32 (S-32) (Fig. 21-6). The energy (Q) available to this decay is 1.71 MeV, which is the maximum energy β⁻ particles can carry,

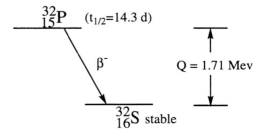

**FIG. 21-6.** Phosphorus 32 decaying to sulfur 32.

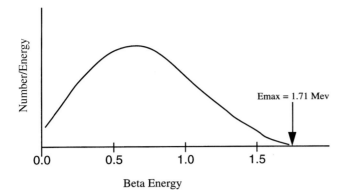

FIG. 21-7. Distribution of β⁻ particles with different energies in the decay of ³²⁰P. (Adapted from Jensen et al. Phys Rev 1952;85:112.)

$E_{\beta max}$. The average energy of the β⁻ particles, $E_{\beta ave}$, is 695 keV. The beta spectrum of P-32 decay is shown in Fig. 21-7.

Other radionuclides useful in nuclear medicine are I-131 and Mo-99. These have more complicated negatron decay schemes, involving emission of several β⁻ particles as well as several gammas.

### Positron Decay

Positron (β⁺) decay involves neutron-deficient nuclides (with excess number of protons; see Fig. 21-2), wherein a proton is transformed to a neutron with the emission of a positron and a neutrino. A positron, the antiparticle of an electron, was proposed by Dirac based on the observation that electronic wave equations have solutions corresponding to electrons in both negative and positive energy states. Dirac reasoned that the unobserved negative energy states are normally filled, but, with enough energy, an electron in these states can be lifted to a positive energy state, thereby simultaneously producing an electron as well as a "hole" in the negative energy states. This hole would have the properties of a positively charged electron, called a *positron*. Positrons were first detected by Anderson in cosmic rays; later, positrons were also detected in radionuclide decay. Positron decay requires that the unstable nucleus have

excess energy (Q value of reaction) at least equivalent to the combined mass of 2 electrons or 1.022 MeV, which in Dirac's formulation is needed to promote an electron in the negative energy state to a positive energy state. Energy in excess of 1.022 MeV is then shared as kinetic energy by the positron and neutrino as both speed away from the nucleus. Being an antiparticle of an electron, the positron, after it exhausts its kinetic energy, combines with an electron at the end of its 1- to 2-mm track and annihilates, to give two gamma rays each with an energy of 511 keV, the mass of an electron. To conserve momentum, this pair of 511-keV annihilation photons are emitted 180 degrees to each other. The colinearity of this photon pair allows the quantitative imaging in humans of the distribution of compounds labeled with positron-emitting radionuclides by positron emission tomography (PET), which is discussed further in Chapter 24. An example of positron decay is that of fluorine-18, the most common radioisotope in PET imaging (Fig. 21-8).

The energy, Q, available to this decay is 1.655 MeV, of which 1.02 MeV is used to create an electron and a positron. Similar to β⁻, positrons are emitted in a spectrum of energies. The maximum β⁺ energy ($E_{\beta max}$) for F-18 positrons is 0.635 MeV; $E_{\beta ave}$ is 250 keV. The shape of the energy distribution of F-18 positrons is similar to that of P-32 negatrons (see Fig. 21-7). Other short-lived, positron-emitting radionuclides useful in PET are oxygen 15 (O-15; half-life [T-1/2], 2 minutes), nitrogen 13 (N-13; T-1/2, 10 minutes), and C-11 (T-1/2, 20 minutes).

### Electron Capture Decay

In EC decay, an orbital electron is captured by the unstable nucleus followed by the emission of a monoenergetic neutrino with energy equal to the mass difference between parent and daughter nuclei. EC competes with positron decay in neutron-deficient nuclides. In nuclides that undergo both β⁺ and EC decays, the same transmuted stable daughter is formed. Because of the energy threshold for positron decays, EC is the sole pathway for the decay of neutron-deficient radionuclides when the energy available (Q value) is <1.022 MeV. The capture of an orbital electron by the

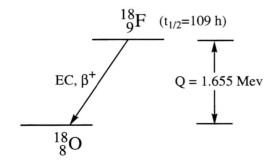

FIG. 21-8. Positron decay of fluorine 18.

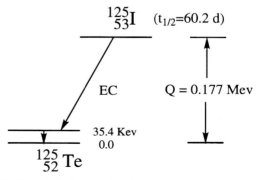

FIG. 21-9. EC decay of iodine 125.

nucleus can be explained in quantum mechanical terms by the fact that the wave function for electrons has finite amplitudes at the nucleus. Furthermore, because this amplitude is largest for the innermost K shell electrons, K shell EC is most probable compared to the capture of electrons from other shells. EC decay of I-125 is shown in Fig. 21-9.

The observable radiations from the decay of I-125 are electrons, x-rays, and the 35.4-keV gamma ray, which is observed approximately 7% of the time. The low percentage of gamma emission in this decay is due to a competing decay mechanism for low-energy transitions, which involves electron emissions instead of gamma emission. This mechanism, called *internal conversion,* is discussed further in the next section. Because of its low-energy radiations, which cannot be detected extracorporeally, I-125 is not useful for imaging but is often used for in vitro nuclear medicine procedures, such as radioimmunoassay. Other useful nuclear medicine radionuclides that decay by EC are indium 111 (In-111), gallium 67 (Ga-67), I-123, and thallium 201 (Tl-201).

## Gamma Decay

Gamma decay occurs when a nucleus in an excited state de-excites to the ground state by the emission of electromagnetic energy. The excited nucleus is usually formed after alpha decay, beta decay, or nuclear reaction, wherein a stable nucleus is bombarded and absorbs particles, such as neutrons, protons, deuterons, and alphas, as well as gamma rays. The decay of excited nuclei depends on the initial and final states and follow specific selection rules, in which some transitions are allowed but some are forbidden. Discussion of these selection rules is beyond the scope of this chapter. Suffice it to say that there are stringent rules governing the emission of gamma rays. Gamma rays are very important in diagnostic nuclear medicine because of their relatively long range, which allows extracorporeal detection that in turn allows the acquisition of physiologic images after the administration of the appropriately radiolabeled pharmaceuticals.

## Internal Conversion

Another de-excitation process, which competes with gamma decay, is internal conversion. In this process, instead of emitting gamma radiation, the excess energy of the nucleus is transferred to an electron, which leads to its ejection from its extranuclear orbit. Again this is explained by the finite amplitude of the electronic wave function at the nucleus. Internal conversion is more probable for low-energy transitions (in keV range) and high-Z nuclei. An important requirement for this process is that the energy available is sufficient to (1) overcome the binding energy of the electron, and (2) provide enough kinetic energy for the electron to escape its electronic orbit.

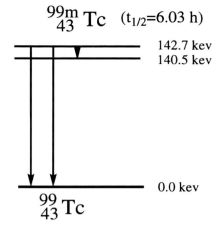

**FIG. 21-10.** Decay of Tc-99m.

## Isomeric Transitions

The gamma transitions described so far are those that occur immediately after a primary (alpha or beta) decay process. Some nuclei are in some metastable excited states, called *isomeric states,* which are excited energy states with measurable lifetimes. Radioisotopes that decay by IT are pure gamma emitters and thus are important in nuclear medicine because the absence of particulate emissions lead to lower radiation doses to subjects given these radioisotopes. An example of IT is the decay of the most important radioisotope in nuclear medicine, technetium 99m (Tc-99m, Fig. 21-10). The main useful radiation from the decay of Tc-99m is the 140.5-keV gamma ray, which is observed in 87.9% of the decay of this radionuclide. Characteristics of this important nuclear medicine radionuclide are discussed under Generators.

## DECAY LAWS

In 1901, Becquerel recognized the temporal characteristics of radioactivity. Consequently, it was only after the application of chemical separation techniques, which allowed the isolation of shorter-lived radioactivities from uranium, that the time dependence of radioactive decay was properly studied. One of these separated activities was called *thorium X* (now known as *radium 234*), which was observed by Rutherford to lose radioactivity with time in a simple exponential manner, as follows:

$$N = N_0 \, e^{-\lambda t}, \qquad (1)$$

where $\lambda$ is the decay constant for thorium X, $N$ and $N_0$ are the number of thorium X nuclei at time $t$ and $t = 0$, respectively. Because $A = \lambda N$, where $A$ is radioactivity with units of disintegrations per second,

$$A = A_0 \, e^{-\lambda t}. \qquad (2)$$

A graphic representation of radioactive decay are the plots of the decay of Tc-99m (Fig. 21-11).

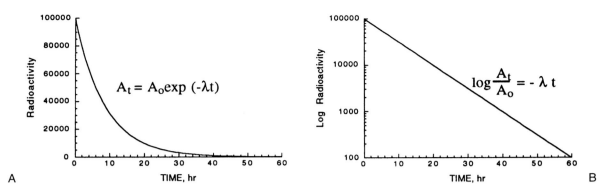

**FIG. 21-11.** Graphs showing the decay of Tc-99m ($A_0$ = 100,000) as a function of time in **(A)** a linear plot and **(B)** a logarithmic plot.

The more common constant to express radioactivity is the half-life, T-1/2, which is the time it takes for $N_0$ nuclei to decay to half of $N_0$.

$$\frac{N_0}{2} = N_0\, e^{-\lambda t}, \qquad (3)$$

which leads to

$$\text{T-1/2} = \frac{\ln 2}{\lambda}. \qquad (4)$$

Another way to express radioactivity is mean lifetime, $\tau$, which is the inverse of the decay constant $\lambda$. Mean lifetime is the measure of radioactive decay most useful in radiation dosimetry calculation.

### Units of Radioactivity

The unit of radioactivity introduced in 1910 was the curie. At that time, the curie was defined as the radioactivity of radon found in radioactive equilibrium with 1 g radium. In 1948, a curie was officially accepted as $3.7 \times 10^{10}$ disintegrations per second. At present, the internationally accepted unit for radioactivity is the becquerel, which is defined as 1 disintegration per second. Both the curie and the becquerel are used in the United States, but most countries using the metric system use becquerels exclusively. Because the curie

(Ci) is a relatively large number compared to the becquerel (Bq), which is small in normal usage of radioactive sources, subunits of the curie are used: nanocurie (nCi, $10^{-9}$ Ci), microcurie (μCi, $10^{-6}$ Ci), millicurie (mCi, $10^{-3}$ Ci). The commonly used subunits of the becquerel are kilobecquerel (KBq, $10^3$ Bq), megabecquerel (MBq, $10^6$ Bq), and gigabecquerel (GBq, $10^9$ Bq).

### Half-Life Determination of Mixed Radioactivities

For a sample containing a mixture of several radioactivities, one characteristic that can be used to identify the constituent radioisotopes is half-life. A curve-stripping scheme (Fig. 21-12) for radioisotope identification is available in simple computer programs. This method is difficult to use for radioisotope identification, however, if the half-lives of the constituent radionuclide are very similar, in which case radiochemical separations may be necessary. The hypothetic sample shown in Fig. 21-12 is composed of three radioisotopes, with initial activities of 1,000; 5,000; and 10,000 counts and half-lives of 10 hours, 1 hour, and 2 hours, respectively. In this analysis, the sample is counted using any radiation detector without energy discrimination until only the nuclide with the longest half-life remains. The half-life and initial activity of this long-lived nuclide can be obtained from the graph,

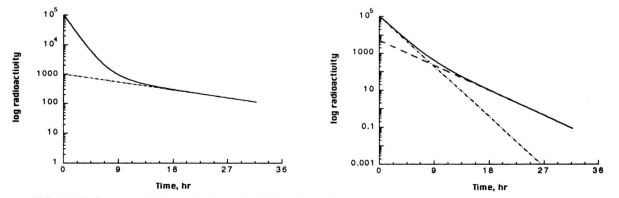

**FIG. 21-12.** Curve-stripping to obtain the half-lives of the three components of a mixture of radionuclides.

and its contribution to the total activity of the mixture can be subtracted from the data, as shown in Fig. 21-12A to obtain the aggregate counts of the two remaining radionuclides shown in Fig. 21-12B. The data in Fig. 21-12B can then be similarly resolved to obtain half-lives and initial activities of the remaining two radionuclides in the mixture. Simple computer programs can also be used to resolve this mixture into its individual components.

## DECAY OF PARENT-DAUGHTER RADIOISOTOPES

Several radioisotopes decay to daughters that are themselves radioactive. An example is U-238, which decays in a chain of successive decays, in which the daughter straddles the line of stability (see Fig. 21-2) until the stable Pb-206 is reached. This uranium series, which is one of three naturally occurring radioactive families or series, consist of eight alpha decays and six beta decays. The semi-empiric mass equation previously mentioned can also be used to explain the decay of these series.

In the simplest of a radioactive family, wherein a parent nucleus decays to a radioactive daughter, which then decays to a stable nucleus, the rate of change in the amount of daughter nuclei, $N_d$, is as follows:

$$\frac{dN_d}{dt} = -N_d\lambda_d + N_p\lambda_p, \qquad (5)$$

where $N$ is number of nuclei and $\lambda$ the decay constant; subscripts $p$ and $d$ refer to parent and daughter. Differentiation gives the number of daughter nuclei at any time $t$, as follows:

$$N_d(t=0) = N_p(t=0)\left(\frac{\lambda_p}{\lambda_d - \lambda_p}\right)(e^{-\lambda_{pt}} - e^{-\lambda dt})$$

$$+ N_d(t=0)\,e^{-\lambda dt} \quad (6)$$

From this equation, three types of equilibrium between parent and daughter can result. The first situation is that the daughter's half-life is very short compared to the parent's half-life. This leads to secular equilibrium, wherein the number of daughter nuclei reaches equilibrium with the parent, and both decay at the same rate if the mixture is left undisturbed. In the second situation, the half-life of the parent is shorter than that of the daughter, in which case no equilibrium is reached. In the third situation, the half-life of the daughter is not much shorter than that of the parent. In this case, a transient equilibrium is reached wherein, after some time, the number of daughter nuclei is the same as the parent nuclei but then exceeds it by the factor $[\lambda_p/(\lambda_d - \lambda_p)]$. If left undisturbed, the daughter decays at the same rate as the parent. Parent-daughter pairs whose decays can be described either by secular or transient equilibria have been useful in nuclear medicine as generators of radioisotopes, which have enabled clinics to have short-lived radionuclides from longer-lived parents purchased from distant production facilities. An example of a generator is the Mo-99–Tc-99m generator (see Chapter 22).

## STATISTICAL NATURE OF RADIOACTIVE DECAY

Radioactive decay is a statistical process in the sense that it is difficult to predict the decay of a single nucleus even if its half-life is known. Radioactive decay is the bulk property of several nuclei and is best described using the laws of statistics. Because the unstable nucleus either does or does not decay in a certain time period, binomial distribution can describe the statistics of decay. In most applications, the number of radioactive nuclei (or the number of trials) involved are in the thousands or more, therefore, the binomial distribution is approximated by the Poisson distribution. This law of distribution best describes radioactive decay. In Poisson distribution, the standard error or variance is the square root of the counts, $\sqrt{N}$. Thus, the higher the number of counts obtained, the lower the percent error ($\sqrt{N}/N$). This standard error is useful in determining the reliability of counting equipment because deviation of a set of repeated counts should approximate the square root of the average counts if the equipment is properly functioning. It should be made clear that this definition of standard error holds only for measured counts and not count rate ($R = N/t$), which involves a constant: the counting time $t$ needed to obtain $N$ counts. In the case of count rates, the standard error ($\sigma$) is calculated as follows:

$$\sigma = \frac{\sqrt{N}}{t} = \frac{\sqrt{R}}{t} \qquad (7)$$

When counts are added or subtracted, the $\sigma$ of the sums or differences of counts $N_1$ and $N_2$ can be obtained as follows:

$$\sigma = \sqrt{N_1 + N_2}$$

$$\%\sigma = \frac{100\sqrt{(N_1 + N_2)}}{(N_1 \pm N_2)} \qquad (8)$$

For example, to subtract background from a count, $N_g$:

$$N_n = N_g - N_b, \qquad (9)$$

where $N$ is the number of counts, and subscripts $n$, $g$, and $b$ refer to net, gross, and background. The $\%\sigma$ is calculated like this:

$$\%\sigma = \frac{100\sqrt{(N_g + N_b)}}{(N_g - N_b)} \qquad (10)$$

In terms of count rates, the $\%\sigma$ is found with this equation:

$$\%\sigma = \frac{100\sqrt{[(R/t)_g + (R/t)_b]}}{[(R/t)_g + (R/t)_b]} \qquad (11)$$

When a count $N_1$ is multiplied or divided by another count $N_2$, the $\%\sigma$ is found this way:

$$\%\sigma = \sqrt{(\%\sigma \text{ of } N_1)^2 + (\%\sigma \text{ of } N_2)^2} \qquad (12)$$

The rules on propagation of errors are applicable to all situations encountered in the counting of radiation. For further examples of counting statistics, see the textbook by Sorenson and Phelps mentioned in the Suggested Reading at the end of this chapter.

## CHEMICAL EFFECTS OF RADIOACTIVE DECAY

The transformation of a radioactive nucleus to a more stable configuration via a radioactive decay process has the following chemical consequences:

1. A change in chemical identity occurs; for example, alpha decay leads to (Z – 2) daughter, $\beta^-$ decay leads to (Z + 1) daughter, and both $\beta^+$ and EC decay lead to (Z – 1) daughter.
2. A charged daughter forms; for example, $\alpha$ decay leads to a daughter with a –2 charge, $\beta^-$ decay leads to a +1 daughter, and $\beta^+$ and EC lead to a –1 daughter.
3. To conserve momentum, the daughter nucleus recoils opposite the direction of emitted radiation. This recoil energy in most instances is greater than the bond energy of the atom, leading to the breakup of the molecule.
4. Electronic excitation due to sudden change in nuclear charge leads to ionization, wherein one or more electrons are "shaken off."

In nuclear medicine, the radioisotope is usually attached to a molecule or radiopharmaceutical, which gives it selectivity toward its target organ. The net consequence of these four nuclear and electronic changes is that the daughter nucleus breaks its chemical bonds to its parent molecule, which generally leads to the fragmentation of the molecule. Although these radiopharmaceutical molecules are given in very minute (tracer or subpharmacologic) amounts, the fragmentation after radioactive decay ensures the loss of biological activity of the molecule after decay of the radiolabel.

Another interesting effect of radioactive decay modes (e.g., EC and internal conversion) that result in inner electronic shell vacancy is that the ensuing rearrangement of electrons to fill the vacancy created by radioactive decay results in the emission of x-rays and electrons. This process of electronic rearrangement is called the *Auger effect*. The transition of a higher orbital electron to fill the lower shell vacancy is accompanied by the release of an x-ray whose energy is the difference between the energies of electronic levels involved in the transition. A competing process to this x-ray release is the emission of an electron, called an *Auger electron*, whose kinetic energy is that which the x-ray would have had minus the binding energy of the Auger electron. The emission of the Auger electron leaves another electron shell vacancy in addition to the initial vacancy. These vacancies are then filled by electrons from higher orbitals, which are then also accompanied by emission of other x-rays or Auger electrons. The release of x-rays and Auger electrons continues until the vacancies reach the outermost shell of the atom; this leads to an ion with multiple positive charges. Because the time frame of these electronic rearrangements is shorter than vibrational times, this multiple positively charged ion, if it were bound in a molecule, draws electrons from other atoms in the molecule. The momentary result is a molecule made up of positively charged atoms, which then fragment due to coulombic repulsion. The low-energy x-rays

and Auger electrons emitted in this process have been found to be highly cytotoxic, especially when localized in the highly sensitive cell nucleus. Radioisotopes such as I-125, which decays by EC, and bromine 80m, which decays by internal conversion, have been found to be very toxic to cells in vitro when incorporated into the cells' DNA. Using Auger electron–emitting isotopes attached to a suitable target-seeking ligand has been suggested as possible therapy for some neoplastic diseases. The radiobiological consequences of this effect has led to the re-evaluation of the dosimetry of radionuclides that undergo the Auger process.

## INTERACTIONS OF RADIATION WITH MATTER

It is important to understand the interactions of radiation with matter for reasons of safety, for purposes of detection and measurement, and for accurate dose calculations.

Radiations can be classified into particulate and nonparticulate radiations. Particulate radiations include charged particles, such as the heavy charged particles (e.g., alpha particle, proton) and electrons ($e^-$, $\beta^-$, $\beta^+$), and the uncharged neutron. Nonparticulate radiations are energetic electromagnetic radiations, including gamma rays and x-rays. Particulate and nonparticulate radiations interact with matter via different mechanisms, described separately below.

Atomic volume is essentially defined by the electronic shell. Atomic radii are on the order of $10^{-10}$ m, whereas nuclear radii are approximately $10^{-15}$ m, so radiation is more likely to interact with electrons than the nucleus of an atom. These electronic interactions include ionization (knocking out of valence electrons and inner shell electrons from their orbits), excitation, and elastic and inelastic scattering processes. Interaction of radiation with target nuclei may involve nuclear excitations or reactions that lead to radioactive nuclei. Interaction with the nuclear field alone may result in emission of radiation (bremsstrahlung), or, in the case of energetic gammas, lead to the creation of matter (electron-positron pair).

### Particulate Radiation Interactions

Charged particles, such as alpha particles and electrons, cause ionizations and excitations as they encounter atoms in their track. Because it's a heavy particle, an alpha particle causes high ionization density along its path; the level of ionization increases as it slows down toward the end of its track. A beta particle, being of smaller mass than an alpha particle, is more easily deflected from its track. Beta particles have a more tortuous path and, thus, less predictable ranges. In addition to ionizations and electronic excitations, a beta particle can interact with the electric field of nuclei in its path by accelerating or decelerating, depending on its charge ($\beta^-$ or $\beta^+$). In this interaction, beta particles lose energy by emitting x-rays called *bremsstrahlung* (braking radiation). In some cases, such as with yttrium 90 (Y-90), these x-rays can be imaged. Alpha

## Photoelectric Effect    Compton Scattering    Pair Production

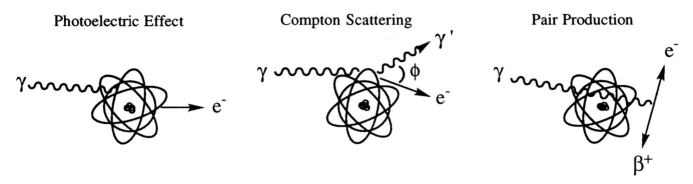

**FIG. 21-13.** Diagrammatic representation of the three main types of gamma interactions with matter.

and other heavy particles also interact with nuclei in a similar manner, but because of their heavier mass, loss of energy by bremsstrahlung is minimal. Both alpha and beta particles can cause ionizations, wherein the ejected electron has energy high enough to cause secondary ionizations. These energetic electrons are called *delta* (δ) *rays*.

### Nonparticulate Radiation Interactions

Gamma rays are important in the production of images of radiotracer localizations in nuclear medicine procedures. The major electronic interactions of photons with matter are photoelectric effect and Compton scattering. A third gamma interaction with matter, called *pair production,* involves gamma-nucleus interaction (Fig. 21-13).

#### Photoelectric Effect

Photoelectric effect involves the complete transfer of photon energy to an orbital electron, which is then ejected as a photoelectron with energy equal to the energy of the photon minus the electron's binding energy. The binding energy of electrons is small, usually in the electron volt (eV) range, whereas γ energies useful in nuclear medicine are in the hundreds of kiloelectron volt (KeV) range. The kinetic energy of the photoelectron then is essentially equal to the energy of the incident gamma. Because gamma energy is an identifying characteristic of the emitting radionuclide, gamma spectrometry using solid state detectors, which measures photoelectron energies, can be used to identify unknown radionuclides.

#### Compton Scattering

Compton scattering involves the incomplete deposition of photon energy, wherein a Compton electron and a scattered photon of reduced energy escapes the absorber atom. The angle φ between the direction of the electron and scattered γ′ defines how the energy of the incident γ is shared between the Compton electron and the scattered photon, γ′.

#### Pair Production

When the photon energy is >1.022 MeV, a third interaction, pair production, between the photon and the nuclear electric field produces an electron-positron pair. The 1.022-MeV threshold is required to provide the mass of the electron-positron pair, and the gamma energy >1.022 MeV is shared by the pair.

The relative probabilities of each of these three photon interactions depends on photon energy and atomic number, Z, of the absorber. Photoelectric probability, τ, decreases rapidly with increasing photon energy but increases with increasing absorber Z. Compton scattering probability, σ, decreases slowly with increasing photon energy and also increases with increasing absorber Z. Pair production probability, κ, starts at zero at the 1.022-MeV threshold and increases logarithmically with increasing photon energy and absorber Z. In the context of radionuclide imaging, photoelectric effect is what produces images of radiotracer localization, and Compton scattering degrades or blurs the image. For optimal photon detection and thus better images, radionuclides are selected on the basis of photon energies optimized for high photoelectric probability, τ, and low Compton probability, σ. The radionuclide must also have sufficiently high energy to get out of the body yet be stopped by the external detector (gamma camera), which uses high-Z materials.

### RADIOISOTOPE PRODUCTION

In the early years of nuclear medicine, the available selection of radioisotopes was very limited due to the limited knowledge of radioisotope production techniques. Although Lawrence developed the cyclotron in 1932, only simple radioisotopes, such as P-32, were available. For some time, the most commonly available radioisotopes were fission daughters of uranium, notably I-131. Because of the unique iodine-sequestering property of the thyroid, the use of radioiodine for imaging and therapy was a major application in the early days of nuclear medicine. After World War II, principally because of advances made in the Manhattan Project on nuclear reactions and radiochemical separation tech-

**TABLE 21-2.** *Examples of radioisotopes produced via neutron reactions in a nuclear reactor and some of their useful properties*

| Radioisotope | Decay mode | Half-life | Production route | % Natural abundance of target isotope |
|---|---|---|---|---|
| $^{14}$C | $\beta^-$ | 5,730 yrs | $^{14}$N + n $\rightarrow$ $^{14}$C + p | 99.63 |
| $^{18}$F | $\beta^+$ | 109.8 mins | $^6$Li + n $\rightarrow$ $^7$Li $\rightarrow$ $^3$H + $^6$O $\rightarrow$ $^{18}$F + n | 7.5 |
| $^{24}$Na | $\beta^-$ | 15 hrs | $^{23}$Na + n $\rightarrow$ $^{24}$Na + $\gamma$ | 100 |
| $^{32}$P | $\beta^-$ | 14.3 days | $^{31}$P + n $\rightarrow$ $^{32}$P + $\gamma$ | 100 |
| $^{35}$S | $\beta^-$ | 87.4 days | $^{35}$Cl + n $\rightarrow$ $^{35}$S + p | 75.77 |
| $^{42}$K | $\beta^-$ | 12.36 hrs | $^{41}$K + n $\rightarrow$ $^{42}$K + $\gamma$ | 6.73 |
| $^{45}$Ca | EC | 165 days | $^{44}$Ca + n $\rightarrow$ $^{45}$Ca + $\gamma$ | 2.09 |
| $^{51}$Cr | EC | 21.7 days | $^{50}$Cr + n $\rightarrow$ $^{51}$Cr + $\gamma$ | 4.35 |
| $^{59}$Fe | $\beta^-$ | 44.6 days | $^{58}$Fe + n $\rightarrow$ $^{59}$Fe + $\gamma$ | 0.29 |
| $^{64}$Cu | EC, $\beta^-$, $\beta^+$ | 12.7 hrs | $^{63}$Cu + n $\rightarrow$ $^{64}$Cu + $\gamma$ | 69.2 |
| $^{65}$Zn | EC, $\beta^-$ | 244.1 days | $^{64}$Zn + n $\rightarrow$ $^{65}$Zn + $\gamma$ | 48.6 |
| $^{75}$Se | EC | 118.5 days | $^{74}$Se + n $\rightarrow$ $^{75}$Se + $\gamma$ | 0.87 |
| $^{82}$Br | $\beta^-$ | 35.34 hrs | $^{81}$Br + n $\rightarrow$ $^{82}$Br + $\gamma$ | 49.3 |
| $^{90}$Y | $\beta^-$ | 64.1 hrs | $^{89}$Y + n $\rightarrow$ $^{90}$Y + $\gamma$ | 100 |
| $^{99}$Mo | $\beta^-$ | 66 hrs | $^{98}$Mo + n $\rightarrow$ $^{99}$Mo + $\gamma$ | 24.1 |
| $^{131}$I | $\beta^-$ | 8 days | $^{130}$Te + n $\rightarrow$ $^{131}$Te $\rightarrow$ $^{131}$I | 34.5 |

n, neutron; p, proton.

**TABLE 21-3.** *Radioisotopes produced in accelerators and some of their useful properties*

| Radioisotope | Decay mode | Half-life | Production route | % Natural abundance of target isotope |
|---|---|---|---|---|
| $^{11}$C | $\beta^+$ | 20.38 mins | $^{11}$B + p $\rightarrow$ $^{11}$C + n | 80.3 |
| | | | $^{14}$N + p $\rightarrow$ $^{11}$C + $\alpha$ | 99.63 |
| $^{13}$N | $\beta^+$ | 9.96 mins | $^{12}$C + d $\rightarrow$ $^{13}$N + n | 98.89 |
| | | | $^{13}$C + p $\rightarrow$ $^{13}$N + n | 1.11 |
| $^{15}$O | $\beta^+$ | 122 secs | $^{14}$N + d $\rightarrow$ $^{15}$O + n | 99.63 |
| | | | $^{15}$N + p $\rightarrow$ $^{15}$O + n | 0.366 |
| $^{18}$F | $\beta^+$ | 109.8 mins | $^{20}$Ne + d $\rightarrow$ $^{18}$F + $\alpha$ | 90.51 |
| | | | $^{18}$O + p $\rightarrow$ $^{18}$F + n | 0.204 |
| $^{22}$Na | $\beta^+$ | 2.6 yrs | $^{23}$Na + p $\rightarrow$ $^{22}$Na + 2n | 100 |
| $^{52}$Mn | EC, $\beta^+$ | 5.59 days | $^{52}$Cr + p $\rightarrow$ $^{52}$Mn + n | 83.79 |
| $^{67}$Ga | EC | 78 hrs | $^{67}$Zn + p $\rightarrow$ $^{67}$Ga + n | 4.10 |
| $^{68}$Ga | $\beta^+$ | 68 mins | $^{68}$Zn + p $\rightarrow$ $^{68}$Ga + n | 18.8 |
| $^{89}$Zr | EC, $\beta^+$ | 78.4 hrs | $^{89}$Y + p $\rightarrow$ $^{89}$Zr + n | 100 |
| $^{111}$In | EC | 2.83 days | $^{111}$Cd + p $\rightarrow$ $^{111}$In + n | 12.8 |
| $^{123}$I | EC | 13 hrs | $^{124}$Te + p $\rightarrow$ $^{123}$I + 3n | 4.6 |
| $^{201}$Tl | EC | 73 hrs | $^{201}$Hg + d $\rightarrow$ $^{201}$Tl + 2n | 13.3 |

n, neutron; $\alpha$, alpha particle; p, proton; d, deuteron.

niques, more radioisotopes became more readily available for medical applications.

### Reactor-Produced Radioisotopes

With nuclear reactors in the postwar era producing usable quantities of neutrons for nuclear reactions, new radioisotopes for use in medicine became more available. Some radioisotopes produced in nuclear reactors commonly used in biomedical research and some of their properties are listed in Table 21-2.

### Accelerator-Produced Radioisotopes

Most of the radioisotope production methods using the nuclear reactor are based on the $^A_Z X(n,\gamma)$ $^{A+1}_Z X$ reaction, wherein the target $^A_Z X$ nucleus absorbs a thermal neutron, promptly emits gamma radiation, and results in the product $^{A+1}_Z X$ nucleus. If one considers specific activity, which is defined as the amount of radioactivity per the total number of molecules of that element, a disadvantage of using the $(n,\gamma)$ reaction for radioisotopes production is that in most cases low–specific activity products are obtained. This is because the product radioisotope is the same element as the target. There are, however, other neutron reactions, such as the $(n,p)$ reaction, which are useful in the production of high specific activity radionuclides. A general method to produce high–specific activity radioisotopes involves the use of a charged particle accelerator such as a cyclotron. In this case, product nuclei are usually different from the target nuclei and are usually chemically separable from the bulk target material. Common particle beams obtained from current accelerators are beams of protons, deuterons, He-3, and alpha particles. Table 21-3 lists some examples of accelerator-produced radioisotopes and some of their properties.

## Generators

The development of generators made it easier and more practical for many clinics to perform radionuclide imaging in sites distant from a reactor or a cyclotron. The most widely useful generator is the Mo-Tc generator. As it turned out, technetium (element 43), which is not present in nature and represented by an empty box in the chemical periodic table before its discovery in 1937 by Segre, is the most ideal radioisotope for nuclear medicine imaging. The characteristics of Tc-99m that make it ideal include the following:

- It decays by isomeric transitions and emits a single major gamma ray without particulate emissions, thus the radiation dose is minimized.
- The gamma energy of 140 Kev is in the optimal energy range for external detection. Gammas with lower energies would undergo more scattering and attenuating processes before emerging from the body for external detection by gamma cameras, whereas gammas with higher energies would have longer ranges but higher probability of escaping detection by zipping through the detector without interacting.
- A variety of compounds with different target organs have been developed that can be labeled with Tc. These clinically useful Tc radiopharmaceuticals can be prepared from commercially available kits.
- The 6-hour half-life of Tc is sufficiently matched to most imaging applications.

- Generators are available that reach transient equilibrium in approximately 1 day. These can isolate fresh batches of Tc-99m by "milking" the Mo-99m "cow" daily to correspond to the maximum Tc-99m activity in the generator.

These optimal characteristics of Tc-99m as imaging label have proved to be self-perpetuating for this radionuclide, which is now the workhorse of nuclear medicine. A large segment of the nuclear medicine industry is involved in optimizing the production of Tc-99m, in developing technetium compounds for a variety of physiologic applications as well as the easy preparation of these new agents using simple kits, and in developing gamma cameras that are optimally designed to detect the 140-keV gamma ray of Tc-99m.

In the last half-century, developments in nuclear medicine procedures resulting in more effective methods to diagnose and treat disease have established this field as a common clinical subspecialty. The improved cost-benefit ratio of procedures have allowed nuclear medicine to flourish despite unfounded fears of low levels of ionizing radiation and competition with other imaging modes, such as x-ray CT and MRI. Visualization of biochemical and physiologic functions is still the domain of nuclear medicine and will remain so for a long time to come.

## SUGGESTED READING

Friedlander G, Kennedy JW, Macias ES, Miller JM. Nuclear and Radiochemistry (3rd ed). New York: Wiley, 1981.

Kane, G. The Elementary Particle Garden: Our Universe as Understood by Particle Physicists. Reading, MA: Addison-Wesley, 1995.

Sorenson JA, Phelps M. Physics in Nuclear Medicine (2nd ed). New York: Grune & Stratton, 1987.

*Textbook of Nuclear Medicine,*
edited by Michael A. Wilson.
Lippincott–Raven Publishers, Philadelphia © 1998.

# CHAPTER 22

# Radiopharmaceuticals

Michael A. Wilson and Richard J. Hammes

Substances given to patients are defined as drugs or pharmaceuticals. Section 201g of the Federal Food, Drug, and Cosmetic (FDC) Act defines drugs as "articles intended for use in the diagnosis, cure, mitigation, treatment or prevention of disease in man or animals" and "articles (other than food) intended to affect the structure or any function of the body of man or animals." Note that it is the intended use, and not the article itself, that makes it a drug.

Radiopharmaceuticals (RPs) are drugs that contain one or more radioactive atoms and are used for diagnosis and treatment. All RPs are legend drugs (as opposed to over-the-counter drugs) and are subject to all the regulations that apply to other legend drugs, including state medical and pharmacy practice acts, in addition to the regulations of the U.S. Food and Drug Administration (FDA), which enforce the FDC act. Because they are radioactive, they are regulated by state boards of radiologic health. If they include fission by-product material covered by the Atomic Energy Act, they are also regulated by the Nuclear Regulatory Commission (NRC).

A key characteristic of all RPs is that they are administered in *tracer* amounts. The mass amount administered is low enough to have no intrinsic pharmacologic effect. For diagnostic use, it is imperative that the tracer does not perturb the physiologic parameter it is measuring. For therapeutic use, it is the radiation and not the pharmacologic effect of the labeled molecule that produces the desired therapy. Sometimes, the RPs are actually the radioactive atoms (radionuclides) themselves. In these drugs, the radionuclide defines the biodistribution, for example, radioiodines (iodine 131 [I-131] and I-123) in thyroid studies and the inert gases (xenon 133 [Xe-133], Xe-127, and krypton 81m [Kr-81m]) used in ventilation imaging. More often, the RP is a combination of the radionuclide, which provides a detectable signal, and a ligand, which determines the biodistribution.

RPs provide the uniqueness of nuclear medicine imaging and explain why nuclear medicine exists as an imaging modality when the resolution is a full order of magnitude less than that of computed tomography, magnetic resonance imaging, ultrasonography, or plain films. The exploitation of the difference in normal physiology and pathophysiology provides a functional perspective that is important clinically.

Milestones in the early history of RPs are shown in Table 22-1. Apart from the obvious importance of the work of Becquerel, Hevesy, and others, it was only with Siedlin's successful treatment of thyroid cancer with I-131 that the peace-time use of radioactivity became popular and received considerable financial support. Neither the successful commercial production of the gamma camera nor the molybdenum 99m–technetium 99m (Mo-99/Tc-99m) generator immediately revolutionized nuclear medicine. Rather, it was the introduction of the "instant kit" using the stannous ion reduction method that provided a general labeling technique and allowed the widespread dissemination of Tc-99m RPs establishing nuclear medicine as a viable clinical specialty.

## DEFINITIONS

Although often used interchangeably, the words that follow have the specific meanings provided:

- *Nuclide:* individual atom described by specific number of neutrons and protons
- *Isotope:* nuclides with the same number of protons but different numbers of neutrons
- *Radioactivity:* the process of emitting particles or electromagnetic radiation (gamma or x-rays) characteristic for each radionuclide
- *Radionuclide:* a radioactive nuclide
- *Radioisotope:* radionuclides with the same number of protons (e.g., iodine 123 [I-123], I-125, I-131)
- *Pharmaceutical:* substance given to patients for medical reasons (i.e., drug)
- *Radiopharmaceutical:* a radioactive pharmaceutical used for diagnostic or therapeutic procedures
- *Tracer:* a readily detected substance that can be followed through a biological process without affecting the process
- *Radiotracer:* a radioactive tracer
- *Specific activity:* radioactivity per unit mass of a nuclide

**TABLE 22-1.** *Early history of radiopharmaceuticals*

| Researcher | Year | Event |
|---|---|---|
| Becquerel | 1896 | Discovers radioactivity |
| Hevesy | 1923 | Establishes tracer method |
| E. Lawrence | 1931 | Invents cyclotron |
| Joliet and Curie | 1934 | Discover artificial radio-activity |
| Perrier and Segre | 1937 | Locate technetium for space 43 |
| J. Lawrence | 1938 | Uses P-32 in leukemia therapy |
| Seaborg | 1938 | Discovers I-131 |
| Hertz | 1938 | Measures thyroid uptake (I-128) |
| Hamilton and Soley | 1939 | Use I-131 in humans |
| Hertz and Roberts | 1941 | Use I-131 to treat hyper-thyroidism |
| Fermi | 1942 | First sustained nuclear reaction |
| Manhattan Project | 1946 | Fission radionuclides (I-131) available |
| Siedlin | 1946 | Treats thyroid cancer with I-131 |
| Cassen and Curtis | 1949 | First scintillation scanner |
| Richards | 1957 | Suggests role of Tc-99m generator |
| Anger | 1958 | First scintillation camera |
| Nuclear Chicago | 1961 | First commercial gamma camera |
| Med. Consult. Corp. | 1965 | First commercial Tc-99m generator |
| Stern et al. | 1966 | Tc-99m SC produced by thiosulfate method |
| Eckelman | 1970 | DTPA by $Sn^{+2}$ (instant kit) method |
| Subramanian | 1971 | Polyphosphate by $Sn^{+2}$ kit |
| Lebowitz | 1975 | Tl-201 for heart imaging |

- *Specific concentration:* radioactivity per unit weight or diluent volume

## THE IDEAL RP

Selection of the appropriate RP is fundamental to the practice of nuclear medicine, which is based on the physiologic processing of these radiolabeled drugs. Because the goal of diagnostic studies is to provide detectable photons with minimal biological effect, the criteria for an ideal diagnostic agent are quite different from those for a therapeutic RP where cytotoxic effects are desired. In both cases there are some common goals: achieving a high target-to-nontarget ratio in the pathologic tissue and minimizing radiation exposure to normal organs. As a result, many of the desirable attributes of diagnostic RPs apply to therapeutic RPs.

### Diagnostic RPs

The criteria for the diagnostic RP of choice include the following categories: nuclear properties, biological properties, chemical properties, economics, and regulatory status. The goal in most diagnostic applications is to obtain an image of pathologic tissue. In a few applications, the goal is merely the quantification of activity by counting an organ (with a probe) or a blood or urine sample (in a well counter). The desirable qualities of the RP are as follows:

- Easily detectable and quantifiable with the available instrumentation
- Localizes in the tissue of interest and clears from others
- Appropriate physical and biological half-life
- Chemical stability during preparation and in vivo
- Approval by regulatory agencies
- Available at a cost-effective price

**TABLE 22-2.** *Common radionuclides with their physical characteristics and production methods*

| Radionuclide | Physical half-life | Principal decay mode | Principal energy (keV) | Abundance (%)* | Production method |
|---|---|---|---|---|---|
| O-15 | 2 minutes | $\beta^+$ | 511 | 200% | Cyclotron |
| N-13 | 10 minutes | $\beta^+$ | 511 | 200% | Cyclotron |
| C-11 | 20 minutes | $\beta^+$ | 511 | 200% | Cyclotron |
| F-18 | 110 minutes | $\beta^+$ | 511 | 194% | Cyclotron |
| Tc-99m | 6.02 hours | IT | 140 | 89% | Generator |
| I-123 | 13.2 hours | EC | 159 | 100% | Cyclotron |
| Mo-99 | 66 hours | $\beta^-$ | 740 | 14% | Reactor |
| In-111 | 67 hours | EC | 173, 247 | 184% | Cyclotron |
| Tl-201 | 73 hours | EC | 69–81 | 93% | Cyclotron |
| Ga-67 | 78 hours | EC | 90, 190, 298 | 82% | Cyclotron |
| Xe-133 | 5.3 days | $\beta^-$ | 83 | 37% | Reactor |
| I-131 | 8.05 days | $\beta^-$ | 361 | 81% | Reactor |

$\beta^+$, positron decay; $\beta^-$, beta decay; IT, isomeric transition; EC, electron capture.
*Abundance of the principal energies listed.

### Nuclear (Physical) Properties

Four physical properties (Table 22-2) of the radionuclide must be considered:

1. Physical half-life
2. Decay mode
3. Emitted photon energies
4. Availability

### Half-Life

A radionuclide's half-life must be long enough to allow the synthesis, administration, biological localization, and background tissue clearance of the RP. If the radionuclide is too long-lived, unnecessary body irradiation occurs. A rule of thumb is that the physical half-life should be approximately equal to the time it takes to prepare the RP, administer it, and complete the imaging. It must be noted that an important modifier is the biological rate of uptake and clearance of the RP. If the biological uptake and clearance of a particular RP are very fast, as with lung ventilation studies, the radionuclide's physical half-life is inconsequential from a dosimetry point of view.

In determining the overall, or *effective*, half-life, the effects of both the physiologic and physical half-lives are included. The resultant effective half-life is always less than the shorter of the physical and physiologic half-lives.

$$T_{eff} = \frac{T_p T_b}{T_p + T_b}, \qquad (1)$$

where $T_{eff}$ is the effective half-life, $T_b$ is the biological half-life, and $T_p$ is the physical half-life.

The metabolic fate, including route of excretion, helps to determine the biological half-life. Renal excretion routes often are important, which explains why the bladder is often the critical organ (organ with the greatest radiation dose). RPs preferentially excreted by the gastrointestinal (GI) tract have the bowel as the critical organ. RPs with long half-lives that are partially excreted into the bowel often have high doses to the large bowel because of the prolonged residence time (e.g., although gallium 67 [Ga-67] citrate is predominantly excreted renally, the large bowel is the critical organ).

### Decay Mode

Imaging procedures require an electromagnetic photon (gamma ray or x-ray) to produce an image. It is desirable that the photon be emitted in high abundance and be monoenergetic. Particulate radiations such as beta or alpha rays are not detected. These radiations produce a high density of ions per unit path length and hence result in significant tissue damage, though they do not penetrate tissue more than 1 or 2 cm. It follows that for diagnostic use, a pure gamma-emitting decay mode would be desirable, but it must be recognized that there are no pure electromagnetic radiation decay modes. Radionuclides that decay by isomeric transition (IT) (e.g., Tc-99m, Kr-81m) or electron capture (EC) (e.g., thallium 201 [Tl-201], Ga-67, indium 111 [In-111], I-123) are the most useful and diagnostic. With IT, for the energy range we are concerned about, there is always some production of conversion and auger electrons. With EC, there are always auger electrons and some conversion electrons. These secondary electrons are as highly ionizing as beta particles. Nonetheless, radiation exposure is acceptable when using a radionuclide that decays by one of these modes.

The exception is positron decay, the basis of positron emission tomography (PET) technology. In PET, a particle (a positron) is emitted and interacts with an electron and results in a pair of annihilation 511-keV photons. In this case, the ideal positron radionuclide would emit only positrons and not electromagnetic photons.

### Photon Energy

One of the big tradeoffs in nuclear medicine involves the balance between resolution and sensitivity. This is a major concern when designing gamma camera system crystals, collimators, and electronics because the design is strongly dependent on photon energy. The energy must be high enough that it escapes the body without being attenuated too much, but it must also be low enough to undergo a photoelectric interaction in the camera crystal. The gamma camera electronics are conventionally set up to detect radiation in the 60- to 400-keV range, but this needs to be extended for PET to allow detection of the 511-keV annihilation photons. Making the crystal thicker increases the probability of an interaction but degrades the resolution. With higher-energy photons there is more separation between the photoelectric peak and Compton scatter, which allows better resolution, but the higher-energy photon is more likely to pass right through the crystal, thus giving decreased sensitivity (Table 22-3). Higher-energy photons require thicker-walled collimators, which further decrease sensitivity. For an optimal balance between resolution and sensitivity with current Anger cameras, the energy of the RP emission should be in the range of 100 to

**TABLE 22-3.** *Photon detection efficiency in half-inch NaI (TI) detector*

| Radionuclide | Energy (keV) | Efficiency (%) |
|---|---|---|
| Tc-99m | 140 | 86 |
| In-111 | 173 | 73 |
|  | 247 | 43 |
| I-131 | 364 | 12 |
| Positron | 511 | 8 |

200 keV. In this regard, the ideal radionuclides are Tc-99m (140 keV) and I-123 (159 keV).

When multiple same-day studies are required (e.g., lung ventilation and perfusion studies or stress and rest myocardial perfusion imaging) two approaches are possible. If there is a mixture of radionuclides with different photon energies, it is best to use the lower-energy RP first, followed by the higher-energy RP study. If using Xe-133 (80 keV) for ventilation studies, the ventilation scan should be done before the Tc-99m (140 keV) macro-aggregated albumin (MAA) perfusion scan. This is problematic because only one ventilation scan view can be obtained with a single dose of inert gas, and it would be helpful to know which projection best shows the perfusion defect (see Chapter 4). The Tc-99m pentetate aerosol is the most popular RP for ventilation studies because it is readily available and reasonably priced, gives multiple views, and has all the inherent advantages of Tc-99m (i.e., physical half-life, energy, decay mode). Because it is the same energy as the Tc-99m MAA, it is given before the perfusion scan in a total dose of approximately 0.5 mCi. The Tc-99m MAA is then given at a dose of 4 mCi (eight times as much as the ventilation scan dose) to flood out the pentetate activity.

*Availability*

One key criterion for an ideal RP is availability. If it is unavailable, no matter how ideal it may be in other respects, it will not see widespread use. The most readily available non–Tc-99m radionuclides decay by $\beta^-$ decay, but for diagnostic use, nonparticulate radiation is preferable and occurs with electron capture (EC) decay. EC radionuclides are characterized by an excess of protons over neutrons in their nuclei. They are typically produced by bombardment in a proton accelerator, usually a cyclotron.

The most readily available radionuclide is Tc-99m, because this is eluted from a Mo-99/Tc-99m generator. A generator is nothing more than an ion-exchange column that separates the daughter technetium from the parent molybdenum. The parent Mo-99 decays by $\beta$ decay, with a half-life of 66 hours, resulting in a shorter-lived (6-hour) daughter (Tc-99m). A new generator is purchased once a week and supplies all the Tc-99m needed for that week, available 24 hours a day. This availability, along with its nearly ideal half-life, decay mode, and gamma energy, has resulted in Tc-99m being the workhorse radionuclide for RP production.

**Biological Properties**

The nuclear properties of the radionuclide determine the usefulness of an RP for detection by imaging or counting, but the biological properties of the RP determine its localization and fate after administration. Some RPs localize

because of the radionuclide's own elemental state (inert gases of ventilation scanning, e.g., Xe-133) or ionic state (thyroidal uptake of I-123 as iodide). Most clinically useful RPs are taken up because of the localization mechanisms (Table 22-4). The ideal RP should do the following:

- Localize rapidly and exclusively in the organ of interest
- Localize more in pathologic tissue than in normal tissue
- Be metabolically inert unless metabolism determines targeting
- Clear rapidly from background tissues
- Be rapidly excreted after the study is completed

The ideal RP should also be pharmacologically inert, so it does not perturb the system it is measuring; have no side effects; require minimal patient preparation; and have few drug interactions.

*Mechanism of Localization*

The actual uptake mechanism covers a large range of specific and nonspecific processes that involve chemical, physical, receptor, and physiologic properties (Table 22-5). Similar Tc-99m RPs have their biodistribution decided by

**TABLE 22-4.** *Types of radiopharmaceuticals*

| Type | Example |
|---|---|
| Elemental | Xe-133, Kr-81m |
| Simple ions | I-131 as I$^-$, Tc-99m as TcO$_4^-$ |
| Small molecules | I-131 OIH, Tc-99m DTPA |
| Macromolecules | Tc-99m HSA, In-111 MOAB |
| Particulate | Tc-99m SC, Tc-99m MAA |
| Cellular elements | In-111 WBC, Tc-99m RBC |
| Isotopic substitution | C-11 in methionine or glucose |

**TABLE 22-5.** *Localization mechanisms*

| Functional | Mechanical |
|---|---|
| Passive transfer (diffusion) | Capillary blockage |
|   Tc-99m TcO$_4^-$ for blood-brain barrier |   Tc-99m MAA in lung perfusion scan |
|   Tc-99m DTPA for glomerular filtration | Phagocytosis |
| Active transport or uptake |   Tc-99m SC for liver-spleen scan |
|   I-123 in thyroid | Sequestration |
|   Tc-99m IDA in liver |   Heat-denatured Tc-99m RBCs for spleen |
| Metabolic trapping | Compartmental space localization |
|   F-18 FDG scanning |   In-111 DTPA for CSF flow |
| Receptor binding |   Tc-99m RBC for cardiac function studies |
|   In-111 pentetreotide |   Xe-133 for ventilation scan |
| Antibody binding | Abnormal extravasation |
|   Tc-99m arcitumomab |   Tc-99m IDA in bile leaks |
|   In-111 satumomab pendetide |   Tc-99m RBC in GI bleeding |

very minor ligand changes; for example, the different renal excretion according to minor structural changes (15%, 9%, and 1% renal excretion) for the three FDA-approved hepatobiliary agents (lidofenin, disofenin, and mebrofenin).

Pharmacologists have investigated specific physiologic receptor sites by using radioactive tracers. It was a small extension to label the receptor-specific drugs with imaging radionuclides for diagnostic use. The first FDA-approved receptor-specific RP was In-111 pentetreotide, approved in 1994. This agent binds to somatostatin receptors, which are expressed by many neuroendocrine tumors. The nonlabeled analog is octreotide, which is used therapeutically for these same tumors. Approval of In-111 pentetreotide was followed closely by the approval of I-131 iobenguane (meta-iodobenzylguanidine [MIBG]) for use as a norepinephrine analog in pheochromocytomas and neuroblastomas.

Many other receptor-specific RPs have been synthesized for clinical research purposes, including agents for the dopamine receptor, serotonin receptor, estrogen receptor, progesterone receptor, and benzodiazepine receptor. These have often been labeled with one of the positron emitters (fluorine 18 [F-18], carbon 11 [C-11], or nitrogen 13 [N-13]), but single-photon radionuclides, such as I-123, have also been used. This is an area of major expansion in the use of RPs. Closely related to this area is the development of molecular recognition units. Molecular recognition units are essentially the amino acid sequence structures responsible for the antibody-antigen reaction and the current ongoing investigations in antisense RPs based on radiolabeled DNA nucleotide sequences. The diagnostic potential of this technology is unlimited.

### Route of Administration

The absorption and route of administration often determine the localization characteristics of RPs. Lung ventilation can be studied by inhalation of an aerosol or gas, whereas pulmonary perfusion is studied by the intravenous injection of labeled particles. The vast majority of RPs are administered intravenously. By selecting the route of administration, totally different biodistributions and kinetics can be obtained: Tc-99m sulfur colloid (SC) injected intravenously concentrates in the reticuloendothelial system, injected subcutaneously is cleared by the lymphatics, and administered orally is confined to the GI tract.

### Target Uptake

It is axiomatic that the agent with a better target uptake is a superior imaging agent. The rate of uptake is also important, and the time of imaging depends on it. It is generally preferable to get earlier images for patient convenience; examples include I-123 sodium iodide (NaI) versus Tc-99m pertechnetate ($TcO_4^-$) for thyroid imaging. The thyroid can be imaged at 20 minutes with $TcO_4^-$ but not until 4 to 6 hours with I-123 NaI.

### Tracer Excretion

Just as the rate and extent of RP uptake is important, so is the rate of clearance. Organ visualization is better when the background tissues have less uptake than the target uptake and background level determines the target-to-nontarget ratio and kinetics. The RP must clear from blood and background tissue to achieve high contrast. This is especially true with small lesions. The rate of renal clearance is often a function of the amount of protein binding in plasma because only unbound drug is eliminated by glomerular filtration. The other major excretion routes are the GI tract and the hepatobiliary route.

## Chemical Properties

Because the nuclear properties criteria tend to favor radionuclides with short half-lives, it becomes necessary to synthesize the final product in-house or at a nearby commercial nuclear pharmacy. This mode of synthesis has become routine for the convenient Tc-99m–based RPs, usually from ready-to-use commercial reagent kits. It is also necessary to compound other products locally, such as In-111–labeled monoclonal antibodies (MOABs), labeled blood elements, positron RPs, and the new In-111 pentetreotide somatostatin receptor agent. In some cases, such as In-111 pentetate, I-131 iodide, or Tl-201 chloride, the products are chemically stable and the physical half-life is long enough that the synthesis and required quality control (QC) are completed by manufacturers. This greatly simplifies their use at the hospital level.

### Ease of Preparation and Availability

As mentioned earlier, RP availability is paramount in clinical practice. When RPs require radionuclides that must be ordered, the test must be delayed.

### Stability and Expiration

The best Tc-99m kit formulations give products that are stable for at least 6 hours after preparation, and some are stable for as long as 24 hours. Given the amount of effort that must be expended to synthesize and perform QC on a preparation, it is advantageous to have a product that can be used all day. Stabilized bone scan (medronate) kits (Bracco/Squibb, Princeton, NJ, or Amersham/Medi-Physics, Arlington Heights, IL) are preferable to nonstabilized kits (DuPont, North Billerica, MA, or Mallinckrodt, St. Louis, MO) if multiple doses are injected over the course of the day. The worst RPs are very unstable, and in the past, some had expiration times of 30 minutes or less (e.g., the original formulations of dimercaptosuccinic acid

[DMSA] and hexamethylpropyleneamine oxime [HMPAO]). Amersham/Medi-Physics has invested many resources to produce stabilized DMSA and HMPAO kit formulations, and these recently received FDA approval.

### Formulation

Different formulations of the same chemical product can have a significant effect. The stabilizer in medronate is an antioxidant, ascorbic acid, which prevents the reoxidation of the technetium and stabilizes the tin as stannous ion. The result is less pertechnetate impurity in the preparation along with an extended stability (as long as 12 hours or more) and an increased capacity in terms of the maximum Tc-99m that can be added to the kit (≤500 mCi). In the absence of ascorbic acid, as soon as 4 hours after preparation, pertechnetate levels are high enough to be seen accumulating in the stomach, thus degrading the image. Using a stabilized formulation, many more doses can be obtained from a vial over a 12-hour day. This formulation reduces costs per dose and produces higher-contrast images. The new stabilized formulation of HMPAO contains a buffer and the antioxidant methylene blue. As a result the HMPAO can be labeled with up to 50 mCi (instead of 30 mCi) Tc-99m and is stable for up to 5 hours (instead of 30 minutes).

### Cost and Regulatory Status

Economics is a reality of current health care practice and must be considered when selecting the appropriate RP. The impact of cost has been magnified in recent years by the tremendous increases in the prices for new agents, which commercial suppliers claim are the result of research and stringent regulatory requirements. Strontium 89 (Sr-89, $2,200 per dose); I-131 MIBG ($800 to $1,200 per dose); In-111 pentetreotide, satumomab pendetide, and capromab pendetide ($800 to $900 per dose); Tc-99m ethylcysteinate dimer (ECD) and HMPAO ($260 per dose); Tc-99m mercaptoacetyltriglycine (MAG3) ($90 to $110 per dose); and Tc-99m sestamibi ($50 to $80 per dose) exemplify the inflation in the cost of new RPs. Contrast these to the older RPs, such as Xe-133, Tc-99m methylene diphosphonate [MDP], diethylenetriamine pentaacetic acid [DTPA], and MAA, which cost in the range of $1 to $20 per dose. It is obvious that attention must be paid to this parameter when selecting an RP and a particular vendor or brand and when making the clinical decision to perform a particular study.

The high cost of new agents has undoubtedly hindered their introduction into current practice and has been a major headache for those responsible for budgeting and inventory control of RPs. With the new era of capitation and the associated emphasis on patient outcomes, it is necessary that these new agents be shown to be cost-effective in the overall care of the patient, if they are to be used. The competitive market place has been effective in holding down costs when there are alternatives that can be competitively bid (e.g., Mo-99/Tc-99m generators, MDP kits, MAA kits, DTPA kits, SC kits, ventilation aerosols, Tl-201, and Ga-67).

One cannot select on the basis of cost alone. The quality of the product needs to be considered, along with stability, formulation, biological properties, and other factors that may make one brand of RP more cost-effective, even though the bid dollar cost is more. Significant differences between commercially available DTPA kits have been shown in terms of stability in plastic syringes and in terms of protein-binding. The penta-sodium formulation of Medi-Physics (now also available from Bracco/Squibb) is preferred for glomerular filtration rate (GFR) quantitation because it is more stable than alternative formulations. Cost is therefore secondary when using Tc-DTPA for this indication.

### Therapeutic RPs

Use of therapeutic RPs dates back to 1911, when radium 226 (Ra-226) was used ineffectively to treat lupus. In 1939, phosphorus 32 (P-32) phosphate was used to treat leukemia in the first medical use of an artificially produced radionuclide, predating conventional chemotherapy. In 1942, Sr-89 was used to treat metastatic bone lesions in prostate cancer, predating the FDA approval by 50 years. In the same year, I-131 was produced and subsequently used to treat thyroid cancer effectively. In 1953, gold 198 colloid was used to treat malignant effusions, and this role is continued with P-32 chromic phosphate. The future is bright for therapeutic MOABs, and already advanced B-cell non-Hodgkin's lymphomas have been effectively treated when other therapies have failed.

RP therapy has significant advantages over chemotherapy and external beam irradiation:

- The carrier-free nature of RPs allows the therapeutic effect to be accomplished without pharmacologic effect. This minimizes side effects and allows the targeting of very low-concentration receptors.
- RP therapy exposes neighboring malignant cells to lethal irradiation even if the nuclide is not bound to them, whereas, with chemotherapy, the drug molecule must be taken up by the cell to be lethal.
- RP therapy is selective; that is, a high target-to-nontarget ratio can be achieved. External beams irradiate all the tissues in its path, and chemotherapy targets all fast-growing cell populations. With Sr-89, ratios of metastatic to normal bone uptake as high as 36:1 have been documented.
- One can select the range in tissue by using radionuclides with different energy emissions. For large tumors, more range is needed, whereas for circulating malignancies, such as leukemias, a very short range is needed. If a nuclide is localized intracellularly within the nucleus, an ultra–short-range auger electron emitter, such as I-125, with a range of 10 nm, can be used. I-125 MIBG is being investigated to treat neuroblastomas, the cells of which may be interspersed with normal bone marrow cells.

- RP therapy delivers a hyperfractionated dose compared to external beam irradiation. Fractionation, or spreading out of radiation over time, has been shown to be more effective against tumors with less side effects to normal tissue.

As a result of these advantages, a significant research effort is being expended on therapeutic RPs, and it promises to be an area with significant expansion in the future.

### Nuclear Properties

Because the desired effect is lethality to the target tissue rather than imaging, criteria for RPs differ from those for diagnostic use, especially in terms of the nuclear properties.

### Half-Life

A shorter physical half-life means there is a higher dose rate and therefore a greater biological effect. On the other hand, a longer half-life would give greater fractionation of the dose and a longer duration of action, provided the RP is not cleared or metabolized by the tumor cells. The half-life must be long enough to localize in diseased cells and clear from normal cells. Waste disposal becomes more of a problem with RPs with long half-life.

The half-life must be long enough to allow synthesis, formulation, and delivery of the RP, which in most situations is at least 12 hours to facilitate preparation and localization in the patient. If the half-life is <4 to 5 days, >33 mCi needs to be administered to get an adequate exposure, and that means the patient may have to be treated as an inpatient.

### Decay Mode

Particulate radiation with high–linear energy transfer is desirable for maximum exposure and damage to tissue. Historically, beta emitters have been used (all approved therapeutic RPs [I-131, P-32, Sr-89] are beta emitters), but alpha emitters and auger electron emitters (EC decay mode) have potential and are being investigated. The optimal decay mode depends on the range in tissue desired for a particular application. Beta particle ranges are in millimeters, alpha particle ranges are in micrometers, and

**TABLE 22-6.** *Processes important in tumor therapy*

| Physical processes | Half-life allows localization |
|---|---|
| | High LET particles |
| |   Alpha: micrometer (monoenergetic) |
| |   Beta: millimeter (spectrum of energies) |
| |   Auger: nanometer (monoenergetic) |
| Biological processes | Rapid blood clearance |
| | Good tumor localization |
| | Long residence time |
| | Nontumor RP quickly excreted |
| Chemical processes | Radionuclide binds to localizing ligand |
| | Chemical stability |
| | High specific activity |

auger electron ranges are in nanometers (Table 22-6). An advantage of alpha particles and auger electrons is that they are monoenergetic, as opposed to beta particles, which have a continuous energy spectrum up to their characteristic maximum energy ($E_{max}$).

### Energy and Range

The optimal particle range depends on the size of the tumor with large tumors requiring more range. A radionuclide is then selected that has particle emission with an energy that provides the optimal range. For beta particles, the average energy is approximately one-third of the $E_{max}$. Table 22-7 gives the maximum and average range in water (equivalent to soft tissue) for some radionuclides.

### Gamma Energy and Abundance

It is desirable to have a gamma ray of imageable energy to allow in vivo verification of the localization of the RP and possible patient-specific dosimetry calculations with a gamma camera. In addition, dose calibrator measurements are much easier and more accurate if there is a gamma emission. In the absence of a gamma ray, the dose calibrator is measuring bremsstrahlung radiation, which is very dependent on the RP container and detector construction material and geometry. The optimal radionuclide would have a gamma ray of 150 keV in approximately 10% abundance.

**TABLE 22-7.** *Common therapeutic radiopharmaceuticals and their physical attributes*

| Therapeutic radionuclide | Half-life (days) | Decay process | Energy (keV) max/mean | Range (mm) max/mean |
|---|---|---|---|---|
| I-131 | 8.05 | β | 606/190 | 2.4/0.95 |
| Sr-89 | 50.50 | β | 1,470/583 | 8.0/2.92 |
| P-32 | 14.30 | β | 1,709/694 | 8.7/3.47 |
| Sm-153 | 1.95 | β | 804/233 | 3.0/1.16 |
| Rh-186 | 3.77 | β | 2,116/766 | 5.0/1.75 |

*Stable or Long–Half-Life Daughter*

To minimize exposure to normal tissue after decay and subsequent biological clearance, it is best if the progeny of the radionuclide is stable or has a very long half-life.

### Biological Properties

It is axiomatic that the ideal therapeutic RP localizes preferentially in the target tissue (see Table 22-6). The longer it stays there (residence time), the higher the dose delivered. It is equally important that it get there quickly to minimize exposure to normal tissue. If it localizes in normal tissue it should be minimal and clear quickly. I-131 iodide has been very effective for thyroid therapy because of the highly efficient trapping mechanism in thyroid tissue: Excess iodide is cleared quickly by glomerular filtration, resulting in minimal normal tissue uptake. It has been successful in thyroid tumors, which concentrate iodide.

### Metabolism and Excretion

Ideally, the RP should not undergo any metabolism because the organ involved with metabolism would get a high radiation exposure. A faster rate of metabolism decreases exposure to the organ involved and may also be useful if it contributes to faster elimination or faster target uptake. As a general rule, renal excretion is rapid, and, if present, it reduces blood levels and whole-body, and marrow exposures. Liver biliary excretion is slower and leads to higher GI exposure and longer whole-body exposure. With GI excretion there is also the potential for reabsorption into the blood, which would further delay blood clearance and contribute more to whole-body exposure. The liver is the usual organ involved in metabolism of the RP. One of the problems with therapeutic MOAB agents is their liver metabolism, which leads to dose-limiting hepatic exposure.

Other routes of administration that result in localization are useful. Intracavitary administrations have been used successfully for symptomatic relief of malignant effusions and for articular radiation synovectomy. Intra-arterial administration of labeled microspheres has shown some promise in tumors with rich blood supply, especially if the blood supply is distinct (soft-tissue sarcomas).

### Chemical Properties

The chemical properties are identical to those of diagnostic RPs.

### Future

Although there is a rich history of the therapeutic use of RPs, we have just seen the tip of the iceberg. Many potential applications are under investigation, and this will be an area of nuclear medicine growth. There is also a need for clinical research to identify the optimal mix of therapy. For example, it is possible that a cocktail of different bone-seeking agents with different ranges, half-lives, and activities will be more effective than a single therapeutic agent. The possibility that these bone pain therapies may be curative is still to be tested, but significant remissions have been induced by rhenium 186 ethylenehydroxydiphosphonate, and samarium 153 has produced cures in primary bone sarcoma in dogs at high doses. Most research with RPs done so far has been done in terminal patients who have failed other therapies. RP therapy is expected to be most effective in killing small micrometastases rather than large tumor masses.

## PRODUCTION OF RADIOPHARMACEUTICALS

Naturally occurring radionuclides have long half-lives and are therefore unsuitable for medical use. Radionuclides used in medicine are artificially produced in reactors or cyclotrons. Radionuclides available in generators have their parents produced in reactors or cyclotrons.

Most medical radionuclides are manufactured by bombarding a stable nucleus with subatomic particles (e.g., neutrons, protons) produced in a nuclear reactor or particle accelerator. The process of all radionuclide production is described by this general equation format: Mo-98$(n,\gamma)$Mo-99. The target element is on the left, and the bombarding particle used is on the left inside the bracket. The product is on the right, and emission is on the right in the bracket.

Radionuclides are formed by three primary means:

- Separation from fission products; these radionuclides generally decay by beta emission (e.g., I-131, Xe-133, Mo-99)
- Irradiation of target nuclei with low-energy neutrons in a reactor (formerly used to make Mo-99)
- Irradiation of target nuclei with charged particles to make neutron-deficient radionuclides that decay by EC (I-123, Ga-67, In-111, Tl-201) or positron emission (F-18, oxygen 15 [O-15], N-13, C-11)

Both nonfission reactor and cyclotron methods of radionuclide production require a target. Pure metals are the best targets because they can sustain the high temperatures that exist in these devices. Some radionuclide productions do not use metal foils but, rather, high-pressure gases (Xe-124 for I-123) and liquids (O-18 for F-18).

### Reactor-Produced RPs

Three processes are in use by which reactors produce radionuclides.

### $(n,\gamma)$ Reaction

Low-energy thermal neutrons (~0.025 eV) irradiate stable nuclei to produce neutron-rich radioisotopes of the original target. These radionuclides generally decay by β⁻ emission, often with accompanying gamma emissions that may be useful for imaging. The product radioisotope has the same chemical properties as the target, so chemical separation is not possible unless the product rapidly decays to another radionuclide. Because of this, the (n,γ) reaction generally results in the production of low–specific activity radionuclides.

### (n,p) Reaction

In (n,p) reactions the neutron energy is higher than in the (n,γ) reaction. This extra energy results in an intermediate nucleus, where a proton gains sufficient energy to overcome the nuclear binding energy and to escape from the nucleus, producing an isobar (same atomic number, A) rather than the isotope (same number of protons) produced in the (n,γ) reaction. Chemical separation is then possible, and high–specific activity radionuclides result.

### (n,f) By-Product Reaction

Neutron bombardment of fissionable material results in the production of an intermediate nucleus that rapidly breaks into fission products that can be readily separated by chemical means. In practice, uranium (the principal isotopes and their natural abundance are U-238 [99.3%] and U-235 [0.7%]) is the fissionable material used. To facilitate this reaction, natural uranium is enriched with U-235 (to ~93%). When U-235 captures a thermal neutron, the intermediate nucleus is very active and fissions into radioactive fragments immediately. Each U-235 fission results in more neutrons (on average, 2.4 neutrons), and so a chain reaction can develop. These neutrons can be slowed by moderating media (heavy water or graphite), and the moderators of thermal neutrons (boron or cadmium rods) control the fission rate. Pulling out the graphite rods results in a fast reaction, and pushing the rods in causes a shutdown in the reaction. Heat generated by the reactor can be carried off for electric power generation. In reactors made for radionuclide generation, windows are provided so target material can be inserted.

The fission products are numerous and have atomic masses between 70 and 170 with mass numbers that peak at 90 and 140. These can be separated chemically and currently serve as the major sources of Xe-133, I-131, and Mo-99.

### Cyclotron RPs

This technique is used for the production of a wide range of radionuclides. The principle of operation is the acceleration of charged particles toward an oppositely charged electrode. In cyclotrons these electrodes are two semicircular devices (called "Dees") that accelerate the particle. The polarity of each Dee is reversed by a radiofrequency oscillator, and the charged particle increases in speed by the rapidly changing (~10⁷ times per second) polarity of the electrodes. These Dees are placed in a large evacuated chamber that is enclosed in an electromagnetic field, and the accelerated charged particles assume a circular orbit that gradually increases in radius with speed. Once the particle energy is great, and the path reaches the periphery of the Dees, the particle exits and is directed onto a target. This same process can be accomplished in a linear fashion in a linear accelerator.

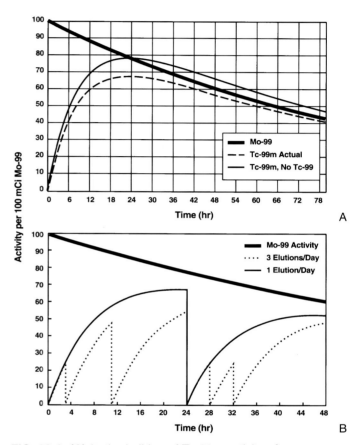

FIG. 22-1. **(A)** In the buildup of Tc-99m activity after a generator elution, the y axis represents the Tc-99m activity per 100 mCi of Mo-99 present at the time of elution. The peak of Tc-99m activity occurs at 23 hours. At 66 hours, the half-life of Mo-99, Mo-99 activity has decreased to 50 mCi. Equilibrium occurs at 70 hours, after which the Tc-99m curve parallels the Mo-99 line. The actual Tc-99m activity is then equal to 95% of the current Mo-99 activity. If Mo-99 did not decay directly to Tc-99 14% of the time, there would be more Tc-99m activity than Mo-99 activity (110% at equilibrium). This is a characteristic of transient equilibrium.

**(B)** This graph compares Tc-99m activity eluted with several elutions per day to 1 elution per day after 24 hours of buildup. A total of 224 mCi of Tc-99m is eluted per 100 mCi Mo-99. The single daily elution yields Tc-99m of 68 and 57 mCi, for a total activity eluted of 125 mCi. Multiple elutions yield 79% more total Tc-99m over the 2 days, whereas the first elutions each day were only reduced by 21%. A 100% elution efficiency is assumed. In practice, actual yields may vary due to radiolytic chemical phenomena on the column forming insoluble reduced species of technetium that are not eluted. Typical yields are >90% of the total available technetium.

**TABLE 22-8.** *Practical secular equilibrium generator systems*

| | | |
|---|---|---|
| Ge-68 (287 days) | → | Ga-68 (68 mins) |
| Sn-113 (114 days) | → | Sn-113m (99 mins) |
| Sr-82 (25 days) | → | Rb-82 (1.3 mins) |
| Rb-81 (4.7 hours) | → | Kr-81m (13 secs) |

## Generators

A generator is a system that provides a radionuclide by radioactive decay. This system usually produces a relatively short–half-life product (daughter) that otherwise could not be delivered reliably by the manufacturer on a daily basis. Convenience is enhanced when the parent source has a suitably long half-life to make at least weekly deliveries. Although the user is responsible for some of the radionuclidic and radiochemical QC parameters, many of these QC responsibilities remain with the commercial supplier. The ubiquitous Mo-99/Tc-99m generator is the classic example of a transient equilibrium generator system in which the parent half-life is approximately 10 times that of the daughter half-life. In general, at equilibrium, generators that decay completely to a single daughter result in activity levels slightly in excess of the parent (Fig. 22-1). The Mo-99/Tc-99m generator does not do this because 14% of Mo-99 decays directly to Tc-99 rather than through the desired daughter, Tc-99m. Examples of secular equilibrium when the half-life of the parent is approximately 1,000 times longer than the daughter half-life are described in Table 22-8. All these secular generator systems have been, or are, commercially available.

### Mo-99/Tc-99m Generator

This generator system has revolutionized the practice of clinical nuclear medicine. Before the description (1957) and first commercial introduction (1965) of this generator system, and the shake-and-bake kits for Tc-99m RPs (1970), higher-energy radionuclides (e.g., I-131 or Sr-87m) dominated the clinical applications and dictated the need for thick (1- to 3-inch) NaI(Tl) crystals used in rectilinear scanners. With the introduction of a large number of practical Tc-99m RPs in the early 1970s, individual nuclear medicine departments purchased Mo-99/Tc-99m generators and gamma cameras, and nuclear medicine became an important imaging specialty.

The Mo-99/Tc-99m generator fulfills all the requirements of a clinically useful system:

- Cost-effective, safe, and simple to use
- Sterile, pyrogen-free, and isotonic eluate
- High radionuclidic and chemical purity
- Tc-99m produces numerous useful RPs
- Parent half-life of 66 hours allowing weekly delivery

The Mo-99/Tc-99m generator is typical of most generator systems, with a chromatographic column (alumina) that the parent (Mo-99) is strongly adsorbed to, and for which the daughters have a lesser affinity. It is important to use high–specific activity Mo-99 because the extraction efficiency of Tc-99m is proportional to alumina thickness. The Mo-98(n,γ)Mo-99 reaction was the early reactor method of production of the generator parent, but, because of the low–specific activity product, Mo-99 is now produced by the (n,f) fission reaction. Carrier-free Mo-99 is possible with fission Mo-99 production because good chemical extraction techniques are available to separate molybdenum from other elements. Alumina is prepared, heated, and activated, and then acidified Mo-99 is added to the column as molybdate ($MoO_4^{2-}$). While on the column, Mo-99 as $MoO_4^{2-}$ decays to Tc-99m $TcO_4^-$ with a change in chemical properties. Consequently, $TcO_4^-$ exchanges with chloride ($Cl^-$) in the saline eluate, so Tc-99m $NaTcO_4$ is readily eluted while $MoO_4^{2-}$ remains attached to the column.

### Elution Efficiency

Typically, >90% of the technetium on the column is eluted on a single elution, with approximately 95% of the total activity coming off in the second and third milliliter of eluate. The amount of Tc-99m on the column is a function of the amount of Mo-99 activity and the time since the previous elution. The Tc-99m activity can be calculated using the following equation:

$$A_{Tc\text{-}99m} = \frac{\lambda_{Tc\text{-}99m}}{\lambda_{Tc\text{-}99m} - \lambda_{Mo\text{-}99}} \times 0.86 \left[ e^{-(\lambda_{Mo\text{-}99} \cdot t)} - e^{-(\lambda_{Tc\text{-}99m} \cdot t)} \right]$$
$$\times A_{Mo\text{-}99} \quad (2)$$

where $\lambda_{Tc\text{-}99m} = \dfrac{\ln 2}{6.0 \text{ hrs}}$,

$\lambda_{Mo\text{-}99} = \dfrac{\ln 2}{65.92 \text{ hrs}}$,

$t$ is the time since previous elution, and $A_{Mo\text{-}99}$ is the activity of Mo-99 at the previous elution (Table 22-9; see Fig. 22-1).

The time of peak Tc-99m activity can be calculated by setting the first derivative of this equation with respect to time equal to zero and solving for $t$.

**TABLE 22-9.** *Available Tc-99m activity as percent of Mo-99 activity at various times after previous elution*

| Time (hrs) | % of Mo-99 activity at previous elution | % of current Mo-99 activity |
|---|---|---|
| 2 | 17.5 | 17.9 |
| 4 | 31.1 | 32.4 |
| 6 | 41.5 | 44.2 |
| 12 | 59.7 | 67.8 |
| 23 | 67.6[a] | 86.2 |
| 70 | 45.3 | 94.6[b] |

[a] Peak.
[b] Equilibrium.

$$t \text{ peak} = \frac{\ln\lambda_{Tc} - \ln\lambda_{Mo}}{\lambda_{Tc} - \lambda_{Mo}} = 23 \text{ hours} \qquad (3)$$

Hence the maximum Tc-99m activity is available 23 hours after the prior elution. This activity is 67.6% of the Mo-99 activity at the previous elution (23 hours prior) or 86% of the current Mo-99 activity (see Table 22-9). If the generator is not eluted for 70 hours, a dynamic equilibrium occurs; the available Tc-99m activity equals 94.6% of the Mo-99 activity and decreases with the half-life of the Mo-99. This is an example of transient equilibrium (see Fig. 22-1).

Note that 94.6% is equal to the value of the constant terms in this equation:

$$\frac{\lambda_2}{\lambda_2 - \lambda_1} \times 86\% \qquad (4)$$

If Mo-99 decayed to Tc-99m 100% of the time, this value would be 110%, and there would be more daughter activity than parent.

Scrutiny of Fig. 22-1 and Table 22-9 shows that the Tc-99m activity buildup is very rapid and exponential early after elution: 26% of the maximum is available at 2 hours and 46% of the maximum after 4 hours. Hence a generator may be eluted frequently during the course of a day. If at least 12 hours of buildup is allowed, the available activity the next morning will be reduced by only approximately 10%. The problem with frequent elutions is that the activity concentration may be too low for good bolus injections. Most generators require approximately 3 ml to elute most of the technetium. Because it is possible to fractionally elute a generator in 1-ml increments, the second and third increments have the highest concentrations, and this may overcome some concentration problems when preparing RP after generator elutions.

### Tc-99 Content of Eluate

The longer the Mo-99/Tc-99m generator is not milked, the greater the proportion of Tc-99 in the eluate. Tc-99 accumulates by direct decay from Mo-99 (14%) and via Tc-99m (86%) decay. When the generator is milked, both Tc-99m and Tc-99 are eluted because of their identical chemical properties. Because of the shorter half-life of Tc-99m, the ratio of Tc-99m to Tc-99 continuously

**TABLE 22-10.** *Tc-99m/Tc-99 eluate ratio at various times after elution*

| Hours since elution | % of Tc-99m | % of Tc-99 |
|---|---|---|
| 3 | 77 | 23 |
| 6 | 62 | 38 |
| 9 | 53 | 47 |
| 24 | 28 | 72 |
| 48 | 13 | 87 |
| 72 | 8 | 92 |

decreases with time, as shown in Table 22-10. This can create a problem with labeling efficiencies of Tc-99m RPs, especially if the labeling reaction is marginal, as with Tc-99m labeling of red blood cells (RBCs) and HMPAO. With HMPAO the generator must have been previously eluted within 24 hours, and the eluate must be <2 hours old or else poor tags result.

### Generator Types

Two types of Mo-99/Tc-99m generators are sold: wet-column devices, which have a self-contained saline source and are eluted using evacuated vials, and dry-column devices, in which the user plugs in a saline source with each elution and elutes with an evacuated vial at the collection port.

### Radionuclide Purity

The major radionuclidic impurities are those of Mo-99 and Tc-99. The most important contaminant is that of Mo-99, with its 66-hour half-life and beta decay, and its potential for significant "breakthrough" from the alumina column. Tc-99 is not a clinically important contaminant, with its 214,000-year half-life.

Mo-99 decays by $\beta^-$ emission to Tc-99m and Tc-99 and gives off two high-energy gamma rays, 740 and 778 keV, which have an abundance of 14% and 4%, respectively. The NRC requires the measurement of this contaminant on every elution used. The most common method of measuring this is differential attenuation. The test routinely performed uses a special lead container supplied by the dose calibrator manufacturer, with walls approximately 6 mm thick. The half-value layer (HVL) in lead of the Tc-99m photon (140 keV) is approximately 0.2 mm, whereas the HVL of the high-energy Mo-99 photons (740, 778 keV) is approximately 6 mm. The Tc-99m photon is attenuated very efficiently by the 30 HVL of lead, resulting in virtually no passage of Tc-99m photons because 99.999995% are attenuated. In contrast, only 50% of the Mo-99 photons are attenuated by the single HVL of lead. There are effectively eight orders of magnitude difference in attenuation, so if the eluate is measured both with and without the lead container, the amount of Mo-99 breakthrough can be measured for compliance with the NRC regulations. There should be <0.15 µCi of Mo-99 per 1 mCi of Tc-99m at the time of administration. Trace amounts of other fission products may contaminate the generator, but these are present in minuscule amounts. The manufacturer must assure the user at delivery that there are <2.5 µCi total other radionuclidic contaminants per elution.

### Chemical Purity

The U.S. Pharmacopeia (USP) and NRC require testing for aluminum ($Al^{+3}$), which can be washed off the alumina column. This material is not toxic but may affect the biodistribution of $TcO_4^-$ by allowing colloid formation and possible hepatic visualization. A flocculent precipitate may also form by precipitating aluminum phosphate from phosphate buffers in SC and pyrophosphate (PYP) kits. This precipitate localizes in the lungs and liver. $Al^{+3}$ must be tested for with each generator elution by using a paper aurin tricarboxylic acid colorimetric strip that turns purple when $Al^{+3}$ is present. The intensity of the color is compared to a standard that contains the USP limit of 10 µg/ml $Al^{+3}$. With the better methods of preparing high–specific activity Mo-99 now used, large alumina columns are not needed, and there is virtually no risk of this impurity. We have not seen this column problem for >20 years, but it has been observed when needles with aluminum hubs are used.

### Radiochemical Purity

The USP requires that 95% of Tc-99m be in the VII state (i.e., Tc-99m $TcO_4^-$). This test is not required, but it should be performed if labeling problems occur in preparing routine Tc-99m RPs.

### Pyrogenicity and Sterility

Problems of pyrogenicity and sterility are addressed by the commercial supplier and not tested by the user, although aseptic technique in elution and compounding is mandatory for patient safety.

### Other Generator Systems

Numerous generator systems have been produced. The most commonly used, practical, commercially available system is the Sr-82/Rb-82 positron system used in myocardial perfusion imaging. This is supplied complete with delivery system. In addition, a Rb-81/Kr-81m system is FDA approved for lung ventilation imaging.

## TC-99M RPS

The space for technetium in the periodic table among the transition metals was left by Mendeleev, who called it *eka manganese*. The name for this element derives from the Greek, *technetos*, meaning artificial. Effectively, all the technetium isotopes in the earth's crust have decayed to other elements, and the only technetium available is manufactured. There are many technetium isotopes, including Tc-94m, a positron emitter used here at University of Wisconsin (UW)-Madison. Because technetium is a transition metal, it exists in many oxidation states and can combine with a variety of electron-rich substrates.

Tc-99m RPs are ideal because of the:

- Ideal energy of 140 keV (patient exit and crystal interaction)
- Low patient dose (absent particulate radiation)
- Acceptable physical half-life (for RP preparation and clinical application)
- Generator source and modest cost (weekly delivery, cheapest radionuclide)

### Tc-99m RP Preparation

Technetium was discovered in 1937, the first generator system Tc-99m source was described in 1957, and the first commercial source made Tc-99m available in 1965. This radionuclide did not revolutionize nuclear medicine, even though modern gamma cameras were commercially available in 1961. Before then, thicker crystal imaging devices (rectilinear scanners) were used because most clinically useful RPs were not based on Tc-99m despite the fact that the generator eluate, Tc-99m $TcO_4^-$ in the heptavalent state (VII), was an excellent thyroid and brain scanning agent. In these clinical situations the focused rectilinear scanner was a satisfactory imaging device.

It was not until 1970, when the stannous ion reduction method of Tc-99m DTPA production as an "instant kit" was described, that a simple and convenient shake-and-bake preparation of numerous Tc-99m RPs was possible and nuclear medicine was revolutionized. Within 3 years, instant kits of Tc-99m–labeled albumin, RBCs, polyphosphate, PYP, and diphosphonate RPs were available.

### Tc-99m Reduction

The most stable aqueous form of technetium is the VII state of $TcO_4^-$, but this oxidation state combines only with Tc-99m SC, a heptasulfide ($Tc_2S_7$) liver-spleen imaging agent. $TcO_4^-$ has to be reduced to various charged species to combine with other ligands, and the stannous ion is the primary reducing agent in clinical use.

Tc-99m reduced to the III, IV, or V state combines with many chelating agents. In conventional kits, the ligand is provided in lyophilized form, and stannous ion is included to reduce the added $TcO_4^-$ to a reactive state. In most reactions, the commercially provided vial and the $TcO_4^-$ eluate are merely shaken together. These first-generation Tc-99m RPs include DTPA, DMSA, glucoheptonic acid (GH), phosphates, and phosphonates; all had a significant effect on the practice of medicine. In these RPs, the Tc-99m is merely a label attached to the chelate, and the radionuclide does not have a role in the localization process.

Second-generation RPs have been developed in which the Tc-99m is incorporated into the RP molecule. These include MAG3, ECD, HMPAO, and methoxyisobutylisonitrile (common name MIBI, generic name sestamibi). Tc-99m sestamibi is unique because the $TcO_4^-$ is reduced to the I state for incorporation into the RP.

### Reoxidation Problems

The shake-and-bake process is delightfully simple but can be readily compromised. Only a small amount of introduced oxygen can cause reoxidation of the Tc-99m to the VII state, resulting in a vial containing impurities, such as Tc-99m $TcO_4^-$ and other forms of the Tc-99m ligand in addition to the desired Tc-99m RP. The most common example is the bone scan, in which free $TcO_4^-$ results in visualization of the thyroid, stomach, and salivary glands, and the formation of other diphosphonate moieties results in unusual biodistributions (see Fig. 1-5). To prevent this, the reaction vial is often filled with nitrogen to ensure complete reduction of the $TcO_4^-$, and antioxidants are added to prevent changes after RP preparation, when oxygen can result in the reformation of $TcO_4^-$. RPs in which the ligand bonds weakly with the technetium are more susceptible to subsequent oxidation of the technetium back to the VII state, so antioxidant stabilizers are often added, for example, ascorbic acid in some commercial Tc-99m medronate bone scan kits. Radiolysis of the eluate can result in peroxides that can cause oxidation of the RP with similar results.

Oxidation of the stannous ion from the II state to the IV state can result in lower reducing capacity, with subsequent $TcO_4^-$ presence and altered RP moieties. To prevent this, stannous ion is nearly always provided in excess.

### Abnormal Colloid Formation

Another frequent problem with ill-prepared RPs is the formation of colloids that are phagocytosed by the liver and result in hepatic visualization. This occurs when there is low concentration of ligand and reduced or hydrolyzed technetium ($TcO_2$) is formed. Excess stannous ions can also create a colloid of tin ($Sn[OH]_2$). These occurrences highlight the need for very careful design of Tc-99m RP kits and the need for strict adherence to the manufacturer's instructions and QC procedures.

### Carrier Tc-99

As described previously, carrier Tc-99 is common in all generator eluates. This Tc-99 is chemically identical to Tc-99m and so competes in all chemical reactions resulting in a nonimaging pharmaceutical. Because some Mo-99 decays directly to Tc-99 (14%) and all Tc-99m decays to Tc-99, this nonimaging Tc-99 is routinely available in three times the concentration of Tc-99m in a typical radiopharmacy operation with daily elutions of the Mo-99/Tc-99m generator (see Table 22-9). In generators not eluted over the weekend, or newly delivered generators from the manufacturer, the proportion of Tc-99m can be <10% of the total technetium eluted.

The longer the eluate is stored before use, the greater the amount of Tc-99. This is true because Tc-99m decays with its physical half-life of 6.0 hours, whereas for practical pur-

poses Tc-99 does not decay (half-life, 214,000 years). In the formulation of RPs with significant amounts of ligand and stannous ions (the strong ligands), this phenomenon has no effect. In RP preparations in which the ligand binding is weaker or when reagents must be in limited supply, however, decreased labeling or stability can ensue, as with Tc-99m–labeled RBCs, HMPAO, and MAG3.

Other factors that affect labeling efficiency include pH, ligand concentration, temperature of reaction, and reaction times. Optimization of these parameters is decided by the kit manufacturer, which supplies specific preparation instructions to ensure the optimal reaction conditions.

### QC of Tc-99m RPs

Depending on who does the final preparation, the RP preparer is responsible for some QC parameters, the manufacturer for others (e.g., sterility, pyrogenicity, and radionuclidic purity of the generator eluate and sterility, pyrogenicity, and chemical purity of the kit). When unit doses are provided by a commercial radiopharmacy, no QC is required by the user except to ensure that the correct patient gets the appropriate RP and dose. Even with this lack of legal requirements for patient safety, the individual dose should be inspected for any untoward appearance. In nearly all cases the RP should be clear, with no particulate matter present. Note that stabilized Tc-99m HMPAO is blue. Expiration times must be honored unless end-user testing validates the RP quality at later times.

In summary, QC of generator Tc-99m $TcO_4^-$ eluate is as follows:

- Radiochemical purity: USP requires 95% (preparer responsibility)
- Radionuclidic purity:
  <0.15 µCi Mo-99 per mCi Tc-99m (preparer responsibility)
  <2.5 µCi other radionuclides (manufacturer responsibility)
- Chemical purity: <10 µg $Al^{+3}$ per ml eluate (preparer responsibility)
- pH, pyrogenicity, sterility: manufacturer (all) and preparer (pH) responsibility

### Radiochemical Purity

The radiochemical purity is usually measured by chromatography. Chromatography is a method of separating in which a mixture is applied as a narrow initial zone to a stationary porous sorbent (solid) phase, and the components undergo differential migration by the flow of the mobile (solvent) phase. The many different permutations of chromatography are characterized by the physical configuration and nature of the stationary phase.

In clinical nuclear pharmacy, thin-layer and paper chromatography are usually used, in which the solid, stationary phase is either silica gel (SG) or paper. Each RP component to be tested has a distinctive migration (Rf value), depending on the particular system and brand used. The Rf value is defined as the distance the compound moved divided by the distance the solvent moved and varies between zero and 1.0. The Rf is zero for the components that are insoluble in the solvent and remain at the solid phase origin. The Rf is 1.0 if it moves with the solvent front. The Rf value is characteristic for a given combination of compound, media, and solvent.

Column chromatography is also used. The development of miniaturized, prepackaged columns, such as Sep-Pak columns (Millipore Corporation, Bedford, MA), has facilitated the use of this technique. The principles are the same, but columns are characterized by the retention volume (the volume of solvent required to elute the components from the column) instead of the Rf value.

### First-Generation Tc-99m RPs

The older Tc-99m RP preparations are either water-soluble (DTPA, PYP, GH, MDP, hydroxymethylenediphosphonate [HDP]) or insoluble particulates (SC, MAA). With the exception of SC (which does not involve the reduction of the $TcO_4^-$), the FDA-approved kit vials supplied by the manufacturer contain the stannous ion, the ligand, and sometimes various stabilizers and buffers. When the $TcO_4^-$ solution is added to the vial, it is reduced by the stannous ion and subsequently binds to the ligand. Water is the most prevalent molecule in the vial and reacts slowly (via hydrolysis) with reduced technetium to produce an insoluble compound called *hydrolyzed technetium* ($TcO_2$). There is the potential for three main chemical forms of technetium:

- The desired Tc-99m RP
- Unreduced Tc-99m $TcO_4^-$
- Hydrolyzed or Tc-99m $TcO_2$

To separate the three components for QC purposes, we use two solvent-media chromatography systems: an aqueous solvent (normal saline) to separate the water-soluble products ($TcO_4^-$ and RP) from the water-insoluble $TcO_2$, and an organic solvent (acetone or methylethylketone) to separate the $TcO_4^-$ from the RP. Instant thin-layer chromatography with solid-phase SG (ITLC-SG) (Gelman, Sciences Inc., Ann Arbor, MI) and Whatman (Maidstone, England) paper are the stationary phases used. Paper with saline does not give adequate separation with some Tc-99m RPs (GH, PYP), whereas the ITLC-SG works for all these products with both solvents.

At UW-Madison, we use ITLC-SG for both solvents to simplify the process. $TcO_4^-$ is soluble in both acetone and saline and moves near the solvent front in both systems. $TcO_2$ is insoluble in both solvents and stays at the origin in both systems. The water-soluble Tc-99m RPs move with the solvent front in saline and stay at the origin in acetone. The strips are cut and the activity in each piece

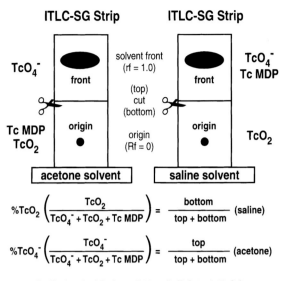

$$\%TcO_2 \left( \frac{TcO_2}{TcO_4^- + TcO_2 + Tc\ MDP} \right) = \frac{bottom}{top + bottom} \text{ (saline)}$$

$$\%TcO_4^- \left( \frac{TcO_4^-}{TcO_4^- + TcO_2 + Tc\ MDP} \right) = \frac{top}{top + bottom} \text{ (acetone)}$$

Radiochemical Purity = 100% − (% $TcO_4^-$ + % $TcO_2$)

**FIG. 22-2.** Two ITLC-SG strips are set in solvent baths. The solvents migrate along the strips, and $TcO_4^-$ moves with the acetone, but the RP (Tc MDP) and reduced or hydrolyzed technetium ($TcO_2$) remains at the origin. In saline, both Tc MDP and $TcO_4^-$ migrate with the solvent front. The scissors show where the strip is cut for placement in the well counter. The calculation is shown below.

counted (Fig. 22-2) with a dose calibrator or well counter, or the whole strip is scanned with a camera or chromatography scanner, and a histogram of activity is generated. The percentage of RP present is determined by subtracting the percentage at the solvent front in the acetone or methylethylketone ($TcO_4^-$) and the percent at the origin in the saline ($TcO_2$) from 100%.

With the particulate products (SC, MAA) it is not possible to separate the $TcO_2$ from the desired RP, so just one system is used to quantify the $TcO_4^-$. $TcO_2$ behaves similarly to technetium SC (phagocytosed by the reticuloendothelial system), and therefore small amounts are not clinically significant. Likewise, small amounts of liver-spleen activity are not problematic for pulmonary imaging with Tc-99m MAA. The kit manufacturer is required by the USP monograph to do in vivo biodistribution studies in animals to show that each batch of MAA kits produces a product with <5% liver uptake and >80% lung uptake at 5 to 10 minutes after injection.

### Newer Technetium RPs

The chemistry of the newer Tc-99m RPs is much more sophisticated, and consequently, the chromatographic analysis of these products is more complex. In many, the technetium atom is a required component of the final molecule so as to achieve the desired biodistribution; that is, the precursor does not localize the same as the labeled complex

(MAG3, MIBI). The preparation may require an additional step of ligand exchange (MAG3, ECD, boron adducts of technetium dioximes), and stereo isomers may give different localizations (MAG3, HMPAO, ECD). As a result, more potential impurities must be accounted for in the chromatographic analysis to ensure optimal imaging. In addition, the newer products may have more lipophilic properties and less aqueous solubility, requiring different solvents and systems than the older first-generation, water-soluble products. At the manufacturing level, high-performance liquid chromatography is often used, but this technology is beyond the capabilities of the average hospital nuclear medicine facility. Many institutions prefer to buy unit doses of these agents rather than deal with the more complex preparation and QC analysis. Following is a brief discussion of some of the newer agents.

### Hepatobiliary Agents

The hepatobiliary iminodiacetic (IDA) agents require a different system because they are only partially water soluble. ITLC with solid-phase silicic acid with 20% NaCl quantifies the percent of $TcO_4^-$ (percent at solvent front) because $TcO_2$ and the RP do not migrate. ITLC-SG with $CH_3CN$ 75% and water quantifies the hydrolyzed (percent at origin) because both $TcO_4^-$ and the RP migrate.

### Brain Agents

The new lipophilic brain perfusion agents hexametazime (HMPAO [Ceretec]) and bicisate (ECD [Neurolite]) require three different systems if it is necessary to quantify the percent of each individual impurity components ($TcO_4^-$, $TcO_2$, and hydrophilic technetium). Because the original HMPAO had only a 30-minute expiration time and it was difficult to complete these tests before expiration, a one-strip method was devised. This method did not give the percentage of each individual impurity but did tell the percentage labeled HMPAO. This technique used paper strips with either ethyl acetate or ether as the solvent. ECD is tested using SG with ethyl acetate, drying the spot for 5 minutes before proceeding with the test. With both of these systems, only the desired lipophilic labeled compound moves near the solvent front.

### Cardiac Agents

The cardiac agent, sestamibi, also requires a special system, which is described in the package insert. We developed a simpler column technique using Sep-Pak alumina columns. The column should be pre-eluted with approximately 5 to 10 ml of the solvents before the analysis. If the amount of $TcO_4^-$ present is required, it can be calculated by eluting the column first with 10 ml normal saline, fol-lowed by 10 ml ethanol. The sestamibi is in the ethanol fraction, the $TcO_4^-$ is in the saline fraction, and the hydrolyzed material remains on the column. Care must be taken to apply the starting material (0.05 to 0.10 ml) onto the column and to elute with the solvents slowly, drop by drop. The ethanol must be 100%, not 95%, as the presence of any water leads to migration of the $TcO_4^-$ and underestimation of the RP purity.

### Renal Agent

Mertiatide (MAG3) is also analyzed by a column technique. It uses C-18 Sep-Paks with two solvents, ethanol and saline 1:1 and 0.001 N HCl. C-18 Sep-Paks must be pre-eluted with an organic solvent before a polar solvent can be used. Before adding the sample, 10 ml of 100% ethanol is run through the column, followed by 10 ml of the HCl solution. The sample is then applied to the column, and water-soluble impurities are eluted with 10 ml of 0.001 N HCl slowly into a tube. The mertiatide is then eluted into a second tube using the ethanol-saline mixture, and $TcO_2$ material stays on the column.

### Technical Considerations

Many factors may influence the separation and the Rf values on any given chromatographic separation, including the following:

- Purity of the solvent
- Humidity (solvent and media)
- Concentration of sample
- Shape of strip
- Direction of grain in strip
- Length of strip and solvent migration
- Air flow in development chamber
- Temperature
- Sample application and spot size
- Column packing
- Radiation detection technique

The person performing the analysis must be aware of these factors and make every effort to keep the technique constant, or separation is not reproducible. Ideally, one should end up with a compact peak for each component on the developed chromatogram. In practice, the zones are often distorted and erroneous results occur. The most common errors leading to artifacts in the analysis are as follows:

- Sample spot distorted or too large or too small
- Counting geometry, statistics and dead-time problems
- Strip cut in wrong place
- Spot placed near edge of the strip
- Spot immersed in the solvent
- Wrong solvent or media used
- Solvent splashed on sides of development chamber

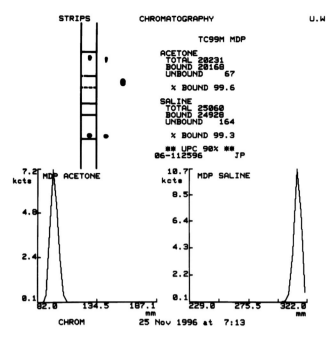

**FIG. 22-3.** The upper portion shows the gamma camera image of the radioactivity on three pairs of spots in different strips. The left strip is "gridded," showing the MDP-acetone system (top half) and the MDP-saline system (bottom half). The other spots represent different QC procedures performed at the same time. In the bottom portion of the image, the left peak shows the acetone system with nearly all the activity at the origin (mostly Tc-99m MDP and some Tc-99m $TcO_2$). The right peak shows the saline system with nearly all the activity having migrated with the solvent front (mostly Tc-99m MDP and some Tc-99m $TcO_4^-$). The top right numeric data demonstrate that only 0.4% of the radioactivity migrates in acetone (i.e., this is Tc-99m $TcO_4^-$) and that 0.7% does not migrate in saline (i.e., this is neither Tc MDP nor $TcO_4^-$). The Tc-99m MDP radiochemical purity is 100% minus (0.4% + 0.7%), or 98.9%.

- Solvent contaminated
- Water (humidity) in solvent or media
- Solvent not equilibrated with atmosphere in chamber

Of these, the most common problem relates to the size of the spot. The radioconcentration of RPs is sufficiently high that very small (1 to 5 μL) spots can be made and give adequate count rates for sodium iodide detectors. In fact, even the smallest spots often give count rates that are too high for typical well counters. The result is overestimation of impurities due to dead-time losses in counting the higher activity pieces of the strip (the portions containing the labeled RP). This can be corrected by using constant geometry and counting the strip pieces at a fixed distance from the detector.

Many institutions use dose calibrators to quantify the activity. Dose calibrators are not very accurate at activities <100 μCi (3.7 MBq) and have a great deal of variation and error <10 μCi (0.37 MBq). One microliter of an RP with a typical RP concentration of 40 mCi (1,480 MBq)/ml yields 40 μCi (1.48 MBq). If an impurity is present at levels of 10% (typical required RP purity is 90%), only 4 μCi (0.15

MBq) of impurity is present. Sufficient activity is required for counting a larger spot, and these larger spots may result in separated peaks that become too broad, and the tail end may inadvertently be clipped when cutting the strip. At UW-Madison, we have made a Lucite phantom that holds up to 12 strips and allows reproducible placement on a gamma camera. The gamma camera computer prints a histogram and does the computations, automatically displaying the areas counted in each peak (Fig. 22-3). The camera and collimator combination can easily handle the count rates involved, so dead-time losses are not significant, and yet the system is sensitive enough that the smallest possible spots can be used.

Whenever an analysis indicates unacceptably low radiochemical purity, it should always be repeated by an experienced chromatographer with fresh solvent before an RP preparation is rejected. Nine times out of 10, poor results are due to the chromatography technique rather than a truly bad preparation. It is very rare to get a bad tag with most RPs. The preparations with the lowest purity in our experience have been HMPAO, sestamibi, and MAG3.

The USP requires that the Tc-99m RPs in most cases radiochemical purity be >90% (Table 22-11). In the case of Tc-99m SC, the USP required radiochemical purity is 92% ($TcO_2$ acts as SC and cannot be separated chromatographically or in patient images, hence the $TcO_2$ is added to the RP total, making it 92%). In the case of $TcO_4^-$, the USP requires that radiochemical purity be 95%. Because $TcO_4^-$ is the precursor of all Tc-99m RPs, it should be of higher purity. Some RPs have <90% required radiochemical purity, and in each case this is the result of the difficulty of RP preparation.

It is important to realize that these values represent minimum standards. In the routine RPs, the average radiochemical purity is excellent (e.g., annual mean purity of Tc-99m MDP was 99.7% at UW-Madison), whereas with other RPs, it may be difficult to reach even the minimum standard (e.g., Tc-99m HMPAO, where 85% radiochemical purity was difficult to achieve before the recent introduction of the stabilized form).

### *Other QC Requirements*

The radionuclidic purity QC of these Tc-99m RPs is provided when the eluate purity is checked at the time of gener-

**TABLE 22-11.** *USP radiochemical purity requirements for Tc-99m RPs*

| | |
|---|---|
| Pertechnetate | 95% |
| Sulfur colloid | 92% |
| MAA, GH, MDP, HDP, DTPA, PYP, HSA, MIBI*, IDA, MAG3* | 90% |
| DMSA | 85% |
| HMPAO* | 80% |

*Package insert (FDA) requirements.

ator elution. The chemical purity, sterility, and pyrogenicity QC responsibility lies with the generator manufacturer and kit supplier. Proper attention to aseptic technique during preparation and dispensing, including the use of sterile laminar flow hoods, is mandatory.

## NON–TC-99M RADIOPHARMACEUTICALS

Because of the excellent physical attributes of Tc-99m, Tc-99m RPs are the preferred RPs for nuclear medicine. If a Tc-99m RP is not used, a Tc-99m ligand has not yet been produced as a substitute or the localization or clearance requires a radionuclide with a longer half-life. These non–Tc-99m radionuclides can either be RPs in their own right (e.g., Tl-201, Ga-67, I-131, I-123, and the inert gases) or in combination with ligands (e.g., In-111 combined with antibodies, receptor agents, or blood cell elements). In the former cases, the RP is supplied by the commercial source ready to use, but in the latter, the local commercial radiopharmacy or the nuclear medicine department must prepare the radionuclide-ligand combination and do the required QC.

## Thallium 201

Tl-201 is made by exposing pure natural Tl-203 to a high-energy proton beam that results in Pb-201 (Tl-203 [p,3n] Pb-201), which has a half-life of 9.4 hours. This Pb-201 is chemically separated from the target Tl-203 and allowed to stand to decay to Tl-201; the Tl-201 is then chemically separated from the Pb-201. The Tl-201 is sold with the manufacturer's guarantees of radionuclidic purity (<1% Tl-200, <1% Tl-202, and <0.25% Pb-203) (1) and that the RP is in the 1+ valence state for appropriate biodistribution. The USP requirement is that 95% is thallous chloride as Tl-201 (Table 22-12). The user merely injects this RP.

Tl-201 decays by EC to mercury 201 with a half-life of 73 hours and gives off mercury-characteristic x-rays (69 to 80 keV) with 95% abundance and two usable gamma rays of 135 and 167 keV, with a combined abundance of 12%.

**TABLE 22-12.** *USP or package insert radiochemical purity of non-Tc diagnostic radiopharmaceuticals*

| Radiopharmaceutical | Required |
| --- | --- |
| I-131 OIH | 97% |
| I-125 albumin | 97% |
| Tl-201 (thallous chloride) | 95% |
| Iodine radioisotopes | 95% |
| I-131 NP-59 and MIBG | 95% |
| In-111 labeled proteins | 90% |
| Ga-67 (gallium citrate) | 85% |

## Radioisotopes of Iodine

Radioiodine can substitute into many iodine pharmaceuticals (e.g., orthoiodohippurate [OIH]), and, when oxidized (e.g., by chloramine T), can attach itself to aromatic rings (e.g., tyrosine) to make RPs. The ability to obtain very high–specific activity I-123 provides the potential for developing receptor agents that can be used in single photon emission computed tomography (SPECT) imaging. Many PET RPs developed already have available I-123 SPECT alternatives.

### Iodine 131

I-131 is obtained as a by-product of uranium fission. It decays by beta emission with a half-life of 8.05 days to Xe-133. The transition energy between I-131 and the Xe-133 ground state is 971 keV, and although several beta transitions occur, the principal ($\beta_5$) results in 607 keV to the beta (with neutrino) and a 364-keV photon. Fourteen gamma rays are emitted, the most important, with abundance (%), being 364 keV (82%), 637 keV (7%), 284 keV (6%), and 723 keV (2%). The 364-keV gamma is the major one used diagnostically, even though the high-energy photon is difficult to image because of the poor stopping power of the NaI(Tl) crystal and septal penetration problems.

I-131 is used in adrenal imaging using iodomethyl-norcholesterol (NP-59) or MIBG (iobenguane) and has a role in thyroid imaging of metastatic cancer as NaI when the potential for thyroid therapy is being evaluated. The absorbed thyroid dose is approximately 1 rad/μCi (1 cGy/37 KBq) with normal thyroid uptake. Thus, this radioisotope is no longer used for thyroid imaging, and saturated solution of potassium iodide is administered with I-131 RPs that may result in I-131 elution (NP-59, MIBG, OIH) to block thyroidal uptake of I-131. A limited role remains for I-131 OIH, but this renal tubular agent is rapidly being replaced with Tc-99m MAG3. The USP radiochemical purity of I-131 as NaI is 95%, as I-131 OIH is 97%, and as the adrenal imaging agents is 95%.

### Iodine 125

I-125 can be produced by the Xe-124(n,γ)Xe-125 reaction, where the Xe-125 decays by EC to I-125. I-125 decays by EC with a half-life of 60 days, giving off a 35-keV gamma ray (7% abundance) and characteristic tellurium (Te) x-rays from 27 to 32 keV (140% abundance). I-125 is sold as I-125 albumin and iothalamate, which are used in small doses for plasma volume and GFR measurement, respectively. In these RPs, the long half-life is an advantage for prolonged shelf life in these infrequently used agents. The USP requires 97% radiochemical purity of I-125 albumin.

## Iodine 123

I-123 is the preferred thyroid iodine imaging agent, imparting 1% of the thyroid dose per microcurie when compared to I-131. Despite I-123 being a virtually ideal RP with excellent physical and biological characteristics, many institutions prefer Tc-99m $TcO_4^-$ for thyroid imaging. I-123 decays by EC with a 13-hour half-life, the major radiation being an ideal imaging 159-keV photon with 83% abundance. A cerebral perfusion agent (iofetamine) was available but has been withdrawn by the manufacturer.

The 13-hour half-life of this RP makes it tempting to use the day after delivery, but with the passage of two half-lives (25% of the original I-123 dose), the contaminant with the longer half-life (I-125, 60 days) may contribute significant patient doses. The USP radiochemical purity required is 95%. USP radionuclidic purity required is 85%, but given the long half-lives of the iodine contaminants, the I-123 purity should be higher than the USP standard. This is the case with the commercial supplier's package insert standards. Even when the radionuclidic purity is 97% at delivery, 12.5% of the radioactivity will be contaminants at expiration time, 30 hours after calibration (Mallinckrodt package insert data).

There are several methods of preparing I-123. The initial method of Medi-Physics used the Te-124(p,2n)I-123 reaction, which yielded a radionuclidic purity of 94.7% I-123. The radiocontaminants were I-124 ($\leq$4.8%) and I-125, I-126, I-130, Na-24, and Te-121 ($\leq$0.5% in total). Because the contaminants have long half-lives, at expiration the purity was only 85.5%. This is the product on which the USP standards were based.

The next production method produced a product with higher radionuclidic purity (99.6%). This method used the I-127(p,5n)Xe-123$\rightarrow$I-123 reaction, which requires 60- to 70-MeV protons. There are very few cyclotrons in the world capable of that high an energy. The contaminants in this technique are I-125 and Te-121, mostly I-125.

The current production uses the following reactions using 31-MeV protons, which are attainable on many cyclotrons:

$$\text{Xe-124(p,2n)Cs-123} \xrightarrow[\substack{6\text{ mins}}]{\substack{B+,EC}} \text{Xe-123} \xrightarrow[\substack{2\text{ hrs}}]{\substack{EC,B+}} \text{I-123} \quad (5)$$

$$\text{Xe-124(p,pn)Xe-123} \xrightarrow[\substack{2\text{ hrs}}]{\substack{EC,B+}} \text{I-123} \quad (6)$$

There is <0.1% I-125 and virtually no other contaminants with this method, and it is still >98% pure at expiration (30 hours). All current suppliers use this method, and both Medi-Physics and Mallinckrodt products are >99.9% pure. Note that the dosimetry and specifications in current package inserts are based on a conservatively low radionuclidic purity. Medi-Physics uses 99.5% at calibra-

tion and 98.3% at expiration. Mallinckrodt uses 97% at calibration and 87.2% at expiration because it has not updated its package insert after converting to the new method. Because they do not specify the production reaction in the package insert, the FDA does not require modification of the package insert.

## Indium 111 RPs

In-111 is produced by the Cd-111(p,n)In-111 reaction in a cyclotron and results in a 67-hour half-life radionuclide that decays by EC as a pure gamma emitter with 173-keV (89% abundance) and 247-keV (94% abundance) photons.

In-111 DTPA is available commercially for cerebrospinal fluid (CSF) flow studies, and the manufacturer assures sterility and apyrogenicity. Apyrogenicity is essential in CSF studies, and the manufacturer must establish that there will be no pyrogen reaction in the concentration recommended for use.

The most common use of In-111 oxine is in labeling blood cell elements (white blood cells [WBCs] and platelets) and proteins (MOABs and pentetreotide). In protein labeling it is important that the correct specific concentration of In-111 is used, and in the approved RPs the manufacturer may indicate which In-111 radionuclide source should be used to result in optimal radiochemical purity. These differences in purity result from changes in the buffer, pH, and trace metal ion concentrations that effect labeling yields. Chelating reactions typically require up to 30 minutes to complete; this applies to MOABs, peptides, and blood cell products.

In the case of In-111–labeled WBCs, the plasma transferrin competes for the In-111 and reduces labeling efficiency because In-111 binds with greater efficiency to transferrin than WBCs. With poor labeling the blood pool is visualized (labeled transferrin), and the liver is well seen because of transchelation from serum transferrin to the liver. In the labeling of proteins, the protein is first bound to DTPA. DTPA binds with the terminal-amide ($NH_2$) groups of proteins and any exposed amide at other sites (e.g., amino acids lysine and phenylalanine). This provides a general protein labeling technique and explains the common finding of the generic word *pendetide* in package inserts of these RPs (a reference to the DTPA-amide coupling). The DTPA then chelates In-111 when it is added to the mixture as $InCl_3$.

## Gallium 67 Citrate

Ga-67 is produced by a cyclotron Zn-68(p,2n)Ga-67 reaction. Ga-67 decays by EC with a half-life of 78 hours with a series of imageable gamma rays from 91 to 400 keV, with cumulative abundance of approximately 85%. It is delivered as Ga-67 citrate from the manufacturer in unit doses. The USP-required radiochemical purity is 85%.

## Inert Gases

Inert gases are used to add specificity to lung scanning for the diagnosis of pulmonary embolism. These gases use reactor (Xe-133), cyclotron (Xe-127), and generator (Kr-81m) production, with varying physical features resulting in different image techniques (Xe-133 preperfusion imaging, Xe-127 postperfusion imaging, and Kr-81m, where the ultrashort half-life allows simultaneous planar and SPECT ventilation and perfusion scans). Despite this range of features, Tc-99m DTPA aerosol is becoming the major ventilation RP, and improved Tc-99m RPs are being developed (see Chapter 4).

### Xenon 133

Xe-133 was initially used for ventilation scans. It is a by-product of uranium fission and has a 5.3 day half-life with 35% abundance of 81-keV photon. This photon energy requires the ventilation scan to be performed before the Tc-99m MAA perfusion scan.

### Xenon 127

Xe-127, reported in 1973, has a half-life of 36 days, a 68% abundant 203-keV gamma ray, and fewer 172- and 375-keV photons, allowing the ventilation scan to be performed after the Tc-99m MAA perfusion scan. This tracer was produced in a linear accelerator from Brookhaven, but it is no longer commercially available because of the inconsistent supply, high cost, and low demand.

### Krypton 81m

Another inert gas is Kr-81m, which has an ultrashort half-life of 13 seconds with excellent 191-keV photon with 66% abundance. This agent is supplied in generator form, but the 4.5-hour parent half-life is somewhat impractical for clinical use because weekend and night use is not possible.

### QC of Non–Tc-99m RPs

The unit-dose RPs supplied by the manufacturer or commercial radiopharmacy do not need specific user QC processes. The In-111 kit sets that are reconstituted on site need QC, and the manufacturer's recommendations supplied in the package insert should be followed. In each case, the radionuclide-ligand complex is compared to free radionuclide to determine radiochemical purity. In WBC or platelet labeling, the unbound radionuclide is eliminated at the end of the labeling procedure. Extreme care must be taken during the labeling of patient cells to ensure that they are reinjected into the same patient to prevent the accidental transmission of blood-borne infectious diseases. Aseptic technique and use of laminar flow sterile hood is necessary.

## PET RADIOPHARMACEUTICALS

Many PET RPs have been produced, but only 25 are regularly used in clinical and research practice. The advantage of PET over other imaging techniques is the fact that the positron emitters include elements (e.g., C, O, N, and Fl) that can be substituted into many biological agents without altering their function. In addition, PET can be quantified, and with the short half-lives of these RPs, they can be administered with acceptable patient radiation doses.

The PET RPs are usually produced in accelerators, and some can also be obtained from generators. For clinical applications, F-18 fluorodeoxyglucose (FDG) is most widely used. It constitutes approximately half of all PET research studies and virtually all clinical PET studies. FDG is also produced as unit doses in regional distribution centers, and conventional SPECT scanners can be modified for positron use.

The short physical half-lives of PET RPs constrain the radionuclidic, radiochemical, and chemical purity, as well as sterility and pyrogenicity QC procedures. Local institutions making PET RPs can utilize the chromatographic techniques used in preparation and adsorbent cartridges to remove some impurities, but sterility and pyrogenicity studies can be performed only after the patient has received the RP. This diligent retrospective review of the QC data provides evidence that the process is safe.

At the local institutional PET center level, all manufacturing and QC responsibility lies with the center. The FDA is currently seeking New Drug Applications (NDA) for PET RPs not produced under an existing investigational new drug (IND) application. New users are required to provide all the good manufacturing practices (GMP) specified by the FDA.

## DOSIMETRY

Dosimetry of RPs is covered in individual organ systems chapters and in Chapter 27. Several relevant topics are repeated here, especially as they relate to RPs.

### Effective Dose Equivalent

The effective dose equivalent (EDE) is powerful for explaining internal and external radiation risks to the population, although this concept is not widely endorsed. Patient dosimetry is usually calculated using the standard medical ionizing radiation dosimetry (MIRD) technique. This technique allows the calculation of accurate and specific organ doses in nuclear medicine but does not allow the comparison of risks, which would enable patients to better understand the radiation dose disclosure that is part of informed consent in their own medical management. By allowing varying organ doses to be expressed as a single equivalent whole-body dose, the EDE is a powerful tool for providing

**TABLE 22-13.** *Weighting factors in calculation of EDE*

| Organ | Weighting factor |
|---|---|
| Gonads | 0.25 |
| Breast | 0.15 |
| Red marrow | 0.12 |
| Lung | 0.12 |
| Thyroid | 0.03 |
| Bone | 0.03 |
| 5 remaining tissues* | 5 @0.06 |

*The 5 remaining organs with highest dose.

**TABLE 22-14.** *EDEs for various common radiation exposures*

| Source | EDE |
|---|---|
| General background | 0.30 |
| Worker "allowable" | 5.00 |
| CXR | 0.10 |
| Lumbar spine | 0.13 |
| Barium enema | 0.41 |
| Chest CT | 0.48 |
| Tc-99m MDP | 0.44 |
| Tc-99m RBC | 0.65 |
| In-111 WBC | 1.20 |
| Ga-67 citrate | 10.00 |

comparisons between nuclear medicine tests and other radiologic and environmental exposures.

To determine the EDE, each organ is weighted by a factor (Table 22-13), the weighted dose equivalent is obtained, then these are added. The weighing factors are a function of each organ's radiosensitivity for fatal cancers or genetic effects. Examples of EDEs for various common radiation exposures are provided (Table 22-14). This concept should not replace individual organ doses, which are critical for full evaluation of patient dosimetry.

## Worker Radiation Limits

The Code of Federal Regulations (CFR) contains all the federal regulations that apply to different situations. In Title 10, all regulations relating to civilian radiation use are to be found; parts 19, 20, and 35 are relevant to radiation workers. Ten CFR Part 19 provides minimum instructional standards to workers, and 10 CFR Part 20 defines the occupational dose limits. If a female worker declares herself pregnant, a whole-body annual dose limit of 0.5 rem for the term of the pregnancy is applied. For radiation workers, the annual limit is as follows:

- Whole body: 5 rems (50 mSv)
- Organ, skin, or extremity: 50 rems (500 mSv)
- Lens of the eye: 15 rems (150 mSv)

## Patient Doses

With Tc-99m RPs, the radiation dose to the patient is modest, so protocols are designed to optimize images, that is, they allow sufficient activity to be administered to prevent patient-movement degradation of the image. Most tracers that distribute throughout the body (Tc-99m MDP in bone scans) are prescribed in 15- to 30-mCi (555 to 1,110 MBq) doses. RPs that sequester in an organ require lower doses (e.g., Tc-99m SC liver-spleen scans and Tc-99m MAA lung perfusion scans) of 4 to 6 mCi (148 to 222 MBq) to obtain excellent images. RPs that partially sequester in an organ (e.g., Tc-99m $TcO_4^-$ in thyroid imaging) require intermediate doses of approximately 10 mCi (370 MBq).

With non–Tc-99m RPs, the dose administered is determined by the radiation burden imparted given the particular physical characteristics of the radionuclide, the biodistribution, and the organ radiosensitivity. A good example of this is In-111: When administered as labeled WBCs, the dose is limited by organ radiation (the spleen) to 0.5 mCi (18.5 MBq), whereas, as a labeled MOAB, 5.0 mCi (185 MBq) can be used. In these non–Tc-99m studies, the image acquisition is nearly always compromised by patient dose.

In children and adults of unusual size, the RP dose should be modified. However, the individualization of patient doses is wasteful of effort. Many departments decide to individualize the RP doses based on weight only if the patient is outside the 45- to 90-kg or 45- to 125-kg range. The intent is to ensure adequate statistics for images while ensuring that the radiation dose to the patient is as low as possible.

## Pregnancy

The dose to a fetus results mainly from bladder and colon RP activity, often as part of the route of excretion. Few human data are available to assess the risk of fetal irradiation, but two sources exist: pregnant women irradiated for gynecologic cancers (~250 rads [2.5 Gy]) in the 1920s and Japanese A-bomb data. Fetal malformations were found in the gynecologic cancer group. In the A-bomb data, microcephaly and mental retardation were found in 40% of offspring when the fetus received 100 rads (1 Gy) during the 8- to 15-weeks interval of pregnancy. This risk was small when the A-bomb dose was <10 rads (10 cGy). No increase in childhood cancer or teratogenetic effects was seen, regardless of dose.

Animal experiments suggest teratogenesis occurs in the equivalent of 1 to 7 weeks of human pregnancy (the period of organogenesis), but this effect has not been documented in any described population. It is established that the risk of radiation-induced teratogenesis is negligibly small when compared to the natural rate of 4% to 6%.

The Oxford survey of childhood cancer (2) suggests an increase in leukemias and solid cancers, especially from irradiation during the first trimester. This survey also suggests that the relative risk of fatal cancer before age 16 from this diagnostic in utero radiation is 1.4. At most this would account for no more than 7% to 8% of all childhood cancer cases. The American College of Radiology (ACR) believes that this question is not settled because the increased risk has not been seen in A-bomb survivors and in several small prospective studies. It is probably best to consider the risk of in utero exposure no more than that of an adult or infant to the same exposure.

What practical steps should be taken to prevent the unnecessary radiation of a fetus? The Joint Commission on Accreditation of Healthcare Organizations requires that each female patient of childbearing age having a scan or x-ray should be asked whether she is pregnant, and this should include a redundant method of questioning. We do this by prominently displaying signs asking patients to inform staff if they are pregnant, and each time an RP is administered, the technologist administering also checks by direct questioning.

### Pregnancy Tests

In patients in whom significant doses would be imparted to the fetus (e.g., I-131 therapy) or any radionuclide that readily crosses the placental membrane (e.g., Tl-201), the procedure should be performed after the patient's next menstrual period begins, if possible. The most sensitive pregnancy test is the quantitative serum human chorionic gonadotropin (HCG) measurement, which confirms pregnancy 5 to 7 days after fertilization, 4 to 5 days after implantation, that is, barely before the patient's next menstrual period. The serum test becomes positive at 5 mIU/ml, whereas the urine test becomes positive when the serum level is effectively 40 mIU/ml. For each doubling of the HCG, 1 to 2 days must elapse; so the urine test becomes positive 7 to 11 days after implantation, that is, at the start of the expected menstrual period. Neither test is efficient at detecting pregnancy before the next expected period, so pregnancy tests do not safeguard against giving pregnant patients RPs. A patient whose period is late is a suitable candidate for a serum or urine pregnancy test.

### Known Pregnant Patients

In patients known to be pregnant, a risk-benefit analysis is done to weigh the need for the test against the potential hazard to the fetus. In each case, the decision depends on the clinical presentation: The bone scan is excellent for diagnosing early stress fractures, but the patient can be treated without confirmation, or an x-ray can make the diagnosis without significant fetal irradiation. On the other hand, where a scan is essential, as with ruling out pulmonary embolism, then the benefit outweighs the risk and the scan can be modified to lower the risk even further, for example, by eliminating the ventilation scan or reducing RP dose and imaging for a longer time.

Some patients return to the nuclear medicine service after a diagnostic test or therapy with the information that, unbeknownst to them, they were pregnant when they received the RP. In this case, the fetal dose should be calculated and dis-cussed with the patient. With bone scans, Ga-67, In-111 WBC, Tl-201 scans, and I-131 therapy, the fetus would receive between 0.5 and 5.0 rads (0.5 to 5.0 cGy). A rule of thumb called the *Danish rule* suggests that fetal doses of <1.0 rad (1 cGy) are of no concern, doses of 1 to 10 rads (1 to 10 cGy) might make one think of therapeutic abortion only in extenuating circumstances, and doses >10 rads (10 cGy) are an indication for considering therapeutic abortion (3). The ACR is against this rule because thousands of normal pregnancies would need to be terminated for each defect prevented by abortion. Very few radiologists or nuclear physicians suggest a therapeutic abortion for any diagnostic nuclear medicine test.

### Lactation

Many times, nuclear medicine physicians are asked to determine the role of a scan in patients who are breast-feeding their infants. The important factors are as follows:

- Whether RP concentrates in milk ($TcO_4^-$ and $I^-$ as NaI do)
- Effective half-life of radionuclide in milk (hours or days)
- Volume of milk produced (volume and dose ingested by child)
- Frequency of breast-feeding (can breast be pumped and the milk stored?)
- Actual dose imparted to child (should not exceed 0.5 rem [5 mSv])

Various reports on this subject are available but are difficult to compare because of different methods used. Perhaps the most widely quoted study is that of Mountford and Oakley (4); it is modified significantly in Table 22-15.

### REGULATION OF RP ADMINISTRATION

### Regulatory Status

RPs are not generally available until they receive FDA approval as safe and effective. Moreover, the Health

**TABLE 22-15.** *Secretion of radioactivity in human breast milk*

| Routine doses of various RPs | Effective half-life in milk | Instructions concerning breast-feeding |
|---|---|---|
| Tl-201, Ga-67, I-131 as NaI, In-111 peptides | 3–15 days | Discontinue breast-feeding* |
| $TcO_4^-$ and I-131 OIH | ~6 hrs | Stop 1–2 days |
| Tc MAA, Tc RBC, I-123 NaI | ~6 hrs | Stop 6–12 hrs |
| Other Tc-99m ligands | ~6 hrs | Continue feeding |

*If mother strongly desires to continue breast-feeding, the administered dose may be modified, breast milk stored before RP administration for use as a replacement source during procedure, and the expressed milk after the scan can be measured for radioactivity content to indicate when breast-feeding can recommence (after ensuring adequate detector sensitivity).

Care Financing Agency does not authorize reimbursement for an unapproved indication or drug for Medicare/Medicaid patients. Considering that we usually read about new agents in the literature many years before they are approved, the impact of this becomes obvious. Very often, the new agent is significantly superior to existing alternatives, but unless it is available and reimbursable, the average nuclear medicine department does not use it. The state pharmacy laws, Department of Transportation (DOT), FDA, and NRC all claim jurisdiction over some part of the administration of RPs. Each component of the DOT, FDA, and NRC laws are well defined in the CFR.

## Nuclear Regulatory Commission

The NRC regulates those who produce and use reactor-produced RPs by licensure of the user, defines these requirements well, and provides regulatory guides on how this is accomplished (see Chapter 29). In general, 10 CFR part 19 describes notices, instructions, and reports to workers and the inspection processes. Ten CFR Part 20 describes the standards for protection against radiation, including occupational dose limits. The average occupational dose is 195 mrem (1.95 mSv) in nuclear medicine practices that receive unit doses and 342 mrem (3.42 mSv) where the doses are prepared in-house using the same technologists for imaging and RP preparation (5). Posting, room labeling, and waste disposal (on-site decay is possible if half-life is <65 days) is discussed there. In 10 CFR Part 35, the medical use of by-product material is described. This includes supervision, survey instrument checks, survey requirements, safety precautions, and the release of therapy patients.

The NRC has no role in the interpretation of nuclear medicine scans or tests but has every role in the administration of RP. This role dates back to 1954 and the Atomic Energy Commission. With the abolition of this agency, the NRC was born. Strictly, the NRC rules apply only to by-product materials (e.g., Mo-99, I-131, Xe-133), but the states are required to enforce similar rules for other RPs. All patient RP uses are treated similarly.

The NRC has jurisdiction over the following:

- Routine use of RPs
- Nonroutine uses of RPs
- Misadministrations (defined in Table 22-16)
- ALARA (as low as reasonably achievable) limits
- Quality Management Plan (I-125 and I-131 as NaI and therapy uses)
- Records of clinical practice, such as
  Personnel dosimetry
  Radionuclide receipt
  Surveys and wipe tests
  Tc-99m eluate records
  RP dose records
  Disposal of radionuclides
  Instrumentation QC

The NRC can transfer its regulatory function to the states and has done so in 29 states; four states are in the process of seeking this local control. At the time of writing, the Institute of Medicine has suggested that the role of the NRC in the practice of nuclear medicine can be safely returned to the states, and should be. The NRC's vigorous application of the standards appears to be appropriate for the nuclear power industry but inappropriate to the practice of medicine. For instance, the NRC requires that the RP therapy prescription not only be signed but also dated in the physician's own hand, whereas with conventional pharmaceuticals this level of regulation is rivaled only by Schedule II controlled drugs, and then the date can be typed or written by someone else. The costs of NRC licensure are provided in Chapter 29. The NRC recently relaxed its restrictions on unindicated uses of RPs and the compounding and administration of non-FDA approved agents or modifications of approved preparation procedures. Their regulatory guide for implementation for this is still in development at this time, however, and an early draft had significant procedural obstacles to these types of unapproved uses.

**TABLE 22-16.** *Types of incidents considered to be misadministrations or recordable events in a nuclear medicine department*

| Procedure | Recordable event | Misadministration |
|---|---|---|
| Therapeutic RPs | Administered dosage differs by >10% than prescribed | Wrong patient or wrong RP |
| | Without written directive | Wrong route of administration |
| | Without daily dosage record | >20% variation from prescribed dose |
| Sodium iodide RPs (>30 μCi I-125 or I-131) | >10% variation from prescribed dosage *and* >15 μCi | Wrong patient or wrong RP |
| | Without written directive | >20% variation from prescribed dose *and* >30 μCi |
| | Without daily dosage record | |
| All diagnostic RPs (<30 μCi I-125/I-131 as NaI) | No defined recordable event | Wrong patient, RP, route, or dose *and* 5 rems to organ or 50 rems to body |

## Food and Drug Administration

The FDA initially believed that the NRC should control RPs. In the 1970s, the FDA realized that RPs were really little different from other drugs, so in 1975, it revoked its exemption of RPs. The FDA is concerned with the safety of RPs, their manufacture, and diagnostic efficacy, and all investigational and research use of RPs falls under its jurisdiction. The NRC staunchly claims its authority over the routine use of RPs. In 1975, the FDA required commercially produced RPs to have either an NDA or IND application approved.

The major difference between RPs and conventional drugs is related to the presence of a radionuclide and the desired absence of a pharmacologic effect. Although diagnostic RPs are generally prescribed in microscopic doses and for one-time use, some RPs can have pharmacologic effect, especially if the preparation and purification process is defective. Adverse drug reactions do occur, which establishes that the pharmacologic effect of RPs is not absent. Virtually all RPs used have NDA approval, but the application of the standard drug approval requirements is a severe hindrance to the development of new RPs. The NDA process has been estimated to cost between $10 and $70 million for each new RP approval. Given that only 24 million RP procedures are performed worldwide annually, with a total projected annual expenditure of $1 to $2 trillion, it represents a substantial risk for drug companies to embark on a new diagnostic RP investigation.

The FDA is currently attempting to extend its jurisdiction in the PET field by insisting that all clinical use PET RPs be produced under NDA approval and follow GMPs. GMPs are designed for large-scale drug production and appear inappropriate for small PET centers, where only several patient prescriptions per day are compounded. This new interpretation of the FDA role appears in contrast to other physician or pharmacist compounding, which is allowable for other RPs and drugs. There is also a move by the FDA to require that approved INDs be replaced by NDAs, which would then require GMPs. This added cost could potentially cease small-scale PET imaging and end its potentially important role in clinical medicine.

## U.S. Adopted Names Council

The nomenclature of RPs appears confusing, with chemical names, biochemical names, code names (groups of numbers or letters, e.g., RP-30 and MIBI for sestamibi and IDA for hepatobiliary iminodiacetic acids), and trademark names. The U.S. Adopted Names (USAN) Council generates nonproprietary names that are selected through a formal process involving the manufacturer. This expert committee is jointly sponsored by the American Medical Association (AMA), the USP, and the American Pharmaceutical Association (APhA).

The drug company comes forward with a proposal that includes chemical structure, chemical name, code designations, source of material, pharmacologic activity, or therapeutic usefulness, and trademark name applied for. The USAN council

**TABLE 22-17.** Common RPs with official name, common name, and some brand names

| Official name | Code name | Brand names |
|---|---|---|
| I-125 albumin (human) | IHSA, RISA | Isojex, IHSA I-125 |
| Tc-99m albumin (human) | HSA | Tc-99m HSA - Squibb |
| Tc-99m albumin (macroaggregated) | MAA | AN-MAA, TechneScan MAA, Tc-99m MAA, Pulmolite, Macrotec |
| Tc-99m arcitumomab | Anti-CEA MOAB | CEAScan |
| Tc-99m bicisate | ECD | Neurolite |
| In-111 capromab pendetide | CYT 356 MOAB | ProstaScint |
| Co-57/58 cyanocobalamin | Co-57/58 B-12 | Dicopac kit, Rubratope 57 |
| Tc-99m disofenin | DISIDA | Hepatolite |
| Tc-99m exametazine | HMPAO | Ceretec |
| Tc-99m gluceptate | GH or GHA | GlucoScan, TechneScan gluceptate, glucotec |
| In-111 indium chloride | InCl₃ | Indiclor (use with satumomab) |
| I-131 iobenguane sulphate | MIBG | I-131 MIBG |
| I-131 iodohippurate | IOH | Hipputope, Hippuran |
| I-123 iofetamine | IMP | Spectamine |
| I-125 iothalamate | I-125 iothalamate | Glofil |
| Tc-99m lidofenin | HIDA | TechneScan HIDA |
| Tc-99m mebrofenin | TMBRIDA | Choletec |
| Tc-99m medronate | MDP | Osteolite, AN MDP, MPI MDP, TechneScan MDP, MDP Squibb |
| Tc-99m mertiatide | MAG3 | TechneScan MAG3 |
| Tc-99m nofetumomab merpentan | Anti-SCCA MOAB | Verluma |
| Tc-99m oxidronate | HDP | TechneScan HDP, OsteoScan HDP |
| In-111 oxyquinoline (WBC) | In oxine (WBC) | In-111 oxyquinoline (WBC) |
| In-111 pentetate | In DTPA | MPI Indium DTPA |
| Tc-99m pentetate | Tc DTPA | Techneplex, AN-DTPA, MPI-DTPA |
| In-111 pentetreotide | In-111 octreotide | OctreoScan |
| Tc-99m pertechnetate | TcO₄⁻ | UltraTechneknow, Tc-99m generator |
| Tc-99m pyrophosphate | PYP | TechneScan-PYP Cis-Pyro, AN-Pyrotec, pyrolite, phosphotec |
| Tc-99m red blood cells | Tc RBC | UltraTag RBC |
| In-111 satumomab pendetide | Anti TAG-72 MOAB | OncoScint |
| Tc-99m sestamibi | MIBI or RP-30 | Cardiolite |
| Sr-89 strontium chloride | SrCl₂ | Metastron |
| Tc-99m succimer | DMSA | MPI DMSA |
| Tc-99m sulfur colloid | Tc SC | AN Sulfur Colloid, TechneColl, Tesuloid |
| Tc-99m tetrofosmin | Tetrofosmin | Myoview |

must search for a distinctive nonproprietary name that does not conflict with established drugs and trademarks. It is expected that the drug company will not select a trademark that capitalizes on the generic name as approved. The selected name is forwarded to various cooperating agencies worldwide and is finally published in the *Journal of the American Medical Association*.

In 1938, the FDC Act (precursor of FDA) stipulated that "the common or usual name" be used on labels, and in the absence of this sanctioned name, the chemical name should be used. In 1962, the FDA was then given the authority to designate official names, and now the FDA acts in concert as the USAN Council (one representative each from the AMA, APhA, FDA, and USP, with an additional at-large member). If this council does not decide on a name, the commissioner of the FDA can select one.

The general rules include a preference for single words with not more than four syllables, and only under compelling circumstances is a name acceptable with more than one modifier (RPs are an exception, e.g., satumomab pendetide [OncoScint]). The official name is designed to reflect chemical or pharmacologic characteristics, and simple stem elements are used in all members of a group of common characteristics (e.g., *-mab* in MOABs, *-fenin* in hepatobiliary agents).

A group of such names is supplied in Table 22-17. One can also see that several manufacturers' proprietary names have common elements that make them identifiable for that particular company:

- AN-MAA, AN-glucotec, AN-MDP, AN-DTPA, AN-pyrotec: CIS (Bedford, MA)
- Pulmolite, Microlite, Hepatolite, Osteolite, Pyrolite: DuPont-Pharma (North Billerica, MA)
- TechneScan MAA, OsteoScan HDP, TechneScan gluceptate, TechneScan PYP, TechneScan MDP, TechneColl: Mallinckrodt (St. Louis, MO)
- MPI MDP, MPI DTPA, and MPI DMSA: Medi-Physics/Amersham (Arlington Heights, IL)
- Phosphetec, Choletec, Macrotec: Bracco/Squibb (Princeton, NJ)

### State and Other Laws

State laws regarding the practice of medicine and pharmacy apply to RPs. The states control non–reactor-produced RPs (i.e., cyclotron products, such as PET agents, In-111, Tl-201, and Ga-67) and follow the same requirements of the NRC. Their supervision and inspection requirement for x-ray and RP radiation safety, however, have not been as unnecessarily rigorous as that of the NRC. State and DOT rules must be followed when transporting diagnostic and therapeutic RPs.

### State Law and Nuclear Pharmacies

Nuclear pharmacies that sell RPs to users are licensed by both the NRC and the state boards of pharmacy and require a state-approved and licensed pharmacist or radiopharmacist. The state board of pharmacy licensure is not required for a hospital-based nuclear pharmacy operating under an NRC physician-authorized user. These physician-authorized pharmacies are not allowed to distribute RPs beyond their institution, although distribution is possible between broad licenses if the establishments are very closely situated.

Initially, commercial nuclear pharmacies merely compounded commercially available RPs with NDA status. With the development of in-house PET RPs, the FDA considers these pharmacies manufacturers and therefore subject to GMPs and the laws governing large pharmaceutical manufacturers. The nuclear medicine fraternity believes the practice of pharmacy and medicine to be the preparation of an RP using a prescription for an individual patient. It is generally agreed, however, that if the RP is prepared by a physician in one establishment and administered in another, this is effective manufacturing.

## USER RESPONSIBILITY

Regardless of source of RP, the user is required to ensure that the proper dose of the proper RP is administered to the proper patient by the proper route and at the proper time. The person injecting the RP should ensure that this dose is appropriate, and to do this, the person must read the label. The simple problem of failure to read the label accounts for 75% to 90% of all RP administration errors. The user should read the label before administering the RP, at the time of administration, and immediately after RP administration.

The user is also required to assay the RP dose if >30 μCi are administered, and this measurement should be assayed in the dose calibrator to within 10% of the prescribed dose. Simple visual inspection of the RP is prudent because cloudy or particulate matter in the injectate is fair warning of preparation problems. Color may also be useful in certain RPs: P-32 supplied as $NaHPO_4$ is clear (therapy of blood dyscrasias), whereas P-32 colloid is blue-green (intracavitary therapy).

The user must also understand the shelf life of the prepared RP. Most RPs have shelf life of 6 to 8 hours unless special stabilizers have been added, but some have much more limited lives, especially if quantitation is used, as with Tc-99m DTPA for absolute GFR quantification.

All these varied responsibilities are discharged when the nuclear medicine staff member who injects the RP adheres to all the departmental directives. We have described in our protocols (see Chapter 30) the 15 functions this individual must do. Here, we re-emphasize the most important duties:

- Ensure nuclear medicine physician approval.
- Confirm that the prescribed dose appears appropriate for the test indicated.
- Remeasure the dose in the dose calibrator, and check that patient name, dose, and RP are the same on the request

form and the dose shielding (i.e., the dose is checked against the request form).

- Verify the patient's identity by requiring the patient to spell out his or her name and date of birth or by other means as appropriate (i.e., the patient is checked against the dose and the request form).
- Specifically ask all women of childbearing age if they are pregnant or breast-feeding.
- Advise the patient of appropriate actions to enhance RP uptake, decrease body burden by enhanced excretion, or prevent inappropriate RP administration. Examples include
  Low-iodine diet prior to I-131 therapy to improve uptake
  Increased fluid intake and urine voiding to improve bone scan quality
- Prevent inappropriate RP administration.
  Ensure stable iodine is given to patients receiving I-131 OIH, NP-59, or MIBG (to reduce the thyroid burden) before administering RP.

## Extravasation of Dose

Extravasation of injected RP doses is relatively common but only identified if whole-body images are obtained relatively soon after injection. During quality assurance studies, it is common (20% to 30% incidence) to find evidence of mild extravasation, and it is reported that approximately 2% of patients have demonstrable lymph node visualization that usually occurs with significant extravasation (see Fig. 1-15). The extravasation can significantly alter the results of some procedures, especially glomerular filtration measurements and stress myocardial perfusion scans by reducing the immediate availability of the RP.

The safety significance of the extravasation depends primarily on whether the RP has particulate irradiation as part of the radionuclide decay scheme. For Tc-99m RPs, this is generally not a problem, but for Tl-201, I-131 as NP-59 or MIBG, and all therapeutic RPs, it can be a significant complication. Extravasation can be checked for using a Geiger-Müller survey meter and passing this over the injection site from distal to proximal. Because the RP is often distributed through the body, one expects to identify activity in the arm, but there should not be a significant increase of tracer (two- or threefold) localized to the actual injection site. In many cases, especially with Tl-201, there may be localization of RP to the vein walls and a detectable increase, but this should be apparent diffusely over the vein's proximal path rather than localized to the injection site.

Once extravasation is identified, the first step is to attempt to estimate the local irradiation burden using the administered dose, administered volume, and specific dose factor (Table 22-18). If the dose and volume of a particular RP indicates that the worst-case local dose could be >2,000 rads (20 Gy) (total local deposition of dose), an estimate of the portion extravasated and the biological half-life at the extravasation site are required to determine the likely local dose.

**TABLE 22-18.** *Specific dose factors*

| Radionuclide | Specific dose factor (rad ml/mCi) |
| --- | --- |
| Tc-99m | 321 |
| I-123 | 1,147 |
| In-111 | 7,521 |
| Tl-201 | 9,467 |
| Ga-67 | 9,715 |
| I-131 | 114,012 |

Source: Shapiro B, Pillay M, Cox PH. Dosimetric consequences of interstitial dose extravasation following IV administration of a radiopharmaceutical [short communication]. Eur J Nucl Med 1987;12:513–522.

Extravasation is usually identified by patient complaint of pain, sudden onset of local swelling, lack of blood return into the needle and syringe, or by a change in the flow rate of the intravenous line. Once recognized, the individual administering the dose should try to aspirate the injectate back into the syringe or intravenous administration line, mark the site carefully, and seek assistance from experienced personnel. The first priority is to determine the portion of RP extravasated. One method is to image the patient quickly and determine the relative portions at extravasation site and target organs. Such estimates (with varying attenuations) are crude but valuable. With this estimate and the specific dose factor, the extent of potential damage can be estimated. It is agreed that doses <2,000 rads (20 Gy) are unlikely to cause significant injury. The wash-out rate from the extravasation site should also be monitored. This rate determines whether intervention (local heat, massage, hyaluronidase) is required to accelerate dispersion of the extravasated RP.

It was formerly believed that the only potential problems could occur with therapeutic, Ga-67, and Tl-201 RPs. Recently, it has been appreciated that larger doses of In-111 (labeled peptides) and some Tc-99m and I-123 RPs have the potential for injury (6).

## Adverse Drug Reactions

Adverse drug reactions (ADRs) are defined as unexpected responses to the administration of an RP; these are usually in response to the RP ligand because the radionuclide is present in too small a quantity to engender a reaction. The only ADRs requiring reporting are of those RPs used under a physician or commercially sponsored IND. The Society of Nuclear Medicine (SNM) has maintained an ADR registry since 1970, and similar registries exist in the United Kingdom, Australasia, and Europe. Most nuclear medicine studies are free of problems, and while most of these reactions are due to the ligand there are examples of the radionuclide itself causing pruritus, rashes, and flushing reactions despite the minuscule doses of chemicals used, for example, Tl-201.

As drugs, RPs are very safe, mild reactions are uncommon, and severe reactions very rare.

### ADR Rates

Over the last two decades, the reported ADR rate has decreased, perhaps as a result of improved formulation and commercial supplier QC measures. The ADR rate estimated in the United States over the last 20 years is between 1 and 6 per 100,000 administrations, but this is considered to be a 10-fold underestimation of the true ADR rate (~0.04%). This 10-fold underestimation is presumed because more than one-half of nuclear physicians are unaware of a reporting system, and that although 14% of physicians surveyed had observed an ADR, only one-fifth of these physicians had reported it.

This low ADR rate (0.04%) compares very favorably with nonradioactive drugs, in which estimates of 1.0% to 35.0% inpatient error and ADR rates have been reported. The true incidence of ADR rate may be only 1.0%, a rate still 10 times greater than that of RPs.

Over the years of voluntary RP ADR reporting to the SNM, there has been a significant change in the distribution of reported ADRs. The majority (90%) are now due to these drugs:

- Tc-99m diphosphonates (30%)
- Tc-99m colloids (15%)
- Tc-99m particulates, such as MAA (15%)
- Ga-67 citrate (10%)
- I-131 as NaI, Tc-99m DTPA, and Tc-99m GHA (each 5%)

The general classification of ADRs is described in Table 22-19. The real problem is in determining whether the ADR is due to the administered RP or other medications the patient is receiving. To determine that the patient's symptom complaints are not due to an ADR, the complaint must be classified as merely a vasovagal response or it must be established that the reaction

- Did not follow a reasonable time sequence after administration

**TABLE 22-19.** *Types of adverse drug reactions and associated symptoms*

| Reaction | Symptom complex |
| --- | --- |
| Vasovagal (at injection) | Faintness, paleness, sweating, diaphoresis |
| Anaphylaxis (immediate onset) | Nausea, vomiting, hypotension, incontinence, flushing, tachycardia, syncope |
| Allergic (delayed onset) | Rash, urticaria, pruritus, dyspnea, chest pain, palpitations, tachycardia |
| Pyrogen* | Fever and headaches |

*All patients injected with the same batch of RP are at risk for this reaction.

- Did not follow a known response pattern to the suspected RP
- Could have been produced by the patient's clinical state or other medications
- Does not recur or worsen with retesting

### Common ADRs

#### Bone Scanning

The typical ADR to bone scanning RPs has often been reported with Tc-99m MDP: The patient describes a rash and itching that appears 2 to 24 hours after injection, sometimes associated with nausea and vomiting.

#### Colloids and Particulate Tc-99m Ligands

These reactions occur quickly after injection, when the patient presents with flushing, itching, and a rash. When microspheres were available, there was a high incidence of side effects, including anaphylaxis and anaphylactoid reactions.

#### Ga-67 Citrate

This reaction occurs 1 day after injection and usually presents with rashes, hives, and tachycardia.

#### I-131 NP-59 (Iodocholesterol)

This rarely used drug is available under a physician-sponsored IND, so all ADRs must be reported. This reaction rate is believed to be 3 to 5 per 1,000 and is presumed due to the Tween-80 carrier rather than the RP. The symptoms occur immediately, last 5 to 20 minutes, and consist of dyspnea, palpitations, nausea, and dizziness.

#### Cisternography Agents

The ligand in these RPs is DTPA, and the USP stipulates that this should be administered in very small concentrations, as supplied by the manufacturer, to prevent pyrogen reactions. In-111 DTPA is the USP-recommended cisternography RP because the pyrogen concentration is guaranteed by the commercial supplier to be sufficiently small to prevent pyrogen reaction. We have used Tc-99m DTPA for cerebrospinal flow shunt and leak studies for years because of the better photon flux and preferred photon characteristics. Using the supplier's DTPA kit and the USP-permitted pyrogen concentration, and provided high–specific activity Tc-99m $TcO_4^-$ is used in the labeling process, the pyrogen concentration of Tc-99m DTPA is less than that of the USP-approved In-111 DTPA CSF agent.

## CLINICAL SITUATIONS

### Preparation Problems

Many clinical examples of RP problems are provided in the relevant clinical chapters and in previous portions of this chapter. Several common examples are provided below.

### *Bone Scanning*

The most commonly recognized problems in bone scanning relate to the radiochemical impurities resulting in occasional visualization of the stomach (see Fig. 1-5), thyroid, and salivary glands due to the presence of Tc-99m $TcO_4^-$ and visualization of the liver and spleen due to reduced or hydrolyzed Tc-99m ($TcO_2$), which can result either from improper preparation or storage or from abnormal eluate and kit components (e.g., $Al^{+3}$ or excess $Sn^{+2}$). When the labeling procedure is perturbed, unusual diphosphonates or other Tc-99m–labeled moieties may be prepared that disturb the desired biodistribution and so affect imaging. Tc-99m diphosphonates have been studied most, and they have the benefit of stabilizers added by some manufacturers. These image abnormalities should be prevented by routine QC procedures, except when oxidation of the prepared RP is allowed to occur after the QC has been performed.

### *RBC Labeling*

Another excellent example of the myriad of things that can go wrong is the labeling of RBCs with Tc-99m by the in vitro technique using UltraTag kits. Generally, excellent labeling efficiency occurs (≥95%), and this has now become the standard method. The process is sensitive to multiple chemical reaction constraints during both the RBC harvesting and the labeling process. Heparin is the preferred anticoagulant used in the collection process because the use of anticoagulant citrate dextrose (ACD) requires very strict concentration limits to prevent interference with labeling. Changing the following components results in significantly decreased labeling efficiency:

- Excess Tc-99 (e.g., age of $TcO_4^-$ eluate or first elution of new generator)
- Decreasing the blood volume
- Decreasing incubation times
- Decreasing incubation temperature
- Increasing ACD concentration (if used)

It has also been reported that increasing the amount of Tc-99m activity, decreasing the $Sn^{+2}$ in the vial, using certain commercial sources of saline, and the incorrect order of reagent mixing (adding the stannous ion scavenger hypochlorite to the vial before $TcO_4^-$) also reduce labeling efficiency, but to a lesser extent.

### *WBC Labeling*

Another example of blood element labeling problems is the preparation of labeled WBCs for scanning purposes. In the case of In-111 oxine–labeled WBCs, there is poor efficiency if either plasma transferrin or excess RBCs and platelets are present in the sample. In the case of Tc-99m HMPAO–labeled WBCs, the labeling efficiency is generally much lower than with In-111 (50% to 70% vs. 97%). The labeling efficiency decreases in these instances:

- The pH increases from 7.5 to 8.0.
- Short incubation times are used.
- Inadequate numbers of WBCs are present.

The efficiency increases significantly if the concentration of HMPAO is increased (e.g., if the HMPAO vial volume is reduced to one-fourth or one-third). ACD is preferred to heparin in the labeling of WBCs (the opposite to RBC labeling) to prevent WBC adherence to plastic, but excess ACD can decrease labeling efficiency.

Yet another example of blood element labeling problems is Tc-99m impurities that can be formed during the HMPAO WBC labeling process. These HMPAO-labeled moieties are either excreted renally (small, non–protein-bound molecules) or by hepatobiliary clearance (small, lipophilic, and polar molecules). These result in urinary and GI tract visualization, with an incidence that is inversely related to the measured binding efficiency (see Figs. 8-5 and 8-6).

### Kit Component Problems

### *Mo-99/Tc-99 Eluate Problems*

Three major problems are related to $TcO_4^-$ eluates in TC-99m RP kits: $Al^{+3}$ excess, radiolysis products and oxidants, and the specific activity of Tc-99m.

### *$Al^{+3}$ Excess*

Alumina in the Mo-99/Tc-99m generator is the most common potential source of $Al^{+3}$ in Tc-99m RP preparation, although in some reactions very sensitive to $Al^{+3}$, the use of aluminum needles can be problematic. The generator source has not been a problem for many years because generators are now made using fission-produced, high–specific activity Mo-99, which requires smaller alumina columns. The first elution from the generator has the highest $Al^{+3}$ levels, and USP requirements are that there be <10 μg/ml eluate. This level of $Al^{+3}$ would result in the formation of a colloid when preparing diphosphonate bone scanning RPs, with subsequent visualization of the liver. Much lower levels can cause flocculation of Tc-99m SC, with subsequent pulmonary visualization, because these larger particles are trapped in the pulmonary capillaries.

## Radiolysis

Radiolysis of water in the Mo-99/Tc-99m generator produces hydrogen peroxide, a strong oxidizing agent that can react with $Sn^{+2}$ in the kit to produce $Sn^{+4}$, resulting in lower labeling efficiencies. Other generator oxidizing agents can do this, too, and can change the oxidation state of $TcO_4^-$ in the eluate. These agents (hydrogen peroxide, hydroperoxy free radicals, oxygen, oxidants from generators, and some oxidants introduced into specific kits) can interfere with virtually all Tc-99m RPs (SC, MDP, human serum albumin [HSA], MAA, RBCs, IDA, HMPAO, DTPA, GH, DMSA, MAG3, sestamibi).

## Specific Activity of Tc-99m

Carrier Tc-99 is inevitable in Mo-99/Tc-99m generator eluates, with 14% coming directly from Mo-99 decay, the remainder from Tc-99m decay. As the eluate decays, the proportion of carrier Tc-99 continues to rise relative to the Tc-99m. The kit sets used in RP preparation have fixed amounts of stannous ion and ligand (reducing and chelating components), so in preparations where the chemical proportions are critical, the amount of useful technetium (Tc-99m) can be important. After a weekend with no elution of the generator, the proportion of Tc-99 rises dramatically compared to other days (see Table 22-10), and this can adversely affect Tc-99m RPs (GHA, HSA, RBCs, HMPAO, DTPA, and MOABs). Similarly, the use of aged eluate (i.e., eluate used hours after elution) decreases the efficiency of MAG3, MIBI, HMPAO, and MOABs labeled with Tc-99m. Too high a concentration of Tc-99m can also affect the labeling of RBCs, MAG3, and HMPAO.

### Stannous Ion Problems

The stannous ion method of reduction of $TcO_4^-$ to a reactive form is nearly universal among Tc-99m RPs, with current exceptions being SC (using thiosulfate method) and the as-yet-unapproved cardiac agent (furifosmin). Insufficient $Sn^{+2}$ results in decreased labeling and residual $TcO_4^-$,

whereas excess $Sn^{+2}$ can result in colloidal impurities. In most Tc-99m kits, $Sn^{+2}$ is supplied in excess, but in some kits this excess can be a problem (UltraTag for RBCs, ECD, MAG3, and HMPAO).

## Non–Tc-99m RPs

Significant radionuclide impurities can be present in certain cyclotron-produced radionuclides in general use, especially at their expiration time (Table 22-20).

The source of In-111 chloride in the labeling of pentetreotide (OctreoScan) and the anti-TAG-72 MOAB (satumomab pendetide [OncoScint]) is important in these two peptide labeling procedures. Each RP manufacturer requires that a particular supplier of In-111 be used because of pH and trace metal constraints and urges that only the appropriate commercial source be used. In the case of pentetreotide, the manufacturer even provides the needle to transfer the In-111 from the radionuclide source vial to the reaction vial because $Al^{+3}$ from standard needle hubs may interfere with the reaction.

## Physical Configuration

Several RPs are particulate, colloidal, or delivered to the patient as aerosol. The size of these particles or droplets determines the biodistribution. Large denatured RBCs (heated to 49°C to 50°C) are sequestered in the spleen permanently, providing very specific spleen scans, and activated WBCs disturbed during the labeling procedure ex vivo sequester temporarily in the pulmonary capillaries. Larger protein molecules that have been aggregated together to form solids in the 10- to 90-μm range (Tc-99m MAA) impact in the smaller arterioles and capillaries and provide images of organ perfusion, as in pulmonary and hepatic arterial perfusion scans.

Colloidal material is phagocytosed by the reticuloendothelial system and produces images of the liver, spleen, and bone marrow. By manipulating the size of these particles, preparations can be made to better identify the spleen or bone marrow. Slightly larger colloidal suspensions visualize the spleen; slightly smaller particle suspensions visual-

**TABLE 22-20.** *Impurities in cyclotron-produced radionuclides*

| Radionuclide (calibration %) | | Primary contaminant (calibration %) | | % other contaminants | Primary contaminant (expiration %) | |
|---|---|---|---|---|---|---|
| I-123 | (97.0) | I-125 | (<2.90) | <0.10 | I-125 | (12.50)[a] |
| I-123 | (99.9) | I-125 | (<0.10) | <0.10 | I-125 | (0.46)[b] |
| Tl-201 | (98.0) | Tl-202 | (<1.00) | <1.00 | Tl-202 | (2.50)[a] |
| In-111 | (99.9) | In-114 | (<0.06) | <0.06 | In-114 | (0.25)[c] |
| Ga-67 | (99.9) | Ga-66 | (<0.01) | <0.01 | Ga-66 | (<0.01)[d] |

[a] Mallinckrodt package insert.
[b] Actual impurities of Xe-124 (p,2n) and Xe-124 (p,pn) reactions used.
[c] DuPont-Pharma package insert.
[d] Medi-Physics package insert.

**TABLE 22-21.** *Common drug-radiopharmaceutical interactions*

| Radiopharmaceutical (effect) | Drugs interacting with radiopharmaceutical |
|---|---|
| Tc-99m bone scans (increased renal visualization) | Adriamycin, cyclophosphamide, and vincristine |
| Tc-99m RBC (decreased RBC labeling and increased ejection fraction) | Adriamycin, digoxin, hydralazine, methyldopa, nifedipine, prazosin, propranolol, and quinidine |
| I-131 NaI (decreased uptake and therapy) | Amiodarone, contrast agents, expectorants, kelp, health foods, seafood, and sushi |
| Ga-67 citrate (increased skeletal uptake, poor liver [and possibly tumor] uptake) | Cisplatin, hemodialysis, significant hemolysis, methotrexate, and XRT |

ize the bone marrow. Tc-99m SC is the preferred liver-spleen scanning agent (10 to 1,000 nm), and Tc-99m antimony SC (~10 nm) was used for bone marrow imaging. The last-named colloid was used also for lymphoscintigraphy, but with the demise of its supply company, the smaller colloid has been approached by passing Tc-99m SC through a 100-nm Millipore filter.

The Tc-99m RPs used in aerosol ventilation imaging can be changed to produce certain subtle changes in physiology. Tc-99m DTPA is generally used and results in 2% to 3% of the dose reaching the alveoli. Tc-99m PYP results in 3% to 5% reaching the alveoli. When the aerosol is used to evaluate ciliary function, Tc-99m SC or MAA is preferred. These slightly larger droplets are deposited more proximally, and instead of being absorbed, they are swept proximally to the oropharynx by ciliary action.

**Drug Interactions**

Just as drugs interact with each other, drugs can interact with RPs. In some cases, the drugs cause specific organ changes that result in RP uptake. For example, bleomycin or nitrofurantoin pulmonary damage results in lung uptake of Ga-67, and digoxin or spironolactone can cause male breast hypertrophy and uptake of bone scanning agent. The more important considerations are scan pattern alterations without established pathophysiologic explanation, which can impair

scan interpretation. The best and most common examples include intense renal visualization on bone scans in patients with recent chemotherapy, poor RBC labeling in multigated cardiac studies in patients on chemotherapy interfering with the accurate measurement of cardiac function, iodine intake affecting radioiodine thyroid uptake measurement and therapy, and the effect of chemotherapy and x-ray therapy on the biodistribution of Ga-67 and possible decreases in sensitivity of lymphoma patients (Table 22-21). The adrenal imaging RPs are particularly sensitive to various prescribed and over-the-counter drugs that can invalidate the scan (see Chapter 18).

**REFERENCES**

1. Package insert A12010 thallous chloride Tl-201 injection. St. Louis: Mallinckrodt Medical, revised June 1993.
2. Knox EG, Steward AM, Kneale SW, Gilman E. Prenatal irradiation and childhood cancer. J Soc Rad Prot 1987;7:177–189.
3. Hammer-Jacobsen E. Therapeutic abortion on account of x-ray examination during pregnancy. Dan Med Bull 1959;6:113–122.
4. Mountford PJ, Oakley AJ. A review of the secretion of radioactivity in human breast milk: data, quantitative analysis and recommendations. Nucl Med Commun 1989;10:15–27.
5. Sources and Magnitude of Occupational and Public Exposures from Nuclear Medicine Procedures. Recommendations of the National Council on Radiation Protection and Management. NCRP Report No. 124, 1996.
6. Shapiro B, Pillay M, Cox PH. Dosimetric consequences of interstitial dose extravasation following IV administration of a radiopharmaceutical [short communication]. Eur J Nucl Med 1987;12:513–522.

*Textbook of Nuclear Medicine,*
edited by Michael A. Wilson.
Lippincott–Raven Publishers, Philadelphia © 1998.

# CHAPTER 23

# Radiation Detection

Michael A. Wilson, Jesus A. Bianco, Raymond K. Tu, and Louis V. Zager

## INTERACTION WITH MATTER

The production of an image in nuclear medicine depends on the interaction of a photon emitted from the patient's organ system with the detector system. As a photon passes through any media there is a probability that it will interact with that media; this probability is a function of photon energy, media composition, and media thickness. These interactions occur primarily in three sites: the photon source (the organ of interest), the tissues around the source (the patient), and the detector system and its surrounds (crystal, collimator, and detector enclosure).

### Possible Interactions

There are five possible interactions of photons with matter (see also Chapter 21). In order of importance to nuclear medicine, they are

1. Photoelectric absorption
2. Compton scattering
3. Pair production
4. Coherent scattering
5. Photodisintegration

### *Photoelectric Absorption*

Photoelectric absorption (PE) results from total absorption of the incident photon by the media. PE absorption is the primary process of interaction of most photons used in nuclear medicine imaging when interacting with sodium iodide (NaI) crystals and lead (Pb) collimators. Few thallium 201 (Tl-201) (5%), technetium 99m (Tc-99m) (1%), or positron emissions (0.02%) interact in the body tissue by this process. The photon is absorbed by an inner electron shell and a photoelectron is ejected with an energy equal to the incident photon less the ejected electron's binding energy. With the loss of the inner shell electron the atom

becomes an ion, and an outer shell electron drops down to replace the ejected electron. This de-excitation process is achieved by the emission of characteristic x-rays (inner shells) or auger electrons (outer shells). The entire process takes approximately 1 microsecond to complete. The probability of PE absorption increases with low-energy gamma rays and in media with higher atomic numbers (Pb > NaI > bone > tissue). The likelihood of PE absorption varies with the third power of Z of the medium and decreases with the third power of energy: For NaI crystal versus tissue, this is a factor of 400; for lead versus tissue, this is a factor of 1,000. Thus, the lead shielding of the detector and the NaI detector itself favors complete absorption of the gamma ray, but this is not the case in the patient.

These photoelectric events are responsible for creating high-quality images because they come directly from the organ and are not scattered. High-quality imaging requires that photoelectric photons are maximized and all others minimized by good collimation, proper energy windows, and small detector-to-organ distance.

### *Compton Scattering (Incoherent Scattering)*

The incident photon interacts with a loosely bound outer shell electron and is deflected through a scattering angle. The electron receives energy from the incident photon and recoils forward in the same general direction as the incoming photon. Thus, the photon gives up some of its energy to the recoil electron. The angle of the electron recoil depends on the change in incident photon direction. Each scattered photon can scatter again or undergo the photoelectric effect, but, as a result, positional information is misrepresented to the detector. Conservation of energy and momentum rules allow calculation of the angle of the deflected photon for the entire range of energy transfers to the recoil electron. In this way a distribution of deflected photon energies can be calculated, and the angles of deflection that are likely to be measured by the NaI scintillation detector imaging system can be estimated. This Compton (incoherent) scattering process occurs especially in materials with low atomic mass (e.g., tissue, where the effective Z is 7). Compton interactions are likely with intermediate photon energies typical in nuclear medicine (70 to 400 keV) and decrease with increasing incident photon energies. The probability of their occurrence is proportional to the electron density of the scattering medium. In tissue this is the primary photon interaction that occurs.

Compton scattered photons degrade image quality. Significant angular deflections are routinely recorded in the photon's photopeak. They are minimized by setting "tight" energy windows designed to accept photoelectric events but discriminate against Compton scattered photons. Despite this, conventional window settings result in significant scatter angles being accepted as photoelectric events; for example, for Tl-201 with a 28% window scatter, angles up to 100 degrees are accepted and 30% of all accepted events are scattered. Current strategies for correcting the radionuclide scatter during high-resolution single photon emission computed tomography (SPECT) imaging use methodology such as multiple energy window scatter compensation.

### Pair Production

Pair production requires incident photons in excess of 1.022 MeV, and this interaction forms the basis of positron emission tomography (PET). The interaction occurs between the incident photon and the electric field associated with the nucleus (this is described in Chapter 24).

### Coherent Scattering

In coherent scattering, there is no energy loss, but the direction of the photon changes slightly. This occurs as the photon interacts with all the electrons of the atom, setting them into coherent oscillation. Fortunately for imaging, this only occurs at very low photon energies (e.g., I-125, 35 keV), below those used for imaging.

### Photodisintegration

Photodisintegration occurs with photons in excess of 7 to 10 MeV and so does not apply to nuclear medicine imaging.

### Half-Value Layer

The half-value layer (HVL) is that thickness of media or absorber that reduces the number of unscattered transmitted photons by half. This attenuation occurs by both photoelectric absorption and Compton scattering, and both of these are proportional to electron density, which is in turn related to absorber density. The HVL varies for each gamma ray energy and each medium. The HVL provides an easy method of determining how thick a material must be to provide ade-

**TABLE 23-1.** *Half-value layer (HVL)*

| Nuclide | Energy (keV) | HVL (cm) | | |
|---------|--------------|----------|-----|------|
| | | Water | NaI | Lead |
| Tl-201 | 70 x-ray | 3.85 | 0.048 | 0.006 |
| Tc-99m | 140 gamma | 4.60 | 0.270 | 0.017 |
| I-131 | 364 gamma | 6.35 | 1.500 | 0.300 |
| Mo-99 | 740 gamma | 35.50 | 2.500 | 0.620 |

quate shielding from gamma rays of a known energy. One HVL decreases incident rays (and exposure) to 50%, two HVLs to 25%, three HVLs to 12.5%, and so forth. Thus, seven HVLs decrease exposure to <1% of the unshielded level. Given that the HVL for Tc-99m with lead is 0.18 mm, shielding to <1% of the incident radiation would require only 1.3 mm of lead. Shielding of I-131 to the same level requires 15 mm (42 mm for Mo-99). The HVL for typical radionuclides in water, NaI, and lead is shown in Table 23-1. By definition, the HVL (in centimeters) is related to μ (total linear attenuation coefficient) by this formula:

$$HVL = \frac{0.693}{\mu_1} \qquad (1)$$

where $\mu_1$ is the linear attenuation coefficient and $\mu_1$ is equal to $\mu_{mass}$ ($cm^2/g$) × density ($g/cm^3$).

## RADIATION DETECTORS

Radiation detectors used in clinical nuclear medicine include ionization detectors, used primarily in radiation safety efforts, and crystal scintillation detectors, used mainly in imaging and laboratory procedures.

### Ionization Detectors

Gas-filled chambers are used in clinical nuclear medicine in three different configurations:

1. Ionization chambers, "cutie pie" survey meters, dose calibrators, pocket dosimeters
2. Proportional counters
3. Geiger-Müller (GM) counters

All these gas-filled detectors are vital to the preparation and safe use of radiopharmaceuticals, and the principle of these detectors is common to each detector class. They rely on the interaction of the incident radiation with a gas that is contained within a chamber producing ionization of the gas. When ionizing radiation produces ion pairs in the gas, electrons are attracted to the anode and the positive ions are attracted to the cathode (Fig. 23-1). The ordinarily nonconductive gases in the chamber permit conduction of electrons, which results in current that is detectable by the instrument electronics. Gas-filled chambers give one electrical pulse for each successful interaction of incident radiation with the

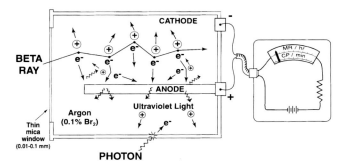

**FIG. 23-1.** This diagram shows an idealized Geiger-Mueller counter (see text), with an incoming beta ray penetrating the thin mica window, causing multiple subsequent events leading to the measurement of an electrical pulse. (+, ions; –, electrons.)

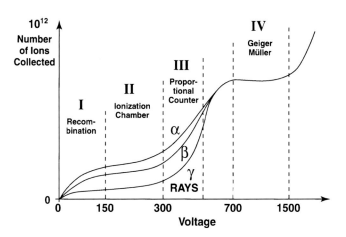

**FIG. 23-2.** An idealized plot of voltage versus count rate for an ionization detector (see text), with the various regions clearly demarcated.

chamber gas. Ion pair production depends on the irradiation itself: least with photons because a gas is a very poor photon absorber, and increasing significantly with particulate radiation (beta and alpha rays).

The behavior of the electrons and positive ions once produced in the gas detector is determined by the voltage applied to the detector's electrodes, which in turn determines the type of gas-filled detector. If the voltage is low (<100 V), the electrons and ions recombine locally and, as a result, do not reach the oppositely charged electrodes and so do not produce a signal. This region is not used in radiation detection (region I of Fig. 23-2).

In region II of Fig. 23-2, with voltages of approximately 200 to 300 V, is the "ionization chamber plateau" or saturation level, where all the ion pairs produced in the gas are collected by the electrodes, and none recombine in the detector volume. This is the first useful region of the curve and is used for pocket dosimeters, survey meters such as "cutie pies," and dose calibrators. This area is useful because the current produced by the ionization is proportional to the number of ion pairs. These detectors are very insensitive,

and radiation that produces more ion pairs in the gas (e.g., alphas and betas) works best; for gamma rays the efficiency is <0.1%, but this is still useful.

### Pocket Dosimeters

These personal dosimeters can be charged and reset by the department using a charging kit. They are used in limited applications for short-term situations; for example, a nurse caring for a single patient receiving radionuclide therapy. In this device the dosimeter is charged, and with incident radiation this charge is lost, and the loss is proportional to the amount of radiation detected. They usually measure 100 to 200 mR (0.1 to 0.2 cGy) and are useful for energies from 50 keV to 2 MeV.

### Personal Radiation Monitoring

The routine badge and ring dosimeters worn by radiation workers are not gas-filled detectors but thermoluminescent devices, which are described briefly here because of their similar function to pocket dosimeters. In crystals of thermoluminescent material (e.g., lithium fluoride), electrons jump from the valence band to the conduction band by absorbing energy from ionizing radiation impinging on the crystals. Some electrons remain trapped in these intermediate energy levels as a result of impurities in the crystals. The trapping of these electrons is a function of the energy absorbed by the phosphor. On heating, the trapped electrons are released and electrons return to the valence band. Light is liberated during this process, which can be quantitated back at the commercial suppliers to produce the personnel dosimetry measurements. The useful linear dose range is from 1 mrad to 1,000 rads (0.01 mGy to 10 Gy).

### Cutie Pie Survey Meters

The cutie pie device is used to measure beta particles and gamma rays or x-rays over a wide range of exposure (0 to 5,000 mR [0 to 50 mGy]/hour, or 0 to 50 R [0 to 0.5 Gy]/hour). In general this device can measure higher dose rates than standard GM devices (discussed later), so they are used in I-131 therapies or PET scanning applications where high photon flux rates are the standard.

### Dose Calibrator

The dose calibrator—a requirement in nuclear medicine practice—is an ionization chamber that contains argon at 25 to 30 atm of pressure. In this device, the current produced by a given radioactive source in a given detector's geometric arrangement is directly proportional to the radioactivity of the source. However, different radionuclides with the same amount of radioactivity produce different amounts of current. This difference results from differences in the radionuclide emission spectra. Thus, the device is not able to discriminate energies or types of radiation and so cannot distinguish between radionuclides, and the equipment supplier provides a calibration factor for each radionuclide to be measured. The calibration factors are determined by using a pure source of the radionuclide of known activity in a standard glass ampule. The useful range is a thousandfold: The RadCal device can measure from 1 µCi to 2 Ci (37 MBq to 74 GBq) and has an applied voltage of 300 V, whereas the Capintec device measures from 1 µCi to 5 Ci (37 MBq to 184 GBq) and operates at 150 V.

Exposure (E) directly measured (in roentgens) can be related to activity (in mCi) by means of the formula:

$$E = \frac{A\Gamma}{d^2} \quad (2)$$

where $E$ is exposure rate, $A$ is activity in millicuries, $d$ is distance (e.g., in centimeters), and $\Gamma$ is radionuclide's specific gamma ray constant for the voltage applied (roentgens per hour per millicurie at 1 cm).

The particular radionuclide-predefined calibration factor must be selected for the dose being inserted into the device, and appropriate calibration factors convert the measured gas ionization to an appropriate activity level. The calibration is critical for each radionuclide and depends on the type, number, and energies of each emission component of the specific radionuclide decay scheme as well as interaction of these with the radiopharmaceutical container (e.g., plastic syringe or glass vial) and the construction material and geometry of the calibrator itself. The detector geometry is nearly 360 degrees because the sample when inserted into the chamber cylinder is almost completely surrounded by the ionization chamber.

NRC requirements for dose calibrators include the following:

1. Accuracy tests annually: Use National Institute of Standards Technology certified standards over the clinically used range (cobalt 57 [Co-57], 122 keV; barium 133 [Ba-133], 356 keV; cesium 137 [Cs-137], 662 keV; Co-60, 1.17 and 1.33 meV). The device must be accurate to within ±10%.

2. Linearity tests quarterly: These are done by decaying short-lived nuclide (i.e., Tc-99m) or using a set of attenuation sleeves supplied commercially. This must also be accurate to within ±10%.

3. Constancy test daily: Each day the calibrator is used it must be tested, including nights and weekends. (At University of Wisconsin-Madison [UW-Madison], we alternate daily use of sources Co-57 [half-life 270 days, 122 keV] and Cs-137 [half-life 30 years, 662 keV].) The test must be performed on all commonly used calibrator settings unless limitation to one setting is a condition of the facility's license. This must be accurate to within ±10%.

4. Re-evaluation of geometry at installation or whenever the ionization chamber is repaired or the calibrator is moved. The volume containing radionuclide, the container material and thickness, and the Perspex carrier supplied for holding the radionuclide can all affect the measurement of the dose rate being delivered. For routine agents, such as technetium 99m (Tc-99m) and iodine 131 (I-131), these absorption problems introduce differences of only approximately 1%, but with radionuclides that decay by electron capture, they represent a problem, especially for I-123 and indium 111 (In-111), because of the low-energy characteristic x-rays emitted. The NRC allows this geometry test to be done with Tc-99m, but geometry problems do not occur with this radionuclide. Allowable accuracy is ±10%.

The disadvantages of dose calibrators include the following:

- Inefficiency: <1% incident photons, such as gamma and x-rays, are measured.
- Photon absorption that occurs before the photon interaction with the gas detector. The liquid solute containing the radionuclide, the walls of the radiopharmaceutical container, the plastic sample holder, the plastic chamber insert, and the metal ionization chamber walls all generate bremsstrahlung from particulate radiation.
- Pure beta emitters do not penetrate the chamber, and only the bremsstrahlung is measured. (This is a practical problem when measuring phosphorus 32 [P-32] and strontium 89 [Sr-89] therapy doses.)

Despite these limitations, dose calibrators are functional and accurate over a wide range of activity and radionuclides, and they provide the means to ensure a safe environment for our patients.

### Proportional Counter

The next curve region (see Fig. 23-2) is called the *proportional region* (III). In this region, the charge collected increases as the voltage increases for the same incident radiation flux. This increase in voltage from a 400-V to an 800-V region results in acceleration of the electrons, which then causes additional ionizations within the chamber. These secondary and tertiary ionizations cause a local avalanche effect, producing thousandfold to millionfold increases in amplification (i.e., improved sensitivity), but the current produced is proportional to the initial ionizing radiation, hence the name *proportional counter*. The collection rate of electrons is rapid (millions per second), so high counting rates are achieved. The size of the pulse is proportional to the energy deposited, so it can be used for energy discrimination, whereas other ionization detectors cannot. These proportional counter devices are only used in research involving alpha and beta detection.

### GM Counters

The next curve region (see Fig. 23-2) is the GM region (IV). The applied voltages here are high (800 to 1,500 V), and tertiary processes develop so that the entire gas is activated with each ionization process. The gas used most often is argon (like the dose calibrator), and every measured event results in the same current output (i.e., plateau region of curve) regardless of the type of incident radiation. Amplification is now increased to the millionfold to billionfold range, versus 10- to 100-fold for the ionization chamber and thousandfold to millionfold for proportional chambers. GM counters detect alpha particles and electrons with moderate efficiency, whereas gamma and x-rays are detected with very low efficiency (<1%).

The avalanche effect that occurs in the GM counter results in almost complete ionization of the argon gas. Although the electrons collect quickly at the anode, the positive ions migrate more slowly to the cathode. Because this process is ongoing, the ionized gas chamber remains unresponsive to other incoming radiation. This anion migration takes 200 to 300 microseconds and by itself would result in a significant "dead-time" effect. When the anions approach the cathode, electrons present interact with the positively charged gas, producing ultraviolet light that initiates additional electrons from ionization and thus keeps the chamber's gas discharged and unresponsive. To detect another event, the continuous avalanche discharge induced by the initial and subsequent ionizations must be stopped, which is achieved with a quencher that can absorb electrons without being ionized. Quenchers can be polyatomic ions (alcohols) or halogens. Organic quenchers (xylene, ethyl alcohol, isobutane) have a limited life because the quencher is used up in the quenching process, but halogens, like bromine and chlorine in low concentration (<1%), recombine when the discharge is complete. This halogen recombination makes them less effective quenchers, but their overall longevity makes them the preferred agents used in GM counters.

When quenchers are used, count rates of 20,000 cpm (equivalent to 2 mR [0.05 mGy]/hour), depending on what form of radiation is being counted, can be achieved. Some GM tubes have computers to perform dead-time corrections, and can measure up to 50 R (0.5 Gy) per hour. The gas chambers can also be fabricated in different shapes and volumes to perform different functions: Flat, disclike, thin-window gas chambers ("pancake" probes) are exquisite beta counters, and smaller, cylindric chambers are used for high-flux situations (e.g., therapy applications). Annual calibration is required, and all have an internal standard radioactive source for daily checks before use (these are both NRC requirements). Note that the annual calibration must be recorded, but the daily checks do not need to be recorded for the NRC.

## Scintillation Detectors

Scintillation detectors used in clinical practice are made of solid NaI crystals. Bismuth germanate crystals and other materials can be used for positron detectors, and currently considerable ongoing research is under way in the commercial development of solid-state detectors. Whereas 99% of x-ray and gamma radiations traverse the low-density gas detectors described above, the use of solid, commercially available NaI crystal as detectors in nuclear medicine results

in greater detection efficiency (70% to 90% for Tc-99m). The actual photon absorption is related to the thickness of the crystal. NaI is an excellent absorber, given its density (3.67 $g/cm^3$), and has a Z of 53 (effective density of 1.0 $g/cm^3$) as compared to an effective Z of 7 for soft tissue. The interaction is measured as light, with the scintillation crystal producing a burst of light with an intensity proportional to the energy of the incoming photon. The detector system interaction measures the energy of the primary incoming photon (both photoelectric and Compton scattered interactions), of photons that were Compton scattered previously (in the patient or the collimator), and any background activity.

In the gamma camera crystal detector, the incident photons used in nuclear medicine are predominantly absorbed by the PE effect. The ejected orbital photoelectron of the photoelectric absorption interaction travels a short distance from its source, giving up energy as it comes to a stop. The emitted characteristic x-rays and auger electrons produced during the internal rearrangement that followed photon interaction also gives up energy to the NaI crystal. Photons undergoing Compton scatter give off energy, and the resultant scattered photon either scatters again, loses all its energy in a subsequent photoelectric interaction, or scatters out of the detector system. These multiple combinations of crystal interactions occur so quickly as to be nearly simultaneous.

Thallium impurities are added to the NaI crystal at a molar ratio of 0.1 to 0.4 moles %, and the secondary electrons emitted by the NaI(Tl) crystal are trapped by these thallium activation centers. Thallium activation is required because x-ray and gamma-ray photon interactions do not cause fluorescence in NaI at room temperature. The atoms of thallium form preferred sites in the crystal for the excited electrons to return to the ground state, and the frequency of the light emitted in this thallium de-excitation process is well suited to the spectral sensitivity of the photocathode tubes used in imaging.

The total number of light photons is directly proportional to the photon energy absorbed by the crystal for each gamma-photon interaction. Approximately 12% of the deposited energy is transformed to light; the remainder is transferred to the crystal as heat and vibration. This proportion is very efficient among scintillators and, combined with cost and convenience, explains the widespread use of NaI crystals. Twenty to 30 light photons are emitted for each kiloelectron volt of energy of the incident photon, so for each 140-keV Tc-99m photon, approximately 3,500 light photons are produced. This light production is rapid, reaching a maximum of approximately 30 nanoseconds after photon arrival, then decaying exponentially, with a decay time of 250 nanoseconds. It takes 1.25 microseconds for all the produced light to decay to zero. A 10°C change in crystal temperature can result in a 1% change in light emission.

The NaI(Tl) crystal transmits light well, and it continues to do so while translucent. NaI is hygroscopic, so water must be kept out of the crystal to prevent darkening and decreased transparency. The crystal is enclosed to prevent water

## PHOTOMULTIPLIER TUBE

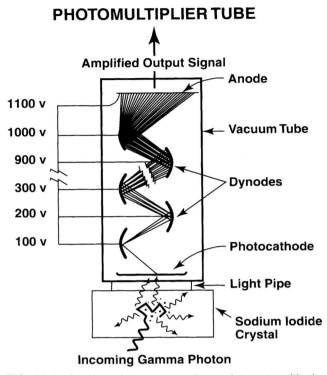

**FIG. 23-3.** An incoming gamma photon interacts with the crystal with several Compton scatters locally before total absorption. This nearly instantaneous reaction produces numerous light photons (*arrowed wavy lines*), some of which leave the crystal and displace an electron from the photocathode. This electron is now accelerated to dynodes and multiplied with each passage on to the next dynode with a million- to billionfold multiplication of the electron cascade.

**TABLE 23-2.** *Absorbed fraction in NaI(Tl) crystals*

| Radionuclide | Energy (keV) | ½ inch | ⅜ inch | ¼ inch |
|---|---|---|---|---|
| Tl-201 | 70 | 1.00 | 1.00 | 1.00 |
| Xe-133 | 81 | 1.00 | 1.00 | 1.00 |
| Tc-99m | 140 | 0.92 | 0.85 | 0.72 |
| I-123 | 159 | 0.83 | 0.74 | 0.57 |
| Ga-67 | 93 | 1.00 | 1.00 | 0.98 |
| | 185 | 0.72 | 0.63 | 0.47 |
| | 300 | 0.26 | 0.20 | 0.14 |
| In-111 | 173 | 0.73 | 0.62 | 0.48 |
| | 247 | 0.40 | 0.32 | 0.22 |
| I-131 | 364 | 0.15 | 0.12 | 0.08 |

absorption and outside light from entering, the surfaces are left rough to decrease reflection, and a very light-transparent coupling is provided from the crystal to the photomultiplier tube (PMT), which is used to amplify the energy obtained in the detector photon-crystal interaction. Polishing this common crystal-PMT interface and using Pyrex and special clear silicone grease connections (Fig. 23-3) ensures excellent transfer of light.

### Gamma Spectroscopy

The scintillation crystal collects light emitted from the incident photon efficiently. In the case of Tc-99m, the 140-keV photon is nearly always stopped within the absorber (72% to 92% for ¼- to ½-inch–thick crystals), and all the energy is deposited within the crystal, regardless of the type of photon interaction. Although 15% of incident Tc-99m photons may pass through a ⅜-inch crystal (Table 23-2), the majority of the photons interact with the crystal and dissipate their energy within the crystal. If the incident photon Compton scatters and then undergoes a photoelectric event, all the photon's energy is collected by the crystal detector virtually

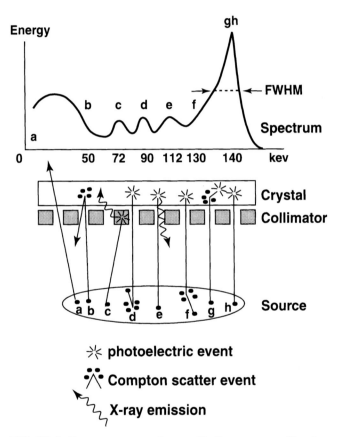

**FIG. 23-4.** Gamma ray spectrum, with the source-collimator-crystal-photon interactions demonstrated from left to right in the figure. (a) Photon is not attenuated by the crystal. (b) Photon backscatters out of the crystal (Compton edge at 50 keV). (c) Photon interacts with the Pb collimator, and Pb x-ray is detected (72 keV). (d) Photon backscatters in source then interacts with the crystal (140 − 50 = 90 keV). (e) Photon interacts with the crystal, but iodine-characteristic x-ray escapes (140 − 28 = 112 keV). (f) Photon scatters in the source at a low angle, then interacts with the crystal (e.g., if 45°, would be 130 keV). (g) Photon Compton scatters in the crystal then interacts by photoelectric effect (140 keV). Energy discrimination is excellent, the spatial location is suboptimal. (h) Photon interacts with the desired photoelectric effect (140 keV).

simultaneously, although it may be somewhat spatially dispersed. Some Compton scattered photons emerge from the crystal detector having given up only some of the incident photon energy. Many photons that enter the crystal may have already undergone Compton scatter in either the patient (Compton scattering is very common in human tissue) or the detector collimator and surrounds within the crystal (a relatively unusual event). In these cases, less than the typical Tc-99m photon energy is deposited in the crystal for each photon-crystal interaction. All these components, when recorded by the crystal and gamma camera electronics, make up the gamma ray spectrum (Fig. 23-4), which is a combination of the various energy contributions and the variations that result during their acquisition and measurement.

### Pulse-Height Spectrum

A photopeak consists of the energy deposited from the total absorption of a gamma ray of a particular radionuclide in the scintillation crystal. It has one or more prominent peaks that correspond to characteristic photon energies of the measured radionuclide: For Tc-99m, it is a single (140-keV) peak; for In-111, it is two (173- and 245-keV) peaks. With an ideal detector system (e.g., solid-state detector), these photopeaks should be sharp and discrete (Fig. 23-5),

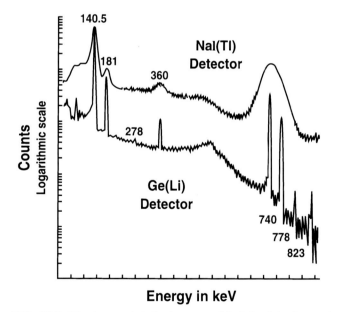

**FIG. 23-5.** The lower plot displays a solid-state detector and the spectrum obtained from an Mo-99 generator, with both Mo-99 and Tc-99m detected. The upper plot is the typical NaI detector spectrum with much wider peaks. Note that the 740- and 778-keV peaks (used in assessing Mo "breakthrough") are recorded as a single blurred peak with NaI but as two discrete peaks with a germanium (lithium) (Ge [Li]) detector. (Modified with permission from Raeside DE, Widman JL. An introduction to pulse electronics for nuclear medicine personnel. Appl Radiol 1977;Jan/Feb:199–205.)

representing the radionuclide's characteristic photopeak. The usual photopeak in an NaI detector is spread because of the following variations:

- The crystal interaction itself
- Proportion of heat versus light production
- The emission of secondary electrons
- Sensitivity of the photocathode
- PMT amplification
- Electronic amplification gains

All these variations make NaI(Tl) a less than ideal scintillation detector, but, despite these compromises, it is a very practical scintillator. This random variation is measured to describe the system energy resolution of the system in terms of full width at half maximum (FWHM), where the width of the photopeak spectra in kiloelectron volts at half the actual photopeak height is expressed as a percentage of photopeak in kiloelectron volts (see Fig. 23-4). In good detector systems, this FWHM is usually 7% of the height. The "window" width selected for routine clinical image acquisition is often double the FWHM. Solid-state detectors have excellent energy spectra, and photopeaks do appear as the expected narrow linear peaks (1% FWHM), but these detectors need to operate at −196°C. Although they do measure the incident photon spectra well, they have not been used successfully in imaging to date.

### Effect of Compton Scatter on Spectrum

The pulse-height spectrum resulting from a particular radioactive source consists of various peaks and valleys that reflect the photopeak and complex lower-energy scatter components. The lower-energy scatter components include

- Interactions occurring in the crystal
- Interactions occurring before the photon reaches the crystal (i.e., in the patient and in the collimator)

Both of these scatter contributors degrade the image. The fraction of the photons that scatter ("the scatter fraction") increases with the distance of the source from the detector, with the amount of scatter material between source and detector, and for large sources compared to smaller sources.

### Within-Detector Scatter

Photons that are scattered within the detector can then be absorbed by the photoelectric effect, undergo further Compton scatter, or scatter out of the detector itself. If the incoming photon Compton scatters in the crystal, it is likely to be absorbed immediately via the photoelectric effect, and the virtually simultaneous energy releases are treated as one, with loss only imparted to the electron (see Fig. 23-4g). The maximum energy that can be transferred to an electron during a single Compton interaction occurs when the incident photon is backscattered out of the crystal, so the energy

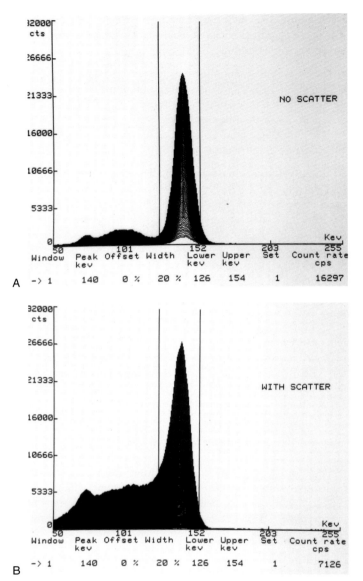

A

B

**FIG. 23-6.** These two spectra are from the same GE gamma camera using Tc-99m without **(A)** and with **(B)** a modest thickness of tissue equivalent attenuating material. **(A)** The no-scatter spectrum shows the lower edge of the photopeak to the right of the lower spectrum limit (126 keV) and little Compton scatter below this. **(B)** The scatter spectrum, which in this case mimics the clinical situation, shows this lower end of the photopeak to be smeared by the low-angle scatter (f of Fig. 23-4), and the filling in of the Compton valley due to a severalfold increase in Compton photons detected when compared to the no-scatter spectrum.

deposited in the crystal comes solely from the ejected electron. This backscatter maximum for Tc-99m is 50 keV and is described as the Compton edge (see Fig. 23-4e).

### Predetector Scatter

Compton scatter events that occur in the patient or in the collimator and detector housing and that then interact with the crystal detector have a wide range of energies, mostly between the photopeak and the Compton edge. The photon energy decrement is proportional to the photon scatter angle but has higher energies than the scatter within the crystal. This is a very significant clinical problem because considerable numbers of scattered photons can be emitted from the patient and form a large contribution to the observed spectrum (Fig. 23-6). Because these Compton scatter photons have only slightly reduced energy levels (i.e., low-angle scatter), they can be measured in the photopeak window (see Discrimination Electronics) and can form a considerable proportion of those events in the desired photopeak region (see Fig. 23-4f). For example, a Tc-99m photon that scatters 45 degrees loses only 7.4% of its energy (10 keV) and so can be measured in the Tc-99m photopeak used clinically. Thirty percent of Tl-201 recorded events in cardiac studies are actually scattered events from the patient or detector.

### Other Spectral Peaks

#### Backscatter Peak

The backscatter peak is the energy of a photon that is scattered 180 degrees before it enters the crystal (the opposite of the Compton edge effect in the crystal) and so has a peak at 90 keV with Tc-99m (see Fig. 23-4d). This scatter could occur in the patient and then pass into the crystal or can result from a photon that passes through the crystal (15% in a typical modern gamma camera) and then is scattered back into the crystal from the detector surrounds.

#### Iodine Escape Peak

This peak is the result of the L shell electron of the NaI crystal atoms filling the K shell vacated by the photoelectron. If this characteristic iodine x-ray (the difference in binding energies of K and L shell iodine electrons) escapes from the crystal (see Fig. 23-4e), it leaves a peak at 112 keV (140 keV less K-shell 28-keV iodine-characteristic x-ray).

#### Lead X-Rays

Just as the characteristic iodine x-ray can be produced, a characteristic lead x-ray can be produced (72 keV) in the collimator, and if this is directed to the crystal, it is included in the scatter spectrum (see Fig. 23-4c).

#### Summation Peaks

The virtually simultaneous arrival of two Tc-99m photons and their absorption would produce a photopeak that had an apparent energy of 280 keV. Similarly, the simultaneous arrival of various scattered photons produces a wide range of detected energies. The random nature of radioactive decay makes summation peaks inevitable, and this likelihood increases with high photon fluxes. Summation peaks, however, are not a significant clinical problem in imaging, except in secondary osteomyelitis, when Tc-99m bone scans and In-111–labeled white blood cell (WBC) scan images are acquired together (see Figs. 8-13 and 8-14).

## IMAGING DEVICES

### Overview

Hal Anger built the first well counter in 1950, described the gamma camera in 1957 (a 4-inch NaI detector with a pinhole collimator for thyroid imaging), built the first whole-body scanner in 1956, and built a positron camera in 1959. The first commercial gamma camera was available in 1964, and in 1971, an 11.5-inch crystal practical gamma camera with 19 photomultiplier tubes was available. Earlier gamma cameras had a liquid mineral oil interface between the crystal and photomultiplier tubes and, as a consequence, could only be used in the horizontal position. Construction of gamma cameras was initially limited by the size of crystal that could be produced, and were most efficiently grown in a round shape. Gamma camera crystal sizes have increased from 8 to 21 inches (20 to 53 cm) as the NaI crystal production process has changed. Crystals are made by melting NaI powder and inducing the NaI to crystallize while recooling. This produces an ingot that is then cut to size. Very large crystals, as are used in whole-body devices, are obtained by reheating the ingot and then forging the parts into the desired size.

### Components Resulting in Image Creation

The ability to produce images from photons emitted from a patient requires a localization technique for the photon-crystal interaction and the production of electrical pulses, which are validated to have the photopeak energy.

The system components that allow this localization include the PMTs, the preamplifiers and amplifiers connected to these, and the pulse height analyzers (PHAs), which discriminate between desired photopeaks and undesirable Compton scatter. Various electronic manipulations then determine the x and y localization for the creation of a two-dimensional image. The overall system comprises the following parts:

- Collimator, to result in a "gamma image" on the crystal
- Crystal, to "convert" gamma photons to light photons
- PMT, to "convert" the light photons to electrical pulses
- High-voltage supply, used to "power" the PMTs
- Preamplifier, to match the impedance of the signal from the PMTs to the rest of the electronics to allow signal passage over a cable without loss or distortion

- Amplifier, to shape and magnify the signal pulse
- Analog or digital circuitry, to position the pulse sources
- PHA, to detect a predefined range of photon energies
- Digital data storage device
- Output device, to display the image components

### Photomultiplier Tubes

The PMT is required to convert the tiny amount of light energy produced in a photon-crystal interaction to a measurable electric pulse (20 to 30 photons are required to produce each electron volt). Approximately 30% of the light photons produced by such an interaction reach the PMT photocathode and dislodge electrons (see Fig. 23-3). It takes several light photons to release a single electron from the cesium-antimony metal photocathode located in the evacuated PMT on the surface closest to the crystal. This process requires very efficient light transfer from the crystal to the PMT cathode. The dislodged electron is then accelerated to another plate (dynode) of higher voltage (a 100-V increment). This results in the dislodgment of several more electrons, which are then accelerated to an even higher voltage plate (another dynode with another ~100-V increment), and so the electron transfer rate is multiplied. There are 6 to 14 dynodes in each PMT, resulting in $10^6$- to $10^8$-fold magnification to produce a measurable voltage pulse. The size of the pulse is proportional to the amount of light reaching the PMT (i.e., the incident photon), but the variations of light photons produced in the crystal, the number of light photons required to dislodge a photocathode electron, and the variable dislodgment of successive dynode electrons help to explain the rather broad photopeak spectrum obtained, compared to the theoretical sharp monoenergetic photopeak desired (see Fig. 23-5).

### Gamma Camera Speed

Preamplifiers on each PMT clip and shape the amplified electrical pulse that the incident light photon has produced. Light emission from the NaI(Tl) crystal after interaction of an incoming photon begins immediately and has a total decay time of approximately 1.0 to 1.5 microseconds. The pulse from the PMT anode is generated over an even longer time period than the light decay, especially if most of the original energy (light) is integrated to improve spatial resolution. The integrated electrical pulse must now be processed, first by the preamplifiers to match subsequent electronics and then shape the rising pulse. The amplifiers both increase the pulse a hundredfold and reshape the pulse, especially the down-sloping portion. The initial light pulse duration (about 1,250 nanoseconds) is reduced to about 1 nanosecond (Fig. 23-7) by this process, thus improving the count rate capability of the gamma camera.

**POWER SUPPLY**

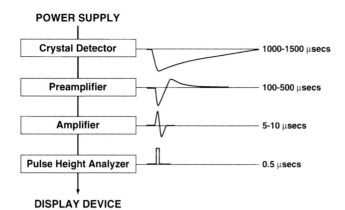

FIG. 23-7. In the crystal detector, most of the light is emitted over 1,000 to 1,500 nanoseconds. The preamplifier reshapes this input and reduces it, the amplifier reduces it further yet. By the time the pulse is processed for possible inclusion in the image, this time has reduced to 0.5 microsecond.

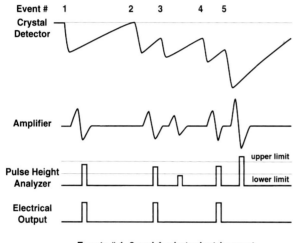

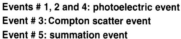

Events # 1, 2 and 4: photoelectric event
Event # 3: Compton scatter event
Event # 5: summation event

FIG. 23-8. The application of the electronic modifications shown in Fig. 23-7 in randomly arriving photons. Without these manipulations there would be significant overlapping of the electronic output. Note the upper and the lower threshold limits set by the pulse height analyzer used to select desired photopeak events.

These pulse manipulations allow higher count rates to be accepted without baseline shifts in the signal or pulse pile-up (where one pulse occurs during the processing time of the previous pulse). Baseline shifts occur when the pulse is distorted by prior and subsequent events (events 3 to 5 in Fig. 23-8). Modern gamma camera can handle pulses arriving in time intervals of 0.5 to 5.0 microseconds, and a realistic maximum count rate for single crystal cameras is 140,000 cps when the average interval between events is approximately 8 microseconds. For faster counting rates

(e.g., as required in first-pass nuclear cardiology procedures), multicrystal cameras are required to permit higher counting rates. Time losses also occur in the subsequent processing steps of energy discrimination and positioning logic (energy and spatial resolution), plus any manufacturer-integrated quality control (QC) processes.

This count rate capability problem is made more difficult by the random nature of radioactive decay, the significant contribution of scattered photons (about half total incident photons), and the pulsatile nature of the gamma camera detector, where each event must be processed before the next event is considered. There are two components to the degradation of temporal processing: The first is related to the crystal, the second to the electronics. The light-crystal interactions are largely paralyzable: An event occurring while light is still being released from a prior event results in summing of the light and the inability of the detector to identify the start, site, and end of these light sources, essentially paralyzing the system until the detector returns to baseline. The electronic processes can manipulate the resultant electrical pulses by dramatic pulse shaping and shortening, enabling the device to discriminate two events (this is a nonparalyzable system).

Methods to increase count rate capabilities include

- Using only a fraction of the light emitted (usually the initial portion)
- Using variable integration times
- Buffering procedures
- Bypassing pile-up and other correction circuits

All these result in spatial and energy resolution compromises while increasing the capability of detecting incoming photons (i.e., sensitivity).

### Discrimination Electronics

The PHA measures the final output voltage of each pulse and is adjusted to accept the preselected energy representing the desired photopeak. In this way, the gamma camera can detect only selected radionuclide photoelectric events, discriminating against many scattered photons (see Fig. 23-8). As many as two-thirds of the events detected by the crystal are scattered photons and not clinically useful. In typical clinical applications using a 28% energy window width with Tl-201, 100-degree Compton scatters are accepted as valid photons, and in Tc-99m with a 20% energy window, 50-degree Compton scatters are accepted as valid photopeak photons. It is possible to exclude even less-scattered photons by only accepting gamma rays above a higher energy threshold—that is, narrowing the window. This lengthens acquisition time significantly. Modern gamma cameras can collect and separate three or more energies and so can identify multiple peaks of one radionuclide, such as the three main peaks of Ga-67, or multiple radionuclides, such as the Tc-99m photopeak and the two peaks of In-111.

### Positioning Logic

Each incoming gamma ray photon interacting with the NaI(Tl) crystal results in the production of light. The light is dispersed isotropically (equally in all directions) within the crystal, with half moving away from the PMT photocathodes. As the thickness of the crystal increases, the dispersal of light increases, so the ability to accurately determine the origin of the gamma ray-crystal interaction (i.e., resolution) decreases. This explains why high-resolution gamma cameras are equipped with thin ¼-inch crystals, whereas gamma cameras designed for use with higher-energy photons (gallium 67 [Ga-67] or I-131) employ thicker (⅜- to ½-inch) crystals, which have greater stopping power (detection efficiency) (see Table 23-2).

Gamma cameras have been equipped with between 7 and 142 PMTs, and modern round gamma cameras have at least 37 PMTs but more commonly 61 or 91 PMTs. These PMTs are packed in tight hexagonal arrays for round crystals, whereas in rectangular crystals, the PMT arrays are linear. Several PMTs receive light from a single crystal-photon interaction, while the rest of the light disperses throughout the crystal. The nearest PMTs receive the most light, the neighboring PMTs receive less light. Integrated and shaped voltage pulses from each PMT are sent to a position-decoding circuit. The outputs of each PMT are weighted in each coordinate direction (x$^+$, x$^-$, y$^+$, y$^-$), and these weighted outputs are summed separately for each coordinate direction, resulting in the location of the scintillation event. The current generated by all the adjacent PMTs represents the total fraction of the light energy received, and it is summed to ensure that this is a desired photopeak interaction. Originally, summing was done using Anger's algebraic method, but recent modifications include digitization. Regionalization of this signal in newer digital gamma cameras can improve processing time and position localization, that is, improved temporal and spatial resolution. Then, individual PMT contributions are analyzed, and by interpolating between PMTs, the x and y coordinates in the crystal can be calculated that correspond to the site of photon interaction with the crystal. These events are located for eventual reconstruction into a two-dimensional image of the patient's three-dimensional organ. By this means, an intrinsic spatial resolution of 2 mm can be obtained, even though the PMTs are spaced 5 cm apart.

### Collimators

The source of radioactivity (the patient organ) emits gamma rays isotropically. Because the final objective is a two-dimensional image of the three-dimensional volume of the organ being imaged, a method of accepting only those photons that produce a useful image is required. The collimator provides the means of producing a "gamma image" on the crystal and assumes a role similar to a focusing lens. This is done by interposing between the photon source and the crystal a device that allows only photons traveling in a

defined direction to pass, the remaining off-axis photons are absorbed. Consequently, only gamma rays traveling within the narrow solid angle of acceptance of the collimator holes can pass undisturbed through the holes to the detector. Collimators are composed of dense materials with high Z values that are opaque to the routine gamma ray photons used in nuclear medicine. These materials include the inexpensive and relatively malleable lead and, in special situations, tungsten or gold. The majority of photon-collimator interactions are photoelectric, so off-axis events are totally absorbed by the collimator, thus decreasing the chance of Compton scatter into the crystal.

Ninety-five percent of all collimators in clinical use are parallel-hole collimators. With the increased use of multidetector SPECT systems, there is an increased interest in the use of fan-beam collimators. High-resolution devices designed for Tc-99m use may have 75,000 to 115,000 holes. High-resolution collimators have small-diameter holes to direct only the desired photons to the crystal. Increasing the length of the collimator septa (hole depth) also improves resolution by accepting only the photons that are most vertical or perpendicular to the crystal (Fig. 23-9). Increasing the number of holes and making them smaller results in the septa becoming proportionately larger, thereby decreasing the number of photons incident to the crystal (the efficiency). This results in an inverse relationship between efficiency and resolution (see Collimator Efficiency).

Three different photon sources are important in image production:

1. The preferred photons that pass directly down the collimator holes to the crystal

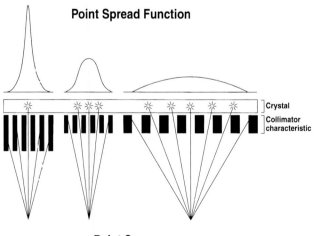

**Point Spread Function**

**Point Sources**

**FIG. 23-9.** The point spread function (PSF: the count-rate profile recorded from a point source) is displayed over a diagrammatic representation of the collimator. The PSF profile is most compact (best resolution) when the collimator has small holes and long "barrels," as seen on the left of figure. PSF is most spread out (poorest resolution) when the holes are larger and the barrel shorter, as seen on the right of figure.

2. The photons that undergo a Compton scatter in the patient or collimator and are scattered down the collimator holes to be recorded (scattered photons)
3. The off-axis photons that pierce the septa but still reach the crystal (septal penetration)

The objective of collimation is to maximize preferred photons and minimize scattered and septal penetrating photons to decrease image degradation. Increasing the thickness of the collimator septa lessens septal penetration, but, as the thickness of the septa increases, the total proportion of accepted incident photons is reduced, thereby decreasing the sensitivity and image statistics. For low-energy photons, such as 140-keV Tc-99m, the typical thickness of lead septa need be only 0.25 mm (~1 HVL); whereas collimators designed for 400-keV photons use septa that are usually 4.5 mm thick.

In low-energy collimators, the septa are usually constructed from sheets of attenuator foil that are glued together, whereas in high-energy collimators, the holes are drilled into blocks of lead. In high-energy photons, a specific "star" pattern occurs during septal penetration, and photons cross over into adjacent holes when the collimator is not designed for adequate performance. If a high-energy collimator is used with the correct septal thickness, a honeycomb pattern usually results as each septum is identified (see Fig. 7-29).

The collimator design represents a series of complex compromises that depend on photon energy, expected photon flux, collimator material used (lead versus tungsten), collimator hole size and depth, and septal thickness. As a rule of thumb, <5% septal penetration is desired, and collimators should be selected for the highest gamma energy that has >5% to 10% abundance. I-131 has a 7% abundant 637-keV photon and Ga-67 a 5% abundant 393-keV photon: These photons contribute significant septal penetration if the higher collimator choice is not selected.

## PRACTICAL IMAGING

### Isotropic Sources

When a bone scanning agent is administered to a patient, only 35% of the tracer localizes in the skeleton; the rest is excreted. If we start imaging the patient 2 to 3 hours after administration, radioactive decay will have reduced this photon flux by a further 20%. If the posterior pelvis is imaged, only 10% of the total body skeletal tracer is at that site. If the image takes 4 minutes, imaging is done while <1% of the total administered radioactivity actually decays. As the patient lies under the crystal, only 20% of the photons from a point source reach the gamma camera collimator surface, the other photons being directed away from the detector. Of the photons that reach the collimator, only 0.02% of them are "desirable" and pass vertically down the collimator holes; all the others should be attenuated by the

**TABLE 23-3.** *Number of photons emitted by the patient to result in light photon hitting the photocathode*

| Source of energy loss in process | Efficiency (loss factor) | Cumulative losses |
| --- | --- | --- |
| Light arrives at photocathode | 1.0000 | 1.00 |
| Crystal light incident on PMT | 0.3500 | 2.86 |
| Crystal efficiency for Tc-99m | 0.8500 | 3.36 |
| Collimator efficiency | 0.0005 | $6.72 \times 10^3$ |
| Photons incident on collimator | 0.2000 | $3.36 \times 10^4$ |
| Soft-tissue attenuation of photon | 0.5000 | $6.72 \times 10^4$ |
| Tc-99m decaying during image | 0.0010 | $6.72 \times 10^7$ |
| Dose decay before imaging | 0.8000 | $8.40 \times 10^7$ |
| Proportion of tracer in pelvis | 0.1000 | $8.40 \times 10^8$ |
| Skeletal uptake of tracer | 0.3500 | $2.40 \times 10^9$ |

lead septa. This ratio of 1:2,000 is in practice remarkably similar for high- and low-energy collimators. Once the photons reach the ⅜-inch crystal, only 85% interact with the NaI crystal; the remaining 15% pass right through it. Finally, of the photoelectric events that occur, a minority (~12%) is transformed to light, and only 35% of the light photons reach the photocathode of the PMT (Table 23-3). This explanation demonstrates that in acquiring a posterior view of the pelvis, only approximately one part in a billion of the available injected radionuclide photons' energy (up to the PMT photocathode) is used to create the electrical impulse that generates the desired image.

### Resolution

Resolution is the ability to faithfully reproduce the image of an object. Spatial resolution is generally defined as the minimum distance between two points that allows both to be detected by the system. This represents a compromise between the resolution of the detector crystal and of the electronics (together called the *intrinsic resolution*), the collimator resolution, and the scatter resolution. In practice, the intrinsic resolution is one-third of the collimator resolution. The overall system resolution is the square root of the sum of the square of the intrinsic, collimator, and scatter resolutions.

$$r_o = \sqrt{r_i^2 + r_c^2 + r_s^2}, \qquad (3)$$

where $r_o$ is the overall resolution, $r_i$ is the intrinsic resolution, $r_c$ is the collimator resolution, and $r_s$ is the scatter resolution.

### Intrinsic Resolution

Intrinsic resolution is degraded by the variations that result in the spread of the gamma ray spectra, including variation due to crystal thickness, number and position of PMTs, optical coupling of crystal and PMT, and all the amplification (PMT, preamplifiers, and amplifiers), position logic, and PHA electronic variations. The thickness of the crystal is important, and with Tc-99m tracers, very thin (¼-inch) crystals have become the norm. This improvement is explained by the decreased dispersal of light from the photon-crystal interaction site to the crystal-PMT interface. Another major factor is the photon energy: Low-energy photons produce less light, which results in lower statistical PMT outputs and lower image resolution. This decrease in light from more remote PMTs is the basis of electronic modifications that improve resolution: Distant tube data are discarded by thresholding PMT outputs (improving location, i.e., spatial resolution), and all tubes are used in summing the incident energy (improving energy resolution). Analog-to-digital converters allow digitization-aided processing (digital cameras). The current intrinsic resolution ranges from 2.8 to 3.5 mm for most manufacturers.

### Collimator Resolution

Collimator resolution is the major determinant of overall image resolution and emphasizes the importance of correct collimator choice and use. In this discussion only the parallel hole collimator is reviewed. Assuming the optimum collimator is chosen, then the most important resolution variable best controlled by the imager is collimator use.

$$r_c = \frac{a\,(l_c + f + b)}{l_c},\qquad (4)$$

where $a$ is the area of the hole, $l_c$ is the length of the collimator, $f$ is the collimator to source distance, and $b$ is the correction factor for crystal thickness.

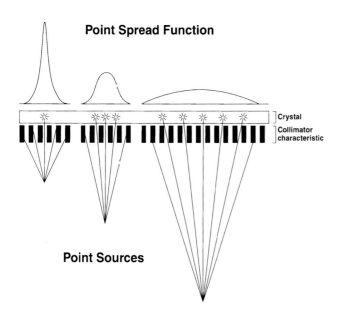

**FIG. 23-10.** The PSF is displayed here for an identical collimator to the one shown in Fig. 23-9, but the distance from point source to collimator is increased twofold, then fourfold. With increasing distance, the PSF is flattened, and resolution deteriorates.

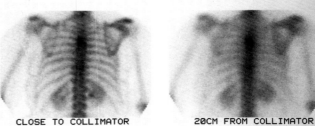

CLOSE TO COLLIMATOR      20CM FROM COLLIMATOR      A,B

**FIG. 23-11.** These posterior thorax images of a patient with subtle T5 and T9 lesions are obtained with a conventional 15% window: The patient-collimator distance is near zero **(A)** and is increased to 20 cm **(B)**. Considerable image resolution deterioration of normal structures has occurred with the greater distance. When whole-body anterior scans are performed, it is possible for the patient-to-collimator distance to approach 20 cm at some regions.

Note that as the collimator score increases, the resolution actually worsens. The formula above indicates that as the collimator hole gets smaller and the hole length (collimator thickness) increases, the resolution improves (see Fig. 23-9). Collimator design and construction are fixed when purchased, but the collimator-to-source distance is the only feature that nuclear medicine technologists can control to ensure optimal imaging. As the distance from the collimator decreases, the flux of the photons incident on the crystal from a point source is greatest along the axis of the collimator hole, and a penumbra of reduced photon numbers permitted by the collimator holes surrounds this axis (Fig. 23-10). The penumbra increases as the source is moved away from the collimator, and the image is degraded (Fig. 23-11) as shown by the point spread function, or the count rate recorded from a point source.

### Scatter Resolution

Scattered radiation from within the patient can interact with the crystal if it is scattered to become incident on the crystal. Provided the Compton scatter angle is no more than 50 degrees in the patient, the PHA accepts a Tc-99m Compton scattered photon (see Fig. 23-4) within the 20% PHA window (126 to 154 keV). These scattered photons can decrease the resolution of the system. It has been stated that 14% to 22% of all "accepted photopeaks" are scattered events in Tc-99m sestamibi myocardial perfusion imaging. For the lower-energy Tl-201, when the window is increased to accept the 69- to 81-keV x-rays, this scattered fraction can reach 30% to 40% of total "accepted photopeaks." With modern cameras, the photopeak window width can be decreased to improve resolution because the FWHM of the system is now typically 10%. Resolution improvement follows from reducing the Tc-99m photopeak window from 20% to 15% in most clinical applica-

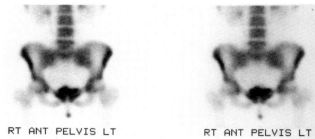

RT ANT PELVIS LT          RT ANT PELVIS LT

10% WINDOW              25% WINDOW

**FIG. 23-12.** These anterior pelvic images of the patient in Fig. 23-11 were acquired with different PHA characteristics. The left image uses a 25% window, the right image a 10% window. Note the slightly sharper image due to less scatter accepted within the narrower window and the better visualization of the vertebral plates with the narrower window.

tions (Fig. 23-12). Corrections for scatter will be required when quantitative SPECT is introduced.

## Collimator Efficiency

The sensitivity or efficiency of a collimator is described by formulae that include a constant due to the collimator hole shape and array configuration. The sensitivity decreases as the square of the collimator hole dimensions (diameter or length) increases, which is the inverse of the formula describing collimator resolution. Other collimator factors that influence sensitivity include septa thickness but not the distance from the photon source to collimator face, which is the single most important and controllable imaging resolution variable. When this formula is compared with the resolution formula, there is an inverse square relationship between sensitivity and resolution: If resolution increases by a factor of 2, sensitivity will decrease by a factor of 4.

$$s = \frac{\text{Open area of holes}}{\text{Total detector area}} = \frac{n\pi\, r^2}{4l_c^2}, \quad (5)$$

where $s$ is the efficiency or sensitivity, $n$ is the number of collimator holes, $r$ is the radius of collimator hole, and $l_c$ is the collimator hole length.

Note that as the number of holes ($n$) increases, septal thickness decreases and septal penetration subsequently increases, thereby adversely affecting resolution. This efficiency formula does not include distance from collimator to point source because parallel-hole collimators have a constant efficiency in air, regardless of the distance from collimator to point source. Although the sensitivity of a single collimator hole decreases inversely with the square of the distance from collimator to source (the inverse square law), as the source is moved away from the source, the number of septal holes that allow photons to interact with the crystal increases, and a greater crystal surface area is exposed (see Fig. 23-10), and overall efficiency is unchanged.

## Counting Rates

The gamma camera response to high count rates is important in nuclear medicine studies that have high photon fluxes (e.g., first-pass cardiac and organ perfusion studies). If each component of the gamma camera detection process (e.g., crystal and electronics) had to return to baseline before the next step was performed, the maximal useful count rate might be less than 10,000 counts per second (cps), and first-pass studies would not be possible.

The dead time, or resolving time, is the time required for the detector system to process each pulse and return to baseline before another individual pulse can be identified. The 1,250-microsecond decay time of the light emission in the crystal is the initial determinant of dead time. This time is increased by integration time of the pulse in the preamplifier and the decay time of the signal in the amplifier. Although it is desirable that this signal return to baseline to obtain the best spatial and energy resolution, for the best temporal resolution the shortest sampling interval practical is of paramount importance. The detector system is therefore a compromise between these competing variables, and typical final system dead times after electronic manipulation are in the 1.5- to 5.0-microsecond range. Current gamma cameras are able to handle counting rates of 140,000 cps in the desired photopeak window with <20% loss of counts due to dead time.

Counting systems can be paralyzable or nonparalyzable. In a paralyzable system, each event adds its own dead time if it arrives within the dead time of a previous event. This makes the dead time of the total system cumulative. If the count rate gets too high, each event occurring during the dead time of the previous event is lost and its additional dead time "tacked on." Ultimately, the system is paralyzed, and no image is recorded at all. In a nonparalyzable system, each new event is not recorded if it arrives during the dead time, but this event does not add to the total dead time of the first event, so some counts are always recorded. A given scintillation camera detector system has both paralyzable and nonparalyzable components. Broadly speaking, the crystal is a paralyzable system, and the electronic components are nonparalyzable.

The dead time of a particular detector system can be determined by counting two sources separately and together. The sources must be of sufficient activity that there are significant count losses when they are counted together but not when counted separately (<20,000 cps per source). Thus, the sum of the individual count rates is greater than the combined count rate. Once the dead time of the system is known, true counting rates can be calculated from observed counting rates.

$$\tau = \frac{R_1 + R_2 - R_{1+2}}{2R_1 R_2} \text{ microsecond}, \quad (6)$$

where $R_1$ is the count rate from source 1, $R_2$ is the count rate for source 2, $R_{1+2}$ is the combined source 1 and 2 count rate, and $\tau$ is the dead time. The true counting rate, $R_t$, can then be computed from the observed count rate, $R_o$ as

$$R_t = \frac{R_o}{1 - R_o \tau}. \tag{7}$$

## Methods to Improve Count Rate

Several methods have been used to improve the count rate in dynamic studies: Initial attempts included bypassing of nonuniformity corrections to improve the electronic response and shortening the integration time of the fluorescent flash. These methods seriously compromised system resolution, but because high-sensitivity (and therefore low-resolution) collimators are typically employed in dynamic flow studies, this loss of intrinsic resolution may not be important. Other methods to improve counting rates without paralysis include clipping of the integration time and, though there is some loss in intrinsic resolution, count rates of 150,000 to 200,000 cps are possible in the 20% useful window. These count rates provide useful first-pass radionuclide angiograms, sufficient for clinical use, although they are not as fast as multicrystal cameras, which are capable of counting 450,000 cps.

## Gamma Camera QC

QC is the periodic inspection of equipment to ensure high-quality images. Numerous organizations (Joint Commission on Accreditation of Healthcare Organizations [JCAHO], Bureau of Radiologic Health, American College of Nuclear Physicians, American College of Radiology, and the U.S. Food and Drug Administration) suggest or mandate imaging equipment QC, but most do not describe explicitly what to do or how frequently to do it. Physicists' associations (American Association of Medical Physicists and Hospital Physicists Association), however, suggest standardized acceptance testing and, specifically, the use of National Electronic Manufacturers Association standards. These very lengthy procedures are done without scattering media, do not simulate normal operating conditions, and require special phantoms and software to perform, thus they are impractical for routine use. Manufacturers have now become the most important advisers on QC for their machines, probably driven by product liability law. The manufacturers' suggestions should be followed because only they can tell us what to do to ensure optimal performance.

The high voltage supply for a gamma camera must be constant, so it is left on continuously. When environmental conditions (heat and humidity) change significantly or when the power is lost temporarily, QC procedures must be repeated. The gamma camera is inherently nonuniform due to these factors:

- Crystal nonuniformity
- Defects in optical coupling

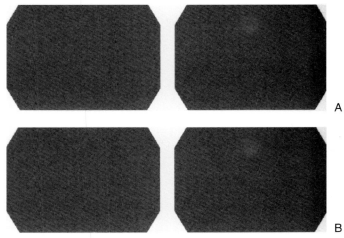

**FIG. 23-13. (A)** Minor abnormality on the flood field image (right) that disappears on the "corrected" image (left). **(B)** This thresholded image better displays the abnormality (right) and confirms that the correction works (left).

- Variations in PMTs
- Nonlinearity of the processing circuitry

At the time of construction, the manufacturer matches the various gamma camera components (e.g., PMTs) to minimize these variations. The user must check for the spatial inhomogeneities that are inherent in the device. A "flood field" technique is used to check for these minor inhomogeneities using a presumed uniform field source. This flood field is stored in a matrix, and each pixel count is divided by the mean so as to obtain a correction factor. Images of the flood field should be obtained daily with and without this correction. The test should be done on weekends and holidays if a clinical study is to be done. Both images should be uniform and normal, and, at the very least, the corrected image should be uniform (Fig. 23-13). If too much correction is required to obtain a uniform field, the device should be serviced.

The energy spectrum should also be measured. Modern cameras do this continuously using very stable light-emitting diodes (e.g., one diode source per PMT) and then apply corrections. Some manufacturers measure the energy spectrum before imaging, others during the image acquisition process. When the energy and uniformity check is performed routinely, images will be accurate. Images of the flood field when the energy window is skewed off peak are shown (Fig. 23-14), but this is not usually a problem with modern equipment. Whether the above-peak setting causes a "hot" or "cold" spot defect over the PMT is a manifestation of the camera design itself, and not the offset direction (above or below peak).

Unfortunately, although QC is done, the results are not always evaluated and acted on. The JCAHO requirement of a physicist inspecting the QC information is testament to their understanding of this human frailty. Various studies of the use of QC data have confirmed frequent lack of recogni-

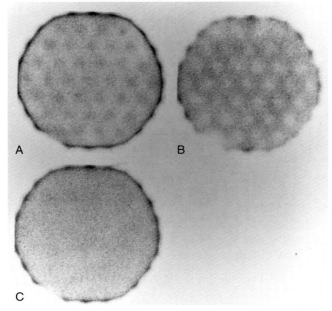

**FIG. 23-14.** This composite image of an older camera shows a below-peak setting **(A)**, above-peak setting **(B)**, and a correct peak setting **(C)**. In this camera, these "off-peak" settings result in hot and cold artifacts respectively. (Courtesy of Dr. Raymond Tu.)

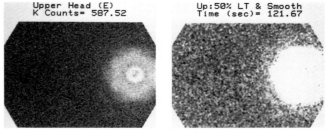

**FIG. 23-15.** This flood field shows a significant abnormality **(A)** on the routine flood that is displayed with 50% lower thresholding **(B)**. **(A)** This image shows the single tube defect, with the effect that this tube has on the light measured by the surrounding tubes. **(B)** The defect is more apparent on the 50% threshold image, where the abnormality affects the central and surrounding six tubes.

tion of equipment shortcomings despite the presence of QC data that establish the problem.

### Uniformity

Uniformity and resolution testing should be performed regularly and can be done with or without the collimator.

The collimator defines extrinsic (source extrinsic to the collimator) and intrinsic (source intrinsic to the collimator) testing. Uniformity requires a uniform test source, and the simplest method is to acquire a source from a manufacturer and require them to guarantee the uniformity. Most centers use Co-57 (122-keV) uniformity phantoms because Tc-99m–filled phantoms are subject to geometric distortion by central bowing. The 6-hour half-life of Tc-99m is too short for repeated use, and a convenient alternative is Co-57 impregnated in a solid plastic material. The 122-keV photon is suitable, and the very long half-life makes it a crude measure of sensitivity if tested with the same collimator in extrinsic measurements. Because uniformity is the first parameter to deteriorate, we at UW-Madison concentrate on checking it, and virtually all nuclear medicine sections perform daily uniformity testing. Count differences should be significant before they are recognized visually, with as much

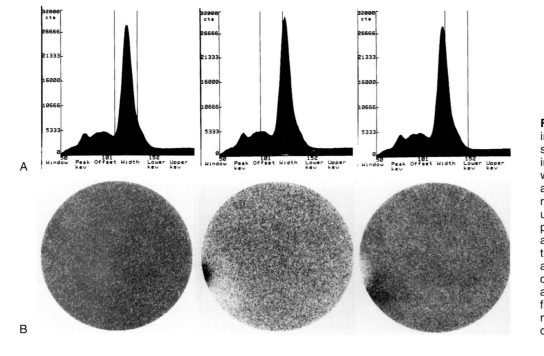

**FIG. 23-16.** This series of images display the acquisition spectrum **(A)** and flood field images **(B)** when the energy windows were deliberately maladjusted (left: correct window; middle: window mispeaked to upper offset; right: window mispeaked to lower offset). In this already suboptimal camera, the adequacy of correction is apparent (left), but when the camera is mispeaked, complex abnormalities develop in the flood field in the region of deteriorating PMT (at 7 o'clock middle and right image).

as 5% to 10% variations required to be able to identify the nonuniformity. For this reason, computer methods are often applied (Fig. 23-15) to enhance early recognition of problems. Most problems are due to PMT or preamplifier gain variations. Minor crystal, PMT, and preamplifier irregularities are better identified with off-peak settings (Fig. 23-16).

### Resolution

Resolution is conveniently checked with a line or bar phantom. A four-quadrant phantom is commonly used for this, and for one of our new GE cameras, the provided test pattern phantom cannot physically be rotated as generally recommended to check the x and y axes in each quadrant. The four-quadrant phantom does allow one to check resolution, provided the manufacturer-supplied slit phantoms are in range of optimal system resolution (i.e., 2 to 4 mm). As a rule, FWHM is usually 1.7 (range, 1.4 to 2.0) times the smallest bars discerned on a phantom. Although one strives to optimize intrinsic resolution, it is better to remember that the spatial degradation from the patient-to-collimator distance is more significant and controllable. Previously, linearity was an important test of QC, but because this is well controlled by manufacturer-determined circuitry and these compensation methods have had a very successful track record for many years, linearity is no longer routinely measured on modern machines. Energy resolution is difficult to measure routinely and so is not done routinely.

### Multiple-Window Resolution

With the use of dual tracer techniques (e.g., Tc-99m MDP and In-111 WBC for secondary osteomyelitis) and two- and three-peak radionuclides (In-111 with 273- and 247-keV photons, Ga-67 with 93-, 185-, 300-, and 394-keV photons) in many clinical tests, the technical limits of our imaging devices are being stressed. Because images created from photons of various energies are of different sizes, the correction circuitry must also compensate for this. Procedures for checking for this size correction are available, but alert physicians might recognize indistinct margins to organs and so anticipate the problem. An easy method in older cameras (without computerized edge-masking devices) shows additional margins at the image edges due to different edge-packing effects for the misregistered or misamplified peaks (see Fig. 23-14).

## IMAGING ARTIFACTS

The differentiation of fact from artifact marks the skill of an experienced radiologist and nuclear medicine physician. Nuclear medicine procedures pose more artifact problems than many other commonly used radiologic modalities. The differentiation of artifact from true abnormality is more than an academic interest, given that misdiagnosis of pathology may lead to unnecessary and potentially harmful intervention and therapy (Fig. 23-17).

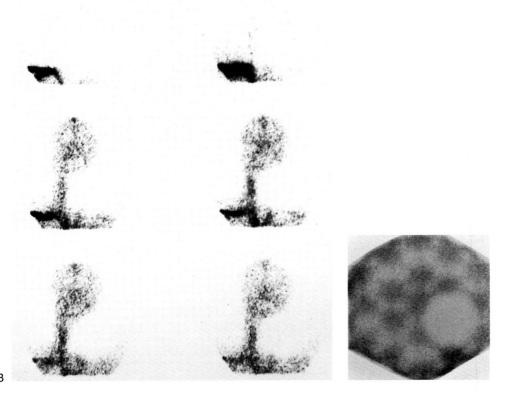

A,B

**FIG. 23-17.** This dramatic image illustrates how a misdiagnosis can occur from improperly functioning instrumentation. **(A)** The brain flow study shows flow from the injected right arm (upper row), then right common carotid arterial flow (lower rows), but no flow in the left common carotid artery. **(B)** The QC flood field shows a tube missing. (Courtesy of Dr. Raymond Tu.)

**TABLE 23-4.** *Artifacts by pattern*

| Artifact | Pattern |
|---|---|
| Diffuse | Bears little resemblance to the anticipated distribution |
| Multifocal | Many areas of altered activity on expected distribution |
| Localized | Focal alteration in otherwise normal distribution |

Five general categories of nuclear medicine artifacts should be considered: planar, SPECT, radiopharmaceutical, administration, and imaging technique. Each contains three scintigraphic patterns: diffuse, multifocal, and localized. Lists of examples of typical artifacts are provided in Tables 23-4 and 23-5.

## Planar Artifacts

Camera QC is vital to ensure reliable images. The following examples show the results of the breakdown of such QC efforts.

### Diffuse Artifacts

Wrong energy window settings for the radiopharmaceutical cause too much scatter, increase soft-tissue activity, produce image nonuniformity, and result in loss of sharp organ outline, although the body or organ still contains marginally recognizable shapes (see Fig. 8-7). The photopeak window setting can be too high or too low, resulting in a nonuniform image. The star pattern results, with septal penetration of high-energy radionuclide energy with a low- or medium-energy collimator setting (see Fig. 7-29). A previous nuclear medicine scan is the most common cause of GI tract activity on a bone scan, especially a prior hepatobiliary scan (Fig. 23-18). Photographic errors, such as underexposure or incorrect display level, may severely degrade image quality, but these problems are easily recognized and corrected. Physiologic causes of soft tissue accumulation of bone scanning agent occurs in edematous soft tissues, espe-

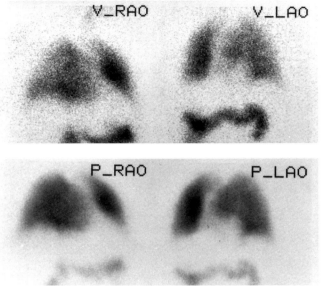

**FIG. 23-18.** These ventilation **(A)** and perfusion **(B)** scans in the RAO (left) and LAO (right) views show a normal ventilation and perfusion scan, but considerable GI activity from a hepatobiliary scan performed the day before. The relative increase in GI activity in the ventilation scan is due to the scan technique, in which less Tc-99m aerosol gets into the lungs than the perfusion agent, and the total overall count rate is lower than the perfusion lung scan. (Therefore the GI activity is relatively increased.)

cially in lymphedema secondary to axillary node dissection (see Fig. 1-24A).

### Multifocal Artifacts

Field nonuniformity may result from voltage drift or the wrong energy peak selection and can cause or exaggerate existing electronic problems (Fig. 23-19). The intrinsic causes of nonuniformity in gamma camera response are the failure of electronic correction circuits to overcome variations in sensitivity across the face of the crystal (uniformity board failure), nonlinearity in the position signals, and spatial distortions. Static electrical discharge may cause many spots of film exposure resulting from faulty grounding of electrical equipment.

**TABLE 23-5.** *Examples of planar imaging artifact*

| Diffuse | Multifocal | Localized |
|---|---|---|
| Wrong energy window | Static electricity | Electronic malfunction |
| Damaged crystal | Electronic malfunction | PMT coupling failure |
| Septal penetration | Photographic error | Movement artifact |
| Prior scan | MAA clumping | Tissue uptake, e.g., breast |
| Drug effect | Urine contamination | Injection extravasation |
| Stannous ion in IV line | Barium enema | Coins, implants, buckles, etc. |

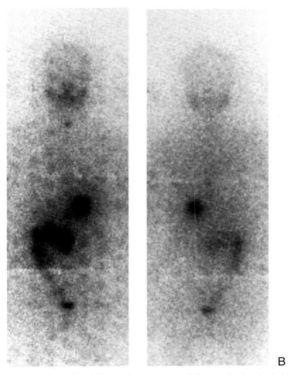

A                                          B

**FIG. 23-19.** Anterior **(A)** and posterior **(B)** whole-body I-131 metastatic survey scans from an outside institution. **(A)** Note the regular hot-spots configuration over the whole image in the anterior view of this whole-body format. The horizontal linear artifacts in the lower thorax and abdomen indicate composite "spot" views combined to make this whole body-image. **(B)** The posterior view does not demonstrate this artifact. These images suggest the wrong energy (radionuclide) flood field correction was applied to the anterior image. The scan report did not indicate a technical problem. Although a thyroid remnant is seen in the neck, this anterior view should not have been used in clinical management decisions.

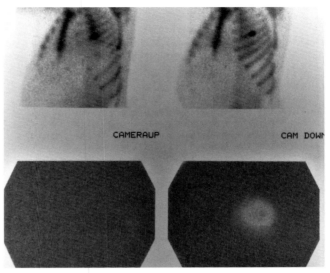

**FIG. 23-21.** A spot LAO view of the chest wall of the patient in Fig. 23-20 shows a central defect when the camera head is above the patient (upper left), but no defect when the same view was obtained with the patient prone and the camera head below the patient (upper right). This position-dependent abnormality can be very difficult to identify when only whole-body images are obtained (see Fig. 23-20) and could be due to uncoupling of the PMT-crystal interface or a loose connection of the PMT preamplifier (as in this case). The lower row shows flood field images obtained with the camera head facing down on the flood source (lower right), which was absent when the camera head was facing up (lower left).

### Localized Artifacts

A damaged NaI crystal can cause cold bands with hot edges on an image. Crystal hydration or cracks from physical trauma are the most common mechanisms of crystal deterioration. Review of daily flood images allows correct identification. Very small cold defects can occur where the collimator septa are displaced to obstruct the normal holes. PMT failure or loss of high-voltage supply or coupling

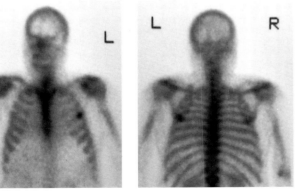

A,B

**FIG. 23-20.** This figure is part of a moving-table, single-camera, whole-body bone scan: **(A)** There is a subtle decrease in uptake in the anterior image only, involving the left facial and anterior chest wall regions with a focal hot lesion in antero-lateral portion of left fourth rib. **(B)** The posterior view, obtained immediately after the anterior view, is normal.

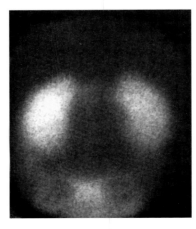

**FIG. 23-22.** This Polaroid image represents a double exposure of a brain scan and renal scan, creating a composite that defies recognition.

between the PMT and crystal can cause cold defects or a nonuniform image (Figs. 23-20 and 23-21). Patient contact with the camera surface may occasionally contaminate it, with residual excreted tracer creating irregular hot artifacts. This can be demonstrated by repeat imaging after decontamination. Photographic errors may result in overexposure or double exposure, creating interesting images that often defy explanation (Fig. 23-22).

## Administration Imaging Artifacts

### Diffuse Artifacts

The presence of stannous pyrophosphate in the intravenous line results in the premature reduction of Tc-99m before entry into the RBC during blood pool labeling procedures. Tc-99m pyrophosphate is thus accidentally created, and the expected blood pool image may not be as good as expected because the patient will have, for all practical purposes, both a labeled RBC and a bone scanning agent. Subcutaneous infiltration of the stannous pyrophosphate dose during Tc-99m labeling of RBCs for multiple gated acquisition at rest precludes adequate labeling and diffusely increased background and results in a suboptimal study. Efficient RBC labeling requires a minimum stannous ion concentration of 10 μg/kg. Drugs such as digoxin, quinidine, methyldopa, and prazosin may cause diminution in ability to

visualize the cardiac chamber border due to poor labeling of RBCs, as a result of dissociation of the label and RBC by unknown mechanisms.

### Multifocal Artifacts

Macroaggregated albumin (MAA) particles used for pulmonary perfusion imaging are irregularly shaped particles between 10 and 90 μm in size. During injection of Tc-MAA, blood should not be allowed to mix with particles. Tracer contamination with blood for even a few seconds produces clumping of the radiopharmaceutical, which appears as hot spots during lung imaging. This artifact has not been seen lately. The last time we found it (Fig. 23-23), it was due to the manufacturer's QC problems because larger-than-usual MAA particles were present in each batch.

### Localized Artifacts

Poor injection technique can result in the extravasation of the radiopharmaceutical into the soft tissues. If significant subcutaneous tracer extravasation occurs, the radiopharmaceutical clears via the lymphatic system. Visualization of axial lymph nodes after subcutaneous injection of a bone agent is seen with a large antecubital deposition (Fig. 23-24). Superimposition of the injection site over the area of interest causes aberrant hot spots.

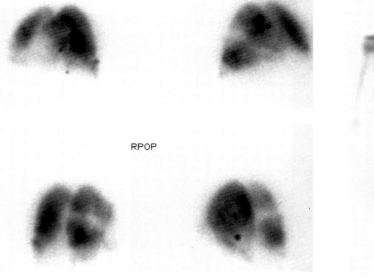

RPOP

**FIG. 23-23.** These two anterior oblique **(A)** and two posterior **(B)** oblique views of a Tc-99m MAA lung perfusion scan show small "hot-spot clumps" of radioactivity within the lungs. This was found to be due to excessively large particles supplied by the manufacturer, rather than clumping (coating of blood with MAA). The manufacturer replaced this radiopharmaceutical lot.

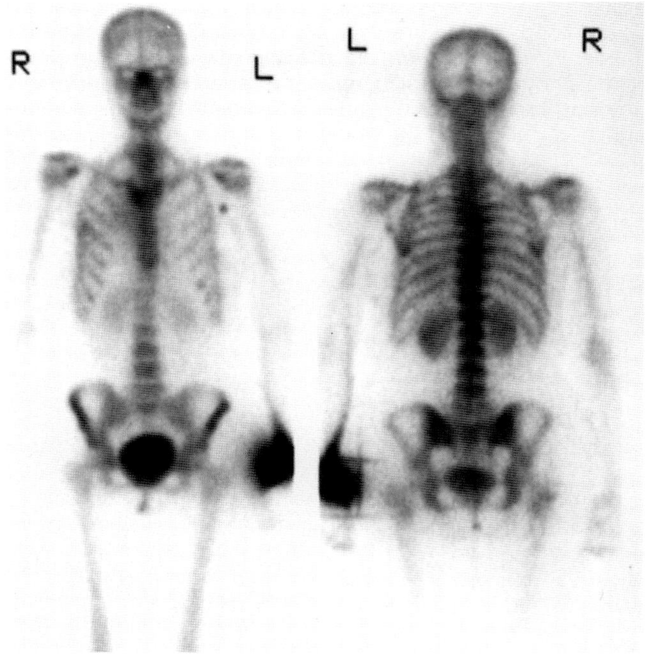

**FIG. 23-24.** The dose has infiltrated the soft tissues, and the draining lymphatic vessel and axillary lymph node are seen. The arm rest causes increased scatter from the infiltrated dose, with visualization of the arm rest struts seen in the posterior image (right).

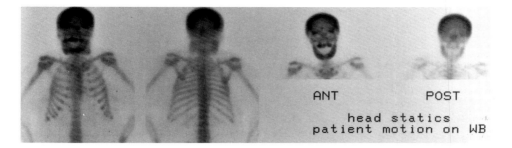

**FIG. 23-25.** This patient has secondary hyperparathyroidism due to renal disease (note absent kidney and soft-tissue activity and diffusely increased skeletal uptake). He moved his head during the whole-body scan acquisition, thus distorting the mandible. The static head images (right) more clearly demonstrate the typical mandible of hyperparathyroidism.

## Imaging Technique Artifacts

### Diffuse Artifacts

Patients must be urged to remain motionless during imaging. Minor movement greatly decreases the resolution of scintigraphy (Fig. 23-25). Patients can usually only tolerate 5 to 10 minutes of sitting and 15 to 20 minutes of lying down without movement. Imaging for >20 minutes per view drastically enhances the risk of motion distortion, with particularly profound effects in image quality.

### Multifocal Artifacts

A common problem in bone scanning is skin and clothing contamination with radioactive urine because >50% of the injected bone tracer is excreted via the kidneys within 3 hours. Oblique views are as helpful as lateral views in establishing contamination (Fig. 23-26). For patients with indwelling catheters or whose urinary tract has been diverted, the technologist must move the catheter and collecting bag outside the imaging field. Highly radioactive

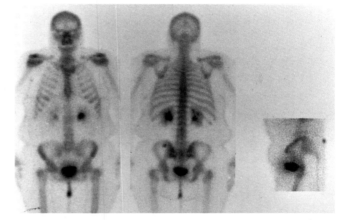

**FIG. 23-26.** This whole-body bone scan shows a prominent abnormality in the left iliac bone seen only in the posterior (middle) image. A lateral view (right) clearly shows this as surface contamination.

urine obscures detail in the imaged regions behind or adjacent to lesions. Contamination with a urine-soaked tampon or bandage is a not uncommon imaging artifact.

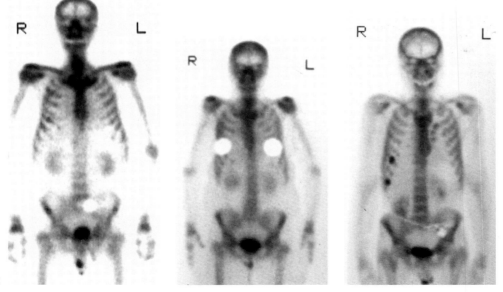

A–C

**FIG. 23-27.** Three whole-body bone scans with metallic artifacts leaving sharply outlined photopenic defects: **(A)** large belt buckle, **(B)** brassiere inserts, **(C)** lock and chain.

### *Localized Artifacts*

Attenuation due to metallic objects, such as belt buckles (Fig. 23-27), earrings, medallions, and coins (see Fig. 1-8), is seen as very well-defined photopenic regions with sharp edges. These artifacts are not infrequent, particularly on outpatient studies. The technologist should always remove metallic objects from the imaging field. Residual barium sulfate in the bowel, dentures, and breast prostheses also cause attenuation. Less obvious artifacts result from less dense materials, and these can make scan interpretations difficult (Fig. 23-28).

## SUGGESTED READING

Anger HO. Scintillation camera. Rev Sci Inst 1958;29:27–33.

Williams LE. Nuclear Medicine Physics. Boca Raton, FL: CRC, 1987.

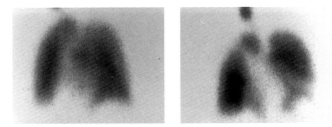

A,B

**FIG. 23-28.** Attenuators equivalent to soft tissues do not leave sharp borders and are difficult to identify as artifacts. In this scan, **(A)** is an LAO lung perfusion scan, **(B)** is another LAO view on the same patient done soon afterward that suggests multiple perfusion defects. The patient's left arm was drawn up across the body and touching the opposite shoulder **(B)**, creating artifactual attenuation effects in perfusion that could be mistaken for defects in the left basal and right anterior upper lobe segments.

*Textbook of Nuclear Medicine,*
edited by Michael A. Wilson.
Lippincott–Raven Publishers, Philadelphia © 1998.

CHAPTER 24

# Emission Tomography

Michael A. Wilson, Jesus A. Bianco, and Robert W. Pyzalski

The history of transmission computed tomography (TCT) and emission computed tomography (ECT) is inexorably linked to pioneers in nuclear medicine (1–4). The idea of tomography (i.e., reconstruction from projections) comes from the 1920s and 1930s, and the very first transmission image reconstruction from projections was performed using an iodine 131 (I-131) source in 1961. Transaxial imaging was introduced by David Kuhl in 1963, and soon thereafter, Kuhl and Edwards constructed the first of a series of single photon ECT (SPECT) scanners (2–4).

Emission scanners are designed for use with either positron (positron emission tomography [PET]) or SPECT radiopharmaceuticals. All these techniques (TCT, PET, and SPECT) produce tomographic images, that is, slices or planes through the patient, where each slice or plane is displayed without the confusing data from above or below that slice. This feature increases object contrast, which is the major attribute of ECT (Fig. 24-1).

Stacking of transaxial tomographic images provides a useful volume-rendering display format for clinical use (Fig. 24-2). This can also be done in the heart in the gated mode (see Fig. 2-10).

In 1977, the detector was first made to rotate around the patient rather than the patient rotating in front of the detector, and the first practical SPECT systems were constructed (5,6). At the same time, PET scanners were being developed. In the interval between Kuhl's description of transaxial imaging and commercial SPECT and PET scanner construction, x-ray TCT (the CT or computerized axial tomography [CAT] scanner) was introduced in 1971, after Cormack and Hounsfield demonstrated that a two-dimensional (2D) map of attenuation coefficients in the body could be reconstructed from transmission projection data (7–9). These inventors went on to receive the Nobel Prize in physiology and medicine in 1979.

Both TCT and ECT produce images of patient organs. The conventional TCT image represents an image of the attenuation of the external x-ray source rotated about the patient and is basically a map of the distribution of densities (electrons), whereas the ECT image is a map of radiopharmaceutical distribution modified by the attenuating effect of the body. This highlights the important differences of the two techniques: TCT is anatomic, and ECT is physiologic.

## SINGLE PHOTON EMISSION COMPUTED TOMOGRAPHY

In TCT, the images represent a 2D reconstruction of the linear attenuation coefficients ($\mu$) of tissues through which x-rays pass. The incident radiation beam in each projection is exponentially decreased by the sum of linear attenuation coefficients of the tissue through which the x-ray passes, and it is measured as it exits the body on the side opposite from the source. In ECT, the source of radiation is a functional radiopharmaceutical, which localizes in body organs. The photon emissions are variably attenuated according to the individual radionuclide source site and the tissue the photon must pass through to exit the body (10). TCT uses a collimated x-ray source that passes through the body in an orderly fashion, whereas the emissive source of ECT radiates isotropically (i.e., in all directions) from the points of origin in a random manner. Tissue attenuation and scattering of the emitted photon in the body means the photons counted do not truly represent radionuclidic tissue concentrations, but if appropriate corrections are applied (relatively simple in PET but difficult in SPECT), quantitative measurements are possible.

### Clinical Utility of SPECT Imaging

At the time of writing, there are >4,000 SPECT units in use worldwide. The established indications in which this technology is particularly useful and significantly improves clinical results include

- Myocardial perfusion imaging
- Brain perfusion imaging
- Gallium 67 (Ga-67) imaging of lymphoma

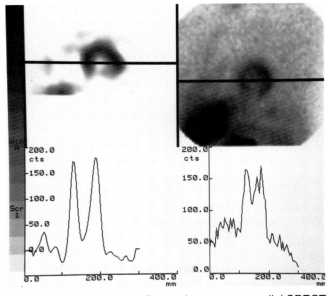

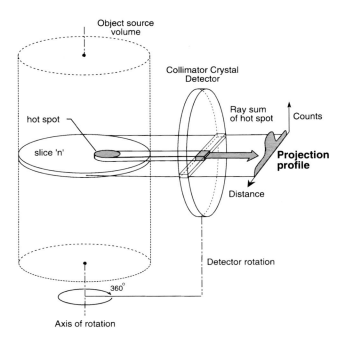

**FIG. 24-1.** This composite figure shows a myocardial SPECT image slice on the left with profile below, and the right shows a planar image with profile below. The profiles show a better target-to-background ratio for the SPECT slice than for the planar image.

**FIG. 24-3.** This simplified image shows a dark hot spot within a cylindrical object source volume with the detector system and axis of rotation shown, a single ray sum, and the resultant profile of slice 'n' through the source and hot spot.

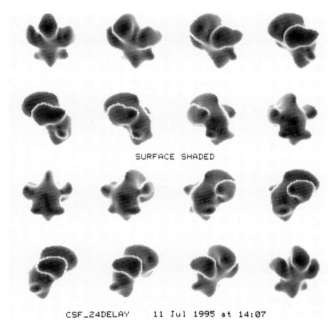

**FIG. 24-2.** A composite view of a rotating surface shaded stacked transaxial SPECT CSF slices showing radionuclide in the cranial ventricular system. These reconstructed views are displayed at 22.5-degree increments. Such a display format, especially when viewed in motion, aids interpretation.

- Bone imaging in lumbar spondylolysis, the pelvis, and temporomandibular joint disease
- Imaging of hepatic hemangioma
- Imaging of labeled peptides (e.g., pentetreotide) and monoclonal antibodies

## Data Acquisition

In SPECT, a gamma camera detector system is rotated around the patient and a set of angular samples (multiple planar images) is collected around the axis of rotation of the detector (10,11). SPECT images are "reconstructed" by a computer, which effectively removes overlying and underlying activities from the planes of interest to produce the desired tomographic planes. The most popular method of reconstruction is the filtered backprojection (FBP) technique. This process uses a complex mathematical algorithm, but the basic idea is that each planar image is divided up into a matrix of picture elements or pixels (typically 64 × 64, with a pixel size of approximately 6 mm, depending on crystal size). Ignoring tissue attenuation, photon scatter, and detector response, it is assumed that the number of counts in each pixel of the planar image is the sum of the counts coming from a single line or ray from the patient, which is perpendicular to the face of the camera and that particular pixel (Fig. 24-3). The combination of all these pixels in the matrix slice is called a projection.

During image acquisition, planar views are obtained at small-angle increments (typically 3- or 6-degree increments) as the gamma camera detector rotates stepwise around the patient. During backprojection for reconstruction, the total counts in each pixel of the planar image are projected back along the line of acquisition, with the counts equally distributed along each projection ray sum because the actual source of the photon is unknown. When this process is repeated for each planar image, a final cross-sectional image of the total

**Emission Profiles Obtained at 30° Intervals**

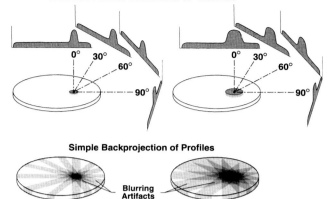

**Simple Backprojection of Profiles**

Blurring
Artifacts

**FIG. 24-4.** The activity profiles of two sources are displayed for four angles (0–90 degrees). When seven activity profiles of each slice are simply backprojected, a reconstructed slice ('n') of the object source and hot spot is obtained. Unfortunately, because the activity in each profile is presumed to be equally distributed along the entire ray sum, the reconstructed image is blurred and indistinct, with star-like blurring artifacts.

volume can be reconstructed. Unfortunately, there are significant blurring artifacts (Fig. 24-4) as a result of the uncertainty of origin of the photon.

Ideally, the sum of counts detected in each ray (the ray sum) of each profile should be the total number of gamma emissions from the radionuclide in the patient, but in reality this is degraded by the following factors (10,11):

- Depth-related attenuation
- Loss of photons by scattering out of the ray
- Detection of undesirable scattered photons from other rays
- Nonuniformity of crystal-detector response
- Misalignment of the detector
- Lesion and organ size (the partial volume effect)
- Patient and organ motion
- Type of SPECT orbit

## Collimation

Collimation is a key issue for ideal planar and SPECT imaging, and it is important to recall that very few of the emitted photons are detected (see Table 23-3). In single-detector SPECT systems, a low-energy, all-purpose collimator is used for imaging with technetium 99m (Tc-99m) radiopharmaceuticals to improve sensitivity, but the recent trend for SPECT imaging is to use a high-resolution collimator (11). Collimator efficiency (and therefore system sensitivity) is important because noise increases significantly as the number of counts in an image decreases. The high-resolution collimator may significantly reduce image counts, but it puts those counts where they belong with an increase in image signal-to-noise ratio that makes this choice practical in many situations.

Collimator resolution worsens linearly with increasing distance from the collimator face, so every effort should be made to minimize patient distance from the collimator face. This is a difficult task when data must be collected from around the entire organ, which, in the case of the heart, is eccentrically located within the chest. The spatial resolution of the reconstructed SPECT image is almost equal across the image, and it approximates the resolution of the camera-collimator system measured at a distance equal to the SPECT system's radius of rotation. This differs from the spatial resolution of the planar system image, which is maximal when the object of interest is at the collimator face and then decreases rapidly as the source is moved away from the collimator surface. Typical single-head SPECT system resolution is 15 to 18 mm at full-width, half-maximum (FWHM) for the body versus 10 mm for planar imaging when the object is near the surface.

Traditionally, SPECT orbits around the patient are circular. Since 1979, a noncircular orbit (body contouring) has been recommended to keep the detectors in close proximity to the body surface. The elliptical orbit has been compared to the circular orbit in nuclear cardiology studies (12), and it was shown that the distance from collimator to the eccentrically located heart can be greater for elliptical orbits than circular orbits. Therefore, the elliptical orbit has the potential to produce artifacts in SPECT myocardial perfusion studies. Some vendors have introduced systems where body contouring is done automatically, with efficient positioning of the detector near the patient body surface at all times.

SPECT imaging of medium- and higher-energy photons is associated with large amounts of septal penetrating and scattered photons. These undesirable photons create a background that degrades image contrast (13,14). This problem exemplifies the need for correct collimator choice in both planar and SPECT imaging when using medium-energy radiopharmaceuticals. Even when using medium-energy collimators (200 to 300 keV), there can be significant Compton scatter contributions from higher-energy emissions; for example, Ga-67 has an approximately 5% abundant 394-keV photon. These gamma rays may not be routinely imaged, yet their Compton scatter photons are included in the selected photopeaks and degrade the image.

### Fan-Beam and Cone-Beam Collimation

Although parallel-hole collimators are most commonly used in SPECT, converging-hole collimators can be used. The converging collimators provide improved detection efficiency (1.5- to 2.0-fold increases) with similar system resolution (Fig. 24-5), gained at the expense of a smaller field of view (FOV). For nuclear imaging of organs that are smaller than the SPECT system's FOV (e.g., brain, heart, or children's organs), it is useful to use converging collimators, with their tradeoff between spatial resolution and sensitivity (15–17). Fan-beam collimators reduce the FOV by focusing to a *focal line* parallel to the axis of rotation on the other side of the

**Projection Profiles**

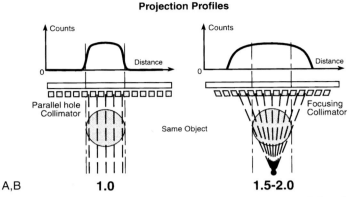

A,B

**FIG. 24-5.** The conventional parallel-hole collimator **(A)** with the activity profile of the object above it. The converging collimator **(B)**, with the activity profile of the same object also shown above. The converging collimator results in magnification and a 1.5- to 2.0-fold increase in detection efficiency.

**TABLE 24-1.** *Facts pertinent to SPECT QC*

| | 32 × 32 | 64 × 64 | 128 × 128 |
|---|---|---|---|
| Matrix size | | | |
| Pixels (round detector) | 804 | 3,217 | 12,868 |
| Required flood counts | $8 \times 10^6$ | $30 \times 10^6$ | $120 \times 10^6$ |
| Counts per pixel | 9,950 | 9,325 | 9,325 |
| Coefficient of variation | 1% | 1% | 1% |

from the collimator (the usual resolution factors in planar imaging, see Chapter 23), it is also a function of hole angulation and the minification to the object plane (the focusing effect). At the time of this writing, fan-beam collimation is recommended for SPECT brain imaging and is being used by some for cardiac imaging, but torso imaging may be associated with truncation artifacts (19).

**Sampling**

For data acquisition to be accurate, it is necessary to detect sufficient radiopharmaceutical concentration that a valid image reconstruction can be performed. These acquisitions are commonly acquired in a *step-and-shoot* mode, where the camera moves and stops, acquiring data during each stop. This simple step-and-shoot acquisition is preferred over the faster continuous acquisition mode, especially if high-resolution collimators are used. In brain or other studies where patient movement may be a problem, multiple rapid acquisi-

patient, at the collimator's focal length. Cone-beam collimators focus on a *focal point* on the other side of the patient. This focusing in both x and y directions can provide further increases in sensitivity at the expense of additional decreases in the FOV (18). With the use of collimators that magnify the organ image, care must be taken that unique detector orbits and appropriate reconstruction algorithms are used.

With these collimators, the resolution is not only a function of hole diameter, bore length, and distance of the object

**TABLE 24-2.** *Typical SPECT acquisition guidelines*

| Study | Radiopharmaceutical (mCi) | Collimator[a] | Acquisition | Image matrix | Angular increment | Orbit shape | Seconds per projection |
|---|---|---|---|---|---|---|---|
| Bone | | | | | | | |
| Hips | Tc-99m MDP (25–30) | LEGP | 360 degrees | 64 | 6 degrees | Contour | 25 |
| Spine, knee, TMJ | Tc-99m MDP (25–30) | LEHR | 360 degrees | 128 | 3 degrees | Contour | 15 |
| Liver | Tc-99m SC (4–6) | LEGP | 360 degrees | 64 | 6 degrees | Contour | 20 |
| | Tc-99m RBC (20) | LEHR | 360 degree | 128 | 3 degree | Contour | 15 |
| Brain | Tc-99m HMPAO/ECD (15–30) | LEHR | 360 degrees | 64 | 6 degrees | Circle | 30 |
| Tumor | Ga-67 citrate (10) | MEGP | 360 degrees | 64 | 6 degrees | Contour | 40 |
| | In-111 MOAB/peptide (5–6) | MEGP | 360 degrees | 64 | 6 degrees | Contour | 40–60 |
| | Tc-99m MOAB fragments (15–30) | LEHR | 360 degrees | 64–128 | 3–6 degrees | Contour | 20–45 |
| | Tl-201 (3) | LEGP | 360 degrees | 64 | 6 degrees | Contour | 25 |
| | Tc-99m sestamibi (20–30) | LEHR | 360 degrees | 128 | 3 degrees | Contour | 20 |
| Infection | In-111 WBC (0.5) | MEGP | 360 degrees | 64 | 6 degrees | Contour | 40 |
| | Tc-99m WBC (20) | LEHR | 360 degrees | 128 | 3 degrees | Contour | 20 |
| | Ga-67 citrate (5) | MEGP | 360 degrees | 64 | 6 degrees | Contour | 40 |
| Myocardial perfusion | Tl-201 chloride (3.5) | LEGP | 180 degrees[b] | 64 | 3 degrees | Circle | 30 |
| | Tc-99m sestamibi | | | | | | |
| | Rest (8) | LEHR | 180 degrees[b] | 64 | 3 degrees | Circle | 25 |
| | Stress or 2-day test (25) | LEHR | 180 degrees[b] | 64 | 3 degrees | Circle | 20 |

[a] LEGP, low-energy general purpose; LEHR, low-energy high-resolution; MEGP, medium-energy general purpose.
[b] 180 degrees in single- or dual-headed devices, 360 degrees with triple-headed devices.
MDP, methylene diphosphonate; TMJ, temporomandibular joint; SC, sulfur colloid; RBC, red blood cell; HMPAO, hexamethylpropyleneamide oxime (Ceretec); ECD, bicisate (Neurolite); MOAB, monoclonal antibody; WBC, white blood cell.
Source: Data from General Electric recommendations and other sources.

tions each of short duration can be acquired, and the data summed in orbits where no movement occurs. If movement occurs, the data sets collected before the movement can be combined, and those subject to movement can be discarded.

*Pixel size* is the useful FOV of the camera divided by the matrix size. The acquisition matrix size is typically $64 \times 64$ and occasionally $128 \times 128$, but when the $128 \times 128$ matrix is selected for improved spatial resolution the number of counts acquired must be increased by a factor of 4 to retain similar count-rate statistics in each pixel (Table 24-1). Note that this count requirement is somewhat smaller when circular crystals are used because the total number of pixels is less. Because of the reprojection process and the redistribution of counts along the entire ray sum because the actual photon source is not known, and the subsequent removal of some pixels by filtering, the images obtained with circular crystals are even noisier than Poisson statistics alone would suggest, resulting in even higher statistical uncertainty in SPECT images.

The angular sampling requirement is important because inadequate sampling (fewer projection profiles used in reconstruction) results in streak artifacts (due to aliasing). The number of angles required is usually $2\pi$ times the number of resolution units across the image.

The acquisition matrix size should be large enough that the pixel size is no more than half the spatial resolution of the tomographic device. With zooming, smaller matrices can be used for imaging small organs. In the reconstruction process, the pixel size should be the same as that used in the acquisition matrix (11).

If the radionuclide used is activity limited (e.g., thallium 201 [Tl-201] and other non–Tc-99m radiopharmaceuticals), the patient must be immobile for a long time, and patient motion may limit the potential resolution gains of the increased matrix size (decreased individual pixel size). As the number of planar images (orbital increments of the detector head) increases, the time for each acquisition must be held constant to maintain adequate statistics, so the total acquisition time increases proportionally. The individual equipment manufacturer provides practical suggestions for acquisition parameters for each radiopharmaceutical and organ imaged, including the necessary compromises (Table 24-2).

### Single-Head Systems

For a single-head system, 120 (liver, bone) or 60 (brain, heart) individual planar images are obtained at 3- or 6-degree increments around the organ of interest for subsequent reconstruction into SPECT images. In cardiac studies, 180-degree acquisitions are performed (12), with the recognition that this is a compromise that is unique for the eccentrically placed heart in the thorax. It is said that the time advantage of 180-degree SPECT and increased image contrast (most of the profiles acquired contain the heart) makes this acquisition practical. However, the 180-degree technique may result in distortion and artifacts not seen with 360-degree acquisitions.

### Multidetector Systems

For a 180-degree SPECT study of the myocardium, one optimal configuration is two detectors arranged 90 degrees apart. In this system, the full 180-degree orbit may be acquired in half the time with only 90 degrees of motion (20,21). For triple-headed gamma cameras, 360-degree acquisitions are used, with each detector moving 120 degrees during acquisition (21).

A significant advantage of 360-degree acquisitions is the potential for obtaining the arithmetic or geometric mean (square root of the product of opposing ray sums), which can be helpful in preprocessing attenuation correction algorithms. A triple-headed SPECT system has improved sensitivity for the same acquisition time as single- or dual-headed systems, and ultra–high-resolution collimators can be used that have a spatial resolution of 7.5 mm at a radius of rotation of 15 cm (10,11). Another advantage of multidetector systems is the ability to perform emission and transmission studies simultaneously (see Attenuation Correction).

## Image Reconstruction

An image reconstruction algorithm is required to take the measured projection planar images (with counts in x and y coordinates, i.e., spatial domain) and reconstruct them into a three-dimensional (3D) image for clinical use. The most popular reconstruction method is the FBP or Fourier method (10,11), which transforms the acquired projection sets into the frequency domain (defined below). This is done because of computational advantages that come from processing data in the frequency domain. Therefore, routine SPECT reconstruction is relatively simple compared to more complex iterative algorithms that are being developed for quantitative SPECT.

### Spatial Versus Frequency Domain

Any function may be considered in two ways. One is the form of a graph where the function $f(x)$ is plotted on one axis and the value along the other axis. This is referred to as the *spatial* domain. The other way is to represent the function as the sum of different periodic functions (sines and cosines) of differing frequencies, amplitudes, and phases. Any wave from a simple square wave to very complex waveforms can be represented successfully in the *frequency* domain. This can be displayed as a spectrum that plots amplitude versus frequency (Fig. 24-6) and has the advantage of being readily manipulated mathematically. The image in the spatial domain is familiar to us, but when it is transformed into the frequency domain, it no longer looks anything like the original image.

## Uniform Source in Matrix

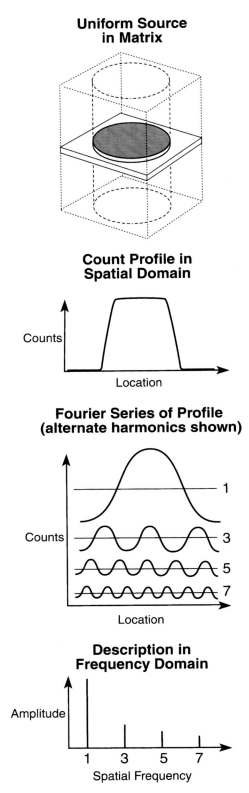

**Count Profile in Spatial Domain**

Counts

Location

**Fourier Series of Profile (alternate harmonics shown)**

Counts

1

3

5

7

Location

**Description in Frequency Domain**

Amplitude

1    3    5    7

Spatial Frequency

**FIG. 24-6.** A uniform source and a squarish waveform in the slice profile are shown above the combination of cosine waves of the fundamental frequency and harmonics that can recreate the waveform. The simple frequency and amplitude spectrum (bottom) contains all the parameters needed to describe the frequency domain of the waveform and source.

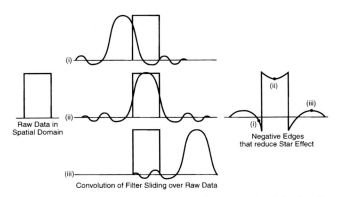

(i)

Raw Data in Spatial Domain

(ii)

(iii)

Convolution of Filter Sliding over Raw Data

(ii)

(iii)

(i)

Negative Edges that reduce Star Effect

**FIG. 24-7.** The raw square wave is shown on the left, the filter convolution is shown being passed over the square wave (but done in the frequency domain), with resultant negative tails that sharpen the edge in the reconstruction process.

These manipulations include convolutions, which are simply multiplications in the frequency domain (Fig. 24-7). Such manipulations in the spatial domain would be very complicated and relatively more time-consuming.

The Fourier transformation is a mathematical way of relating these two forms of the function. By use of the Fourier transform, the various frequency components (frequency, amplitude, phase) can be found for a function in the spatial domain. Figure 24-8 shows the inverse transformation for the common ramp filter used in FBP. The inverse Fourier transform takes a series of periodic functions in the frequency domain and "puts them together" to create the function in the spatial domain.

When considering an image in nuclear medicine, one usually refers to the number of counts per pixel or the number of counts per unit time. Thus, the number of counts may be considered as a function of distance or time. This would be a representation in the spatial (or time) domain. It is also possible (though much less intuitive) to consider an image in the frequency domain. In this domain, one considers how "fast," or how "much," the number of counts changes from pixel to pixel (a measure of frequency). The Fourier transformation can be used to relate these two means of looking at the image and can be used to look at an image in terms of different frequency components, which can then be easily manipulated.

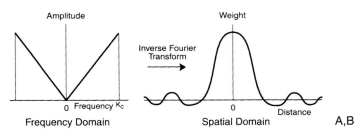

Amplitude

Weight

Inverse Fourier Transform

0   Frequency $K_c$

0         Distance

Frequency Domain

Spatial Domain

A,B

**FIG. 24-8.** The simple ramp filter is displayed in the frequency domain **(A)** and in the spatial domain **(B)**. This transition between the frequency and spatial domain is achieved through Fourier transformation. $K_c$ is the frequency where the filter cuts to zero.

The advantage of the frequency domain is that certain frequencies typically contain the background while other frequencies contain the noise components that we desire to eliminate from our scans. The more uniform background activity is represented by lower frequencies. The frequency domain component of noise, which varies from pixel to pixel in the projection image, is represented by higher frequencies. Unfortunately, the high-frequency values of the frequency spectrum also contain many of the important image details and edges important in image formation.

### Backprojection

The SPECT projection data are stored as sinograms, with each portion of the sinogram representing the projection data acquired at each stop around a particular slice (*n*) of the source volume (Figs. 24-9 and 24-10). There are as many sinograms stored as there are slices, that is, 64 in a 64 × 64 matrix, 128 in a 128 × 128 matrix.

If the measured projection values from a point source are simply backprojected along their acquisition trajectories, then because the assumption is made that the detected photon sources are evenly spread along the ray sum (22), the

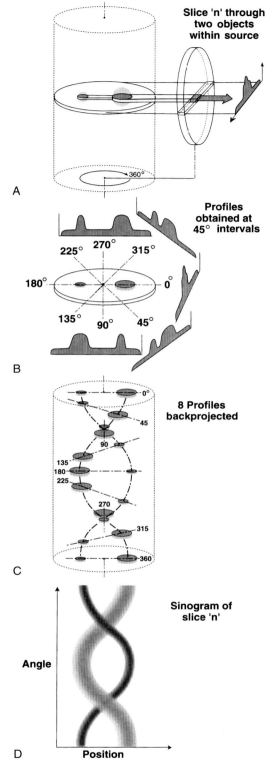

**FIG. 24-9.** The creation of a sinogram for a single slice of the object source with two rounded hot spots (one large, one small) **(A)**. In this display, the projection profiles are obtained at 45-degree increments **(B)** and reprojected into a 3D volume **(C)**, thus making the familiar sinogram **(D)**. For each slice of the object there is an appropriate sinogram. The final image is reconstructed from the sum of all sinograms.

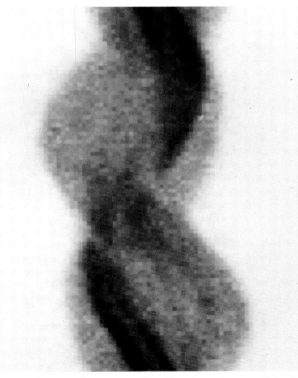

**FIG. 24-10.** This sinogram of a slice through a cardiac study was acquired on a triple-headed detector system (TRIAD, Trionix, Cleveland, OH). The dark portion is the cardiac uptake, the lighter represents hepatic activity in the sinogram slice displayed.

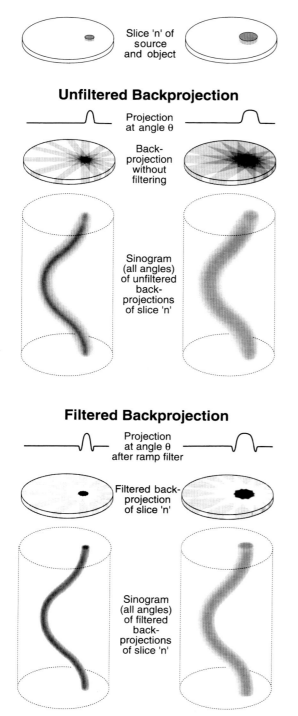

## Unfiltered Backprojection

Slice 'n' of source and object

Projection at angle θ

Back-projection without filtering

Sinogram (all angles) of unfiltered back-projections of slice 'n'

## Filtered Backprojection

Projection at angle θ after ramp filter

Filtered back-projection of slice 'n'

Sinogram (all angles) of filtered back-projections of slice 'n'

**FIG. 24-11.** This figure is similar to Fig. 24-4, with the addition of the unfiltered profile and subsequent sinogram (unfiltered backprojection); below the projection data is modified by the ramp filter and a filtered and backprojected sinogram (filtered backprojection) is obtained. The ramp filter function results in "deblurring" of the sinogram. This deblurring is achieved by the negative edges of the spatial domain representation of the ramp filter (see Fig. 24-7), which subtracts the tails of the backprojection nearest the reconstructed image of the sources to sharpen the image of the object. The sinogram confirms this sharpening, and the image reconstructed from the multiple sinograms will also be sharper.

reconstructed image looks like a number of lines or columns that intersect centrally (see Fig. 24-4). When a more complex data source (e.g., brain perfusion image) is backprojected, there is a large central blob where these wide columns intersect. The superimposition of these reconstructed profiles does not reproduce the radioactive source accurately, leaving "star" artifacts and significant background activity in the reconstructed image. The application of the ramp filter results in elimination of much of the star effect about the source by restoring the edge features lost in the backprojection process (Fig. 24-11).

Because of noise and statistical fluctuations associated with radioactive decay, compounded by acquisition compromises, such as suboptimal sampling inevitable in SPECT and the effects of attenuation, scatter, and collimator and detector constraints, the ramp filter alone does not result in an acceptable reconstructed image of the source. This is compounded because both noise and fine anatomic details are located in the high spatial frequency range, so appropriate additional filters must be used to optimize the image while suppressing noise.

### Filters

If one could eliminate (or reduce) the undesirable low- and high-frequency components of an image, one would be able to lessen the effects of background and noise. This is the task of a filter: to reduce image components of "undesirable" frequency. The major problem with simply "eliminating" high-frequency noise components is that image detail (such as edges) is also a high-frequency component of the image because the number of counts may "change rapidly" at an edge. Thus, a filter must be chosen to eliminate high-frequency noise but not high-frequency image detail. Such a tradeoff is in practice quite difficult to accomplish.

The basic method of action of a filter is relatively simple. Because an image can be treated as a sum of different-frequency components, if one multiplies each frequency component by a certain value and then recreates the image (by inverse Fourier transformation) one can control how much weight each frequency component has. Filters are characterized as *low-pass* if they reduce high frequencies and allow the lower frequencies to pass (Fig. 24-12). To do this, filters set the high frequencies to zero or a small number to minimize these in an image.

A *high-pass* filter emphasizes the higher frequencies (see Fig. 24-12). The ramp filter is the most common high-pass filter used in nuclear medicine and other imaging FBP methods. The most common low-pass filters in use are the Hamming, Hanning, Butterworth, and Parzen filters. The Parzen window tends to emphasize somewhat lower frequencies than the Hamming or Hanning windows (and may be better for low-count studies such as a Ga-67 scan). The Butterworth filter tends to emphasize somewhat higher frequencies (and is better for higher-count studies or studies of organs and diseases that need higher spatial resolution, such as the brain and the heart).

## Original Waveform

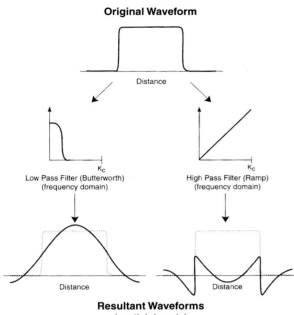

**FIG. 24-12.** Here the original square waveform (top) is filtered by the ramp function on the right, which emphasizes the edges by the enhancement of the high-frequency components. A low-pass filter enhances the lower frequencies and therefore assumes a sinusoidal shape (left). The effect of these filters is shown in the resultant waveforms in the spatial domain. ($K_c$, cutoff frequency.)

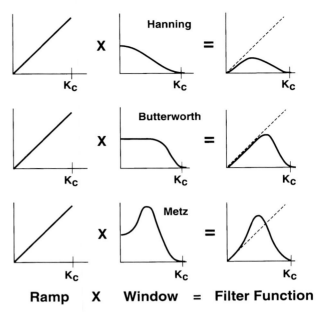

**Ramp  X  Window  =  Filter Function**

**FIG. 24-13.** Combination of the ramp and "window" filters (simply multiplied together in the frequency domain) to produce commonly used filter functions. The Hanning filter enhances the lower and middle frequencies, and the Butterworth filter enhances the higher frequencies. The Metz filter actually amplifies the midrange frequencies, as seen when the filter function is compared to the dotted ramp function. ($K_c$, cutoff frequency.)

Some guidelines (provided by General Electric, Waukesha, WI, and other equipment suppliers) are given in Table 24-3. The Hamming and Hanning window functions are very similar and some use them interchangeably, but the Hanning window is actually a specific form of the Hamming window with one of the coefficients in the mathematical description being set equal to 0.5.

It is very common to combine a ramp filter with one of the low-pass filters (by multiplying them together) to create a form of *band-pass* filter, which emphasizes frequencies within a certain range and minimizes the high and low frequencies. This is often termed a *window* function. For example, a ramp filter is combined with a Hanning window to produce a ramp-Hanning filter (Fig. 24-13). The resulting band-pass filter acts to suppress low-frequency background

**TABLE 24-3.** *General data reconstruction guidelines for commonly performed SPECT studies*

| Study | Radionuclide | Slice thickness (pixels) | Suggested window function | Frequency cutoff (critical; cm⁻¹) | Power | Attenuation correction |
|---|---|---|---|---|---|---|
| Bone | Tc-99m MDP | 1–2 | Hanning | 0.7–0.8 | — | No |
| | Alternative | 1–2 | Butterworth | 0.4–0.5 | 15 | No |
| Liver | Tc-99m SC | 1–2 | Butterworth | 0.4 | 10 | Optional |
| | Tc-99m RBC | 1–2 | Hanning | 0.7–0.8 | — | — |
| Brain | Tc-99m HMPAO/ECD | 1 | Butterworth | 0.4 | 10 | Optional |
| Tumor or abscess | Ga-67 citrate | 2 | Butterworth | 0.3 | 5–10 | Optional |
| | In-111 MOAB/peptide | 2 | Butterworth | 0.5 | 5–10 | Optional |
| | Tc-99m MOAB fragment | 1–2 | Butterworth | 0.4–0.5 | 5 | Optional |
| | Tl-201 | 2 | Hanning | 0.8 | — | Optional |
| | Tc-99m sestamibi | 1–2 | Butterworth | 0.4 | 5 | Optional |
| Infection | In-111 WBC | 2 | Butterworth | 0.3 | 5–10 | No |
| | Tc-99m WBC | 1–2 | Butterworth | 0.4 | 5 | No |
| Myocardial perfusion imaging | Tl-201 chloride (stress test) | 1 | Hanning | 0.8 | — | No |
| | Tc-99m sestamibi (stress/rest) | 1 | Butterworth | 0.5 | 5 | No |

and high-frequency noise, while preserving (as much as possible) the useful image data.

### Nyquist Frequency

In the frequency domain, the number of cycles of the sine wave is described per unit distance. This means the distance can be described in terms of metric measure (centimeters) or in terms of pixel size. The pixel size is described by the crystal size (10 to 40 cm) and acquisition matrix ($64 \times 64$, or $128 \times 128$). When a pixel size is 0.5 cm, then 1 cycle per pixel and 1 cycle per 0.5 cm are equivalent descriptions of frequency units.

The Nyquist frequency is a confusing term, but it describes the frequency that can be measured with a given pixel size. To be able to measure a periodic function it must be sampled at least twice during the function period. The highest frequency that can be measured is therefore 0.5 cycle per pixel, so for a given sampling interval (pixel size) there is a limit to the frequency that can be determined, and all frequencies higher than the Nyquist frequency do not contribute to the image.

$$1.0 \text{ Nyquist} = 0.5 \text{ cycle/pixel}$$
$$= 0.5 \text{ cycle/cm (if 1 pixel = 1 cm)}$$
$$\text{or } 1.0 \text{ cycle/cm (if 1 pixel = 0.5 cm)}$$
$$\text{or } 1.5 \text{ cycles/cm (if 1 pixel = 0.33 cm)}$$

### Cutoff Frequency

Although the basic shape of a filter is set by the particular mathematical description that describes it, modifications can be introduced by the user. One of these is the cutoff frequency. This is the frequency at which the filter window is set to zero; it is a tradeoff between image noise and image spatial resolution desired. Projection data with high noise should have a low-frequency cutoff, and data with low noise should have a high-frequency cutoff. Because the Nyquist frequency is the highest frequency of possible use, there is no point to making the cutoff frequency any higher, but it usually may be set to any lower value. The lower the cutoff frequency is set, the more high-frequency image components are eliminated, causing a smoother image (and lowering the image resolution). For example, if the filter is set at 0.2, then 80% of the upper frequencies are discarded.

### Butterworth Filter

The Butterworth filter window is a special case in that there are two user-selectable modifications. The critical frequency is defined as the frequency at which the window value is 0.707 (i.e., $1/\sqrt{2}$) and is similar in function to the cutoff frequency. Just as with the cutoff frequency, lowering the critical frequency produces a smoother image.

The order of a particular Butterworth filter window is changed by altering an exponent in the mathematical description; this defines how quickly the window value falls (steepness of the slope). This, in turn, determines how much weight certain low and midrange frequencies have. Higher orders produce smoother images.

### Preconstruction Versus Postreconstruction Filtering

Filtering can be performed before reconstruction (preconstruction) or after reconstruction (postreconstruction). The prereconstruction filter is most frequently used because it is done rapidly in the frequency domain. Filtering done after reconstruction is preferable because the statistical variations are potentially reduced in the reconstructed image that uses all the combined projections, but it requires extensive computational capacity and so is not widely used.

### Restoration Filtering

Restoration filters are sometimes used and have frequency values in excess of unity in the low and mid ranges, but the usual cutoff is in the high-frequency range. Therefore, if noise is low and maximum spatial resolution is desired, one can try a Wiener or Metz filter (see Fig. 24-12).

The selection parameters for SPECT filters are quite critical, and they include the following:

- Radiopharmaceutical (photon abundance)
- Organ (radiopharmaceutical uptake)
- Normal anatomy (e.g., the rapid normal changes in the brain due to perfusion differences in white and gray matter)
- Disease process (small vs. large defects)
- Other constraints of data acquisition (patient obesity or patient movement)

Each manufacturer supplies suggestions for which filter should be used for each scanning device and procedure (see Table 24-3), but the user must decide when to vary these suggestions to suit the particular patient and image viewed. It is very likely that the perception of a reader for an optimal image is a function of experience with image interpretation. This influences the selected tradeoff between spatial resolution and smoothing of images.

### Attenuation Correction

The issue of attenuation correction for SPECT has been discussed by many in the recent past (10,19). In Chapter 23, the interactions of radiation with matter are fully discussed. Effective atomic numbers, physical densities, linear attenuation coefficients, and half-value layers for Tl-201 and Tc-99m in air, muscle, lung, and bone are presented in Table 24-4 (19). It is important to point out that if the attenuator is made up of a number of different mate-

**TABLE 24-4.** *Effective atomic number, physical density, and linear attenuation coefficient (HVL) for various materials for Tl-201 73 keV and Tc-99m 140 keV photons*

|  | Air | Lung | Muscle | Bone |
|---|---|---|---|---|
| Effective atomic number | 7.6 | 7.4 | 7.4 | 13.8 |
| Density (g/cm³) | 0.0013 | 0.33 | 1.0 | 1.85 |
| µ for Tl-201 | 0.0002 | 0.063 | 0.191 | 0.479 |
| HVL for 73 keV | 3,465 | 11.0 | 3.6 | 1.45 |
| µ for Tc-99m | 0.0002 | 0.051 | 0.153 | 0.286 |
| HVL* for Tc-99m | 3,465 | 13.6 | 4.5 | 2.4 |

*HVL = cm⁻¹.

rials, the attenuation of photons is a function of the sum of attenuation coefficients for each material that the photons pass through times its thickness. This effect is common to TCT, SPECT, and PET techniques. Before backprojection, data needs to be corrected for attenuation because, for each centimeter of tissue, 15% of Tc-99m photons are attenuated. Without this correction, as much as three-fourths of the counts of a large deeper organ (e.g., liver) are not recorded.

In SPECT, the attenuation depends on the amount of absorber between the detector and the point source producing the photon. The source can be located anywhere within the FOV, and the actual photon absorption and required attenuation correction vary according to this origin. The FBP reconstruction technique is based on the assumption that the measured photon source can be located anywhere through the object and that the photon has an equal probability of arising from any part of the ray sum. This assumption invalidates attenuation correction in conventional FBP reconstruction of all but uniform-source distributions, but some approximations are possible.

### Uniform Attenuation

In preprocessing attenuation correction methods, conjugate counting techniques are used to produce the geometric mean to correct for body thickness. These methods work when attenuation is uniform through the body and the source distribution is also uniform. A postprocessing attenuation correction method developed by Chang assumes known body contours and a uniform attenuation coefficient; it works well with small point sources (23). The data are first subject to FBP, then every point in the image is corrected by the attenuation coefficient to obtain the first-order corrected image. This is reprojected to generate new projection data. This process continues with production of new projection data, calculation of error projections, and repeated backprojection and attenuation correction. With noisy data, this process is limited to one or two iterations. The method has been clinically successful but has never resulted in quantitative SPECT.

### Nonuniform Attenuation

The compensation for organs in the chest demands algorithms that include nonuniform attenuation because of the large differences in attenuation that occur with different tissues (see Table 24-4). An effective method is the Chang algorithm, which includes the actual attenuation distribution in the calculation of the correction factor. This is fast, and good accuracy is achieved with a single iteration. Iterative reconstruction methods used in quantitative SPECT can also do this type of attenuation correction well; they are discussed below in Quantitative SPECT.

### Compton Scatter Correction

Scatter is the second most important problem with SPECT and is inexorably linked with attenuation. Furthermore, deeper regions in the patient, which are most attenuated, have much more scatter contribution in the detected rays. Without scatter correction, quantitation and optimal image reconstruction is difficult. The major effect of Compton scatter on SPECT imaging is to effectively reduce contrast. Scattered photons that undergo small-angle or moderate-angle scatter lose only a small amount of energy and are detected in the photopeak window, effectively causing blurring of the image. This is especially so because photoelectric absorption of Tc-99m photons in tissue is low (<1%), and Compton scatter is the major photon-tissue interaction. As described in Chapter 23, these scattered photons form a significant proportion of events accepted by the pulse-height discriminator. Photons that are scattered multiple times or are scattered at large angles lose enough energy to render them suitable to rejection by pulse-height analysis. In a typical 20% Tc-99m window, single scatter events of up to a 50-degree angle are accepted in the photopeak, and a significant number of photons that scatter twice are also accepted. This is especially so in Tl-201 scans, in which a 28% window is typically used to include the various 69- to 80-keV characteristic x-rays, and as many as 40% to 60% of detected photons in the photopeak window are actually scattered photons. In older camera systems with photopeak resolution of 12% to 15% (FWHM), narrowing the window reduces sensitivity significantly because many true photoelectric events are also not detected in the narrower windows. Newer cameras with 8% to 10% FWHM energy resolution have lower proportions of scatter angles accepted in the photopeak. If energy resolution was capable of 3% further, scatter correction would be unnecessary.

The scattered photons primarily lie in the lower half of the photopeak window because they lose energy during the scatter process. This energy loss can be used to help correct for the scatter process, and if multiple energy windows are created, the lower photopeak windows can be used to assess scatter. This is the principal design feature used by equipment manufacturers to reject scatter. One method of scatter correction is to use an asymmetric window, using only the higher unscattered portion of the window in image construction. Narrowing the window can have dramatic effects in the performance of a camera system, because although narrowing the acceptance window improves scatter rejection, this can be accompanied by very significant sensitivity losses, and gamma camera systems perform differently with off-peak settings (see Fig. 23-14).

The most common approach to deal with the scatter problem is to use the counts measured simultaneously in one or more energy windows located at other positions within the spectrum (24–26). These techniques estimate the distribution of scattered photons in the photopeak, which can then be corrected. The imaging device must be robust enough to provide excellent spatial alignment (registration) between the photopeak and scatter data and to provide excellent detector uniformity with these off-peak settings. Published scatter correction methods most commonly use from 1 to 32 windows acquired simultaneously to encompass the photopeak. The parameters that characterize these procedures are the number, location, and width of energy windows used and the modeling-enabling estimation of the photopeak scatter. The dual energy window subtraction technique (25) consists of subtracting a fraction of the image data recorded within a lower energy window from the image data recorded within the primary photopeak energy window. This method is affected by varying source geometries as well as the characteristics of the imaging system, that is, the energy resolution and actual settings of the two energy windows (27).

### Partial Volume Effects

The partial volume effect is well known to TCT users and is just as important in ECT (20). This phenomenon results in a decrease in detected radionuclide counts for object sizes less than twice the spatial resolution. For example, assuming that SPECT has a spatial resolution of 1.5 cm for cardiac studies, it is impossible that SPECT can measure endocardial (~3 mm) or epicardial (~3 mm) myocardial counts.

### Quantitative SPECT

There is an ongoing attempt to develop quantitative SPECT imaging techniques by all equipment manufacturers. Any method that helps in the development of quantitation also improves routine SPECT image quality by improving image resolution and contrast. This is achieved despite the facts that tomographic nuclear imaging generally results in noisier images than planar views and that SPECT resolution is poorer than planar resolution.

Although it is agreed that quantitation methods improve SPECT imaging, it is important that clinical users do not use these modifications if they cannot recognize the artifacts associated with the new methods. Institutions without in-house physicists might be better served by concentrating on quality control (QC) procedures to improve SPECT image quality rather than incorporating newer quantitation tech-

niques. However, as more and more manufacturers develop these methods, they will become incorporated into standard nuclear medicine practice with adequate manufacturer-suggested safeguards and QC (28).

The trend in research toward quantitation has been associated with hardware and software improvements in gamma camera technology. Manufacturers now offer (28) analog-to-digital converters at each photomultiplier tube ("digital" cameras) and nonuniform attenuation correction, scatter correction, and resolution recovery techniques. For attenuation correction, most manufacturers appear to be offering line sources (25 to 800 mCi [825 to 29,600 MBq] gadolinium 153 [Gd-153]) for calculating simultaneous or sequential transmission attenuation maps, using a variety of iterative (maximum likelihood expectation minimization [MLEM], iterative preconstruction with ordered subsets expectation minimization [OSEM], and FBP with iterative corrections [Chang]) algorithms. Double-, triple-, and multiple-window scatter correction methods are now offered, and several manufacturers offer quantitative brain and gated myocardial SPECT programs for clinical use (28). This demonstrates the rapid progression of SPECT research techniques into the clinical field.

### Iterative Reconstruction Methods

Iterative reconstruction techniques have been available since 1974 (29). The major strategy for these techniques is the inclusion of models of the imaging process to compensate for system degradations, such as the effects of scatter, attenuation, and camera system response characteristics. The computationally less demanding FBP method in general clinical use cannot correct for all these parameters.

The reconstruction and image restoration in SPECT is performed by two general methods. Both methods require that in each projection slice the photon source in the body at a given angle results in an event detected at a particular pixel in the camera detector. To create an image from projection data, the equation below must be solved:

$$P_i = \Sigma w_{ij} Y_j, \qquad (1)$$

where $P_i$ is the projection data for slice at angle $i$, $Y_j$ is the activity in pixel $j$, and $w_{ij}$ is the weighting factor of the contribution of pixel $j$ to the projection $i$. Note that this solution can only account for processes that occur in the projection ray, and the weighting factors are constant (equally weighted) along the entire length of the ray. FBP is a member of the class of solution that assumes the photon source can occur anywhere along the projection ray and that reprojects the data with the probability distributed equally along the backprojection ray. This means that during the reconstruction process one cannot account for photon scatter or attenuation.

If

$$P_i = \Sigma C_{ij} Y_j, \qquad (2)$$

$C_{ij}$ is now the weighting factor of $w_{ij}$ of equation 1, $C_{ij}$ can now include the effect of the physics of radioactive decay, interaction of photons with matter, detector response, and scatter in and out of the projection ray. A model of attenuation, scatter, and detector response can be included in the reconstruction, and it allows for quantitation and improved images. This can be done by an iterative process, in which the collected data are repeatedly recalculated against a model that includes the physics, a presumed body configuration, and an assumed radiopharmaceutical distribution (often considered uniform). This process matches the initial measured reconstructed image projections to the model-estimated projection of the object source distribution, the imaging process, and the image-degrading factors. In this circumstance, the $C_{ij}$ is different from $w_{ij}$ used in FBP because the physics solutions are included. The weighting factor $C_{ij}$ can now differ for each potential site of photon origin in the body (rather than being distributed equally along ray sum) and for each crystal interaction according to various physical or distribution hypotheses (e.g., to allow for nonuniform attenuation, as occurs in the chest).

Using various statistical tests, the difference between the actual measured data and the model is used to update the initial estimated image, which is then used to create a new set of data for comparison with the measured data. This is repeated (iterated) until there is a minimal difference between the original measured and continuously calculated data. Compensation for the image-degrading effects is included in the projection and backprojection steps of the iterative reconstruction algorithm. The important SPECT problems (attenuation and scatter) can be directly incorporated into the algorithms, something that cannot be done with FBP techniques.

The major problem with this technique is the extensive computational requirements, which explain why early iterative reconstruction methods on CT scanners were replaced by FBP methods. The first head CT scanners used iterative reconstruction techniques and created uniform attenuation throughout the FOV by the use of water bags applied to the patient's skull, which made the computations simpler. Computers now allow the use of iterative approaches, and they are quickly being incorporated by gamma camera manufacturers.

Another limitation is that many of these iterative techniques (e.g., MLEM) are sensitive to the initial solution. Why not start with the FBP and then apply iterative techniques? If this is done, the initial FBP artifacts persist. In practice, in the iterative approach, the reconstructed image is used to calculate an estimate of the measured sinogram. The measured sinogram is compared with the calculated sinogram. The image pixel values are iteratively adjusted until the difference between the calculated and measured sinogram reaches an acceptable minimum value.

In the MLEM method, the data are adjusted to maximize a likelihood function, using the calculated and observed values of the projection data to evaluate the function. At the present time, most commercial vendors of SPECT systems that incorporate nonuniform attenuation correction methods use iterative reconstruction methods (28). MLEM is computationally

intensive, but a new method that offers interesting possibilities is the OSEM (30), in which the projection data are divided into subsets, thus allowing significant computer time saving.

### Attenuation Correction

Attenuation methods can assume that attenuation is constant through the portion of the body imaged (e.g., the head), but this assumption is not always valid. Measured attenuation compensation is readily incorporated into iterative reconstruction quantitative SPECT. An attenuation coefficient map or image must be created, and it may be defined by gamma ray CT using a transmission source.

The attenuation data (the transmission scan) must be obtained simultaneously or sequentially with the emission data (31). This prevents misregistration errors between transmission and emission data sets. Transmission imaging consists of positioning a source of radiation on one side of the patient and a detector on the other side to measure the transmitted intensity. By taking the ratio of the transmitted intensity to the intensity without the patient present ("blank" scans), the transmitted fraction (TF) is computed. The linear attenuation coefficient μ is determined by Equation 3:

$$\mu = \frac{\ln\left(\frac{1}{TF}\right)}{X}, \tag{3}$$

where $X$ is the attenuator thickness. The reconstruction algorithm can now include the attenuation for each pixel. Crossover corrections are needed to correct cross-contamination of the transmission and emission data.

For SPECT to be quantitative, one needs to account for attenuation by calculating a map showing the spatial distribution of attenuation coefficients in any region of interest (ROI). A method that uses fan-beam collimators with a stationary line source is available from Picker as a simultaneous transmission-emission protocol (STEP). Many other manufacturers are preparing similar systems for market. In these systems, three-headed scanners are used with line sources of either Gd-153, cobalt 57 (Co-57), or Tc-99m and an iterative reconstruction algorithm.

Photons can be attenuated by structures, such as breast tissue, that result in variation in sensitivity with site of emission, so an outline of the body contour is required. Manglos et al. (32,33) demonstrated anisotropic (not equal in all directions or three dimensions) attenuation caused by variations in the depth of the source (resulting in different photon path lengths) and depth-dependent (nonstationary) spatial resolution that occurs in gamma cameras. These deficiencies of the imaging system result in geometric distortion of imaged objects that are greater in 180-degree reconstructions than 360-degree reconstructions (34). Besides attenuation, there also occurs enhancement of count densities in areas close to regions with high counts as a result of scatter effects.

## Compton Scatter

The attenuation problem is increased by Compton scatter. When photons undergo Compton scattering, they change direction and lose an amount of energy proportional to the scatter angle. These photons can scatter out of the ray sum, and other photons can scatter into the ray sum. The effect of Compton scattering (19) is to modify the equation for TF that is used to describe attenuation of photons from

$$TF = e^{-\mu X}, \qquad (4)$$

where $\mu$ is the linear attenuation coefficient and $X$ is the thickness of the attenuator, to

$$TF = B(\mu X)^{e^{-\mu x}}, \qquad (5)$$

where $B$ is the buildup factor or relative increase in counts due to scattered photons.

The fraction of scattered photons added to photopeak events is a function of location of the radioactive source in the attenuator, the geometry and composition of the attenuator, photon energy, energy resolution of the detector, and energy window used for imaging (19). In sum, the photopeak spectrum at each voxel (volume unit) needs to be computed before reconstruction and incorporation into the reconstruction process.

This energy loss associated with scatter can be used to help correct for the scatter process, and if multiple energy windows are created (24–26), the lower-energy ones can be used to assess and correct for scatter. Ichihara et al. (35) reported a triple-energy window (TEW) scatter compensation method for determining position-dependent Compton scatter. The method estimated the count of primary photons at each pixel in the acquired images using a 24% main window centered at the photopeak energy and 3-keV windows on both sides of the main window. Clinical projection data are acquired in two windows, and the scatter components can be removed from each pixel. This method, or a similar methodology, is being evaluated for use in current systems that have quantitative SPECT capability.

## SPECT Quality Control

As described in Chapter 23, the user is required to perform QC by several organizations, including the Joint Commission on Accreditation of Healthcare Organizations, the U.S. Food and Drug Administration, and the Bureau of Radiological Health, but none indicate a particular QC protocol to follow. Each user's practice should be established individually with input from the manufacturers, who know their machines best and provide standards that are designed to protect them from product liability laws. These companies provide adequate QC parameters to achieve this protection.

Graham (36) has addressed this topic recently, and a suggested QC schedule is provided in Table 24-5. Usually, commercial manufacturers' recommendations concerning

**TABLE 24-5.** *QC testing and intervals*

| | |
|---|---|
| Energy peaking | Daily |
| Extrinsic uniformity (flood) | Daily |
| Intrinsic bar phantom | Weekly |
| Center of rotation | Monthly |
| Uniformity correction map (all collimators used) | Monthly |
| Multipurpose phantom | Monthly |
| Pixel sizing | Quarterly |
| Line source resolution | Quarterly |
| Detector head alignment | Quarterly |

SPECT acquisition, reconstruction, and QC are best followed. These recommendations vary with the organ imaged, radiopharmaceutical dose, collimation employed, acquisition matrix size, angular frequency of acquisition stops, acquisition times, as well as reconstruction method, filtering techniques, and QC procedures. QC of the gamma camera is critical for SPECT because any imperfection is magnified greatly during the tomographic reconstruction process. The basic planar QC measures are performed using more rigorous standards, and additional special QC measures must also be performed, including center of rotation (COR) correction, x and y gain calibration, and detector head alignment.

The acceptance testing procedure performed on the delivery of new equipment is essential to this QC process. It provides the opportunity to ensure that the device supplied meets the manufacturer's own specifications and forms a benchmark baseline for future clinical QC methods. Testing should include the collimator, which is especially important in SPECT, particularly the high-resolution devices where minor construction hole alignment aberrations can result in major reconstruction misalignments. These image distortions often produce abnormalities in normal patient organ images. In a small user practice, it would probably be wise to employ the services of a consultant physicist to oversee the acceptance testing (well-described National Electronic Manufacturers Association standards exist that are endorsed by medical physicist societies). This consultant can help to plan an ongoing QC program and demonstrate how to review the data specific to the equipment and clinical applications.

### Uniformity Correction

A 1% nonuniformity in the planar image can be amplified to a 20% nonuniformity in parts of the final reconstructed SPECT image. This dictates why detector uniformities of 1% are required for SPECT imaging, although 5% uniformity is sufficient for planar imaging. The photon source used for uniformity correction must itself be uniform, and statistical fluctuations in this source distribution must be sufficiently small to allow its use as the standard. Most services now use Co-57 (half-life, 270 days; 120 keV) flood-field sources, for which the manufacturer guarantees >1% uniformity. The use of Tc-99m sources (ideal for Tc-99m imaging) is compromised by Plexiglas liquid source holders that bulge slightly when filled and problems with staff irradiation associated with the daily filling and mixing of the sources.

The 30-million count requirement for SPECT uniformity correction derives from the need for each pixel to have only a 1% error for uniformity corrections of SPECT data. Poisson statistics dictate that the standard deviation (SD) of a given number of counts is the square root of the number. For the SD to reach 1% of the total counts, 10,000 counts per pixel is required. With a $64 \times 64$ square matrix, to get 10,000 counts in each pixel, a total of 40 million counts (30 million if detector is round) is required; with a $128 \times 128$ matrix, 160 million counts are required (120 million if detector is round). These acquisitions take 20 to 30 minutes, require very uniform sources, and, with multiheaded cameras, are very time-consuming. The camera must be decommissioned or the procedure done after hours because of both the time commitment and the need to prevent nearby patients with injected radiopharmaceutical influencing the acquisition. It would be ideal if the equipment service organization did uniformity correction. Currently, we have it built into the cost of the service contract, so this QC is performed without machine downtime and without external contamination from the presence of adjacent patient radioactivity.

With this calibration flood-field acquisition, the average pixel count is determined. Each individual pixel is then compared to the average to obtain a correction factor and create a uniformity correction map that can be used during the image acquisition and SPECT reconstruction process. A high-count uniformity correction is usually performed monthly, although some users prefer to do it weekly. The manufacturer's specifications should be followed, because it has data on the particular device's stability and other factors important in this decision. A lower acquisition (3 to 10 million counts) is performed daily to identify gross problems before routine clinical use.

Uniformity correction is important because any regional aberration in detector sensitivity is amplified many times during the reconstruction process. Regional variations in the center of the FOV are affected most, with the production of the worst ring artifacts (Fig. 24-14), because every reprojected ray passes through that part of the reconstructed image. Peripheral field uniformity variations are reconstructed into multiple image sites, and their effect is often not discernible. The intensity of this artifact is inversely proportional to the distance of the nonuniformity from the axis of rotation, but the axis of rotation may not be the center of the reconstructed image in off-axis organs, such as the heart. The width of the ring artifact is determined by the size of the nonuniformity, and degree of ring artifact intensity is also related to the degree of the regional defect. The ring abnormality can be either hot or cold, depending on whether the crystal-collimator nonuniformity is over- or undercorrected by the renormalization process that occurs at reconstruction.

Ring artifacts are difficult to discern in many clinical images, and in multiheaded SPECT devices the "rings" are only arcs (part of a ring) and may not be perceived even in the worst cases by even the most careful observers. Careful scrutiny of the daily flood-field data (3 to 10 million counts) and the monthly correction flood-field maps (30 to 160 million counts) is necessary. When minor abnormalities are perceived, they are often only detected with use of software programs (Fig. 24-15) to determine integral (global) uniformity, which is measured by this formula:

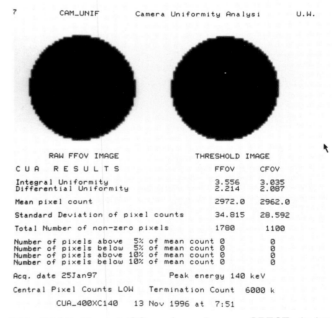

FIG. 24-15. Normal QC performed on a SPECT device shows excellent uniformity of the detector. The differential and integral uniformity is calculated using the manufacturer's (General Electric, Waukesha, WI) QC software.

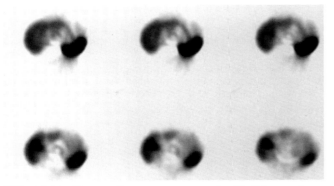

FIG. 24-14. Ring artifacts are apparent with this medium-energy acquisition of a pentetreotide study. Artifacts were due to inappropriate uniformity maps.

$$100 \times \frac{\text{Max (high) counts} - \text{min (low) counts}}{\text{Max (high) counts} + \text{min (low) counts}} \quad (6)$$

and differential (regional) uniformity, which is performed using a $5 \times 5$–pixel region and using essentially the same formula (see Fig. 24-15). These measurements are performed over the central FOV (CFOV) (25% to 30% of detector area), the useful FOV (50% to 60% of detector area), but not the peripheral area (10% to 20% of detector area). The CFOV is usually defined as having a radius (round detector) of 75% of the useful FOV (UFOV) radius. The action level of these measurements is set by the manufacturer. For the displayed instrument, the number of pixels outside the accepted range should be <8% for the free FOV and <5% for the CFOV. When these figures lie outside the recommended levels, a new field-uniformity correction map is obtained; if this results in normalization (results lower than thresholds supplied), the instrument can be used. If normalization does not occur, then service is required. These differential and integral uniformity measurements are plotted in a control chart fashion to follow QC parameters.

Although the normalization process is essential to good SPECT imaging, extreme caution must be applied to ensure that the appropriate (most recent) map is used. The most common cause of uniformity problems is the instability of the photomultiplier tubes, and daily extrinsic floods of 3 to 10 million counts reveal any significant crystal-collimator changes. This problem is particularly prevalent in infrequently used camera and radionuclide combinations.

When radionuclides other than Tc-99m are used, the ideal method would be to test the collimator-crystal combination with a liquid sheet source containing the appropriate radionuclide, such as Ga-67 or indium 111 (In-111). This is not practical for radiation safety and cost reasons, given the relatively short half-life of the radiopharmaceuticals. Some manufacturers recommend acquisition of intrinsic flood-field (uses more readily available and cheaper point sources of appropriate radionuclide) maps and extrinsic Co-57 flood fields to compute the extrinsic flood values for different energies.

### Center of Rotation

For the reconstruction process to work properly, it is important that as the detector moves around the patient, the COR of the detector orbit corresponds to the center of the matrix of pixels of the image. This is done by placing a point or line source at the COR, imaging it, then reconstructing the data to determine whether the point source is imaged in the same pixel location at all angles. Minor offsets of the COR result in mere blurring (loss of resolution) of the line source, whereas major offsets result in a ring artifact in the reconstructed image. This discrepancy in the COR testing is especially obvious when the projections are 180 degrees apart.

Small COR offsets result in blurring of the reconstructed image and are not discernible apart from otherwise unexplained resolution losses, as might occur with inadequate dose or excessive distance between the detector and patient organ. Signifi-

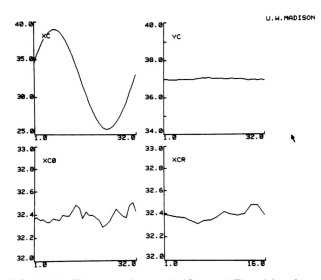

**FIG. 24-16.** This manufacturer's (General Electric) software display demonstrates that the detector is correctly aligned with expected display in the x and y axes for the degree of offset used (upper row). The display is for a $64 \times 64$ matrix and shows that the COR is at 32.4 pixels (bottom row) and no correction is required.

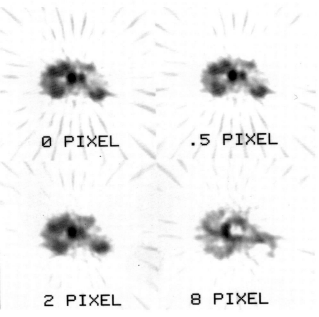

**FIG. 24-17.** This clinical pentetreotide study displays the same transaxial image with the COR deliberately offset to show the decrease in intensity of the left prevertebral lesion with the 2-pixel offset, and the bizarre image seen with an 8-pixel offset.

cant COR offsets result in unrecognizable organ images. Unrecognizable images also result from inappropriate step location assignment in multiheaded devices, where images result from misplaced projection data used in backprojection.

Each manufacturer suggests the appropriate method for determining the COR, with software packages available.

These use either a line or a point source imaged by the detector system. The COR data that correctly align the point source for backprojection reconstruction result in a sharp dot or line in the image. The manufacturer's software provides a sinogram of the point source when displayed on the x axis perpendicular to the axis of rotation, and a straight line on the axis parallel to the axis of rotation (Fig. 24-16). These protocols indicate where the display axis of rotation is and how to correct for it. The normal COR for a 64 × 64 matrix should be 32.5 pixels, and 64.5 pixels in a 128 × 128 matrix.

The display COR should be no more than 0.5 pixel from the acquisition COR, otherwise offsets should be added each time reconstruction is performed (Fig. 24-17). The machine geometry needs to be modified if the offset requirement exceeds 2 to 4 pixels.

### X and Y Gain Calibration

To calculate appropriate attenuation correction factors, attenuation correction programs require correspondence between the size of a pixel and true distances. This calibration is made when the software is installed. A pixel is typically 6 mm for a 64 × 64 matrix and a 40-cm detector head. The calibration should be checked by imaging two point sources placed a known distance apart, and then confirming how many pixels apart they are in the image.

### Detector Head Alignment

To produce accurate images, the planar views must be obtained in planes perpendicular to the camera's axis of

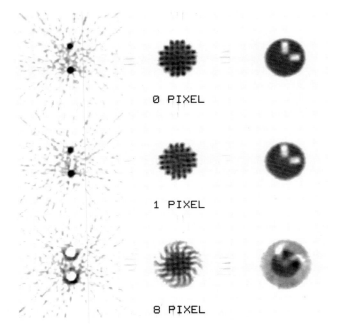

**FIG. 24-19.** For dramatic display, the effect of deliberate COR displacement on part of the same phantom in Fig. 24-18. The true image is on the top row, a 1-pixel displacement in the middle row, and 8-pixel displacement in the lowest row. The point source region of the phantom is in the left column, multiple hot sources in the middle column, and cold defects in a uniform source in the right column. The undisplaced data are fine. The 1-pixel displacement shows minimal central disarray of resolution in the view of multiple hot sources (middle). With large (8-pixel) displacements, the point sources become rings (left), and bizarre "pinwheel" shapes occur with larger sources (middle and right).

rotation, requiring proper alignment of the camera face. A 1% tilt at a distance of 14 cm from the detector produce a shift of approximately 1 pixel in a 64 × 64 matrix. Camera head tilt should be assessed quarterly. This can be done by imaging a point source, or more simply by using a carpenter's (bubble) level when the camera is at the 12 o'clock and 6 o'clock positions.

### Routine Phantom Study

An excellent method of evaluating SPECT performance is the imaging of a phantom that tests all components of the SPECT acquisition and reconstruction package (Figs. 24-18 and 24-19).

### QC for Patient Procedures

Patient motion should be assessed at each patient acquisition. This is best performed by inspection of a movie of the planar projections, a stacked transaxial 3D representation, or evaluation of the sinogram (Fig. 24-20).

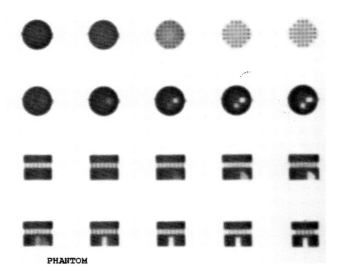

**PHANTOM**

**FIG. 24-18.** Image of a phantom shows the system is working well. Transaxial images (upper 2 rows) show good delineation of hollow tubes filled with radionuclide (upper row right) and cold defects in a hot background (second row right). In the lower two rows, the same regions in sagittal slices with the tubes and photopenic defects are again well demonstrated.

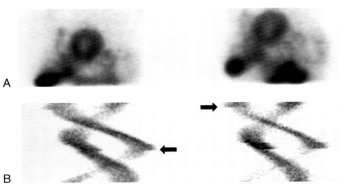

A

B

**FIG. 24-20. (A)** The first and last projections of a cardiac patient (imaged with Tc-99m sestamibi) with significant displacement of the heart due to "upward creep" during the acquisition. **(B)** The sinograms of a renal patient (imaged with Tc-99m DMSA) acquired on a dual-headed camera displayed at two different thresholds, with sudden movement toward the end of the acquisition, demonstrated by staggering (*arrows*) of the sinograms at two different sites (dual-headed camera). These movements were not identified during routine scanning acquisition despite close observation of the patient by the technical staff. In both cases, repeat acquisition provided images without artifacts.

### SPECT Imaging Artifacts

Just as in planar imaging, unique SPECT artifacts can be considered in several broad categories. All the previously described planar artifacts apply to SPECT, but the following additional artifacts also occur.

### *Diffuse Artifacts*

When imaging higher- or lower-energy radioisotopes, such as Tl-201 or In-111 and Ga-67, separate specific floods are needed for each radionuclide to produce uniformity cor-

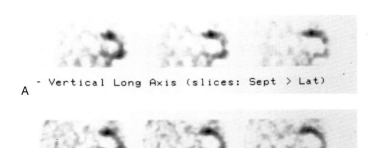

A

B

**FIG. 24-21.** Three vertical long-axis slices of a single-head SPECT Tl-201 acquisition at stress **(A)** and rest **(B)**. Note multiple symmetric cold spots, two of which are affecting the apex in the stress images. Because of changes in positioning at rest, these cold spots lie at different sites respectively in the rest and stress images.

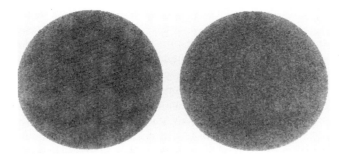

**FIG. 24-22.** When the images of Fig. 24-21 were obtained, the QC of the instrument was checked. The Tl-201 uniformity map was old (this device is rarely used for Tl-201 imaging) and now abnormal (left) and was reacquired (and normalized) on the right.

rection maps. The equipment often defaults to the Tc-99m correction table or potentially to an earlier flood of the appropriate radionuclide, and the failure to apply the appropriate translation table of the radionuclide being used produces diffuse hot and cold defects in the acquisition data. These defects are even more obvious in the reconstructed images (Fig. 24-21). To investigate this, the appropriate translation table map should be inspected, because the routine Tc-99m floods appear normal (Fig. 24-22). Eccentrically placed organ abnormalities are very difficult to recognize in this circumstance.

### *Multifocal Artifacts*

Most SPECT systems are able to cope with COR discrepancies <2 mm from the center of the matrix. COR misalignment >3 mm (typically half a pixel) significantly alters the quality of the reconstructed images. Such a SPECT acquisition malfunction can produce disastrous effects on images, making them uninterpretable. Apparent misalignment of myocardial lateral and septal walls results when the COR is incorrect, and a linear band may extend throughout the myocardium, creating an apparent defect. COR misalignment is particularly likely to occur in cardiac studies, where 180-degree acquisitions are common. The problem is inherent in the FPB process currently used in SPECT software. Hot or cold streaks also can result from COR misalignment.

### *Localized Artifacts*

The best-known cardiac focal artifact is breast attenuation. Soft-tissue attenuation results in areas of apparent decreased myocardial perfusion on cardiac SPECT studies. This is seen as an anterior or anterolateral fixed defect when caused by the breast. The severity and location of the defect depends on the thickness, density, and position of the breast. A planar view can readily delineate the breast's location and confirm the defect as breast artifact.

## SPECT IMAGING OF POSITRON EMITTERS

### High-Energy Collimators

Recently, Burt et al. (37) and Martin et al. (38) have imaged fluorine 18 (F-18) fluorodeoxyglucose (FDG) with two- or three-headed SPECT cameras fitted with high-energy collimators (39). The SPECT systems need to be capable of holding the heavy (400-lb) collimators. Such collimators, designed for 511-keV detection, are very inefficient (approximately 50% of the surface area is lead septae), so the sensitivity of the system is reduced along with even greater reductions in sensitivity that stem from the thin gamma camera crystal (91% of 140-keV photons lead to photopeak interaction in a half-inch crystal versus 17% for the 511-keV photon). Although a multiheaded SPECT unit may be 10 to 15 times less sensitive than a PET unit, the modified 511-keV SPECT units are 50 to 100 times less sensitive. This means lesions seen with 511-keV SPECT systems must have significant size (1 to 2 cm) and uptake to be detected. These devices are clinically useful in myocardial studies identifying FDG lesions and in larger oncology lesions (e.g., 2-cm solitary pulmonary nodules).

### Coincidence Detection

Another area of research is SPECT imaging of positron emissions using dual detector scintillation cameras without collimators. Image acquisition is similar to SPECT imaging, with the detectors rotating around the patient and acquiring a series of projections. These coincidence detection systems are designed to be used for conventional SPECT imaging with collimators in place. They can yield a spatial resolution in the range of 5 to 7 mm for 511-keV imaging and increased sensitivity (four times higher than that achieved with 511-keV collimated imaging).

Coincidence imaging without collimation depends on the fact that when a positron decays, two 511-keV annihilation photons are emitted simultaneously on the same line nearly 180 degrees apart. This colinear property can be used to collimate the photons by high-speed electronic timing (40), similar to PET scanner imaging. The two annihilation gamma photons derived from the positron decay (see Positron Emission Tomography, below) must interact within 10 to 15 nanoseconds to be considered coincident events. The true coincident events in PET are <1% of the single rate, which approaches 500,000 to 1,000,000 cps. Using multiple crystals in a typical PET scanner, this rate is possible, but with the two large crystals of a SPECT scanner, the current counting rate needs to be improved significantly. Many manufacturers are already working on these problems, and commercial dual purpose (PET and SPECT) scanners are being sold.

## POSITRON EMISSION TOMOGRAPHY

PET provides quantitative functional information about metabolic processes in the body. This information is

**TABLE 24-6.** *Positron-emitting radionuclides*

| | Half-life (mins) | Maximum positron energy (MeV) | Maximum positron range (mm) |
|---|---|---|---|
| F-18 | 109.7 | 0.6 | 2.4 |
| C-11 | 20.3 | 1.0 | 5.0 |
| N-13 | 10.0 | 1.2 | 5.4 |
| O-15 | 2.0 | 1.7 | 8.2 |
| Ga-68 | 68.3 | 1.9 | 9.1 |
| Rb-82 | 1.3 | 3.1 | 16.0 |

Source: Ho ZH, Chan JK, Ericksson L, et al. Positron ranges obtained from biologically important positron-emitting radionuclides. J Nucl Med 1975;16:1174–1176.

extracted from the spatial distribution of an injected radiopharmaceutical. Therefore, PET is similar to SPECT in principle, but it uses different radiopharmaceuticals and a more complex acquisition method.

PET radiopharmaceuticals contain short half-life radionuclides that decay, emitting positrons. In a few nanoseconds, these positrons migrate a short distance in tissue (Table 24-6), dissipate some of their energy, slow down, and annihilate by colliding with electrons present in the surrounding tissue. The annihilation process converts the positron-electron pair into two gamma photons, each with an energy of 511 keV. The momentum conservation principle requires that the two rays be generated along the same geometric line and diverge in opposite directions. However, a small deviation of the order of about a half degree from the common geometric line may occur due to residual kinetic energy of a

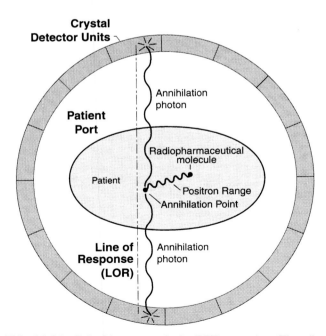

**FIG. 24-23.** Coincidence mode in PET scanning. The diagram shows the origin of positron and annihilation photons. Note that the definition of the LOR is based on the center points of two opposite detectors, but photons may interact anywhere within the detector volume.

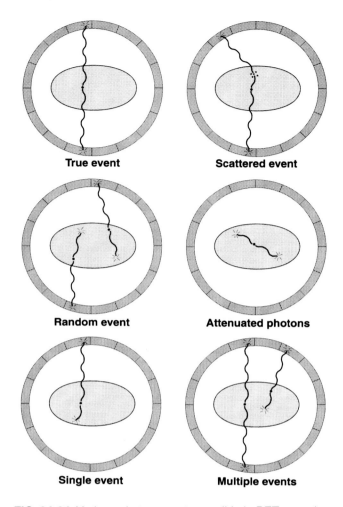

**FIG. 24-24.** Various photon events possible in PET scanning. Photons not reaching detectors represent absorbed photons, but note that random or single events can also happen when photons escape the gantry region undetected (not shown). Single and multiple events are rejected in real time during acquisition.

positron at the time of annihilation. This energy depends on the particular positron radionuclide and determines the mean free path of positrons before annihilation. The higher the residual kinetic energy, the larger the positron range and slightly larger angular deviation. Angular deviation is deviation from colinearity and has the effect of decreasing spatial resolution. The positron range also lowers spatial resolution by causing annihilation in a location at a distance from the site of the radiopharmaceutical molecule.

In modern PET scanners, the detection system has a ring of individual detector units encircling the patient on the scanner bed. Detecting one gamma photon by an individual detector is called a *single event*. Thus, two single events are needed to detect annihilation, and they have to be registered during the few nanoseconds necessary for the gamma rays to travel across the gantry. This time period, called the *coincidence window*, includes some intrinsic delay due to the nature of the detecting

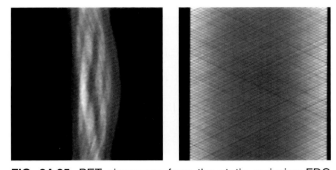

**FIG. 24-25.** PET sinograms from the static emission FDG study of the brain **(A)** and from the transmission blank scan acquired for daily QC **(B)**. Note some nonuniformities in the count distribution of the blank sinogram. They are corrected by normalization. Both sinograms were obtained on the GE Advance PET whole-body scanner.

system. Such two-photon detection is said to be in the *coincidence mode,* and the result is called a *true (coincidence) event*.

The location of two detectors involved in the true event define the direction of the *line of response* (LOR). Every LOR recorded during PET acquisition provides information about the location of the origin of radiation, and at the same time, about the radiopharmaceutical location (Fig. 24-23). Each region of the patient that contains radiopharmaceutical becomes a source of many such LORs. The number of true events along the LOR is related to the radiopharmaceutical concentration and forms the basis of quantitation.

Not all pairs of single events acquired in the period of the coincidence mode represent a single annihilation. There is always a fraction of data that comes from scattered photons and random coincidences (Fig. 24-24). These contribute to the noise and lowering of contrast in the final images, and usually some corrections are applied to minimize their impact.

The acquisition yields an array of raw PET data, called a *sinogram*, that contains the number of true events along all available LORs (Fig. 24-25). The location of the count value in the sinogram is related to the orientation of the LOR. The sinogram is raw PET data, and it has to be processed to yield an image of the radiopharmaceutical distribution. This computational processing is called *reconstruction*, and it is usually done by a dedicated, fast computer with array processors. Typically, PET images provide transaxial views, presented on a high-resolution color monitor of the computer workstation. Most PET systems provide software that also reformats the data to other orientations.

## PET Equipment

In general, every PET scanner consists of four main elements:

1. Gantry with the patient port and detecting system
2. Patient bed

3. Electronics for data processing and scanner control
4. Operator console

The detectors are scintillation crystals that convert gamma radiation into ultraviolet (UV) light connected to photomultipliers that convert the UV light into electrical signals (see Chapter 23). The kind of scintillator material greatly influences the scanner's major characteristics: sensitivity and maximum counting rate. Bismuth germanate is the most common PET scintillator because of its excellent detection efficiency of the high-energy annihilation photons and its high signal-to-noise level. Among other materials, cesium fluoride and barium fluoride have excellent time resolution capability. They are used in *time-of-flight* PET scanners, where the difference in photon arrival times is measured and used as additional information to localize the radiopharmaceutical source position along the LOR. Sodium iodide, used mostly in older scanners, has high light output but low stopping power for these high-energy annihilation photons. This scintillation material is likely used more in clinically oriented devices because of the potential dual role of SPECT and PET in some scanners.

The size of the detector crystals is one of the main factors that determine the spatial resolution of the scanner. They cannot be very small due to limitations of the photomultiplier tube diameter. Considering the circular form of the detecting ring and the finite distance between opposing crystals, the number of LORs that can be detected is greatest in the center of the gantry. Therefore, the resolution is highest in the center of the gantry and slowly decreases as the distance from the gantry center increases. This nonuniform spatial resolution through the detector volume is a result of the scanner design and cannot be avoided (see review of PET instrumentation [41]).

All PET scanners can acquire emission scans in the 2D mode, where the orientations of LORs are limited to transaxial planes or very close to them. Some newer scanners can also acquire scans in 3D mode. The angular limitation of LORs is significantly relaxed in the 3D mode, and the total counts acquired are far greater than those of an equivalent 2D scan. Therefore, a 3D scan may deliver higher-quality data than a 2D scan, or alternatively, data of similar quality can be acquired in a shorter time. 3D imaging is possible from increased axial sampling resulting from removal of septa (used in 2D acquisition mode) between the rings of detectors. It should be noted, however, that although septa removal increases the true events by 2 to 5 times, it also increases the scatter by up to 50%.

Since the early 1970s, when the first PET images were generated, PET scanners have evolved significantly. Resolution has been improved from 1 to 2 cm at that time to approximately 4 mm, which is close to the theoretical limits of approximately 1.8 mm for the head and 2 mm for the body. The detector axial width has been extended by adding more rings of detectors, and it has increased from a few cm to approximately 15 cm. Therefore, modern scanners can acquire data from the entire head or heart in a single bed position. At the same time, additional features have been introduced, such as whole-body scanning, 3D acquisition mode, quicker reconstruction times, and data processing. Several procedures have been simplified, most notably transmission scans used for attenuation correction. This is now done on the newest scanners by orbiting radioactive rods about the patient (older scanners required large cylindrical radioactive sources inserted into the gantry port). A comprehensive list of the currently available PET cameras is included in the Technology Report by University Hospital Consortium (42).

## Characterization and QC of the Detecting System

Maintaining high quality in PET scanning involves several procedures, most of which deal with quality of the detecting system. Temperature changes and aging of the detector crystals and electronics elements cause slow drift of the detection parameters. They need new characterization (also called calibration) every few weeks to few months. The several hundred detecting units comprising the PET system must have similar sensitivity, and their ability to determine locations of LORs must be well characterized to avoid image artifacts. The following parameters can be calibrated: photomultiplier gain, position mapping, energy thresholding, and coincidence window. Full calibration of a PET scanner is usually done based on the manufacturer's recommendation. Typically, it is necessary once every few months or when some parts of the detecting system are replaced.

For all detectors, small deviations from uniform response are still present after the calibrations described above. An additional correction is applied, called the *normalization procedure*. A scan of long duration (usually 12 hours) of a uniform phantom or orbiting radioactive source is required for this step, and counts are found for all LORs. An average count per LOR is computed, and an array of coefficients is generated to normalize the count along each LOR. The results are stored as normalization correction data and applied to every sinogram acquired for each patient scan. In this aspect, the QC is similar to planar and SPECT devices. Reconstruction of a sinogram without normalization may lead to image artifacts. Raw patient data should always be archived with the appropriate normalization correction so that another data reconstruction at a later time is possible without compromising image quality.

Status of the detecting system has to be controlled every day before beginning of scanning. It is usually done by a short acquisition from a uniform phantom or by acquiring a blank scan from orbiting radioactive rods. A uniform image of the sinogram from such a scan is expected in a well-working scanner (see Fig. 24-25). Practice of QC may require some statistical analysis of the sinogram data to reveal trends in the parameters of the detector system.

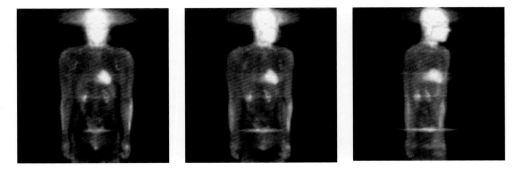

**FIG. 24-26.** Three views generated by 3D volume-rendering software from the whole-body PET FDG study. Note particularly the axillary and cervical lymph nodes in this AIDS patient. No attenuation correction was applied. Note the minimal overlapping of individual frames obtained as the scanner bed is incremented through the detector gantry. More obvious streaks occur across the image in regions of high tracer concentration (head, heart, renal pelvis, and bladder). Displaying these views in sequence (animation) aids in depth perception and is helpful in anatomic localization of metabolic findings.

Some considerations for PET QC can be found in the literature (27,43,44).

### Radiopharmaceuticals

PET radiopharmaceuticals must be labeled with positron-emitting radionuclides having a half-life short enough to minimize the patient radiation exposure yet long enough to allow incorporation into the required biologic molecules. Only a limited number of radionuclides can be used for PET. F-18 is used most often, but nitrogen (N-13), carbon (C-11), oxygen (O-15), and rubidium (Rb-82) are also used frequently (see Table 24-6).

Fortunately, this short list of radionuclides includes those that are biologically important, and a large number of radiopharmaceuticals can be produced from them. FDG, an analog of sugar, is one of the agents most commonly used to study glucose metabolism in the brain, heart, and other organs. It is also used to localize malignant tumors with increased glycolytic metabolism. Several other F-18 radiopharmaceuticals are applied for neuroreceptor mapping. Ammonia is a common blood-flow radiopharmaceutical with N-13 and is often used for cardiac perfusion studies, and when used with FDS can assess myocardial viability. Water with O-15 is used as a blood flow radiopharmaceutical in neurology and cardiology. C-11 can be used in many radiopharmaceuticals when incorporated into biological molecules to measure fatty acid and glucose metabolism, protein synthesis, and neuroreceptor mapping.

The short half-lives of PET radionuclides require production in close proximity to the PET facility or in a cyclotron that is part of the PET center. All of the described isotopes can be produced from targets like water (e.g., F-18, N-13) or stable nitrogen (e.g., C-11, O-15). The radionuclides have to be incorporated into biologically active molecules in a radiopharmacy, which is a part of the facility. The short half-lives of these radionuclides require special techniques, and automated (robotic) devices for the radiopharmaceutical

synthesis are available. The usual rules of good manufacturing practice and QC must be performed to ensure the purity of the radiopharmaceutical.

### Patient Scanning Modes

#### Emission Scans

Emission scans are the most important PET scans and can be acquired in several ways. In all of them, radiation from the patient is detected.

##### Static Scan

A static scan is taken from one bed position, and the entire scan forms one set of data (one frame). It may take anywhere between 5 and 20 minutes, depending on the part of body, amount of radiopharmaceutical injected, and the pathophysiology of the organ being evaluated.

##### Dynamic Scan

A dynamic scan consists of a series of static emission scans (frames) over time. It allows observation of the radiopharmaceutical uptake and associated metabolic or functional processes as a function of time. The duration of the frames varies from a few seconds to minutes depending on the half-life of the isotope, the physiology, and phase of the process of interest. Correction for radionuclide decay is needed in the dynamic scan mode.

##### Whole-Body Scan

A whole-body scan consists of several frames, like a dynamic scan, but each subsequent frame is acquired after moving the bed by the length of axial width of the scanner. The motion of the bed is computer controlled. The frames are then reconstructed into a single image set that covers the entire body or a large part of it (Fig. 24-26).

*Gated Heart Scan*

A gated heart scan (a scan synchronized to the beating heart) collects emission data into several sinograms instead of one. A separate sinogram is used for each segment of the cardiac cycle, and this series of images may be displayed in a cine mode, just as seen in gated planar ventriculograms and gated SPECT myocardial perfusion imaging. Although the effect of cardiac motion can be reduced by gating, the number of counts per frame may be prohibitively low.

*Transmission Scans*

The transmission mode of scanning collects radiation that comes from an external source, not from the patient. The scans are taken to measure attenuation of the annihilation photons by the patient's body. In newer scanners, the source is a small radioactive rod that can orbit the patient. The source generates pairs of annihilation photons. One photon from the pair goes directly to the adjacent detectors, and the second penetrates the patient body along an LOR and is attenuated appropriately. A major advantage when using rotating transmission sources is that one can perform transmission scanning after the radiopharmaceutical has been injected, either immediately before or after the emission scan, or even concurrent with emission scanning. The emission contamination is measured and subtracted from the transmission data (27,44–47).

In the past, contamination of the transmission scan by radiation from the patient was avoided by performing the transmission scan before the radiopharmaceutical injection. However, because of the radiopharmaceutical uptake time, the emission scan often could not be acquired immediately after the transmission scan, so the patient had to stay on the bed motionless from the time of the transmission scan to that of the emission scan or be repositioned just before the emission scan. The repositioning was a source of many image artifact errors.

*Rectilinear Scans*

The rectilinear scan mode is available on some PET scanners to aid patient positioning before emission or transmission scans. Image from rectilinear scans is not tomographic (no reconstruction involved) and is formed in the same way as in conventional gamma camera imaging. Emission as well as transmission images may be obtained in this mode.

## Data Acquisition

Running a modern PET scanner is greatly simplified due to automation brought by computers. Dedicated hardware and software control, acquisition parameters, bed motion,

and patient positioning provides checks of resources available for the scan, and allows fast data processing and archiving. Often, a learning mode is included, which allows the operator to record all steps involved in a scan and its processing. Such recorded procedures can be replayed to run the next scan or provide a convenient template for later scans.

The computer environment of a PET scanner is usually multitasking. It contributes to better usage of the scanner by allowing several processes to proceed at the same time. In a multiframe scan, like a dynamic acquisition, frames already completed can be reconstructed as others are still being acquired. Data processing can therefore be interleaved with the data acquisition. Computer networking allows remote data access and distribution of images.

During the scan acquisition, the operator must pay close attention to patient motion, because it may lead to image artifacts and blurring. Any repositioning of the patient during a scan by a distance larger than half of the spatial resolution causes some image quality degradation. The problem is less significant when the movement happens close to the very beginning or very end of the scan. Very comfortable patient positioning on the scanner bed is crucial to minimize patient motion. Repositioning of the patient during the scan after movement may reduce the impact of motion on data quality, provided that the original patient position can be re-established. Laser beams together with patient body markers can be helpful in this role. Some patient motion is unavoidable: thoracic cyclic motion due to breathing and the beating heart always leads to some degradation of cardiac image quality by smearing anatomic details. An electrocardiographic gated study eliminates most of the cardiac effect but has no effect on the degradation due to respiratory motion.

## Corrections to the Raw Data

The raw data acquired in any emission or transmission scanning mode is saved in a series of sinograms. Usually the sinograms need several corrections before they can be reconstructed into an image set (44).

*Attenuation Correction*

Correction for attenuation of gamma rays by the tissue has the most significant impact on the image quality. Radiation attenuation cannot be avoided, and it may significantly affect the quality of data. For example, in the chest, up to 80% to 90% of the coincident photons do not make it out of the body without being absorbed or scattered out of FOV. Without attenuation correction, the images exhibit gradually reduced concentrations of radiopharmaceutical from outer to inner regions of the body. Such images may be still useful in some instances, but they cannot be quantitated.

Precise attenuation correction can be obtained in PET because, in the coincidental mode of the acquisition, the amount of attenuation is independent of the localization of the radiopharmaceutical along any LOR, depending only on the overall absorption along the given LOR. Based on this property, the amount of attenuation can be measured in the transmission scan. The patient transmission scan is supplemented by a blank scan, which is acquired under the same conditions but without the patient in the gantry. The ratios of the blank count to the transmission count for all LORs provide data about attenuation by the patient body along every LOR, and are applied to the emission sinograms to compensate for attenuation.

The measured attenuation correction is very accurate, but it requires an additional scan and prolongs the study. Orbiting radioactive sources used in many modern PET scanners have the potential to acquire transmission data simultaneously with emission data, but this method is not yet ready for routine use (48). In the case of the brain, because of the relatively uniform attenuation and simple and reproducible shape of the head, the measured attenuation method can be substituted by a calculated attenuation correction method. The absorption is computed assuming an ellipsoid head shape and uniform tissue density. Until recently, this method was not used for other body parts because of tissue nonuniformities and different body shapes. However, recent work brings new approaches that combine a very short transmission scan with calculated attenuation correction for the whole-body scans by applying image segmentation (49,50). This would be an important improvement because whole-body scanning with conventional measured attenuation correction is very time-consuming and may require the patient to stay motionless on the bed for up to 2 hours.

### Random Events Correction

The random coincident events are caused by chance detection of photons from unrelated annihilation events within the coincidence timing window (see Fig. 24-24) and increase at high counting rates. These random events can be decreased by using shorter coincidence-resolving times. The random events can be measured in real time (i.e., during the scan) by delayed coincidences, or from the single's rates. No more than 50% of the measured coincidences should be random because they decrease image contrast. The measured random coincidences are subtracted from the measured coincidence data before image reconstruction.

### Scatter Correction

The scatter coincidences can originate from within or outside the imaged plane, and, because they arise from common annihilation events, they cannot be eliminated by using shorter coincidence-resolving times. In most PET imaging studies, scattered coincidences are 10% to 25% of the total counts. They are manifest in a slowly varying background activity level in the image. Scatter events are reduced in 2D acquisition mode due to septa between the rings of detec-

tors. Because scattered coincidences cannot be distinguished from true coincidences electronically, no exact correction for scatter is possible (44).

### Dead-Time Correction

Dead-time correction compensates for count losses due to the inability of the detector to operate immediately after a prior event. Because the losses originate from several places in the detection process, dead-time correction may have several components. One component is usually directly related to the detector block, and another corrects for losses in the electronics (see Chapter 23).

## Reconstruction and Image Processing

Corrected sinograms are reconstructed to PET images. The reconstruction can be based on one of several tomographic algorithms, of which the filtered backprojection (FBP) method is used most often, for 2D as well as 3D acquisitions. Images obtained from the reconstruction may be viewed by a display software provided with the scanner. However, often they are further processed to obtain quantitative images or to enhance some features present in the data.

### Quantitation

Pixel values in the reconstructed images do not represent true counts, but accurate attenuation correction leads to images that can be quantified. In the simplest approach, the quantitation involves multiplication of all pixel values in images by a constant factor, which converts the pixel values into isotope activity or radiopharmaceutical concentration. The quantitation factor can be calculated based on data acquired from a phantom with known radioactivity. There are several reasons why this simple quantitation schema is not sufficient in many cases. One of the most common problems is related to the *partial volume effect*. This causes objects of less than twice the size of the intrinsic resolution of the detectors to be only partially represented in the reconstructed images. There is no universal method to correct this problem, which applies to all CT radiologic techniques (SPECT, CT, and MRI).

More complex quantitation algorithms are also required to obtain parametric images that represent specific variables related to physiologic processes. For example, brain images obtained with FDG may be converted into images of regional cerebral glucose metabolic rates using mathematical modeling. Brain PET scans for such analysis are associated with the drawing of several blood samples and measuring their radioactivity as a necessary part of this modeling process (see Chapter 17). Different kinds of problems have to be solved to quantitate myocardial perfusion scans, where corrections for the *spillover effect* from one anatomic or physiologic compartment to another (e.g., from the ventricular blood pool into the myocardium) must be included. A review of quantitation principles and limitations can be found in reference 51.

### Reconstruction Filtering

Some filtering is an integral part of any tomographic reconstruction. The reconstruction filters remove a fraction of the noise that is always present in the raw data. Selection of the filter is a compromise between resolution and the amount of noise to be left in the image. For example, the ramp filter does not affect the resolution significantly, but image quality is perceived as worse than that of other filters because noise is still present in the images. The Hann filter, one of the most commonly chosen for PET data, leads to smooth images with slightly lower resolution. Reconstruction software provides the filters for the user selection. The ability of a filter to remove noise can be modified by the cutoff frequency. A larger value of this parameter leads to greater reduction of noise.

### Color Maps and Display Filters

Part of the image preparation for viewing and medical interpretation of PET scans is the selection of a color map. Typically, a variety of color maps are provided with the image display software. A properly chosen color map may enhance perceived contrast in images and at the same time may camouflage low-count noisy background always present in PET images.

Independent of the reconstruction filters, a variety of filters also may be applied to smooth or sharpen images after reconstruction. A smoothing effect can be achieved by low-pass filters, which reduce noise and blur edges. High-pass filters enhance edges and improve contrast.

Features of color maps and filters need to be well understood, and user experience is required to use them properly. Wrong color maps may introduce high contrast to the image details, which can be due to either unimportant biological variations or merely noise in the data. In the opposite case, it may obscure some important aspect of the images. Improper application of filters may create image artifacts and lead to overall degradation of image quality. Both problems lead to misinterpretation of images.

### Data Reformatting

Reformatting of the original transaxial views to other projections can be very helpful in extracting maximum information from the images. Coronal and sagittal views are most convenient for the interpretation, especially for brain and whole-body studies. Heart images may need special oblique orientation related to the heart axis. 3D volume rendering provides the most comprehensive method of viewing PET data and may also contribute to anatomic localization, especially in whole-body studies (see Fig. 24-26). In general, however, any attempt to localize a feature in the PET scan

has to be done with great care because this imaging modality is not anatomic. The resemblance of the PET images to anatomic images can be misleading. This problem can be eliminated by coregistering PET images with MRI or CT images of the same patient, a method requiring special software that finds a common reference coordinate system for both sets of images and displays them together.

## COMPARISON OF PET AND SPECT

Both PET and SPECT provide tomographic images that map radiopharmaceutical distribution. Due to electronic collimation, PET images can be easily corrected for photon attenuation and quantitated. In SPECT, both attenuation correction and quantitation are very difficult and inaccurate. Both techniques use different radionuclides and radiopharmaceuticals; therefore, SPECT image interpretation differs from PET.

PET and SPECT have several physical and technical similarities. The detector modules use the same main principle of converting high-energy radiation interaction in scintillation crystals into UV or visible light, which is then detected by photomultipliers. Raw data are collected into sinograms in both modalities, although the structure of the PET sinogram is different in 3D PET acquisition mode. Some data corrections, such as detector dead time or scatter, are similar in both modalities.

### PET Advantages

PET scanning has several advantages over SPECT: improved resolution and the ability to use coincidence detection (10 to 20 times improved sensitivity over SPECT) and to perform attenuation correction (allow quantitation). Because the common PET radionuclides include the body's main constituents (e.g., carbon, nitrogen, and oxygen), they can be readily substituted into biologically important molecular radiopharmaceuticals (e.g., glucose, methionine, and fatty acids), and quantitation of perfusion and important metabolic pathways can be performed in vivo. These offer enormous potential for research and clinical applications. In some cases, the high resolution of PET studies does not provide qualitatively different information from SPECT to justify their higher cost.

### SPECT Advantages

A SPECT scanner is smaller, simpler in technical details, and cheaper to produce than PET equipment. SPECT radiopharmaceuticals are often cheaper, are accessible without an on-site cyclotron, emit less penetrating radiation, and involve simpler and more effective radiation protection. Relative radiopharmaceutical distributions are possible in SPECT but not quantitation. Much work is being done on attenuation correction to improve this.

In the last decade, considerable advances have been made in SPECT and PET imaging devices and in the development of new radiopharmaceuticals. Both SPECT and PET scanners are rapidly approaching their theoretical resolution limits: 1.8 mm for the head and 2 mm for body PET images, and 4.0 mm for dedicated head SPECT units and 6.0 mm for whole-body SPECT. The clinical applications of both modalities have advanced significantly the role of nuclear medicine in clinical situations by the very tomographic nature of the images.

## REFERENCES

1. Anger HO. Multiplane Tomographic Gamma-Ray Scanner. In Freedman GS (ed), Medical Radioisotope Scintigraphy. Vienna: International Atomic Energy Agency, 1969;203–216.
2. Kuhl DE, Edwards RQ. Image separation radioisotope scanning. Radiology 1963;80:653–662.
3. Kuhl DE, Edwards RQ. Cylindrical and section radioisotopes scanning of the liver and brain. Radiology 1964;83:926–935.
4. Kuhl DE, Edwards RQ. Reorganizing data from transverse section scans of the brain using digital processing. Radiology 1968;91:975–983.
5. Jaszczak RJ, Murphy PH, Huard D, Burdine JA. Radionuclide emission computed tomography of the head with $^{99m}$Tc and a scintillation camera. J Nucl Med 1977;18:373–380.
6. Keyes JW, Orlandea N, Heetderks WJ, et al. The humogotron: a scintillation camera transaxial tomography. J Nucl Med 1977;18:381–387.
7. Cormack AM. Representation of a function by its line integrals, with some radiological applications. J Appl Phys 1963;34:2722–2727.
8. Cormack AM. Reconstruction of densities from their projections, with applications in radiological physics. Phys Med Biol 1973;18:195–207.
9. Hounsfield GN. Computerized transverse axial scanning (tomography). I. Description of the system. Br J Radiol 1973;46:1016–1022.
10. Jaszczak RJ, Tsui BMW. Section 1, General Principles: Single-Photon Emission Computed Tomography (SPECT). In Wagner HN, Szabo Z, Buchanan JW (eds), Principles of Nuclear Medicine. Philadelphia: Saunders, 1995;317–328.
11. Keyes JW. Section 3, Operational Guidelines: Single-Photon Emission Computed Tomography (SPECT). In Wagner HN, Szabo Z, Buchanan JW (eds), Principles of Nuclear Medicine. Philadelphia: Saunders, 1995;332–341.
12. Cullom SI. Principles of Cardiac SPECT. In DePuey EG, Berman DS, Garcia EV (eds), Cardiac SPECT Imaging. New York: Raven, 1995;2.
13. deVries DJ, Moore SC, Zimmerman RE, et al. Development and validation of a Monte Carlo simulation of photon transport in an Anger camera. IEEE Trans Med Imag 1990;9:430–438.
14. Moore SC, Kouris K, Cullom I. Collimator design for single photon emission tomography. Eur J Nucl Med 1992;19:138–150.
15. Jaszczak RJ, Chang LT, Murphy PH. Single-photon emission computed tomography using multi-slice fan beam collimators. IEEE Trans Nucl Sci NS 1979;26:610–619.
16. Jaszczak RJ, Floyd CE, Manglos SM, et al. Cone beam collimation for single-photon emission computed tomography: analysis, simulation, and image reconstruction using filtered backprojection. Med Phys 1987;13:484–489.
17. Tsui BMW, Gullberg GT, Edgerton ER, et al. Design and clinical utility of a fan beam collimator for SPECT imaging of the head. J Nucl Med 1986;27:810–819.
18. Datz FL, Gullberg GT, Zeng GL, et al. Application of convergent-beam collimation and simultaneous transmission emission tomography to cardiac single-photon emission computed tomography. Semin Nucl Med 1994;24:17–37.
19. King MA, Tsui BMW, Pan TS. Attenuation compensation for cardiac single-photon emission computed tomographic imaging. I. Impact of attenuation and methods of estimating attenuation maps. J Nucl Cardiol 1995;2:513–524.
20. Garcia EV. Quantitative myocardial single-photon computed tomographic imaging: quo vadis? (Where do we go from here?) J Nucl Cardiol 1994;1:83–93.
21. Faber TL. Multiheaded rotating gamma cameras in cardiac single-photon emission computed tomographic imaging. J Nucl Cardiol 1994;1:292–303.
22. Madsen MT. Introduction to emission CT. Radiographics 1995;15:975–991.
23. Chang LT. A method for attenuation correction in radionuclide computed tomography. IEEE Trans Nucl Sci 1978;25:638–643.
24. Jaszczak RJ, Greer KL, Floyd CE, et al. Improved SPECT quantitation using compensation for scattered photons. J Nucl Med 1984;25:893–900.
25. King MA, Hademenos GJ, Glick SJ. A dual photopeak window method for scatter correction. J Nucl Med 1992;33:605–612.
26. Ogawa K, Harata Y, Ichihara T, et al. A practical method for position-dependent Compton-scatter correction in single photon emission CT. IEEE Trans Med Imag 1991;10:408–412.
27. Jaszczak RJ, Hoffman EJ. Section 3, Scatter and Attenuation: Positron Emission Tomography (PET). In Wagner HN, Szabo Z, Buchanan JW (eds), Principles of Nuclear Medicine. Philadelphia: Saunders, 1995;362–377.
28. Slowka P, Dey D. Review of instrumentation developments at the SNM 1996 Annual Meeting. J Nucl Med 1996;37:25N–33N.
29. Budinger TF, Gulberg GT. Three-dimensional reconstruction in nuclear medicine emission imaging. IEEE Trans Nucl Sci 1974;21:2–20.
30. Pan TS, Luo DS, King MA. Influence of ordered subset reconstruction and elliptical orbits on SPECT 3D spatial resolution. J Nucl Med (in press).
31. King MA, Tsui BMW, Glick SJ, Soares EJ. Attenuation compensation for cardiac single-photon emission computer tomographic imaging. Part 2. Attenuation compensation algorithms. J Nucl Cardiol 1996;3:55–63.
32. Manglos SH, Jaszczak RJ, Floyd CE, et al. Nonisotropic attenuation in SPECT: Phantom tests of quantitative effects and compensation techniques. J Nucl Med 1987;28:1584–1591.
33. Manglos SJ, Jaszczak RJ, Floyd CE, et al. A quantitative comparison of attenuation-weighted backprojection with multiplicative and iterative postprocessing attenuation compensation in SPECT. IEEE Trans Med Imag 1988;7:128–134.
34. Knesaurek K, King MA, Glick SJ, Penney BC. Investigation of the causes of geometrical distortion in 180-degree and 360-degree angular sampling SPECT. J Nucl Med 1989;30;1666–1675.
35. Ichihara T, Ogawa K, Motomura N, et al. Compton scatter compensation using the triple-energy window method for single- and dual-isotope SPECT. J Nucl Med 1993;34:2216–2221.
36. Graham LS. Quality control for SPECT systems. Radiographics 1995;15:1471–1481.
37. Burt RA, Perkins OW, Oppenheim BE, et al. Direct comparison of fluorine-18-FDG SPECT, fluorine-18-FDG PET and rest thallium-201 SPECT for detection of myocardial viability. J Nucl Med 1995;36:176–179.
38. Martin WH, Delbke D, Patton JA, Sandler MP. Dectection of malignancies with SPECT versus PET, with 2-(fluorine-18)-fluoro-2-deoxy-D-glucose. Radiology 1996;198:225–231.
39. Patton JA, Sandler MP, Ohana I, Weinfeld Z. High-energy (511 keV) imaging with the scintillation camera. Radiographics 1996;16:1183–1194.
40. Muehllehner G, Geagan M, Countryman P. SPECT scanner with PET capability. J Nucl Med.1995;36:223P.
41. Budinger TF, Derenzo SE, Huesman RH. Instrumentation in positron emission tomography. Ann Neurol 1984;15:S35–S43.
42. University Hospital Consortium. Technology Report: Positron Emission Tomography. Oakbrook, IL: University Hospital Consortium, March 1994.
43. Spinks T, Jones T, Heather J, Gilardi M. Quality control procedures in positron tomography. Eur J Nucl Med 1989;15:736–740.
44. Ter-Pegossian MM. Section 1, General Principles. Daube-Witherspoon ME. Section 2, Operational Guidelines: Positron Emission Tomography (PET). In Wagner HN, Szabo Z, Buchanan JW (eds), Principles of Nuclear Medicine. Philadelphia: Saunders, 1995;342–361.
45. Ho ZH, Chan JK, Ericksson L, et al. Positron ranges obtained from biologically important positron-emitting radionuclides. J Nucl Med 1975;16:1174–1176.
46. Carson RE, Daube-Witherspoon ME, Green MV. A method for

postinjection PET transmission measurements with a rotating source. J Nucl Med 1988;29:1558–1567.

47. Ranger NT, Thompson CJ, Evans AC. The application of a masked orbiting transmission source for attenuation correction in PET. J Nucl Med 1989;30:1056–1068.

48. Meikle SR, Bailey DL, Hooper PK, et al. Simultaneous emission and transmission measurements for attenuation correction in whole-body PET. J Nucl Med 1995;36:1680–1688.

49. Meikle SR, Dahlbom M, Cherry SR. Attenuation correction using count-limited transmission data in positron emission tomography. J Nucl Med 1993;34:143–150.

50. Smith RJ, Karp JS. Attenuation correction in whole-body PET using short transmission scans. J Nucl Med 1996;37:172P.

51. Hoffman EJ, Phelps ME. Positron Emission Tomography: Principles and Quantitation. In Phelps M, Mazziotta J, Schelbert H (eds), Positron Emission Tomography and Autoradiography: Principles and Application for the Brain and Heart. New York: Raven, 1986.

*Textbook of Nuclear Medicine,*
edited by Michael A. Wilson.
Lippincott–Raven Publishers, Philadelphia © 1998.

CHAPTER **25**

# Fourier Mathematics and Filters

Joseph Bellissimo

High-level mathematics plays an important role in modern noninvasive imaging. This is especially true for tomographic techniques, such as single photon emission computed tomography (SPECT), computed tomography, and magnetic resonance imaging. Fourier mathematics as well as other related techniques are used extensively and are in fact essential for the creation of these images.

It is nearly impossible to comprehend the full meaning of these images without some understanding of the powerful mathematics behind them. This is because the mathematical manipulations, although necessary to create the images, have the potential to delete or alter important information and as a result to affect the appearance of the images obtained. It is important, therefore, that individuals interpreting these images have at least a conceptual understanding of how the original data have been processed and manipulated to produce the final image. Typically, most of these techniques, especially Fourier mathematics, have been beyond the level of training for most clinicians.

The purpose of this chapter is to give the reader with a limited background in mathematics a very basic introduction to the concepts of Fourier mathematics along with examples of its applications in nuclear medicine. It is not intended to present a rigorous discussion of the complex mathematics of image reconstruction; there are entire books dedicated to this. But before discussing Fourier mathematics, it is important to understand the concept of the spatial and frequency domains and how they are related.

## COORDINATE SYSTEMS

Scientific data and mathematical functions typically need to be described in terms of a coordinate system. Usually this takes the form of spatial coordinates (e.g., x, y, z) and time. These are also known as the *spatial* and *time domains*, or together as *real space*. This is not the only way to organize such information, however.

In the mind of a Fourier mathematician, many of the functions and signals of interest can be considered the sum of an infinite series of sine or cosine functions, in which each term has its own frequency and amplitude. Under these circumstances an alternative coordinate system can be devised in which the signals are described in terms of the amplitude and frequency of the individual sine and cosine terms. This new coordinate system is known as the *frequency domain*, or as *Fourier space*. Some simple examples will demonstrate how these different coordinate systems are related.

A simple cosine function in the general form of Equation 1 is plotted in the time domain in Fig. 25-1A. In this example,

- Amplitude, $A$, is equal to 1
- Frequency, $\omega$, is the reciprocal of the cycle length, $T$ ($\frac{1}{2}\pi$ in this example)
- Phase lag, $\phi$ (to be introduced shortly), is 0

$$y(t) = A\cos(\omega t + \phi) \qquad (1)$$

Although quite different in appearance, the same information is plotted in the frequency domain (i.e., amplitude vs. frequency) in Fig. 25-1B. In this format one can easily determine that the signal of interest comprises a single cosine function with amplitude 1 and frequency of $\frac{1}{2}\pi$.

In any format there must be a mechanism to handle the case when the cosine function contains a phase lag, that is, the maximum value of the signal occurs at some time other than zero. As shown in Fig. 25-2A, this information is a natural part of the time domain plot. In the frequency domain, although the amplitude versus frequency plot remains the same, an additional plot of phase lag versus frequency is required to handle this information (Fig. 25-2B).

For this simple example with a single frequency there is practically no advantage to the frequency domain because all the information of interest is readily available in the time domain. Its utility becomes more apparent as the signals become more complex.

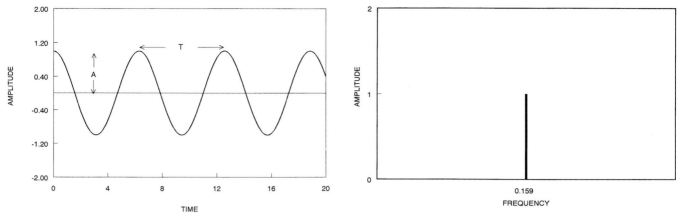

**FIG. 25-1. (A)** This plot shows a simple cosine function with amplitude $A$ and frequency $1/T$. **(B)** This plot shows the same cosine function in the frequency domain; the amplitude is 1 and the frequency is $\frac{1}{2}\pi$, or 0.159.

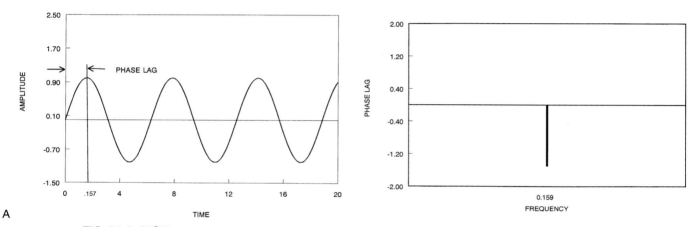

**FIG. 25-2. (A)** The same cosine function as Fig. 25-1, with a phase lag of $-\pi/2$ introduced. **(B)** The frequency domain plot of the phase lag versus frequency.

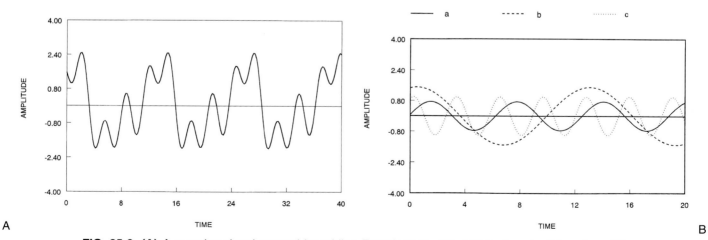

**FIG. 25-3. (A)** A complex signal created by adding Equations 2a, 2b, and 2c (see text) together, **(B)** which are plotted individually.

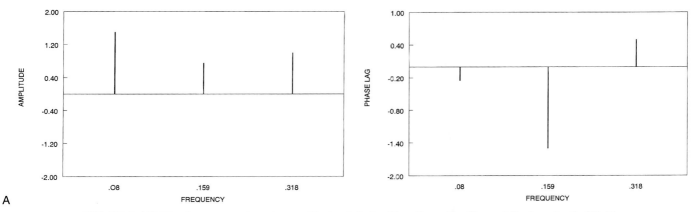

**FIG. 25-4. (A)** The frequency domain amplitude plots for Equations 2a, 2b, and 2c (see text). **(B)** The frequency domain phase plots for the same equations.

The signal shown in Fig. 25-3A was created through the addition of the three cosine functions shown in curves a, b, and c in Fig. 25-3B. They are described in Equations 2a, 2b, and 2c, below, where it can be seen that each function has its own amplitude, frequency, and phase lag. If presented only with the complex summed signal, most people would find it quite difficult to determine the individual components.

$$y(t) = 0.75 \cos(t - 1.5) \qquad (2a)$$

$$y(t) = 1.5 \cos(\tfrac{t}{2} - 0.25) \qquad (2b)$$

$$y(t) = \cos(2t - 0.5) \qquad (2c)$$

When presented as amplitude and phase plots in the frequency domain (Fig. 25-4), it is easy to distinguish the individual components on the basis of their frequencies, amplitudes, and phase lags. In general, the more complex the signal, the more useful it can be to work in the frequency domain with regard to frequency analysis.

## FOURIER SERIES

Jean Baptiste Joseph Fourier was a politician, historian, scientist, and engineer in France during the reign of Napoleon. He is best remembered now primarily for his work as a mathematician. The concept now known as the *Fourier series* came out of work he did concerning the characterization of heat conduction problems. The basic premise on which the Fourier series is based is that any periodic function (i.e., any function with a regular repeating pattern), fulfilling certain criteria, can be thought of as the sum of an infinite series of sine or cosine functions. In the framework of this concept, the frequencies of the sines and cosines in the series must all be integer multiples, or harmonics, of the fundamental frequency (i.e., the overall repeating frequency of the function; e.g., in the case of a radionuclide ventriculogram, this would be the heart rate).

The general expression for the Fourier series can be written in a number of ways. One example is shown in Equation 3:

$$y(t) = a_0 + a_1\cos(\omega_0 t + \phi_1) + a_2\cos(2\omega_0 t + \phi_2) +$$
$$\ldots + a_i\cos(i\omega_0 t + \phi_i) + \ldots, \qquad (3)$$

where $y(t)$ is the amplitude of a signal as a function of time, $\omega_0$ is the fundamental frequency, $i\omega_0$ is the harmonic frequencies, $\phi_i$ is the phase lag associated with each frequency, and $a_i$ is the amplitude coefficient for each frequency.

To create a Fourier series for any given signal, the individual amplitude and phase coefficients must be determined for each frequency, which is often a difficult and tedious task. Fortunately, for many applications it is not necessary to know how to do this because the coefficients have been determined and tabulated for a number of commonly used functions.

In general, the higher the number of terms included in the series (i.e., the higher the frequencies that are included), the more closely the original signal is approximated by the series. There is a practical limit to this concept, however, because the series are infinite and in general the number of terms to be included is determined by the particular application and the degree of precision required. For a fairly straightforward application of Fourier series in nuclear medicine, the creation of phase and amplitude images from radionuclide ventriculography data is considered.

## PHASE AND AMPLITUDE IMAGING

In the process of determining the left ventricular ejection fraction during radionuclide ventriculography, a time-activity curve (TAC) is generated in which the number of counts in the left ventricle is plotted as a function of time (Fig. 25-5). This curve resembles a straightforward cosine function to a fair degree and as a result is adequately characterized by a simple Fourier series.

Due to the close resemblance to a cosine function and the fact that only gross characteristics of the curve are required

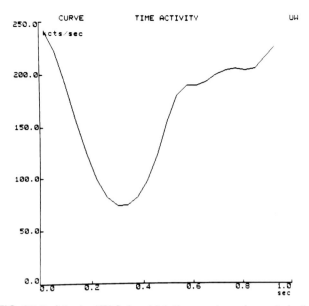

**FIG. 25-5.** A typical TAC, in which the number of counts in the left ventricle is plotted as a function of time.

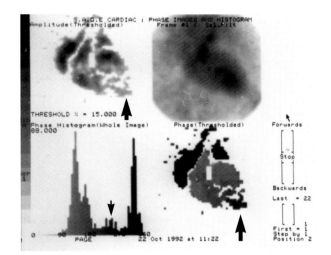

**FIG. 25-6.** The upper right image is of a dilated left ventricle. The lower right corner is the phase image from the same patient, demonstrating significant dyskinesis in the apical region (*arrow*). The lower left corner is the phase histogram, showing the relative number of pixels at each phase angle, with the dyskinetic pixels (*small arrow*) between the atrial (*dark*) and ventricular (*light*) peaks. The upper left corner is the amplitude image, representing the local ejection fraction, which suggests significant apical dysfunction. Motion (amplitude) is present in the apex, corresponding with the abnormal phase (*arrow*). The region around this dyskinesis shows no phase or amplitude, indicating the absent wall motion around the dyskinetic segment.

for analysis in this application, one needs to include only the first two terms of the Fourier series to achieve an adequate approximation of the TAC (Equation 4).

$$y(t) = a_0 + a_1\cos(\omega_0 t + \phi_1) \qquad (4)$$

By keeping the expression simple, the coefficients all take on physical significance:

$y(t)$ = number of counts as a function of time

$a_0$ = average number of counts over one cycle

$a_1$ = amplitude coefficient, representing the maximum deviation in counts above and below the average

$\omega_0$ = fundamental frequency, which in this case is equal to the heart rate

$\phi_1$ = phase lag, that is, the time from the R wave on the electrocardiogram to the peak number of counts in the cycle

Usually, it is not necessary to perform this type of analysis for the ventricle as a whole because the ejection fraction and other characteristics can be obtained directly from the TAC. It is more interesting to realize that a similar TAC exists for each pixel, or picture element, and that an expression similar to Equation 4 can be written for each one. Each of these equations has its own values for $a_0$, $a_1$, and $\phi_1$ ($\omega_0$, however, stays the same because it is equal to the heart rate). Being able to determine the values of the coefficients can be useful because they convey information about local ventricular function. To illustrate this point, a brief description of phase imaging follows.

The normal left ventricle, to a certain degree, contracts as a unit; therefore, nearly all the pixels that represent the left ventricle are in phase (i.e., the phase lags, $\phi_1$s, are approximately equal). When wall motion abnormalities exist (such as after a myocardial infarction) or conduction abnormalities

are present (such as with left bundle block), there can be a significant change in the local phase lag. Some insight into the severity of local dysfunction can be achieved by evaluating the degree of phase shifting that has occurred. This information is usually assessed in the form of the phase image.

The typical gated radionuclide ventriculogram is a series of static images which, when played back in a cine format, give the illusion of a beating heart. In each of the static images, reflecting the number of counts present in the left ventricle at a particular point in the cardiac cycle, the computer is being instructed to display the number of counts present in each pixel either as a color or a shade of gray. To create a phase image, the computer is merely instructed to display the phase angle, $\phi$, as determined for each pixel rather than the number of counts.

The phase lag is determined initially in terms of absolute time (e.g., seconds). This makes it difficult to put the value into perspective outside the study in which it was obtained because the R-R interval on the electrocardiogram (the basis for determining the phase lag) may be different. To avoid this difficulty, the phase lag is converted to a *phase angle*, a term expressing the phase lag as a fraction of the duration of the cardiac cycle.

To accomplish the conversion, the R-R interval is defined to be equal to 360 degrees, removing the units of absolute time. The phase angle is then calculated as a fraction of 360. For instance, if the R-R interval is 1 second (corresponding

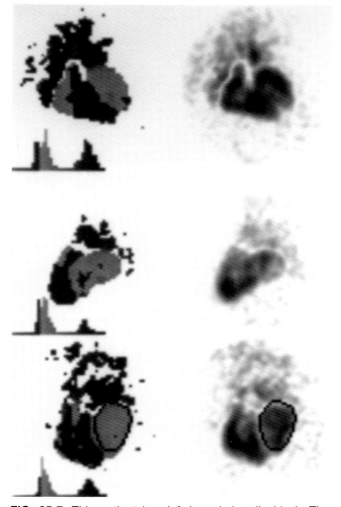

**FIG. 25-7.** This patient has left branch bundle block. The phase (left column) and amplitude images (right column) are shown for the anterior (upper row), left lateral (middle row), and best septal (lower row) views. The ventricular phase histograms are biphasic, and the right ventricle (*black*) in each view contracts before the left ventricle (*gray*), and this is clearly shown in this image. The phase histograms are biphasic, in keeping with the images. The left ventricle is outlined in the best septal view.

Figure 25-6 comes from a patient with severe left ventricular dysfunction and dyskinetic wall motion in the apex of the left ventricle. The dilated heart in end-diastole, taken from the radionuclide ventriculogram, is in the upper right corner of the figure. The phase diagram, just beneath it, shows the apex to be significantly out of phase with the remainder of the left ventricle, manifested by the darker colors assigned to the pixels in this region. The corresponding phase histogram, in the lower left corner of the figure, indicates the number of pixels with a given phase angle. The large peak to the left of the histogram represents the majority of the left ventricle; the large peak to the right represents primarily the atria; and the smaller peak in between represents the dyskinetic portion of the left ventricle. The amplitude image from the same patient is in the upper left corner of the figure. The relatively lighter shading in the apical region of the ventricle suggests that the local ejection fraction, and hence the function, in this region is diminished.

Figure 25-7 is the phase image and histogram from a patient with left bundle branch block. In this image, during the early part of the activation sequence in the ventricles, it can be seen that the septum and the right ventricle are slightly out of phase with the majority of the left ventricle, which is a result of the delayed activation of the left ventricle seen in left bundle branch block.

## FOURIER TRANSFORMS

In the previous section, the concept of the Fourier series was introduced, whereby a periodic function could be represented by the sum of a series of sine or cosine functions. Many real situations involve more complex signals or functions that are not periodic in nature. It has been demonstrated that even these functions (if they fulfill certain criteria) can be regarded as the sum of an infinite series of sine and cosine functions.

In contrast to the case with periodic functions, where the frequencies of the individual terms in the series had to be harmonics (or integer multiples) of the fundamental frequency, the frequencies used to represent nonperiodic functions may potentially include any possible value between zero and infinity. One way this difference is manifested is in the frequency domain representations of the functions. As seen earlier, periodic functions represented in the frequency domain tend to be discontinuous, whereas nonperiodic functions tend to be continuous in this domain.

In many circumstances, it is useful either to know which frequencies make a significant contribution to a particular signal or to be able to modify a signal on the basis of the frequencies that are present (such as in the filtering of tomographic images). In either case, the ability to determine the frequency domain representation (i.e., the spectrum or frequency content) of a signal is required; and this is what the Fourier transform does.

The determination of the Fourier transform for a particular signal is usually quite involved, and unless the signal is very simple, the use of specialized numerical computing

to a heart rate of 60 beats per minute) and the phase lag (time to the peak number of counts in the pixel) is 0.25 second, the corresponding phase angle is 0.25 × 360, or 90 degrees. A color or shade of gray is assigned to each range of phase angles (e.g., pink for 0 to 30 degrees, blue for 31 to 60 degrees). Each pixel then displays the color corresponding to its phase angle to create the phase image.

A similar plot can be constructed by displaying the amplitude coefficient, $a_1$, as determined from the TAC, for each pixel. This quantity is generally regarded as a local ejection fraction, giving some insight into local ventricular function. Examples of gray scale phase and amplitude images are shown in Figs. 25-6 and 25-7.

techniques, such as the fast Fourier transform, is required. These algorithms attempt to minimize the time and number of calculations needed while minimizing the data lost through the sampling errors that are typical of digital processes. Although these calculations are indeed complex and involved, the basic concepts are fairly straightforward. With a simplified example, the general ideas behind how and why the Fourier transform works can be made clear.

In a similar fashion to the Fourier series, assume that the signal, which this time is nonperiodic, may be adequately represented by a series of cosine or sine functions, or both, and that there are no restrictions on the allowable frequencies for the terms in the series. To keep things relatively simple for the purpose of this illustration, it is assumed that the series contains only cosine functions, as in Equation 5:

$$y(t) = a_1\cos(\omega_1 t + \phi_1) + a_2\cos(\omega_2 t + \phi_2) + \ldots + a_i\cos(\omega_i t + \phi_i) \quad (5)$$

This expression is further simplified for this demonstration by assuming that the phase lag, $\phi_i$, is zero for each frequency, yielding Equation 6:

$$y(t) = a_1\cos(\omega_1 t) + a_2\cos(\omega_2 t) + \ldots a_i\cos(\omega_i t) \quad (6)$$

The amplitude and frequency coefficients in this expression, $a_i$ and $\omega_i$ respectively, are constants whose values need to be determined. The frequency domain representation then, as discussed under coordinate systems, is nothing more than a plot of the amplitude coefficients versus the frequency coefficients. The next step is to show how the Fourier transform determines these values.

This is accomplished by inserting Equation 6, the simplified expression representing a nonperiodic function, into the general expression for the Fourier transform. Through a series of substitutions and further simplifications, it can be seen that the Fourier transform is applying a simple mathematical test to each frequency to determine if, and to what degree, that frequency is present in the signal in question.

The general expression for the Fourier transform is given in Equation 7:

$$Y(\omega) = \int y(t)e^{-j\omega t}dt \quad (7)$$

This formidable expression states that when a function, $y(t)$, in the spatial domain is subjected to the process shown, one obtains the frequency domain representation of that function, $Y(\omega)$, as the amplitude presented as a function of frequency. In the case of Equation 6, where phase is not an issue and there are no sine terms, the Fourier transform can be simplified quite a bit to yield Equation 8:

$$Y(\omega) = \int y(t)\cos(\omega t)dt \quad (8)$$

After inserting the expression in Equation 6 for $y(t)$, it becomes Equation 9:

$$Y(\omega) = \int [a_1\cos(\omega_1 t) + \ldots a_2\cos(\omega_i t) \ldots ]\cos(\omega t)dt \quad (9)$$

Keep in mind that all the subscripted coefficients have fixed values (although at this point in the analysis we may

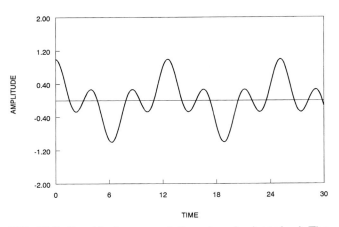

**FIG. 25-8.** Graphical representation of $\cos(\omega_1 t)\cos(\omega_2 t)$. The area under the curve contains both positive and negative values, which tend to cancel one another out.

not know what they are) and that the nonsubscripted frequency, $\omega$, is a variable. Equation 9 can then be evaluated for a wide range of values of $\omega$ to determine what contribution, if any, a particular frequency makes to the function or signal of interest. To see why this works, it is helpful to rearrange Equation 9 to yield a series of integrals, as in Equation 10:

$$Y(\omega) = a_1\int \cos(\omega_1 t)\cos(\omega t)dt + a_2\int \cos(\omega_2 t)\cos(\omega t)dt + \ldots \quad (10)$$

Each of these integrals has an interesting property: When the integral is evaluated between 0 and $2\pi$, or as in this case, between minus infinity and plus infinity, the value of the integral is 0 unless the coefficient $\omega_i$ is equal to the value of the variable frequency, $\omega$, currently being evaluated. The reason that this is true is illustrated in Fig. 25-8.

Recalling that the integral of a function is the area under a curve representing the function, note that in Fig. 25-8, when $\omega_i$ and $\omega$ are not equal, there is area both above (positive area) and below (negative area) zero. Over the long run, the positive and negative areas cancel one another out, and the resulting net area is zero. On the other hand, when $\omega_i$ and $\omega$ are equal the function being integrated is $\cos^2(\omega t)$, and as seen in Fig. 25-9, the area under this curve is always positive. In this way, the Fourier transform tests frequency after frequency to determine whether or not a given frequency is present in the signal. If it is present, the amplitude coefficient may be calculated from the resulting area. Because the series being dealt with is infinite, it is again not practical or even possible to solve for $a_i$ for every possible value of $\omega$. In most circumstances it is possible, however, to limit the number of calculations by limiting the range of frequencies evaluated, and within that range by limiting the number of frequencies sampled. This results in a more reasonable number of calculations that must be performed. It is accomplished, however, at the cost of sacrificing some data as a result of sampling.

In many applications, getting the data into the frequency domain is only half of the problem. After some manipulation

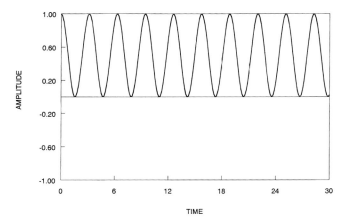

**FIG. 25-9.** A plot of $\cos(\omega_1 t)\,\cos(\omega_1 t)$. The area under the curve is always positive.

of the data in the frequency domain, such as with the application of a filter, it is necessary to get the data back into real space. This is accomplished through the use of the inverse Fourier transform, which is quite similar to and essentially undoes the original transform process. Similarly, the necessity of limiting the number of calculations by sampling results in the loss of some information each time a transform process is performed. Fortunately, the amount of information lost is usually tolerable.

## APPLICATIONS OF FOURIER TRANSFORMS: FILTERING

Fourier transforms are frequently used as a part of image reconstruction. In nuclear medicine, the most common situation for clinicians to encounter Fourier transform is the filtering of SPECT images. SPECT image reconstruction is complex. By the time an image is ready for viewing, there have been numerous calculations and corrections for such things as geometry, attenuation, scatter, and detector nonuniformity; many of these steps are proprietary. In most systems, however, the interpreter is given some choice of how the final images will appear through the selection of filters. Before continuing with this brief introduction to filtering, it is important to have an understanding of a key concept in image processing, spatial frequency.

Most people have a good grasp of the concept of frequency when it is discussed in the context of sound or electromagnetic waves. The concept of *spatial frequency* is more abstract and usually a bit more difficult to understand. An analogy to the pointillist painting style of Georges Seurat can be helpful in making this concept seem more concrete. Seurat created images with small dots of paint. The amount of detail that can be achieved in a given picture is directly related to the size and spacing of the dots. To achieve a high degree of detail, small dots spaced close together are required. In other words, the spatial frequency, or the number of dots per centimeter, is high. By contrast, with fewer dots

per centimeter, the spatial frequency is lower and the level of detail that can be achieved is lower as well.

In essence then, the spatial frequency is the rate at which image characteristics, such as contrast or color, change. In Seurat's paintings, the dots are of a fairly uniform size and consequently, the available range of spatial frequencies is limited. This translates into a limited ability to portray fine detail and define edges.

The nuclear medicine equivalent to the pointillist's dot size is the size of the pixel matrix; it determines the range of usable spatial frequencies and limits the level of resolution that can be achieved. In contrast to Seurat's paintings, the images obtained in nuclear medicine contain a complex mixture of high- and low-frequency information. The basic shape and contours of an image tend to be defined primarily by low spatial frequencies, whereas edge definition and detail tend to be defined in the higher frequencies.

Returning to the discussion of filtering: Tomographic imaging with SPECT techniques is plagued by noise and reconstruction artifacts, especially when count levels are low. Image quality can theoretically be improved if these effects can be selectively removed or attenuated. This is the aim of filtering.

Filters in this context are mathematical constructs rather than mechanical or electronic devices. Mechanical filters remove particles from a mixture on the basis of their size, but these mathematical filters remove or attenuate signals contributing to an image on the basis of their spatial frequency. For the most part, filtering is aimed at two areas of concern: low-frequency artifacts introduced as part of the backprojection reconstruction process and high-frequency noise.

Because filters operate on the basis of frequency, filtering is demonstrated in the most straightforward fashion in the frequency domain. Data, however, are collected in the spatial domain, and it is here that the Fourier transform is used to reformat the data in the frequency domain. Once in the frequency domain, the original image data are multiplied by a weighting factor at each frequency, determined by the individual filter. The newly revised data set is then put back into the spatial domain for display through the use of the inverse Fourier transform.

Filtering in this fashion can actually be carried out at any point in the reconstruction process and may actually be somewhat more efficient if it is performed early at the initial backprojection stages. In most instances, filtering to reduce reconstruction artifacts is done at this stage because it is almost universally applied to SPECT images. Noise reduction filtering is usually done at or near the end of processing to allow the viewer to optimize filter use without having to completely reprocess the data after each filter is tried.

The backprojection technique by its very nature introduces a significant amount of low-frequency artifact into the images. Through experience it has been demonstrated that most of this artifact can be corrected through the use of a ramp filter (Fig. 25-10) to attenuate the signal in a linear fashion with decreasing frequency.

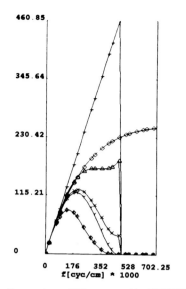

**FIG. 25-10.** Examples of filters used in SPECT imaging. They vary from ramp filter (uppermost plot), primarily used to attenuate low-frequency artifacts, to the Parzen filter (lowermost plot), which severely attenuates higher frequencies. The filters between, from top to bottom, are Butterworth, General Hamming, Hamming, and Hanning. The cutoff frequency is 0.46, except for the Butterworth filter, which is 0.702.

Noise, in contrast to most reconstruction artifacts, tends to be more of a high-frequency phenomenon that becomes increasingly important as the count levels decline. Situations in which filtering may be considered vary considerably: from those with high count data (e.g., technetium sestamibi cardiac imaging with a multi-headed camera requiring little if any noise reduction filtering) to those with low count data (e.g., single-detector thallium images requiring significant filtering to obtain reasonable images). To handle this wide

spectrum of imaging conditions, a variety of filters have been developed. Examples of some commonly used filters are displayed in Fig. 25-10.

The filters shown are distinguished primarily by the degree to which they attenuate higher frequencies. These examples range from the ramp filter that minimizes low frequencies and actually emphasizes high frequencies to the Parzen filter, which severely attenuates the higher frequencies. The effect that changing filters has on image quality is shown in Fig. 25-11. As expected, filters that attenuate high frequencies (like the Parzen) produce smoother-appearing images with less noise but also with less detail. The ramp filter by contrast produces images that are not so smooth, have more noise, but also have more detail and better edge definition. Caution must be exercised in the application of these filters because noise is not the only information present in the higher frequency ranges: There is also much of the information concerning edge definition and detail. As a result, when images are filtered, there is the potential to lose important information.

As shown in Fig. 25-10, there is a certain *cutoff* frequency for each filter, above which it does not operate (i.e., the weighting factor becomes 0). In most systems, the user may designate the cutoff frequency, but the best images are usually obtained when it is set at approximately 0.5 cycle per pixel (the actual number of cycles per centimeter depends on the size of the pixel matrix being used). This is not a random value but rather is a product of the Nyquist sampling theorem.

The Nyquist theorem states that, to adequately characterize a frequency contained in a signal, the signal must be sampled at a rate that is at least twice that of the frequency of interest. In nuclear medicine, the maximum frequency that can be characterized is ultimately determined by the size and spacing of the pixels. For example, if there are $x$ centimeters between pixels, the highest frequency that one

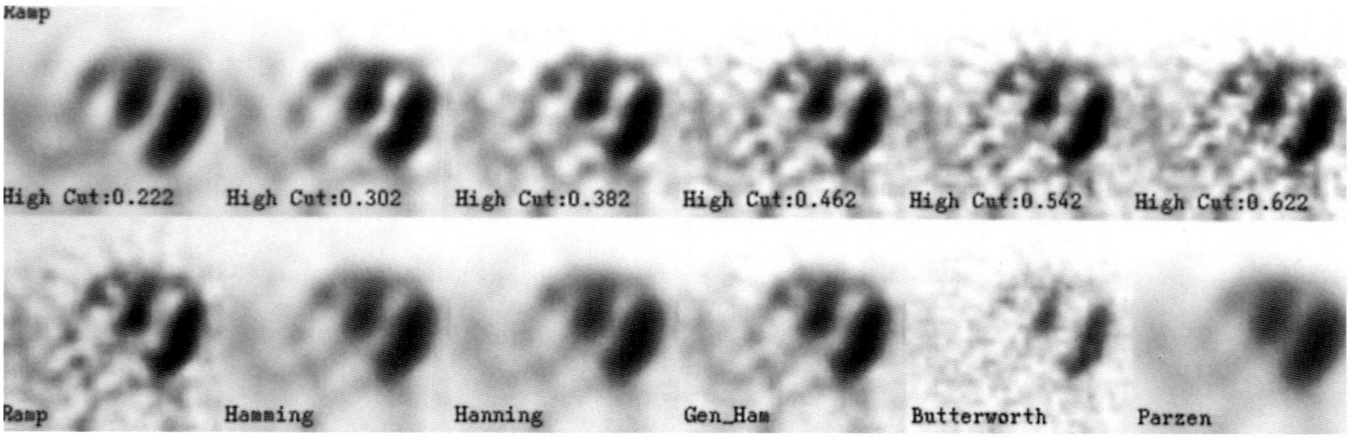

**FIG. 25-11.** Examples of the effects on image quality caused by variations in the filters and cutoff frequencies used. The upper row of images shows that progressive increases in the cutoff frequency of the ramp filter result in noisier images. The bottom row demonstrates that filters (same as in Fig. 25-10) that more severely attenuate the higher spatial frequencies result in images that are smoother, with less detail and more poorly defined borders.

could characterize would be $\frac{1}{2}x$ cycles per centimeter, corresponding to 0.5 cycles per pixel. Including frequencies above this level cannot improve image quality because the instrument is not capable of displaying them, and to do so may actually degrade image quality by adding noise and sampling errors related to the extra calculations. Conversely, setting the cutoff frequency too low has the same effect as a high-frequency filter, resulting in smoother, less detailed images (Fig. 25-11).

Whenever filtering is used to improve image quality, the benefits of an image with less noise need to be weighed against the potential loss of information that occurs as a consequence of the process. In the ideal setting, the degree of filtering and other processing to be performed should be evaluated on a case-by-case basis to maximize the amount of information obtained from the data. In the real world, that goal is not often achieved for practical reasons, and much of the time a constant level of processing is applied to all studies with the hope that the results are adequate most of the time.

## CONVOLUTION

Filtering, as described in the previous section, is easier to understand when it is discussed in terms of the frequency domain. It is possible, however, to achieve essentially the same result in the time domain, without the use of Fourier transforms, by using a technique commonly used in spectroscopy: *convolution*. These two techniques are intimately related in that the convolution of two functions in the spatial or time domain is equivalent to the multiplication of their Fourier transforms in the frequency domain. Although the process is not as easy for most people to follow intuitively, in actual practice convolution is often preferred over filtering in the frequency domain because it makes more efficient use of the available computing capacity.

As discussed previously, filtering removes noise from a signal by attenuating the frequencies where noise occurs, the result being a smoother signal. Convolution accomplishes the same result by directly smoothing the original data in the spatial or time domain, using a special type of averaging function, the convolution kernel, which dictates how the smoothing is to be done. In this type of filtering application,

the kernel is the inverse Fourier transform of the corresponding filter function that would have been used had the filtering been done in the frequency domain. The general expression for the convolution of a function, y(t), and a kernel, h(τ) is shown in Equation 11:

$$Y_0(t) = \int h(\tau)y(t)d\tau = h \otimes y \qquad (11)$$

As was the case with the Fourier transform, it is really not necessary for most people involved with interpreting images to know in detail what this expression means and how to manipulate it, but it is helpful to have some idea of how this technique is used to modify image data. With any of these techniques, it is important to realize that as a result of the sampling errors introduced to perform these procedures digitally, there is the potential to lose important information if they are not applied carefully.

## SUMMARY

The aim of this chapter is to give the reader with a limited mathematical background some insight into the basic concepts of Fourier mathematics along with examples of how they can be applied to imaging problems. The concepts of spatial, time, and frequency domains lead to the idea of using Fourier series to describe periodic functions and the Fourier transform to determine the frequency domain representation of nonperiodic functions. Filtering is one application of Fourier transforms in SPECT imaging. The topic of convolution was mentioned to illustrate that these processes can be done in either the spatial or time domains.

## REFERENCES

1. Croft BG. Single-Photon Emission Computed Tomography. Chicago: Year Book, 1986.
2. Oppenheim BE, Appledorn CR. Single Photon Emission Computed Tomography. In Gelfound MJ, Thomas SR (eds), Effective Use of Computers in Nuclear Medicine. New York: McGraw-Hill, 1988.
3. Sorenson JA, Phelps ME. Physics in Nuclear Medicine. Orlando, FL: Grune & Stratton, 1986.
4. Rogers LW, Clinthorne NH. Single Photon Emission Computed Tomography (SPECT). In Williams LE (ed), Nuclear Medical Physics, vol. III. Boca Raton, FL: CRC Press, 1987;1–47.
5. Parker JA. Image Reconstruction in Radiology. Boca Raton, FL: CRC Press, 1987.

*Textbook of Nuclear Medicine,*
edited by Michael A. Wilson.
Lippincott–Raven Publishers, Philadelphia © 1998.

# CHAPTER 26

# Radioimmunoassay and Immunoradiometric Assay

Ian H. Carlson

## HISTORIC DEVELOPMENT OF IMMUNOASSAYS

In 1956, a serendipitous discovery by Berson and colleagues (1,2) led to a plethora of analytical techniques based on the quantitative relationships between an antigen and its antibody. They established that insulin labeled with iodine 131 (I-131) reacted with antibodies generated against insulin. Since that time, numerous immunoassay techniques have evolved using antigens labeled with a wide variety of radionuclidic, fluorescent, enzymatic, and other labels. Another fortuitous discovery of Berson and colleagues' was that the human host produces antibody against injected bovine insulin. The response of the immune system against foreign protein in terms of antibody production has been exploited to produce a wide variety of antibodies for analytical, imaging, and drug delivery applications.

Soon after the Berson group's announcement of the radioimmunoassay (RIA), Ekins (3) and Murphy (4) used naturally occurring hormone-binding globulins for thyroxine ($T_4$) and cortisol measurement. This expanded the assay technique to include nonantibody competitive protein binding (CPB) assays. The discovery by Jensen et al. (5) of the binding characteristics of uterine receptors for estradiol led to the development of the radioreceptor assay (RRA) and a variation on that theme presently being applied in the form of immunocytochemistry of breast tumor tissue receptors. The generation of antibodies against small nonantigenic molecules, such as steroids, using hapten-protein conjugates (6) to generate antibodies against the steroid (hapten) provided more specific and sensitive assays than the available CPB assays.

The clinical value of these techniques was not overlooked, nor was their commercial significance. How to raise large quantities of highly avid, specific, polyclonal antibodies was a challenge. Initially, herds of large domestic animals with their larger blood volumes were the source of

antibodies. Further impetus to provide large amounts of antibodies was provided by the description of a direct or noncompetitive immunoassay technique by Miles and Hales (7), known as the *immunoradiometric assay* (IRMA) system. This technique used excess antibody, which was often in short supply but offered significant benefits in terms of sensitivity, assay range, and ease of separating free and bound fractions.

A remarkable feat of bioengineering by Kohler and Milstein (8) involving the fusion of a specific antibody-producing cell with a myeloma cell line to form a hybridoma resulted in the continuous supply of a large amount of highly specific antibody. These discoveries have led to an explosion of immunologically based techniques, as reviewed by Gosling (9) and Nakamura et al. (10), and have expanded the vistas of basic, applied, and clinical research, as well as treatment opportunities.

## THE ANTIGEN-ANTIBODY REACTION: LAW OF MASS ACTION

Quantitative competitive immunoassays, protein-binding assays, and receptor assays have common reaction characteristics that can be used in a number of important ways.

Under appropriate conditions, the antigen (Ag)-antibody (Ab) reaction follows the law of mass action:

$$\text{Ag} + \text{Ab} \underset{k_2}{\overset{k_1}{\rightleftharpoons}} \text{AgAb} \qquad (1)$$

Rate of AgAb formation = $R$

$$R = k_1(\text{Ag})(\text{Ab}) - k_2(\text{AgAb})$$

At equilibrium, $R = 0$

$$k_1(Ag)(Ab) = k_2(AgAb)$$

$$\frac{k_1}{k_2} = \frac{(AgAb)}{(Ag)(Ab)} = K$$

where $k_1$ is the association rate constant, $k_2$ is the dissociation rate constant, $K$ is the equilibrium constant, and (Ag), (Ab), (AgAb) are in moles per liter.

These relationships are used to establish quantitative analytical systems that allow us to determine concentrations of the antigen in question (immunoassays) or to characterize the binding behavior of the antibody, binding protein, or receptor used in the reaction (various immunoassay uses but also including labeled antibody imaging applications).

## COMPETITIVE RADIOIMMUNOASSAY

To perform the classic competitive radioimmunoassay, the following are required:

- Ag, the analyte of unknown concentration in a known volume of specimen
- Ag*, the radionuclide-labeled analyte of known specific activity
- AgCal, a series of known analyte concentrations used to establish a calibration or standard curve
- Ab, a constant known amount of antibody that is specific for the analyte
- Buffer (a complex solution that provides the appropriate matrix for the reaction)
- Incubation system, such as a temperature-controlled waterbath
- Separation system, such as charcoal slurry and centrifuge
- Detection system (a counter that will detect radioactive decay for a variety of radionuclides)

### Method

When a constant amount of buffer is added to a 12 × 75–mm plastic tube, followed by the Ab, Ag, and Ag*, and is then mixed and incubated at 37°C for a specified period of time, the following reaction occurs:

| Added | | Free | | Bound |
|-------|---|------|---|-------|
| Ag | | Ag | | AgAb |
| Ag* | $\rightleftharpoons$ | Ag* | + | Ag*Ab |
| Ab | | Ab | | |

### Separation Techniques

Separation of the free and bound forms is accomplished by addition of a charcoal slurry, followed by centrifugation. Other separation techniques can be used. Counting the bound fraction (supernatant) in the counter gives the number of counts for the bound fraction.

Because the amount of radioactive analyte added is known, the percent of the radioactive analyte bound (%B) can be determined by:

$$\%B = \frac{CPM\ bound}{CPM\ added} \times 100 \qquad (2)$$

### Standard Curve

If this procedure is repeated for a number of tubes using known quantities of an analyte (AgCals), the relationship between %B and quantity of analyte added to the reaction mixture can be determined. This relationship allows the plotting of a standard curve from which the quantity of unknown analyte in a specimen that is subject to a similar process can be read from the %B calculated for that specimen. Control substances are included for quality control purposes (see Quality Control).

Table 26-1 shows a typical radioimmunoassay setup and the parameters usually encountered. Notice that the highest number of bound counts are found in the tubes containing the zero calibrator and, as the concentrations of the calibrators increase, the number of bound counts decrease. This is the signature of a competitive radioimmunoassay: increased competition for antibody binding sites between the labeled and unlabeled analyte as the concentration of the unknown analyte increases.

A distinction between standard and calibrator must be made. A *standard* is defined as an authentic analyte of known concentration if analyzed by the most accurate method possible and would therefore reflect the true concentration. All diagnostic kits use calibrators rather than true standards to establish the calibration curve. A calibrator yields a curve similar to that of a standard and gives the desired results when assaying a reference preparation but, if

**TABLE 26-1.** *RIA calibration data*

| Tube | Calibrator (ng/ml) | CPM bound | % Bound[a] | % B/B$_0$[b] | Concentration (ng/ml) |
|------|--------------------|-----------|-----------|-------------|----------------------|
| 1, 2 | Total cts | 13,444 | 100.0 | — | — |
| 3, 4 | 0.0 | 5,994 | 44.5 | 100.0 | — |
| 5, 6 | 62.5 | 4,482 | 33.3 | 74.7 | — |
| 7, 8 | 125.0 | 3,372 | 25.1 | 56.3 | — |
| 9, 10 | 250.0 | 2,319 | 17.2 | 38.7 | — |
| 11, 12 | 500.0 | 1,340 | 9.9 | 22.4 | — |
| 13, 14 | 1,000.0 | 715 | 5.3 | 11.9 | — |
| 15, 16 | 2,000.0 | 402 | 2.9 | 6.7 | — |
| 17, 18 | Control 1 | 3,965 | 29.5 | 66.3 | 85.6 |
| 19, 20 | Control 2 | 1,387 | 10.3 | 23.1 | 489.3 |
| 21, 22 | Patient 1 | 2,156 | 16.0 | 35.9 | 274.5 |

Note: Average for two tubes.

[a] $\% \text{ Bound} = \dfrac{CPM\ bound}{Total\ counts\ added} \times 100$

[b] $\% \dfrac{B}{B_0} = \dfrac{\% \text{ Bound}}{44.5} \times 100$

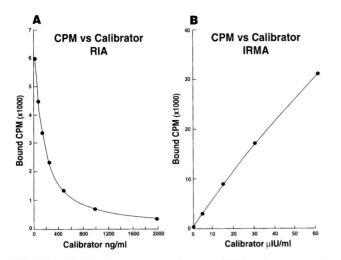

**FIG. 26-1.** Calibration curves showing **(A)** the inverse and **(B)** direct relationships of CPM versus concentration.

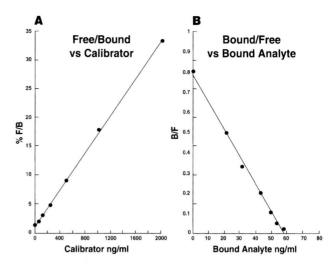

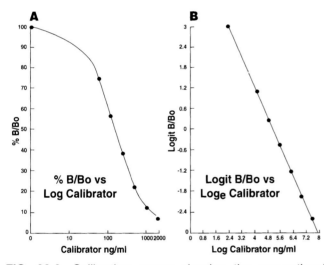

**FIG. 26-2.** Calibration curves showing the conventional handplot of **(A)** $B/B_0$ versus log concentration and **(B)** a logit log transformation that results in linearization of the curve.

**FIG. 26-3.** Calibration curves showing **(A)** free/bound versus concentration and **(B)** bound/free (B/F) versus concentration of bound analyte. The B/F versus bound is the Scatchard plot, used in radioreceptor assays.

and concentration is observed (Fig. 26-1B). The simple hand plot of $B/B_0$ versus concentration on semi-log graph paper linearizes the curve over the useful assay range (Fig. 26-2A) and is the classic plot used. Transformations such as logit of $B/B_0$ versus log concentration usually linearize the entire curve (Fig. 26-2B). Less frequently used transformations include free/bound versus analyte concentration (Fig. 26-3A), and bound/free versus bound analyte concentration (as seen in the Scatchard plot in Fig. 26-3B) commonly used in RRAs.

### Distinguishing Features of RIA

What distinguishes individual RIAs? Initially, the main differences between RIAs was the isotope used. I-131 was commonly used for $T_4$, protein, and polypeptide assays. Hydrogen 3 (H-3) and even carbon 14 (C-14) were used in CPB assays for steroids, and cobalt 57 (Co-57) and I-125 for a combined vitamin $B_{12}$ folate assay. This has changed, and now I-125 is generally the isotope of choice, especially with its favorable low-energy gamma emission and long shelf-life ($T_{1/2}$ of 60 days). Some assays still use H-3, particularly the gold standard RRAs, although I-125 is now being substituted.

Another distinguishing feature of RIA systems is the method of separation of free and bound. The use of second antibodies to precipitate the analyte-antibody complexes superseded dextran-coated charcoal, whereas other mechanisms, using immobilized second antibodies on tubes, beads, or magnetic particles, helped to eliminate a time-consuming centrifugation step. Many of the separation techniques became proprietary trademarks of certain manufacturers of diagnostic kits. The author's laboratory uses most of the separation techniques listed, including the classic dextran charcoal for estrogen and progesterone receptor-binding assays.

assayed by the most accurate method, may yield results slightly different than expected. Calibrators are constituted so that differences in the performance of a diagnostic immunoassay kit are minimized from lot to lot.

Several other outcomes are possible when establishing a calibration curve: The bound fraction can be plotted as counted; these values can be expanded by plotting $B/B_0$ (dividing the bound counts for each calibrator by the number of bound counts in the zero calibrator); and there are a number of options to transform the calibration plot.

When bound radioactivity is plotted against calibrator concentration in an RIA (a competitive reaction), an inverse curvilinear relationship between bound counts and concentration results (Fig. 26-1A). For an IRMA (see Immunoradiometric Assay), an almost linear relationship between bound counts

## IMMUNORADIOMETRIC ASSAY

The IRMA, developed by Miles and Hales (7), is an antibody excess assay that provides a direct measure of the analyte. The most common form uses a first antibody, directed against the analyte, which is usually immobilized on the surface of a tube, well, sphere, or magnetic particle, and a second labeled antibody directed against another epitope (binding site) of the analyte. This is called a *two-site IRMA*. After a specified incubation time, the excess second antibody is washed off and discarded. The remaining complex (first antibody-analyte-second antibody-label complex) is very simply measured without the need for additional complicated separation techniques.

Because this assay format uses considerable amounts of antibody, the breakthrough by Kohler and Milstein (8) providing large quantities of monoclonal antibodies of high specificity through hybridoma technology has made this technique the method of choice today. The attractive features of the IRMA include the substitution of a centrifugation step by a simple and easily automated wash step to separate free and bound fractions. The whole process lends itself well to a robotic microtiter plate assay format, where many of the steps are completely automated using a computer, an x-y robotic arm, a wash station, a microtiter plate holder, a counter that accepts microtiter plates, and software that drives the system and processes the counter output. The IRMA format allows one to label the second antibody with enzymes, fluorescent molecules, or chemiluminescent compounds for improved sensitivity and convenience while eliminating the need for disposal of radioactive waste.

The relationship between the analyte and the second antibody is almost directly linear in nature (see Fig. 26-1B). The extreme sensitivity of IRMA has provided the clinician with a spectrum of sensitive assays that were previously not possible. The utility of thyrotropin (TSH) IRMA as a single best thyroid function test is one of the outcomes of a well-designed IRMA (see TSH Assays).

## ASSAY PERFORMANCE

The three fundamental performance characteristics of precision, sensitivity, and accuracy are of paramount importance in our world of increasing regulation.

### Precision

Precision is the ability of a system to repeat an analytical measurement and produce results that are as close to identical as the assay system allows. Generally, precision is expressed as the standard deviation (SD) of the mean and commonly expressed as the coefficient of variation (CV) of the mean:

$$CV = \frac{SD}{Mean} \times 100 \qquad (3)$$

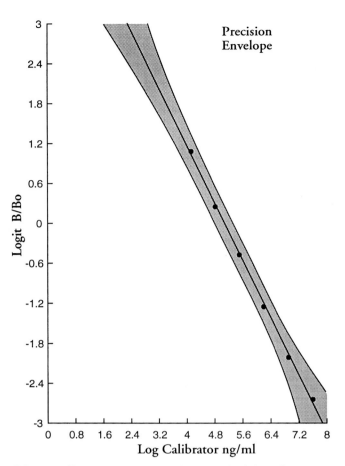

**FIG. 26-4.** Precision envelope about the logit-log plot showing the greater variance at the extremes of the assay (twice that of the central portion of the assay range).

The CV is conveniently expressed as a percent and therefore allows rapid comparison of different assays with different absolute values of SD. Manual RIA systems show within-run CVs from 4% to 10%. Robotic RIA systems show within-run CVs from 2% to 4%. We typically express precision in terms of the series of measurements we make, and the ideal precision is determined within a single run (intra-assay) of 20 consecutive measurements. This within-run figure, although somewhat artificial, provides a standardized way of determining the performance of a method. More realistically, the between-run (interassay) precision of a series of measurements made in sequential assay runs better reflects the performance of a method as used in daily analysis. Between-run or between-day precision values are usually 1% or 2% higher than within-run values.

In RIAs and IRMAs, precision is influenced by many factors that must be optimized individually. These include all the quantitative steps associated with the following:

- Delivery of reagents
- Timing of the reactions

- Control of temperature of the reaction chamber
- Counting of the radionuclide

Precision within an individual assay varies over the measurement range. At the low- and high-concentration extremes of an assay, variance is greater than the midrange (Fig. 26-4). Yalow and Berson (11) and Ekins and colleagues (12–14) have discussed this issue and concluded that the best precision is located at the point of maximum slope of the calibration curve, which is ideally the midpoint of the assay range.

## Sensitivity

Sensitivity depends on precision and can be looked on as a special case of precision. The accepted definition of sensitivity is the ability of an analytical system to distinguish, with a certain amount of statistical certainty, the smallest amount of analyte from the zero analyte. This is usually characterized by determining the precision of the assay at a very low analyte concentration, and determining the concentration equivalent to two standard deviations from the zero analyte concentration. Ekins (13) recognized the importance of the precision profile and has suggested its use for determining sensitivity from within-run measures. A variation of this approach by Bayer (15) used a between-run precision of 10% to determine the lower limit of the assay range because the precision profile showed a sharp increase in CV at the extremes of the assay curve (Fig. 26-5). These approaches provide an operationally reasonable means to define sensitivity.

There is a difference between competitive RIAs and IRMAs at low concentrations. RIA systems have high counts at the low end of the assay range, and the counting error is minimal. IRMA systems have low counts at the low end of the assay range and are more prone to effects of counting error. The magnitude of this error can be calculated based on the Poisson nature of radioactive decay, where the standard deviation is defined as $\sqrt{N}$.

$$CV = \frac{SD}{x} \times 100 \qquad (4)$$

$$= \frac{\sqrt{N}}{N} \times 100$$

For: 100 counts     CV = 10.0%
       1,000 counts     CV = 3.16%
       10,000 counts     CV = 1.0%

It would be prudent for the operator to set the counter for a predetermined number of counts rather than preset times to minimize the counting error at low concentrations in an IRMA and at high concentrations in an RIA. Clinically, this would be most significant for an IRMA measuring TSH, where maximum sensitivity is in the clinically desired low dose range for hyperthyroidism.

## Accuracy

Accuracy is the ability of an analytical system to determine the concentration of an analyte equal to, or as close as possible to, the true value of the specimen analyte. Accuracy of the immunoassay can be compromised by the authenticity of the calibrators used to establish the calibration curve. Ideally, the structure of the calibrator should be identical to that of the analyte. For small molecules, such as cortisol and $T_4$, this is possible. Thienpont and coworkers (16) report on the availability of serum reference materials that may be used to validate steroid assays. Protein hormones, such as growth hormone, insulin, and parathyroid hormone (PTH), also have their structures characterized and can be produced synthetically, so that standardization of calibrators is less difficult than it was in the past.

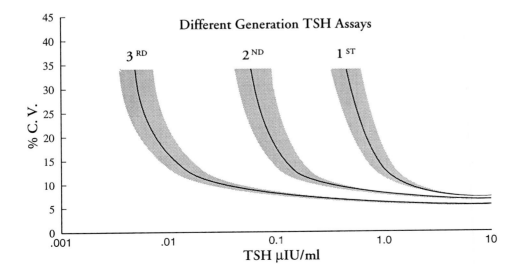

**FIG. 26-5.** Precision envelopes for first-, second-, and third-generation TSH assays using the 20% cutoffs. One can see that the minimal detectable dose is about 1.0, 0.1, and 0.01 µIU/ml respectively.

## Other Assay Characteristics

### Cross-Reactivity

Immunoassays have a number of special considerations that are unique. Antibodies recognize molecules that are close relatives of the measured parent molecule. This is known as *cross-reactivity*. For example, human chorionic gonadotropin, thyrotropin, luteotropin, and folliculotropin assays are developed to detect the beta subunits of their respective molecules because their alpha subunits are virtually identical. Miller and Valdes (17) outline five methods for evaluation of cross-reactivity in immunoassays.

### Interfering Reacting Substances

Monoclonal antibodies can reduce effects due to cross-reactivity to a great degree but are by no means ideal. Papers by Boscato and Stewart (18) and Kricka et al. (19) represent numerous reports on the interferences caused by heterophile antibodies, particularly in IRMA assay systems, that are based on murine hybridoma reagents. The specimens from patients receiving murine antibody imaging materials, such as OncoScint, can react with murine-based in vitro diagnostic reagents and give false values. This phenomenon of humans generating antibodies to foreign antibodies, such as OncoScint, is infrequent, but it requires caution on the part of the laboratory staff. Table 26-2 lists assay systems using murine-based antibodies, which may be influenced by human antimouse antibodies (HAMAs) that develop in response to murine monoclonal antibody imaging pharmaceuticals, such as OncoScint. More than 80% of the immunoassays in the author's laboratory are subject to this type of interference. Vadia and Beatty (20) proposed use of $F(ab')_2$ conjugates and polyclonal mouse immunoglobulin G (IgG) to eliminate HAMA interference in patient specimens. Kricka et al. (21)

**TABLE 26-2.** *Immunoassays using mouse antibodies in author's laboratory*

| Assay | Technology |
| --- | --- |
| B$_2$ microglobulin | EIA |
| CEA | EIA |
| FSH | EIA |
| LH | EIA |
| HCG quantitative | EIA |
| HCG urine | EIA |
| HCG serum | EIA |
| Prolactin | EIA |
| HGH | RIA |
| PSA | EIA |
| TT$_4$ | FIA |
| TSH | EIA |
| HBsAg | EIA |
| Anti-HAV-IgM | EIA |
| Ca-125 | RIA |

EIA, enzymeimmunoassay; RIA, radioimmunoassay; FIA, fluorescence immunoassay.

described a qualitative technique to determine the presence of HAMA in specimens using a proprietary sandwich (two-site IRMA) immunoassay, much like the ICON R rapid pregnancy test, which gives a response in <10 minutes and indicates if the patient's serum contains HAMA.

## DETERMINING ACCURACY

There are several methods by which accuracy of an assay can be determined. The first is by direct comparison of performance against reference standard preparations.

The second involves addition of reference standard material to a patient specimen of known concentration. This approach is known as the *standard addition* or *recovery method*. With this method, we know what the result should be, so any variance from that value is an estimate of assay inaccuracy. These approaches test the calibrators and the linearity of the assay.

A third approach is to perform a serial dilution of a reference preparation or a patient specimen of known high concentration. Ideally, if we plot values obtained against expected values, we should get a straight line with a slope of 1.0. Any deviation from this linearity is an estimate of inaccuracy. This approach tests the effect of specimen matrix on the assay system. Sometimes, interferences of lower binding activity may influence the result. Dilution of the specimen results in a reduction of the interferant to a point where it no longer interferes with the assay. Quantitative methods have been described to evaluate linearity by the National Committee for Clinical Laboratory Standards (NCCLS) in their guidelines NCCLS-EP6-P (22). Emancipator and Kroll (23) have proposed that very precise methods and heteroscedastic assays, such as RIAs, may fail linearity tests despite clinical acceptability. These authors propose an operational definition for the quantitative measurement of nonlinearity based on curve-fitting routines.

A fourth way of characterizing assay performance involves comparing the behavior of the assay to a reference method. The monograph by Westgard et al. (24) is recognized as an authoritative source on the topic. Linnet's comments on regression analysis (25) are also instructive. Essentially, a series of patient specimens with a wide range of values are assayed by the method in question and a reference method. The values obtained for the reference method and the method in question are plotted. A regression line for the points plotted is determined. The slope of the line, the y intercept, and the distribution of the experimental points around the line give estimates of errors associated with the assay in question.

## REGULATORY AGENCIES

Increased regulatory demands in recent years have required the laboratory to verify the performance of immunoassay systems. The Clinical Laboratory Improvement Act of 1988 (CLIA-88) (26) requires laboratories to verify or validate and document, for each method, the performance specifications for accuracy, precision, analytical sensitivity, analytical specificity, effect of interferences, reportable range of test results, and reference ranges. This must be done before diagnostic services are offered using RIA or IRMA methods. An effective approach to verifying an assay system is to use the method comparison approach by Westgard et al. (24). Those studies, along with an assessment of within-run and between-run precision, sensitivity, linearity, analytical range, and reference range, are adequate to validate a method. There is the assumption that a reference method is available. Operationally, if the RIA laboratory has a method already in place, it can serve as the reference method with the realization that it may have performance inadequacies. If the laboratory does not have a method to refer to, another laboratory of recognized stature may be approached to collaborate in the reference study.

**Proficiency Testing**

Assurance of the quality of a diagnostic method is an increasingly more important demand. CLIA-88 (26) requires diagnostic laboratories not only to participate in external quality assurance programs but also to have identified performance standards that must be met, otherwise penalties may be levied. Professional organizations, such as the College of American Pathologists, American Association of Clinical Chemistry, and state or regional programs provide materials and infrastructure. Generically, these programs are referred to as *proficiency testing* (PT) programs and have been the subject of an historical perspective by Sunderman (27). Boeckx has addressed increased government regulation of diagnostic laboratories and the potential for better quality (28).

Regardless, proficiency testing is here to stay, and we are obliged to participate. The question arises: How well must we perform to provide the level of quality expected? Ehrmeyer et al. (29) provide insight into this issue. Because the immunoassay laboratory is considered a subspecialty, a new Centers for Disease Control–Health Care Financing Agency rule (30) requires a laboratory to have 80% of all PT results correct. Because the likelihood of passing such a performance requirement decreases as the menu of tests increases, the shrewd laboratorian would be rewarded for selecting a limited menu of methods, with good precision and little bias. An unwritten rule is to select methods that many others use because PT performance is based on peer group consensus rather than accuracy, so likelihood of failure is reduced as the number of peer participants increases.

Complying with CLIA-88 has been addressed in the spring 1993 issue of the *Journal of Clinical Immunoassay* (31). Other strategies, using total quality management philosophies of continuous quality improvement of processes, discussed by Westgard and Barry (32,33), result in fewer PT failures and higher-quality diagnostic procedures.

**Quality Control**

To ensure that diagnostic immunoassays are performing acceptably, a mechanism to monitor performance is necessary. Quality control is the process by which the performance of an analytical system is monitored. Statland and Westgard (34), in a seminal presentation, have expanded this concept to quality management. The traditional process has been to use appropriate control products in each assay run and follow their values by a Shewhart plot (35) or a Levey-Jennings (36) control chart with 2-SD limits. Depending on the analyte, the laboratory may choose one, two, or three levels of controls to be included in each run. The choice of the number of controls can be determined by the number of medical decision levels that must be made. For example, for TSH, one may choose a control in the hyperthyroid range, the euthyroid range, and the hypothyroid range. The standard for appropriate interpretation of control rules is found in the paper by Westgard (37). Further contributions by Westgard (38) are charts of operational specifications (OPSpecs Charts). With OPSpecs Charts, which are available as a software package (39), one can determine the precision and accuracy requirements for a desired level of quality assurance as provided by a specific quality control rule.

*Corrective Actions*

Once it has been determined that an analytical run is suspect and the values compromised, what action should be taken? Examination of the duplicates of the controls and calibrators may indicate that a single point may be questioned. Elimination of the errant point and recalculation of the run may rectify the problem. Repeating the run may be necessary. Examination of the original specimen and knowledge of the patient may indicate that interferences due to hemolysis, matrix effects, drugs, or endogenous materials have compromised the assay and require the operator to acquire another specimen. Good laboratory practice dictates that corrective actions be recorded and reviewed frequently. Repeated corrective actions may require the laboratory to consider another assay method.

*Reporting While Troubleshooting*

When problems with assays are encountered, the patient's attending physician should be notified that there are suspicions about a particular result and the laboratory is attempting to rectify the problem. Providing notification of the assay problem is important for appropriate patient management and medical decision making. The acquisition of another specimen, the selection of an alternate diagnostic procedure, or consultation with a colleague may be necessary. Consultation with the manufacturer of the product or another laboratory that uses the same product is an important adjunct to effective troubleshooting. Documentation of all these steps is important and helps to reduce risk to the patients and to the organization.

## NEW DIRECTIONS AND DEVELOPMENTS

RIAs and IRMAs have matured and are being replaced by nonradionuclide label methods because of concerns about radioactivity and its disposal. The more common assays for thyroid hormones, gonadotropins, and tumor markers (e.g., carcinoembryonic and prostate-specific antigens) are now commonly performed by nonradioactive means, such as polarized fluorescence immunoassays, microparticle enzyme immunoassays, immobilized antibody fluorescence immunoassays, enzyme-multiplied immunoassays, and enzyme-linked immunosorbent assays of the microtiter plate format. Many RIAs and IRMAs will continue to be used because of their lower volumes. These will be joined by newer RIAs, IRMAs, and RRAs because radionuclide-labeled assays are easier and less costly to develop.

## RECEPTOR ASSAYS

RRAs have been in use for some time, but a resurgence of interest in the technique is occurring because of the rapidly expanding field of receptor study. The initial observation was by Korenman (40), followed by Korenman and Dukes (41), with CPB assays using a uterine macromolecule as the binding protein and a dextran-coated charcoal separation technique. They successfully measured steroids and detected breast tumor receptors.

Quantitation of receptors by a binding study uses the Scatchard plot (42) (see Fig. 26-3B). The same plot is used to measure receptor densities in positron emission tomography scanning. The ratio of percent bound to percent free against concentration of bound hormone yields a plot with a negative slope, the value of which, if multiplied by –1, is the affinity constant ($K_a$) of the binding protein or receptor. The reciprocal of the affinity constant is the dissociation constant ($K_d$). The interception on the x axis by the slope measures the concentration of the hormone at maximum binding (usually expressed in femtomoles per milliliter).

By convention, the receptor concentration is considered equal to the hormone concentration at maximum binding and is also expressed in femtomoles per milliliter. Receptors can be located in the nucleus, on membranes, or on cell surfaces. To standardize receptor preparations, the cytosol protein content in milligrams per milliliter is determined using an appropriate protein measure, as described by Lowry et al. (43). This allows one to express the receptor concentration in terms of milligrams of cytosol protein rather than that of wet weight of tissue.

## SCATCHARD ANALYSIS

Scatchard analysis is a variation of the setup of a calibration curve of CPB or RIA systems. Equal aliquots of the receptor preparation are incubated in duplicate tubes, at six levels of increasing concentration of radiolabeled ligand or hormone, of known specific activity (disintegrations per minute [DPM] per femtomole per milliliter). To correct for nonspecific binding (NSB), an additional six tubes in duplicate of buffer and radiolabeled ligand are also prepared. After an appropriate incubation time, the reaction is stopped by addition of cold dextran charcoal suspension to each tube, followed by mixing and centrifugation. The supernatant or bound fraction is counted (bound DPM). To determine the specific binding, NSB DPM is subtracted from bound DPM for each receptor tube. Free DPM is determined by subtracting bound DPM from total DPM added to each receptor tube. To arrive at the bound-to-free ratio (B/F), the concentration of bound ligand, and the receptor concentration in terms of femtomole per milliliter of cytosol protein, the following calculations are made:

$$\frac{B}{F} = \frac{(\text{Bound DPM} - \text{NSB DPM})}{(\text{Total DPM}) - (\text{bound DPM} - \text{NSB DPM})} \quad (5)$$

Calculation of bound ligand:

$$[\text{Bound ligand}] = \frac{(\text{Bound DPM} - \text{NSB DPM})}{(\text{DPM/fmol/ml})} = \text{fmol/ml} \quad (6)$$

$$(\text{DPM/fmol/ml}) = \text{specific activity}$$

Then plot:

y = B/F vs. x = concentration bound ligand (fmol/ml)
x intercept = ligand concentration at maximum binding
y intercept = receptor concentration fmol per ml
Slope = $-K_a$ = affinity constant
$\frac{1}{K_a}$ = dissociation constant

To calculate standardized receptor concentration in lieu of wet tissue:

$$\frac{\text{Receptor concentration (fmol/ml)}}{\text{Cytosol protein (mg/ml)}} = \text{Fmol/mg} \quad (7)$$

Receptor studies of hormones, growth factors, and cytokines are becoming more commonplace as adjuncts to cellular molecular studies. Because it is relatively easy and cost-effective to use radiolabels in such studies, there is a bright future for radionuclides in RRAs. Nuclear medicine departments have the knowledge and skills to manage radionuclides that many other hospital departments presently avoid. With the advent of molecular-based imaging techniques it would seem reasonable that a resurgence of RIA, IRMA, and RRA systems will occur within nuclear medicine departments.

## CLINICAL APPLICATIONS

### Thyroid Measurements

More than 40% of the adult population will exhibit some form of thyroid disease, mostly nodular thyroid disease. Approximately 1% of the population develop hyperthyroidism or hypothyroidism, and tests evaluating thyroid function and diseases are requested frequently. The challenge lies in the appropriate selection and interpretation of those procedures. The American Thyroid Association (ATA) guidelines for nomenclature have been documented and reported by Larsen et al. (44). Guidelines promulgated by the ATA on the use of laboratory tests in thyroid disorders have been reported by Surks et al. (45). More recently, ATA guidelines on TSH measurements and the assessment of $FT_4$ have been reported by Hay et al. (46). Additional information regarding use and misuse of the sensitive TSH assay has been reviewed by Nicoloff and Spencer (47). Hay and Klee (48) have discussed the relationship between medical needs and performance goals for thyroid function tests. With the above guidelines in mind, following are the suggested procedures of choice for evaluating thyroid function.

### TSH Assays

TSH assays have been classified by Nicoloff and Spencer (47) in terms of first-, second-, third-, and fourth-generation procedures. First-generation assays were RIA procedures sensitive to 1.0 mIU/liter. Second-generation TSH procedures were IRMAs, and these lowered the sensitivity to 0.1 mIU/liter, whereas third-generation TSH IRMAs were sensitive to 0.01 mIU/liter (see Fig. 26-5). A fourth-generation of TSH assay has become available that is sensitive below 0.001 mIU/liter. The more sensitive third- and fourth-generation TSH assays are typically enhanced fluorescent or chemiluminescent techniques. Second-generation TSH assays are considered to be the test of choice for thyroid dysfunction, readily differentiating between euthyroid and thyrotoxic subjects and monitoring patients on thyroid hormone replacement. Sensitive TSH (s-TSH) assays are considered inappropriate as the only screening test in patients with pituitary or hypothalamic disease, thyroid function screening of hospitalized patients with either nonthyroidal illnesses or acute psychotic disorders, and for monitoring the treatment of hypothyroidism or hyperthyroidism without a sufficient time interval (i.e., 6 weeks) for the response to drug therapy (e.g., $T_4$) to occur. TSH is a sensitive indicator of pituitary function, however, and warrants careful consideration because linear changes in $FT_4$ levels during replacement therapy result in logarithmic changes in TSH (49,50).

### Free $T_4$ Index and Free $T_4$ Estimate

$T_4$ is bound to $T_4$-binding globulin, albumin, and prealbumin while circulating in the bloodstream. Only 0.03% of total $T_4$ is free to react with end organ receptors. Because the proteins that bind thyroxine may vary in amount, a measurement of total $T_4$ may be misleading. To compensate for the variation in binding proteins, an assessment of the $T_4$ bound to those proteins is determined by the triiodothyronine uptake ($T_3U$) test. The product of $T_4 \times T_3U$ per 100 is known as the *free thyroxine index* ($FT_4I$).

Because the $FT_4I$ does not equal the free $T_4$ level nor give a value that reflects the total $T_4$ value, attempts were made to normalize the measurement by comparing $T_3U$ to a normal control population specimen that gives a $T_3U$ ratio (see below). The free $T_4$ estimate ($FT_4E$) is calculated using the $T_3U$ ratio and gives a value that more closely relates to total $T_4$.

$$FT_4E = T_4 \times \frac{T_3U \text{ patient}}{T_3U \text{ control}} \qquad (8)$$

$FT_4I$ and $FT_4E$ are procedures commonly performed by automated chemistry profile instruments or automated batch analyzers, are cost-effective, and are very competitive with s-TSH in terms of predictive value. The national Blue Cross/Blue Shield Association favors $FT_4I$ rather than s-TSH as the first-choice test of thyroid function. An extensive review by Helfand and Crapo (51) supports this position.

### $FT_4$ by Dialysis

Conceptually, the measurement of $FT_4$ would appear to be an ideal to achieve. This concept has been recently discussed by Ekins (52), who leaves considerable doubt about the ability of $FT_4$ assays to achieve consensus values on reference specimens. Although the ATA has recommended that $FT_4$ and s-TSH be the two principal tests for thyroid disease, a discussion by Hay et al. (46) raises some doubts as to whether there is clear resolution of this issue. $FT_4$ by the classic equilibrium dialysis method or the minidialysis chamber method is time-consuming and does not lend itself to high-volume routine laboratory applications and is most often sent out to reference laboratories, even from tertiary care centers such as the University of Wisconsin Hospital.

### $FT_4$ by Analog and Two-Step Immunoassays

Methods such as two-step immunoassays or analog immunoassays are advantageous because of their wide availability, speed, and reduced cost. They perform equally well as dialysis methods on normal, hyperthyroid, hypothyroid, pregnant, and estrogen-treated subjects but perform less well on patients with extreme binding abnormalities, as seen in late pregnancy and patients with severe nonthyroidal illness. $FT_4$ analog and two-step methods need to be more standardized before they can be strongly recommended as a viable replacement for the less costly $FT_4I$ and $FT_4E$.

### Total $T_3$

Measurement of total $T_3$ by RIA is a useful procedure to confirm thyroid disease in cases where $T_4$ measurements are equivocal. $T_3$ levels can be selectively elevated in patients having goiter due to iodine deficiency, in the early stages of hypothyroidism, and $T_3$ toxicosis, which occurs in subjects with multinodular goiter who occasionally exhibit elevated $T_3$ with normal $T_4$ levels. Patients with a single autonomous nodule can show preferential elevations of $T_3$. The $T_3$ level can be influenced by other circumstances external to the thyroid gland; for example, the peripheral conversion of $T_4$ to $T_3$ can be reduced by glucocorticoids, propranolol, amiodarone, iopanoic acid, sodium ipodate, and the thiouracils (45).

### Reverse $T_3$

Severely ill patients have depressed $T_3$ levels that correlate with their likelihood of survival and have increased levels of reverse $T_3$ ($rT_3$). The measurement of $rT_3$ has been more of an academic curiosity than a mainstream diagnostic test and is unlikely to be widely used.

### Tests for Autoimmune Thyroiditis

A diffuse firm goiter, normal $T_4$ and $T_3$, slight elevation of TSH, and significant elevation of microsomal and thyroglobulin antibodies are definitive indicators for autoimmune thyroiditis or Hashimoto's disease. The methods of choice are IRMA or RIA for thyroglobulin antibodies determinations and hemagglutination for microsomal antibodies because of their high sensitivities of 95% (53). Patients with the fibrous variant demonstrate thyroglobulin antibodies more frequently than patients with the hypercellular form. There is a positive correlation between TSH levels and sensitivity of assays for antibodies to thyroglobulin and microsomes. For TSH levels >20 µIU/ml, tests for thyroglobulin and microsomal antibodies are equally sensitive. For TSH levels <20 µIU/ml, the sensitivity of the IRMA assay for thyroglobulin antibodies falls to 50%, whereas the sensitivity for microsomal antibodies remains >70%. This suggests that microsomal antibodies appear earlier in the development of the disease and that both tests are relatively insensitive in early Hashimoto's thyroiditis.

## PTH Measurements

### Primary Hyperparathyroidism

Primary hyperparathyroidism is the result of a parathyroid adenoma and is documented by inappropriately elevated levels of PTH in the presence of hypercalcemia. The method of choice in these cases is the N-terminal intact (residues 1 to 85) PTH IRMA assay, although the C-terminal mid-molecule (residues 35 to 84) assays give equally useful information.

### Secondary Hyperparathyroidism

Secondary hyperparathyroidism is the result of renal disease and is documented by elevated levels of PTH and low normal or reduced serum calcium levels. The method of choice in well-established disease is the N-terminal intact PTH IRMA. Because the C-terminal fragments are cleared less rapidly in patients with renal disease, elevations of C-terminal fragments may not give a true reflection of parathyroid activity. Elevated levels of intact N-terminal PTH, and hypercalcemia in patients with renal disease reflect increased parathyroid function and the potential for glandular hypertrophy or hyperplasia that may need to be treated surgically.

### Tertiary Hyperparathyroidism

Tertiary hyperparathyroidism is encountered in renal transplant patients whose graft is somewhat refractory to PTH. This is documented by elevated levels of PTH and a spectrum of serum calcium levels from low to elevated. The method of choice is the N-terminal intact PTH IRMA, which reflects glandular function as opposed to changes in renal clearance seen in fragment assays. Surgical intervention may be indicated in those cases where high N-terminal intact PTH levels are observed, suggesting glandular hypertrophy and adenomatous transformation.

### Renal Osteodystrophies

Renal osteodystrophies include osteitis fibrosa as a result of excess PTH, and osteomalacia as a result of aluminum deposition or reduced availability or action of 1,25 dihydroxy vitamin D. Increasing levels of intact PTH and reductions of 1,25 dihydroxy vitamin D are indicators of early renal failure and the onset of bone disease, as Pitts and colleagues observed (54). In adults, high levels (>500 pg/ml) of intact PTH IRMA are diagnostic of osteitis fibrosa, whereas levels of 300 pg/ml are associated with a sensitivity of 85% and are considered the cutoff point for this disease. In children, intact PTH IRMA levels twice the upper limit of the normal range are diagnostic of bone lesions.

### Hypercalcemia of Malignancy

Hypercalcemia of malignancy is documented by low, or low normal, levels of parathormone and significantly elevated serum calcium as a result of a PTH–like peptide, secreted by squamous cell tumors of the head and neck and occasionally by other malignancies of the lung or ovary. The N-terminal sequence (residues 1 to 14) of the related peptide is sufficiently similar to that of PTH to react with the PTH receptor, but not reactive with antibodies used to measure PTH. Instead, an IRMA specific for the PTH-related peptide is now available to investigate suspected hypercalcemia of malignancy.

## REFERENCES

1. Berson YA, Yalow RS, Bauman A, et al. Insulin I-131 metabolism in human subjects: demonstration of insulin binding globulin in the circulation of insulin treated subjects. J Clin Invest 1956;35:170.
2. Berson YA, Yalow RS. Kinetics of insulin and insulin binding antibody. J Clin Invest 1957;36:873.

3. Ekins R. The estimation of thyroxine in human plasma by an electrophoretic technique. Clin Chem Acta 1960;5:433.
4. Murphy BEP. Some studies of the protein-binding of steroids and their application to the routine micro and ultramicromeasurement of various steroids in body fluids by competitive protein-binding radioassay. J Clin Endocrinol 1967;27:973.
5. Jensen EV, DeSombre ER, Jungblut PW. Estrogen Receptors in Hormone-Responsive Tissues and Tumors. In Wissler RW, Dao TL, Wood S (eds), Endogenous Factors Influencing Host-Tumor Balance. Chicago: University of Chicago, 1967;15.
6. Lieberman S, Erlanger BF, Bieser SM, Agate FJ Jr. Steroid-protein conjugates: their immunochemical and endocrinological properties. Recent Prog Horm Res 1959;15:165.
7. Miles LEM, Hales CM. Labelled antibodies and immunological assay systems. Nature 1968;219:186.
8. Kohler G, Milstein C. Continuous cultures of fused cells secreting antibody of predefined specificity. Nature 1975;256:495.
9. Gosling JP. A decade of development of immunoassay methodology. Clin Chem 1990;36:1408.
10. Nakamura RM, Tucker ES, Carlson IH. Immunoassays in the Clinical Laboratory. In Henry JB (ed), Clinical Diagnosis and Management by Laboratory Methods. Philadelphia: Saunders, 1991;848.
11. Yalow RS, Berson SA. Introduction and General Considerations. In Odell WD, Daughaday WH (eds), Principles of Competitive Protein Binding Assays. Philadelphia: Lippincott, 1971;9.
12. Ekins R, Newman B. Theoretical Aspects of Saturation Analysis. In Diczfalusy E (ed), Karolinska Symposia on Research Methods in Reproductive Endocrinology and Symposium: Steroid Assay by Protein Binding. Supplement no 147, Acta Endocrinologica (KBH), 1970;17.
13. Ekins R. The Precision Profile: Its Use in Assay Design, Assessment, and Quality Control. In Hunter WM, Corrie JET (eds), Immunoassay for Clinical Chemistry. Edinburgh: Churchill Livingstone, 1983;76.
14. Ekins R, Chu FW. Multianalyte microspot, immunoassay-microanalytical compact disc of the future. Clin Chem 1991;37:1955.
15. Bayer M. Performance criteria for appropriate characterization of highly sensitive thyrotropin assays. Clin Chem 1987;33:630.
16. Thienpont L, Siekmann L, Lawson A, et al. Development, validation, and certification by isotope dilution gas chromatography-mass spectrometry of lyophilized human serum reference materials for cortisol (CRM 192 and 193) and progesterone (CRM 347 and 348). Clin Chem 1991;37:541.
17. Miller JJ, Valdes R Jr. Methods for calculating cross-reactivity in immunoassays. J Clin Immunoassay 1992;15:97.
18. Boscato LM, Stuart MC. Heterophilic antibodies: a problem for all immunoassays. Clin Chem 1988;34:27.
19. Kricka LJ, Schemerfeld-Prus D, Senior M, et al. Interference by human anti-mouse antibody in two-site immunoassays. Clin Chem 1990;36:892.
20. Vadia HC, Beatty BG. Eliminating interference from heterophilic antibodies in a two site immunoassay for creatine kinase MB by using F(ab')$_2$ conjugate and polyclonal mouse IgG. Clin Chem 1992;38:1737.
21. Kricka LJ, Nozaki O, Goodman DBP, Ji X. Simple quantitative immunoassays of human anti-mouse antibodies evaluated. Clin Chem 1992;38:2559.
22. National Committee for Clinical Laboratory Standards. Evaluation of the Linearity of Quantitative Analytical Methods: Proposed Guideline. Villanova, PA: NCCLS Publication EP6-P, 1986.
23. Emancipator K, Kroll MH. A quantitative measure of nonlinearity. Clin Chem 1993;39:766.
24. Westgard JO, deVos DJ, Hunt MR, et al. Method Evaluation. Bellaire, TX: American Society for Medical Technology, 1978.
25. Linnet K. Evaluation of regression procedures for methods comparison studies. Clin Chem 1993;39:424.
26. Medicare, Medicaid, and CLIA programs. Regulations implementing the clinical laboratory improvement amendments of 1988. U.S. Department of Health and Human Services, Fed Reg 1992;57:7002.
27. Sunderman FW Sr. The history of proficiency testing/quality control. Clin Chem 1992;38:1205.
28. Boeckx RL. Government regulation: can it guarantee quality in the clinical laboratory. Clin Chem 1992;38:1203.
29. Ehrmeyer SS, Laessig RH, Leinweber JE, Oryall JJ. 1990 Medicare/CLIA final rules for proficiency testing: minimum intralaboratory performance characteristics (CV and bias) needed to pass. Clin Chem 1990;36:1736.
30. Centers for Disease Control and Health Care Financing Agency. Proposed Uniform Proficiency Testing for Clinical Laboratory Act of 1967 and Medicare Laboratories. U.S. Department of Health and Human Services, Fed Reg 29590. August 5, 1988; 29590-632.
31. Nordbloom G (ed), Theme: Complying with CLIA '88. Wayne, MI: Clinical Ligand Assay Society, 1993.
32. Westgard JO, Barry PL. Cost-Effective Quality Control: Managing the Quality and Productivity of Analytical Processes. Washington, DC: American Association of Clinical Chemistry, 1986.
33. Westgard JO, Barry PL. Total quality control: evolution of quality management systems. Lab Med 1989;20:377.
34. Statland BE, Westgard JO. Quality Management. In Henry JB (ed), Clinical Diagnosis and Management by Laboratory Methods. Philadelphia: Saunders, 1991;81.
35. Shewhart WA. Economic Control of Quality of Manufactured Products. New York: Van Nostrand, 1931.
36. Levey S, Jennings ER. The use of control charts in the clinical laboratory. Am J Clin Pathol 1950;20:1059.
37. Westgard JO, Barry PL, Hunt MR, Groth TA. Multi-rule Shewhart chart for quality control in clinical chemistry. Clin Chem 1981;27:493.
38. Westgard JO. Charts of operational process specifications ("OPSpecs Charts") for assessing the precision, accuracy, and quality control needed to satisfy proficiency testing performance criteria. Clin Chem 1992;38:1226.
39. Westgard JO. QC Validator Program Manual. Ogunquit, ME: Westgard QC, 1993.
40. Korenman SG. Radio-ligand binding assay of specific estrogens using a soluble uterine macromolecule. J Clin Endocrinol Metab 1968; 28:127.
41. Korenman SG, Dukes BA. Specific estrogen binding by the cytoplasm of human breast carcinoma. J Clin Endocrinol Metab 1970; 30:639.
42. Scatchard G. The attractions of proteins for small molecules and ions. Ann N Y Acad Sci 1949;51:660.
43. Lowry OH, Rosebrough NJ, Farr AL, Randall RJ. Protein measurement with the folin phenol reagent. J Biol Chem 1951;193:265.
44. Larsen PR, Alexander NM, Chopra IJ, et al. Revised nomenclature for tests of thyroid hormones and thyroid related proteins in serum. J Clin Endocrinol Metab 1987;64:1089.
45. Surks MI, Chopra IJ, Mariash CN, et al. American thyroid association guidelines for use of laboratory tests in thyroid disorders. JAMA 1990;263:1529.
46. Hay ID, Bayer MF, Kaplan MM, et al. American thyroid association assessment of current free thyroid hormone and thyrotropin measurements and guidelines for future clinical assays. Clin Chem 1991;37:2002.
47. Nicoloff JT, Spencer CA. The use and misuse of the sensitive thyrotropin assays. J Clin Endocrinol Metab 1990;71:553.
48. Hay ID, Klee GG. Linking medical needs and performance goals: clinical and laboratory perspectives on thyroid disease. Clin Chem 1993;39:1519.
49. Klee GG, Hay ID. Biochemical thyroid function testing. Mayo Clin Proc 1994;69:469.
50. Stockigt JR, Topliss DJ. Assessment of Thyroid Function: Current Strategy. In Stockigt JR (ed), Fellowship Affairs. Endocrine Society of Australia, June 21, 1992.
51. Helfand M, Crapo LM. Screening for thyroid disease. Ann Intern Med 1990;112:840.
52. Ekins R. The free hormone hypothesis and measurement of free hormones. Clin Chem 1992;38:1289.
53. Gupta MK. Autoimmune thyroiditis (AIT): humoral aspects of thyroid autoimmunity. The American Society of Clinical Pathologists Check Sample Continuing Education Program. Immunopathology 1987;11:88.
54. Pitts TO, Pirano BH, Mitro R, et al. Hyperparathyroidism and 1,25 dihydroxy vitamin D deficiency in mild, moderate, and severe renal failure. J Clin Endocrinol Metab 1988;67:876.

*Textbook of Nuclear Medicine,*
edited by Michael A. Wilson.
Lippincott–Raven Publishers, Philadelphia © 1998.

CHAPTER **27**

# Biological Effects of Radiation

John F. Fowler

---

The hazards from ionizing radiation are minimal to staff and patients in a well-run nuclear medicine department. Nevertheless, questions always arise from the use of radioactive substances because injurious effects are delayed and random.

Chromosomes can be damaged by radiation, but at low dose rates there is only a small probability of genetic mutation or malignant transformation leading to cancer many years later. The main hazard appears to be cancer in the irradiated individual. No genetic effects (i.e., those passed to a future generation after irradiation of the parents) have been observed in the human population offspring of irradiated patients.

There is a separate hazard to the fetus with irradiation of a pregnant woman when the fetus is between 8 and 15 weeks old. In this circumstance, the development of the fetal central nervous system (CNS) might be compromised, with possible loss of intelligence in the offspring. This chapter gives some recent estimates of probabilities, based on human and animal data.

## UNITS OF RADIATION DOSE

The traditional unit of radiation dose for hazard estimation is the rem (rad equivalent man). In the radiation risk literature, the term is changing to the sievert (Sv). One rem equals one rad multiplied by the quality factor, Q. For the radiation commonly used in nuclear medicine—gamma rays (photons), x-rays (low-energy photons), beta rays (electrons), and positrons (positively charged electrons)—Q is 1.0, so 1 rem is equal to 1 rad. The equivalent Système International d'Unités (International System of Units) units are 1 Sv and 1 gray (Gy), equal to 100 rems or rads, respectively. The value of Q rises to 10 for neutrons and to 20 for alpha particles. Alpha particles are used rarely in medicine, and then only for radioimmunotherapy. Neutron-emitting or alpha-particle–emitting radionuclides have been used only to treat cancer patients. However, alpha particles are emitted by radon gas diffusing out of

earth and rocks, which delivers about one-half of the natural background radiation dose.

Table 27-1 gives conversion factors and describes the population background exposure from all sources, of 100 to 600 mrem (1 to 6 mSv) per year, depending on the locale and housing. An average figure is approximately 360 mrem (3.6 mSv) per year in the United States. This is the figure to bear in mind, because a practical way of expressing an occupational or diagnostic dose is to say how many months or years of background radiation would give the same dose. This is the background equivalent radiation time (BERT), and it is particularly useful for nonspecialists (1).

For example, a particular diagnostic test delivers an average whole-body dose of 360 mrem (3.6 mSv), which is equivalent to a BERT of 1 year. Nuclear medicine tests generally deliver very low doses of this order to most of the body and higher doses to specific organs.

## GENERAL PRINCIPLES

Radiobiological theory indicates that at low doses, the risk of a biological lesion being formed (e.g., in DNA) should depend linearly on the dose if a single event is required, or on the square of the dose if two events are required. It is commonly held that densely ionizing radiation (alpha particles and neutrons) can cause lesions by the traversal of a single particle. These latter are called *high-LET* (linear energy transfer) radiations. For low-LET radiation (electrons, gamma rays, and x-rays), either one or two photons might be required. At low doses, the induction of mutations or malignant transformations is predominantly linear. At higher doses, where the effect might increase with the square of the dose, radiation causes cell sterilization or death, which competes with the process of malignant transformation. The probability of avoiding cell death at yet higher doses follows the usual laws of cell survival, which indicate that it should

**TABLE 27-1.** *Units of dose and background exposure rates*

### Definitions

| | |
|---|---|
| 1 rem | = 1 rad $\times$ Q |
| 1 sievert | = 1 gray (Gy) $\times$ Q |
| Q | = 1.0 for gamma and beta rays |
| | 10 for neutrons |
| | 20 for alpha particles |

### Conversions

| | |
|---|---|
| 1 rem | = 1 centisievert (cSv) |
| 1 rad | = 1 centigray (cGy) |
| 1 gray | = 100 rads |
| 1 sievert | = 100 rems |

### Background exposure estimates for U.S. general population

| | mrem | mSv |
|---|---|---|
| Natural background, radon | 200 | 2.00 |
| Natural background, other | 100 | 1.00 |
| Medical diagnostic x-rays | 39 | 0.39 |
| Nuclear medicine | 14 | 0.14 |
| Consumer products | 10 | 0.10 |
| Nuclear industry | <1 | <0.01 |
| Airline travel | 6 | 0.06 |
| Total background (varies from 100–600 mrem) | 369 | 3.69 |

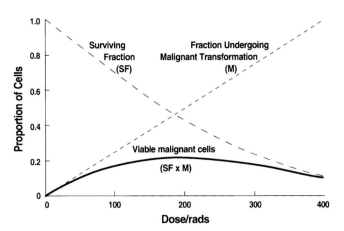

**FIG. 27-1.** Schematic diagram showing (full curve) the decrease of cancer incidence with increasing radiation dose after a maximum at several hundred rads (several gray). At low doses the increasing induction of malignant cells predominates, but at high doses the cell killing eliminates all cells. The full curve is the product of the two dashed curves.

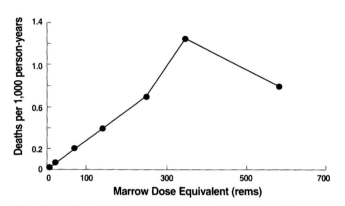

**FIG. 27-2.** Cumulative leukemia mortality in Hiroshima and Nagasaki plotted against the estimated dose equivalent to bone marrow, using the 1986 revised dose calculations. (Redrawn from BEIR V Report: Health Effects of Exposure to Low Levels of Ionizing Radiation. Washington, DC: National Academy Press, 1990; Fig. 5-1, p 243.)

have a decreasing dependence on dose or the square of dose (again, depending on whether one or two events are needed). When these principles are combined, one obtains a general dose-response model for cancer induction, which rises to a flattish maximum at a few grays of dose and then falls as cell killing predominates (Fig. 27-1). In nuclear medicine we are interested in the low-dose rising part of this curve.

There is still uncertainty about whether dose-response curves should be considered linear or supra-linear (linear quadratic). The 1990 Biological Effects of Ionizing Radiation (BEIR) V report (2) concludes that linearity, with no threshold, gives the best fit to data, except possibly for leukemia incidence, and even those data do not exclude linearity (Fig. 27-2). A further uncertainty arises concerning acute versus chronic (low dose-rate or fractionated) irradiation. With few exceptions, the human carcinogenic effects of radiation on the bone marrow, breast, thyroid gland, lung, stomach, colon, ovary, and other organs have been reported only after relatively high doses and dose rates. It is therefore very important for the back-extrapolation to very low doses whether a linear or a curving (dose-squared) response is assumed and whether any threshold dose is assumed. The linear no-threshold assumption is the safest assumption, that is, the worst-case scenario.

Accumulation of a low-LET dose over weeks or months is expected to appreciably reduce the lifetime risk of future carcinogenesis, possibly by a factor of two or three. This allowance is not made in any of the tables in this chapter. Some critics of the BEIR V report believe that

such an allowance should be made, which would reduce the risk probabilities quoted by a factor of two or three. The amount of reduction varies greatly from one type of cell, or tissue, to another. No such reduction in effect occurs with high-LET radiation. Although a reduction in the effect due to chronic administration (low dose rate) is certain in cell kill, it is less certain in carcinogenesis and unlikely in mutations.

Another factor that might reduce the risk of very low radiation dose is radiation hormesis. This can be considered radiation-induced repair, which makes cells more resistant to further radiation damage after they have received a minimal "triggering" dose. This subject is both scientifically and politically controversial, and the reader is encouraged to be alert to further developments. Studies of populations chronically exposed to low-level radiation, such as those residing in regions of four to six times natural background radiation, have not shown consistent or conclusive evidence of an increase in risk of cancer, although more chromosome abnormalities and T-lymphocyte activity are observed. To be on the safe side, the BEIR V report and the values of risk quoted here make no allowance for radiation hormesis.

## SOURCES OF DATA

The currently most up-to-date and authoritative estimates of health effects induced by low-LET radiation, such as x-rays and gamma rays, are published in the 1990 BEIR V report of the National Academy of Sciences (2), which is quoted extensively here. The author's indebtedness to that report is acknowledged.

The human data on cancer induction by radiation are extensive. The most comprehensive studies are those of the survivors of the atomic bombings of Hiroshima and Nagasaki, tuberculosis patients examined repeatedly with x-rays, and patients irradiated during treatment of ankylosing spondylitis, cervical cancer, or tinea capitis. Both the natural incidence and the radiation-induced incidence of cancer depend on the site of cancer, the age at irradiation, and other factors, such as hormonal status. As mentioned above, there are difficulties in extrapolating from the high doses given by the atomic bombs or the radiotherapy treatments to the low doses and low dose rates that concern us here.

Radiation injury in humans is classified as either somatic or genetic. Radiation effects are *somatic* if they occur in the exposed individual, or *genetic* if they are expressed in the individual's descendants. Regarding genetic disorders, considerable progress has been made in our understanding of the mutation process on genes and chromosomes, but there is no direct evidence of any increase in human heritable effects resulting from radiation exposure, including that from Hiroshima and Nagasaki. Estimates of genetic risks can be made, but they are based primarily on experimental data from laboratory animals, with the usual reservations about extrapolations from mouse to man. The risks are often expressed in terms of the *doubling dose,* which is the unit of radiation estimated to cause a doubling of the spontaneous background rate. The higher the estimated doubling dose, the safer is any given dose of radiation.

## RADIATION EFFECTS

The doubling dose for mutations in humans from low-LET radiation is now estimated to be close to 100 mrem (1 Sv). This is one or two orders of magnitude larger than the usual organ doses from diagnostic procedures. Much larger doses

**TABLE 27-2.** *Approximate thresholds for nonstochastic effects in adult humans*

| Tissue and effect | Total acute dose (rem/cSv) |
|---|---|
| Testes | |
| Oligospermia | 15 |
| Permanent sterility | 350 |
| Ovaries | |
| Permanent sterility | 250–600 |
| Lens of eye | |
| Detectable opacities | 50–200 |
| Cataracts | 500 |
| Bone marrow | |
| Depression | 50 |
| Fatal aplasia | 150 |
| Skin (limited area) | |
| Erythema | 900 |
| Moist desquamation | 2,000 |

Sources: ICRP Publication 41. Nonstochastic Effects of Ionizing Radiation. New York: Pergamon, 1984; and skin data from author's experience.

can cause more immediate "radiation sickness" in irradiated individuals. Such signs and symptoms are generally seen only in cases of radiation accidents or cancer therapy.

The effects of irradiation may also be classified as either stochastic or nonstochastic. *Stochastic* effects are those for which the probability of occurrence of an effect, rather than its severity, increases with dose. Genetic effects and carcinogenesis are stochastic. It is assumed that any dose, no matter how small, may increase the probability of such effects occurring, even if the majority of the population experience no effect. No threshold dose is postulated for stochastic effects. Nonstochastic effects are those for which the severity of the pathologic effect increases with dose, and most individuals would experience the effect at doses above some threshold level. Relatively high levels of dose are necessary to produce such effects. Erythema, epilation, cataracts, cell depletion of the bone marrow, and impaired fertility are nonstochastic effects, and there exist threshold doses below which these effects do not occur.

## NONSTOCHASTIC EFFECTS

### Radiation Syndrome

Table 27-2 lists the threshold doses estimated by the International Commission on Radiation Protection (ICRP) (3) for various pathologic end points in human subjects, plus erythema and desquamation of skin from the author's experience.

Table 27-3 lists the signs and symptoms of acute radiation syndrome after whole-body exposure. These high doses are only relevant to radiation accident situations, not to the questions concerning biological effects after diagnostic procedures in nuclear medicine or radiology.

**TABLE 27-3.** *Radiation syndrome: serious injury to human individual due to radiation accident or nuclear war*

| Dose | Effect |
|---|---|
| <50 rads (<0.5 Gy) | Generally no clinical effect; subject is asymptomatic |
| 50–100 rads (0.5–1.0 Gy) | Mild nausea in some; WBCs increase (↑), then decrease (↓) |
| 100–200 rads (1–2 Gy) | Nausea and vomiting (NV); fatigue; WBCs ↑, then ↓ Recovery in 2–4 days |
| 200–400 rads (2–4 Gy) | 2–3 days of NV and fatigue; WBCs ↓↓ and platelets ↓ Recovery period 1–3 weeks Epilation, diarrhea, bleeding Some die in 4–6 weeks |
| 300–500 rads (3–5 Gy) | $LD_{50}$ (dose lethal to 50% of people exposed) |
| 400–600 rads (4–6 Gy) | Severe NV and diarrhea, sore throat; WBCs and platelets ↓↓ Recovery period brief or absent Symptoms recur, hemorrhages Death in most in <30 days |
| 600–1,000 rads (6–10 Gy) | Severe and continuing NV and diarrhea Death in most in 1–10 days |
| >1,000 rads (>10 Gy) | Severe illness, disorientation, ataxia, burning sensation, shock All die, most in 10–36 hours |

Time scale of effects: gastrointestinal and electrolyte: 1–10 days; marrow, blood counts, bleeding: 2–6 weeks; central nervous system (>10 Gy): 10–36 hours.

## STOCHASTIC EFFECTS

### Genetic Risk

Data from experiments on fruit flies and mice suggest a curvilinear relationship between mutation induction and low-LET dose, with a reduced effect at lower doses and dose rates. This is still controversial because other data from cell culture suggest a linear nonthreshold relationship. A large body of data on frequencies of induced mutations, both for individual gene loci and for more complex effects, such as skeletal stunting, suggest median doubling doses for mice 100 to 114 mrems (1.0 to 1.14 Sv). These doses are similar to the lower 95% confidence limit of doubling dose for the Japanese bomb survivors (4). Only lower limits of doubling dose (corresponding to higher limits of risk) could be derived there because *there was no significant effect* among 75,000 births, of which 38,000 had at least one parent exposed to radiation. Radiation-induced effects were probably not detectable in a population of that size because they would not be different from naturally occurring mutations. The doses received could produce only a small increase in the number of deaths, diseases, and disabilities above the spontaneously occurring rate of up to 10.7% of live-born humans (5).

Mutations normally enter the gene pool at low rates, and deleterious mutations leave the pool at low rates. In undis-turbed populations, the rates of entry and elimination are about equal. This results in a more or less constant but small fraction of the gene pool being mutant in an equilibrium situation. This mutant fraction is called the *mutation burden* or *load*. Almost all genetic mutations are harmful, and damaged genes are eliminated quickly from the population because afflicted individuals are less likely to reproduce successfully. On the other hand, mutations with mild effects may disappear only gradually over many generations.

The spontaneous mutation rate figure of 10.7% of all live births is controversial, depending greatly on the definition of *disability* and the completeness of data collection. The recent BEIR V report (6) revises its previous estimate of 9% downward to 3% of all live births (excepting congenital dislocation of the hip in Hungary). This figure, together with the overall doubling dose for low-LET radiation of 100 rem (1 Sv), enables approximate risks to be estimated. The higher the doubling dose, the lower the risk. The higher the estimate of spontaneous disadvantageous mutations, the higher the absolute risk, but the relative risk does not depend on the baseline rate (be it 10% or 3%).

To illustrate, let us assume that a man was exposed to 10 mrem (0.1 Sv) of gonadal irradiation during three treatments with iodine 131 (I-131) for hyperthyroidism (5). Several years later, he and his wife want to have children, and the couple are concerned about the possibility of congenital malformation. From the figure above of a doubling dose of 100 mrem (1 Sv), the 10 mrem (0.1 Sv) received would be expected to increase the risk by (ln 2) × 10/100, which is 0.069, or 7%. The 7% increase in risk on top of the background 10.7% would lead to a possible risk of 11.4%. If the background were 3%, this would lead to a possible risk of 3.2%. These are small increases, and they may be smaller still by a factor of two or three because the 10-mrem (0.1-Sv) dose was delivered in three separate fractions, each at low dose rate over several days or weeks.

An index of the presumed genetic impact of radiation exposure to a whole population is the *genetically significant dose* (GSD). This is defined as the dose that, if received by every member of the population, would be expected to produce the same number of genetic abnormalities as are produced by the actual doses received by the various individuals. The dose that matters here is not the total dose, but the dose to the gonads of people who later produce children (5). The GSD for natural background radiation is approximately 360 mrem (3.6 mSv) per year, including the dose from radon. Medical x-rays contribute approximately 40 mrem (0.4 mSv), and nuclear medicine procedures approximately 14 mrem (0.14 mSv) to the GSD (see Table 27-1) (5).

### Irradiation of Embryo or Fetus

The effects of relatively large doses of prenatal irradiation on the growth and development of the mammalian embryo

**TABLE 27-4.** *Severe mental retardation in those exposed in utero*

| Fetal dose (rads/cGy) | Gestational age | | |
|---|---|---|---|
| | 8–15 weeks | 16–25 weeks | All ages |
| 25 rads | 3% (0-10)* | 0% (0–2) | 0% (0–4) |
| 70 rads | 25% (13–45) | 0% (0–16) | 10% (4–19) |
| 140 rads | 75% (52–100) | 37% (16–66) | 46% (32–62) |

*(90% confidence interval)

Sources: UNSCEAR Report E 86. IX.9. Genetic and Somatic Effects of Ionizing Radiation. New York, NY: United Nations, 1986; and BEIR V Report. Health Effects of Exposure to Low Levels of Ionizing Radiation. Washington, DC: National Academy Press, 1990;354–362.

and fetus are mediated through direct radiation injury (cell killing leading to organ depletion). These include gross structural malformations, growth retardation, embryo lethality, sterility, and CNS abnormalities. Major malformations have been observed in all species by irradiation during early organogenesis; however, the time of maximum susceptibility is sharply circumscribed. In contrast, retardation of postnatal growth has been produced over a broad range of gestational ages in experimental animals and humans.

The most definitive human data concerning the effects of large single doses of prenatal irradiation are those relating to brain development (7). Among the 1,598 Japanese atomic bomb survivors who were irradiated in utero, a prevalence of mental retardation and small head size was found to increase with the uterine dose. Thirty of these children were diagnosed before the age of 17 to have severe mental retardation.

Gestational age was an important factor, with 8 to 15 weeks being an especially sensitive period because it is the period of rapid CNS development (Table 27-4). Some uncertainties are associated with the risk estimates in Table 27-4, but the effect is sufficiently large and clearly related to increasing fetal dose. The possibility of a threshold dose of 10 to 40 rems (0.1 to 0.4 Sv) could not be either excluded or confirmed. It can be

seen from Table 27-4 that the risk from an exposure of 0.1 Sv is small, even if no threshold is assumed.

Intelligence tests of these children at age 10 to 11 years showed significantly low IQ scores only for those irradiated at 8 to 15 weeks (8). A higher frequency of maladjustment and psychiatric disorders was also recorded in two groups of tinea capitis patients (mean dose, 130 rems [1.3 Sv]) and in a group of patients treated for childhood leukemia with brain irradiation to doses of 1,000 to 2,000 rems (10 to 20 Sv) (8).

### Radiation-Induced Cancers

The main risk to consider from small doses of radiation is an increase in the incidence of cancer. Radiation, like chemical carcinogens, can induce cancer in any organ, roughly in proportion to the natural incidence. Age at exposure, sex, cancer type, hormonal status, smoking habits, and unknown environmental and genetic factors can all influence the radiation induction of cancer.

For the purpose of risk assessment, the BEIR V report (9) considers the population-weighted average lifetime excess risk of cancer death after an acute low-LET dose equivalent to all body organs of 10 rems (28 years of BERT) to be 0.8%. This lifetime risk varies considerably with age at the time of exposure. It is important to remember that accumulation of low-LET radiation dose over weeks or months may reduce the risk appreciably, possibly by a factor of two or three. The BEIR V estimated lifetime risks do not allow for this. The estimated lifetime risks are similar overall for males and females, although they differ in specific organs. The risk from exposure during childhood is about twice as large as the risk for adults (9).

This 0.8% increase in the absolute risk of cancer is equal to an increase in relative risk of 4% on the baseline risk of "spontaneous" cancer incidence of approximately 20% in a lifetime: 20% × 4% = 0.8%. The 90% confidence range on the 0.8% estimate for an acute whole-body dose of 10 rems (0.1 Sv) is 0.5% to 1.2% (mean, 0.77%) for males of all ages and 0.6% to 1.2% (mean, 0.81%) for females of all ages (9).

**TABLE 27-5.** *Major characteristics of the data sets used for model fitting for risk estimates of cancer induction*

| | | Cancer sites | Total cases | Total person-years |
|---|---|---|---|---|
| Atomic bomb survivors | Mortality | All | 5,936 | 2,185,335 |
| | Incidence | Breast | 376 | 940,000 |
| Ankylosing patients | Mortality | Leukemia | 36 | 104,000 |
| | Mortality | Nonleukemia* | 563 | 104,000 |
| Canadian patients | Mortality | Breast | 482 | 867,541 |
| Massachusetts fluoroscopy | Mortality | Breast | 74 | 30,932 |
| NY postpartum mastitis | Incidence | Breast | 115 | 45,000 |
| Israel tinea capitis | Incidence | Thyroid | 55 | 712,000 |
| Rochester thymus treatment | Incidence | Thyroid | 28 | 138,000 |

*Except colon cancer.

Source: Table 4-1 in BEIR V Report: Health Effects of Exposure to Low Levels of Ionizing Radiation. Washington, DC: National Academy Press, 1990;164.

A linear no-threshold model is currently proposed to fit the data best, in the dose range below 400 rems (4 Sv). The influence of age at exposure and sex on the carcinogenic response to radiation by humans has been characterized to a limited degree, as shown in Table 27-5, but changes in response due to dose rate and LET have not been quantified. Table 27-5 summarizes the human data used by the BEIR V report for testing the fit of various statistical models used to predict the variation of cancer incidence and mortality with age at irradiation. The largest numbers to study come from the atomic bomb survivors. For solid cancers, there is an induction period of at least 10 years before the radiation-induced incidence begins to rise; for leukemias, the induction period is <2 years. Carcinogenic effects of radiation on the bone marrow, breast, thyroid gland, lung, stomach, colon, ovary, and other organs reported for atomic bomb survivors are similar to findings reported for other irradiated human populations.

Figures 27-3 and 27-4 and Table 27-6 give the BEIR V Committee's estimates for the increase in risk of cancer induction for the remaining lifetime of individuals irradiated with 0.1 Sv (10 rems) at the ages shown. Although young children are certainly more sensitive to cancer induction, as shown by the total curve in the figures, the estimated risks at these young ages are less reliable than those for irradiation at middle age because of the smaller numbers available for analysis. Table 27-6 indicates the uncertainties by presenting the 90% confidence intervals in brackets. These estimated risks, reproduced with permission from the BEIR V report (2), present the best values likely to be available for the next few years. They assume a linear no-threshold dose response curve, which is the most cautious (worst-case) assumption.

It is clear that the solid tumors (dashed curves in Figs. 27-3 and 27-4) show the highest risk for the irradiation of

**TABLE 27-6.** *Excess risk estimates from 10 rems (0.1 Sv) acute exposure to 100,000 males of each age*

| Age at exposure | Leukemia (95% CI) | Nonleukemia (95% CI) |
|---|---|---|
| 5 | 111 (20–455) | 1,165 (673–1,956) |
| 15 | 109 (21–450) | 1,035 (642–1,775) |
| 25 | 36 (8–87) | 885 (534–1,442) |
| 35 | 62 (21–134) | 504 (272–947) |
| 45 | 108 (43–223) | 492 (257–883) |
| 55 | 166 (59–338) | 450 (217–815) |
| 65 | 191 (65–369) | 290 (137–572) |
| 75 | 165 (56–316) | 93 (38–233) |
| 85 | 96 (33–183) | 14 (5–44) |

Source: Table 4D-4, BEIR V Report: Health Effects of Exposure to Low Levels of Ionizing Radiation. Washington, DC: National Academy Press, 1990;203, with permission from the National Academy of Sciences Press. These figures are to be added to the approximately 20,000 representing the 20% risk of "spontaneous" cancer.

children and young adults. These estimated values are high because uncertainties make cautious estimates necessary. The risk diminishes with age because of the diminishing period at risk (shorter life expectancy) and because of the long delay between irradiation and cancer incidence for solid tumors. The total risk is mostly due to the risk of solid tumors.

The risk-versus-age function is different for leukemia, which is why it is shown separately. The leukemia risk for irradiated children is higher than for young adults, and it increases again for older adults. This shape reflects the natural incidence of leukemias.

It is emphasized that the "excess risk percentages" are to be added to the risk of spontaneous cancer, which is approximately 20% for a full lifetime. Thus, the total risk of any

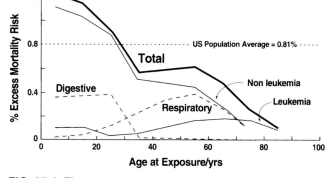

**FIG. 27-3.** The estimated increase in risk of cancer occurring in the remainder of the lifetime of males exposed at various ages to a dose of 10 rems (0.1 Sv). These percentages should be added to the approximately 20% "spontaneous" incidence. See Table 27-6 for the 90% confidence ranges. (Based on BEIR V Report: Health Effects of Exposure to Low Levels of Ionizing Radiation. Washington, DC: National Academy Press, 1990; Table 4-3, p 175.)

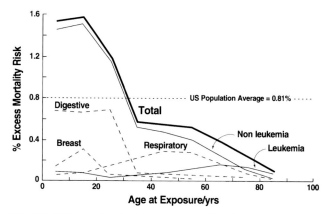

**FIG. 27-4.** The estimated increase in risk of cancer occurring in the remainder of the lifetime of females exposed at various ages to a dose of 10 rems (0.1 Sv). These percentages should be added to the approximately 20% spontaneous incidence. See Table 27-6 for the 90% confidence ranges. (Based on BEIR V Report: Health Effects of Exposure to Low Levels of Ionizing Radiation. Washington, DC: National Academy Press, 1990; Table 4-3, p 175.)

**TABLE 27-7.** Weighting factors ($W_T$) for specific gains, for calculation of effective dose equivalent

| Tissue | $W_T$ |
|---|---|
| Gonads | 0.25 |
| Breast | 0.20 |
| Red marrow | 0.12 |
| Lungs | 0.12 |
| Thyroid | 0.03 |
| Bone surface | 0.03 |
| Skin | 0.01 |
| Other organs | 0.05 each |

Source: International Commission on Radiological Protection Publication 53. Radiation Dose to Patients from Radiopharmaceuticals. New York: Pergamon, 1988;1–377.

cancer, whether solid or leukemia, for a male irradiated (10 rems [0.1 Sv]) at age 45 is 0.6% plus 20%, equal to 20.6% (see Fig. 27-3). For a girl aged 5 (see Fig. 27-4) the same dose is associated with a lifetime total cancer risk of 20 + 1.53 = 21.5%. Of this excess, <0.1% is due to the risk of leukemia (see Fig. 27-4).

## LIMITED VOLUME DOSES

Figures 27-3 and 27-4 and Table 27-6 quote the risks estimated by the BEIR V report for a uniform whole-body exposure to a dose of 10 rems (0.1 Sv). However, most medical irradiation procedures give measurable doses to only a limited volume of the body. An arbitrary approach to allowing for such nonuniformity has been made for radiation workers (10). Weighting factors have been assigned by the ICRP to organs and tissues that represent the fraction of the total stochastic risk (i.e., fatal cancer and serious inherited disorders) resulting from the irradiation of that organ or tissue when the total body is irradiated. If only that organ is irradiated to a stated dose, as is likely in many diagnostic and nuclear medicine procedures, we may consider the probabilities in the whole-body tables above to be reduced by multiplying by the weighting factors in Table 27-7. It should also be remembered that low dose rates and low total doses might reduce these probabilities by a factor of two or three.

## Leukemias

The increased incidence in leukemias was significant at 2 years after irradiation, peaked in the first 5 years, and then declined but remained significant for over 15 years with little change at longer times. The relative risk (relative to the natural incidence of leukemia in the unirradiated population) depended little on age, but was higher in males. "An excess number of cases of leukemia have been observed in children who were exposed to diagnostic x-irradiation in utero; the excess is larger per unit dose than in children who were irradiated during postnatal life . . . it has been estimated that

approximately 1% of all leukemia cases in the general population may be attributable to diagnostic radiography" (11).

## Breast Cancer

The sensitivity of the mammary gland to the carcinogenic effects of ionizing radiation was first demonstrated in x-irradiated mice in 1936 and confirmed in other species. An increase in the incidence of breast cancer in irradiated humans was first recognized in 1965 in women who had received repeated fluoroscopic examinations, and subsequently in the Japanese atomic bomb survivors in 1968. A strong linear component is seen in the dose-response relationship, with little evidence of sparing by fractionation. Radiation-related cancers are similar in age distribution and histopathologic types to breast cancers resulting from other or unknown causes. No radiation-associated breast cancers have been reported as appearing before the age of 25, the earliest age at which breast cancer appears in the general population. Age at exposure strongly influences susceptibility. Women who are irradiated before the age of 20, and especially at puberty, are more at risk than those irradiated at 20 to 40. For women over age 40 at exposure, the relative risk estimate is reduced. There is no evidence that radiogenic breast cancers appear during the first 10 years after exposure, but after this the incidence rises rapidly, peaking at 15 to 20 years after irradiation, with mortality peaking 5 years later.

The effects of diet, and hence of body weight and fat, are likely to be hormonally mediated. The incidence of breast cancer in North America and northern Europe is five to six times that of Asia and Africa. Recent experimental evidence suggests that total caloric intake is a more important risk factor for breast cancer than is the fat concentration in the diet. Fatty tissues contain aromatizing enzymes that convert adrenal androgens into estrogens. This leads to continued hormonal stimulation of the mammary glands after menopause, and likely accounts in part for the greater risk among the generally heavier postmenopausal women of North America and northern Europe than the lighter Asian population.

These findings are consistent with the conclusion that radiogenic initiation and subsequent development into overt mammary cancer are under hormonal control. Conditions that induce functional mammary differentiation, and hence that reduce target cell numbers (e.g., early and multiple pregnancies and lactation), reduce the risk of breast cancer. Conditions that reduce or block full functional differentiation and increase mitogenesis (e.g., nulliparity and glucocorticoid deficiency) increase the risk of breast cancer (12).

## Lung Cancer

Data come from Japanese atomic bomb survivors, but also from patients treated for ankylosing spondylitis and from uranium miners and other miners exposed chronically to high-LET (alpha) radiation from inhaled radon and its progeny. The ankylosing spondylitis patients received approximately 2 Gy (200 rads) to 80% of the lung in multiple fractions. Lung cancers became obvious beginning approximately 9 years after the first treatment and continued at an elevated level up to 20 years or more. The relative risk was 1.21. The risks to underground miners are considered in detail in the separate BEIR IV report (13). They relate to inhaled or ingested radionuclides, for which the dosimetry is difficult.

Absolute radiogenic risks of radiation-induced lung cancer are similar for both sexes, although baseline cancer risks are higher for males. Data suggesting interactions between radiation and smoking are equivocal, but the two appear to be additive (14).

**Thyroid Cancer**

The incidence of thyroid cancer was evaluated in two groups of patients treated with external x-irradiation for benign conditions: children in Israel in the Tinea Capitis (ringworm) Study and the Rochester Thymus Study (see Table 27-5). Radiation-induced thyroid cancers were not seen until 5 years after exposure, the risk increasing somewhat with time after irradiation. The risk appeared greater for a westernized lifestyle, as demonstrated by differences in Israeli subgroups, being estimated as an eightfold increase in the background risk for a dose of 1 Gy.

The effect of internally deposited I-131 and other iodine radionuclides is lower, however, probably because of nonuniform uptake at the cellular level. It has been studied in three categories of human subjects:

- Patients who received large doses of I-131 for therapeutic purposes (mostly thyrotoxicosis)
- Patients who received much smaller diagnostic doses of I-131
- Those on the Marshall Islands during fallout from the Bikini bomb test in 1954

Data from the high–therapeutic dose group is difficult to interpret because thyrotoxic patients have a higher baseline incidence of thyroid cancer and because the very large doses cause extensive cell death, which can itself reduce cancer risk (see Fig. 27-1). The estimates of relative risk vary widely from a ninefold increase to no significant increase.

For the diagnostic I-131 dose patients, with a mean radiation dose of approximately 50 rads (0.5 Gy), a total of 50 thyroid cancers were found in 35,000 Swedish subjects (80% women), compared to an expected number of 39.4, yielding an overall incidence ratio of 1.27 (95% confidence interval 0.94 to 1.67, that is, not significantly different from no increase). Two-thirds of the cancers occurred among the minority of subjects who had received a diagnostic dose of I-131 because of an already suspected thyroid cancer. Nearly half of those cancers became clinically apparent as

soon as 5 to 9 years after exposure, suggesting that they were occult at the time of the diagnostic test rather than the result of radiation from the test. These data do not support the conclusion that diagnostic doses of I-131 significantly increase the risk of thyroid cancer.

In the Marshall Islands, the doses were large enough to cause nausea or partial epilation, indicating significant total body and surface doses (see Table 27-3). By 8 years after irradiation, two boys who were 1 year of age when irradiated were diagnosed with myxedema. Nine years after exposure, the first thyroid nodule was noted in a 12-year-old girl. Although the dose estimation is open to question, the prevalence of hypothyroidism, thyroid nodules, and proven thyroid cancer appears to increase with the dose.

The thyroid status has been followed in school children in Nevada and Utah who lived there as infants from 1952 to 1955, when there was fallout from bomb tests. Cumulative radiation doses to the thyroids of children could have averaged as much as 100 rads (1 Gy). Although there was, up to 14 years later, no increase in thyroid cancer, there was a suggestive 20% to 30% greater prevalence of all thyroid abnormalities in exposed children; but the 90% confidence interval of the prevalence ratio included 1.0, so no strong radiogenic risk was demonstrated in that population.

The National Council on Radiation Protection and Measurements reviewed the data on radiation-induced thyroid cancer that were available through 1985 and recommended the use of a specific risk estimate (15). Females are roughly three times as susceptible to radiogenic, as well as nonradiogenic (baseline) thyroid cancer, as males. Hence, relative-risk estimates do not differ by sex. The risk of radiation-induced thyroid cancer is two to three times greater in children than in adults. Only about 1 in 10 thyroid cancers is potentially lethal (16). Cancers in other sites, such as kidney and bladder, after I-131 treatment for hyperthyroidism, have shown no increase during the 24 years after the therapy, in spite of relatively high doses to the urinary tract (17).

**Kidney, Bladder, Colon, Rectum, Ovary, Uterus, CNS, Bone, and Other Cancers**

Data from the Japanese atomic bomb survivors showed significant increases of these types of cancer that appeared to be dose related in most sites. Data from animal experiments have demonstrated radiation-induced cancers in all tissues.

**CONCLUSIONS**

The estimated human risks are summarized in Figs. 27-3 and 27-4 and Table 27-6. No mammalian tissues or organs are exempt from carcinogenic risk, but the radiogenic risks from carefully administered applications of medical radiation are low compared with the baseline incidence of cancer.

## REFERENCES

1. Cameron JR. The BERT: a radiation unit for the public. Physics Society 1991;20:2.
2. BEIR V Report: Health Effects of Exposure to Low Levels of Ionizing Radiation. Washington, DC: National Academy Press, 1990;1–421.
3. ICRP Publication 41. Nonstochastic Effects of Ionizing Radiation. New York: Pergamon, 1984.
4. BEIR V Report. Health Effects of Exposure to Low Levels of Ionizing Radiation. Washington, DC: National Academy Press, 1990;102, 125.
5. Siegal BA, Kirchner PT (eds). Nuclear Medicine: Self-Study Program I. Radiobiology and Radiation Protection. New York: Society of Nuclear Medicine, 1988;3–33.
6. BEIR V Report. Health Effects of Exposure to Low Levels of Ionizing Radiation. Washington, DC: National Academy Press, 1990;85–86.
7. UNSCEAR Report E 86. IX.9. Genetic and Somatic Effects of Ionizing Radiation. New York: United Nations, 1986.
8. BEIR V Report. Health Effects of Exposure to Low Levels of Ionizing Radiation. Washington, DC: National Academy Press, 1990; 354–362.
9. BEIR V Report. Health Effects of Exposure to Low Levels of Ionizing Radiation. Washington, DC: National Academy Press, 1990;6.
10. International Commission on Radiological Protection Publication 53. Radiation Dose to Patients from Radiopharmaceuticals. New York: Pergamon, 1988;1–377.
11. BEIR V Report. Health Effects of Exposure to Low Levels of Ionizing Radiation. Washington, DC: National Academy Press, 1990;247.
12. BEIR V Report. Health Effects of Exposure to Low Levels of Ionizing Radiation. Washington, DC: National Academy Press, 1990;266–267.
13. BEIR IV Report. Health Effects of Exposure to Low Levels of Ionizing Radiation. Washington, DC: National Academy Press, 1988;602.
14. BEIR V Report. Health Effects of Exposure to Low Levels of Ionizing Radiation. Washington, DC: National Academy Press, 1990;278.
15. NCRP Report No. 80: Induction of Thyroid Cancer by Ionizing Radiation. Bethesda, MD: National Council on Radiation Protection and Measurement, 1985.
16. BEIR V Report. Health Effects of Exposure to Low Levels of Ionizing Radiation. Washington, DC: National Academy Press, 1990;287–298.
17. BEIR V Report. Health Effects of Exposure to Low Levels of Ionizing Radiation. Washington, DC: National Academy Press, 1990;321.

*Textbook of Nuclear Medicine,*
edited by Michael A. Wilson.
Lippincott–Raven Publishers, Philadelphia © 1998.

CHAPTER 28

# Nuclear Medicine Quality Improvement

Janet Endorf-Olson, Kristine M. Leahy-Gross, and Michael A. Wilson

## QUALITY IMPROVEMENT

Maintaining and improving quality is a high priority for health care organizations as they seek to fulfill their responsibility for ensuring quality health care, respond to purchasers (business, government, and managed care entities), remain competitive, and meet the requirements of accrediting bodies. Quality improvement (QI) is no longer limited to the review of quality, but now includes cost-effectiveness and access. Quality, cost-effectiveness, and access (together known as *value*) are three issues fueling the demand for changes in health care. Health care organizations and departments within organizations are now challenged to enhance quality, improve cost-effectiveness, and increase accessibility to the health care system without losing existing strengths. Providers can use QI programs to raise their level of performance and document their progress toward excellence (1).

As individual health care organization leaders understand the concept of QI, they need to provide direction for their QI activities. These efforts are already resulting in significant changes affecting almost every area of the delivery system, including individual hospital practice guidelines, economic credentialing of procedures, public profiling of hospitals, and an emphasis on consumerism and advocacy for value. Such efforts result from increased collaboration within and among health delivery systems, such as capitation and the move away from fee-for-service payment systems. Preparation for survival in this rapidly changing health care environment includes remaining informed on health care reform; participating in clinical and administrative outcome studies, functional assessments, and practice guidelines development; surveying consumers; and intensifying comparative studies on indicators (a measurement of practice quality) and practitioner profiles (2). All the while, health care organizations must keep in mind QI and issues of quality, cost-effectiveness, and access.

## THE QUALITY MOVEMENT

The quality movement in health care has evolved from traditional quality assurance (QA) to continuous quality improvement (CQI) and total quality management (TQM). The following definitions highlight the differences among these approaches.

- *Quality assurance* is a systematic, organization-wide approach to ensuring a specified standard of care. QA traditionally focused on individual variance and a few individuals detecting and solving problems. QA monitoring and evaluation activities typically focused on outliers of a documented standard, with the results based on an individual's performance. This type of quality review demanded perfection and assumed quality, with little emphasis on improvement.
- *Continuous quality improvement* is a systematic, organization-wide approach to improving the overall quality of care that emphasizes performance improvement as well as a specified standard of care. CQI is process focused and relies on a data-driven, problem-solving approach. QI monitoring and evaluation activities focus on the process of a standard of care or practice and on what can be done to improve the process. This approach promotes a mindset and involvement among all employees of identifying improvement opportunities and solutions. CQI techniques have been widely accepted by business corporations, especially in Japan under the tutelage of Demming. They have also been accepted by many successful progressive hospitals.
- *Total quality management* is a management philosophy that influences an organization's infrastructure, policies, and protocols. It is a fundamental change in the way in which patient care is delivered and management operates. TQM embraces features of both QA and CQI (3).

The widely held belief that an organization would have fewer problems if only the workers did their jobs well has been disputed by Dr. Joseph M. Juran, who asserts that improving the systems under which the work is performed can prevent problems. A rule of thumb states that at least 85% of problems can be corrected by changing systems, and <15% of problems are under an individual's control (4). Once it is recognized that systems create the majority of problems, QI is not perceived by the staff as a punitive process directed against individuals. Routine monitoring of existing systems help to identify areas for improvement and results in the development of new and better systems. Process improvement monitors in nuclear medicine (NM) and radiology may focus on diagnostic accuracy, appropriateness of requested imaging study, image quality, and patient or referring physician satisfaction. Such monitoring is designed to identify opportunities for process improvement rather than personnel deficiencies. As a result, improvements can occur without the need to identify suboptimally performing individuals, the outliers sought by the traditional QA approach.

In addition to intra-service and hospital-wide demands for patient-centered QI, outside regulating agencies have begun to accept, and in some cases promote, the concept of improvement through systems evaluations. For example, the Joint Commission on Accreditation of Healthcare Organizations (JCAHO) has turned their emphasis to CQI and performance improvement. Other agencies, such as the Nuclear Regulatory Commission (NRC) and the U.S. Food and Drug Administration (FDA), require similar proof of ongoing QI effort within imaging specialties, such as the NRC-mandated Quality Management Plan (QMP) and the Congress-mandated and FDA-regulated Mammography Quality Standard Act.

## FRAMEWORK FOR CONTINUING QUALITY IMPROVEMENT

Recognizing the need for QI, the JCAHO emphasizes two dimensions of performance: *doing the right thing* and *doing the right thing well*. These dimensions provide a framework for executing an improvement plan that facilitates efforts in meeting internal and external demands for QI (Table 28-1).

Many of the practices learned during the evolution of CQI are applicable to future QI activities. Of particular value are the practices of effective leadership, the realization that opportunity for improvement exists, the identification of a scientific method of approach, maintaining a systems perspective, and collaboration among individuals and disciplines.

### Leadership

During this time of uncertainty about the ultimate direction of health care, there must be a management framework to ensure that an organization remains focused on QI efforts while positioning itself for possible changes. As the level of uncertainty rises, organizations may detect fear among employees, and the leadership may become frustrated with the lack of immediate results and be tempted to abandon the long-term vision and improvement efforts it has accepted. Then, more than ever, leadership must provide an emphasis on goals, continuous monitoring of systems and processes, and empowering staff to influence change. This leadership must be present at all levels of the health care organization, down to and including each individual department, division,

---

**TABLE 28-1.** *Definitions of dimensions of performance*

1. Doing the right thing
   The *efficacy* of the procedure or treatment in relation to the patient's condition
      The degree to which the care of the patient has been shown to accomplish the desired or projected outcome(s)
   The *appropriateness* of a specific test, procedure, or service to meet the patient's needs
      The degree to which the care provided is relevant to the patient's clinical needs, given the current state of knowledge
2. Doing the right thing well
   The *availability* of a needed test, procedure, treatment, or service to the patient who needs it
      The degree to which appropriate care is available to meet the patient's needs
   The *timeliness* with which a needed test, procedure, treatment, or service is provided to the patient
      The degree to which the care is provided to the patient at the most beneficial or necessary time
   The *effectiveness* with which tests, procedures, treatments, and services are provided
      The degree to which the care is provided in the correct manner, given the current state of knowledge, to achieve the
         desired or projected outcome(s) for the patient
   The *continuity* of services provided to the patient with respect to other services, practitioners, and providers, as well as over time
      The degree to which the care for the patient is coordinated among practitioners, among organizations, as well as over time
   The *safety* of the patient (and others) to whom the services are provided
      The degree to which the risk of an intervention and the risk in the care environment are reduced for the patient and
         others, including the health care provider
   The *efficiency* with which services are provided
      The relationship between the outcomes (results of care) and the resources used to deliver patient care
   The *respect and caring* with which services are provided
      The degree to which the patient or a designee is involved in his or her own care decisions and to which those providing
         services do so with sensitivity and respect for the patient's needs, expectations, and individual differences

Source: Joint Commission on Accreditation of Healthcare Organizations. 1997 Comprehensive Accreditation Manual for Hospitals. Improving Organizational Performance. Oakbrook Terrace, IL: JCAHO, 1997;P1–4.

and section with their individual physician, administrator, technologist, and clerical support staff leaders.

The responsibility of the senior health care organization leadership is to establish a system-wide plan. Ideally, this vision is created with an understanding of patient and community needs and is consistent with the organization's strategic plan for meeting those needs. To realize this vision, the administrative, departmental (e.g., radiology), and sectional (e.g., NM) leadership must actively participate in the development of the entire organization's strategic plan, in the decision-making processes, and in ensuring ongoing organization-wide improvement efforts. Effective communication of the organization's vision provides guidance for program development and daily activities among employees; creates a culture that rewards innovation, improvement, and growth; and fosters a unity of purpose and a commitment among employees throughout the organization. This is most successful when the organization's vision is shared and understood by all employees.

## Opportunity for Improvement Exists

The greatest barrier to QI is satisfaction with the status quo. A basic principle of improving care is the realization that opportunities for improvement do exist. We need to recognize that despite our best efforts, some of the care we provide is inappropriate. A few examples of inappropriate care may include selecting the most expensive imaging test when a less expensive modality is as effective, performing the wrong test or a test that was not indicated, delay in providing the appropriate test due to system obstacles (scheduling), and delay in providing test reports to the referring physician. Opportunities for improvement may be identified through a variety of sources: evaluation of performance expectations of the departmental mission and vision; customer (referring physician and patient) judgments about the quality of the test performance and information provided; sources or standards available from scientific and professional organizations, such as the Society of Nuclear Medicine (SNM) and American College of Nuclear Physicians (ACNP); and available databases in the literature.

## Scientific Method of Approach

QI activities require a scientific approach, with organization-wide acceptance. An example of a QI approach includes PDCA (i.e., plan, do, check, act). With the implementation of a common scientific problem-solving method to improve care, the improvement process will proceed smoothly and quickly.

QI efforts must be driven by data to be effective; therefore, measurement is vital to the improvement design. Monitoring tools should identify potential process improvement, and CQI principles should enhance the improvement effort. The health care organizations and their NM departments that apply these principles will fare better than others in times of health care reform. Initially, the interpretation of collected data by QI professionals provides information about the performance level and stability of existing functions, processes, and outcomes. Based on this information, improvement opportunities may be identified and prioritized, and, using conventional statistical tools, improved processes can be designed. The JCAHO standards suggest that performance measurements include processes and outcomes, which affect a large volume of patients, place patients at serious risk, are problem prone, promote patient satisfaction, and guarantee safety of the care environment (5).

Once new processes have been designed and implemented, evaluation through remeasurement can determine whether improvement has occurred.

## Systems Perspective

Referring to the observation that at least 85% of problems can be corrected by changing systems and <15% are under an individual's control, organizations are called on to change their focus from individual to organization performance. Frequently, it is the system in which one works that inhibits efficiency and effectiveness. W. Edwards Demming referred to this as suboptimization: a condition where system components work against each other. Therefore, it seems logical that a systems perspective and cross-departmental analysis become a major requirement when evaluating the delivery of care (6).

## Collaboration

Many existing processes are complex, arbitrary, and poorly understood. Realizing that many problems and opportunities for improvement derive from process weaknesses, it becomes clear that QI activities should involve the individuals closest to the activity. People are the driving force behind processes and cannot be separated from the processes in which they participate (7). Hence, QI activities typically involve collaboration among individuals and disciplines and the development of multidisciplinary teams. Such collaborative efforts to improve performance are more likely to succeed when there is a perceived need for change, an accepted scientific approach, and a systems perspective.

It is recommended that organized groups evaluating performance understand what will be studied and recognize the importance of confidentiality throughout the assessment process. This ensures a level of trust and commitment to the study process and profiles obtained. Assessment must be performed without censure or blame, and data must be presented in a nonthreatening manner. This is especially so in peer review, when individual medical practitioners may feel very sensitive and threatened about their professional performances. When these personal reservations are successfully overcome, the process can be very educational and produce significant quality gains.

Change within an organization may not occur easily. A sensitivity to everyone's position is essential. Change and improvement are more likely to occur when the laws of organizational change are followed:

- Understand the history behind any problem before attempting to improve on it.
- Avoid intuitive solutions and use scientific methods.
- Listen to and involve the affected people in every step of the improvement effort.

Embracing change with a vision and positive outlook will enhance the health care facility's survivability during the coming health care revolution.

## DRIVING FORCES IN QUALITY IMPROVEMENT

The departmental or sectional QI plan integrates functions and processes, the dimensions of performance, quality indicators, and quality controls for the year. It allows for the tracking or identification of indicators that are developed by a department, as well as indicators that are developed as a result of ongoing CQI activity (8).

The QI plan in an NM section must ensure that imaging studies are of high quality, accurate, provided in a radiation-safe environment, appropriate, and efficacious to patient outcome. In the past, medical imaging was fueled by a fee-for-service payment system that encouraged the introduction and widespread use of imaging, virtually regardless of its incremental benefit to patient management. New technologies are now considered expense items in the institutional budget. In a managed care environment, the institution's recovery of imaging expenses may be possible only if there is evidence of significant patient gain by outcome measures. This requires a positive and measurable test effect that has an impact on patient care; for example, the investigation of a particular differential diagnosis is concluded or a particular treatment is initiated. If the outcome of imaging is merely to order another diagnostic procedure, it will be very difficult to show that the particular study performed had enough impact to warrant continued reimbursement.

Uncertainty makes patient care expensive. It is important that the imaging physician understand the clinical problem, so that before performing the study, the imager can determine whether the study is likely to have an impact. If it is unlikely that the image will help, the study should not be performed. NM physicians are the most fortunate among imagers because NRC regulations mandate that a physician must agree that the test is appropriate before allowing a radiopharmaceutical to be administered. As a result, the NM physician is generally provided with better clinical data than other imagers and is thus able to behave as an imaging consultant. Judicious use of imaging enhances NM's cost-effectiveness, a clearly important quality-of-care issue at this stage of health care reform. Using this judgment, appropriate alternatives can be communicated to the ordering physi-cian, or the procedure can be modified to maximize clinical utility of the procedure, such as using a different procedure, a different modality, or additional views of the current study.

At present, numerous organizations provide guidelines to improve quality. These include professional specialty and subspecialty organizations, such as the SNM, the ACNP, and the College of American Pathologists (CAP). These programs contribute by providing continuing medical education (SNM); voluntary proficiency testing programs, such as the ACNP Practice Certification Program; and the testing program pioneered by CAP and now jointly managed by the ACNP and SNM.

Educational organizations contributing to QI include the American College of Graduate Medical Education (ACGME) and the American Board of Nuclear Medicine (ABNM). These organizations contribute to quality by providing accreditation of training programs (ACGME) and the examination of trainees (ABNM).

Several federal agencies exert control over NM. These include the NRC, which requires a QMP for therapeutic radiopharmaceuticals and diagnostic I-131 and I-125 studies using sodium iodide in doses >30 μCi. The QMP was introduced in NRC-regulated states on January 27, 1992, and is required in agreement states as of January 1, 1995. A form provided by Myron Pollycove, M.D. (a visiting medical fellow to the NRC at that time) is a useful method of recording all the NRC QMP requirements. At the University of Wisconsin Hospitals and Clinics (UWHC), we have added the contents of this form to the back of our prescription form so that all NRC QMP requirements can be easily recorded and kept at one site available for audit (Fig. 28-1).

The FDA influences the quality of NM practice by its role as gatekeeper to new technology, preventing unsafe or ineffective products, and facilitating medically appropriate technologies. FDA regulation has expanded from x-ray machines to medical devices and now to medical software. The FDA has also been directly involved in quality control (QC), with an interest in single photon emission computed tomography (SPECT). In the 1992 Mammography Quality Standard Act, Congress mandated the FDA to regulate the quality of equipment and users of mammography equipment. The FDA may potentially extend its requirements to other imaging modalities if directed by Congress.

The JCAHO is a complex nonfederal organization that originated in 1913, when the American College of Surgeons (ACS) initiated an evaluation of hospital operating rooms. This evaluation was eventually extended to all categories of care delivery and, in 1950, shifted from an emphasis on minimum standards to optimum achievable standards. Beginning in 1986, the JCAH embarked on an initiative to reshape its accreditation process in an effort to address quality issues. In 1987, the organization modified its name and broadened its emphasis from just hospitals (JCAH) to health care organizations (JCAHO). In 1994, it began to allow direct public access to health care organization performance results and commentaries. Currently, the JCAHO accredits

_____________________ HOSPITAL
NUCLEAR MEDICINE QUALITY MANAGEMENT FORM
(Therapeutic or Radioiodide Doses in Excess of 30 μCi)
Hospital Number:
Patient Name:
Location:

| Written Directive | Inpatient | Outpatient |
|---|---|---|
| Date | | |
| Radiopharmaceutical | | |
| Dose (millicurie) | | |
| Route of Administration | | |
| Male ☐ Female ☐ Pregnant? Breast Feeding? | Yes ☐ No ☐<br>Yes ☐ No ☐ | Yes ☐ No ☐<br>Yes ☐ No ☐ |
| Signature (Authorized User) | | |
| Patient Confirmation | Check Two | Check Two |
| Name | | |
| Birthdate | | |
| Hospital I.D. | | |
| Relative/Friend | | |
| Wrist Band | | |
| Before Dosing, Confirm: | | |
| Followed Directive | Yes ☐ No ☐ | Yes ☐ No ☐ |
| After Dosing, Confirm: | | |
| Radiopharmaceutical | | |
| Dose | | |
| Route of Administration | | |
| Signature | | |
| Date | | |

Place Labels Here

A

| University of Wisconsin Hospital & Clinics Nuclear Medicine Dept 600 Highland Avenue Madison, Wisconsin | Rx Number | |
|---|---|---|
| | Filled by: | Activity: |
| | Date: | Time: |

| | |
|---|---|
| Patient Name | |
| Med Rec Number | |
| Radiopharmaceutical Chemical & Physical Form | |
| Dose in mCi | |
| Route of Administration | |
| Signature of Authorized MD | Date Signed |

NUCLEAR MEDICINE QMP WRITTEN DIRECTIVE

BEFORE ADMINISTERING DOSE TO PATIENTS:

| Patient ID - 2 methods must be used: | | Informed consent obtained & written radiation safety instructions provided: Yes ☐ No ☐ |
|---|---|---|
| Name | | |
| Birthdate | | Estimated maximum dose to an individual exposed to patient. ________ mRem |
| Address | | |
| Clinic Card | | |
| Hospital ID | | Table 2, DG-8015 was used for dose calculation (15.33 mRem/mCi for I-131) Yes ☐ No ☐ |
| S.S. Card | | |
| Other (explain) | | |

Male ☐ Female ☐ Pregnant: Yes ☐ No ☐
Breastt Feeding: Yes ☐ No ☐

CONFIRMATION OF ADMINISTRATION & PT. RELEASE

Written directive understood and followed: Yes ☐ No ☐

| | |
|---|---|
| RPh | Admin. Date |
| Dose | Admin. Time |
| Admin. Route | Pt. released at time of administration: |
| Admin. by | Yes ☐ No ☐ |

B

**FIG. 28-1.** This composite figure shows the form **(A)** suggested by Dr. Myron Pollycove (visiting medical fellow to NRC). The two UWHC forms on the right **(B)** are the prescription (upper) and the QMP requirements (lower) use Dr. Pollycove's suggestions and comply with all current and anticipated NRC requirements. This form is retained for at least 3 years.

5,300 hospitals and other health care organizations. The JCAHO Board of Commissioners include members of the following organizations: ACS, American Hospital Association, American Medical Association (AMA), American College of Physicians, and American Dental Association. Although the JCAHO gets credit for pushing the quality aspects of its user institutions, it plays no role in developing policies and procedures and does not attempt to accredit individual physicians, which remains the traditional function of the profession itself.

The AMA also believes strongly in the quality paradigm and considers its contribution to be the quality continuum of science-education-service-outcome. The AMA attempts to influence the education of health care providers through graduate and continuing medical education while providing physicians with an ethical milieu.

## JCAHO EXPECTATIONS

One impetus for the move to QI in hospitals is the JCAHO's agenda for change, which includes four underlying concepts:

1. Patient outcomes are influenced by all activities within a health care organization.
2. Continual improvement in the quality of care should be a priority goal for a health care organization.

3. The JCAHO should focus on health care organization activities that are most important to providing quality care.
4. Traditional standards compliance assessments should be complemented by the JCAHO collecting, analyzing, and providing feedback on key activities of accredited organizations.

Such concepts have prompted creation of new objectives and new activities since 1990. Most significant is the JCAHO's development of standards that place greater emphasis on continual improvement (3).

The JCAHO agenda for change initiative hit full stride in 1995, marking the transition from assessment of capabilities to assessment of actual performance. The overall goal of the JCAHO standards is to improve patient care through improved organizational performance. Because organizational performance is emphasized, the emphasis shifts from individual staff performance or variance to that of organizational systems and processes. The 1995 JCAHO standards emphasize the role of organization leaders in establishing, directing, and sustaining QI programs; methodologic requirements for systematic broad-based QA and QI activities; and effective management of information that supports QA and QI activities. Clearly, if a hospital wants to be accredited by the JCAHO, it must comply with its standards, a paradigm that demands a CQI approach (3).

The JCAHO's *Comprehensive Accreditation Manual for Hospitals* (CAMH) provides an evaluation process that can be used to measure, assess, and improve the hospital or imaging service's performance (5). The suggested methodology for improving performance is provided: flowcharts, process diagrams, or fishbone diagrams—the classic tools of CQI and TQM. This methodology includes continuous loops of design, measurement, assessment (including statistical analyses and comparison with data from other facilities), improvement, and redesigning the process, as necessary.

Because the JCAHO believes that process improvement requires multidisciplinary teamwork and involves many departments and services, the standards were reorganized as an integrated manual. The previous vertical hierarchy of departmental requirements has been changed into a horizontal or cross-departmental function. This facilitates organization-wide ownership and requires that each service know the entire organization's function and structure and how the service fits into this. The JCAHO now appears to require four or five larger multidisciplinary interdepartmental CQI projects rather than individual departmental projects. The 1995 manual contains six new chapters, all of which apply to NM. To comply with the standards, a review of the entire 599-page manual was recommended by JCAHO. Fortunately, the 1996 manual is smaller. Previously, staff in individual services, such as NM, could read the chapter on NM in the manual and check their performance against the required standards. The shift to performance-based functionally organized standards represents a substantial change. In 1997, the JCAHO requires detailed outcome assessment.

The JCAHO survey process has also been changed. Much information is exchanged between the health care organization and the JCAHO surveyor before the visit. During the interactive part of the survey, JCAHO surveyors interview hospital and departmental leadership and review documentation of QA activities. Surveyors may spend up to half their time visiting areas of patient care, interacting with many hospital staff, and comparing their performance against the described policies and procedures previously reviewed.

## PRACTICAL APPROACH TO JCAHO

In general, there are several distinct facets of QI that individual NM sections must address for continued JCAHO approval. The need for an equipment QC process and an official physicist or equivalent review is essential for JCAHO, just as the QC of in-house preparation of radiopharmaceuticals is required by the NRC. The customer service needs of the patient and referring physician staff must be met, and a method of documenting this must be established and monitored. Federal or state organizations with jurisdiction must also be addressed, including the FDA, NRC QMP, and Clinical Laboratory Improvement Act of 1988 (CLIA-88). It is important to realize that the JCAHO surveyors are now looking for data, not policy, and that they expect the completion of the PDCA process with documentation of the success of the effort.

### Annual Review

On an annual basis, the NM QI chairperson and committee should examine the current JCAHO accreditation manual to determine the requirements and scoring system that apply to one's service. Using the published guidelines to evaluate compliance is identical to the process that surveyors use in evaluating your department. It is important to use automated computer-based evaluation methods to decrease staff time commitment to the process, but it is equally important to obtain useful information. Spreading the data acquisition across the entire service involves all members, promoting their QI commitment, but does not overburden any one group. QI should be a service-wide commitment of physicians, administrators, technologists, clerical workers, and support staff.

### Peer Review

Another general classification that requires individual unit design is peer review. Peer review, its documentation, and the application of the results to the credentialing process is important. In the cross-departmental emphasis of CQI, peer review remains the most important clinical departmental function in the latest JCAHO standards. Although the introduction of peer review has elicited individual concern about

```
┌─────────────────────────────────────────────────┐
│            NUCLEAR MEDICINE QA                    │
│            PHYSICIAN MONITOR                      │
├─────────────────────────────────────────────────┤
│ Procedure _____   Patient # _____    │
│                                                   │
│ Scan Date _____   Review Date _____   │
├─────────────────────────────────────────────────┤
│ REASON FOR REVIEW:                                │
│ Good Case Conference _____  Coronary Angiogram _____ │
│                                                   │
│ Pulmonary Arteriogram _____  Monthly Review _____ │
│                                                   │
│ Endocrine Conference _____  PET Study _____     │
│                                                   │
│ Focused Review _____  OTHER (specify) _____     │
├─────────────────────────────────────────────────┤
│ CLINICAL INDICATION:                              │
│ Appropriate Request _____ Yes _____ No          │
│                                                   │
│ Test Approved by Physician _____ Yes _____ No   │
│                                                   │
│ Information From _____ Request form _____ NM physician │
│                                                   │
│ Test Changed/Modified _____ Yes _____ No        │
├─────────────────────────────────────────────────┤
│ IMAGE QUALITY:                                    │
│ Satisfactory _____ Yes _____ No                 │
├─────────────────────────────────────────────────┤
│ IMAGE REPORT:                                     │
├─────────────────────────────────────────────────┤
│ PEER REVIEW:                                      │
│ Reader _____ A _____ B _____ C _____ Original report │
│                                                   │
│ Correlation _____ Exact _____ Similar _____ Discrepant │
├─────────────────────────────────────────────────┤
│ AVAILABILITY OF REPORT:                           │
│ Preliminary Report in NM Insert _____ Yes _____ No │
│                                                   │
│ Final Report Present _____ Yes _____ No         │
│                                                   │
│   If no _____ Days since dictated _____ In computer system │
│                                                   │
│ Dictated Day Done _____ Yes _____ No            │
│                                                   │
│   If not , is it after-hours study _____ Yes     │
│                                                   │
│ Time from dictation to transcription _____ Hours │
│                                                   │
│ Final report answers clinical question _____ Yes _____ No │
└─────────────────────────────────────────────────┘
```

**FIG. 28-2.** Skeleton of the UWHC form used for peer review purposes, for both routine and correlative imaging sessions.

the validity and fairness of this subjective performance assessment, it is surprising how much improvement in physician interpretation can result. Interobserver variability can be assessed retrospectively by reviewing an adequate sample size of films to determine subjectively if the initial read was accurate. A standardized form (Fig. 28-2) can be used to indicate the presence of appropriate clinical information, image quality, availability of report, and the peer review over-read.

In imaging and in peer review, one question prevails: How do we determine the truth? The review can compare individual physician reports to a gold standard (histology, autopsy, coronary angiograms, pulmonary arteriograms, and correlative imaging), although the gold standard may not always be pure gold. This sort of analysis is much easier in a teaching environment, with the use of good case conferences and research activities aimed at establishing the role of imaging in diagnosis. Many research publications from a department can be used in the QI process. Because NM is relatively unique in the amount of research done even in private practice, many NM sections can use this approach.

The easier component of ongoing physician peer review is how well the physician readers agree with one another. As early as 1934, Garland was ridiculed when he reported a 20% disagreement in reading pulmonary nodules on chest x-rays, but this is now the accepted standard. Similar discrepancies are expected in NM over-reads. This explains why peer review forms (see Fig. 28-2) use "similar" and "discrepant" categories: Many of the reading differences stem from individual physician fears of false positives and false negatives, a very individual and personal trait. The JCAHO recommends that one over-read a representative sample of cases for any particular study. In NM sections where a range of 70 individual tests are available, it seems reasonable to review 100% of the rare studies because these are usually more problem prone. Many over-reads must be performed if physicians have 20% disagreement rates because hundreds of studies are necessary to see if an individual differs from the accepted 20% misread rate.

One way of assessing such differences may be the kappa test (9). In this statistic, there is perfect agreement if the result of physician comparisons is near 1, absolute disagreement if the result is −1, and no correlation if the result is 0. Excellent agreement is present if the value is >0.75, good agreement if the value is 0.4 to 0.74, and poor agreement when <0.4. Here the test results are evaluated for observer agreement and contrasted with chance agreement. The kappa statistic is as follows:

$$K = \frac{P_o - P_c}{1 - P_c}, \qquad (1)$$

where $P_o$ is the proportion of observer agreement and $P_c$ is the proportion of chance agreement.

The kappa figure is derived from a $2 \times 2$ table of readings in which one reader (reader A) is compared with another (reader B) and four agreement-disagreement combinations are possible. The agreement is calculated from this table by adding the proportion when there is agreement that the test is abnormal (a) or normal (d), that is, agreement total of (a + d). The chance agreement is calculated by adding the marginal proportions $P_1 \times Q_1$ and $P_2 \times Q_2$.

|  |  | First reader | | |
|---|---|---|---|---|
|  | Test | + | − |  |
| Second reader | + | a | b | $P_1$ |
|  | − | c | d | $P_2$ |
|  |  | $Q_1$ | $Q_2$ | 1.0 |

The kappa score can then be calculated by this formula:

$$K = \frac{(a + d) - (P_1 \times Q_1 + P_2 \times Q_2)}{1 - (P_1 \times Q_1 + P_2 \times Q_2)} \quad (2)$$

In this way, differences between readers may be identified. In practice, few if any centers use such an approach.

## EXAMPLE OF A QI PLAN

At the UWHC, the NM department is a section of the Department of Radiology and reports annually to the Radiology Quality Improvement Committee. The Radiology QI Committee then reports annually to the hospital-wide QI Committee. The section of NM at UWHC meets monthly for discussion of all aspects of quality care and section function. This requires a significant amount of time, but it facilitates problem solving and prevents minor problems from becoming major issues of quality failure. This activity includes NM physicians, clericals, and technologists and results in an additional 1.5 full-time equivalent effort performing: equipment and radiopharmaceutical QC, physician over-reads, data collection for monthly reports, writing and reading of minutes, and updating of clinical protocols.

## QI Indicators

The radiopharmacist generates a monthly QC report of the appropriate radiopharmaceuticals, listing the individual, mean, and standard deviation of the QC parameters. The procedure protocols are also updated when new techniques or modifications are introduced during the year by article review, continuing medical education, or scientific program attendance. Ideally, protocol revision is accomplished by the entire team of physicians, technologists, clerical staff, and support staff. However, it is acceptable for an individual to revise protocol and report back to the committee for approval.

Ongoing departmental monitors include patient satisfaction questionnaires, documentation of arrival of correlating x-rays, and the availability of imaging service to patients in a timely fashion; for example, percent of total studies added on that day and percent of inpatient studies performed on the day requested. Where possible, this is done electronically through integration of the hospital information system and the radiology file system.

We divide the year into 12 monthly reviews. In each month, a particular organ system or procedure type is reviewed separately:

| | |
|---|---|
| January | Renal (nontransplant) |
| February | Nonthyroid endocrine |
| March | Abscess and tumor detection |
| April | Equipment QC |
| May | Laboratory tests, CLIA-88 |
| June | Cerebral |
| July | Thyroid and therapies (QMP) |
| August | Transplant procedures |
| September | Bone |
| October | Ventilation-perfusion scans |
| November | Gastrointestinal |
| December | Cardiac |

For each system, a physician is assigned to peer review the month's procedures. Using a form (see Fig. 28-2), the physician reviews the indications, technical quality, diagnostic accuracy, timeliness of study, timeliness of dictation and transcription, availability of the final report, and other pertinent issues. In viewing a dictated report, it is important to determine whether the reader knew what information the referring physician desired from the study. We have developed two very simple questions to elicit this:

- Diagnosis or reason for study?
- Specific information required?

Previously we used five questions to direct physicians who hand wrote requests, but we found that the carefully designed, simple form (with just two questions) improved the clinical information provided (10,11).

When reviewing the reading physician's final written report, it is important to determine whether the following were described:

- Scan findings
- Disease and probability statement
- Comments, qualifications, and recommendations to the referring physician, as necessary

To accomplish this review, clerical staff obtain a random selection of patient studies that is predetermined by the QI program. In September, this might include 25 whole-body bone scans, 15 limited bone scans, 15 triple-phase bone scans, and 15 SPECT studies for a total of 70 studies (overall, 12% of the total bone scan workload). In tests rarely done, such as laboratory tests, all the year's procedures may be reviewed and the total number of reviews may still be only 10. The clerical staff use our pharmacy management database to randomly select the actual studies to be reviewed. It is helpful to choose the studies for review from different days and weeks to sample different physicians and technologists. The data sources used in the review include the NM request data sheet (order form generated at time of request) that is retained in the NM insert of the x-ray jacket, which establishes that the relevant clinical information was available before the test was done and that an NM physician approved the study before the start. The scan is then reread and documented on the review form. The official copy of the report is then evaluated for the other logistic information about timeliness of request, reading, and transcription. The official report is then compared with the over-read just performed and also used to determine whether the clinical question was satisfactorily answered. Peer review can now be performed as the official report is compared with the over-read. These peer review requirements are not specifically outlined for NM in the CAMH but are gleaned from the medical staff portions of the manual. We document the monitor results monthly and maintain annual summaries. Individual physician peer review is recorded in a coded fashion, readily available for credentialing purposes, and forwarded to the department chairperson for this purpose.

A teaching institution is given additional opportunities for peer review. We independently reread interesting cases and myocardial perfusion scans at two separate weekly teaching conferences, where correlating clinical and test data (e.g., coronary arteriograms for myocardial perfusion studies) are reviewed for a definite diagnosis using non-NM reference sources. Other possible correlations use autopsy reports, histology reports of surgical specimens, referring physician queries or complaints, and radiologist reviews or rereads of previous studies, when they perform routine reading to compare old studies with a current procedure.

The challenge is to find a nonthreatening means of reviewing someone else's work and communicating slight dissimilarities and discrepancies without provoking animosity. The problem is usually in setting up this procedure rather than the review process itself. Most concerns evaporate as the review process proceeds and individuals recognize that major improvements in scan reading and information transfer to the referring physician. This is especially so in infrequently performed, difficult technical procedures, where the actual technical performance of the procedure can limit diagnostic information. We have found that strict adherence to a protocol has improved the diagnostic performance considerably in infrequently performed, problem-prone procedures, such as CSF shunt studies.

## Annual Reports

Annual reports are prepared of the ongoing monitors and peer review, including focused reviews or modifications of sectional policies and procedures. The annual report includes data to answer these fundamental questions:

- Are the quality performance improvement activities appropriately focused?
- Is the department meeting all applicable external standards?
- Has the department identified opportunities for improvement in care and service?
- Has the necessary action been taken?
- Have measurable improvements been made?
- Have the effectiveness of actions taken in this and past reporting periods been evaluated?
- Are the performance improvement and peer review processes clearly documented?

It is likely that significant ongoing QI is occurring if all these questions are answered affirmatively.

## CONCLUSION

NM, like all physician services, must do the following:

- Prevent duplication of tests and services
- Prevent overtreatment
- Decrease the practice of defensive medicine

All these measures are an attempt to ameliorate rising costs. NM must continue to introduce useful diagnostic and therapeutic procedures while concentrating on procedures that produce meaningful information and materially affect patient management. For years, the imaging specialty generally believed it only had to introduce tests that supported the presumptive diagnosis and, if enough tests were performed, the final diagnosis was ultimately determined. For a test to be introduced in these times, it must be highly accurate and either rule in or rule out a diagnosis or treatment. The unique functional attributes of NM put us in this position for some diseases, such as liver hemangiomas and acute cholecystitis. Our imaging modality can exclude or establish these diagnoses with considerable accuracy using a single test. To date, NM procedures have been underrated in the medical community, and it is hoped that many of our procedures will acquire increased status as a result of cost-efficacy studies.

## REFERENCES

1. Pine M. The quality encounter between purchasers and providers: what to ask and how to answer. Managed Care Q 1993;1(2):4–12.
2. Gibbons B. Healthcare reform and the healthcare quality professional: understanding and preparing for the change. NAHQ News 1993/1994; Winter:1, 4.
3. Carefoote R. Implementing TQM/CQI at rehabilitation hospitals: a survey. J Healthcare Quality 1994;16(3):34–38.
4. Scholtes P. The Team Handbook. Madison, WI: Joiner Associates, 1989;2–8.
5. Joint Commission on Accreditation of Healthcare Organizations. 1995 Comprehensive Accreditation Manual for Hospitals. Improving Organizational Performance. Oakbrook Terrace, IL: JCAHO, 1997;P1–4.
6. McDaniel GL. Applying a systems perspective to quality improvement training. J Healthcare Quality 1994;16(2):6–8.
7. Rice WR. Motivation: the most basic process in TQM/CQI. J Healthcare Quality 1993;15(3):38–42.
8. Lathrop CB. Coordinating functional chapters of the Joint Commission and performance for departments and teams. J Healthcare Quality 1995;17(1):14–18.
9. Ker M. Issues in the use of kappa. Invest Radiol 1991;26:78–83.
10. Wilson MA. Improvement in referral practices elicited by a redesigned request format. Radiology 1983;146:677–679.
11. Fischer HW. Better communication between the referring physician and the radiologist [editorial]. Radiology 1983;146:845.

*Textbook of Nuclear Medicine,*
edited by Michael A. Wilson.
Lippincott–Raven Publishers, Philadelphia © 1998.

CHAPTER 29

# Nuclear Regulatory Commission License Application

Ronald R. Bresell

## BACKGROUND

A century ago, radioactivity and x-rays were discovered. Initially, the scientific community investigated these energy forms and in a matter of months, radiation was first used in medical diagnosis (1–3). Because the x-ray techniques used were relatively crude (perhaps 20 kV, 2 to 33 mA, 30-minute exposure time), the potential for radiation to damage living cells was noted and documented (4). Some of the detrimental effects documented in these early studies, such as Evans' study of the effects of radium (5,6) and the prenatal effects documented by Stewart and Kneale (7), are still referenced in the literature. Thus, it should not be surprising that as use of radiation has increased, there should be a desire to regulate the exposure from that radiation to ensure that the risk from radiation use is balanced by the benefit derived from that use.

Under the Atomic Energy Acts of 1946 and 1954, Congress established the Atomic Energy Commission (later to become the Nuclear Regulatory Commission [NRC] by the Energy Reorganization Act of 1974), empowering that agency to regulate the processing and use of *source material* (natural uranium [U] and thorium), *special nuclear material* (U-233, enriched uranium [higher percentage of U-233 or U-235 than occurs naturally], and plutonium), and *by-product material* (radioactive material produced through the operation of a nuclear reactor).

Although it may appear that the NRC makes the rules and regulations regarding radiation exposure, it is the Federal Radiation Council (established in 1959 [8] and in 1970 consolidated into the Environmental Protection Agency (EPA]) that "advise the President with regard to radiation matters directly or indirectly affecting health" (8). When the EPA's radiation protection guides (RPG) are approved by the President, they have the force and effect of law because all federal agencies are required to follow these guides. Thus, the regulations of the NRC that are applicable to its licensees

must be consistent with the RPGs. Other federal agencies and their special areas of radiation regulation include the following:

- The U.S. Food and Drug Administration (FDA) approves new radioactive drugs and devices under Title 21, Code of Federal Regulations (CFR).
- The EPA regulates the emission of radioactive material to the environment under Title 40 CFR.
- The Department of Transportation (DOT) regulates the transportation of radioactive materials under Title 49 CFR.
- The Occupational Safety and Health Administration (OSHA) regulates workplace exposures to radiation under Title 29 CFR.

When areas of jurisdiction overlap, conflicts are usually resolved by agreements (memoranda of understanding) between the governmental parties involved via division or delegation of authority. An example of such conflict involved the use of radiopharmaceuticals in nuclear medicine. These materials are radioactive drugs and are governed by both the FDA and the NRC. On February 9, 1979, the NRC published its policy, *Regulation of the Medical Uses of Radioisotopes; Statement of General Policy* (9).

## REGULATORY AGENCIES

Many federal and state agencies regulate exposure to radiation and radioactive material. The NRC promulgates its regulations in Title 10 CFR. Title 10 CFR has various parts dealing with specific areas of by-product material use, for example:

Part 19  Notices, Instructions, and Reports to Workers; Inspections
Part 20  Standards for Protection against Radiation
Part 21  Reporting of Defects and Noncompliance

507

Part 30  Rules of General Applicability to Licensing of By-Product Material
Part 35  Human Uses of By-Product Material

Because the congressional statute that established the NRC specified that the NRC may regulate only certain radioactive material, to include reactor-generated by-product radioactive materials (i.e., radioactive materials produced in nuclear reactors), naturally occurring radionuclides (e.g., radium) or accelerator-or cyclotron-produced radionuclides (e.g., fluorine 18, cobalt 57 [Co-57]) are not under the control of the NRC. These are normally regulated by state governments. Some (a total of 29 as of 1994) states have assumed the responsibility of regulating radioactive material and radiation devices within the state. This leads to several categories of regulation of radioactive material by states:

- *Nonagreement states* allow the NRC to regulate by-product material use within their boundaries. These states may regulate naturally occurring, cyclotron-produced, and other machine-produced (e.g., x-ray) sources. The following are currently nonagreement states: Alaska, Connecticut, District of Columbia, Delaware, Hawaii, Idaho, Indiana, Michigan, Minnesota, Missouri, Montana, New Jersey, Ohio, Oklahoma, Pennsylvania, South Dakota, Vermont, Virginia, West Virginia, Wisconsin, and Wyoming and territories of Guam, Puerto Rico, and the Virgin Islands.
- *Agreement states* have entered into an agreement with the NRC allowing them to regulate by-product material within the state using regulations that are at least as stringent as the NRC's regulations. Before becoming an agreement state, the state must demonstrate to the NRC that it has the capabilities to assume the NRC's mission within its borders and that the intended regulations are consistent with NRC rules and regulations. Massachusetts is the most recent state to move from being a nonagreement state to an agreement state.
- *Licensing states* are states that regulate all sources of ionizing radiation (e.g., by-product material, cyclotron-produced, naturally occurring, machine-produced) within their borders. Most, but not all, licensing states are agreement states. The unofficial Conference of Radiation Control Program Directors (CRCPD) produces a uniform set of suggested regulations that may be used by state departments of radiologic health as guidance for formulation of state law. Agreement state status is approved by the NRC CRCPD. Licensing states apply the same level of oversight to all non–by-product material as well as machine-produced sources of radiation within their borders. There are 15 licensing states; Illinois is one.

Whether your facility is in a nonagreement (NRC) state or an agreement state will determine the specifics of obtaining a license to use radioactive materials in nuclear medicine. Although there may be some differences in the forms used, because the purpose of licensing is to assure the appropriate regulatory agency that you and your facility have the neces-

**TABLE 29-1.** *Radioactive materials commonly used under a general license*

| Isotope | Limits (µCi)* per sample |
|---|---|
| Hydrogen 3 | 50 |
| Carbon 14 | 10 |
| Iodine 125 | 10 |
| Iodine 131 | 10 |

*The general license shall not possess at any one time, at any one location of storage or use, a total amount of I-125, I-131, Se-75, and/or Fe-59 in excess of 200 µCi.

sary skills and equipment to use the requested material safely in diagnosis and treatment, the basic information needed in either case will be similar. Approximately 22,000 licenses are issued for medical, academic, and industrial use. Of these, approximately 2,000 are administered by the NRC; the rest are administered by the agreement states.

## TYPES OF LICENSES

The type of work anticipated and the quantities of radioactive materials that a facility desires to use will determine the type of (NRC) by-product material license. There are two basic types of licenses: general and specific.

### General License

A general license allows physicians, clinical laboratories, and hospitals to use specific small quantities (defined in 10 CFR 31.11) in certain in vitro clinical or laboratory testing. Such a license may be used by small radioimmunoassay labs or other labs, with specific limits of some commonly used radioactive materials (Table 29-1).

A general license is normally obtained by completing a Form NRC-483, "Registration Certificate for In Vitro Testing with By-Product Material Under General License." The benefit that a general license bestows on a department or clinic is that it exempts them from some specific requirements of 10 CFR 19, 20, and 21.

### Specific License

A general license does not allow sufficient radioactivity (e.g., <200 µCi of iodine 125 [I-125]) for an average-sized laboratory, and it does not allow for the administration of material to humans. If larger quantities of material or human use is desired, one of two types of specific licenses is needed. The user requests a specific license for human use under 10 CFR 35 by completing a Form NRC-313 (Fig. 29-1), Application for Material License, for use of the designated materials at specified areas and locations.

A specific license is issued to the named applicant after the NRC has reviewed and approved the application that the

| NRC FORM 313 | U. S. NUCLEAR REGULATORY COMMISSION | APPROVED BY OMB: NO. 3150-0120 EXPIRES 6-30-96 |
|---|---|---|
| (10-94) 10 CFR 30, 32, 33 34, 35, 36, 39 and 40 | | ESTIMATED BURDEN PER RESPONSE TO COMPLY WITH THIS INFORMATION COLLECTION REQUEST: 9 HOURS. SUBMITTAL OF THE APPLICATION IS NECESSARY TO DETERMINE THAT THE APPLICANT IS QUALIFIED AND THAT ADEQUATE PROCEDURES EXIST TO PROTECT THE PUBLIC HEALTH AND SAFETY. FORWARD COMMENTS |
| **APPLICATION FOR MATERIAL LICENSE** | | REGARDING BURDEN ESTIMATE TO THE INFORMATION AND RECORDS MANAGEMENT BRANCH (T-6 F33), U.S. NUCLEAR REGULATORY COMMISSION, WASHINGTON, DC 20555-0001, AND TO THE PAPERWORK REDUCTION PROJECT (3150-0120), OFFICE OF MANAGEMENT AND BUDGET, WASHINGTON, DC 20503. |

**INSTRUCTIONS:** SEE THE APPROPRIATE LICENSE APPLICATION GUIDE FOR DETAILED INSTRUCTIONS FOR COMPLETING APPLICATION. SEND TWO COPIES OF THE ENTIRE COMPLETED APPLICATION TO THE NRC OFFICE SPECIFIED BELOW.

| APPLICATION FOR DISTRIBUTION OF EXEMPT PRODUCTS FILE APPLICATIONS WITH: | IF YOU ARE LOCATED IN: |
|---|---|
| DIVISION OF INDUSTRIAL AND MEDICAL NUCLEAR SAFETY OFFICE OF NUCLEAR MATERIALS SAFETY AND SAFEGUARDS U.S. NUCLEAR REGULATORY COMMISSION WASHINGTON, DC 20555-0001 | **ILLINOIS, INDIANA, IOWA, MICHIGAN, MINNESOTA, MISSOURI, OHIO, OR WISCONSIN, SEND APPLICATIONS TO:** |
| **ALL OTHER PERSONS FILE APPLICATIONS AS FOLLOWS:** | MATERIALS LICENSING SECTION U.S. NUCLEAR REGULATORY COMMISSION, REGION III 801 WARRENVILLE RD. LISLE, IL 60532-4351 |
| **IF YOU ARE LOCATED IN:** | |
| **CONNECTICUT, DELAWARE, DISTRICT OF COLUMBIA, MAINE, MARYLAND, MASSACHUSETTS, NEW HAMPSHIRE, NEW JERSEY, NEW YORK, PENNSYLVANIA, RHODE ISLAND, OR VERMONT, SEND APPLICATIONS TO:** | **ALASKA, ARIZONA, ARKANSAS, CALIFORNIA, COLORADO, HAWAII, IDAHO, KANSAS, LOUISIANA, MONTANA, NEBRASKA, NEVADA, NEW MEXICO, NORTH DAKOTA, OKLAHOMA, OREGON, PACIFIC TRUST TERRITORIES, SOUTH DAKOTA, TEXAS, UTAH, WASHINGTON, OR WYOMING, SEND APPLICATIONS TO:** |
| LICENSING ASSISTANT SECTION NUCLEAR MATERIALS SAFETY BRANCH U.S. NUCLEAR REGULATORY COMMISSION, REGION I 475 ALLENDALE ROAD KING OF PRUSSIA, PA 19406-1415 | NUCLEAR MATERIALS LICENSING SECTION U.S. NUCLEAR REGULATORY COMMISSION, REGION IV 611 RYAN PLAZA DRIVE, SUITE 400 ARLINGTON, TX 76011-8064 |
| **ALABAMA, FLORIDA, GEORGIA, KENTUCKY, MISSISSIPPI, NORTH CAROLINA, PUERTO RICO, SOUTH CAROLINA, TENNESSEE, VIRGINIA, VIRGIN ISLANDS, OR WEST VIRGINIA, SEND APPLICATIONS TO:** | |
| NUCLEAR MATERIALS LICENSING SECTION U.S. NUCLEAR REGULATORY COMMISSION, REGION II 101 MARIETTA STREET, NW, SUITE 2900 ATLANTA, GA 30323-0199 | |

PERSONS LOCATED IN AGREEMENT STATES SEND APPLICATIONS TO THE U.S. NUCLEAR REGULATORY COMMISSION ONLY IF THEY WISH TO POSSESS AND USE LICENSED MATERIAL IN STATES SUBJECT TO U.S.NUCLEAR REGULATORY COMMISSION JURISDICTIONS.

| 1. THIS IS AN APPLICATION FOR *(Check appropriate item)* | 2. NAME AND MAILING ADDRESS OF APPLICANT *(Include Zip code)* |
|---|---|
| A. NEW LICENSE B. AMENDMENT TO LICENSE NUMBER _____ C. RENEWAL OF LICENSE NUMBER _____ | |

| 3. ADDRESS(ES) WHERE LICENSED MATERIAL WILL BE USED OR POSSESSED | 4. NAME OF PERSON TO BE CONTACTED ABOUT THIS APPLICATION |
|---|---|
| | TELEPHONE NUMBER |

SUBMIT ITEMS 5 THROUGH 11 ON 8-1/2 X 11" PAPER. THE TYPE AND SCOPE OF INFORMATION TO BE PROVIDED IS DESCRIBED IN THE LICENSE APPLICATION GUIDE.

| 5. RADIOACTIVE MATERIAL. a. Element and mass number; b. chemical and/or physical form; and c. maximum amount which will be possessed at any one time. | 6. PURPOSE(S) FOR WHICH LICENSED MATERIAL WILL BE USED. |
|---|---|
| 7. INDIVIDUAL(S) RESPONSIBLE FOR RADIATION SAFETY PROGRAM AND THEIR TRAINING EXPERIENCE. | 8. TRAINING FOR INDIVIDUALS WORKING IN OR FREQUENTING RESTRICTED AREAS. |
| 9. FACILITIES AND EQUIPMENT. | 10. RADIATION SAFETY PROGRAM. |
| 11. WASTE MANAGEMENT. | 12. LICENSEE FEES *(See 10 CFR 170 and Section 170.31)* FEE CATEGORY \| AMOUNT ENCLOSED $ |

13. CERTIFICATION. *(Must be completed by applicant)* THE APPLICANT UNDERSTANDS THAT ALL STATEMENTS AND REPRESENTATIONS MADE IN THIS APPLICATION ARE BINDING UPON THE APPLICANT.

THE APPLICANT AND ANY OFFICIAL EXECUTING THIS CERTIFICATION ON BEHALF OF THE APPLICANT, NAMED IN ITEM 2, CERTIFY THAT THIS APPLICATION IS PREPARED IN CONFORMITY WITH TITLE 10, CODE OF FEDERAL REGULATIONS, PARTS 30, 32, 33, 34, 35, 36, 39 AND 40, AND THAT ALL INFORMATION CONTAINED HEREIN IS TRUE AND CORRECT TO THE BEST OF THEIR KNOWLEDGE AND BELIEF.

WARNING: 18 U.S.C. SECTION 1001 ACT OFJUNE 25, 1948 62 STAT. 749 MAKES IT A CRIMINAL OFFENSE TO MAKE A WILLFULLY FALSE STATEMENT OR REPRESENTATION TO ANY DEPARTMENT OR AGENCY OF THE UNITED STATES AS TO ANY MATTER WITHIN ITS JURISDICTION.

| CERTIFYING OFFICER -- TYPED/PRINTED NAME AND TITLE | SIGNATURE | DATE |
|---|---|---|
| | | |

**FOR NRC USE ONLY**

| TYPE OF FEE | FEE LOG | FEE CATEGORY | AMOUNT RECEIVED $ | CHECK NUMBER | COMMENTS |
|---|---|---|---|---|---|
| APPROVED BY | | | DATE | | |

NRC FORM 313 (10-94)                                                                 PRINTED ON RECYCLED PAPER

**FIG. 29-1.** Application for NRC material license.

requester has submitted. The application contains the stated radionuclides, the maximum quantities to be possessed at any one time, the proposed uses of these radioactive materials, laboratory facilities and handling equipment, training and experience of users, radiation detection equipment available, external and internal personnel monitoring procedures, and radioactive waste disposal procedures. Additionally, maintaining radiation exposure to as low as reasonably achievable (ALARA) and quality management plans (QMPs) must be submitted. These requirements essentially establish the licensee's or user's radiation protection program.

The user (either individual or facility) is responsible for compliance with the statements made in the license application. Normally, a facility conducts the radiation safety program under the authority of a Radiation Safety Committee (RSC) as implemented by the Radiation Safety Officer (RSO).

There are two types of specific licenses.

### Specific License of Limited Scope

The licensee is allowed to use specific radiopharmaceuticals approved by the FDA or specific nuclides in a specific procedure, or both. The NRC has divided medical uses of radionuclides into groups or categories, depending on type of medical use, and specified the use in various subparts of 10 CFR 35. That is, the use of radiopharmaceuticals for diagnosis involves measurement of uptake, dilution, and excretion; imaging and localization; therapy; and use of sealed-source nuclides (currently, cesium 137, Co-60, gold 198, iridium 192 [Ir-192], strontium 90 [Sr-90], I-125, gadolinium 153 [Gd-153]) in brachytherapy, teletherapy, and diagnosis. A specific license of limited scope is usually used by private nuclear medicine practitioners and smaller hospitals.

### Specific License of Broad Scope

If an institution or organization desires also to engage in research and development, the limitations of a group-specific license are often too confining. A broad scope license does not limit radionuclides to specific uses, rather it allows the facility to review use applications from individual staff members and to authorize use of radionuclides on its own initiative. Obviously, such a broad licensure requires the facility to demonstrate to the NRC that it has the staffing, experience, facilities, and controls necessary to safely and properly manage such use. This license is used by large hos-

pitals and research institutions and represents approximately 3% of the 6,700 NRC-controlled licenses.

## HUMAN USE OF RADIOACTIVE MATERIAL

As noted, human use of radioactive material requires a specific license. In most instances, the license is issued to the medical institution where the material is to be used. The use is limited to specific physicians named on the license or, in the case of a broad scope license, the institution's (Medical) Radiation Safety Committee may be authorized by the licensing agency to approve physicians for human use based on some previously submitted approving criteria. Regardless, the physician users must satisfy the training and experience criteria established in 10 CFR 35 for their desired use.

When requesting a license to administer radioactive materials to humans for diagnosis or therapy, the user submits the Form NRC 313 (see Fig. 29-1). NRC Regulatory (Reg) Guide 10.8, "Guide for the Preparation of Applications for Medical Use Programs" (8) or, for broad scope licenses, Reg Guide 10.5, "Applications for Licenses of Broad Scope" (9) is invaluable in the preparation of Form 313 and the license application. Not only do these discuss the information needed for each part of a license application, but, in various appendices and exhibits, they also provide model procedures that may be cited to satisfy various licensing aspects.

### Application Form NRC 313

This application requires certain information. Each paragraph (item) is discussed in detail.

### Radioactive Material and Purpose (Items 5 and 6)

Items 5 and 6 on Form NRC 313 require the applicant to specify the radioactive material, amount desired, and purpose. If the application is for one or more of the six medical use groups specified in 10 CFR 35.100 to 35.500 (use of a teletherapy device requires a separate license application), this section need merely reference the appropriate part of the regulations (Table 29-2).

Broad scope medical users may also simply request "any by-product material with atomic numbers 3 through 83 for medical use." The licensee must specify that medical uses and users will be approved by various approved standing

**TABLE 29-2.** *Items 5 and 6 on Form NRC 313*

| Item | By-product material | Amount | Item | Purpose |
|------|---------------------|--------|------|---------|
| 5.a | Material in 35.100 RP for uptake, dilution, and excretion | As needed | 6.a | Medical use |
| 5.b | Material in 35.200 RP for imaging and localization (generators and kits) | As needed | 6.b | Medical use |
| 5.c | Material in 35.300 RP for therapy | As needed | 6.c | Medical use |
| 5.f | Material in 35.500 sealed sources for diagnosis | As needed | 6.f | Medical use |

RP, radiopharmaceutical.
Note: 35.400 is Use of Sources for Brachytherapy.

committees that are empowered to authorize human use of radioactive materials or ionizing radiation. The committees that authorize such uses include these:

- FDA-approved New Drug Application (NDA) radiopharmaceutical or device: Medical Radiation Safety Committee (MRSC)
- FDA-approved Investigational New Drug (IND) or Investigational Drug Committee (IDC): MRSC and Human Subjects Committee (HSC)
- Non–FDA-approved investigational protocols: MRSC, HSC, and Radioactive Drug Research Committee (RDRC)

If other radioactive materials are needed, separate entries for each item are made. However, note that Part 35.57 authorizes the licensee certain calibration and check sources, so these need not be specifically requested. Additionally, if some of the material listed in a Part 35 paragraph is not desired, the items you do not wish to possess must be listed line by line.

### Individuals Responsible for Radiation Safety Programs— Their Training and Experience (Item 7)

Because a purpose of regulating radionuclide use is to protect the patient against the risk of unnecessary exposure, one of the application's key items is to ensure that the user is qualified by training and experience to use the requested radioactive materials for the purposes requested, in such a manner as to protect health and minimize danger to life or property. Subpart J of Part 35 (i.e., 35.900 to 35.972) delineates the acceptable training and experience requirements for authorized users for medical use and for the RSO.

### Authorized User for Medical Use

Although there may be many people using radioactive material in the facility (e.g., technicians, staff physicians), these persons are "using" the material under the supervision of an authorized physician user, who bears the responsibility for these workers' omissions. Thus, it is important that the authorized user for medical use be qualified. Each authorized "group" has specific training requirements, including professional board certification (e.g., American Board of Nuclear Medicine, American Board of Radiology) or classroom or laboratory training. These qualifications may be documented in several ways: copy of board certification, previous license number or license (if authorized by other NRC or agreement state license), or prior training and experience and a preceptor's statement to document appropriate training for those without appropriate board certification.

For a nuclear medicine department, this training and experience can usually be satisfied if the physician has spent 6 months in nuclear medicine as part of a training program approved by the Accreditation Council for Graduate Medical Education. Such a requirement is normally satisfied by an approved 4-year radiology residency program or other structured internal medicine residency programs that are tailored to satisfy the NRC requirements. These requirements have changed as human use has expanded. Before July 1, 1984, the NRC training requirement was satisfied by a 3-month rotation in nuclear medicine. Physicians who trained under such a program are considered to meet the current training requirements.

In some facilities, treatment of thyroid problems with I-131 may also be performed in a different department (e.g., internal medicine). For these physicians, in lieu of board certification, the following is required: 80 hours of classroom or laboratory training and clinical experience under the supervision of an authorized physician user and documented on a Preceptor Statement that the physician has performed (a) for therapeutic use of unsealed byproduct material, use of I-131 for diagnosis of thyroid function and treatment of hyperthyroidism or cardiac dysfunction in 10 individuals and use of I-131 for treatment of thyroid carcinoma in three individuals; (b) for treatment of hyperthyroidism, use of I-131 for diagnosis of thyroid function and treatment of hyperthyroidism in 10 individuals; and (c) for treatment of thyroid carcinoma, use of I-131 for treatment of thyroid carcinoma in three individuals.

A preceptor's statement may also be required for treatment of thyroid problems with I-131 by certain physicians who are board certified, if they are board certified by the American Board of Radiology in Diagnostic Radiology. This is because the training requirement under Part 35.930, Training for Therapeutic Use of Radiopharmaceuticals, specifies board certification by the American Board of Radiology in Radiology or Therapeutic Radiology but does not mention Diagnostic Radiology. However, some agreement states require preceptor's statements for individual therapies even for physicians board certified in nuclear medicine (e.g., Texas). Alternatively, these states may require only the applicant's name on a previous license as evidence of authorized user status.

Besides having the appropriate training and experience, the non–board-certified applicant must demonstrate either that the training was recent (within the past 5 years) or that the applicant has continued to maintain expertise through related continuing education and experience.

### Visiting Authorized User

If you are in a clinic that has only one authorized physician, there are provisions to allow for visiting authorized physicians to use radioactive materials for medical use under your license for a maximum of 60 days each year (e.g., to give your physician a vacation). Specifically, the visiting physician must have permission from the hospital's management and RSC, and you must have a copy of the visiting user's radioactive materials license showing what procedures they are authorized to perform under that license. This visiting physician is then authorized to perform the same procedures (if your license allows the procedures to be performed) at your facility. Thus, if the visiting physician were authorized to use xenon 133 (Xe-133) in lung function studies, but your license does not allow for the use of Xe-133, then the visiting physician would not be allowed to use Xe-133 at your hospital.

### Radiation Safety Officer

In small facilities, the RSO may also be the authorized user. In more complex facilities, the management may designate a different person as RSO to manage many or all aspects of radiation safety at the organization. Such persons must also submit their qualifications, such as certification by an appropriate board (e.g., American Board of Health Physics, American Board of Radiology, American Board of Nuclear Medicine, American Board of Science in Nuclear Medicine, or Board of Pharmaceutical Specialties in Nuclear Pharmacy), classroom or laboratory training, or experience as an RSO under another medical use license.

It is desirable that the RSO be a full-time employee of the organization; however, a consultant meeting the qualifications of RSO may be employed to assist the organization. In such instances, the management of the institution is still responsible for complying with the radiation safety program required in the license.

### Radiation Safety Committee

Except for small, single-physician licenses where the physician is also RSO and head of the clinic, medical institutions must establish an RSC to oversee the medical use of by-product material. This committee must have at least three members, including an authorized user for each type of use permitted by the license, the RSO, a nursing service representative, and a representative of management who is neither an authorized user nor an RSO. Other members may be appointed to the RSC, as appropriate to the size and complexity of the program. The committee must meet at least quarterly, convening with a quorum of at least one-half of the membership, to include the RSO and management's representative. Committee minutes must be written, a copy provided to each member, and one copy must be kept for the duration of the license.

The basic task of the RSC is to oversee the use of licensed material in the licensee's facility, with the aim of keeping radiation exposure to workers and patients ALARA. The RSC accomplishes this by reviewing the training and experience of persons who desire to become authorized users and also the RSO or the teletherapy physicist. The RSC may also perform safety reviews of minor radiation safety changes, review incidents involving radioactive material, maintain and review radiation exposures of workers, and (annually) evaluate the status of the radiation safety program.

### Radioactive Drug Research Committee

The NRC and FDA agreed that, as of January 1, 1995, the NRC would only regulate the radiation safety aspects of by-product radiopharmaceuticals and defer to the FDA in matters of clinical use and research. Under FDA regulations, research involving human use of radiopharmaceuticals can only be accomplished if it has an NDA, if an industry-sponsored IND application has been filed, or it has been approved (preclinical basic science research) by an FDA-approved RDRC.

The development and marketing of a new drug is a long and expensive project. Typically, costs of $10,000,000 to $70,000,000 are incurred in the development of a new radiopharmaceutical. A new radiopharmaceutical drug product must be approved by the FDA as safe and effective before it can be sold for clinical use, and the developer must submit a Notice of Claimed Investigational Exemption for a New Drug (IND) to the FDA and conduct research in phases to obtain an NDA for general use. These phases are defined below, as described in Department of Health, Education, and Welfare publications:

- Phase I: Clinical pharmacology is intended to include the initial introduction of a drug into humans. Phase I studies may be in the usual "normal" volunteer subjects to determine levels of toxicity and, when appropriate, pharmacologic effect, and be followed by early dose-ranging studies in patients for safety and, in some cases, early evidence of effectiveness. For some new drugs, for ethical or scientific considerations, the initial introduction into humans is more properly done in selected patients. The number of subjects and patients in phase I will, of course, vary with the drug but may generally be in the range of 20 to 80 subjects on the drug.
- Phase II: Clinical investigation consists of controlled clinical trials designed to demonstrate effectiveness and relative safety. Normally, these are performed on closely monitored patients of limited number. This phase seldom goes beyond 100 to 200 patients on the drug.
- Phase III: Clinical trials are the expanded controlled and uncontrolled trials intended to gather additional evidence of effectiveness for specific indications and more precise definition of drug-related adverse effects.
- Phase IV: Postmarketing clinical trials are of several types:
  - Additional studies to elucidate the incidence of adverse reactions, to explore a specific pharmacologic effect, or to obtain more information of a circumscribed nature
  - Large-scale, long-term studies to determine the effect of a drug on morbidity and mortality
  - Additional clinical trials similar to those in phase III, to supplement premarketing data where it has been deemed in the public interest to release a drug for more widespread use before acquisition of all data that would ordinarily be obtained before marketing
  - Clinical trials in a patient population not adequately studied in the premarketing phase, such as children
  - Clinical trials for an indication for which it is presumed that the drug, once available, will be used

Often certain basic research studies attempt to determine whether a drug localizes in a particular organ or fluid space and to describe the kinetics of that localization. Many of these studies may be done without filing an IND if they are conducted under the auspices and approval of an FDA-approved RDRC. These studies are limited to using radioac-

**TABLE 29-3.** *RDRC allowable adult radiation doses within 1 year*

| | Description | Dose |
|---|---|---|
| Radiosensitive organs* | Single dose | 3 rems (0.03 Sv) |
| | Annual and total | 5 rems (0.05 Sv) |
| Other organs | Single dose | 5 rems (0.05 Sv) |
| | Annual and total | 15 rems (0.15 Sv) |

*These organs are the whole body, active blood-forming organs (including liver and spleen), lens of the eye, and gonads.

tive drugs in human research subjects. The RDRC must consist of a minimum of five members, including a nuclear medicine physician, a radiopharmacist, and a radiation safety representative. It reviews all radioactive drug protocols for limits on pharmacologic and radiation dose. The radiation dose to an adult from a single study or cumulation of studies conducted within 1 year must not exceed the specified limits (Table 29-3).

The RDRC may routinely approve protocols involving no more than 30 adult subjects. If more research subjects are desired or if some research subjects are <18 years old, the FDA must be notified. This development route cannot be used for clinical tests.

Often, the IND is used to generate information on a drug's safety and efficacy as a prelude to the sponsor's submitting an application for FDA approval to market a new drug (NDA). The NDA provides a complete analysis of the studies and suggests that the FDA approve the radiopharmaceutical's use for specific indications.

### Training for Individuals Working in or Frequenting Restricted Areas (Item 8)

The applicant must also describe the training program for persons who will work with or around radioactive materials (to include nursing staff who may tend patients receiving therapeutic quantities of radiopharmaceuticals) as well as for people who may be exposed to radioactive materials but are not working with the materials themselves (e.g., those transporting patients to and from the clinic, custodians, secretaries). An acceptable training program can be found in Appendix A of Reg Guide 10.8 (8).

### Facilities and Equipment (Item 9)

Applicants should submit an annotated drawing of the room or rooms and adjacent areas where by-product material will be used. This drawing should include room numbers and the use of each room or area (e.g., waiting, hot lab, radioactive waste storage), any shielding available, and additional safety equipment (e.g., fume hood, area monitors). Facilities using radioactive gases must document that the areas where these gases will be used are designed to prevent accidental exposures (see Radiation Safety Program [Item 10], below).

Other items that must be described (and for which appropriate Reg Guide 10.8 appendices exist) include the following:

- Survey instrument calibration (Appendix B)
- Dose calibrator calibration (Appendix C)
- Personnel monitoring program (Appendix D)

If the purpose of the license is to provide a mobile nuclear medicine service, the applicant must also include procedures for checking the equipment to ensure that it has not been damaged in transit from one site to the next. Reg Guide 10.8, Appendix E, details the model procedure for checking equipment used in a mobile nuclear medicine service (8).

### Radiation Safety Program (Item 10)

The NRC requires that the licensee have established appropriate administrative procedures to ensure control of procurement and use of radioactive materials. In large facilities, this would take the form of a radiation safety procedures manual. In small facilities, the appendices provided in Reg Guide 10.8 may be used or augmented to compile an appropriate procedures manual (8).

Except for physicians individually licensed who are both RSO and RSC, and licensees authorized only to use diagnostic sealed sources (e.g., a bone mineral density lab with I-125 and Gd-153 sources licensed under 10 CFR 35.500), the licensee must describe the RSC and the authority delegated to the RSO. Because these are the two institutional agencies responsible for the radiation safety program, they must have sufficient authority to perform that function. Reg Guide 10.8, Appendix F, contains the model radiation safety committee charter and radiation safety officer delegation of authority.

Except for licenses issued under 35.500 (e.g., bone mineral density labs), all activities must submit an ALARA program document. The ALARA program describes the organization's philosophy about radiation workers' exposure and the various quarterly action levels for exposure. Reg Guide 10.8, Appendix G is a template of a model program for maintaining occupational radiation exposure at medical institutions ALARA. The annual review conducted by the RSO and presented to the RSC is done to ensure that all exposures exceeding various ALARA action levels (Table 29-4) have been investigated and that all users have made reasonable efforts to keep individual and collective radiation exposures ALARA.

**TABLE 29-4.** *ALARA investigational levels*

| Type of exposure | Investigational levels (mrems/calendar quarter) | |
|---|---|---|
| | Level I | Level II |
| Whole body, head and trunk, active blood-forming organs, gonads | 125 | 375 |
| Hands, forearms, feet, ankles | 1,250 | 3,750 |
| Skin of whole body | 1,250 | 3,750 |
| Lens of eyes | 375 | 1,125 |

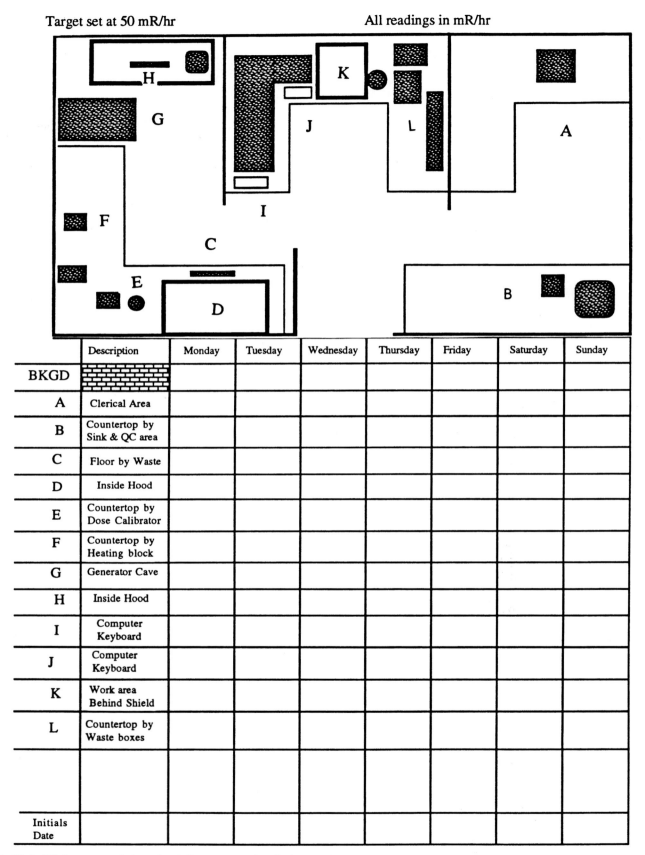

Target set at 50 mR/hr                    All readings in mR/hr

| | Description | Monday | Tuesday | Wednesday | Thursday | Friday | Saturday | Sunday |
|---|---|---|---|---|---|---|---|---|
| BKGD | | | | | | | | |
| A | Clerical Area | | | | | | | |
| B | Countertop by Sink & QC area | | | | | | | |
| C | Floor by Waste | | | | | | | |
| D | Inside Hood | | | | | | | |
| E | Countertop by Dose Calibrator | | | | | | | |
| F | Countertop by Heating block | | | | | | | |
| G | Generator Cave | | | | | | | |
| H | Inside Hood | | | | | | | |
| I | Computer Keyboard | | | | | | | |
| J | Computer Keyboard | | | | | | | |
| K | Work area Behind Shield | | | | | | | |
| L | Countertop by Waste boxes | | | | | | | |
| | | | | | | | | |
| Initials Date | | | | | | | | |

**FIG. 29-2.** Clinic map and chart for daily surveys of radiation and radioactive contamination.

Exposures less than level I values usually require no further action. Doses between levels I and II should be reported to the RSC, but no action is required unless directed by the RSC. Exposures higher than level II values must be investigated and reported to the RSC.

Other items that must be described (and for which appropriate Reg Guide 10.8 Appendices exist) include the following:

- Leak test (Appendix H)
- Safe use of radiopharmaceuticals (Appendix I)
- Spill procedures (Appendix J)
- Ordering and receiving radioactive material (Appendix K)
- Opening packages that contain radioactive material (Appendix L)
- Unit dosage, multidose vial, and molybdenum concentration (Appendix M.1, M.2, and M.3)
- Area survey procedures (Appendix N)
- Radiopharmaceutical therapy (Appendix P)

*Area Surveys*

Surveys for radiation and radioactive contamination are one of the key methods to keep exposures ALARA. Reg Guide 8.23 (10) provides a thorough discussion of survey considerations. The clinic must use a radiation detection survey meter that is calibrated to detect dose rates as low as 0.1 mR per hour and, at the end of each day, survey all areas where radiopharmaceuticals are routinely prepared or administered, and weekly survey all areas where radiopharmaceuticals and radioactive waste are stored. Additionally, a weekly wipe survey of all areas where radiopharmaceuticals are routinely prepared for use, administered, or stored must be performed to check for removable contamination. The wipe media must be analyzed on a detector system capable of detecting a minimum of 2,000 disintegrations per minute (dpm) on the sample.

Reg Guide 10.8, Appendix N, suggests that a map of the clinic be constructed and the points to be surveyed identified on the map. Below the map a grid can be used to document the daily survey results (Fig. 29-2). The form should include the date of the survey, the instrument used for the survey or sample analysis, and the initials of the person performing the survey. The columns should include the survey results (in either millirads per hour or dpm, as appropriate) for each of the identified points.

*Trigger Levels*

The survey forms should designate trigger levels in millirads per hour or dpm, enabling the person performing the survey to compare the survey and notify the RSO if either a dose rate or contamination exceeds the trigger level. These levels are established based on the type and energy of the emitted radiation. Suggested trigger levels for dose rate surveys is 5 mR per hour at 30 cm (the definition of a Radia-

**TABLE 29-5.** *Trigger levels of removable contamination*

| Radiopharmaceutical | Unrestricted areas (per 100 cm$^2$) | Restricted areas (per 100 cm$^2$) |
|---|---|---|
| P-32, Sr-89, In-111, I-123, I-125, I-131 | 200 dpm | 2,000 dpm |
| Co-57, Ga-67, Tc-99m, Tl-201 | 2,000 dpm | 20,000 dpm |

tion Area). When analyzing radiopharmaceutical contamination, the results must be converted into units of activity (e.g., mCi or dpm) from cpm. This is accomplished by using the appropriate efficiency for the radioisotope involved, or using a worst-case efficiency (i.e., the lowest efficiency of your counter for any of the radionuclides used in the pharmacy). Reg Guide 10.8 contains suggested trigger levels for removable contamination (Table 29-5).

*Gases or Aerosols*

If the applicant wants to use noble gases or aerosols, procedures to control air concentrations of these radioactive materials must be submitted. These are detailed in Reg Guide 10.8, Appendix O, and consist of items such as estimating worker dose from submersion in noble gases or aerosol concentrations, estimating aerosol and gas concentration in effluents, and calculating spilled gas clearance times.

*Iodine 131*

Special precautions must be taken with I-131 because of its ease of metabolism and incorporation into thyroid tissue. Appendix P of Reg Guide 10.8 discusses considerations for inpatient radioiodine therapies. Essentially, any patient who receives 33 mCi (1,221 MBq) or more of I-131 must be treated on an inpatient status until the level of I-131 in the body is <33 mCi (1,221 MBq). The patient's room must be restricted from general use until a survey by the hospital staff reveals no contamination in excess of 200 dpm per 100 cm$^2$. Additionally, all absorbent paper, wastes, and linens must be treated as radioactive waste. Measurements of thyroid uptakes (i.e., bioassay) must be performed on any worker who handles unsealed I-131 and I-125 in quantities exceeding those listed in Reg Guide 8.20, Applications of Bioassay for I-125 and I-131 (11).

**Waste Management (Item 11)**

Most of the radionuclides used in nuclear medicine are relatively short lived. Except for I-125, which has a 60-day half-life, most commonly used radioisotopes have half-lives <8 days. Given this, most clinics segregate their radioactive waste into half-life groups of short (technetium 99m [Tc-99m], I-123), medium (gallium 67, indium 111, I-131, thallium 201), and long (chromium 51, Sr-89, I-125). To dispose

**TABLE 29-6.** *Types and costs of medical licenses*

| Type of fee application | 7A teletherapy | 7B broad scope | 7C nuclear medicine | 2B source material |
|---|---|---|---|---|
| New | $3,600 | $3,900 | $1,800 | $130 |
| Amendment | $400 | $740 | $460 | $290 |
| Annual | $10,300 | $23,500 | $4,700 | $490 |

of these wastes without regard to their radioactivity, clinics must hold their radioactive waste for a minimum of 10 half-lives to allow for decay. After surveying the container with a radiation survey meter to verify decay and after defacing all radioactive labels, the user must dispose of the waste as either medical waste or normal trash. Most clinics that receive molybdenum 99/Tc-99m generators hold these generators for decay, and they are usually returned to the manufacturer. Reg Guide 10.8, Appendix R, describes the model procedure for waste disposal. The only exception to radioactive waste requirements is that excreta from patients administered radioactive materials is not regulated unless that excreta is collected. Items contaminated by radioactive excreta, such as urinary catheters or absorbent pads, are not exempt.

Aqueous liquids that are readily soluble in water and that do not contain hazardous chemical, biological, or infectious constituents may be disposed of through the sanitary sewer, provided that local sewer regulations are met. The daily and monthly sewer limits are based on the total sewage flow of the facility and the allowable activities listed in Tables 2 and 3 of Appendix B, 10 CFR Part 20. Usually the number of gallons of sewage per day can be obtained either from the plant engineers or from the sewer bill from the municipality. Except for patient wastes, records (date, radionuclide, and activity) must be kept for all radioactive aqueous liquids disposed through the sanitary sewer. In addition to the concentration limits, the total activity a licensee is allowed to dispose in 1 year cannot exceed >1 Ci of all radionuclides, except hydrogen 3 and carbon 14, for which the individual limits are 5 Ci and 1 Ci, respectively.

### License Fees (Item 12)

Congress has mandated that the NRC recoup expenses through fees for actions and services. Two types of fees are collected from licensees in nonagreement states. License fees are the fees charged for new license applications and amendments. Annual fees are the fees charged each licensee on the anniversary month for their particular medical license. Both sets of fees are based on the type of license and are specified in 10 CFR 170 and 171, respectively. The NRC categorizes licenses into several categories; human use is category 7. The license fees for each category remain relatively constant from year to year. Annual fees are collected to enable the NRC to recoup expenses and these can fluctuate significantly (e.g., the annual fee for a type 7B license was $30,900 in 1994, but only $23,300 in 1995). These annual fees are calculated to make up the difference of expenses minus expected income from license fees. The total is then rated over all active licensees except for the categories of licenses that are exempt (e.g., public educational institutes, etc.). Licensees fear that, as medical users give up their licenses (700 did in 1992–1993), and as more states become agreement states, these fees will increase for the remaining licenses.

Comparing the three types of medical licenses (teletherapy, nuclear medicine, and broad scope), you can see that cost depends on the level of use (Table 29-6).

Some teletherapy devices use depleted uranium as a shield in the teletherapy head or collimator, and some nuclear medicine generators are shielded with depleted uranium. Because depleted uranium is a radioactive substance, it must be listed in Item 5/6 on the license as a separate item, and the licensee must include the appropriate fees for that category of license, Category 2B (possession and use of source material for shielding).

## QUALITY MANAGEMENT PROGRAM

Each medical licensee must have a written QMP. The administration of by-product material to patients can be a complex process involving many workers throughout the clinic. When the use is of high activities of material for therapeutic purposes, the consequences of errors may be too grave to be left to chance. The goal of a QMP is to ensure that by-product material is administered as directed by the authorized user. Reg Guide 8.33, Quality Management Program (12), provides considerations and suggested policies and procedures for certain therapeutic by-product material uses. This topic is discussed in the chapter on quality improvement, but one point must be emphasized: The authorized user must sign and date the therapeutic prescription personally. Elsewhere in medicine, this personalized date requirement is not necessary. The definition of therapeutic radionuclide includes doses of I-131 >30 μCi, so diagnostic scans for metastatic thyroid cancer are also under this regulatory umbrella.

## RECORDKEEPING

One key to demonstrating continued incident-free operation is good recordkeeping. The Joint Commission on Accreditation of Healthcare Organizations describes most of the concepts and requirements for records. A rule of thumb is that, if you do it, you should have a procedure describing how to do it and you should keep records showing it was done. The NRC requires users to maintain records of the receipt, use, transfer, and disposal of radioactive materials for a period of 3 years. All letters, requests, and so forth pertaining to the NRC license should be maintained for the duration of the license. Records pertaining to sealed sources should be maintained for at least 3 years after the source has been disposed. Records of personnel exposure to ionizing radiation should be maintained for the life of the license and then placed in long-term record storage. Records relating to patients are probably governed by the administrative requirements of each individual facility.

## TRANSFERRING RADIOACTIVE MATERIALS: INTERLICENSE TRANSFERS

The NRC license issued to your facility requires that you handle radioactive materials in a responsible fashion. Other facilities, if they desire to use radioactive material, must have an appropriate (NRC, state, or Department of Energy) license. The NRC allows a licensee to transfer radioactive materials to other licensed facilities. However, the NRC does not allow the selling or manufacturing of radioactivity unless your facility has a specific license or authorization to do so. Before transferring radioactive material to any facility outside of your license, you must first obtain a copy of the other facilities' license to use and possess radioactive materials and verify that they have indeed authorized the type and quantity of radioactive materials you intend to send them. The copy can usually be obtained by contacting that facility's RSO. If you send material to some facility not authorized to receive the radioactive material, you will be in violation of your license. Once you have verified that the requesting organization is licensed for the radioactive material, you must prepare the item for shipment according to the DOT rules and regulations (49 CFR). Normally, your RSO can assist you in complying with these regulations.

## CURRENT EVENTS

Because of the way rules and regulations come into existence (e.g., petition for rule making, proposed change), the various regulations affecting an organization continually change. All persons at an organization (RSO, pharmacist, physician) must review regulations and ensure that they keep abreast of these changes. Some of the more recent or pending actions are discussed below.

### Radioactive Waste Disposal Facilities

The Low-Level Radioactive Waste Policy Act (1980) and Amendments (1985) shifted responsibility for waste disposal from the federal government to the states. Individual states, or groups of states (called *compacts*), are now responsible for providing for the safe disposal of low-level radioactive wastes. Although most states and compacts (nine exist currently) are making progress toward implementing these regulations, the June 30, 1994, deadline passed with few states having access to low-level radioactive waste sites. This problem highlights the need for each licensee to implement a viable, aggressive program to reduce radioactive waste volumes and to adequately manage wastes once generated.

### Revised 10 CFR 20

In 1980, the NRC completely revised 10 CFR 20 to bring it into line with international guidance. Unfortunately, this revision became victim of the federal government's attempt to reduce the federal bureaucracy and was not implemented. During the interim, the NRC reviewed EPA and international radiation protection guidance and rewrote and revised 10 CFR 20, making the changes effective January 1, 1994. For most day-to-day nuclear medicine operations, this revision has little impact. Affected areas include the following:

- Survey of all incoming packages that are not exempt from Radioactive I, II, or III labeling
- Annual whole-body radiation limit changed to 5 rems per year
- Radiation doses from external and internal (e.g., I-131) radiation sources must be considered. Implementation of ICRP 30 guidance for radiation exposure includes assigning a weighing factor to internal exposure, summing of internal and external doses, providing annual reports to workers, and so forth.
- Changes in effluent levels

### Patient Release

The revised 10 CFR 20 mandates that members of the general public not be exposed to >100 mrem in 1 year. It is possible that certain patients receiving radioactive materials in therapeutic procedures could have residual radioactivity sufficient to expose nonpatients to levels in excess of 100 mRem. The past policy for release of therapy patients is based on guidance found in the National Council on Radiation Protection and Measurement (NCRP) Report 37, Precautions in the Management of Patients who Have Received Therapeutic Amounts of Radionuclides. The NRC allows patients who receive <30 mCi of radioiodine to be treated on an outpatient basis, and patients receiving 30 mCi or more to be treated on an inpatient basis.

Because this procedure may allow for some members of the general public to receive doses >100 mrem (but probably <500 mrem) from the patient, the NRC revised patient release procedures for those receiving therapeutic quantities of gamma-emitting radionuclides. The requirements are again based on the exposure rate from the patient at 1 m and will require additional documentation for patients receiving therapeutic doses of I-131 >6.5 mCi. The clinic will need to perform a rough calculation of the maximum dose to a member of the general public based on the ratio 15.33 mrem per 1 mCi of I-131. Patients with >33 mCi of I-131 must be hospitalized until the exposure rate decreases to <7 mrem per hour at 1 m. The NRC has suggested guidance and forms in Draft Reg Guide DG 8015, Release of Patients Administered Radioactive Materials, to enable nuclear medicine clinics to document their evaluation of each case and the guidance presented to the patient and persons likely to be exposed.

This rule is perhaps indicative of regulatory problems. Publishing the rule would not substantially change the practice of patient release (i.e., at 30 mCi), but clinics would need to document many more iodine safety briefings for all patients receiving doses between 6.5 and 30 mCi. Clinics also might need to reduce doses for diagnostic scans merely not to be forced to document the briefing. Thus, many negative comments were received and, although the revision was supposed to be published in final form in January 1996, because of the widespread comments received, the publication date was extended. The rule was finalized May 29, 1997.

### Institute of Medicine Report

In late 1992, several high-profile events (e.g., Indiana, Pennsylvania High Dose Rate Afterloading device misadministration; *Cleveland Plain Dealer* series on radiation in medicine; the U.S. Senate investigation into radiation medicine), the NRC solicited the Institute of Medicine (IOM) to "conduct a detailed independent review and make recommendations for needed changes" in (1) policy issues underlying regulation of medical radioisotopes, (2) overall risks from radiation medicine compared to other medical risks, and (3) assessment of the regulatory framework for regulation of medical uses of by-product material. The IOM report, *Radiation in Medicine* (13), is the result of the 2-year study conducted by the 16-member IOM committee.

Apparently the medical professionals operating under NRC licensure are frustrated because they perceive a lack of flexibility in the NRC. Although mistakes in medicine are regrettable, errors happen in any operation. Given an error rate of 1% to 5% in many medical arenas and a serious event rate of 0.02% (1 per 5,000 patients), the fact that the rate of serious errors in NRC-licensed medical activities—0.002% (approximately 2 per 100,000 administrations)—is not lauded but criticized seems to indicate unrealistic expectations. The same rules apply to megacurie nuclear reactors as to millicurie medicine and research, even though there is 1,000,000,000 times less radioactivity involved.

In addition to the seeming over-regulation of NRC materials in medicine is the fact that this form of radiation accounts for only 10% of the use of radiation in medicine. For this regulation, each licensee pays both license and annual fees but seems to have no voice in the regulatory process. For example, even though the NRC's proposed QMP (10 CFR 35.32 and 35.33) was reviewed negatively by nearly all licensees, and the Office of Management and Budget (13) stated that "reporting and recordkeeping requirements will have little if any practical utility furthering the goal of reducing injuries from misadministrations," the NRC commissioners voted to implement the regulations.

The IOM committee recommended the following measures: (1) Remove the NRC from regulating medical uses and revoke Part 35, (2) shift guidance for this source of radiation to the FDA's Department of Health and Human Services, and (3) encourage states to assume this regulatory role using the guidance of the CRCPD. Such a drastic recommendation must be a manifestation of the frustration in the medicine community.

### REFERENCES

1. Wright AW. Experiments upon the cathode rays and their effects. Am J Sci 1896;1(15):235–244.
2. Thomson E. Roentgen rays act strongly on the tissues. Elect Engineer 1896;22:534.
3. Rollins W. X-light kills. Boston Med Surg J 1901;144:173.
4. Walsh D. Deep tissue traumatism from roentgen ray exposure. BMJ 31 July 1897:272.
5. Evans RD. Radium poisoning: a review of present knowledge. Am J Public Health 1933;23:1017–1023.
6. Evans RD. The radiation standard for boneseekers—evaluation of the data on radium patients and dial painters. Health Phys 1967;13:267–278.
7. Stewart A, Kneale GW. Radiation dose effects in relation to obstetric x-rays and childhood cancers. Lancet 1970;1:1185–1187.
8. U.S. NRC Regulatory Guide 10.8, Revision 2, Guide for the Preparation of Applications for Medical Use Programs. Washington, DC: Nuclear Regulatory Commission, August 1987.
9. U.S. NRC Regulatory Guide 10.5, Revision 3, Applications for Licenses of Broad Scope. Washington, DC: Nuclear Regulatory Commission, August 1991.
10. U.S. NRC Regulatory Guide 8.23, Revision 1. Radiation Safety Surveys at Medical Institutions. Washington, DC: Nuclear Regulatory Commission, January 1981.
11. U.S. NRC Regulatory Guide 8.20, Revision 1. Applications of Bioassay for I-125 and I-131. Washington, DC: Nuclear Regulatory Commission, September 1979.
12. U.S. NRC Regulatory Guide 8.33. Quality Management Program. Washington, DC: Nuclear Regulatory Commission, October 1991.
13. Gottfried KD, Penn G (eds). Radiation Medicine: A Need for Regulatory Reform. Washington, DC: National Academy Press, 1996.

*Textbook of Nuclear Medicine,*
edited by Michael A. Wilson.
Lippincott–Raven Publishers, Philadelphia © 1998.

CHAPTER 30

# Clinical Protocols

Michael A. Wilson

These protocols in this chapter are the University of Wisconsin's nuclear medicine procedure protocols used at the Clinical Health Sciences Center in Madison. They are arranged in 14 groups, in order of the chapters in the text. Although throughout the book doses have been included as both millicuries and megabecquerels, in this chapter only millicuries are used. It is important to understand that these protocols represent a single institution's standard protocols, and are a consequence of the expertise and equipment available. Other sources of protocols include the Society of Nuclear Medicine Procedure Guidelines Manual 1997, from the Commission on Health Care Policy and Practice, Guidelines and Communications Committee.

These protocols are provided in a standard format: They begin with the appropriate current procedural terminology (CPT) code and appropriate patient indications. They then indicate patient preparation and departmental scheduling requirements (time, radiopharmaceutical, imaging device), and then the imaging procedure (data acquisition and display) for the technologist. Helpful interpretation hints are then provided. Special forms and aids are also included as figures. Included in Appendix B is the dose adjustment (for size) nomogram.

The order of the protocol groups follows that of the individual chapters, and page numbers are as follows:

## Administrative Protocols

### ADMINISTRATION 1: ADMINISTRATION OF RADIOPHARMACEUTICALS

Before the radiopharmaceutical is administered, these tasks must be performed:

1. Order and prepare the dose if not already prepared by radiopharmacy staff.
2. Ensure that the dose is adjusted for the stated patient weight where appropriate.
3. Complete radiopharmacy computer input as necessary.
4. Confirm that prescription printout is correct for patient.
5. Verify (assay) dose and document on the prescription, confirming that dose, time, patient name, weight, and radiopharmaceutical appear to be appropriate for the patient.
6. Identify the patient by at least two methods, which may include name, medical record number, birth date, or wrist band.
7. Ask female patients whether they are pregnant or nursing. If so, inform nuclear medicine (NM) physician immediately so that an informed medical decision can be made concerning risks and benefits of the procedure. After discussion with the patient and sometimes the

referring physician, possible modifications of the procedure, including cancellation, ensue.

8. Explain the procedure to the patient.
9. Examine the consultation request form, and verify that this test and dose are suitable for the patient and patient history as supplied. Any questions raised should be discussed with NM physician staff.
10. Administer the dose.
11. Affix the sticker to the consultation request form.
12. Ensure that dose, radiopharmaceutical, time, site, route of injection, and the initials of the person administering the dose are recorded on the consultation request form.
13. Discard needles, gloves, trash, and so forth.
14. Direct the patient on what to do next (e.g., have a seat, return at a later time, eat/don't eat).
15. Remove or deface the label from the syringe or holder.

Individuals authorized to administer radiopharmaceuticals include all radiology residents, all cardiology fellows, and all physicians with nuclear cardiology reading privileges.

## ADMINISTRATION 2: BIOASSAY TESTS, THYROID COUNTS

1. Thyroid counts for iodine 131 (I-131) will be performed on all technologists in NM at weekly intervals and within 3 days of handling >30 mCi of I-131.
2. The radiopharmacist and radiopharmacy technician will have a thyroid count performed at weekly intervals for I-131 and within 3 days of handling >30 mCi of I-131.
3. Any NM staff physicians and residents (and any other personnel involved) who administer therapy doses of I-131 will have a thyroid count at least at weekly intervals and within 3 days of handling >30 mCi of I-131.
4. The results of these counts, the background count, and the standard count are recorded in a log book kept with the uptake probe.

**Comment:** Maximum permissible thyroid burden for I-131 is 70 nanocuries. Any count >2× background must be converted to nanocuries and rems and reported to radiation safety department.

## ADMINISTRATION 3: EMERGENCY VENTILATION-PERFUSION SCAN FOR PULMONARY EMBOLISM

Ventilation-perfusion (V/Q) scans will be provided after hours to on-call physicians if the NM resident or staff physician on call determines that it is clinically indicated as an emergency study. Otherwise, the scan will be performed as early as possible the next day, preferably as the first study of the next day.

The general philosophy is to reduce the number of after-hours studies because they may be of limited quality due to their often being done bedside. In addition, an after-hours surcharge significantly increases the patient cost.

It is anticipated that patients suspected of PE will be bolused with heparin by the time the request for a V/Q scan is made. This policy is approved by the Pulmonary Section for most clinical situations because therapy is begun several hours earlier than otherwise possible. The Pulmonary Section invites the referring physician to obtain a pulmonary consult should there be controversy about the necessity for an emergency V/Q scan.

If anticoagulation is contraindicated and the NM physician on call determines that the scan is indicated, an emergency study is done as early as possible. A current chest x-ray is mandatory. There might be occasions when other diagnoses are likely, and the scan might be clinically indicated to allow the referring physician to continue the diagnostic workup that would otherwise be halted pending the result of the V/Q scan. In these unusual circumstances, a V/Q scan is done immediately. Scan requests after 1:00 AM are generally deferred until the next morning.

Both ventilation and perfusion scans are required to diagnose PE with high specificity. Bedside ventilation scans are not offered.

### Contraindications to Anticoagulation

Contraindications to anticoagulation may be absolute or relative. Absolute contraindications of anticoagulation are the following:

- Recent intracranial surgery or bleed
- Recent (<48 hours) orthopedic or other surgery
- Active gastrointestinal (GI) bleeding
- Severe hypertension (malignant)
- Pregnancy
- Hemorrhagic blood dyscrasia

Relative contraindications include a history of recurrent GI bleeding and surgery that is recent (but >48 hours old).

## ADMINISTRATION 4: EMPTY INTRAVENOUS SOLUTION

The NM technologist calls to inform the referring service that the IV solution will be empty before the patient's study is finished. If nursing personnel cannot come to NM and replace or switch the patient's IV, the NM technologist hangs a bag of 5% dextrose on a keep-vein-open rate.

## ADMINISTRATION 5: INVASIVE PROCEDURES

NM has three minimally invasive (low-risk, low-volume) procedures:

- Cerebrospinal fluid (CSF) shunt patency study (CPT 78645)

- CSF leak or flow study (CPT 78650 and 78630)
- Peritoneal-venous shunt patency study (CPT 78291)

**Outline of Procedures**

*CSF Shunt Evaluation: CPT 78645*

This procedure is performed by the neurosurgical physicians while NM assists by providing the radionuclide and imaging, so NM does not contribute to the invasive portion of the procedure. The neurosurgical team should follow up this procedure, and the informed consent and description of the procedure in the patient chart is provided by the neurosurgical team member (resident or staff physician). No immediate neurologic complication is likely with this procedure, but the chance of nosocomial infection is remotely possible. Approximately half of these patients have obstructed shunts and will have surgical revision within 24 hours. The remaining patients are often discharged after the test. Any readmission for central nervous system infection occurs in <30 days and is monitored by the complication review process. Any nosocomial infections of other inpatients should be detected by the discharge analyst as a complication. These are referred to the neurosurgical quality assurance (QA) program, and NM is made aware of the complication by way of incidence reports.

*CSF Flow Study: CPT 78650 and 78630*

These procedures are performed by NM personnel after the intent and nature of the procedure is explained by the referring physician. NM physicians explain the lumbar puncture (LP) and the imaging procedure and note informed verbal consent in the body of the report. The patient's neurologic status and resultant changes are monitored by the physician performing the LP. The only distant complication is that of nosocomial infection, and that can be expected to be recorded as a complication if it caused hospital admission when the procedure was done to an outpatient. Hospital QA checks can be expected to identify these complications, and NM is informed by way of incidence reports.

*CPT 78291*

This procedure is minimally invasive, and the invasive portion of the procedure is performed by NM staff. Possible complications would include needling a viscus or organ in the peritoneal cavity. If such an event is detected (e.g., withdrawal of bowel contents or sudden complaint of significant pain), the procedure is terminated and the patient observed for 30 minutes. The patient's physician should be contacted and the appropriate follow-up done as a result of this con-

sultation. Other possible complications include secondary infection of the peritoneal cavity, which would be detected from readmission of the patient. Hospital QA checks can be expected to identify these complications, and NM would be informed by way of incidence reports.

**ADMINISTRATION 6: LUMBAR PUNCTURE**

**Preprocedure**

Informed consent should be supplied by the referring physician, but NM should confirm that the patient knows the lumbar puncture (LP) will be performed and describe the imaging protocol.

**Procedure**

The preprocedure note should include the following information:

1. That verbal informed consent was obtained
2. Position of patient
3. Vertebral interspace used
4. Number of attempts
5. Opening pressure
6. Amount of CSF removed and radiopharmaceutical administered
7. Condition of patient after the procedure
8. Name (legible) of clinician performing procedure

If difficulty occurs in successfully performing the LP, Special Procedures should be contacted to perform the LP under fluoroscopy.

**Postprocedure**

If requested by the patient's referring physician, NM supplies the tubes of CSF. If any immediate neurologic change occurs, the referring physician should be informed and the patient returned to the ward. On delayed imaging, the condition of the patient should be noted and documented in the NM report.

**ADMINISTRATION 7: SEDATION FOR NUCLEAR MEDICINE STUDIES**

NM will adhere to the hospital-wide policy on sedation.

Adult patients requiring sedation will be supervised by the referring service.

Pediatric NM studies are similar to other imaging studies in which patient cooperation is essential to prevent motion artifacts. Sedation for most pediatric patients is essential for patient cooperation during the imaging procedure. Therefore, sedation of pediatric patients is the responsibility of the department with the greatest familiarity with the patient (in most instances, this is the referring pediatric service). There is a hospital-wide pediatric sedation team available, and all NM tests will be scheduled through or with this team. Administration of sedation should be done before transport to NM but may be done after the patient arrives in the NM module.

Regardless of whether sedation is administered on the ward or in NM, the study will be canceled if the patient is unable to lie quietly for the study. The patient will be rescheduled for the next day, depending on the time of the study and the volume of other patient studies for that day.

## ADMINISTRATION 8: TECHNOLOGIST ROTATION

### Rotations

Technologists will routinely be assigned weekly rotations through each imaging station. Laboratory procedures will be performed by the technologist assigned to the radiopharmacy for administering doses. If the person is unavailable, the procedure will be assigned to the most available technologist according to workload. Some laboratory procedures require CLIA-88 certification and are limited to those technologists approved.

### Pregnancy

Technologists who declare themselves pregnant will do the following:

- Rotate through all areas, including call
- Not draw I-131 doses for metastatic surveys or radioiodine therapies or open packages of same
- Be issued a personal dosimeter that can be checked immediately. Each month the radiodosimetry report will be reviewed by the pregnant technologist and supervisory staff, and an investigation will be conducted when 125 mR is accumulated during the pregnancy.

This policy is determined from long-term follow-up of radiation dosimetry records that demonstrate no significant body doses to personnel, certainly much less than maximum safe doses suggested by the Nuclear Regulatory Commission (NRC). Because I-131 can result in internal contamination, the restrictions for larger doses (metastatic surveys and therapies) are applied.

# Musculoskeletal Protocols

## MUSCULOSKELETAL 1: WHOLE-BODY BONE SCAN

CPT code: 78306
**Indications:** This examination detects the presence and distribution of bone lesions in a variety of disorders, including the following:

- Primary and secondary cancer
- Benign bone tumors
- Osteomyelitis
- Arthritis
- Avascular necrosis
- Trauma
- Occult fractures
- Stress fractures
- Other sports injuries
- Child abuse
- Bone graft viability
- Unexplained bone pain

Most bone scans are done to survey patients for presence of metastatic disease (documenting progression or regression of metastases), sports injuries, and other orthopedic indications.
**Patient preparation:** Pediatric patients need an IV in place at time of arrival for injection. Those between the ages of 1 and 5 years probably need to be sedated at time of scan. A urinary catheter with collection bag should be in place at time of scan for sedated and non–toilet-trained children.

Adult patients need no patient preparation.
**Scheduling:** Allow 45 minutes on dual-headed camera, 60 minutes on single-headed camera at 3 hours after injection, unless otherwise specified. When imaging the distal extremities, the preferred imaging time is 4 to 6 hours after injection.
**Radiopharmaceutical and dose:** 24 to 36 mCi technetium 99m methylene diphosphonate (Tc-99m MDP). Dose will be adjusted for patients ≤17 years of age and ≤45 kg. If an adult patient weighs ≥127 kg, consult with NM physician.

After injection, patient should drink four 8-ounce glasses of liquid before returning for the scan.
**Imaging device:** Gamma camera with low-energy, high-resolution (LEHR) collimation for planar imaging. Multiheaded device with LEHR collimation for single photon emission computed tomography (SPECT).
**Imaging procedure:** Patient should be asked decorously to empty his or her bladder just before being imaged. The patient should be scanned as follows, keeping the scanning speed as slow as possible and yet keep the patient immobile:

1. Use whole-body mode when available. Keep collimator as close to patient as possible.

2. If patient is unable to empty bladder completely, obtain 15- to 30-degree posterior oblique views to view the sacrum, or perform delayed views.
3. When doing spot films only (e.g., for claustrophobic patients), acquire these views:
    a. Spot view of anterior chest for 1,000 K counts. Record time. Use 800 K counts or time for all other views.
    b. Anterior spot views from head to toes.
    c. Posterior spot views from head to pelvis.
    d. Spot views of arms, forearms, and hands.
4. Child abuse: In cases of child abuse, perfect limb symmetry is required to identify long bone fractures, especially those at bone ends. This may mean that individual bones are imaged separately, that is, the views should include correctly oriented femurs, tibias, and so on. To optimize resolution in infants, scan patient directly on the collimator.

**Display:** Display the whole-body images using the dual display: the first anterior and posterior images using the maximum count as determined in the upper one-third of the body (excluding renal activity), and in the second set of images the posterior image with –15% intensity, the anterior image with +15% intensity.

**Interpretation:** In general, abnormalities on bone scans are hot. This represents reactive new bone formation, a nonspecific response to any noxious stimuli. Occasionally, abnormalities are cold spots, such as hemangioma (this can also be hot) and tense packed lesion (e.g., tumor or osteomyelitis) with no blood flow to the lesion.

## MUSCULOSKELETAL 2: LIMITED BONE SCAN (SPECIFIC REGIONS)

CPT code: 78300
**Indications:** This scan is requested for examinations limited to a specific region. Typical examples include the following:

- Trauma or sports injuries (e.g., stress fractures); no flow study is required.
- Benign primary tumor (e.g., osteoid osteoma, simple cyst, aneurysmal bone cyst, giant cell tumor); this may require a flow study.
- Any expected localized lesion where there is no need to do a whole-body scan.

**Patient preparation, scheduling, radiopharmaceutical and dose, and imaging device:** Same as for whole-body bone scan (CPT code 78306)
**Imaging procedure:** Patient should be asked decorously to empty his or her bladder just before being imaged.
  The patient should be scanned as follows:

1. Position the area of interest, ensuring that the affected area (and opposite extremity if a limb) are firmly against the collimator (tape can be used to immobilize).

2. Place a radioactive marker on the collimator next to the lateral aspect of the right extremity or region.
3. Obtain tangential and orthogonal views of the lesion site and the opposite extremity or region. A minimum of two different views are needed to best define area of interest.
4. When imaging the distal extremities, image at 4 to 6 hours after injection (the preferred imaging time).

**Special Considerations**

- If the patient has a history of cancer, be sure to include a whole-body scan as well as the limited regions.
- If the patient has a stress fracture, sports injury, or trauma of lower extremities, include views from the pelvis to the toes.
- If the patient has knee pain, image the lower back and pelvis as well as knees (rule out referred pain).
- If the patient has foot pain, always acquire plantar views in addition to appropriate orthogonal views.

**Interpretation:** Same as for bone scans generally.

## MUSCULOSKELETAL 3: BONE SPECT

CPT code: 78320
**Indications:** This examination is done to "SPECT" particularly sites where planar imaging might be normal but the patient has a lesion. The classic indications are these:

- Spondylolysis
- Avascular necrosis (AVN) of hip
- Temporomandibular joint disease
- Patellar disease or other knee derangements
- In patients with a question of vertebral metastases, where SPECT is more sensitive than planar views and characterizes the lesion better

**Patient preparation, scheduling, radiopharmaceutical and dose, and imaging device:** Same as for whole-body bone scan (CPT code 78306)
**Imaging device:** Single and multiheaded camera with LEHR collimation (the multiheaded detector camera is preferred)

**Image Acquisition**

### Single Head

Matrix: 128 × 128
Acquisition: Contoured, 6-degree stops of 25 to 40 seconds
Filter: Butterworth, cutoff 0.4 to 0.5, power 15
Display: 1- to 2-slice thickness

### Dual Head

Matrix: 128 × 128
Acquisition: Contoured, 6-degree stops of 25 to 40 seconds

Filter: Butterworth, cutoff 0.4 to 0.5, power 15
Display: 1- to 2-slice thickness

### Triple Head

Matrix: 128 × 128
Acquisition: Contoured, 4-degree stops of 45 seconds
Filter: Butterworth, cutoff 0.5 to 0.6, power 10
Display: 1- to 2-slice thickness
**Interpretation**: Occasional cold spots occur (especially with AVN, in the first few days). In suspected metastatic disease, the location of the focal abnormality is critical: Involvement of vertebral body and posterior process is typical of metastatic disease.

## MUSCULOSKELETAL 4: TRIPLE-PHASE BONE SCAN

CPT code: 78315
**Indications:** This scan is requested for examination of blood flow to a specific region and to determine whether the bone scan lesion is associated with hyperperfusion.

Conditions always requiring triple-phase bone scans (TPBS) include

- Infection (acute osteomyelitis or septic arthritis)
- Cold injury (frostbite)
- Reflex sympathetic dystrophy

Conditions that may require TPBS include

- Trauma (e.g., stress fractures and tendonitis)
- Benign primary tumor (e.g., osteoid osteoma, aneurysmal bone cyst, giant cell tumor)
- Malignant primary tumor
- Soft-tissue tumors (to determine whether adjacent bone is involved)
- Other skeletal lesions with expected associated flow abnormalities

**Patient preparation:** As for whole-body bone scan (CPT code 78306)
**Scheduling:** The test is a two-part test, with flow and blood pool images obtained first. Allow 30 minutes for flow study. Allow 60 minutes for delayed images at 3 hours after injection for axial skeleton, 4 to 6 hours after injection for extremities.
**Radiopharmaceutical and dose, imaging device:** As for whole-body bone scan (CPT code 78306).

### Imaging Procedure

1. Position the area of interest, ensuring that the affected area and opposite extremity are firmly against the collimator (tape can be used to immobilize). In the case of foot symptoms, the plantar aspect is preferred for the flow study unless otherwise indicated by the NM physician. Distal tibia or fibula lesions should preferably be flowed posteriorly unless otherwise indicated by the NM physician. Place a radioactive marker on the collimator next to the lateral aspect of the right extremity.
2. Do a flow study by injecting the Tc-99m MDP followed by a 15-ml saline flush as a bolus injection. Obtain computer acquisition of flow study using 1-second images for 60 seconds.
3. Do an immediate blood pool image for 2 minutes. Obtain additional tangential and orthogonal views of the lesion site and opposite extremity. Record counts.

   A minimum of two orthogonal views (90 degrees to each other) are required to define the area of interest.
4. Special views: If the patient has cancer, perform a whole-body scan, too. For cold injury (frostbite), perform 24-hour–delay images of affected areas.

**Display:** The flow images are routinely displayed at 5-second intervals (sometimes shorter) with blood pool images of the same size on the same film. The delayed images should also have a blood pool image displayed on the same piece of hard copy, at the same size, to allow comparison of flow, blood pool, and delayed images.
**Interpretation:** The purpose of this scan is to compare the perfusion and blood pool images with the delayed images.

Acute osteomyelitis (OM) is the most common indication. An abnormal scan suggesting acute OM requires an intense focal abnormality on delayed images and a concordant abnormality in both early flow images (first or second image) and blood pool image. Study is abnormal 7 to 10 days before x-ray changes develop.

In reflex sympathetic dystrophy, the scan is very sensitive when the disease is early (before atrophic skin changes) and generally has increased flow and an unusual but characteristic periarticular pattern of increased uptake. Some patients (~15%, especially children or lower limb involvement) have reduced flow and reduced bone uptake.

Bone tumors have increased flow (and blood pool) as their malignancy increases; benign lesions have normal flow unless additional processes occur (e.g., fracture of simple cyst).

## MUSCULOSKELETAL 5: BONE SCAN WITH WHITE BLOOD CELL SCAN FOR "SECONDARY" OSTEOMYELITIS

CPT code: 78306 Bone Scan, 78193 WBC Scan
**Indications:** To rule out secondary osteomyelitis or septic arthritis. This study is limited to situations with possible secondary infections (infection associated with trauma, surgery, fracture, prosthesis, Charcot's joints, past osteomyelitis, and superimposed cellulitis or skin ulceration).
**Patient preparation:** As for whole-body bone scan (CPT code 78306). If skin ulceration is present, ask the patient to have dressing changed before arrival and to bring a fresh dressing change to all appointments.

**Scheduling:** Schedule either:

- First choice: Both a TPBS (begin at 8 AM with delays at 3 PM) and same-day indium 111 white blood cell (In-111 WBC) scan.
- When In-111 is not available: TPBS (begin at 8 AM with delays at 3 PM); 2 days later, perform a Tc-99m WBC scan (or an In-111 WBC scan).

**Radiopharmaceutical and dose**:

- In-111: 400 to 600 μCi
- Tc-99m MDP: 24 to 36 mCi

Adjust dose for patients ≤17 years of age and ≤45 kg. If an adult patient weighs ≥127 kg, consult with an NM physician.

After injection, patient should drink four 8-ounce glasses of liquid before returning for the scan.

**Imaging device:** Gamma camera with

- Medium-energy (ME) collimation for In-111 scan with or without simultaneous bone scan
- LEHR collimation for Tc-99m scan

**Data acquisition:** Images are obtained in the position that best separates the putative infected site from the prosthesis, old fracture site, skin ulcer, or soft tissue inflammation. Orthogonal views are then obtained and other views as required.

*First-choice procedure* (TPBS and In-111 WBC scan):

Day 1
1. At 8 AM:
   a. Draw blood for In-111 WBC scan.
   b. Perform Tc MDP flow study.
2. Reinject patient with WBC's immediately after labeling.
3. At 3 PM, obtain combined Tc-99m and In-111 images. Use these energy windows:
   a. Tc-99m = 140 keV, 20%
   b. In-111 = 247 keV only, 20%
Day 2: At 24 hours, obtain delay images of TPBS and In-111 WBC scan. Use energy windows:
1. Tc-99m = 140 keV, 20%
2. In-111 = use 247 keV only, 20%.

*Second-choice procedure:*
Day 1: Do the triple-phase bone scan (TPBS).
Day 3: Do Tc-99m WBC or In-111 WBC scan. Use 20% 247- and 173-keV windows for In-111.

**Data analysis:** The following sets of images are produced for each day:

1. TPBS images
2. In-WBC (247 keV only) images in combined In-111/Tc-99m scans.

The GE software RIRR allows markers to be placed in the simultaneously acquired and separate WBC and bone scan images for correlation.

**Interpretation:** Decision concerning the presence or not of In-111 WBC focus is made (uptake occurs at bone scan), then a decision is made as to whether this is in bone or soft tissue by correlation of WBC and bone scans.

## MUSCULOSKELETAL 6: JOINT SCAN

CPT code: 78306

**Indications:** To establish multifocal inflammatory joint disease (including but not limited to possible multisite septic arthritis, rheumatoid arthritis, acute synovitis, and other inflammatory joint diseases).

**Patient preparation:** Pediatric patients need an IV line in place at time of arrival for injection. Those between the ages of 1 and 5 years probably need to be sedated at time of scan. A Foley catheter with collection bag should be in place at time of scan for sedated and non–toilet-trained children.

Adult patients require no patient preparation.

**Scheduling:** Allow 45 minutes at time of injection and 1 hour (45 minutes for dual-headed camera) 3 hours after injection.

**Radiopharmaceutical and dose:** 24 to 36 mCi Tc-99m MDP. Dose will be adjusted for patients ≤17 years of age and ≤45 kg. If an adult patient weighs ≥127 kg, consult with an NM physician.

After injection, the patient should drink four 8-ounce glasses of liquid before returning for the scan.

**Imaging device:** Single-headed or dual-headed gamma camera with LEHRP collimation to include entire skeleton.

**Imaging procedure:**

1. Perform a TPBS of the most symptomatic or involved region.
2. Five minutes after injection, acquire whole-body images of all symptomatic joints. If multiple joints are symptomatic, a whole-body scan in posterior view is appropriate.
3. At 3 hours after injection, obtain a whole-body scan on the same device. Additional images (including orthogonal views) of symptomatic joints may also be required.

**Interpretation:** Abnormalities are shown by blood pool and static images: increased flow to synovia of affected joints in blood pool image and increased uptake to periarticular regions of affected joints.

## MUSCULOSKELETAL 7: BONE MARROW SCAN

CPT code: 78104

**Indications**

- Determination of extent of marrow (myeloproliferative disorders)
- Detection of ischemic or infarcted regions (sickle-cell disease, dysbaric osteonecrosis, AVN)

- Detection of asymmetric marrow distribution (e.g., tumors such as myeloma and Hodgkin's disease)
- Assessment of regional differences in marrow (e.g., metastatic disease)
- Confirmation of effect of cytokine

**Patient preparation:** No patient preparation
**Scheduling:** Allow 105 minutes total (75 minutes camera time).
**Radiopharmaceutical and dose**: 8 to 12 mCi Tc-99m sulfur colloid (SC) (this radiopharmaceutical can be filtered like the lymphoscintigraphy agent to enhance marrow uptake). Adjust the dose for patients ≤17 years of age and weight ≤45 kg. If adult patient weighs ≥127 kg, consult with an NM physician.
**Imaging device:** Gamma camera with LEHRP collimation.
**Imaging procedure:**

1. Perform a standard six-view liver-spleen (L/S) scan at 30 minutes after injection.
2. Obtain whole-body image. The liver or spleen should be shielded with lead to prevent scatter.

**Interpretation:** The distribution of marrow that takes up tracer is normally limited to the axial skeleton, with some localization in the proximal femurs. Generally the distribution is symmetric, but frequently, activity in the femoral heads is asymmetric. With expanded active marrow, this distribution is increased into the appendicular skeleton. With focal replacement of marrow, defects are seen. As focal disease (solid or marrow tumors) increases, the number of lesions increases and extends to involve the appendicular skeleton. An agent likely to replace this is the labeled monoclonal antibody (MOAB) to WBC precursors (currently available in Europe).

# Gastrointestinal Protocols

## GASTROINTESTINAL 1: HEPATOBILIARY SCAN (INCLUDING GALLBLADDER EJECTION FRACTION)

CPT code: 78223
**Indications**

- Diagnosis of acute cholecystitis (both calculous and acalculous disease)
- Determination of patency of common bile duct (CBD) when ultrasound examination is not diagnostic (e.g., very early obstruction)
- Evaluation of hepatic function
- Assessment of intrahepatic biliary duct patency
- Evaluation of biliary dyskinesia and spasm of sphincter of Oddi (gallbladder ejection fraction [GB EF] test)
- Identification of biliary leaks
- Evaluation of liver transplants
- Differentiation of biliary atresia from neonatal hepatitis
- Evaluation of presence or absence of spleen (with Tc-99m SC liver scan [CPT 78215])
- Not indicated for chronic cholecystitis

**Patient preparation**

- Patient should be fasting (NPO) for a minimum of 2 hours before this test.
- In patients fasted for >24 hours, on parenteral nutrition, or with a history of alcoholic liver disease, cholecystokinin (CCK-8: dose 0.04 µg/kg) should be administered prior (~20 minutes) to tracer injection.
- Record any meperidine (Demerol) or morphine used in last 12 hours.

- In some infants when differentiation between neonatal hepatitis and biliary atresia, pretreatment with phenobarbitone may be required.

**Scheduling:** The routine test takes 60 minutes of imaging. Modified protocols are required for bilirubin >30, GB EF (requires 2 hours) and for critically ill patients.
**Radiopharmaceutical and dose:** 4 to 6 mCi Tc-99m mebrofenin. Dose will be adjusted for patient weight if ≤45 kg or ≥90 kg.
**Imaging device**

- Gamma camera with LEHR collimation
- Portable camera with diverging collimation

**Imaging procedure:** The following protocol should be used.

1. Patient should be supine under the camera.
2. Imaging should be started immediately after injection.
3. A dynamic acquisition rate of 1 frame per minute for 60 minutes.
4. Watch the acquisition to determine if and when to give morphine. Morphine administration (dose of 0.04 mg/kg) is to be considered when there is visualization of the CBD and duodenum but no visualization of the GB at 30 minutes. Morphine should be administered (0.04 mg/kg) 40 minutes after tracer injection. The duodenum should demonstrate decreased and changing activity to confirm that the sphincter of Oddi has contracted. Gastric reflux often (60%) occurs with morphine. At 20 minutes after morphine, the GB should visualize in normals and those with chronic cholecystitis. A physician is to slowly administer the morphine over a 2-minute period. This IV use of mor-

phine has been exempted from conscious sedation policy requirements.

5. Images are continued to 60 minutes after radiopharmaceutical injection or until the GB is visualized (a right lateral and oblique views may be taken at physician's discretion).

**GB EF protocol:** If the GB EF is to be measured, wait 60 minutes before injecting CCK-8. Ensure that the GB is separated from duodenum; if not, reposition the patient (LAO view preferred). Collect data for 20 minutes after slow (3 minutes) IV infusion of CCK-8 (0.02 μg/kg). A double dose (0.04 μg/kg) may be administered if no GB contraction occurs with first injection.

**Modified protocol:** If bilirubin (BR) >30, the protocol should include a larger dose and more prolonged study: 30 minutes of acquisition should be obtained at the time of injection, and 10 minutes of imaging at 2 to 4 hours and the next morning.

**Critically ill patient protocol**: Critically ill patients with sepsis require a prolonged IV administration of CCK-8 (over 30 minutes by slow IV infusion) prior to scan and possibly larger doses of morphine (0.08 mg/kg) with delayed images (30 minutes vs. the more usual 20 minutes after morphine).

**Interpretation:** Nonvisualization of the GB indicates obstruction of the cystic duct: This is the NM physiologic requirement of acute cholecystitis.

The GB is normally visualized at 17 ± 15 minutes with mebrofenin, somewhat slower in the postprandial state (21 ± 25 minutes), and even later after CCK-8 preadministration.

If there is poor visualization of the intrahepatic biliary ducts or delayed blood clearance, hepatocyte dysfunction is likely. The BR should be reviewed, and later imaging will be required to diagnose diseases.

In acalculous cholecystitis, the cystic duct can be patent, resulting in a false negative test, but this is unusual (<10% of patients). To decrease the number of false positives in acute acalculous cholecystitis, the following modifications are suggested: slow IV pretest infusion of CCK-8 over 30 minutes, double dose of morphine to contract sphincter of Oddi, and delayed postmorphine images to continue for 30 minutes (see Scheduling, above).

When using morphine, watch for emptying of the duodenum as evidence of spasm of sphincter of Oddi. Morphine results in increased intra-CBD pressure and therefore fills the GB in chronic cholecystitis and possibly acalculous cholecystitis.

The hepatobiliary scan can diagnose obstruction of the CBD before ultrasound (but this occurs only in the first 4 or 5 days). To diagnose obstruction, image for 60 minutes and then obtain delayed (4- to 5-hour) views. With obstruction, intra-CBD pressure rises; as this increases and becomes persistent, CBD and later intrahepatic biliary duct dilatation occurs. Ultrasound detection is then very sensitive. With this passage of time, back pressure on the hepatocyte causes the

biliary tract not to be visualized, but then hepatocyte dysfunction is documented by delayed plasma clearance of tracer.

In biliary dyskinesia and in measuring GB EF, watch for patient movement and ensure small or large bowel activity does not enter the GB region of interest (ROI) used to calculate EF. Tight ROIs should be created around the GB at 60 minutes, then at 10 and 20 minutes after CCK. Without attention to this detail, false negative and positive scans may occur. (The GB EF is the total EF, i.e., dose II value numerator with original dose I denominator.) The literature indicates that male EF should be >50%, female EF >20% to be normal, but most institutions use a GB EF of >35% as normal regardless of patient sex.

In biliary atresia, there is minor urinary excretion (more with disofenin than mebrofenin) but no GI tract excretion. Severe neonatal hepatitis can emulate biliary atresia, but preadministration of phenobarbitone (5mg/kg/day in two divided doses for 3 to 5 days) results in increased hepatobiliary excretion and so distinguishes these two conditions.

## GASTROINTESTINAL 2: GI BLEEDING SCAN

CPT code: 78278
**Indications:** This examination is performed in an attempt to identify the location of active GI hemorrhage.

- Patients with active hemorrhage (bright red blood per rectum and transfusion requirements) are candidates for this examination on an emergency basis.
- Patients with melena are candidates for a more prolonged study with delayed imaging (see below).
- The study is not recommended as the initial test for upper GI bleeding studies (in this case endoscopy is performed).
- In patients with portal hypertension and abdominal collaterals, the optional Tc-99m SC procedure is used.

**Patient preparation:** No patient preparation
**Scheduling:** Before scheduling patients for this study, an NM staff or resident physician should be consulted because there are some times when the test is better modified. The best example is when there is evidence of recurrent bleeding with previous unsuccessful attempts at localization of bleeding site, so the study is started in the morning of a working day, continued during the routine hours, and additional images are obtained as appropriate.

Allow 30 minutes for the labeling process, 60 minutes for imaging, and time for possible delayed views. Always schedule a 10-minute image the next morning. This delayed image acquisition may only be canceled by an NM staff physician.
**Radiopharmaceutical and dose:** 16 to 24 mCi Tc-99m pertechnetate ($TcO_4^-$) for labeling autologous red blood cells. Use in the following cases:

- UltraTag technique (see Laboratory Tests)

- Modified in vivo technique (see Laboratory Tests)
- Labeled Tc-99m SC method (see below)

*Optional procedure in patients with abdominal collaterals:* In patients with established cirrhosis and abdominal collaterals, the labeled RBC method is inappropriate. Ten mCi of Tc-99m SC should be prepared, and four separate 2.5 mCi doses injected slowly with continuous imaging during injection and for 10 minutes after each injection. The injection site should be as far from the abdomen as possible. This procedure allows four opportunities to identify GI bleeding.

Dose will be adjusted for patient weight if ≤45 kg or ≥90 kg.

**Labeling efficiency (average):**

1. Modified in vivo = 92%
2. UltraTag = 97%

**Imaging device:** Gamma camera with LEHR collimation (preferably largest field-of-view [FOV] camera to include entire abdomen).

**Imaging procedure:** Use a predefined study (a movie of 10-second images acquired for 1 hour) plus additional images at longer intervals (at the discretion of the NM physician) and the next morning.

If the stomach is visualized, image neck to document free pertechnetate in the thyroid gland, and image and inspect gastric aspirate if a nasogastric tube is in place.

*Optional procedure with Tc-99m SC:* Begin imaging immediately on injection of the radiopharmaceutical, obtaining 1-minute images for 10 minutes. Cranial tilt may be required to better view the infrahepatic region. If no bleeding is identified, repeat injections of the divided radiopharmaceutical can be administered (up to four separate injections).

**Image display:** The display format will be 5-minute images for the period of the study. If a physician determines that 10-second or 1-minute images better demonstrate a bleed, rebleed, or multiple sites of bleeding, these hard copy images will be required for the relevant portion of the study to demonstrate the bleeding site.

*Optional procedure:* The images can be displayed in 2.5-minute frames (up to a total of 16 frames) for four injections.

**Interpretation:** The study establishes the presence of GI bleeding during the period from tracer injection to imaging. This very sensitive test can detect bleeding sites of 0.2 to 0.5 ml per minute. Because of the frequent retrograde or anterograde passage of tracer, however, the bleeding site may not be accurately localized unless 10-second or 1-minute images are viewed in cine format. Once GI bleeding is confirmed, the study must continue until the site is localized. Once the site is seen, enough time must be allowed to see the passage of tracer and identify whether it is of small or large bowel origin.

It has been established that if a focus of tracer is found in the bowel, its intensity (less than, equal to, or greater than liver) is an indication of the blood transfusion requirements and the need for endoscopy or operative intervention (when greater than liver).

*Optional procedure:* Abnormal scans are characterized by activity foci away from the liver, spleen, and bone marrow. This technique actually detects lesser bleeding rates (0.1 to 0.2 ml per minute), but because the circulating tracer is present for shorter time periods (half plasma disappearance time of radiopharmaceutical is 2.5 minutes), the sensitivity for bleeding detection is less than the labeled RBC method.

## GASTROINTESTINAL 3: GASTRIC EMPTYING

**CPT code:** 78264
**Indications:** This examination

- Can demonstrate abnormal gastric emptying and response to drug therapy (e.g., metoclopramide)
- Is indicated in patients with diabetes and those with complaints of nausea, vomiting, and early satiety

**Patient preparation**

- Patient should be fasting a minimum of 4 hours (depends on feeding interval in infants).
- Insulin may be taken as usual.
- Food sensitivities are to be noted, and changes in test meal must be confirmed with the NM physician.

**Scheduling**

Adult

- Requires 2.5 hours' presence: 0.5 hour to eat and 2 hours for imaging.
- This study has a strict food intake for adult patients of two scrambled eggs, toast, and orange juice. If patient cannot comply, changes are to be arranged with the NM physician.
- The test meal should be prepared after patient arrives in the department. Therefore this test cannot be scheduled before 8:30 AM each day.

Pediatric

- The patient's own formula is used. Volume is same as used for a normal feeding and timing is determined by normal feeding interval.

**Radiopharmaceutical and dose:** Tc-99m SC

Adult: 0.4 to 0.6 mCi added to two beaten eggs, and scrambled in the radiopharmacy. Dose is adjusted for patient weight if ≤45 kg or ≥90 kg.

Pediatric and infant: Adjust the dose for weight with minimum dose of 100 μCi.

**Imaging device:** Gamma camera with LE collimation
**Data acquisition**

- A predefined study sets up files to acquire dynamic 1-minute images for 15 minutes and static 1-minute images every 15 minutes for 120 minutes.

- A predefined study then processes and displays the study.

**Imaging procedure**
Adult

- Have the patient eat all the test meal as quickly as possible. If all the food cannot be eaten, the patient should eat all the eggs (containing the radiopharmaceutical) and as much of the rest of the test meal as possible.
- Image the patient for 15 minutes.
- During delayed imaging, allow the patient to get up and walk around between acquisitions.

Pediatric and infant

- Tc-99m SC is mixed with two-thirds of patient's formula or milk, leaving the remainder unlabeled. The unlabeled portion is used to wash down residual esophageal activity.
- The test is scheduled to start so that it is completed before the next normal feeding (to prevent crying from hunger).
- Feed the patient in an upright position.
- If patient is unable to drink, have the ward or clinic personnel insert a nasogastric tube. This tube is pulled after feeding before test commences.

**Data analysis:** A half emptying time is determined. This identifies the maximum count in the first 15-minute study. To get the half-life, a line is fitted between this and the delays.

Note: If small bowel is lying over the ROI, place the patient in a left lateral decubitus position for 2 minutes and then slowly roll back to a supine position for imaging.

**Interpretation:** The mean gastric emptying half-time for adults is 90 minutes; the upper limit of normal is 120 minutes; lower limit is 60 minutes.

## GASTROINTESTINAL 4: GASTROESOPHAGEAL REFLUX

CPT code: 78262
**Indications:** To determine the presence or absence of gastroesophageal reflux or pulmonary aspiration
**Patient preparation:** The patient must be NPO (nothing by mouth) for 4 hours prior to test. In infants, this time may need to be reduced (to coincide with normal feeding schedule). In infants, if a gastric tube is required for dose instillation it must be in place (placed by referring ward or clinic) and NM allowed to pull it after instillation of dose.
**Scheduling:** Allow 1 hour, in the morning.
**Radiopharmaceutical and dose:** 0.8 to 1.2 mCi Tc-99m SC in 150 ml of orange juice mixed with equal volume of 0.1 N hydrochloric acid (HCl). For infants, give the weight-adjusted dose in the infant's usual formula. Adjust dose for patient weight if ≤45 kg or ≥90 kg.
**Imaging device:** Gamma camera with LEHR collimation
**Imaging procedure:** For adults, imaging begins 15 minutes after ingestion of the radiopharmaceutical preparation; the time delay allows for complete esophageal emptying. For infants, when a nasogastric tube is used, imaging begins immediately.

Adults

- Standing: Check to see if esophagus is clear. If not, an additional 50 to 100 ml of liquid (equal amounts of orange juice and HCl) should be given to clear esophagus.
- Supine: Use the intravenous pyelogram (IVP) binder available in Radiology. Place the folded thigh cuff on top of the patient's abdomen at belt level, and tape in place. Wrap the Radiology IVP binder around the patient with the plastic block over the thigh cuff. The IVP binder has an extension for larger patients. The thigh cuff can now be inflated at the following manometer settings:
  - 0 mm Hg for 60 seconds
  - 20 mm Hg for 60 seconds
  - 40 mm Hg for 60 seconds
  - 60 mm Hg for 60 seconds
  - 80 mm Hg for 60 seconds
  - 100 mm Hg for 60 seconds

  *N.B. Binder is not used in children <12 years of age.*
- Delayed images: Lungs may be imaged immediately after study and at 4 to 6 hours to identify pulmonary aspiration.

Images are obtained in 128 × 128 matrix, 10 seconds per frame for 1 hour.

Infants

- As soon as formula is swallowed or instilled via the gastric tube, the tube is pulled and the infant is laid supine and images obtained (128 × 128 matrix, 10 seconds per frame for 1 hour) to detect GE reflux.
- Before instilling dose via a nasogastric tube, check to see if it is correctly located. Binders are not used. It is routine to obtain views of lungs at 60 minutes. Delayed images may be obtained at 4 to 6 hours.

**Data analysis:** Each 20-mm increment of pressure represents approximately a 5-mm pressure rise at the gastroesophageal junction. Gastroesophageal reflux is quantitated in each frame in the following way using computer-acquired data:

$R$ = Gastroesophageal reflux
$E$ = Esophageal counts during 60-second frame
$E_b$ = Esophageal background counts during 60-second frame
$G$ = Gastric counts during 60-second frame

$$R = \frac{E - E_b}{G} \times 100$$

**Interpretation:** Abnormal results include

- $R \geq 4\%$ (positive for gastroesophageal reflux)
- Evidence of pulmonary aspiration in infants (or adults)

The test is much more sensitive for gastroesophageal reflux than barium studies, which have a 15% to 20% sensitivity. Acidification of the test material increases the sensitivity of the nuclear medicine test as the acidity of the orange juice–HCl mixture delays gastric emptying and lowers the lower esophageal sphincter pressure. Using the above criteria (visual or quantification) gives a test sensitivity of about 90%.

## GASTROINTESTINAL 5: ESOPHAGEAL TRANSIT

CPT code: 78258

**Indications:** These studies are indicated to identify esophageal motility disorders, such as

- Amotility of achalasia or scleroderma
- Hypomotility of presbyesophagus
- Hypermotility of diffuse esophageal spasm

Most esophageal disorders are readily diagnosed with barium and manometry studies, and esophageal radionuclide studies are reserved for patients in whom the screening tests were unhelpful.

**Patient preparation:** Patient should be fasting a minimum of 4 hours.

**Scheduling:** Allow 1 hour for the test: 15 minutes for acquisition, the remainder for readying and processing.

**Radiopharmaceutical and dose:** Tc-99m SC, 1 mCi placed in a test tube with a small amount of water (10 to 15 ml)

**Imaging device:** Gamma camera with a LEHR collimator

**Data acquisition:** Data are acquired in $128 \times 128$ dynamic mode with 1-second frames for 2 minutes, then 15-second frames for 10 minutes (for a total of 160 frames).

**Imaging procedure**

1. Position patient supine with head turned to one side, with the FOV extending from nose to stomach.
2. Have the patient swallow the contents of the test tube using a single swallow. A straw is used to sip the tube contents, and the patient is instructed to swallow after the acquisition has started. Practice swallows without radioactivity are recommended before administering the dose.
3. Instruct the patient to then "dry swallow" once each 15 seconds for the duration of the test (~10 minutes, a total of 60 swallows).

**Image processing:** A cine is made, and an ROI is drawn about the esophagus, the initial oral contents, and the gastric contents, and a chest background ROI away from the mouth, esophagus, and stomach. Esophageal emptying is expressed as a percent of the maximal activity using the formula:

$$\% \text{ Emptying} = \frac{\text{Esophageal}_{max} - \text{Esophageal}_{time}}{\text{Esophageal}_{max}} \times 100$$

In a more refined study, esophageal ROIs are created at the upper, middle, and lower portions for regional time-activity curves, while the mouth and stomach are monitored for delayed swallowing and gastroesophageal reflux. In this case, the initial swallow is followed by subsequent "dry swallows" begun after 30 seconds for a combined esophageal evaluation.

**Display:** Each entire study (total or regional analysis) should be displayed on one sheet, with the ROIs identified. The regional study should be displayed in 2-second images, the total emptying study in 1-minute frames.

**Interpretation:** Esophageal emptying: Usually 90% of the tracer clears from the esophagus with the second swallow, and 96% has cleared by 10 minutes. The literature has reported 100% sensitivity for detecting manometrically proven achalasia, esophageal spasm, and scleroderma.

The regional analysis should show a smooth progression in the bolus through the proximal then middle and distal esophagus. It is possible to differentiate achalasia from scleroderma by studying the distal esophagus, whereas esophageal spasm shows poor bolus passage through the entire length of the esophagus.

## GASTROINTESTINAL 6: SALIVAGRAM

CPT code: 78258

**Indications:** This study is performed on neonates, infants, and children to determine if there is evidence of pulmonary aspiration of saliva that might explain recurrent pneumonias.

**Patient preparation:** The patient should be fasted for 4 hours, but in infants on formula feeding, the suggested schedule time is 1 hour before the next expected feeding.

**Scheduling:** Allow 1 hour of imaging time, with delayed images at 2 hours for 30 minutes.

**Radiopharmaceutical and dose:** A weight-adjusted dose of 1 mCi (no less than 300 µCi) Tc-99m SC instilled into the mouth in a small volume (0.1 ml) via a syringe. The radiopharmaceutical should be placed on or near the base of the tongue.

**Imaging device:** Gamma camera with LEHR collimation

**Data acquisition:** With the patient supine (on gamma camera if infant), posterior images should be obtained in 30-second $128 \times 128$ frames for 1 hour. A delayed 30-image sequence at 2 hours should also be obtained.

**Data analysis:** A movie should be constructed as well as a hard-copy display of 5-minute images of early and delayed acquisition.

**Interpretation:** In the first part of the study there should be only oral, esophageal, and gastric tracer, with no pulmonary activity. Abnormal scans show tracer localization in the trachea, bronchi, and lungs.

## GASTROINTESTINAL 7: LIVER-SPLEEN STUDY

CPT code: 78215 Liver-Spleen, 78205 Liver SPECT

**Indications**

- Confirm presence of Kupffer cells (benignity) for lesions seen by other imaging modalities (e.g., focal nodular hyperplasia)

- Confirm presence of spleen (with SPECT or hepatobiliary scan, CPT code 78223)
- Assess splenomegaly
- Assess diffuse hepatic disease
- Identify focal defects (cysts, metastases, abscesses, hemangiomas, etc.)
- Identify hepatic and splenic trauma

**Patient preparation:** No patient preparation
**Scheduling:** Allow 1 hour patient time.
**Radiopharmaceutical and dose:** 4.8 to 7.2 mCi Tc-99m SC. Adjust dose for patient weight if ≤45 kg or ≥90 kg (refer to Appendix B).
**Imaging device:** Multiheaded gamma camera with LEHR collimation
**Imaging procedure**

Wait 10 to 15 minutes after injection of tracer to allow sequestration before imaging.

Planar: Anterior, posterior, right anterior oblique (RAO)
Right lateral and left lateral (± left posterior oblique)
Each 800 K count views
SPECT
Matrix: 128 × 128
Acquisition: Contoured, 6-degree stops for 30 seconds
Filter: Hanning 0.8
Uniformity correction: Used
Display: 1- to 2-pixel thickness

**Display format:** Hard copy of anterior (± anterior with size marker), posterior, RAO, right lateral, and left lateral 800 K count planar images or planar plus SPECT transaxial, sagittal, and coronal images.
**Interpretation:** Abnormalities present as cold spots regardless of etiology (tumor, abscess, cyst, trauma, etc.). Infarcts occur as wedge-shaped lesions.

Diffuse hepatic dysfunction is manifest, with these signs appearing progressively as disease severity increases: relative increase in size of left lobe of liver, generalized hepatomegaly, nonhomogeneous hepatic tracer distribution, increase in relative splenic uptake, increase in size of spleen, increase in bone marrow uptake, increase in lung uptake and ascites (separation of liver and bone or lung activity), and decrease in size of liver as cirrhotic scarring becomes significant.

## GASTROINTESTINAL 8: SPECIFIC SPLEEN SCAN (HEAT-TREATED RED CELLS)

CPT code: 78185 Spleen Imaging, 78205 Liver SPECT
**Indications:** To determine the presence of the spleen. This test can be used to identify asplenia and polysplenia. It is reserved for instances in which planar and SPECT Tc-99m SC images do not demonstrate a spleen, and when a combined Tc-99m SC and Tc-99m mebrofenin study does not identify splenic tissue (seen on SC but not mebrofenin).

**Patient preparation:** No patient preparation
**Scheduling:** Allow 60 minutes for labeling process. The radiopharmacy must be given, at a minimum, 60 to 90 minutes' notice to stabilize the heating block to the correct temperature. Imaging can be done 2 hours after injection. Allow 60 minutes of camera time.
**Radiopharmaceutical and dose:** 4 to 6 mCi Tc-99m TcO$_4^-$. Adjust dose for patient weight if ≤45 kg or ≥90 kg.

Red cell preparation using UltraTag:

1. Check with pharmacist to make sure the temperature of the heating block is stabilized to 49° to 50°C.
2. Use UltraTag labeling technique.
3. Treat denatured RBCs by heating at 49° to 50°C for 30 minutes.

**Imaging device:** Multiheaded camera with LEHR collimation
**Imaging procedure:** Obtain planar images in anterior, posterior, and left lateral views first (800 K counts).
SPECT
Matrix: 128 × 128
Acquisition: Contoured, 6-degree stops for 30 seconds
Filter: Hanning 0.8
Uniformity correction: Used
Display: 1- to 2-pixel thickness
**Image display:** Display all planar and SPECT images.
**Interpretation:** The presence of a spleen is documented by greatly increased uptake, exceeding the prominent cardiac blood pool and major vessel visualization.

## GASTROINTESTINAL 9: HEPATIC HEMANGIOMA STUDY

CPT code: 78216, 78205 Liver SPECT
**Indications:** Hepatic hemangioma (SPECT scan also required)
**Patient preparation:** No patient preparation
**Scheduling:** The test requires 15 to 20 minutes for a flow study, and a further 30 minutes for the SPECT study (at 45 to 60 minutes after injection).

The site of the lesion in question must be known in advance, therefore the appropriate computed tomography (CT) or ultrasound scan must be available at time of approval of study by NM staff. This study is ideal for hemangiomas if a triple-headed scanner is used and the lesion is >1.4 cm and is not near portal vessels. If lesion is small or near major vessels, suggest magnetic resonance imaging (MRI) as the primary imaging modality to confirm hemangioma.
**Radiopharmaceutical and dose:** 16 to 24 mCi Tc-99m RBCs (see RBC labeling protocol). Adjust dose for patient weight if ≤45 kg or ≥90 kg.
**Imaging device**

- Flow study: gamma camera with LEHR collimation

- SPECT: multiheaded scanner with LEHR collimation.

**Imaging procedure:** A flow study is performed in the view selected to best display the hepatic lesion (anterior or posterior view but determined from other imaging studies).

The flow study is performed, acquiring 1 minute of 1-second images followed by 1-minute acquisitions. Longer imaging times are sometimes required. A SPECT liver study is then obtained.

    SPECT

        Matrix: 128 × 128

        Acquisition: Contoured, 6-degree stops for 30 seconds

        Filter: Hanning 0.8

        Attenuation correction: Used

**Display format:** The flow study is displayed in 5-second images, then in 5-minute frames. The SPECT images are displayed separately.

**Interpretation:** Hemangiomas are typically initially hypovascular, filling in over time to become hypervascular in the delayed views. A common differential diagnosis is a solitary hepatoma, which is typically hypervascular. Some hemangiomas do not demonstrate early hypovascularity, but the typical increase over time is present and diagnostic.

## GASTROINTESTINAL 10: MECKEL'S DIVERTICULUM STUDY

CPT code: 78290

**Indications:** To establish the presence of Meckel's diverticulum

**Patient preparation**

- Patient must be NPO for a minimum of 4 hours. In infants, the NPO period should equal the usual feeding interval, minus the study duration (30 minutes). No thyroid-blocking agent (e.g., perchlorate ion or saturated solution of potassium iodide) should be given within the previous 48 hours.
- CT scans or bowel contrast studies can affect the scan for the next 48 hours, so NM should know of such procedures.
- Pretreatment with cimetidine (300 mg [adjusted for age] 6 times hourly for 24 hours) has been suggested. In difficult cases, it should be considered when repeat studies are contemplated (increases gastric uptake and reduces release of tracer into the bowel). Glucagon, by decreasing peristalsis, may also enhance identification of Meckel's.

**Scheduling:** Allow 60 minutes of camera time.

**Radiopharmaceutical and dose:** 8 to 12 mCi Tc-99m as pertechnetate injected intravenously. Adjust dose for patient weight if ≤45 kg or ≥90 kg.

**Imaging device:** Gamma camera with LEHR collimation

**Imaging procedure:** The patient is asked to void before the study. Patient is placed in a supine position under the camera. Images should include the stomach and bladder area and are acquired as follows: Anterior images are obtained at 1-minute intervals for 15 minutes, then 500,000-count anterior and right lateral images should be obtained at 15 and 30 minutes after injection.

**Interpretation:** Patients with this anomaly may develop serious complications of ulceration and hemorrhage when gastric mucosa lines the diverticulum (50% of Meckel's diverticula have gastric mucosa). This examination is designed to identify the presence of the Meckel's diverticulum by virtue of the presence of gastric mucosa (Tc-99m pertechnetate localizes in the mucus-secreting cells), which actively traps the radiopharmaceutical. Sensitivity of 85% and specificity of 95% are reported. Meckel's diverticulum occurs in 1.5 to 3% of the population, but clinical symptoms appear in only 25% to 30% of these patients.

The activity in Meckel's occurs simultaneously with gastric appearance, whereas common confusing sites (renal pelvis, inflammatory bowel lesions, intussusceptions, polyps) accumulate later.

**False positives:** Barium studies and proctoscopy can cause false positives. Radiopharmaceutical may be seen in the renal pelvis and duodenum, and these can be difficult to separate. If the right renal pelvis is suspected, look for the left renal pelvis, which will be partially obscured by the gastric activity. Posterior views at 15 minutes will show the paired nature of the renal pelvis. Lateral views will help separate duodenum from the kidney.

## GASTROINTESTINAL 11: PERITONEAL SHUNT (LEVEEN OR DENVER)

CPT code: 78291

**Indications:** To check the patency of the LeVeen or Denver shunt

**Patient preparation:** No patient preparation

**Scheduling:** Allow 1 hour.

**Radiopharmaceutical and dose:** 1.6 to 2.4 mCi Tc-99m macroaggregated albumin (MAA). Adjust dose for patient weight if ≤45 kg or ≥90 kg.

**Imaging device:** Gamma camera with low-energy all-purpose (LEAP) collimation

**Imaging procedure:** Patient is injected by a physician intraperitoneally (typically left lower quadrant) under aseptic conditions. This is an operative or invasive procedure and requires appropriate credentialing and appropriate quality improvement and QA follow-up.

With the Denver shunt, it is necessary for the patient to pump the system vigorously after peritoneal injection (as the patient must for normal shunt function).

With patient supine, image

- Abdomen, 3-minute static. Record counts and time.
- Chest and neck, 3-minute static. Record counts and time.

Acquire these static images at 15, 30, and 45 minutes after injection.

**Data display:** Provide anterior views at 15, 30, and 45 minutes of abdomen and chest.

**Interpretation:** If the shunt is working, the lungs should be visualized within 1 hour after injection. If not, delays will be needed at 2 to 4 hours after injection.

**Invasive procedure:** This procedure is minimally invasive. The patient will be observed during the procedure to ensure no ill effects occur, such as inadvertent invasion of a viscus. The risk is low given the presence of ascites. This will be the only monitoring done by NM staff.

The patient will generally be an inpatient, so monitoring will be continued by the patient's ward. Secondary infection as a result of the "stick" will be detected at a later date by the need for readmission to hospital by QA staff.

## GASTROINTESTINAL 12: SALIVARY GLAND SCAN WITH LEMON

CPT code: 78231
**Indications**

- To differentiate Warthin's tumor from other malignant or benign salivary tumors
- To evaluate salivary gland function, especially after head and neck irradiation

**Patient preparation:** Patient should not have been given thyroid-blocking agents (e.g., iodide or perchlorate) within 48 hours preceding the scan.
**Scheduling:** Allow 90 minutes camera time.
**Radiopharmaceutical and dose:** 8 to 12 mCi Tc-99m $TcO_4^-$. Adjust dose for patient weight if ≤45 kg or ≥90 kg.

**Imaging device:** Gamma camera with LEAP collimation
**Imaging procedure**

1. Dynamic study: With patient supine, position in the anterior view with neck extended. Obtain one image per second for 60 seconds, 128 × 128 matrix.
2. Static study: 15 minutes post injection acquire static images, 128 × 128 matrix, 3 minutes per view, with anterior and left and right lateral views of parotid and salivary glands. Record counts and time.
3. Lemon: Saturate gauze with a lemon extract concentrate or lemon juice, and place on both sides of the mouth, packed between cheek and gums. Leave gauze in place for 5 minutes, and give patient a basin to expel excess saliva into. Remove gauze after 5 minutes. Patient should be given a glass of water before imaging post lemon statics to wash out excess oral saliva.
4. Static: 5 minutes after lemon, repeat these three static views at 15 and 30 minutes after lemon.

**Data analysis:** Draw ROIs around the thyroid, submandibular gland, and parotid gland on the appropriate lateral views. Record statistics, and repeat on all sequential timed images for salivary function evaluation.
**Display format:** Display flow study (4 × 5-second images) and pre- and post-lemon views (anterior, right lateral, left lateral, and marker images).
**Interpretation:** Malignant (Warthin's) tumors are unique in that they show a tendency to retain tracer within the mass. Normal salivary glands show a significant decrease in activity after lemon administration.

# Myocardial Protocols

## MYOCARDIAL 1: MYOCARDIAL PERFUSION IMAGING, SPECT OR PLANAR, STRESS AND REST

CPT code: 78461, 78465, 78478
**Indications**

- Diagnosis of coronary artery disease (CAD), especially in patients with moderate or high pretest probability of CAD
- Evaluation of patients with potential false-positive stress electrocardiogram (ECG)
- Diagnosis of CAD in patients with abnormal resting ECG
- Management and prognosis of CAD
- Evaluation of patency of coronary artery bypass graft (CABG) and percutaneous transluminal coronary angioplasty (PTCA)
- Evaluation of left ventricular (LV) disease

**Patient preparation**
*General*
- Patient should be NPO for 4 hours.

- Female patients should change into hospital gowns and remove their bras.
- If it is a 1-day study, patient may eat a light meal between the exercise and delayed images. No nicotine or dairy products are allowed.
- Place a catheter in a peripheral vein of the forearm or antecubital fossa.

*Exercise studies*
- The patient should be off beta-blockers and calcium channel blockers for at least 2 days. Studies to determine medical therapy efficacy can be done with the patient on these medications.
- Bring comfortable shoes and clothes to allow treadmill exercise.

*Dipyridamole or adenosine test*
- The patient should be off theophylline for 3 days, aminophylline for 2 days, and pentoxifylline for 1 day.

- The patient should be off caffeine, cigarettes, and chocolate for 24 hours before study and until after completion of all images.

*Dobutamine:* No drug restrictions

**Radiopharmaceutical and dose:** Tl-201 as thallous chloride: 2.4–3.6 mCi. Adjust dose for patient weight if ≤45 kg or ≥90 kg.

Tc-99m sestamibi requires two separate injections:

- 1-day protocol: First dose 6.4 to 9.6 mCi, second dose 17.6 to 26.4 mCi.
- 2-day test: Each dose (rest and stress): 18 to 24 mCi. Adjust dose for patient weight if ≤45 kg or ≥90 kg.

**Stress procedure**

*Exercise stress:*

1. Obtain a baseline ECG. Either exercise the patient to maximal tolerance by treadmill protocol (preferably Bruce) or by bicycle ergometry. Inject the radiopharmaceutical 60 seconds (Tl-201) or 90 seconds (Tc-99m sestamibi) before peak exercise, and continue stress to ensure optimal myocardial uptake. If exercise cannot be performed, pharmacologic stress will be performed.
2. The physiologic end point is determined by:
   a. Severe anginal type pain (>8 on 10 scale)
   b. Fatigue, dyspnea, claudication
   c. Attainment of 100% maximal predicted heart rate
   d. Systolic hypertension >250 mm Hg
   e. Marked ST depression of 4 mm with normal resting ECG
   f. Fall of 20 mm Hg in absolute units of the systolic blood pressure (BP)
   g. Significant arrhythmias

*Adenosine/Dipyridamole stress:*
IV adenosine = 0.14 mg/kg/min × 4 to 6 minutes
IV dipyridamole = 0.14 mg/kg/min for 4 minutes
These pharmacologic stress tests result in acceptable sensitivity rates compared to exercise stress testing.

1. Monitor the patient with continuous 12-lead ECG.
2. Inject the radiopharmaceutical 2 minutes before completion of infusion of adenosine pharmacologic vasodilation and 4 minutes after completion of dipyridamole infusion.

Dobutamine Stress: In patients who cannot exercise sufficiently, or in those patients with significant limitations for pharmacologic stress in the setting of bronchospastic lung disease. Recent documented clinical experience has suggested that dobutamine stress may be a useful alternative.

1. Monitor the patient by continuous 12-lead ECG.
2. Monitor BP prior to infusion, and at 2 minutes into each stage.
3. Set pump and prepare IV line (can be done by NM technologist):

   a. Enter patient weight in kg.
   b. Dilute dobutamine to 5 mg/ml.
   c. Enter initial dose at 10 μg/kg/min. An initial dose of 5 μg/kg/min may be used, as decided by cardiology staff.
   d. Press Purge, then Start to purge the line.
   e. Insert an 18-gauge needle in the injection port of the IV (IV should be free flowing).
4. When the infusion is to be started, increase the IV rate to approximately 5 ml/min. Start the pump at 10 μg/kg/min.
5. At the end of 3 minutes, increase the infusion to 20 μg/kg/min. To increase the dose, press the Dose key, then increase the dose level to 20, and press Enter.
6. Thereafter, increase the dobutamine infusion by 10 μg/kg/min at 3-minute intervals as directed until:
   a. The patient has achieved 85% of the age predicted maximal heart rate.
   b. The infusion has reached a maximum dose of 40 μg/kg/min.
   c. The BP has reached a maximum of >230 mm Hg systolic or >110 mm Hg diastolic.
   d. A drop in systolic BP of >20 mm Hg has occurred.
   e. A ≥2 mm depression of ST segments in two ECG leads has occurred.
   f. A serious arrhythmia (as deemed by the physician present) has developed.
   g. Angina of a severity that the patient would usually take sublingual nitroglycerin has developed.
7. If the dobutamine infusion reaches the 30 μg/kg/min infusion rate without achieving any of the above end points, then the cardiology staff will administer 0.2 mg atropine IV. Continue to monitor the patient for an additional 3 minutes at 30 μg/kg/min.
8. Increase the dose to 40 μg/kg/min, depending on the response. Further doses of atropine 0.2 mg will be given, depending on heart rate response.
9. Maintain the heart rate for 1 minute.
10. Inject the radionuclide (e.g., thallium, sestamibi) IV when patient reaches any of the above end points. Terminate the dobutamine at that point.
11. Scan the patient when heart rate is <100 beats per minute (bpm) for thallium. Scan sestamibi 30 minutes after injection.

**Patient supervision:** Patients who develop prolonged chest pain or other symptoms and those whose ECG changes are persistent should be referred to the cardiology fellows and staff. The stress is carried out under the supervision of cardiologists or cardiology fellows, who monitor and report on the stress testing. The images are obtained under the supervision of NM.

**Data acquisition**

Timing thallium: Monitor the patient for 2 to 5 minutes, and obtain stress images at 5 minutes. Obtain rest redistribution images 4 hours later.

Sestamibi: Images are obtained before (1-day protocol) or after (2-day protocol) stress. All images are obtained 30 minutes after injection.

If there is excessive hepatic or gastrointestinal uptake obscuring the inferior wall, then repeat acquisition is indicated (especially in rest sestamibi imaging).

Multiheaded SPECT: 64 × 64 matrix, 360-degree acquisitions

- Stress thallium: Low-energy general-purpose (LEGP) collimation, 25 seconds per stop, 4-degree stops
- Rest thallium: LEGP collimation, 35 seconds per stop, 4-degree stops
- Stress sestamibi gated (preferred): LEHR collimation, 50 beats per stop, 6-degree stops
- Stress sestamibi : LEHR collimation, 15 seconds per stop, 4-degree stops
- Rest sestamibi : LEHR collimation, 20 seconds per stop, 4-degree stops

Single-headed SPECT: LEGP collimation, 180-degree acquisition, 32 6-degree stops, 1.33 zoom, 64 × 64 matrix

- Stress and rest thallium: 40 seconds per stop
- Stress Tc-99m sestamibi: 30 seconds per stop
- Rest Tc-99m sestamibi: 40 seconds per stop

Planar: Three static images are taken for 8 minutes: 45-degree LAO, 80-degree LAO view in the right lateral decubitus position, and anterior views.

**Image display**

Multiheaded SPECT: Display rows of stress-rest images, with eight images per row, horizontal long axis on top, vertical long axis in the middle, and short axis on lower rows. All images on one sheet of film.

Single-headed SPECT: Display short-axis, vertical long-axis, and horizontal long-axis images on separate sheets of film.

Planar: Display stress images normalized to maximal pixel count of the three images. Portray delayed images at same maximal pixel count as stress images and normalized to themselves (two sets of images). Display images 4-on-1 format. Display the lung-to-heart ratio.

**Interpretation:** The stress test is interpreted according to physiologic stress level attained and the ECG changes.

The images are examined for perfusion defects and to determine whether they are present only at stress (ischemia) or both at rest and stress (infarct). With large ischemic defects, the referring physician should be contacted to determine patient disposition.

In Tl-201 imaging, if there is a change in ventricular cavity size from stress to rest or the appearance of lung activity in the stress images, both indicate extensive coronary disease, and the referring physician should be contacted immediately.

## MYOCARDIAL 2: ACUTE CHEST PAIN SCAN

CPT code: 78460 Planar, 78464 SPECT

**Indications:** Resting myocardial perfusion images can be used to define the presence, location, and extent of acute infarction or significant myocardial scar and to determine changes in perfusion with resting chest pain.

**Patient preparation:** These patients are usually done emergently, so preparation is not possible.

**Scheduling:** Allow 60 minutes.

**Radiopharmaceutical and dose**

- 16 to 24 mCi sestamibi, SPECT or planar
- Adjust dose for patient weight if ≤45 kg or ≥90 kg.

**Imaging device**

- Multiheaded gamma camera with SPECT and LEHR collimation
- Single-headed gamma camera with LEHR collimation
- Portable camera to study patients in critical care units, but only with prior approval of NM staff

**Imaging procedure**

1. Inject the patient with Tc-99m sestamibi.
2. Perform rest images 30 minutes later. SPECT is performed using established acquisition and display protocols (CPT 78460, 78464).
3. Multiheaded SPECT images: 25 seconds per stop, 64 stops per 360 degrees, 4 degrees per stop
   Single-headed SPECT: 25 seconds per stop, 32 stops per 180 degrees, 6 degrees per stop

**Image display:** Display the rest images in the horizontal long-axis, vertical long-axis, and short-axis projections.

**Interpretation:** Defects seen may be due to the current clinical presentation (ischemia or acute infarction) or past episodes (old infarction). If no defect is seen, it is unlikely the patient has a myocardial infarction and so can be discharged. Abnormal scans require admission or follow-up with delayed rest images.

## MYOCARDIAL 3: REST-ONLY VIABILITY SCAN

CPT code: 78460 Planar, 78464 SPECT

**Indications:** Resting thallium is used in the determination of myocardial viability (the syndrome of dysfunctional hypoperfused myocardium, which improves in function after revascularization).

**Patient preparation:** NPO 4 hours before study. Light meal before the redistribution images for thallium imaging: soup, salad, or sandwich (two of the three choices), no sugar, no dairy products. Female patients should change into hospital gowns and remove their bras.

**Scheduling:** Allow 60 minutes.

**Radiopharmaceutical and dose**

- Tl-201 as thallium chloride. SPECT = 2.4 to 3.6 mCi.
- Dose will be adjusted for patient weight if ≤45 kg (= 1.6 to 2.4 mCi) or ≥90 kg (= 3.2 to 4.8 mCi).

**Imaging device**

- Multiheaded gamma camera with SPECT and LEHR collimation
- Single-headed gamma camera SPECT with LEGP collimation
- Portable camera to study patients in critical care units using LEGP collimator, but only with prior approval of NM staff

**Imaging procedure**

1. Inject patient with Tl-201. Begin imaging 5 to 10 minutes after injection. Images are performed with patient in the supine position.
2. a. Multiheaded SPECT images: 35 seconds per stop, 4 degrees per stop
   b. Single-headed SPECT: 35 seconds per stop, 32 stops per 180 degrees, 6 degrees per stop
   c. Planar: 8 minutes per view: LAO, left lateral, and anterior
3. Acquire second image 4 to 6 hours after injection
4. Acquire third image at 24 hours after injection according to ordering physician or NM staff. One to 1.5 mCi Tl-201 is injected after the 4- to 6-hour image for this delayed reinjection study.

**Image display:** Display a row of rest images with the corresponding row of redistribution images below it. This is done for the horizontal long-axis, vertical long-axis, and short-axis projections. The planar images are displayed in conventional rest, septal, anterior, and lateral views.

**Interpretation:** A single resting study may define myocardial viability. Follow-up 4- to 6-hour or 24-hour imaging improves the sensitivity of detecting viable myocardium in initial defects.

## MYOCARDIAL 4: REST-STRESS MULTIPLE GATED ACQUISITION (MUGX) SCAN

**CPT code:** 78473

**Indications:** Evaluation of ventricular function at both rest and stress. Application of stress results in increased sensitivity of the test and is performed when patients are able to be stressed on the bicycle ergometer. Conditions include the following:

- Diagnosis of CAD
- Prognostication in CAD
- Evaluation of effects of cardiotoxic chemotherapy
- Evaluation of cardiomyopathy
- Pre- and post-cardiac transplantation
- Evaluation of valvular disease.

**Patient preparation:** The patient should be NPO for 4 hours before exercise MUGX scan. Suitable clothing should be worn to allow the patient to pedal energetically on a bicycle ergometer while lying supine.

**Scheduling:** Allow 2 hours: 90 minutes acquisition time, 30 minutes processing.

**Radiopharmaceutical and dose:** 20 to 30 mCi $TcO_4^-$. Adjust dose for patient weight if $\leq$45 kg or $\geq$90 kg (refer to Appendix B). The patient's RBCs are labeled using the UltraTag RBC kit.

**Imaging device:** Gamma camera with LEAP collimation. Use the R-wave trigger to gate the acquisition.

**Imaging procedure**

1. Place three electrodes on the patient's chest: upper left, upper right, and lower left.
2. For the rest ventriculography, obtain the anterior and left lateral (LAO 70- to 90-degree) images. With the patient's feet strapped onto the bicycle pedals, obtain the best septal view (approximately 45-degree LAO, tailored to each individual to best display the septum). A 5° to 10° caudal tilt is recommended in this view.
3. With the patient lying flat, determine the patient's ability to bicycle and whether the stress should be initiated at 25 or 50 W (this is done by the technologist and NM physician). A patient who is an experienced bicyclist or who has previously successfully completed the test should start at the 50-W level.
4. Encourage the patient to stress to exhaustion unless cardiac symptoms develop. The patient exercises at each work level until sufficient counts are obtained for statistically valid determinations (e.g., 2,500,000 to 3,000,000 total counts). Urge the patient to continue stressing despite significant leg fatigue or discomfort (except claudication). At each stress level, make and record the patient's BP and ECG. Stop the test with systolic BP >250, hypotension, dyspnea, angina, arrhythmia, cramps, or other noncardiac complications. The patient is brought to rest slowly at the end of the study.

**Data analysis:** Predefined protocols are used to make movies of each view at rest. Global EFs (left and possibly right ventricular), along with diastolic function parameters, and phase and amplitude images are obtained in the best septal view. Phase and amplitude images are obtained in all views to define wall motion abnormalities.

Obtain movies and EFs with diastolic function parameters, in the best septal view at all stress levels.

**Display format:** The display includes all the parameters described above.

**Interpretation:** Generally, the lower limit of normal LVEF is 50% (mean 60%, range 50% to 70%), RVEF 40%. Severe impairment is present when EFs fall below 30%. Regional wall abnormalities suggest CAD. Phase and amplitude images can help diagnose and quantify akinesia and dyskinesia.

The addition of stress can induce abnormalities not seen at rest, increasing the sensitivity for cardiac disease or ventricular dysfunction. With stress there should be a progressive increase in LVEFs, with an increase of 5% absolute units achieved at maximum stress. A 5% fall indicates significant disease regardless of the resting LVEF, particularly a fall below 50% absolute EF from a normal level is abnormal. Stress-induced regional wall motion abnormalities increase the specificity of diagnosis of CAD.

## MYOCARDIAL 5: REST MULTIPLE GATED ACQUISITION (MUGA) SCAN

CPT code: 78472

**Indications:** Evaluation of ventricular function in the resting state. Because of the reduced sensitivity of this study compared to exercise MUGX studies for detection of valvular dysfunction and CAD, it is generally reserved for patients with severe heart failure or those who cannot stress, such as cardiomyopathy or CAD and patients immediately before or after cardiac transplantation. The study is also used in patients where resting indices of cardiac function alone are needed.

**Patient preparation:** As for rest component of Rest-Stress MUGX Scan (CPT code 78473 protocol Myocardial 4).

Allow 60 to 90 minutes of imaging time, 30 minutes processing.

**Display format:** The preformatted display provides images in all three views, with parametric (phase and amplitude) images and describes ventricular acquisition and calculated parameters.

**Interpretation:** As for rest part of CPT code 78473 (protocol Myocardial 4).

## MYOCARDIAL 6: FIRST-PASS TECHNIQUE

CPT code: 78481

**Indications:** The first-pass technique is used to evaluate RV function by another technique besides the conventional rest MUGA or stress MUGX techniques. This technique is said to provide a better assessment of RV function, but it is more difficult. The test is often done with a MUGA or MUGX scan. Etiologies of RV dysfunction include these:

- Chronic lung disease or primary pulmonary hypertension
- RV infarct
- LV dysfunction (chronic, i.e., valvular heart disease, congestive heart failure)
- Atrial septal defect
- Ventricular septal defect
- Cardiomyopathy
- Pulmonic stenosis
- Lung transplantation

**Patient preparation:** Refer to the MUGA scan protocol (CPT code 78473, Myocardial 4) for electrode placement.

**Scheduling:** Allow 30 minutes of camera time.

**Radiopharmaceutical and dose:** 20 to 30 mCi $TcO_4^-$. Volume should be <0.8 ml. Dose will be adjusted for patient weight if ≤45 kg or ≥90 kg.

**Imaging device:** Gamma camera with high count rate capability and high- or ultrahigh-sensitivity collimation.

**Imaging procedure:** The injection technique is very important in this study.

1. Position the patient supine with the collimator as close to the RV as possible (the anterior view). Use transmission imaging as necessary to help position patient accurately.
2. Label the patient's RBCs using an in vivo labeling technique if a MUGA or MUGX scan is to be done also. First inject the patient with cold pyrophosphate (PYP) (at least 0.8 mg of reconstituted stannous ion). Avoid injections through IV lines in place to optimize labeling capacity of the cold PYP.
3. After 20 minutes, place a 19- to 21-gauge catheter in the right antecubital basilic vein or more proximal vein.
4. Bolus of radiopharmaceutical should optimally be <0.8 ml. Radiopharmaceutical should be loaded slowly into tubing and then administered to the patient as a bolus by pushing sodium chloride behind it. The rate of injection (push) should correlate with the capacity of the venous route (5 to 8 ml per second).

**Data acquisition:** Use a predefined study, placing particular emphasis on the bolus by analysis of this in the region of the superior vena cava (SVC).

**Data analysis:** Follow a predefined analysis protocol. Select frames for the gated first pass from the right atrial phase through to the start of the pulmonary phase. Construct a movie of the first pass process, and calculate the RVEF from that portion of the first pass that provides the most statistics.

**Interpretation:** The study provides useful right ventricular data.

## MYOCARDIAL 7: LEFT-TO-RIGHT SHUNT

CPT code: 78428

**Indications:** To quantify left-to-right shunts

**Patient preparation:** No patient preparation

**Scheduling:** Allow 60 minutes for the test, 30 minutes for processing. With younger patients, where cooperation is essential, the procedure may require additional time.

**Radiopharmaceutical and dose:** 20 to 30 mCi $TcO_4^-$. Volume should be <0.8 ml. Dose will be adjusted for patient weight if ≤45 kg or ≥90 kg.

**Imaging device:** Gamma camera with high count rate capability and high or ultrahigh-sensitivity collimation.

**Imaging procedure:** Use predefined protocol to measure the ratio of pulmonary to systemic flow ($Q_P/Q_S$ ratio).

The procedure requires very strict adherence to protocol; in particular, the injection technique must be impeccable to prevent fractionation of the bolus.

1. Insert a large-sized catheter (preferably 16- to 18-gauge) into a large peripheral vein (i.e., the basilic vein).

2. Position the patient by transmission scan for an anterior view to include both lung fields.
3. Inject a small-volume dose (<0.8 ml) followed with a large flushing dose. In some pediatric cases, the pediatrician may be consulted to perform an injection into the SVC.

**Data analysis:** Use predefined study to perform the analysis. It is important to evaluate the bolus by examining the SVC flow to determine whether it is fractionated. Check this by assessing that the full width at half maximum (FWHM) of the SVC curve does not last >2 seconds. If fractionated, the data cannot be used. Draw an ROI in the SVC, including only the SVC and one of the lung fields, which should not overlap any vessels or cardiac structures.

ROIs are drawn in the lung for the evaluation of systemic and pulmonary circulation. From these data, the $Q_P/Q_S$ ratio is derived.

**Interpretation:** The technique, within technical constraints, is otherwise accurate (and indeed the gold standard).

## MYOCARDIAL 8: RIGHT-TO-LEFT SHUNT

CPT CODE: 78428

**Indications:** Right-to-left shunt studies are performed in patients with suspected or known right-to-left shunt. This may happen with some forms of congenital heart disease, such as tetralogy of Fallot, or with an atrial septal defect. This technique can quantify right-to-left shunts.

**Patient preparation:** No patient preparation
**Scheduling:** Allow 60 minutes: 30 minutes of imaging time, 30 minutes for processing.
**Radiopharmaceutical and dose:** 3.2 to 4.8 mCi Tc-99m MAA. Dose will be adjusted for patient weight if ≤45 kg or ≥90. At least 98% radiopharmaceutical purity of Tc-99m MAA is required. The agent should be used within 3 hours of the time of preparation.
**Imaging device:** Gamma camera with LEHR collimation
**Imaging procedure**

1. Inject the radiopharmaceutical IV using a 21-gauge or larger needle. Smaller needles will break down or filter out particles. Be careful not to draw blood into the syringe prior to injection of tracer.
2. Acquire anterior and posterior whole-body views, creating ROIs.

**Calculating right-to-left shunt ratio**

$$\% \text{ Shunt} = \frac{\text{Total body counts} - \text{lung counts} \times 100\%}{\text{Total body counts}}$$

**Interpretation:** The total body image should be evaluated for nonpulmonary activity, and a decision must be made whether this is due to free $TcO_4^-$ (thyroid, stomach, bladder, salivary glands), labeled albumin stabilizer (blood pool, major vessels, kidneys, liver), or systemic flow (brain, thyroid, spleen, and muscle).

This is a good method of quantifying right-to-left shunt. False positive studies may occur, however, if the label is not adequate. Such studies should be suspected if there appears to be renal excretion of the tracer rather than uptake in the organs receiving the major portion of the systemic cardiac output (cerebrum, thyroid, spleen, and muscle).

## MYOCARDIAL 9: SPECT AND PLANAR INFARCT-AVID SCAN

CPT code: 78466 Planar, 78469 SPECT
**Indications**

- Infarct imaging is indicated for the detection of myocardial infarction when the electrocardiogram and the cardiac enzymes are not diagnostic. This occurs in a variety of situations, such as these:
  Intraventricular conduction defects
  Presentation of patient at a time after enzyme levels would have been expected to peak
  After coronary artery bypass
  After cardioversion
  After possible myocardial trauma
- Infarct imaging is also useful in determining the location and size of acute myocardial infarction.
- Tc-99m pyrophosphate imaging has been used 3 to 6 months after myocardial infarction and in patients with unstable angina to provide prognostic information.
- The test is also sensitive for cardiac amyloidosis.

**Patient preparation:** No patient preparation
**Scheduling:** The test is preferably done with SPECT in NM. Occasionally, NM faculty will give permission for a planar study to be done at the bedside (less sensitive and specific). The study should be scheduled for the second or third day after the clinical event.
**Radiopharmaceutical and dose:** Tc-99m pyrophosphate (PYP): SPECT (16 to 24 mCi), planar (12 to 18 mCi). Adjust dose for patient weight ≤45 kg or ≥90 kg.
**Imaging device:** Single-headed or multiheaded gamma camera with LEHR collimation
**Imaging procedure**

1. Begin imaging 4 to 6 hours after injection.
2. Position the patient supine for imaging.
3. Planar studies: 70-degree LAO, best septal, and anterior images.
4. SPECT imaging (preferred): As for myocardial perfusion imaging (CPT code 78464).

**Interpretation:** The test is very sensitive (~100%) for the detection of full-thickness (Q wave) infarction, less sensitive (~70%) in partial-thickness (non–Q wave) infarction. The persistence of activity beyond several days suggests either a ventricular aneurysm or poor prognosis. In the case of a doubtful positive (intensity of uptake is less than ribs), a repeat scan in 1 to 2 days that shows a scan pattern change means that acute infarction is likely.

Tracer accumulation in myocardial infarctions usually occurs maximally from 2 to 6 days after the infarction has occurred. Little accumulation is seen during the first 24 hours, which limits the usefulness of the technique in the differential diagnosis of acute chest pain.

## MYOCARDIAL 10: DRUGS THAT INTERFERE WITH NUCLEAR CARDIOLOGY STUDIES

### Drugs interfering with RBC labeling:

- Heparin
- Methyldopa (Aldomet)
- Hydralazine (Apresoline)
- Quinidine (Quinaglute, Cin-Quin)
- Digoxin (Lanoxin)
- Prazosin (Minipress)
- Propranolol (Inderal)
- Doxorubicin (Adriamycin)
- Contrast media
- Penicillin

### Drugs interfering with MUGA-stress, ETT stress

*Beta-blockers:*

- Betaxolol (Kerlone)
- Pindolol (Visken)
- Sotalol (Betapace)
- Propranolol (Inderal)
- Acebutolol (Sectral)
- Atenolol (Tenormin)
- Labetalol (Normodyne, Trandate)
- Nadolol (Corgard)
- Timolol (Blocadren)
- Metoprolol (Lopressor)

*Calcium channel blockers:*

- Verapamil (Calan, Isoptin, Verelan)
- Amlodipine (Norvasc)
- Diltiazem (Cardizem)

*Nitrates:*

- Nitroglycerin, Isosorbide Dinitrate (Isordil)
- Pentaerythritol Tetranitrate (Peritrate)

### Drugs interfering with dipyridamole/adenosine studies

- Aminophylline
- Theophylline
- Caffeine
- Trental

# Pulmonary Protocols

## PULMONARY 1: LUNG PERFUSION SCAN

CPT code: 78580

**Indications**

- PE diagnosis (with ventilation scan)
- Follow-up PE (perfusion scan only may be valid)
- Regional perfusion before lung resection (requires forced expiratory volume in 1 second [$FEV_1$]) for tumor or various pulmonary diseases (abscess, bronchiectasis)
- Right-to-left shunt (see Myocardial Protocol 8)
- Assessment of relative perfusion in various congenital, degenerative, or iatrogenic diseases, including pretransplantation and lung volume reduction surgery.

**Patient preparation:** Patient must have had a chest x-ray (CXR) within 24 hours of the scan (within 4 hours when acutely ill) if study is to rule out PE. This CXR must accompany the patient to NM. The requesting service must supply the pretest clinical probability of PE if the scan is to rule out PE.

**Scheduling:** Allow 45 minutes of imaging time.

**Radiopharmaceutical and dose:** 3.2 to 4.8 mCi Tc-99m MAA with 200 to 700 K particles per dose. In a volume of 1 ml, dilute with 0.9% NaCl injection if necessary. Dose will be adjusted for patient age if ≤45 kg or ≥90 kg.

**Caution**

- Severe adverse reactions, including death, have been reported when patients with severe pulmonary hypertension were administered Tc-99m MAA. In patients with pulmonary hypertension, the minimum number of particles should be used (<600,000 particles per 4-mCi dose). This may require compounding a new kit. The dose should be injected slowly. Do not draw blood back into the syringe (hot spots can develop from Tc-99m MAA adhering to blood).
- In right-to-left shunt studies, the Tc-99m MAA must be recently prepared and have little free $TCO_4^-$ (98% purity).

**Imaging device:** Gamma camera with LEHR collimation

**Imaging procedure:** Patient should be injected while in supine position. When contraindicated, consult with an NM physician, and make a notation of position used for injection. Before the injection, the patient should take several deep breaths. Imaging may be started immediately after injection. Use predefined acquisition that includes view, time, and counts for each image.

The following eight views are routinely required:

1. Anterior (800 K counts)
2. Posterior (800 K)
3. Right lateral (600 K)

4. Left lateral (600 K)
5. RPO 45 degrees (700 K)
6. LPO 45 degrees (700 K)
7. RAO 45 degrees (700 K)
8. LAO 45 degrees (700 K)

The patient must be positioned at a 45-degree angle to the detector in the oblique views regardless of what the images look like.

**Display format:** The perfusion scan and the ventilation scan images are displayed with corresponding views under each other. The maximum pixel count for the ventilation and perfusion scan is displayed to establish that V/Q mismatches can be identified.

**Interpretation**

- When reporting studies, indicate the prior probability supplied by the referring physician or include symptoms and relevant risk factors. Indicate the scan probability of PE, providing a numeric gestalt. Provide overall PE probability, including both scan and clinical features.
- Indicate which step you believe is most warranted if the diagnosis is not certain, for example, search for deep vein thrombosis (DVT) or refer for pulmonary angiogram.
- Bedside perfusion scans are limited studies. Until 1993, the highest probability estimate suggested in the literature was 80% (requiring lobar defects). If an eight-view perfusion study shows more than two segmental defects, the probability of PE is similar to that of V/Q scan (intermediate probability is more common without ventilation study). (Stein PD, Terrin ML, Gottschalk A, et al. Value of ventilation/perfusion scans versus perfusion scans alone in acute pulmonary embolism. Am J Cardiol 1992;69:1239–1241.)
- If the study is indicated to follow patients with proven or suspected PE, and previous V/Q or perfusion scans are available, then perfusion scanning alone may be appropriate provided there is no reason to suspect mucus plugging or any other factor that might change ventilation.
- In right-to-left shunts, tracer will be in the systemic and pulmonary circulation. Anterior and posterior computer acquisitions will allow quantitation of the degree of shunting. The brain and kidneys are sites easily recognized on the images if shunting is present.

## PULMONARY 2: VENTILATION LUNG SCAN, AEROSOL

CPT code: 78587
**Indications**

- PE
- Evaluation of COPD
- Evaluation of regional obstructive disease, such as cystic fibrosis

**Patient preparation:** No patient preparation

**Scheduling:** Allow 45 minutes of imaging time.
**Radiopharmaceutical and dose:** 16 to 24 mCi Tc-99m diethylenetriamine pentaacetic acid (DTPA) to start (patient dose ~0.5 mCi). Dose is not weight adjusted.
**Imaging device:** Gamma camera with LEAP collimation
**Imaging procedure:** Using the commercial Ultravent aerosol delivery system, perform the following sequence:
**Radioaerosol delivery system**

- Make sure all fittings on radioaerosol delivery system are snug.
- Place delivery components in lead liner.
- Use face mask or mouthpiece, as you deem appropriate for the type of patient. For a patient on a ventilator, use an adaptor.
- Load system with 16 to 24 mCi Tc-99M DTPA, and bring up reservoir volume to 4 ml.
- Hook up system to oxygen outlet.
- Position patient before camera, then place mask or mouthpiece.
- Deliver radioaerosol to patient with oxygen flow rate at 10 to 12 ml per minute. The patient should breathe for 4 to 5 minutes, with occasional deep inhalations. Terminate when count rate is 2,000 cps in the posterior view.
- Turn off oxygen. Have patient continue breathing through system for another 30 seconds.
- Dispose of components in yellow bag. Attach a piece of "Caution Radioactive Material" tape to the bag, along with the name of radioisotope and date.

**Imaging**

- Images may be obtained immediately.
- The predefined study is for 100 K or 3 minutes, whichever is shortest, and this applies to all views.
- The following eight views are routinely required; counts and acquisition time are displayed:
  1. Anterior
  2. Posterior
  3. Right lateral
  4. Left lateral
  5. RPO 45 degrees
  6. LPO 45 degrees
  7. RAO 45 degrees
  8. LAO 45 degrees

The patient must be positioned at a 45-degree angle to the detector in the oblique views regardless of what the images look like.

**Interpretation:** The scan is interpreted in conjunction with a lung perfusion scan. Segmental ventilation-perfusion mismatch is the hallmark of PE.

## PULMONARY 3: QUANTITATIVE LUNG PERFUSION SCAN

CPT code: 78580 Lung Perfusion

## Indications

- Preoperative assessment prior to possible lung resection for lung cancer, chronic infective process, or lung reduction surgery
- Preoperative and postoperative evaluation of lung transplants

**Patient preparation:** Patient must have had a CXR, and this must accompany the patient to NM. If lung resection is contemplated, an $FEV_1$ is required.

**Scheduling, radiopharmaceutical and dose, imaging device, imaging procedure:** Identical to Lung Perfusion Scan (CPT code 78580, protocol Pulmonary 1).

**Results:** A preset program calculates arithmetic means and individual lung $FEV_1$s. Arithmetic means (A and P views summed) are obtained and the right versus left relative contribution is calculated for lung transplant and preoperative scans. Preoperative scans then have individual lung $FEV_1$s calculated.

## Interpretation

- This study is used for preoperative assessment of potential resection of lobe or lung. This requires an $FEV_1$, and we report the individual lung $FEV_1$, assuming worst-case scenario (resection of entire lung). If this is <0.8 liter, the patient may not be weaned off a ventilator after surgery.
- If the defect is lobar, the use of the other views of the same lung together with ROI selection allows estimates of lobar contribution to total perfusion.
- In single lung transplants, the relative perfusion of right and left (native) lungs are calculated by the addition of anterior and posterior views. The pretransplant scan is to help guide which lung is resected in single-lung transplants and which lung to remove first in double-lung transplants (worst lung resected first).
- In posttransplantation imaging, the donor lung typically receives 75% of total perfusion, and rejection is typified by changes of >5% decrease relative to the last test.

# Genitourinary Protocols

## GENITOURINARY 1: RELATIVE TUBULAR FUNCTION WITH MERCAPTOACETYLTRIGLYCINE (MAG3)

CPT code: 78707

**Indications:** This is the primary test of relative renal function of the kidneys and assesses relative tubular function.

**Patient preparation:** The patient should be well hydrated at the time of study and should have ingested 500 ml of fluid in the previous 2 hours.

**Scheduling:** Allow 35 minutes of imaging time.

**Radiopharmaceutical and dose:** 8 to 12 mCi Tc-99m MAG3. Dose will be adjusted for patient weight if ≤45 kg or ≥90 kg.

**Imaging device:** Gamma camera with LEHR collimation

**Data acquisition:** Predefined study that acquires 1-second images for 60 seconds (flow study), 1-minute images for the next 5 minutes, then 5-minute images to 30 minutes (function study).

**Imaging procedure:** Place the patient supine, being sure to include kidneys and bladder in FOV. Begin acquisition at the time of injection, using predefined study. The syringe is measured 3 seconds before and after (with stopcock) administration.

The relative tubular function study is obtained using a predefined study that measures renal uptake of tracer by integration of the uptake within renal ROIs drawn by the technologist. From this, renograms are drawn, and specific parameters measured: time to peak, renal cortical activity at 20 minutes (20 minutes to peak ratios expressed as percentage).

**Display format:** The display provides a renal flow study and renograms with table of time to peak, renal cortical activity at 20 minutes, right-left ratio, and absolute uptake (corrected for body surface area) at 1.5 to 2.5 minutes after injection.

**Interpretation:** The peak of the renogram occurs at about 2.5 minutes in normal studies, and the data are usually displayed in 5-minute images for 30 minutes, at which time >70% of tracer should be in the bladder.

The slope of the renogram in the first through second minute of data acquisition provides a method of relative (right versus left) tubular function assessment.

Normal (body surface area corrected) renal uptakes in the first to second minute are 9% to 15% for each kidney.

## GENITOURINARY 2: RELATIVE GLOMERULAR FILTRATION RATE AND FLOW

CPT code: 78707

**Indications:** This is a right (%) versus left (%) renal function study. It is used in patients with serum creatinine value <4 mg %. These conditions include vascular, renal, and collecting system diseases of many etiologies.

**Patient preparation, scheduling:** The patient should be well hydrated at the time of the study and should have ingested 500 ml of fluid in the previous 2 hours.

**Scheduling:** Allow 35 minutes of imaging time.

**Radiopharmaceutical and dose:** 8 to 12 mCi Tc-99m DTPA. Dose will be adjusted for patient weight if ≤45 kg or ≥90 kg. Very high purity material (>98%) is required.

**Imaging device**: Gamma camera with HR collimation

**Data acquisition**: Use predefined study for computer acquisition of the data. This acquires 60 seconds of 1-second frames and five 1-minute frames for a total of 6 minutes. A 400 K post-flow image is then obtained. The syringe is measured (3 seconds) before and after (with stopcock) administration.

**Data analysis**: Use predefined analysis protocol to calculate right versus left uptake in the first through third minute after injection (integrates this time period). The body surface area corrected uptake reflects absolute renal activity and can be used to calculate total GFR by the Gates method.

**Display format**: The flow study, background subtraction (interpolated method with kidneys and background displayed), and delayed images are presented.

**Interpretation**: In general, the flow study and GFR should parallel each other except in very acute disease. Normal renal uptakes are about 4% to 9% for each kidney. This test has been largely replaced by the Relative Tubular Function Study Using Tc-99m MAG3.

## GENITOURINARY 3: DIURETIC RENAL SCAN

**CPT CODE**: 78707

**Indications**: The scan is designed to differentiate dilated renal collecting systems (calyces, pelves, or ureters) from obstructed collecting systems. A major indication is the follow-up of such patients to determine either change in obstruction or change in function. The site and side of the putative obstruction must be provided before scheduling the study. Without the site and side nominated, the test will not be performed.

**Patient preparation**

- The patient should be well hydrated and should have ingested two glasses or cups of fluid in the preceding 2 hours.
- Have the referring physician indicate whether or not vesicoureteral reflux is possible, and arrange catheterization in those patients. Check with NM physician for the need to catheterize infants.
- Sedation may be required in infants and toddlers to ensure immobilization.
- A decision may have to be made to increase dose of furosemide if renal function is impaired.

**Scheduling**: Allow 90 minutes: 60 patient minutes, 30 processing minutes. At time of scheduling, inform the patient of the 2 glasses or cups (500 ml) of fluid requirements.

**Radiopharmaceutical and dose**

1. Provide IV access, and give 300 ml if patient is not adequately hydrated.
2. 8 to 12 mCi Tc-99m MAG3. Dose will be adjusted for patient weight if ≤45 kg or ≥90 kg. Infant dose 0.5 mCi/kg of body weight.
3. Furosemide: 1.0 mg/kg for neonates, infants, and children (≤6 years); 0.3 mg/kg for older children and adults.

Typically, adult patients receive 20 mg unless the patient has impaired renal function, in which case a higher dose may be necessary.

Furosemide will be administered at 20 minutes after radiopharmaceutical injection, provided the dilated collecting system in question is visualized. If dilated system is not visualized, wait until the nominated site and side are visualized. If the study has been equivocal in the past, it may be repeated with furosemide administered 15 minutes prior to MAG3 (to maximize the effect of the diuretic), called the F-15 procedure.

**Imaging device**: Gamma camera with LEHR collimation

**Imaging procedure**

1. Have the patient void immediately before imaging; note the time. Have patient void at end of test. Use either urinal or "hat" to collect and measure the volume. Obtain a urine flow rate in milliliters per minute by timing the prescan void to postvoid interval and dividing urine volume by time.
2. Position the gamma camera beneath the supine patient. Both the ureter and renal pelvis must be in the image to draw ROIs for analysis.
3. Start an IV if the patient does not have one running. IV flow rates in infants and toddlers need to be determined by the referring physician. Administer 15 ml/kg over 30 minutes, starting 15 minutes before administration of radiopharmaceutical is typical. Rapidly inject 8 to 12 mCi Tc-99m agent as a bolus, with a 15-ml saline flush. Start the computer at the time of injection, using predefined study. Inject furosemide at 20 minutes (check with NM physician before injection).
4. Collect data for up to 90 minutes, but use 20 minutes after furosemide as the end point.
5. Obtain a postvoid image.

**Data analysis**: Use predefined protocol to obtain perfusion and relative ERPF with MAG3 (CPT code 78704). The ROI used should include the putative site of obstruction (renal, pelvis, or ureter).

**Display**: Routine postinjection and postvoid images are provided (the period images should be normalized to the renogram interval images to allow assessment of residual activity). The renogram curves are provided with the half–wash-out times. The dose and time of furosemide is displayed along with the time used to calculate peak of renogram used in half–wash-out time calculation. The urine flow rate is provided.

**Interpretation**: Furosemide is administered to induce a diuresis. The adequacy should be confirmed by the urine flow rate. If there is no obstruction, merely dilatation, then the total activity in the region will reduce and tracer wash-out will occur, either before or with administration of diuretic.

With obstruction, a continued plateau or an increase in tracer will occur within the ROI.

If there is massive dilation of the region then the test may be false negative (false-negative rate is reduced by performing F-15 scan). Half–wash-out times and their meaning have been suggested (>20 minutes being abnormal, <15 minutes normal, 15 to 20 minutes indeterminate). The degree of hydration and renal impairment profoundly affects the test. If renal function is impaired by 75% (renal MAG3 uptake <3% per kidney), the test may be invalid even if the renogram has an obstructive pattern.

When repeat studies are performed, the prior test result should be reviewed and procedure standardized for better comparison.

## GENITOURINARY 4: CAPTOPRIL RENAL SCAN

CPT code: 78707

**Indications:** Renovascular hypertension (HT) affects only 0.5% of the HT population. The clinical presentation, however, can select a population with a higher prevalence. These presentations include the following:

- Accelerated or malignant HT
- Abrupt onset or sudden worsening of HT
- Continuous systolic-diastolic abdominal bruit
- HT refractory to three-drug treatment
- Unexplained renal impairment with HT
- Renal impairment induced by angiotensin-converting enzyme (ACE) inhibitors
- Evidence of other vascular disease
- Smoking history, especially in females

**Patient preparation:** Inform the patient that this may be a 2-day test. The patient should be in a similar physiologic state for both parts of the test, which should be done at similar times of the day, preferably first appointment in the morning. For each part of the examination, the patient must be NPO for 4 hours preceding the test but must consume approximately 400 to 500 ml (2 to 3 glasses) of fluids in the 3 hours before the test.

Captopril-stimulated test: Standard captopril dose is 25 mg, increased in large patients (> 90 kg). When patient is on an ACE inhibitor: If taking enalapril (10 mg) or lisinopril (10 mg), give 25 mg of captopril. If on lesser doses of enalapril or lisinopril (≤5 mg), give 50 mg captopril. Inject furosemide 5 minutes before injecting radiopharmaceutical.

Baseline (patient off ACE inhibitors) test: Patient should be off enalapril or lisinopril for 2 days if renal function is normal, 2 weeks if abnormal. Patient should be off captopril for 1 day if renal function is normal, 1 week if abnormal. The patient should be off diuretics and potassium supplements for 3 days. If this is impractical, ensure that baseline and captopril-stimulated studies are done on identical medications. Other medications are acceptable.

**Scheduling:** Imaging time: 2.5 hours

Schedule the captopril-stimulated (with captopril) test first. Schedule the captopril baseline (without captopril) after the captopril-stimulated test.

**Radiopharmaceutical and dose:** 8 to 12 mCi Tc-99m MAG3. Furosemide dose is 0.3 mg/kg (maximum 20 mg). Dose will be adjusted for patient weight if ≤45 kg or ≥90 kg.

**Imaging device:** Gamma camera with LEHR collimation

**Imaging procedure:** Place the gamma camera under the supine patient 1 hour after captopril ingestion. Measure the patient's BP before captopril administration, then at 15-minute intervals to the end of the study. Inject furosemide 5 minutes before start of imaging procedure. Hypotension is the most likely drug side effect, although 4% to 7% of patients develop a rash (which may be histamine induced because it can occur with first use of the drug, i.e., no prior sensitization). Acquire 1-second frames for 60 seconds, then 1-minute frames for 60 minutes.

**Data analysis and display:** As for Relative Tubular Function Study (CPT Code 78704) to determine the relative function, percent uptake of the dose, and the renal cortical activity (RCA) at 20 minutes.

**Criteria for abnormal Tc-99m MAG3 captopril-stimulated study**

- Asymmetry of renal function >40:60 ratio of tubular excretion rate (TER) evaluation
- Time to peak activity ($T_{max}$) >6 minutes (normal is 3 to 6 minutes)
- Flat or obstructive renogram curves (see grades defined below)
- RCA at 20 minutes (<30% is normal)

If these are abnormal (specificity and sensitivity 70% to 75%), do the baseline study off captopril.

**Abnormal criteria comparing baseline and stimulated tests**

- >5% change in relative TER
- >5 minute change in time to peak of renogram
- >20% change in RCA
- Change of two grades in renogram curve

  Grade:
  I   Normal renogram
  II  Delay in peak to 5 to 11 minutes
  IIa Delay in upslope with excretion
  IIb Delay in upslope without excretion
  III Marked reduction or absence of uptake

If these changes occur (captopril to baseline), then sensitivity and specificity exceeds 90%.

**Interpretation:** In renal artery stenosis (RAS), angiotensin II–induced vasoconstriction maintains GFR. Captopril, an ACE inhibitor, blocks the conversion of angiotensin I to angiotensin II, thus the effect of angiotensin II on the efferent arteriole is diminished, and the GFR falls. This results in decreased transit and wash-out of tubular tracers.

In the animal model, bilateral disease is difficult to diagnose. However, in humans, bilateral disease is common (29%) but is always asymmetric, so that the same scan criteria apply as for unilateral disease. The test is useful in renal impairment.

## GENITOURINARY 5: RADIONUCLIDE CYSTOGRAM

CPT code: 78740

**Indications:** This examination is most commonly performed for patients with suspected reflux of urine from the bladder into the ureter and upper collecting system. The sensitivity of this examination and the identification of ureteral reflux is equal to the radiographic equivalent with far less (0.01) of the radiation burden.

**Patient preparation:** Catheterization is necessary. Inpatients can be catheterized on the ward. Outpatients can self-catheterize, if they routinely do so. Pediatric outpatients should be catheterized by a parent or nurse (contact Pediatric Specialty Clinic) who accompanies the patient. NM staff can catheterize if necessary.

**Scheduling:** Allow 60 to 90 minutes for study.

**Radiopharmaceutical and dose:** Two doses, each 0.8 to 1.2 mCi Tc-99m DTPA (or other Tc-99m agent if DTPA is not available). $TcO_4^-$ may be used only if a Tc-99m agent is not made. Dose will be adjusted for patient weight if ≤45 kg, minimum dose 0.5 mCi.

**Imaging device:** Gamma camera with LEHR collimation

**Imaging procedure: Predefined Study: Cystogram**

1. Lay the patient supine with detector head below the table. Ensure that the bladder and both kidneys are in the FOV.
    Set up with 500-ml bag of saline running.
2. Begin running saline (warmed to room temperature) into the bladder. Inject dose directly into the first port of the line as soon as saline is running properly. Start the acquisition of 1-minute images.
3. Watch computer screen or persistence scope for reflux. Record time and volume instilled when reflux is first seen.
4. When the bladder is filled (volume in bladder should be >200 ml) or when patient complains of discomfort or the need to void, ask the patient to void through the catheter. Check for reflux.
5. Repeat the entire procedure a second time if reflux is not seen on first filling. At maximum filling, clamp the catheter and ask the patient to attempt to void for 2 minutes. Watch for reflux. Then unclamp catheter and ask patient to void "around and through" the catheter while recording images. Expect possible leakage about the catheter.
6. Measure the volume of urine voided. Calculate the residual volume and reflux bladder volume (Fig. 30-1).

**Display:** This protocol sets up as two studies: voiding 1 and voiding 2. Each study contains two data sets with dynamic filling and dynamic voiding images. Display images with a low upper threshold (about one-tenth of maximum pixel count) to identify small leaks.

On all patients, note time and volume when reflux occurs as well as total volume instilled. Also measure the volume of urine voided and calculate residual volume and reflux bladder volume, according to Fig. 30-1.

**Interpretation:** The study is very sensitive for detecting reflux with low radiation dose. The repeat test is required for maximum sensitivity. Any reflux is abnormal.

---

**WORKSHEET**

**Void #1 and #2**

Right reflux at _____ cc saline instilled

Left reflux at _____ cc saline instilled

Total _____ cc saline instilled

Urinary bladder _____ counts pre void

_____ counts post void

Voided volume of urine _____ ml

Residual volume (RV) _____ ml

$$RV = \frac{(Voided\ volume) \times (counts\ postvoid)}{(Counts\ prevoid) - (counts\ postvoid)}$$

**Reflux Bladder Volume**

Reflux volume =

Initial volume + volume instilled to initiate reflux

(initial volume presumed equal to residual volume)

**FIG. 30-1.**

---

**GENITOURINARY 6: KIDNEY SPECT**

CPT code: 78710

**Indications:** This test determines the presence of normal functioning renal tissue. Usual indications include dromedary hump versus renal cancer, pyelonephritis, and renal infarcts.

**Patient preparation:** No patient preparation

**Scheduling:** Allow 60 minutes of camera time. Dimercaptosuccinic acid (DMSA) and glucoheptonate (GHA) are not stocked, so arrange for radiopharmacy to order as unit doses or unit kit for preparation.

**Radiopharmaceutical and dose**

- 2 to 4 mCi Tc-99m DMSA (when available) calibrated for pediatric patients at 50 μCi/kg with a minimum of 300 μCi, *OR*
- 8 to 12 mCi Tc-99m GHA (pediatric patients, 200 μCi/kg, minimum of 2 mCi)

Dose will be adjusted for patient weight if ≤45 kg or ≥90 kg.

**Imaging device:** Multiheaded gamma camera with LEHR collimation

**Data acquisition**

Matrix: 128 × 128

Acquisition: Circular, 6-degree stops for 40 seconds

Filter: Hanning 0.8

Attenuation correction: No

**Imaging procedure**

Tc-99m GHA: At 2 hours after injection, in children, scan the patient to see if the renal collecting system is visualized and whether it will compromise the test. If needed, inject 1 mg/kg IV furosemide to clear the collecting system, and acquire images 4 hours after injection.

Tc-99m DMSA: Acquire images between 2 and 4 hours after injection.

Obtain planar images of the kidneys in the anterior, posterior, LAO/RAO, and RPO/LPO views for 600 K counts each. SPECT images are obtained. Instruct the patient not to talk, to reduce respiratory excursion.

**Display format:** Conventional planar and SPECT images are produced.

**Interpretation**

- If normal radiopharmaceutical uptake is seen in a region thought to be a tumor, it is unlikely to represent renal cancer.
- In patients with pyelonephritis, segmental regions of decreased tracer accumulation is seen. These have been described as oval (early infection) extending to but not through full cortex; round or wedge-shaped, with evidence of swelling ± cortical rim of activity (abscess); or as wedge-shaped defects with kidney shrunken in region (scar secondary to past infections). Although the latter defects are often multiple, renal infarcts are more likely to be single (although similar in appearance to renal scars).

**GENITOURINARY 7: TESTICULAR FLOW**

CPT code: 78761

**Indications:** The scan is used to differentiate inflammation from ischemia in the symptomatic testis. This study is usually done urgently.

**Patient preparation:** No patient preparation

**Scheduling**

- This scan must be done as soon as possible after request, even to the extent that it requires a patient be "bumped" from the schedule.
- Allow 30 minutes imaging time.

**Radiopharmaceutical and dose:** 8 to 12 mCi Tc-99m $TcO_4^-$ injected IV. For emergency studies any Tc-99m agent may be used although Tc-99m $TcO_4^-$ is preferable. Dose will be adjusted for patient weight if ≤45 kg or ≥90 kg.

**Imaging device:** Gamma camera with converging or LEAP collimation

**Imaging procedure**

1. Place the patient in a supine position with scrotum over one thickness of lead foil. The lead should be symmetric and of regular shape, so that visualization of the testes is easy. This should be small enough to allow visualization of the femoral arteries. The penis is taped to the lower abdomen, out of the FOV.

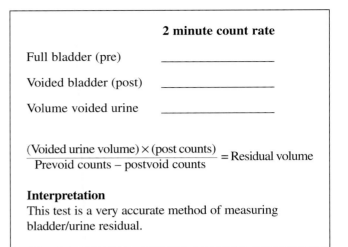

| 2 minute count rate | |
|---|---|
| Full bladder (pre) | _____ |
| Voided bladder (post) | _____ |
| Volume voided urine | _____ |

$$\frac{(\text{Voided urine volume}) \times (\text{post counts})}{\text{Prevoid counts} - \text{postvoid counts}} = \text{Residual volume}$$

**Interpretation**

This test is a very accurate method of measuring bladder/urine residual.

**FIG. 30-2.**

2. Place a cobalt 57 (Co-57) marker to mark each testicle to localize the testes. Then inject the patient with Tc-99m $TcO_4^-$ followed by 20-ml sterile saline flush. Start procedure, then, at the count of 6, inject tracer. Continue acquisition until 60 seconds; acquire two 60-second postflow images. For patients under 2 years of age, use zoom for the static images.

**Display:** Anatomic markers are used to identify both testes. Both flow and blood pool images are then provided. The display protocol provides six 10-second images and two 1-minute static postflow images.

**Interpretation:** The patient presents with a painful testis. If "hot" then infection is likely; if "cold," then ischemia is likely. In "missed torsion," the area about the testis (the dartos muscle of the scrotum) may be hot, but the central region (testis) is cold. This test is not indicated if torsion of the testis is not likely.

**GENITOURINARY 8:**
**BLADDER RESIDUAL PROCEDURE**

CPT code: 78730

**Indications:** The test is used to measure residual urine without urethral catheterization.

**Patient preparation:** No preparation

**Scheduling:** The duration of this study depends on the patient's frequency of urination. The more frequently the patient must void, the shorter time the test will take. Allow 30 minutes camera time.

**Radiopharmaceutical and dose:** 0.8 to 1.2 mCi Tc-99m DTPA or MAG3. Dose will be adjusted for patient weight if ≤45 kg or ≥90 kg.

**Imaging device:** Gamma camera with LEHR collimation with computer

**Imaging procedure**

1. Inject the Tc-99m radiopharmaceutical intravenously. After administration, encourage the patient to drink fluids.

2. One hour after administration or when the patient feels a need to void (whichever time period is shorter), position the detector over the patient's bladder (can be done supine or upright). Acquire a 2-minute image.
3. Have the patient void, collecting all voided urine. Acquire a postvoid image for 2 minutes. Measure all voided urine and record the volume. Calculate residual urine, using counts obtained. Draw an ROI that includes only the bladder. Apply background correction.

**Data analysis:** Use predefined study (Fig. 30-2).
**Interpretation:** The test is a very accurate method of measuring bladder or urine residual.

# Thyroid Protocols

## THYROID 1: THYROID SCAN

CPT code: 78010
### Indications

- Identification of ectopic thyroid tissue, such as lingual or sublingual thyroid and thyroglossal duct tract tissue (Tc-99m $TcO_4^-$ is used initially)
- Postoperatively, localization of residual thyroid tissue
- Differentiation of causes of thyrotoxicosis (subacute thyroiditis vs. Graves' disease and toxic nodules)
- Investigation of thyroid masses
- Determination of whether a palpable thyroid nodule is functional
- Determination of whether thyroid is suppressed by exogenous thyroid in therapeutic situations
- Determination of if a suspected mediastinal mass is thyroid tissue (I-123 may be necessary if blood pool activity is prominent on Tc-99m $TcO_4^-$ scan)
- Differentiation of organification defects from trapping disorders (I-123 and Tc-99m $TcO_4^-$)

### Patient preparation
The patient should comply with the following:

- Be off all thyroid medication, including the following:
  - Propylthiouracil (PTU) or methimazole (Tapazole) for between 3 and 5 days
  - Liothyronine (Cytomel) for at least 10 days
  - L-thyroxine for at least 1 month
- No iodine contrast studies or ingested iodide (e.g., kelp) in the past week (see Protocol 3: Radioactive Iodine Uptake Interactions)
- Complete a thyroid questionnaire on arrival in NM (Fig. 30-3)

**Scheduling:** Technetium thyroid scans are obtained as a routine. Allow 60 minutes: Have the patient arrive 30 minutes before camera time to complete questionnaire and receive dose, then allow 30 minutes' imaging time.
### Radiopharmaceutical and dose

- 8 to 12 mCi of Tc-99m as pertechnetate IV. Dose will be adjusted for patient weight if ≤45 kg or ≥90 kg.
- With NM physician approval (not routine use): 100 to 300 µCi (available as 200-µCi capsules) I-123 as sodium iodide orally

**Imaging device:** Gamma camera with pinhole collimation

### Imaging procedure

*Timing of scan*

- Tc-99m: 20 minutes after dose
- I-123: 4 to 6 hours after dose, and occasionally 24 hours

*Acquisition of images*

- Tc-99m: 100K or 10 minutes
- I-123: 50K or 10 minutes

**Positioning:** With the patient supine, place a pillow under the patient's shoulder blades, extending the patient's neck maximally.
**Views:** Use the pinhole collimator initially at a distance that includes the patient's suprasternal notch and cricoid cartilage (mark both sites on film). Acquire an anterior view with decreased pinhole-to-neck distance so that the thyroid gland nearly fills the entire FOV. The RAO and LAO views are then obtained without markers.

The gland must be palpated by an NM physician and the findings noted, even if the gland appears to be normal. An additional view with markers must be acquired if a nodule is palpable.
**Interpretation:** The scan basically seeks to identify cold nodules (15% chance of malignancy in solitary cold nodule versus 5% for multinodular goiter [MNG] and 1% for hot nodules). Cold nodules or regions occur with carcinoma, colloid nodules, adenomas, cysts, and regions of inflammation (thyroiditis). Discordant iodine and Tc-99m scans indicate regions that trap but do not organify (hot with Tc-99m $TcO_4^-$, cold with radioiodine).

## THYROID 2: THYROID UPTAKE (I-131 OR I-123)

CPT code: 78000
### Indications

- A traditional but seldom used thyroid function test for either hypothyroidism or hyperthyroidism
- To confirm hyperthyroidism prior to therapy (rule out factitious hyperthyroidism or subacute thyroiditis)

Name: _____     Exam: _____
MR #: _____     Date: _____

**Please answer the following questionnaire.** A technologist will be able to help answer any questions if necessary.

1. Why did your doctor order a test of your thyroid?

2. Have you had any thyroid problems in the past? _____ no _____ yes
   If yes, please explain.

3. Is there any history of thyroid problems or goiter in your family? _____ no _____ yes
   If yes, please explain.

4. Have you had any thyroid tests before? _____ no _____ yes
   If yes, please explain.

5. Does your diet include large amounts of sea food, kelp, or health foods? _____ no _____ yes
   If yes, please explain.

6. What medications are your presently taking?

7. Have you had any thyroid surgery? _____ no _____ yes
   If yes, please explain.

8. Have you had any x-ray contrast studies in the past 6 months (e.g., CT scans with intravenous injection, gallbladder or kidney studies, myelogram, arteriogram)?

9. Have you ever had radiation therapy to your neck, head, or chest? _____ no _____ yes
   If yes, please explain.

**For women only:**
Date of first day of last menstrual cycle: _____

I am pregnant: _____ no _____ yes _____ attempting

I am currently breast-feeding: _____ no _____ yes

_____          _____

Patient signature                           Date

_____

Technologist signature

**FIG. 30-3.**

- Calculation of dose of radioiodine to be used in treatment of hyperthyroidism or ablation therapy

**Patient preparation:**

- The patient should be off PTU or methimazole between 3 and 5 (i.e., >3 but <5) days before the uptake is performed. If an uptake is being performed for diagnostic reasons, the patient should be off L-thyroxine and drugs listed in Thyroid Protocol 3.
- The patient can be on beta-blockers.
- The patient must complete a thyroid questionnaire on arrival in NM.

**Scheduling:** This is a 2-day test: dose is administered 1 day and uptake is measured the next (with I-123, a 4- or 6-hour

| | |
|---|---|
| Predose room background (counts/4 minutes) | _____ Counts |
| Predose neck count (counts/4 minutes) | _____ Counts |
| Predose uptake standard (seconds for 10K) | _____ Seconds |
| Predose uptake standard counts | _____ Counts |
| Predose patient dose (seconds for 10K) | _____ Seconds |
| Predose patient dose (counts) | _____ Counts |
| 24-Hour room background (counts/4 minutes) | _____ Counts |
| 24-Hour neck count (counts/4 minutes) | _____ Counts |
| 24-Hour thigh count (counts/4 minutes) | _____ Counts |
| 24-Hour uptake standard (seconds for 10K) | _____ Seconds |
| 24-Hour standard counts | _____ Counts |

**FIG. 30-4.**

uptake is performed). Allow 30 minutes for each visit. The first day's visit should occur midmorning, the uptake measurement early the next morning.

**Radiopharmaceutical and dose**

• I-131 as sodium iodide, 1 to 15 µCi or less PO, from in-house prepared batch of doses. Choose the dose that is closest in activity to the standard for that batch, OR
• I-123 as sodium iodide, 80 to 120 µCi PO (240 to 360 µCi if also scanning the patient)

Dose is *not* adjusted for patient weight.

**Device:** Thyroid uptake probe, peaked appropriately for the nuclide to be used (either I-131 or I-123)

**Procedure**

1. Do a 4-minute predose neck measurement and a 4-minute room background measurement to ensure that no activity from another procedure will contaminate the uptake result. If the predose count is greater than room background, take an additional 4-minute count with the thyroid probe placed over the thigh.
2. Count patient dose and uptake standard for 10 K counts. Record the time and results on the appropriate form (Fig. 30-4).
3. Administer the tracer iodine.

At 24 hours if I-131 is used or at 4 to 6 hours if I-123 is used (note the time interval):

1. Measure each for 4 minutes: room background, patient's neck, and patient's thigh.
2. Count the uptake standard for 10K counts. Record the time and results on the appropriate form.

*Note:* Counts may be made with the patient seated or supine but always with the same detector-to-neck distance of 25 cm from anterior neck to surface of the NaI crystal.

**Interpretation:** Normal uptake is 15% to 30%, with older people having lower uptakes. Hyperthyroid patients have elevated uptakes (Graves' 35% to 95%, mean 60%; MNG 20% to 50%, mean 40%). Near zero or zero uptakes suggest iodine contamination (e.g., kelp tablets, IV contrast large iodine or iodide ingestion, amiodarone), subacute thyroiditis, or replacement suppression therapy.

## THYROID 3: RADIOACTIVE IODINE UPTAKE INTERACTIONS

### Drugs Decreasing 24-Hour Radioactive Iodine Uptake

A. *Sources of iodine*
  1. Nutritional sources, withhold 3 weeks
     a. Seafoods
     b. Kelp and kelp tablets
     c. Vitamin and mineral preparations and nutritional supplements. Brand names:
        Calcidin
        Casec
        Cal-Prenal
        Citratein
        Compleat-B
        Engran-HP
        Flexical
        Filobon
        Gevral Protein
        Instant Breakfast
        Isocal
        Lofenalac
        Lolactene
        Meritene
        Myadec
        Natalins
        Nitrameent
        Nutri-100
        One-A-Day Plus Minerals
        Optilets M
        Paladac & Minerals
        Precision Diets
        Ray-D
        Stuart Formula
        Sustacal
        Sustagen

Theragran M
Unicap Therapeutic
Venthera
Vita Kaps M
Viterra
Vivonex

2. Oral drugs, withhold 3 weeks
  a. Cough preparations
    Calcidrine
    Elixophyllin KI
    Hydriodic acid syrup
    Iodinated glycerol
    Iodo-niacin
    Iophen
    Iophylline
    Iosat
    Organidin
    Myodine
    Mudrane
    Pediacof
    Pima syrup
    Quadrinal
    Saturated solution of potassium iodide
    Strong iodine solution (Lugol's Solution)
    Theophylline KI
    Theo-R-Gen
    Tussi-Organidin
  b. Antiprotozoan, withhold 1 month
    Iodoquinol (Yodoxin); also in shampoo, ointment, and vaginal suppository

3. Topical drugs
  a. Clioquinol a.k.a. iodochlorhydroxyquin (Vioform), withhold 1 month
  b. Iodine tincture, withhold 2 weeks
  c. Povidone-iodine (Betadine, Isodone), withhold 1–9 months
  d. Iodoquinol a.k.a. diiodohydroxyquin (Sebaquin Shampoo, Vytone Cream), withhold 1 month
  e. Iodoform gauze

4. Radiographic contrast agents
  a. Diatrizoate meglumine and diatrizoate sodium, withhold 16 days
    Brand names: Hypaque, Reno-M-Dip, Urovist, Angiovist, Renografin, Cystografin, Gastrovist, MD-Gastroview
  b. Iodipamide (Sinografin), withhold 3–4 months
  c. Ethiodized oil (Ethiodol), withhold 1 year+
  d. Iocetamic acid (Cholebrine), withhold 3–4 months
  e. Iodamide meglumine (Renovue), withhold 16 days
  f. Iodipamide meglumine (Cholografin), withhold 3–4 months
  g. Iopanoic acid (Telepaque), withhold 3–4 months
  h. Iophendylate (Pantopaque), withhold 3 months–years
  i. Iothalamate meglumine (Conray, Cysto-Conray), withhold 16 days
  j. Iothalamate sodium (Conray), withhold 16 days
  k. Ipodate calcium and sodium (Oragrafin, Bilivist), withhold 3–4 months
  l. Metrizamide (Amipaque), withhold 16 days
  m. Propyliodone (Dionosil), withhold 5–6 weeks
  n. Tyropanoate sodium (Bilopaque), withhold 3–4 months

B. *Competing anions,* withhold 1–2 weeks
  1. $TcO_4^-$
  2. $Br^-$
  3. $ClO_4^-$
  4. $BF_4^-$
  5. $SCN^-$
  6. $SeCN^-$
  7. $ReO_4^-$
  8. $At^-$
  9. $NO_3^-$
  10. $IO_3^-$
  11. Sodium nitroprusside—metabolized to thiocyanide ($SCN^-$)

C. *Inhibiting drugs*
  1. Organification inhibitors, withhold 1 week
    a. Propylthiourea (PTU)
    b. Methimazole (Tapazole)
    c. Sulfonylureas high doses >3 g/day
      Tolbutamide (Orinase)
      Chlorpropamide (Diabinese)
    d. Salicylates (high dose)
    e. Antituberculosis drugs
      PAS (para-aminosalicylate)
      INH (Isoniazid)
    f. Antipyrine (Felsol)
    g. Heavy metals (cobalt as $Co-Cl_2$)
  2. Pituitary TSH inhibitors
    a. Thyroid hormone preparations
      1. Desiccated thyroid tablets, withhold 3–4 weeks
      2. Thyroglobulin (Proloid), withhold 3–4 weeks
      3. Liotrix $T_3/T_4$ combination (Thyrolar, Euthroid), withhold 3–4 weeks
      4. Liothyronine ($T_3$) (Cytomel), withhold 1 week (T-1/2 = 1–2 days)
      5. Levothyroxine ($T_4$) (Levothroid, Levoxine, Synthroid), withhold 3–4 weeks (T-1/2 = 6–10 days)
    b. Steroids (also direct depression of thyroid and stimulation of renal clearance of $I^-$, withhold 8 days
      1. Progesterone
      2. Anabolic steroids
      3. Corticosteroids:
        Beclomethasone dipropionate (Beclovent, Vanceril)
        Betamethasone (Celestone)
        Cortisone (Cortone)
        Dexamethasone (Decadron, Mymethasone, Dexone, Hexadrol)

Fludrocortisone (Florinef)
Hydrocortisone (Cortef, Hydrocortone, Solu-
Cortef)
Methylprednisolone (Medrol, Depo-Medrol,
Duralone, Medralone, Methylone, Solu-
medrol, A-methaPred)
Paramethasone (Haldone)
Prednisolone (Prelone, Cortalone, Key-Pred,
Predcor, Articulose, Prednalone, Predate,
Hydeltrasol)
Triamcinolone (Aristocort, Kenacort, Amcort,
Triam-Forte, Triamolone, Trilone, Trisoject,
Aristospan)

c. Phenylbutazone (Butazolidin, Azolid) >800 mg,
withhold 1 week
d. Protein-binding competitors, withhold 1 week
1. Oral anticoagulants (Warfarin, Coumadin)
2. Hydantoins (antiepileptics)
Ethotoin (Peganone)
Mephenytoin (Mesantoin)
Phenytoin (Dilantin)
3. Nonsteroidal anti-inflammatories
Fenoprofen (Nalfon)
Ibuprofen (Motrin, Advil, Midol)
Indomethacin (Indocin)
Ketoprofen (Orudis)
Meclofenamate (Meclomen, Meclodium)
Mefenamic Acid (Ponstel)
Naproxen (Naprosyn)
Phenylbutazone (Butazolidin, Azolid)
Piroxicam (Feldene)
Salicylates, Aspirin (High Doses)
Sulindac (Clinoril)
Tolmetin (Tolectin)
4. Sulfonamides—antibiotics
Sulfasalazine (Azulfidine)
Sulfisoxazole (Gantanol)
5. Penicillin
6. Sulfonylureas—hypoglycemics
Chlorpropamide (Diabinese)
Glipizide (Glucotrol)
Glyburide (DiaBeta)
Tolazamide (Tolinase)
Tolbutamide (Orinase)
7. Thiopental (Pentothal)
e. Morphine
f. Somatostatin a.k.a. octreotide acetate (Sando-
statin)
3. Miscellaneous drugs—inhibition by unknown mech-
anisms
a. Antihistamines
1. Parabromdylamine—not used in United States
2. Chlorpheniramine. Brand names:
Alka Seltzer Plus
Aller-Chlor
Allerest

Chlo-Amine
Chlorafed
Chlortab-4
Chlor-Trimeton
Chlorpro
Co-Pyronil
Co-Tylenol
Codimal
Comhist
Contact
Coricidin
Coryban
Dallergy
Deconamine
Dristan
Duadacin
Extendryl
Fedahist
Histaspan
Naldecon
Novafed
Ornade
Phenetron
Polaramine
Pyrroxate
Resaid
Sine-Off
Sinutab
Teldrin
Triaminic
b. Chlortetracycline (Aureomycin)
c. Chloramphenicol (Chloromycetin)
d. Amiodarone (Cardarone) may increase or
decrease uptake
e. Meprobamate (Equanil, Miltown)
f. Benzodiazepines—tranquilizers
Alprazolam (Xanax)
Chloraepate (Tranxene)
Chlordiazepoxide (Librium)
Diazepam (Valium)
Halazepam (Paxipam)
Lorazepam (Ativan)
Midazolam (Versed)
Oxazepam (Serax)
Prazepam (Centrax)
Temazepam (Restoril)

## Drugs Increasing 24-Hour Radioactive Iodine Uptake

A. Estrogen—variable
B. TSH
C. Lithium—blocks $T_3$ and $T_4$ release and thus stimulates
TSH secretion
Brand names: Eskalith, Lithonate, Lithobid
D. Amiodarone (Cardarone)—may increase of decrease
uptake

## THYROID 4: THYROID UPTAKE AND SCAN (I-123)

CPT code: 78006

**Indications:** Iodine-123 is used in place of Tc-99m pertechnetate only in special situations when the NM physician has approved the use of this radiopharmaceutical in advance. The indications in general are that of a Tc-99m pertechnetate scan (CPT code 78010) and thyroid uptake (CPT code 78000).

- To differentiate between thyroid trapping and organification.
- When thyroid "stunning" is a potential problem in thyroid remnant ablation or thyroid carcinoma metastases therapy, I-123 may be used in doses of ~1.0 mCi with uptake measured in abnormal scan regions (see Metastatic Survey, CPT code 78018).

Appropriate uses of I-123 rather than Tc-99m $TcO_4^-$ are as follows:

- To differentiate organification defect from trapping defect in conjunction with $TcO_4^-$ scan
- When the lesser uptake of $TcO_4^-$ (2.2% vs. 22% with iodide) may compromise the study (e.g., detection of retrosternal masses, evaluation of thyroid remnants or thyroglossal duct tissue) because of adjacent blood pool areas.

**Patient preparation:** Patient preparation is similar to CPT codes 78000 and 78010.

**Scheduling:** This is a two-visit test. Allow 30 minutes for the first visit in the morning for administration of the uptake dose. Allow 60 minutes 6 hours later for the uptake and scan.

**Radiopharmaceutical and dose:** 240 to 360 µCi of I-123 orally as NaI capsule for scan with or without uptake. Dose is not adjusted for patient weight.

**Imaging device:** Same as for CPT codes 78000 and 78010

**Imaging procedure:** Images and uptake measurement should be acquired 4 to 6 hours after dose. Uptake measurements may also be performed at 24 hours. Other features are identical to a thyroid scan (CPT code 78010).

**Interpretation:** If the $TcO_4^-$ scan shows a warm region that is cold on radioiodine (I-123), an organification defect is present.

## THYROID 5: PERCHLORATE WASH-OUT TEST

CPT code: 78003

**Indications:** To determine if there is evidence of thyroid organification defect (enzyme defect, as seen in congenital abnormalities and Hashimoto's disease)

**Patient preparation:** No patient preparation

**Scheduling:** This study is special, and requires personal coordination between the referring physician and NM physician. The time is variable, but because the probe system is used this is not important departmentally; timing is important to the patient, however. Give an early morning slot for the start of the test, and tell the patient that the minimum time is 3 to 4 hours but that the study could take as long as 6 hours.

**Radiopharmaceutical, dose, and device:** Identical to thyroid uptake (CPT code 78000)

**Uptake procedure:** Follow the routine for thyroid uptake (CPT code 78000), with these exceptions:

1. Two hours after administration of dose, the patient's thyroid uptake is determined using the uptake probe (need 10% uptake). If insufficient uptake, remeasure uptake at hourly intervals. Ensure that counting times result in >10,000 counts.
2. One gram of perchlorate or equivalent pharmaceutical is administered orally.
3. Start uptake measurements 30 minutes after perchlorate administration to allow absorption. The patient's uptake is determined at 15-minute intervals post-perchlorate for 2 hours. Check with an NM physician to determine whether this should continue for longer intervals.

*Note:* I-123 can be used when a thyroid scan is required at the same time. The scan would need to be obtained before perchlorate administration.

**Interpretation:** Patients with abnormal organification mechanisms in the thyroid gland have a relative decrease of 50% or more in uptake of dose administered over the 2-hour wash-out period. This often represents an absolute decrease of 5% to 10% because the 2-hour uptake may only be 10% to 20% of the administered dose. In patients with Hashimoto's disease and those with certain enzyme defects, iodine trapped by the thyroid cannot be organified and will be washed out of the gland on administration of perchlorate.

## THYROID 6: THYROID UPTAKE STIMULATION AND SUPPRESSION

CPT code: 78003

**Indications:** To determine whether thyroid tissue (entire gland or region of thyroid) is suppressed, by identification of response to stimulation (with TSH) or suppression by thyroid hormone ($T_3$ or $T_4$). More recently, this test has been replaced with the thyrotropin-releasing hormone (TRH) test.

**Patient preparation:** All patients will be given either TSH or thyroid hormone in preparation for this study. The dose will be determined by an NM staff physician.

**Stimulation test:** Commonly used dose is 10 U of TSH administered intramuscularly on each of 3 consecutive days. For patients in whom metastatic thyroid cancer is a consideration, the dose might be increased to 10 U of TSH on each of 4 consecutive days. Before prescribing TSH, it is important to determine whether this person has had previous TSH injections. Because the current supply of TSH is of bovine origin, there is a likelihood of hypersensitivity reactions with subsequent injections. Acquisition and administration of the TSH is typically handled by the patient's primary

You are scheduled to have a thyroid scan or therapy for thyroid cancer and it is desirable that you avoid iodine for 7 days prior.

Your test is scheduled for _____, and you should implement this diet on _____.

**Avoid**:

1. Any iodine-containing medicines or health foods (e.g., amiodarone, thyroid extracts, cough medicines, but check with your doctor)

2. Iodized salt and dairy products

3. Omit regular bread, cereals, and crackers (iodate stabilizers)

4. Eggs

5. Restaurant and fast food meals

6. Seafood including fish, shellfish, kelp, and seaweed

7. Food containing red dye #3

Check labels for iodized salt, sea salt, iodates, iodides, algin, alginates, agar, and carrageen.

**FIG. 30-5.** (From Lakshmanan M, Schaffer A, Robbins J, et al. A simplified low iodine diet in I-131 scanning and therapy of thyroid cancer. Clin Nucl Med 1988;13:866–868.)

physician. Currently recombinant TSH is being assessed by the FDA.

**Suppression test:** This test is performed after the patient has taken a 7-day course of 25 μg of triiodothyronine (Cytomel) 4 times daily, and the uptake is scheduled for the measurement while the patient is still on suppression therapy.

**Scheduling:** This is a 2-day test: Dose is administered 1 day, and uptake is measured the next. Allow 30 minutes for each visit. The first-day visit should be midmorning, the uptake measurement early the next morning.

**Radiopharmaceutical, dose, device, and procedure:** As for thyroid uptake (CPT code 78000)

**Interpretation:** These stimulated or suppressed uptakes must be compared to a baseline nonstimulated or nonsuppressed uptake result. If there is a portion (or all) of the thyroid gland that is suppressed, then TSH will stimulate this to function, thus confirming autonomous suppression. This study is no longer routinely performed as a TSH measurement; a radioiodine scan (I-123) will provide the same information without the attendant hypersensitivity reactions that can occur with TSH.

If the uptake is suppressed by the exogenous thyroid hormone, then the thyroid gland is not functioning autonomously. This test has also been supplanted by the TRH test and a combination thyroid scan and TSH estimation.

## THYROID 7: THYROID METASTATIC SURVEY

CPT code: 78018

**Indications:** Thyroid carcinoma patients (post-thyroidectomy) to determine whether a thyroid remnant or functioning thyroid carcinoma metastases are present and to quantitate I-131 uptake in identified regions or lesions.

**Patient preparation**

- The patient should be off all thyroid medication: L-thyroxine for 1 month and $T_3$ (Iodothyronine) for at least 10 days. Note the length of time for which the patient has been off replacement thyroid hormone.
- The patient should have a TSH measurement in excess of 60 iUI/ml before scanning (drawn prior, so that result is available on day of scan).
- The patient should be on a low-iodine diet before the survey: Iodide (fish, seaweed, sushi, shrimp, iodized salt, dairy products, eggs, and restaurant food in general) is to be avoided (Fig. 30-5).
- The patient must complete a thyroid questionnaire on arrival in NM.

**Scheduling**

- This is a 2-day test. On the first day, allow 30 minutes (preferably mid-morning) for the patient to receive the radioiodine dose. Two days later, allow 90 minutes (preferably 8 or 9 AM arrival time) for imaging is done early morning, preferably scheduled as the first scan of morning on dual-headed gamma camera.

**Radiopharmaceutical and dose:** 4.8 to 6.5 mCi of I-131 as sodium iodide solution given orally. A written prescription form with the authorized user signature and date, dose, chemical and physical form, route of administration, activity, and double identification verification (e.g., name and date of birth) is required. See the prescription form in Chapter 28.

Advise the patient about radiation safety precautions as necessary. Provide the patient with the departmental pamphlet "Patient Guide to Radioiodine Diagnosis and Treatment of Thyroid Cancer" (Thyroid Protocol 11). Because <6.5 mCi of I-131 is administered, this written radiation safety pamphlet is not an NRC-mandated requirement.

**Imaging device**: Dual-headed gamma camera with HE collimation

**Uptake measurement:** The quantitative neck (thyroid) uptake is done by positioning the patient neck region under the camera and measuring the distance from neck to collimator. Mark the suprasternal notch and the cricoid cartilage on the 5-minute image using the barium 133 (Ba-133) source. Take a 5-minute image on the computer using the predefined protocol. Take a 5-minute image on the computer of the neck phantom with that week's peaking source (50 to 200 μCi I-131) in place, using the same collimator-to-neck distance as used for the patient. Measure the peaking source in the dose calibrator and record the activity (needed in the uptake calculation). In all cases, the thyroid remnant uptake is measured.

**Uptake calculation:**

1. Amount of activity patient received (µCi)
2. Hours from dose to scan
3. Amount of activity in standard (µCi). Place standard in dose calibrator.
4. Total counts in thyroid bed region (protocol uses interpolative background subtraction)
5. Total counts in standard region (protocol uses isocontour to calculate this number)

$$\frac{\text{Activity}}{\text{in neck}} = \frac{\text{Counts in thyroid bed region} \times \text{standard activity}}{\text{Counts in standard}}$$

Correct neck activity for decay.

$$\text{Neck correction} = \frac{\text{Activity in neck}}{\text{Decay factor}}$$

$$\% \text{ of iodine in neck} = \frac{\text{Corrected neck activity} \times 100}{\text{Activity patient received}}$$

If uptake is demonstrated at abnormal sites, proceed to perform a quantitative I-131 uptake of that and any other regions of functioning metastases (e.g., nodes, lung, bones).

**Imaging procedure:** The patient should be recumbent under the camera. Whole-body images are preferred and should be obtained anteriorly and posteriorly. If this is not possible for technical reasons, spot images can be obtained. The spot images should be taken for 10 minutes, recording the counts using predefined study that includes: anterior neck, chest, pelvis, and upper thighs, then posterior chest in two views, including each humerus, and a view of the extremities for abnormalities known to be present.

**Interpretation:** Functioning thyroid tissue in the neck requires ablation with 33-mCi doses. The minimum uptake that requires ablation exceeds in intensity the submandibular gland and nasal activity. This represents an uptake of >0.03% of the administered dose using the above technique.

The physician report should indicate prescan TSH, plan for therapy (if any), when to restart $T_4$ (and dosage), and follow-up plans.

If functioning metastases are seen, the patient is admitted for therapy of 100 to 125 mCi for lymph node metastases, 125 to 175 mCi for pulmonary metastases, and 175 to 250 mCi for skeletal metastases.

The NM physician must have the patient restart thyroid hormone. A follow-up scan or clinic appointment is made.

## THYROID 8: HYPERTHYROIDISM THERAPY

CPT code: 79000 (re-treatments 79001)

**Indications:** Hyperthyroidism (Graves', MNG, solitary autonomous nodule)

**Patient preparation**

- An NM physician will decide whether there is sufficient clinical information for the therapy; if not, then the NM physician should speak with the referring physician.
- A pretreatment 24-hour radioactive iodine uptake is nearly always required but may be deleted by prior approval by NM physician.
- The patient should be off PTU for 3 to 5 days before thyroid uptake or therapy.
- The uptake and therapy are affected by certain medications and iodine agents (e.g., contrast for Radiology procedures, seaweed or kelp products, amiodarone, and some expectorants).
- Patient must complete a thyroid questionnaire on arrival in NM.

**Scheduling**

- The 24-hour uptake dose (1 to 10 µCi) administered 24 hours before therapy.
- The appointment for therapy should be made *only* for the morning. Allow 90 minutes, with uptake measurement taking 30 minutes and therapy taking 60 minutes.

**Therapy calculation:** For Graves' disease, the desired dose to be delivered to the gland is 80 µCi/g; with MNG, 150 µCi/g; and 110 µCi/g for Graves' disease with nontoxic MNG. The prescribed dose is calculated by multiplying the estimated thyroid mass in grams by the "desired dose" and dividing the result by the 24-hour radioiodine uptake.

$$\frac{\text{Size in grams} \times \text{desired dose}}{\text{Uptake at 24 hours}} \times 100 = \mu\text{Ci}$$

For toxic hot nodule, provided there is suppression of the rest of the gland, a suggested empiric dose is 15 mCi. This may be modified by the uptake value when there is not suppression of the remaining normal gland.

**Administration**

- The administering physician must comply with the NRC QMP and personnel bioassay requirements. A written prescription signed or countersigned by NM faculty is required. This is to include radionuclide, dose, physical and chemical forms, and route of administration. NM physicians must sign and date the form in their own handwriting.
- The administering physician must personally measure the therapy immediately before giving it to the patient, supervise the administration, and monitor the administration area with a Geiger-Müller counter for any contamination after patient departs.
- The various forms of therapy available must be described to the patient. The NM physician must determine that the patient understands these options and implications and obtain verbal informed consent. Patient is to be advised about the incidence of retreatment and the incidence of early and late hypothyroidism.

- The patient is cautioned about contact with children and pregnant women over the next few days after therapy administration.
- When >6.5 mCi are administered, written safety instructions are required (see patient guide: Thyroid Protocol 11).

**Interpretation:** This study is reported with the estimated size of the gland, desired dose, uptake measurement result, and actual prescribed dose. The report should also include whether the patient remains on drug therapy (propranolol) or restarts PTU (usually 3 days later) and when he or she should be seen in clinic or at the patient's own physician's office. The report should also advise on the potential for both retreatment and iatrogenic hypothyroidism.

## THYROID 9: REMNANT ABLATION (<33 MCI)

CPT code: 79030
**Indications**

- Ablation of remnant after thyroidectomy for thyroid cancer
- Ablation of thyroid in patients with cardiac disease (to induce hypothyroidism)
- Ablation of thyroid in patients with obstructed airway or esophagus

**Patient preparation**

- The patient should not have received contrast agents, kelp, or other iodine-containing substances in the previous 6 weeks.
- The patient must complete a thyroid questionnaire on arrival in NM.

**Scheduling**

- These patients are ablated only with prior approval of the Chief of NM or designee if it is not done for thyroid cancer. If treatment is for thyroid cancer, any physician can approve.
- In patients with thyroid carcinoma, the ablation is preceded by a metastatic survey. Also, the TSH value has to be elevated, or else the metastatic survey should be deferred until elevated (>60 IU/ml) or until 6 weeks after total thyroidectomy.
- Allow 60 minutes for patient to be in NM. If a thyroid uptake is required, allow an additional 30 minutes.

**Radiopharmaceutical:** I-131 NaI solution PO
**Administration:** The administering physician must comply with the NRC QMP and personnel bioassay requirements.

Generally, doses up to 33 mCi are given for ablation of the thyroid remnant. The dose must be prescribed by the NM physician, recording the dose, the chemical and physical form, the radiopharmaceutical, and the route of administration. The prescription must be signed or countersigned and dated by NM physicians in their own handwriting. The administering physician must personally measure the dose to ensure that the prescribed dose is given the patient. The administering physician must also monitor the administration area with a GM counter for any contamination after patient departs.

The patient is cautioned about contact with children and pregnant women over the next 2 to 5 days. Written safety instructions are provided (see patient guide: Thyroid Protocol 12).

Follow-up metastatic survey recommendations are given the patient if applicable.

## THYROID 10: THERAPY OF THYROID CANCER METASTASES (≥33 MCI)

CPT code: 79035
**Indications:** Thyroid carcinoma with metastases (lymph node, pulmonary, or skeletal)
**Patient preparation:** No patient preparation
**Scheduling**

- Check with NM physician to determine if a metastatic survey and thyroid uptake should be scheduled also (this is frequently a requirement).
- Check with NM physician to determine whether the patient should be on a low-iodine diet (see Fig. 30-5).
- Check before scheduling whether the patient has had any iodine contrast studies within the last 6 weeks because these may affect the therapy.
- Coordinate the admission of the patient with the inpatient unit, the technologist supervisor, and Radiation Safety.
- Confirm the required dose, and ensure that it is ordered.
- Have the patient complete an NM thyroid questionnaire.

**Radiopharmaceutical and dose:** I-131 as NaI solution given PO. In general, lymph node mets require 100 to 150 mCi, lung mets require 150 to 200 mCi, and bone mets require 175 to 250 mCi.
**NM physician:** The following preparations are to be made by the NM physician who will administer the radioiodine:

1. Notify the NM supervisor as far in advance of the therapy as possible. Reserve one of the lead-lined inpatient rooms.
2. Brief the patient about the necessary precautions to be observed:
   - Confinement to room: No items leave the room without NM supervisor or NM physician authorization. Magazines, slippers, socks, and so forth might not be returned.
   - Minimum of visitors and phone calls, preferably no pregnant or young visitors, especially the first day. The telephone will be covered.
   - Side effects (e.g., salivary gland pain, nausea)
   - Bathing: The patient should take bath, shower, and shave before therapy.
   - Eating utensils: All disposable utensils are kept in room.
   - Flushing toilet twice each time used.
3. Brief the nursing staff, and ensure that they are "badged."
4. Ensure that all employees who assist with the administration and subsequent waste removal have satisfied their thyroid counting requirements.

# Nursing Instructions

**Visitor Restrictions:**

_____ No visitors.

_____ No visitors under 18 years or pregnant.

_____ Visitor minutes allowed: Day 1 _____; Day 2 _____; Day 3 _____

_____ Visitors must stay 3 feet from patient.

_____ Visitors may not eat or drink in patient room.

**Nursing Restrictions:**

_____ Patient is restricted to room. *Absolutely nothing* is to leave the room.

_____ Minutes contact per nurse per day: Day 1 _____; Day 2 _____; Day 3 _____

_____ No nurses who are pregnant may render care.

**Patient Care:**

_____ Wear disposable gloves. Wash your hands after caring for patient.

_____ Discard linen, bedclothes, plates, utensils, dressings, etc. in bags in room.

_____ Environmental Services personnel are not permitted in the room.

_____ Only Nuclear Medicine may release room to Admissions.

_____ Wear your radiation monitor when caring for patient. Leave monitor at nursing station at the end of your shift. Use the same monitor on your next shift. Do not share monitors. Call Radiation Safety Officer or designee for additional information or if more monitors are needed.

**In case of emergency, or if you have a question, call:**

Radiation Safety Officer:  Office phone #: _____  Home phone #: _____

Health Physicist:  Office phone #: _____  Home phone #: _____

Chief, Nuclear Medicine:  Office phone #: _____  Home phone #: _____  Pager #: _____

**FIG. 30-6.**

**NM supervisor:** The following preparations are to be made by the NM supervisor on being notified of the impending therapy:

1. Arrange the following for the patient's room with Environmental Services:
   - Remove any waste containers, and remove the paper towels from the paper towel holder.
   - No one from Environmental Services should enter the room from the time the dose is administered (specify date and time) until contacted again by the NM supervisor that the room is released for normal use.
2. Arrange the following with ward personnel:
   - Rubber protective sheets for the mattress
   - Laundry hamper lined with water-soluble plastic bag (to be used for all linens that have been in contact with patient, such as bedding, towels, pajamas, gown, socks, slippers)
   - Gowns for nursing personnel if the patient is not capable of complete self-care
   - Disposable gloves
   - Hamper for other waste materials, disposable food trays, and so on

3. Prepare the room just prior to administration of the therapy dose.
   - Cover the floor of the bathroom and patient's room with plastic-backed absorbent paper, overlapping edges and taping securely.
   - Cover the TV controls, telephone, call button, patient tray, bed rails, and the toilet seat with plastic, securing with tape.
   - Check for the presence of the laundry hamper, garbage hamper, and extra bags.
   - Be certain the following are removed: waste containers, paper towels, blood pressure cuff. A minimum of personal patient effects should remain in the room.
   - Post signs as necessary:
     - Nursing instructions (Fig. 30-6)
     - "Caution: Radiation Area" sign
     - "Nothing to Be Removed" sign.

**Radiopharmacy personnel:** The radiopharmacist preparing the dose will notify Radiation Safety of the therapy before the administration of the dose.

## Radionuclide Therapy Certification

Nuclide administered: _____     Route of administration: _____

Activity administered: _____     Time/date: _____

Chemical and physical form: _____

Remarks:


_____, M.D.     _____
Signature of responsible physician     Office phone number

**Hospital regulation:** This form is to be completed on any inpatient who has therapeutic radiopharmaceuticals. This form is to be signed by the physician who administered the radiopharmaceutical, then placed in the chart.

If the patient expires within 2 weeks of the administration of the isotope, the radioactivity tag must be completed by the physician in attendance at the time of death. This tag is to be attached to the body (preferably the great toe) for the information of the Department of Pathology and the undertaker.

It is the responsibility of the physician in attendance at death of the patient to contact the Radiation Safety Officer (RSO) immediately. During routine work hours, call NM, who will contact the RSO. After hours, call the NM physician on call.

In cases in which the RSO decides that there is an exposure risk, he or she will complete the remaining portion of the radioactivity tag before the body is taken to the morgue.

**FIG. 30-7.** Radioactive drug certification.

## Administration

**NM physician:** The physician administering the dose must reassay the dose, recording the amount and time of the assay and his or her initials on the computer dose ticket. The prescription form used is that of the NRC QMP.

This physician must also complete the radioactive drug certification form (Fig. 30-7) that is to be placed in the patient's chart, along with the physician orders (Fig. 30-8).

Immediately after therapy, with the patient recumbent on the bed, the NM physician records the exposure rates at the following locations:

- Patient surface at neck and abdomen
- Bedside
- One meter from the patient's side
- Two meters from the patient's side
- Bathroom doorway
- Doorway to the hall
- Adjacent rooms on either side of the patient's room (18 inches from the common wall)
- Other locations to be selected by the NM physician

The exposure rates should be recorded daily on the radioiodine therapy checklist (Fig. 30-9) posted inside the patient's room and derived from the table of exposure rates (Table 30-1). From this data, the nursing instruction form is updated.

Immediately on returning to the radiopharmacy after administration of the dose, the administering physician should survey the lead shields for contamination. If contaminated, the shields should be stored as appropriate until they are free of radioactivity. The residual vial activity should be determined using the dose calibrator, and if significant amounts remain (>3%), the therapy form should be modified to reflect the actual administered dose.

**Patient discussions**

1. Emphasize effect of time and distance (the most important discussion to have with patient).
2. No food or drink for 90 minutes after administration, then push fluids to enhance renal clearance of I-131. Obtain hard lemon candies to promote saliva production.
3. Instruct patient on toilet use: Flush toilet two or three times when used, especially in the first 24 hours.

**Discharge of patient:** As a requirement of the NRC, patients who have received >33 mCi of I-131 as therapy must remain hospitalized until the retained activity is <33 mCi. Consistent with this figure, calculations are made and

1. Enter an order to Nuclear Medicine for procedure Thyroid Metastatic Therapy >30 mCi, CPT 79035.

2. Assign patient only to lead-lined inpatient rooms for therapies.

3. Observe nursing instructions on door regarding visitors and nursing care.

4. Medical care will be provided by Nuclear Medicine (NM) physician or designee.

5. Arrange for NM personnel to "paper" the room and post "Caution: Radiation Area" sign and therapeutic administration instructions before therapy is given.

6. Arrange for disposable waste and linen containers.

7. Arrange for a rubberized mattress.

8. Arrange for disposable tableware.

9. Stock patient room with disposable gloves and absorbent paper.

10. Keep patient and objects within the room.

11. Notify Environmental Services not to clean room until notified otherwise.

12. Notify the Radiation Safety Officer (RSO) or designee if the patient dies or has a medical emergency. If the patient vomits in first day, call RSO or designee, prevent spread, but do not dispose of vomitus.

13. Notify the NM supervisory technologist when patient is discharged (for waste removal, survey and decontamination). Only NM can release the room to Environmental Services and Admissions.

14. Keep door open at all times for patient comfort.

15. Have patient flush toilet two or three times after use. Patient may not shower.

Chief, Nuclear Medicine _____, M.D.
office phone # _____ pager # _____
home phone # _____

**FIG. 30-8.** Radioiodine therapies physician orders.

an estimate of activity retained 24, 48, and 72 hours after therapy is determined.

Determining when the patient may be discharged from the hospital is made by the attending NM physician. Information taken into account when making this decision includes the quantity of radioactivity administered, exposure rates after dose, percent excretion, and home situation. The patient may be released without restrictions (10 CFR part 35, effective date 5/29/97) when the body burden has been reduced to <33 mCi of I-131 or exposure rates of <7 mR per hour at 1 m. Written safety instructions are required for patients receiving >6.5 mCi or >7 mR per hour at 1 m.

**NM physician:** Before discharge, the attending NM physician must explain and provide written information concerning necessary precautions to the patient and the patient's family (see patient guide: Thyroid Protocol 12), ensuring that family members' radiation dose not exceed 500 mR and that of nonfamily members of the public not exceed 100 mR.

**NM supervisor:** Once the ward has notified the NM supervisor that the patient has been discharged, it is the duty of the NM supervisor to do the following:

1. Remove all radioactive waste from the room. Double bag and box it, labeling it with a "radioactive waste" sticker for pickup by Radiation Safety.

2. Remove contaminated linen from the room. Double bag and box it, labeling it with a "radioactive waste" sticker for pickup by Radiation Safety.

3. Perform a thorough room survey using a thin-window GM tube to determine if any areas are contaminated.

4. Perform wipe tests on area.

5. Identify areas of contamination (e.g., sink, toilet, bedside table, and so on). Scrub the contaminated items with radiodecontamination solution (Radiacwash, Atomic Products Corp., Shirley, NY) or chlorinated cleanser until the removable contamination has been eliminated. It is desirable not to release the room for use by another patient until all areas show readings of <10 times background and <200 dpm per 100 cm$^2$ on wipe tests. Contaminated cleaning equipment is discarded as radioactive waste.

6. Remove signs posted on the patient's door.

7. Complete the radioactive waste disposal form (Fig. 30-10) and attach to boxed waste.

8. Notify the ward personnel and Environmental Services when the room is released for normal use.

9. Notify Radiation Safety personnel of completion of the room cleanup. Send copies of all paperwork to Radiation Safety.

## THYROID 11: PATIENT GUIDE TO RADIOIODINE TREATMENT FOR HYPERTHYROIDISM

Your doctor has referred you to Nuclear Medicine for diagnosis and possible treatment of your thyroid problem. This brochure addresses the most frequently asked questions and concerns that patients have about this procedure. We hope that it is helpful.

As always, specific questions are best discussed with your doctor or one of our Nuclear Medicine physicians. We will be happy to discuss any concerns you may have.

| Patient | MR # | Room # |
|---|---|---|
| Dose (mCi) | Date and time administered | Administered by |

**Pretherapy checklist**

*Physician*

_____ RSO notified

_____ Patient briefed

_____ Nurses briefed

*Technologist*

_____ Waste set-up

_____ Environmental Services

_____ Laundry

_____ Dietetics

_____ Personnel monitoring

_____ Room preparation

_____ Forms and signs on door

**Routine monitoring (mR/hr)**

| Time | | | | | |
|---|---|---|---|---|---|
| Date | | | | | |
| Instrument used/model # | | | | | |
| Initials of surveyor | | | | | |
| Skin surface, abdomen | | | | | |
| Skin surface, neck | | | | | |
| Patient position in bed | | | | | |
| 1. Bedside | | | | | |
| 2. 1 m from patient | | | | | |
| 3. 2 m from bedside | | | | | |
| Inside room | | | | | |
| 1. Bathroom doorway | | | | | |
| 2. Entry to room | | | | | |
| Outside room | | | | | |
| 1. Hallway | | | | | |
| 2. Adjacent rooms | | | | | |

**Follow-up checklist**

*Physician*

_____ Patient discharge brief

_____ Instructions for family

*Technologist*

_____ Room waste removal

_____ Room survey

_____ Decontamination measures

_____ Release for normal use

or

_____ Restricted as necessary

Comments: _____

**FIG. 30-9.** Iodine therapy checklist.

## What is the thyroid?

The thyroid is a small, butterfly-shaped gland located just below the Adam's apple. It has an important role in controlling the body's metabolism. It produces thyroid hormones, which travel throughout the body.

## What is hyperthyroidism?

Hyperthyroidism is a result of the thyroid gland releasing too much thyroid hormone. This can cause a variety of symptoms, including weight loss, nervousness, heat intolerance, increase in bowel movements, and a fast heart rate (pulse).

**TABLE 30-1.** *Exposure rates for various retained doses*

| Dose rates for various amounts of retained I-131 (mCi) | Time and distance | | | | | |
|---|---|---|---|---|---|---|
| | 3 feet | 0.263 mR/hr/mCi | 6 feet | 0.066 mR/hr/mCi | 10 feet | 0.024 mR/hr/mCi |
| | Hr | Min | Hr | Min | Hr | Min |
| 40 | 2 | — | 8 | — | 22 | 30 |
| 60 | 1 | 20 | 5 | 30 | 15 | — |
| 80 | 1 | — | 4 | — | 11 | 15 |
| 100 | — | 50 | 3 | 15 | 9 | — |
| 120 | — | 40 | 2 | 45 | 7 | 30 |
| 140 | — | 35 | 2 | 30 | 6 | 3 |
| 160 | — | 31 | 2 | — | 5 | 30 |
| 180 | — | 27 | 1 | 50 | 5 | — |
| 200 | — | 25 | 1 | 38 | 4 | 30 |
| 220 | — | 22 | 1 | 30 | 4 | — |
| 240 | — | 20 | 1 | 20 | 3 | 45 |
| 260 | — | 19 | 1 | 15 | 3 | 25 |

Note: These times have been determined using the specific gamma ray constant for I-131 and the inverse square law, and are based on the premise that no individual caring for or visiting the patient should be exposed to more than a total of 100 mR in 7 consecutive work days.

### What can cause hyperthyroidism?

There can be many causes for hyperthyroidism. The most common causes are Graves' disease (an autoimmune disease), overactive thyroid nodule(s), and thyroiditis (inflammation of the thyroid). There are laboratory and Nuclear Medicine tests that can help your doctor to determine the cause for your hyperthyroidism.

### What blood tests will my doctor use?

The most common blood tests are those that measure the levels of certain thyroid hormones in your blood. These include the thyroid hormones ($T_4$ and $T_3$) and thyroid-stimulating hormone (TSH).

### What is the radioactive iodine uptake test?

The radioactive iodine uptake test is an important method of determining how your thyroid gland is working. Iodine is an important building block for thyroid hormone, and the thyroid gland takes it up from the blood. In the uptake test, a small amount of radioactive iodine is given by mouth, and the amount that is taken up by the thyroid is measured 24 hours later; this demonstrates thyroid function.

### How can hyperthyroidism be treated?

The method of treatment may depend on the cause of the hyperthyroidism. Two general forms of treatment can be used: medications (antithyroid or beta-blocker) and definitive treatment (radioiodine or surgery).

### What medications are used?

Antithyroid medications work by preventing the production of thyroid hormone, but they do not treat the underlying cause for the overproduction of the hormone. Two such medications are available in the United States: propylthiouracil (PTU) and methimazole (Tapazole).

Beta-blocker medications work by "blocking" the effect of the thyroid hormones on the body, thereby reducing the symptoms of having too much hormone. They do not affect the thyroid gland itself or reduce the levels of thyroid hormone in the blood.

### What is definitive treatment?

Definitive treatment for hyperthyroidism involves eliminating part of the thyroid gland so that overproduction of hormone will stop. This can be accomplished by giving radioiodine or by surgery. In general, radioiodine treatment is easier and preferred over surgery.

### How does radioactive iodine work?

As mentioned before, iodine is taken up by the thyroid gland normally. One form of iodine, iodine 131, is radioactive and can be used to treat hyperthyroidism. The radioactive iodine enters the thyroid gland and destroys some of the cells. This reduces the size of the gland as well as its ability to produce thyroid hormone. An attempt is made to give an amount of radioiodine that will reduce the production of thyroid hormone to normal levels, thereby curing the hyperthyroidism.

### How long does it take to feel better after receiving radioiodine?

Your symptoms should begin to improve by 1 month after treatment, and the full effect is usually complete by 3

Patient: _____

MR #: _____

Room #: _____

Dose: _____

| | Pre-cleanup mR/hr | Post-cleanup mR/hr |
|---|---|---|
| Room background | | |
| Floor | | |
| Sink | | |
| Table | | |
| Tray | | |
| Bed | | |
| Pillows | | |
| Chair | | |
| TV | | |
| Toilet | | |
| Toilet seat | | |
| Phone | | |
| Door knobs | | |

Trash mR/hr: _____

Linen mR/hr: _____

GM counter: _____

Completed by: _____

Wipe tests by: _____

Attach autogamma printout.

Action level 200 dpm/100 cm$^2$

**FIG. 30-10.** Therapy room cleanup form.

months. Occasionally, the radioiodine treatment needs to be repeated. This happens in about 15% of patients.

**Is radioiodine treatment safe?**

Radioiodine treatment has been used for >50 years and is recognized as a safe and effective method of treating patients with hyperthyroidism. You may have concerns about treatment with radioactivity and the possibility of developing leukemia or thyroid cancer. All the studies done to date show no increased risk of these cancers with radioiodine therapy. In fact, there is a lower rate of thyroid cancer compared to other forms of therapy for hyperthyroidism.

A very rare effect of radioiodine or surgical therapy, called thyroid storm, may occur within the first week after treatment. This can happen if the thyroid gland suddenly releases a large amount of hormone. Thyroid storm produces a very high heart rate (>130 beats per minute) and a high fever (>103°F). If this happens to you, you should contact your doctor or an emergency room. This is a very rare complication of radioiodine treatment.

**What about hypothyroidism?**

Hypothyroidism, the opposite of hyperthyroidism, occurs when not enough thyroid hormone is produced. This is common after treatment with radioactive iodine or surgery. A patient's chance of developing hypothyroidism is 15% to 20% within the first year of treatment. In Graves' disease, there is an additional 2% to 3% chance of hypothyroidism each year thereafter. In 20 years, more than half of patients with Graves' disease will be hypothyroid.

The symptoms of hypothyroidism are vague. You may feel a little bit tired, a little weak, or a little depressed. Therefore, it is important to see your doctor regularly and be tested (with a blood TSH test) to see if you have become hypothyroid.

A simple and effective treatment for hypothyroidism is to replace the thyroid hormone by taking a pill each day. Thyroid pills are inexpensive and are made in many strengths. Your doctor will be able to determine how much replacement hormone you need.

**What precautions should I take after therapy?**

The radioiodine that is not taken up in your thyroid gland will be eliminated from your body within 2 days. The elimination is primarily in your urine, but some is also removed in saliva, sweat, and bowel movement. To promote the removal of the unnecessary radioactivity (which is not in the thyroid gland), it is important to increase your fluid intake and empty your bladder often (approximately every hour or so) for the first day. You should try to have at least one bowel movement each day.

**What about radiation exposure to other people?**

The dose of radioiodine used to treat hyperthyroidism is small, and people around you are at very low risk from the radiation. There are several things that you can do in the first 2 to 3 days to minimize any unnecessary radiation exposure to others:

- Maintain an arm's-length distance from other people if you will be with them for long periods of time. Radiation exposure decreases rapidly with distance.
- Flush the toilet twice after using it. Rinse under the rim of the toilet. If possible, use a different toilet from others.
- Avoid sharing of eating utensils. After use, you can wash utensils as usual.
- If you use a telephone regularly (for example, at work), consider covering it with a latex glove, which you can discard at the end of the day.
- If you think you are pregnant, inform your doctor because radioiodine should not be given to pregnant women. After receiving radioiodine, you should avoid getting pregnant for at least 3 months.
- Radioiodine is secreted in breast milk. Inform your doctor if you are breast-feeding.

These guidelines are of a general nature. We will be happy to discuss your specific situation with you.

**Any further questions?**

We have attempted to answer many of the common questions that patients have about hyperthyroidism and radioiodine treatment. If you have any other questions or concerns, we will gladly help you with them.

## THYROID 12: PATIENT GUIDE TO RADIOIODINE DIAGNOSIS AND TREATMENT OF THYROID CANCER

Your doctor has referred you to Nuclear Medicine for diagnosis and possible treatment of your thyroid cancer. This brochure addresses the most frequently asked questions and concerns that patients have about these procedures. We hope that it is helpful.

As always, specific questions should be discussed with your doctor or one of our Nuclear Medicine physicians.

**What kinds of thyroid cancer are there?**

The two most common treatable forms of thyroid cancer are *papillary* and *follicular* carcinoma. These are also known as *well differentiated*, and they may take up iodine just like normal thyroid tissue.

**What is the treatment for thyroid cancer?**

The primary treatment for thyroid cancer is surgical removal of the thyroid gland and thyroid hormone replacement. Radioactive iodine is frequently used after surgery to ablate (remove) any normal thyroid tissue that could not be removed by surgery. Radioactive iodine is also used to detect any thyroid cancer spread for subsequent treatment with larger amounts of radioiodine. These procedures are performed in a Nuclear Medicine department.

**How does radioactive iodine work?**

As mentioned before, iodine is taken up by the thyroid gland normally and is also taken up by most thyroid cancers. One form of iodine, iodine 131, is radioactive and can be used to diagnose and treat thyroid cancer.

Radioiodine is one of the oldest forms of cancer therapy and is considered the best and most effective treatment for any thyroid cancer that takes it up.

**What is a metastatic survey?**

This is one of the procedures performed in a Nuclear Medicine department for patients with thyroid cancer. It is performed soon after thyroid surgery and at periodic intervals afterward. It is used to find out if there is any thyroid tissue left in your neck after surgery (the "thyroid remnant") or if there is any spread of cancer ("metastases") to other parts of your body.

For the test, you will be given a small amount of radioactive iodine by mouth; this will go to any remaining thyroid tissue and to most thyroid metastases. You will return to the Nuclear Medicine department, usually after 2 days, and images of your body will be obtained. These will show how much thyroid tissue is left in your neck and help to show if there is any spread of the cancer.

**What preparations are there for a metastatic survey?**

If you have been taking any thyroid hormone pills, you will have to stop them about a month before the metastatic survey because they will interfere with the test. You will be instructed on when you should start taking these pills again.

When the metastatic survey is scheduled, you will also be scheduled to have a TSH blood test performed about 2 days before the survey.

You may be asked to maintain a low-iodine diet for a few days to allow the test to work better. This mainly involves avoiding milk products, eggs, seafood, and many seasonings (especially salt, which usually has had iodine added). Most unprocessed fruits, vegetables, and meats are acceptable. Some medications and health foods contain iodine. Ask your physician and check the health food container label for iodine, thyroid extract, seaweed, kelp, or algae content.

**What is thyroid ablation?**

Thyroid ablation is another common procedure performed in a Nuclear Medicine department, usually after a metastatic survey has been done. It is often advisable to remove (ablate) any thyroid tissue that may be left in your neck after surgery. This is easily done by giving you some radioactive iodine by mouth, which goes into the remaining thyroid tissue and destroys it. It is not necessary to remain in the hospital after this form of ablation treatment.

**How is metastatic thyroid cancer treated?**

If a metastatic survey shows spread of thyroid cancer to other parts of your body, it may be advisable to treat with a larger amount of radioactive iodine than that used for simple thyroid ablation. Because of the amount of radioiodine used, you will need to remain in the hospital for a few days. When the amount of radioactivity in your body has fallen to a low level, you will be discharged.

**What precautions should I take after receiving radioiodine?**

The radioiodine that is not taken up in any remaining thyroid tissue (or cancer) will be eliminated from your body within about 2 days. The elimination is primarily in your urine, but some is also removed in saliva, sweat, and bowel movements. To promote the removal of the unnecessary radioactivity, it is important to increase your fluid intake and empty your bladder often (approximately every hour or so) for the first day. You should try to have at least one bowel movement each day.

**What about radiation exposure to other people?**

The dose of radioiodine used to perform a metastatic survey or a thyroid ablation is small, and people around you are at very low risk from the radiation. There are several things that you can do in the first 2 to 3 days to minimize any unnecessary radiation exposure to others:

- Maintain an arm's-length distance from other people if you will be with them for long periods of time. Radiation exposure decreases rapidly with distance.
- Flush the toilet twice after using it. Rinse under the rim of the toilet. If possible, use a different toilet from others.
- Avoid sharing of eating utensils. After use, you can wash utensils as usual.
- If you use a telephone regularly (for example, at work), consider covering it with a latex glove, which you can discard at the end of the day.
- If you think you are pregnant, inform your doctor because radioiodine should not be given to pregnant women. After receiving radioiodine, you should avoid getting pregnant for at least 3 months.
- Radioiodine is secreted in breast milk. Inform your doctor if you are breast-feeding.

These guidelines are of a general nature. We will be happy to discuss your specific situation with you.

**What precautions should I take after metastatic cancer treatment?**

Your Nuclear Medicine doctor will visit you in the hospital and measure the amount of radioactivity remaining in your body. When the radioactivity in your body is low enough, you will be able to leave the hospital. At this point, the amount of radioactivity in your body will be about the same as the amount left after a metastatic survey or thyroid ablation, and you can follow the guidelines given above.

**Any further questions?**

We have attempted to answer many of the common questions patients have about thyroid cancer and radioiodine treatment. If you have any other questions or concerns, we will gladly help you with them.

# Infection Protocols

**INFECTION 1: ABSCESS STUDY (GALLIUM SCAN)**

CPT code: 78806 Planar, 78807 SPECT
**Indications:** For the detection and localization of the following:

- Abscess
- Suspected pulmonary infections (e.g., *Pneumocystis carinii* pneumonia) in human immunodeficiency virus–positive or immunocompromised patients
- Fever of unknown origin

- Activity of known pulmonary inflammatory disease
- Abdominal abscess and inflammatory bowel disease, but WBC scan is preferred in many of these situations
- Vertebral osteomyelitis or disc space infections
- Evaluation and follow-up of granulomatous infections (tuberculosis) or inflammations (sarcoidosis) and drug-induced pulmonary processes (amiodarone)

**Patient preparation:** None. The patient will be instructed on bowel preparation at time of injection (Fig. 30-11).

---

**BOWEL PREPARATION FOR SCANS**

Patient Name: _____

Medical Record #: _____

Planned Scan Date: _____

Please drink plenty of fluids in the days between injection and imaging. You may have a light breakfast on the scan day.

On _____, drink half the supplied bottle of citrate of magnesia (Citroma) in the late afternoon or early evening. If this results in a good bowel movement, drink the remaining half the next afternoon or early evening on _____, the day before the planned scan.

If the first half of the bottle of citrate of magnesia was not effective, buy another bottle and drink the entire bottle. Citrate of magnesia can be stored in the refrigerator.

To ensure your rectum is free of the injected tracer on the day of the scan (this can obscure our imaging), about 30 minutes before leaving home. please use the sodium phosphate enema preparation we provided. This should result in a bowel movement within 20 minutes, and will clear the rectum.

We thank you for your assistance in this delicate matter.

Chief of Nuclear Medicine

---

**Fig. 30-11.**

**Scheduling:** Gallium must be special ordered. Allow 90 minutes for imaging each session. Preferably, schedule in the early morning slot before bone scans.

**Radiopharmaceutical and dose:** 4 to 6 mCi gallium 67 (Ga-67) as gallium citrate. Dose will be adjusted for patient weight if ≤45 kg or ≥90 kg.

**Imaging device**: Gamma camera (preferably dual-headed devices) with medium-energy collimation

**Imaging procedure:**

Planar imaging should be performed 24 hours after injection with possible earlier or later views. Early views at 4 hours may be used in attempting to detect intra-abdominal disease and inflammatory bowel disease (IBD) (before normal bowel excretion), but sensitivity is reduced significantly (to 60% or 70%) compared to 24-hour views. SPECT is commonly used if lesions are suspected on planar images.

In assessing pulmonary activity in sarcoidosis, pneumoconiosis, and other interstitial disease (bleomycin toxicity), 72-hour images are routine.

SPECT imaging:

- Matrix: 64 × 64
- Acquisition: Circular, 6-degree stops per 40 seconds
- Filter: Butterworth, cutoff 0.3, power 5 to 10
- Display: 2-pixel thickness

**Interpretation:** Gallium is excreted renally in the first 24 hours. Visualization of the kidneys at 72 hours is pathologic. At 3 days, Ga-67 is equally divided between liver-spleen, bone, and soft-tissue distributions. Lacrimal and salivary glands and breasts are normally visualized.

Gallium is excreted in the large bowel, so after 24 hours, the colon is visualized.

Gallium lesion uptake can be graded between soft-tissue (grade 0) and hepatic uptake (grade III) and greater (grade IV).

In PCP, the scan is very sensitive (90+%) but nonspecific, because other diffuse inflammatory diseases can emulate it.

**INFECTION 2: IN-111 WBC IMAGING PROCEDURE**

CPT code: 78802 whole-body scan, 78800 limited

**Indications:** This examination is performed to identify the presence and location of abscesses, especially intra-abdominal sepsis. The examination is performed when the cause and site of a patient's septic illness is not apparent, so that anatomic imaging modalities are not applicable. If IBD or acute osteomyelitis is suspected, see protocol modifications.

In-111 WBCs are preferred for more chronic infections because Tc-99m HMPAO preferably labels granulocytes, whereas In-111 labels all WBCs.

**Patient preparation:** Check the patient's white cell count. If <2,500, consider donor WBCs. If 2,500 to 5,000, check with an NM physician before proceeding.

**Scheduling:** Allow 2 hours.

**Radiopharmaceutical and dose:** 0.4 to 0.6 mCi In-111. Dose is adjusted for patient weight if ≤45 kg or ≥90 kg. See Laboratory General 9 for labeling procedure.

**Imaging device:** Gamma camera (preferably dual-headed devices) with MEPH collimation

**Imaging procedure:** At about 24 hours after injection, image the patient using whole-body format. For SPECT imaging, see the Tumor protocols, below.

**Protocol modifications:** When looking for IBD, early images at 4 to 6 hours are indicated (disease-induced diarrhea can result in false localization with later scans because of intestinal shedding and passage of labeled WBCs in bowel). In acute osteomyelitis, see Musculoskeletal Protocol 5.

**Interpretation:** Acute pyogenic abscesses can localize 10% of the injected WBCs. Lesser inflammatory processes result in lesser accumulations of labeled WBCs.

False positives in the bowel occur with GI bleeding and swallowed infective material.

Active IBD demonstrates abnormal collections of tracer in the inflamed bowel regions. Less than 2% of In-111 WBC is excreted via bowel, and about 15% is excreted in IBD. Recent past enemas can mimic inflammation.

## INFECTION 3: TC-99M WBC IMAGING PROCEDURE

CPT code: 78802 whole-body scan, 78800 limited, 78807 SPECT

**Indications:** This examination is performed to identify the presence and location of acute abscesses or in patients with evidence of infection but without suspect site (otherwise, anatomic imaging devices are used: CT and ultrasound).

**Patient preparation and scheduling:** Check the patient's WBC count: If <2,500, consider donor WBCs; if 2,500 to 5,000, check with an NM physician before proceeding.

**Radiopharmaceutical and dose:** 16.0 to 24.0 mCi Tc-99m WBC. Dose is adjusted for patient weight if ≤45 kg or ≥90 kg. See Laboratory General 9 for labeling procedure.

**Imaging device:** Gamma camera with LEHR collimation

**Imaging procedure:** At 1 and 4 hours after injection, planar image using whole-body format. Occasional 24-hour images are performed, especially if significant lung activity is seen.

*For osteomyelitis:* Image at 4 hours after injection only.

### SPECT

- Matrix: 64 × 64
- Acquisition: Contoured, 6-degree stops every 20 seconds
- Filter: Butterworth, cutoff 0.4, power 5
- Display: 1- to 2-slice thickness

**Interpretation:** The labeling efficiency of Tc-99m WBC is less than that of In-111 WBC. This results in significant hepatobiliary (bowel) and renal (bladder) activity in routine imaging after 90 minutes.

# Tumor Protocols

## TUMOR SPECT 1: SCHEDULING INSTRUCTIONS FOR MIBG, GALLIUM, THALLIUM, SESTAMIBI, TC (V) DMSA, OCTREOSCAN, PROSTASCINT, ONCOSCINT, CEA-SCAN, VERLUMA

CPT code: 78802 Tumor Localization, 78803 SPECT

**Indications:** For localization of various tumors

**Patient preparation:** At the time of injection, the patient will be instructed on bowel preparation. If patient has infrequent bowel movement, give patient the preparation instruction sheet (see Fig. 30-11).

A course of SSKI is required for I-131 MIBG, prescribed by the referring physician. Dose is 1 drop tid for 1 day prior and 6 days after MIBG administration. Verify that patient received SSKI before administration of the MIBG.

**Scheduling:** Radiopharmaceutical or kit must be special ordered. Either the referring physician must know which

agent is required (e.g., MIBG, gallium, OctreoScan, ProstaScint, or OncoScint), or the NM physician must confirm that the radiopharmaceutical is appropriate before scheduling the test.

**Radiopharmaceutical and dose:** Doses are adjusted for patient weight if ≤45 kg or ≥90 kg. All but sestamibi must be special ordered.

- Iobenguane (MIBG): 0.8 to 1.2 mCi I-131
- Gallium: 8 to 12 mCi Ga-67
- Thallium: 3.2 to 4.8 mCi Tl-201
- Sestamibi (Miraluma for breast imaging): 20 to 30 mCi Tc-99m
- Tc-99m DMSA (V): 8 to 12 mCi Tc-99m
- Pentetreotide (OctreoScan): 5 to 7 mCi In-111
- Capromab pendetide (ProstaScint): 5 mCi In-111
- Satumomab (OncoScint): 4 to 6 mCi In-111
- Arcitumomab (CEA-Scan): 15 to 25 mCi Tc-99m

- Nofetumomab merpentan (Verluma): 15 to 30 mCi Tc-99m

**Required Purity of Agents**
90%: arcitumomab, capromab pendetide, sestamibi
85%: nofetumomab, satumomab, pentetreotide, DMSA (V)
Supplier responsibility: Ga-67 citrate and thallous chloride
**Imaging:** Dual-headed gamma camera scanners are preferred with appropriate collimation (see individual protocols)
**Imaging times:** Allow 2 hours for imaging with multi-headed camera, 2.5 hours with single-headed device (unless specified). Image at the following intervals after administration of each agent:

- MIBG (Iobenguane): 24 hours (see protocol), then on days 2 and 3
- Gallium: 4 days preferred (3 to 5 days allowed)
- Thallium: start 5 minutes after injection
- Sestamibi: start 5 minutes after injection
- Tc (V) DMSA: planar and SPECT imaging, 2 hours after injection
- Pentetreotide (OctreoScan): 4 hours, then at 1 day (day 2 optional, at NM physician discretion)
- Capromab pendetide (ProstaScint): 30 minutes after injection (allow 1 hour) and at 3 to 5 days later (allow 2 hours).
- Satumomab (OncoScint): 4 days, then possibly days 5 and 6
- Arcitumomab (CEA-Scan): 2 to 5 hours after injection, possible images the next morning
- Nofetumomab merpentan (Verluma): Early the next day after injection (~18 hours)

**Imaging protocol:** This varies with radiopharmaceutical: see appropriate protocol.

## TUMOR 2: TUMOR SCAN WITH GALLIUM

CPT code: 78802 Tumor Localization, 78803 SPECT
**Indications:** For evaluation of tumors in the following circumstances:

- Tumors in which Ga-67 is particularly useful include lymphoma
- Sometimes Ga-67 may be useful in lung cancer, hepatomas, melanoma, seminoma, and head and neck tumors (sensitivity, 85%)

**Patient preparation:** No patient preparation
**Scheduling:** Gallium must be special ordered with the radiopharmacy. Schedule first imaging at 96 hours to include whole-body image and SPECT of chest and abdomen. Allow 120 minutes for imaging each visit with dual-headed gamma camera. Allow 150 minutes for imaging each time with single-headed gamma camera.
**Imaging procedure:** Whole-body scans are obtained at 16 minutes per meter scan speed. Static spot view images are obtained for 1 million counts.

For lymphoma patients, routine SPECT of chest and abdomen is obtained.
**Data acquisition:** SPECT imaging with ME collimation

- Matrix: 64 × 64, 360-degree acquisition
- 6-degree stops for 40 seconds
- Reconstruction: Hanning filter, cutoff 0.8, or Butterworth filter, cutoff 0.3
- Display: 1- to 2-pixel thickness

**Interpretation:** Gallium is excreted renally in the first 24 hours, so visualization of the kidneys at 72 hours is pathologic. Gallium is excreted in the large bowel, so, after 24 hours, the colon is visualized. Normal liver and skeleton are seen in Ga-67 scans, as are salivary glands, lacrimal glands, and breasts.

The study is performed at baseline for Hodgkin's and diffuse large cell lymphoma. Follow-up at 3 months can verify successful treatment if the tumor uptake regresses. Persistent visualization of tumor uptake suggests that more aggressive therapy is required.

## TUMOR SCAN 3: TUMOR SCAN WITH THALLIUM FOR VIABILITY

CPT code: 78607
**Indications**

- For evaluation of tumor viability in patients with brain tumors
- To search for thyroid metastases when serum thyroglobulin is elevated but I-131 metastatic survey is normal.

**Patient preparation:** None. Bowel preparation is not indicated.
**Scheduling:** Allow 120 minutes camera time.
**Imaging device:** Multiheaded gamma camera with LEHR collimation preferred
**Imaging procedure:** Imaging is started approximately 2 to 5 minutes after IV injection of the Tl-201. Local or whole-body images and SPECT are obtained if a specific region is suspect for tumor.
**Data acquisition:** SPECT imaging with LEGP collimation

- Matrix: 64 × 64, 360-degree acquisition
- 6-degree stops for 30 seconds
- Reconstruction: Hanning filter preferred, cutoff 0.8
- Display: 2- (even up to 4-)pixel thickness

**Interpretation:** Tl-201 images should be viewed in all three planes. Low-grade uptake of the thallium corresponds to normal brain uptake (the so-called salt and pepper pattern). Low-grade tumors also may show minimal uptake. Higher-grade tumors show significant uptake of thallium compared to normal brain. Tc-99m sestamibi has a higher uptake of tracer than Tl-201 usually (2- to 5-fold) but displays the choroid plexus. The images should be compared to CT and MRI scans. Uptake is seen in the skull vault as a result of previous surgery.

## TUMOR 4: TUMOR SCAN WITH TC-99M SESTAMIBI

**CPT code: 78607**
**Indications**

- Evaluation of tumor viability in patients with brain tumors
- Search for thyroid metastases
- Potential role in multidrug resistance situations

**Patient preparation:** No patient preparation
**Scheduling:** Allow 120 minutes.
**Imaging device:** Planar camera for breast and thyroid tumor imaging, multiheaded gamma camera with LEHR collimation for brain imaging and special views in thyroid imaging
**Imaging procedure:** Imaging is begun 2 to 5 minutes after injection of Tc-99m sestamibi. When imaging the breast, inject radiopharmaceutical in contralateral arm.
**Data acquisition**

Planar imaging with LEHR collimator: Whole-body images are obtained for thyroid metastasis imaging and special spot images for breast tumor imaging using scintimammography prone breast cushion, which aids in the separation of the breast from adjacent heart, liver, and chest wall structures. In breast imaging, lateral images of the suspect breast are obtained, then the contralateral and lateral views, and finally anterior (patient supine with arms behind the head) views of both breasts (all 10-minute images).

SPECT imaging with LEHR collimation:

- Matrix: 64 × 64
- 360-degree acquisition, 6-degree stops for 30 seconds
- Reconstruction: Hanning filter, cutoff 0.8
- Display: 1- to 2-pixel thickness

**Interpretation:** Similar to tumor scan with Tl-201

## TUMOR 5: TUMOR SPECT WITH TC (V) DMSA

**CPT code: 78802 Tumor Localization, 78803 SPECT**
**Indications**

- Medullary carcinoma of the thyroid
- Soft-tissue sarcomas
- Head and neck tumors
- Highly recurrent benign lesions (e.g., synovial giant cell tumors and aggressive fibromatosis)

**Patient preparation:** No patient preparation
**Scheduling:** Allow 120 minutes at 2 hours after injection for whole-body and SPECT images. The radiopharmaceutical is prepared from the regular Tc (III) DMSA kit with modifications allowed under the practice of pharmacy.
**Imaging device:** Dual-headed gamma camera for planar whole-body scans and dual- or triple-headed SPECT scanner with LEHR collimation
**Data acquisition:** Suggested SPECT acquisition with LEHR collimation

- Matrix: 64 × 64
- 60 stops through 360 degrees
- Reconstruction: Hanning filter, cutoff 0.8
- Display: 1- to 2-pixel thickness

**Interpretation:** The uptake mechanism of Tc (V) DMSA is unknown. Physiologic uptake occurs in the nasopharynx, skeletal muscle, and axial skeleton, so SPECT is helpful in separating this uptake from abnormal uptake in conditions of the head and neck.

## TUMOR 6: TUMOR SCAN WITH PENTETREOTIDE

**CPT code: 78802 Tumor Localization, 78803 SPECT**
**Indications:** Localization of neuroendocrine tumors, including carcinoid, gastrinomas, small cell lung cancer, and paragangliomas where sensitivities approach 95%. Lesser sensitivities (~70%) are seen in medullary carcinoma of the thyroid, lymphomas, paragangliomas, and insulinomas.
**Patient preparation:** No patient preparation
**Precautions**

- Insulinoma patients: Pentetreotide may produce severe hypoglycemia in patients with insulinoma. An IV solution containing glucose should be administered just before and during pentetreotide administration in these patients.
- Concurrent octreotide therapy: Sensitivity of OctreoScan imaging may be reduced in patients receiving therapeutic doses of octreotide acetate.

**Scheduling:** Notify the radiopharmacy to special order the pentetreotide. Schedule patient at 4 hours, then at 1 day (second day optional) after dosing. Allow 120 minutes for imaging on each visit. SPECT of the chest, abdomen, and pelvis is routinely obtained.
**Data acquisition:** Whole-body images are obtained. SPECT is required using MEGP collimation.

- Matrix: 64 × 64
- 360-degree acquisition, 6-degree stops for 50 seconds per stop
- Reconstruction: Butterworth filter, cutoff 0.5, order of 5 to 10
- Display: 1- to 2-pixel thickness

**Interpretation:** Normal physiologic uptake is seen in the spleen, liver, gallbladder, kidney, pituitary gland, thyroid, and urinary bladder. Bowel activity can be present, especially on the later images.

The scan is very sensitive (95%) in carcinoids and gastrinomas. Other diseases with very high sensitivity include small cell cancer of the lung where metastases are well seen and neuroblastomas (but MIBG preferred in neuroblastoma).

## TUMOR 7: TUMOR SCAN WITH CAPROMAB PENDETIDE (PROSTASCINT)

**CPT code: 78802 Tumor Localization, 78803 SPECT**

**Indications:** Patients with clinically localized prostate cancer at high risk for metastases (manufacturers' suggestions):

- Prostate-specific antigen (PSA) >10× upper limit or Gleason score of 3 to 7
- Prostatic acid phosphatase elevated, equivocal lymph node metastases and PSA ≥8× upper limit
- Gleason stage ≥8
- Detection of occult disease (residual or recurrent) after radical prostatectomy when standard imaging techniques are negative or equivocal

**Patient preparation:** A cathartic (citrate of magnesia) is required the day before delayed imaging (3 to 5 days), and a cleansing enema is administered 1 hour before imaging (see Fig. 30-11). The bladder may need to be catheterized the day of the delayed imaging for bladder irrigation.

**Scheduling**

Day of injection: Allow 120 minutes SPECT imaging time to commence 30 minutes after injection to identify blood pool.

Day of delayed imaging: At 3 to 5 days after injection, the patient returns for whole-body and SPECT imaging (total 150 minutes).

**Imaging device:** Multiheaded gamma camera with ME collimation

**Imaging procedure**

Day of injection: SPECT images of the pelvis to obtain a blood pool image

- Matrix: 64 × 64
- 360-degree acquisition, 6-degree stops, 25 seconds per stop
- Reconstruction: Butterworth or equivalent filter, cutoff 0.5, order 5
- Display: 1- to 2-slice pixel thickness

Day of delayed imaging: At 3 to 5 days after injection, the patient returns for planar body images from head to midthigh using a minimum scan time of 35 minutes. Planar spot images should be collected for at least 10 minutes per view.

The SPECT images should include the pelvis and abdomen from the base of the penis to include the liver (often requires two separate collections)

- Matrix: 64 × 64
- 360-degree acquisition, 60 6-degree stops, 50 seconds per stop
- Reconstruction: Butterworth or equivalent filter, cutoff 0.5, order 5
- Display: 1- to 2-slice pixel thickness.

**Interpretation:** The early images are to identify the blood vessels that can be readily confused with lymph node uptake in delayed images. Extreme care must be taken in reading these studies to prevent false positives. Reported to be nonspecifically localized to sites similar to OncoScint (colostomy, degenerative joint disease, aneurysms, inflammatory masses). The technique is not sensitive for skeletal metastases.

HAMA production occurs in 8% after single infusion (with altered biodistribution in 93% of these patients on repeat scans). In 19% of repeat infusions, HAMA is found.

## TUMOR 8: TUMOR SCAN WITH SATUMOMAB (ONCOSCINT)

CPT code: 78802 Tumor Localization, 78803 SPECT

**Indications:** Detection of extrahepatic abdominal cancer in patients with primary tumors (often colon and ovary carcinoma). The test is most useful in patients with rising carcinoembryonic antigen (CEA) levels in which there is no other evidence of metastatic disease. The test is also useful in differentiating postoperative or post-XRT changes from disease recurrence. The test is ideal for documenting peritoneal "studding" (carcinomatosis) in ovarian cancer.

**Patient preparation:** No patient preparation

**Scheduling:** Notify the radiopharmacy to special order satumomab (OncoScint). Preferably, schedule patient at 96 hours after dosing. Allow 120 minutes for imaging. Follow-up imaging is done 1 to 2 days later in some patients.

**Imaging device:** Multiheaded gamma camera with ME collimation

**Imaging procedure**

1. Planar: Slow speed (35 minutes for whole body) or as 1,000 K count spot images
2. SPECT
   - Matrix: 64 × 64
   - 360-degree acquisition, 6-degree stops for 40 seconds
   - Reconstruction: Butterworth filter, cutoff 0.5, power 5 to 10
   - Display: 1- to 2-pixel thickness

**Interpretation:** Physiologic uptake occurs in the liver, spleen, bone marrow, genitalia (men), gluteal fold region, blood pool (early images), colon (15% of patients, which changes over time), and urinary bladder (rare). Uptake can be found at colostomy sites, sites of degenerative joint disease, abdominal aneurysm (organizing), postoperative bowel adhesion, and inflammatory local lesions (IBD, postoperative, post radiation).

Satumomab (OncoScint) localizes in metastatic disease of the colon. Metastatic liver disease may appear as multiple liver photopenic areas on the OncoScint study.

**Special interest:** HAMA occurs in 40% of patients after a single injection. Four to 12 months later, 50% of these patients have persistent HAMA. Repeat administration does not increase the HAMA incidence significantly. HAMA interferes with the biodistribution of the radiopharmaceutical and many murine-based immunoassays, such as CEA and Ca-125.

## TUMOR 9: TUMOR SPECT WITH ARCITUMOMAB (CEA-SCAN)

CPT code: 78802 Tumor Localization, 78803 SPECT

## Indications

- Used in conjunction with standard evaluation of colorectal adenocarcinoma preoperatively for detection of the presence of disease, extent of spread, and postoperatively for disease recurrence
- Evaluation of patients with occult disease (elevated CEA, liver enzymes, or symptoms but conventional imaging studies normal)
- Not indicated as a screening test for colon cancer

**Scheduling:** Allow 120 minutes for multiheaded camera, 150 minutes for single-headed device for whole-body images at 2 to 5 hours after injection with selected patients being reimaged the next morning.

**Radiopharmaceutical and dose:** 30 mCi Tc-99m. Dose will be adjusted for patients ≤45 kg or ≥90 kg.

The radiopharmaceutical is the Fab' fragment and is labeled with 15 to 25 mCi of Tc-99m. QC requires 90% radiochemical purity. The dose should be injected slowly over 5 to 20 minutes in 30 ml of saline.

**Imaging device:** Gamma camera (multiheaded preferred) with HR collimation

**Imaging procedure**

1. Multiheaded scanner with HR collimator: Planar images at 2 to 5 hours after injection: anterior, posterior, lateral head views and anterior and posterior chest, abdomen, and pelvis views with 250 to 500 K counts (early).
2. SPECT imaging
   - Matrix: 64 × 64
   - 360-degree acquisition, 6-degree stops for 30 seconds
   - Reconstruction: Butterworth filter, cutoff frequency 0.4 to 0.5, order 5
   - Display: 1- to 2-pixel thickness

**HAMA response:** One percent of patients develop HAMA. Repeat injections do not result in any significant increase in HAMA response.

**Interpretation:** Sensitivity of the CEA-Scan is comparable or superior to conventional diagnostic imaging modalities. In hepatic disease, equal numbers of lesions are missed and are found by CEA-Scan and CT imaging. Liver lesions are very frequently observed as hot lesions (contrast to In-111 satumomab [OncoScint]).

In patients being evaluated for diagnosis of colon cancer the agent has merit as surgery can be appropriately forgone or extended. In these preoperative patients there is a 40% increase in detecting resectable disease, and a doubling of the identification of nonresectable disease rates.

In occult disease, 81% of patients would have their treatment altered, and there is a 60% decrease in the false negative or equivocal CT scans.

Potential false positive sites include major blood pool regions, sites of antibody fragment elimination, and gallbladder and intestinal activity.

## TUMOR 10: TUMOR SPECT WITH NOFETUMOMAB MERPENTAN (VERLUMA)

CPT code: 78802 tumor localization, 78803 SPECT

**Indications:** Detection of extensive small cell cancer of the lungs in biopsy-proven disease. When limited stage (one hemithorax, bilateral hilar nodes, ipsilateral supraclavicular nodes) disease is detected, then bone scan and other tests are indicated.

**Patient preparation:** Instructions for bowel preparation are provided to patient after injection.

**Scheduling:** Injection in the afternoon, image next morning (optimal imaging time is 14 to 17 hours after injection). Allow 120 minutes for imaging on multiheaded camera, 150 minutes on single-headed device.

**Radiopharmaceutical and dose:** The monoclonal antibody (MOAB) is a Fab fragment of antibody NR-M-10. Two-thirds of the dose is excreted (primarily renal, hepatobiliary secondary) within 24 hours. The dose is at least 15 mCi. Dose will be adjusted for patients ≤45 kg or ≥90 kg.

**Imaging device:** Gamma camera (multiheaded preferred) with LEHR collimation

**Imaging procedure**

1. Acquire 8- to 10-minute spot planar images. If whole-body mode is used, a slow speed is required. Shielding of abdomen is often needed because of hepatic activity.
2. SPECT imaging
   - Matrix: 64 × 64
   - 360-degree acquisition, 64 stops of 40 seconds
   - Reconstruction: Butterworth filter, cutoff 0.4, order 5
   - Display: 1-pixel thick slices

**Interpretation:** Two-thirds of patients presenting with small cell carcinoma of the lung (SCCL) have metastatic spread at presentation, and in these patients surgery is not appropriate treatment. In non–small cell carcinoma of the lung (NSCCL) surgery is helpful if the disease is localized, and this is another major indication for this radiopharmaceutical (early NSCCL).

Nonspecific uptake of nofetumomab occurs in organs of excretion, certain normal tissues (testes, nasal, pituitary, salivary gland, and thyroid), axillary fold, inflammatory lesions, recent surgery, and various other tumor types (adenocarcinomas of breast, ovary, colorectum, and prostate).

In detecting metastatic disease of both SCCL and NSCCL, the technique identifies 75% to 95% of lesions detected by other imaging modalities (CXR, CT chest, CT body). All primary lesions and most metastatic lesions are detected (bone metastases are missed). Lesions <1 cm in size are difficult to detect, and SPECT does not improve sensitivity but helps visualization.

HAMA is elicited in approximately 6% of patients, with return to normal in 3 to 4 months.

## TUMOR 11: LYMPHOSCINTIGRAPHY

CPT code: 78195
**Indications**

- Evaluation of chronic lymphedema of a swollen extremity, where scan is used to differentiate primary or secondary lymphedema (primary [neither lymphatic nor proximal lymph node visualization], secondary [interstitial lymphatic uptake but poor visualization of proximal lymph channels and nodes])
- Identification of patent lymph channels prior to lymphovenous anastomosis
- Determination of lymph node drainage of malignancies, such as truncal or head and neck melanomas and breast cancer
- Determination of internal mammary lymphatic chain in breast cancer
- Evaluation of pelvic and periaortic lymphatic drainage for blockage by trauma or tumor, such as rectal, prostatic, or vulvar cancer

**Patient preparation:** If the patient wears elastic stockings for lymphedema, these should generally be removed 3 to 4 hours before the study. If this cannot be done, it should be noted and considered in the interpretation.

**Scheduling:** Allow 3 hours for initial imaging. Check with the NM physician after initial study to determine if delayed images may be needed. Allow 60 minutes for each delayed imaging.

In the case of internal mammary scintigraphy (breast cancer), injections are performed by NM staff physicians at the start and at 3.5 hours, and images are obtained at 3 and 6 hours.

**Radiopharmaceutical and dose:** Tc-99m SC (colloid suspension contains hyaluronidase to enhance absorption) with a particle size ≤100 nm (by passing through 100-nm Millipore filter). The agent is injected by an NM physician subcutaneously into feet or hands or into the region of tumor (either intradermally around a melanoma, or subcutaneously and adjacent to breast tumor) or into the posterior rectus abdominis muscle sheath (for evaluation of internal mammary chain).

- Adults (>18 years) up to 1 mCi per region
- Children (12 to 18 years) up to 500 μCi per region
- Children (1 to 12 years) up to 350 μCi per region
- Children (0 to 1 year) up to 150 μCi per region

**Injection:** The procedure should be fully explained to the patient.

**Lymphedema:** Tracer is injected subcutaneously in the webs between toes and fingers as desired (two sites per limb, 100 to 250 μCi per site).

**Melanoma:** Tracer is injected intradermally around the tumor or excision site. Four to six injection sites are used, each <0.1 ml with 160 to 240 μCi per site. It is important to be as close as possible (within 5 mm) to the tumor or excision scar site without injecting scar tissue. It is necessary that an NM staff physician be present at injection and for

flow and delayed imaging (i.e., for 20 minutes at injection and 2 hours later).

**Breast cancer:** Tracer is injected subcutaneously in the cardinal quadrants around the tumor. This should be done either by the surgeon or imager if the lesion is palpable, or by a radiologist with ultrasound guidance if the lesion is not palpable.

**Other sites:** At the discretion of an NM physician

**Imaging device:** Gamma camera with LEHR collimation

**Imaging procedure:** Check with an NM staff physician to determine if additional views are indicated.

- *Foot injection:* Inject both feet subcutaneously in the webs between first and second or second and third toes. Acquire 2-minute static of injection sites immediately after injection. At 15, 30, and 90 minutes, acquire anterior whole-body image from feet to head at 12 minutes per meter. Acquire all images with the oldest cobalt sheet transmission source under the table to outline the body.
- *Hand injection:* Inject hand between second and third fingers. Position camera over axilla. Acquire dynamic image 128 × 128 for 1 minute per frame for 1 hour. Repeat imaging procedure at 2 hours. Check with NM staff to determine if additional views are indicated.
- *Rectus abdominis muscle injection:* For breast cancer imaging, the tracer is injected deep in the rectus abdominis muscle using 23-gauge needles, and imaging is performed 3 hours later. At that time, the opposite side is injected, but if the first injection did not display lymph nodes, then this site is reinjected also.
- *Melanoma injection*

  *Lymphatic flow study:* Immediate postinjection (very rapid multi-site injection technique required) imaging (30-second frames for 20 minutes) to identify lymphatic drainage and interval and sentinel lymph nodes. The imaging should include all potential drainage sites.

  *Regional lymph node study:* At 20 minutes, 5-minute images should be obtained of the expected regional nodal sites. Often the patient flow study demonstrates two or more lymphatic draining channels. Where necessary, transmission scan images are obtained with Co-57 markers on appropriate sites.

  a. Axilla: anterior and lateral views to coordinate localization, using skin markers

  b. Neck: anterior, lateral, and oblique views as needed to identify anterior and posterior drainage

  c. Pelvis: anterior and posterior views

  *Delayed images:* At 2 hours, the patient returns for identical images and additional images where appropriate.

  *Presurgery images:* Where surgery is scheduled, delayed images are performed immediately before transfer to the operating room (either the 2-hour images or the next morning):

  a. Site of lymph nodes detected by scanning is clearly identified by indelible marker. Note that it is important that the images be obtained with the patient in the position expected for surgery. This ensures that the orthogonal markers identify the deeper lymph nodes.

b. The Neoprobe is used to identify these nodes.

c. Confirmation of the localization skin markers in the surgical position is required prior to excision.

- *Breast cancer mammary injection:* For mammary injection, the tracer is instilled at 3, 6, 9, and 12 o'clock about the tumor, within 2 to 3 mm of the tumor, at the tumor depth.

*Lymphatic flow study:* Immediately after injection, imaging with 30-second frames should be obtained to identify lymphatic drainage (to axilla, internal mammary chain [ipsilateral or contralateral] and the supraclavicular region) as well as interval and sentinel lymph nodes.

*Regional lymph node study:* At 20 minutes, 5-minute images should be obtained of the expected regional nodal sites. Images should include the axilla, sternum, and supraclavicular regions.

*Delayed image:* At 2 hours, similar images may be obtained.

**Display:** Conventional planar: whole-body and static images.

**Interpretation:** Radiopharmaceutical should promptly ascend up the appropriate lymph node chains. Asymmetry in lymph node uptake may indicate obstruction. The drainage pathways and the first lymph nodes identified should be marked.

# Central Nervous System Protocols

## CENTRAL NERVOUS SYSTEM 1: BRAIN SPECT PERFORMED WITH TC-99M HMPAO OR TC-99M ECD

CPT code: 78607

**Indications:** SPECT is used to evaluate regional cerebral blood flow. These examinations are very useful in evaluating the brain blood flow in a variety of pathologic states, including:

- Epilepsy
- Stroke
- Dementia
- Tumors

**Patient preparation:** No patient preparation

**Scheduling**

- This examination requires 2.5-hour patient presence (50 minute camera time).
- The patient needs to arrive at least 30 minutes before injection.
- A quiet room must be available for the patient at least 1 hour before imaging.

**Radiopharmaceutical and dose**

- 16 to 24 mCi Tc-99m HMPAO (exametazime, Ceretec)
- 16 to 24 mCi Tc-99m ECD (bicisate, Neurolite)

The $TcO_4^-$ needed to reconstitute the kit must have been eluted within the previous 2 hours. The generator must have been eluted within the previous 24 hours. The kit requires greater than 85% tag. The expiration time of the kit is 4 hours. Dose is adjusted for patient weight if ≤45 kg or ≥90 kg.

**Imaging device:** Triple-headed gamma camera with LEUHR collimation (device of choice) or single-headed gamma camera with LEHR collimation

**Imaging procedure:** The patient should arrive 30 minutes before injection. Put the patient in a quiet, dimly lit room. Start an IV drip in the patient. Inform radiopharmacy when

the IV has been placed. Inject agent into the patient using IV. Wait 60 minutes before beginning imaging.

**Data acquisition**

*Triple-headed device*

- Matrix: 128 × 128
- Stops: 360-degree acquisition, 3-degree stops for 25 seconds
- Reconstruction: Hanning filter, 0.9
- Display: 1 pixel

*Single-headed device*

- Matrix: 64 × 64
- Stops: 360-degree acquisition, 6-degree stops for 30 seconds
- Reconstruction: Butterworth filter, cutoff 0.44, power 10
- Display: 1 to 2 pixels

**Interpretation:** Abnormal brain areas, such as those recently suffering a stroke or epileptic foci, demonstrate decreased radiotracer uptake. During an ictus or immediately after ictus, the focal lesion will be hot.

## CENTRAL NERVOUS SYSTEM 2: CEREBRAL FLOW

CPT code: 78615

**Indications:** To determine the presence or absence of intracerebral blood flow

**Patient preparation:** No patient preparation

**Scheduling:** This is a bedside study. It is done emergently, virtually immediately, for valid indications. This test is virtually never denied.

**Radiopharmaceutical and preparation:** 16 to 24 mCi of a Tc-99m agent. The ideal agent is Tc-99m DTPA because it is most rapidly excreted, allowing repeat tests at shorter time intervals. If the study is performed after hours, then $TcO_4^-$ can be used if the DTPA is not available. Dose is adjusted for patient weight if ≤45 kg or ≥90 kg.

**Imaging device**: Mobile camera with LEGP collimation

**Imaging procedure:** Ensure that the patient's head is as straight as possible and that the entire head is in the FOV. With patient positioned and detector head placed, identify the largest vein available, preferably a central line. The imaging protocol is commenced (the computer started), and 6 seconds later (the technologist starts counting aloud 1 through 6 on starting acquisition) the tracer is injected (this provides means of obtaining background activity, which can be subtracted out if radiotracer is present from previous procedure) and ensures the adequacy of the test by documenting carotid and extracerebral blood flow.

**Data acquisition:** Use predefined protocol Brain-Death, which includes 1-second images for 60 seconds and two 1-minute static images (image sets obtained sequentially).

**Data display:** The flow study is displayed in six 10-second intervals, and the two 1-minute images are displayed separately on the same x-ray film.

**Interpretation:** This test does not identify death, it merely identifies absence of intracerebral perfusion. This test does not examine brain stem flow. The absence of activity over the skull vault region (external carotid territory) implies poor injection and invalidates interpretation. The common carotid and the external carotid arterial flow must be documented.

If the "trident" sign is seen (territories of both middle and anterior cerebral arteries), intracerebral perfusion is present. If it is absent, and no sagittal sinus activity is seen in the 1- and 2-minute films, this is the classic scan finding of absent intracerebral perfusion.

Nonvisualization of the anterior and middle cerebral artery territories with some sagittal sinus activity probably means some drainage of the skull vault perfusion into the sinus rather than intracerebral perfusion per se. This does not exclude some minimal intracerebral perfusion, but no patient has made significant recovery from a comatose state with this scan finding.

The test helps the physician to diagnose death by documenting absent intracerebral perfusion. Although the patient is not helped by the study, the patient's family may benefit by discontinuation of life support earlier than otherwise, and there is the opportunity for earlier transplantation.

## CENTRAL NERVOUS SYSTEM 3: CSF FLOW STUDY

CPT code: 78630, 78652 SPECT

**Indications:** The most common indication is in patients with early onset of dementia in whom a diagnosis of normal-pressure hydrocephalus (NPH) is being considered. These patients should have the clinical triad of dementia, dyspraxia, and incontinence. Occasionally, the test is requested to demonstrate the dispersal of a chemotherapeutic agent that is injected intrathecally.

**Patient preparation:** A lumbar puncture (LP) tray and manometer are necessary. Coordinate the study with a staff physician, who will perform the LP and inject the radiopharmaceutical. Have the patient arrive on a cart the first day of the study.

**Scheduling:** Allow the following imaging times:

- Injection time: 10 minutes for planar image
- 4-hours after injection: 1-hour planar images
- 24-hours after injection: 1.5 hours as planar and possibly SPECT
- 48-hours after injection: 1.5 hours as planar and possibly SPECT
- 72-hours after injection (if requested): 1-hour planar images

**Radiopharmaceutical and dose:** 0.4 to 0.6 mCi of In-111 DTPA. Because In-111 DTPA is used, it must be special ordered. Dose is adjusted for patient weight if ≤45 kg or ≥90 kg.

**Imaging device**: Gamma camera with ME collimation. SPECT images may be required at 24 and 48 hours. If the patient is uncooperative, planar images will suffice.

**Imaging procedure:** After injection of tracer, a planar view of the injection site is taken to confirm intrathecal deposition. Planar anterior, lateral view images, and SPECT of the head may be obtained at 4, 24, and 48 hours. Occasionally, 72-hour planar images are obtained.

Occasionally, NM staff tailor the examination to study the flow of a therapeutic agent when different views are required and defined in the request form. In general, this test is performed using the injection volume and technique used by the treating physicians.

**Interpretation:** Injected tracer identifies the patient's CSF flow pathways. The classic and original description of NPH includes ventricular entry of tracer with stasis at or beyond 24 hours, with no flow over the convexities at all, and therefore no aggregation in the sagittal sinus. The other described NPH pattern is ventricular entry and persistence, with slow flow over the convexities and no accumulation in the sagittal sinus. The utility of this test has decreased because it has little predictive value for success of therapeutic shunting.

## CENTRAL NERVOUS SYSTEM 4: CSF SHUNT EVALUATION

CPT code: 78645

**Indications**

- To test for patency of ventriculoperitoneal or ventriculoatrial shunt
- To test for CSF distribution of chemotherapeutic drug when distribution is via reservoir

**Patient preparation:** This study is coordinated with the neurosurgical resident or staff who obtains and documents verbal consent, then inserts the needle into the shunt reservoir under aseptic conditions. An NM physician is present to help as necessary with the protocol and to inject the radio-

pharmaceutical. The x-ray package with shunt series and CTs should be available at the time of the tracer instillation.
**Scheduling:** The study takes 1 hour, and various delayed images (2 to 6 hours) may be required. The necessity for delayed imaging cannot be determined until the early study is obtained.
**Radiopharmaceutical and dose:** 0.4 to 0.6 mCi in 0.3 to 0.5 ml Tc-99m DTPA (activity in the smallest possible volume is desirable)
**Imaging device:** Gamma camera with LEHR collimation
**Imaging procedure:** Use this protocol exactly to reduce interpretation difficulties.

1. When the needle is in place (neurosurgical team), position the patient under the camera (in lateral or anterior position, depending on placement of the shunt). Frequently, the neurosurgical team aspirates 3 to 5 ml of CSF (to confirm that the ventricular side is patent) for flushing and to send to the laboratory. Make sure the entire head is in the FOV. Most times, the distal side of the tubing is occluded manually while the tracer is injected. Start the gamma camera and obtain six 10-second images. At the count of 5 or 6 after starting image acquisition, inject the tracer. Observe the persistence mode to determine that the needle tubing (usually a butterfly needle) has been emptied by the flush of CSF or freshly prepared 0.9% NaCl. After about 30 seconds, release the distal occlusion to determine flow distally.

2. a. Immediately postflow, obtain a 2-minute picture in the same position. Record counts.
   b. Obtain a 2-minute image of orthogonal view to that obtained above. Record counts.
   c. Obtain a 2-minute chest image. Mark sternal notch and xiphoid. Record counts.
   d. Obtain a 2-minute abdominal image. Mark xiphoid and pubic bone. Record counts.

3. Follow with a second series of identical images 20 minutes after injection. Record counts. Do not pump tubing or do any intervention before this second series. If some flow occurs, consider seating or mobilizing the patient, pumping the tubing, then repeating the images.

4. A repeat injection procedure may be required if only one side of the valved reservoir is visualized. Manipulation of the needle is required to place it on the opposite side of the diaphragm from the first injection series.

   If the distal tubing is partially visualized, but no abdominal activity is seen then the physician may request an image while pumping in lieu of reinjection. This can be set up as static images or as a flow study.

5. Follow with a third series of identical images at 2 to 6 hours after injection if necessary (with rolling a bedridden patient or walking a mobile patient between studies), or repeat the entire injection and imaging process as directed by NM physician.

**Display:** Use a predefined study with the intent to obtain all images (flow, immediate, and delayed) on one sheet.

**Interpretation:** The shunt can occlude at either the proximal (ventricular) or distal (atrial or peritoneal) ends. Therefore, during the flow study (injection of tracer), note should be made of whether the tubing is occluded distal to the reservoir (encouraging flow proximally into ventricles). Distal flow should occur when pressure is released. If a reservoir has a flap valve, sometimes the needle may be distal to it, so the proximal site is not tested: A repeat injection can be performed with the needle further advanced (however, if CSF was easily withdrawn, this probably indicates proximal patency). If the first study shows only the proximal (ventricular) side, the needle can be withdrawn slightly and injection repeated with no attempt to occlude tubing.

Obstruction usually occurs at the ventricular and abdominal ends of the shunt, with the abdominal end being more common. Sometimes the tubing can kink or break at other sites along its path.

There may be loculation of tracer around the abdominal end of the catheter without free dispersal through the abdominal cavity. This can mimic normal but slow flow. When this is seen, free flow of tracer is encouraged by walking or moving the patient around (rolling patient from side to side).

When the study is used to determine distribution of a drug injected into a reservoir, the identical procedure to the usual drug injection technique should be employed (same routine with the same flush volume).
**Invasive procedure:** This procedure is minimally invasive; the invasive portion of the procedure is performed by neurosurgeons, remaining in their purview entirely.

## Alternative Procedure

**Indication:** When the physiology of the system is in question (i.e., is the flow rate adequate to remove CSF from the ventricles?).
**Preparation:** The patient must be flat for 2 hours before the test so that the CSF pressure is equilibrated.
**Method:** Using a 25-gauge needle attached directly to the syringe of tracer, inject carefully the smallest possible volume of radiopharmaceutical into the reservoir, but do not flush. Remove needle and image constantly (1-minute images) for 30 minutes.
**Interpretation:** A washout curve is calculated.

## CENTRAL NERVOUS SYSTEM 5: CSF LEAK

CPT code: 78650
**Indications:** To determine the presence of CSF leak. Patients present with past history of trauma or surgery, recurrent CNS infections, such as meningitis, and nasal or otic discharge. In all instances, a physician approves this test in advance and discusses the symptoms with the referring physician and the patient to determine if there is any position more likely to induce the leak.

Patient name: _____

MR number: _____

Appointment at ENT Clinic at _____ (*time*) on _____ (*date*).

Thank you for placing the supplied 1½ × 1½–cm pledgets. These pledgets need to be of uniform size—hence the 1½ × 1½–cm pieces provided by Nuclear Medicine for ENT Service to place. The required positions are the cribriform plate and the sphenoethmoid recess under the middle turbinate.

These need to be bilateral, and to be identifiable when removed (number system provided with pledgets).

Another (a fifth) pledget will be placed by Nuclear Medicine in the buccal mucosa to serve as a background control.

Please return the tubes that the pledgets came in. These are essential for processing the data.

Thank you for your assistance.

**FIG. 30-12.**

| Tube no. | Sample | Counts/ 10 min. | CPM | Net CPM | Empty tube weight (g) | Full tube weight (g) | Net weight (g) | CPM/g |
|---|---|---|---|---|---|---|---|---|
| 1 | Left nostril, low | | | | | | | |
| 2 | Left nostril, high | | | | | | | |
| 3 | Right nostril, low | | | | | | | |
| 4 | Right nostril, high | | | | | | | |
| 5 | 0.5 ml plasma | | | | | | | |
| 6 | Buccal cavity | | | | | | | |
| 7 | Background | | | | | | | |

Date and time of pledget insertion _____     _____

Date and time of pledget removal _____     _____

Total time of pledget absorption _____     _____

Date and time of pledget counting _____     _____

Scale zeroed and calibrated     _____ (initials)

_____

Technologist's signature

**FIG. 30-13.**

**Patient preparation:** The ENT Clinic places pledgets for us for nasal leak (10:30 AM day of injection).

**Scheduling**

- LP is required. Tc-99m DTPA is preferred agent.

- No consent form is required. The test should be explained and consent documented by the person performing LP.
- If a nasal leak is present, verify that an ENT physician is available for 10:30 AM pledget placement at ENT Clinic (Fig. 30-12).

- Schedule:
    - 8:30 Patient injection
    - 10:30 Pledgets placed
    - 12:00 Patient scanned
    - 2:30 Patient scanned
    - 3:00 Pledgets pulled and counted and blood sample taken, spun, and counted
- Images may be required the next day.

**Radiopharmaceutical and dose:** 8 to 12 mCi Tc-99m-DTPA or 400 to 600 µCi In-111 DTPA. When using Tc-99m DTPA consult radiopharmacist to ensure high–specific activity eluate is used to minimize pyrogenicity. Dose is adjusted for patient weight if ≤45 kg or ≥90 kg.

**Technique:** Patient is injected intrathecally by NM staff physician in the department. The dose is followed by a flush with 15 to 20 ml of sterile saline without bacteriostatic agent preparation. This flush material must be newly opened. This step is done to accelerate the time of the test by rapidly putting significant activity in the region of suspected CSF leak. If the suspected leak is nasal, bilateral pledgets are to be used. They should be placed by a physician from the ENT department at both cribriform plates, at each sphenoethmoid recess under the middle turbinate, and one in the buccal mucosa for a control. Contact ENT Service nursing supervisor to arrange this at the ENT clinic 2 hours after injection of tracer. NM removes the pledgets at 5 hours and weighs, then counts them (Fig. 30-13). If an otic leak is suspected, the NM physician places the otic and buccal pledgets.

**Imaging device:** Gamma camera with LEHR collimation for Tc-DTPA, ME collimation for In-111 DTPA

**Imaging procedure:** Images are obtained immediately after CSF injection to document successful intrathecal placement of tracer.

The patient should be positioned with head flexed forward and downward or in a position known to cause rhinorrhea or otorrhea. Anterior and both lateral views are taken at 3 hours and 6 hours (before pledget removal) and, if necessary, the next morning, too.

Pledgets should be removed at the end of the study (6 hours) and counted after weighing. In addition, 0.5 ml of serum is weighed and counted. If the study is to be carried out to 24 hours, images only are obtained.

**Display:** Display images with upper threshold lowered to demonstrate a potential leak. If otorrhea is present, posterior views are included.

**Interpretation:** These studies are notoriously difficult to interpret. To detect small leaks, the upper display threshold must be lowered to demonstrate the leak. The normal nasal secretions contain tracer and hence the use of opposite side (nose or ear), buccal mucosa, and blood to determine what the background activity is per gram of body fluid. Since there is always considerable activity in the serum this measurement is important, and since saliva and nasal fluids concentrate tracer, the leak can only be identified if there is significantly more activity present in the saliva than in the serum. Hence the use of weighed samples and comparison with controls that are normalized for fluid content. At least 3 times the normal body fluid background levels are required for a positive test, and the abnormality should be seen on the images to be called. The pledgets help localize the site of the leak.

**Invasive procedure:** This is a minimally invasive procedure, with very low risk (that of LP). In the event of an outpatient, a complication will be readmission (usually for nosocomial infection). In the event of an inpatient, then attribution of an infection or other complication will be made by the QA monitoring staff (discharge analysts). No special monitoring is required by NM.

# Transplantation Protocols

## ORGAN TRANSPLANT 1: RENAL TRANSPLANT EVALUATION

**CPT code:** 78727

### Indications

- Assessing renal perfusion and function in renal transplant recipients
- Seek surgically correctable lesions (vascular abnormalities, urine leaks, etc.)
- Determining presence of ATN, drug toxicity, or rejection of transplanted organ

**Patient preparation:** Inform technologists if a scan was done in the last 14 days; they will do a background image to determine residual I-131 OIH from prior scans (common in patients with severe rejection and ATN).

**Scheduling:** Allow 90 minutes of camera time

**Radiopharmaceutical and dose:** 8 to 12 mCi of Tc-99m DTPA and 80 to 120 µCi I-131 OIH. Dose is adjusted for children only.

**Imaging device:** Gamma camera with high-energy collimation

### Imaging procedure

- The patient is to receive three drops (35 mg per drop) SSKI PO from technologist prior to scan.
- The patient should be well hydrated.
- The patient should void immediately before the study.

1. If the patient has a Hickman catheter, use it for all injections. If the patient does not have a Hickman, place a 21-gauge butterfly needle (23-gauge if necessary) in the best vein you can find.
2. Place the patient supine and anatomically positioned under the camera to include transplant and bladder regions. Position kidney and bladder in the same FOV. If the patient has a bladder catheter in place, clamp the catheter.
3. Set the camera window for Tc-99m (140 keV, 20% window). Do the kidney flow study. If the entire kidney is not seen in the flow image, move the patient so that the kidney is in the FOV by the second minute (within 60 seconds of flow study).
4. For the I-131 OIH part of the study, obtain a 5-minute background preinjection picture with window set up for I-131 (364 keV, 20% window). Follow with 1-minute frames for 5 minutes, then 5-minute frames for 25 minutes.
5. Obtain 400K Tc-99m image at the end of the study.

**Data analysis:** Use predefined analysis protocol for DTPA flow study and calculate uptake of Tc-99m DTPA in the second through third minute after injection (see Relative GFR protocol, CPT code 78707). The Tc-99m DTPA syringe is measured before and after dose administration. In this analysis, only the transplant organ is analyzed.

Use a predefined renal transplant program for the second part of the study with I-131 OIH.

**Display format:** The renal blood flow is displayed in 10-second images, and the calculated uptake is displayed in the second through third minute. The I-131 OIH 5-minute images are displayed, with renogram and bladder excretion curves.

**Interpretation:** The first postoperative day scan shows the typical ATN features if a cadaveric organ is used (mild decrease in flow, good extraction but poor excretion of OIH). Some drug toxicity scans can also look like ATN. Rejection is identified by decreased flow, extraction, and excretion. Vascular catastrophes are identified by severe decreases in flow. Extravasation of urine often requires delayed imaging to identify.

**Comment:** Tc-99m MAG3 would be an ideal substitute, but as yet the transplant surgeons at this institution still prefer the I-131 OIH study.

## ORGAN TRANSPLANT 2: PANCREAS TRANSPLANT PERFUSION EVALUATION

CPT code: 78445
**Indications:** This examination is performed to assess pancreatic transplant perfusion as an indication of pancreatic function. It is often performed in conjunction with a renal transplant study because many pancreatic transplant patients also have renal transplants.
**Patient preparation:** No patient preparation
**Scheduling:** Allow 30 minutes of camera time.

**Radiopharmaceutical and dose:** 8 to 12 mCi of Tc-99m DTPA. Dose is adjusted for children only.
**Imaging device:** Gamma camera with LE collimation
**Imaging procedure**

1. If the patient has a Hickman catheter, use it for all injections; if the patient does not have a Hickman, place a 21-gauge butterfly needle in the best vein you can find.
2. Place the patient supine and anatomically positioned under the camera to include transplant and bladder regions.
3. Acquire the Tc-99m DTPA flow study, which requires a preadministration injection syringe and stopcock count in special syringe holder for 3 seconds, flow study of sixty 1-second frames and four 1-minute frames for total 5-minute scan acquisition. This is followed by 400 K count postflow image. The postinjection syringe is then counted for 3 seconds. The program then displays flow and postflow images and calculates the percentage uptake in the second through third minute postinjection interval (as for GFR).

**Data analysis:** Use the predefined analysis protocol for a Tc-99m DTPA GFR and flow study. One ROI of the analysis protocol is used for the pancreas region (another is used for the renal transplant, if present). This combined study is easily accomplished because the standard GFR protocol has ROIs for each kidney. The protocol ensures that the correct organ is included in the appropriate analysis.
**Interpretation:** In the immediate postoperative period, the pancreatic perfusion is impaired. The flow maximizes in the first few days, then inexorably, but gradually, decreases with periods of accelerated decreases associated with rejection episodes.

## ORGAN TRANSPLANT 3: RADIONUCLIDE CYSTOGRAM FOR TRANSPLANT PATIENTS

CPT code: 78740
**Indications:** This examination is most commonly performed for patients with suspected urine leak in patients with renal transplants (especially pancreas-renal transplants). The sensitivity of this examination is equal to the radiographic equivalent with far less (0.01) of the radiation burden of the radiologic evaluation.
**Patient preparation:** The referring clinic or unit will catheterize the patient.
**Scheduling:** Allow 90 minutes.
**Radiopharmaceutical and dose:** Two doses, each 0.8 to 1.2 mCi Tc-99m DTPA (may use other Tc-99m agents if DTPA not available)
**Imaging device:** Gamma camera with LEHR collimation
**Imaging procedure**

1. Lay the patient supine with the detector head above the table for transplant patients when looking for leaks. Ensure that the bladder and kidney are in the FOV.

Computer acquisition of data is necessary; use a predefined study. Acquire a series of dynamic 1-minute images for up to 60 minutes.

2. Begin running saline from 500-ml bag of saline (warmed to room temperature) into the bladder. Inject dose directly into the Foley catheter as soon as saline is running properly. Start acquisition.

3. Watch display for reflux. Record the volume instilled and the time when reflux is first seen.

4. When the bladder is filled (volume in bladder should be >200 ml) or when patient complains of discomfort or the need to void, proceed with the next steps.

5. Have the patient void through the catheter. Measure the volume of urine voided.

6. Repeat the entire procedure a second time for transplant patients with no visible leak. Clamp the catheter and ask the patient to attempt to void for 2 minutes (two frames). Watch for reflux or leak. Expect possible leakage about the catheter. Then unclamp the catheter and ask the patient to void through the catheter while recording images. Measure the volume of urine voided.

7. After voiding, take two anterior static images for 3 minutes or 250 K, including the entire abdominal area, to determine if there is a leak. At this point, if a leak is detected, the test is complete.

8. Use the worksheet of the Voiding Cystogram (see Fig. 30-1).

**Acquisition and display protocol:** This protocol sets up two studies: voiding 1 and voiding 2. Each study display contains three data sets: a dynamic filling, a dynamic voiding, and anterior upper and lower abdomen spot views.

Lower the upper window threshold of the films to identify small leaks (lower this to 10% of the maximum pixel count). **Interpretation:** The study is very sensitive for detecting leak with low radiation dose. The repeat test is required for increased sensitivity. In transplant patients, the leak often occurs at the junction of the bladder and duodenal stump for the pancreatic transplant if this technique was used. The leak is often seen to migrate up and around the liver. Note that the second set of anterior images may demonstrate some gastric activity (presumably absorbed free $TcO_4^-$).

# Nonthyroid Endocrine Protocols

## NONTHYROID ENDOCRINE 1: PARATHYROID TUMOR LOCALIZATION

CPT code: 78070

**Indications:** Patients with proven hyperparathyroidism, for the preoperative localization of abnormal parathyroid tissue. This study is performed using the first protocol below. If there is a history of previous parathyroid surgery or if the first study is indefinite (according to NM physician), the patient should have the optional study scheduled.

**Patient preparation:** The referring physician must provide the serum calcium and serum parathyroid hormone measurements at the time of scheduling. The patient must be able to lie flat and still for 90 minutes.

**Scheduling:** Schedule the patient to arrive 30 minutes before camera time for completion of the thyroid questionnaire. The first study (Scan 1) requires 1.5 hours. If the patient returns for the optional study, that scan requires 3 hours.

**Radiopharmaceutical and dose**
*Primary scan:* 2.4 to 3.6 mCi Tl-201 as thallous chloride and 8 to 12 mCi Tc-99m as pertechnetate IV
*Optional scan:* 16 to 24 mCi of Tc-99m sestamibi IV
Dose adjustments

- Tc-99m $TcO_4^-$ and sestamibi: adjusted for patient weight if ≤45 kg or ≥90 kg
- Tl-201: 1.6-2.4 mCi if ≤45 kg; 3.2 to 4.8 mCi if ≥90 kg

**Imaging device**
Primary procedure: Gamma camera with HR collimation for 75 minutes (use 15% Tc-99m and 30% Tl-201 windows)
Optional procedure: Triple-headed camera with LEUHR collimation for 30 minutes, then 2 hours later for 30 minutes (use a 15% Tc-99m window)

**Imaging procedure**
Primary scan

- Make the venipuncture with an Angiocath set for later administration of both thallium and technetium. Position the patient supine beneath the camera with neck extended and head secured with masking tape in the head rest.
- Inject the Tl-201. Position the patient with the thyroid at the top of the FOV so as to image the chest area. Take the 3-minute image (preset: static, 128 × 128 matrix, one frame per minute, zoom 1.33).
- Quickly reposition the patient for the rest of the study by centering the thyroid in the FOV. Explain to the patient that the imaging process is about to begin and how imperative it is that no movement (including talking) occur until you indicate that the procedure is completed. Check that the neck is hyperextended.
- Begin thallium acquisition (preset: dynamic, 1 frame per minute for 15 minutes, 128 × 128 matrix, zoom 2.67).
- At the completion of 15-minute computer acquisition of the thallium study, inject the Tc-99m and begin the computer Tc-99m acquisition immediately (preset: dynamic,

128 × 128 matrix, one frame per minute for 15 minutes, zoom 2.67).

- After completion of the Tc-99m acquisition, have the physician palpate the neck and mark the chin, suprasternal notch, cricoid cartilage and identify thyroid nodules.

Optional scan:

- Inject patient with Tc-99m sestamibi.
- Perform early SPECT on triple-headed camera 30 minutes after injection.
- Acquire 128 × 128 matrix, 25 seconds at 3-degree stops, reconstruct with Butterworth filter cutoff 0.5 and power 10.
- Perform late SPECT, 2 hours after injection, using the same parameters as above.

**Data analysis**

Primary scan: Predefined study includes alignment, normalization, and subtraction of technetium (thyroid) from the thallium (parathyroid and thyroid) images.

1. Check level of subtraction. Determine whether a small number of pixels were completely subtracted:
   - If yes, proceed
   - If no (oversubtracted), redo the normalization, in center of over subtracted thyroid.
2. Check motion analysis set. Edge artifacts should appear and mirror the shift, comparing right to left and upper to lower:
   - If superimposition is OK, proceed.
   - If superimposition is not OK, realign.
3. Note patient motion. If no edge artifacts are identified in the display, there has been significant motion that might possibly be corrected by restarting analysis and using fewer of the 15 thallium or technetium images. However, deletion of too many frames may make statistics too poor to localize adenoma.
4. Note appearance of hot areas (potential adenomas) on each of nine images in motion analysis set:
   - Adenoma in same location in all nine images indicates high confidence in localization (insensitive to ±1 pixel superimposition errors).
   - If adenoma position varies, be very careful. Small adenoma on edge of thyroid is extremely sensitive to ±1 pixel superimposition errors.
5. Separate parathyroid adenomas from other anomalies. Compare location of adenomas to composite thallium and technetium images (upper left quadrant of film). If thyroid is abnormal in appearance, determine whether hot areas are parathyroid adenomas, thyroid adenomas, or other adenomas.

Optional scan: Present early and late SPECT slices, and stack the transaxial slices for rotating cine.

**Interpretation:** Tl-201 localizes in hyperactive parathyroids but is also found in the thyroid, making it difficult to identify the abnormal parathyroid tissue. This dual tracer technique with Tl-201 chloride and Tc-99m pertechnetate uses computerized sub-traction of thyroid (Tc) from thyroid and parathyroid (Tl) to yield an image of parathyroid alone. A critical constraint of this procedure is that the registration of the technetium and thallium image sets be exact (i.e., the patient must not move).

The test is designed to be used only in patients with proven hyperparathyroidism (serum calcium elevated and serum parathyroid hormone inappropriately high) so that specificity is ensured. The images are therefore manipulated to demonstrate the slightest abnormality (maximizing sensitivity).

## NONTHYROID ENDOCRINE 2: ADRENAL CORTICAL SCAN

CPT code: 78075

**Indications:** To distinguish between adenoma and hyperplasia in patients with Cushing's syndrome, virilization, or aldosteronism

**Patient preparation**

- Exclude pregnant and breast-feeding women.
- Dexamethasone suppression is required for hyperaldosteronism and hyperandrogenism but not Cushing's syndrome. Dexamethasone should be prescribed by the referring physician and should be given in a dosing schedule of 1 mg qid for 7 days before the scan and continued throughout the scan period (i.e., 5 or 7 additional days).
- Check with the patient for possible sensitivity to iodine and to determine whether the patient is or is not on dexamethasone or if the patient is to have a barium contrast radiologic examination (if so, this should be deferred until after the iodocholesterol study).
- The uptake of free I-131 by the thyroid should be prevented by the administration of SSKI (one drop tid) beginning 1 day before the dose and continuing for 14 days after the administration of I-131 iodocholesterol. This should be prescribed by the referring physician.
- The patient should be asked about intake of steroids, propranolol, or spironolactone (all decrease iodocholesterol [NP-59] uptake). If so, an NM physician should be consulted. Hypercholesterolemia may also decrease NP-59 uptake.

**Scheduling:** Refer to the NP-59 schedule, which lists shipping dates of first and third Wednesday of each month. Radiopharmacist must order by Tuesday for delivery Thursday. Schedule injection for Friday (day 1). Schedule 90 minutes (dual-headed scanner) or 120 minutes (single-headed scanner) early morning (8 AM) on day 3 (Monday) and day 5 (Wednesday). Occasionally, images at 7 days are required.

**Radiopharmaceutical and dose:** 0.8 to 1.2 mCi I-131 iodocholesterol (NP-59) given intravenously. Dose is adjusted for patient weight if ≤45 kg or ≥90 kg. The dose should be administered under the direction of an NM physician. The injector verifies that the patient is on SSKI and suppression when appropriate. If not, consult an NM physician, who will give and prescribe SSKI. Injection will follow 1 hour after SSKI administration.

This study is performed under an investigational new drug protocol. The examination should be explained to the patient, who must sign three copies of the consent form: (1) kept by patient, (2) put in patient chart, (3) kept in NM.

**Imaging device**: Gamma camera with HE collimation

**Imaging procedure**

1. Obtain anterior and posterior 20-minute spot views. Center the field of view over L2; look for the liver and the hot spots indicating the adrenals. The adrenals should be positioned in the upper half, not center, of the image.
2. At the physician's discretion, if the adrenals are visualized, inject Tc-99m DTPA, and take a 100 K image on the Tc-99m setting with the patient in the same position.
3. Occasionally (e.g., with virilization), additional pelvis views may be required.

**Interpretation:** Autonomously functioning gland or glands visualize when patient is on suppressive doses of dexamethasone. Early visualization is pathologic. Normal glands can "break through" at 5 days (in this case, to correlate kidneys with NP-59 uptake, images at 7 days should also be obtained). Visualization only on days 5 and 7 would indicate breakthrough (30% occurrence rate).

## NONTHYROID ENDOCRINE 3: ADRENAL MEDULLA SCAN

CPT code: 78802

**Indications**

- Diagnosis and localization of adrenal and extra-adrenal functioning paragangliomas (pheochromocytoma and other paragangliomas of the sympathetic and parasympathetic chains). Also useful in adrenal medullary hyperplasia and other apudomas, such as neuroblastoma.
- Evaluation of patients with multiple pheochromocytomas, such as multiple endocrine neoplasia II, neurofibromatosis, or von Hippel–Lindau disease.

**Patient preparation**

- Exclude pregnant and breast-feeding women.
- No bowel preparation is required.
- The following drugs reportedly have the potential to decrease uptake of I-131 iobenguane sulfate in neuroendocrine tumors and may lead to false negative results if administered concomitantly: antihypertensives (labetalol, reserpine, calcium channel blockers), amitriptyline and derivatives, imipramine and derivatives, doxepin, amoxapine, and loxapine, sympathetic amines (phenylephrine, phenylpropanolamine, pseudoephedrine, ephedrine), and cocaine (see Nonthyroid Endocrine Protocol 4). It is unknown whether other

drugs in the same classes have the same potential to inhibit the uptake of I-131 iobenguane sulfate.

The patient should be off all medications such as tricyclic antidepressant drugs, phenothiazine reserpine, cocaine, phenylpropanolamine, other sympathomimetics (e.g., Sudafed, a very common over-the-counter proprietary nasal decongestant), and imipramine for ≥4 weeks, and off labetalol for 3 days before the study.

**Scheduling**

- Imaging time: 90 minutes on dual headed scanners, 120 minutes on other cameras. Schedule at 8 AM for each day.
- Inject on Monday, Tuesday, or Wednesday. Image at 24, 48, and possibly 72 hours (Saturday if Wednesday injection).
- To prevent uptake of free I-131 by the thyroid, the patient should receive one drop tid SSKI (1 g/ml) 1 day before and continue 6 days after the administration of I-131 MIBG. This should be prescribed by the referring physician.
- The radiopharmaceutical has to be special ordered.

**Radiopharmaceutical:** The dose should be administered by or under the direction of a NM staff physician. At the time of administration, verify that the patient is on SSKI. A dose of 0.8 to 1.2 mCi of I-131 MIBG is administered by slow intravenous injection over 15 seconds. The minimum dose should not be <0.25 mCi. Dose is adjusted for patient weight if ≤45 kg or ≥90 kg.

**Imaging device**: Gamma camera with highest-energy collimation. Otherwise consult with NM physician.

**Imaging procedure:** Multiple overlapping images (20 minutes) are obtained at 24 and 48 hours after injection. Generally two anterior images (head to pelvis) and three posterior images (head to knees) are obtained. Imaging may not be necessary at 72 hours.

**Interpretation:** I-131 metaiodobenzylguanidine (I-131 MIBG) is an analog of guanethidine. I-131 MIBG is taken up and stored in tissues in a manner similar to norepinephrine. It accumulates in adrenergic (uptake I mechanism) and nonadrenergic (uptake II mechanism, primarily the liver) tissues. I-131 MIBG has been shown to concentrate in pheochromocytomas, paragangliomas, and hyperplastic adrenal medullary tissue as well as other amine precursor uptake decarboxylation tumors. It is especially useful for detecting ectopic sites and metastatic lesions.

Normal uptake is seen in the salivary glands, liver, and heart. The agent is excreted renally, some of it into the large bowel. In 20% of normal studies, the adrenals are visualized.

## NONTHYROID ENDOCRINE 4: DRUGS THAT INTERFERE WITH I-131 MIBG

Following is a list of drugs that may interfere with the uptake of MIBG. Generic names are given with trade names in parentheses.

**Tricyclic antidepressants and related drugs:** Withhold for 6 weeks before test.

- Amitriptyline (Elavil, Endep, Etrafon, Triavil, Amitril, Emitrip, Enovil)
- Amoxapine (Asendin)
- Desipramine HCL (Pertoframe, Norpramin)
- Doxepin HCL (Adapin, Sinequan)
- Imipramine HCL, Pamoate (Tofranil, Imavate, Janimine, Presamine, SK-Pramine, Tipramine)
- Maprotiline HCL (Ludiomil)
- Nortriptyline HCL (Aventyl, Pamelor)
- Protriptyline HCL (Vivactil)
- Trimipramine Maleate (Surmontil)
- Trazodone HCL (Desyrel)

**Other categories:** Withhold for 2 weeks before test.
- Labetalol (Normodyne, Trandate)
- Bretylium Tosylate (Bretylol)
- Guanethidine (Ismelin)
- Reserpine (Serpasil, Sandril)
- Haloperidol (Haldol)
- Thiothixene (Navene)
- Phenothiazines
  Acetophenazine (Tindal)
  Carphenazine (Proketazine)
  Chlorpromazine (Thorazine, Chloramead, Foypromazine, Promapar)
  Fluphenazine (Prolixin, Permitil)
  Mesoridazine (Serentil)
  Perphenazine (Trilafon)
  Piperacetazine (Quide)
  Prochlorperazine (Compazine)
  Promazine (Sparine, Norazine, Prozine)
  Thioridazine (Mellaril)
  Trifluoperazine (Stelazine)
  Triflupromazine (Vesprin)
- Amphetamines
  Amphetamine (Benzedrine, Edrisal, Biphetamine, Dextrosal Amphaplex, Nobese)

  Benzphetamine (Didrex)
  Chlorphentermine (Pre-Sate)
  Chlortermine (Voranil)
  Dextroamphetamine (Dexedrine, Daro-Tab, Amfedsul, Amsustain, Cendex, Perke-One, Zamitam, Synatan)
  Diethylpropion (Tenuate, Tepanil)
  Fenfluramine (Pondimin)
  Mazindal (Sanorex)
  Methamphetamine (Desoxyn, Methedrine, Methampex)
  Methylphenidate (Ritalin)
  Phendimetrazine (Plegine)
  Phenmetrazine (Preludin)
  Phentermine (Wilpo, Ionamin)
- Nasal decongestants: Most over-the-counter decongestants have either pseudoephedrine, phenylephrine, or phenylpropanolamine. Please check all labels.
  Pseudoephedrine HCL (Halofed, Sudafed, Sudrin, Cenafed, Neofed, Dorcol Pediatric Formula, Neo-Synephrinol Day Relief, Decofed Syrup, Novafed, Cenafed Syrup, Peedee Dose Decongestant)
  Pseudoephedrine Sulfate (Afrinol Repetabs)
  Phenylpropanolamine HCL (also used as an anorexiant) (Propagest, Sucrets Cold Decongestant Formula, Rhindecon)
  Phenylephrine HCL (Neo-Synephrine, Alconefrin, Rhinall, Allerest Nasal, Doktors Nose Drops, Nostril, Coricidin Nasal Mist, Sinex, Sinophen, Sinarest Nasal, Duration Mild)
- Diet control pills
  Phenylpropanolamine HCL (anorexiant) (Diadax, Resolution II Half-Strength, Prolamine, Control, Dex-A-Diet, Dexatrim, Unitrol, Acutrim, Appedrine, Grapefruit Diet Plan with Diadax)
- Cocaine

Source: Courtesy of University of Michigan, Department of Internal Medicine, Division of Nuclear Medicine, Ann Arbor, MI 48109-0028.

# Nonthyroid Therapy Protocols

**NONTHYROID THERAPY 1: SKELETAL METASTASES THERAPY (STRONTIUM 89 OR SAMARIUM 153)**

CPT code: 79400
**Indications**

- Palliation of pain from proven skeletal metastases. Patients may have breast, prostate, lung, or other cancer.

- New treatment protocols are being developed nationwide for therapeutic administrations rather than pain palliation only.

**Patient preparation:** No patient preparation
**Scheduling:** Patient needs to have the following:

1. Hemoglobin, WBC (desire >2,500), and platelet (desire >60,000) counts before scheduling
2. A bone scan in the last 6 weeks and a copy available for NM staff

Date _____ Patient name _____

MR # _____ Age _____ Weight _____

Referring clinic _____ Referring MD _____

Primary care MD _____ Date of last bone scan _____

Primary tumor or type _____

Chemotherapy _____ Last _____

XRT: *yes* _____ *no* _____ Extent _____

**Pretest lab results**

Hb _____ WBC _____ (>2,500)  Platelets _____ (> 60,000)  Date _____

**Interview**

Patient understands transplant aim, and consents _____ Pain consistent with bone scan: ___ yes ___ no

Radiopharmaceutical and dose used _____

Signature of Nuclear Medicine MD _____

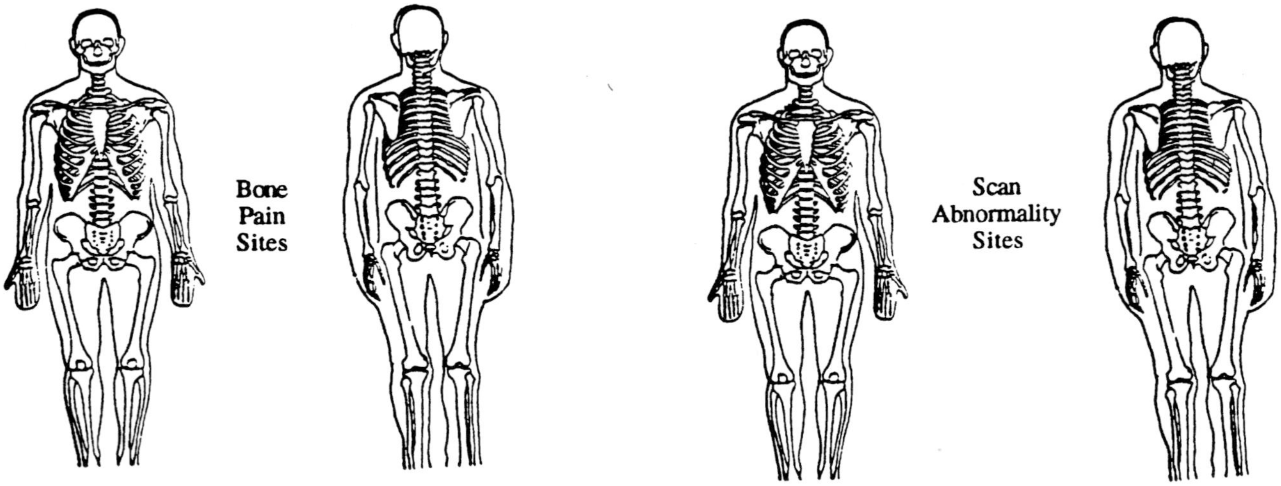

Bone
Pain
Sites

Scan
Abnormality
Sites

**Pain medication**

1. _____ Dose rate _____

2. _____ Dose rate _____

3. _____ Dose rate _____

**Follow-up provided**

Package insert _____

Follow-up laboratory work _____ Follow-up clinical appt. _____

**FIG. 30-14.**

3. Appropriate follow-up appointments for WBC and platelet counts at biweekly intervals for 8 weeks

**Radiopharmaceutical and dose:** Typically, 4 mCi of strontium 89 (Sr-89) as strontium chloride in unit dose form (40 to 60 μCi/kg) or 1mCi/kg of samarium 153 (Sm-153) lexidronam. Doses are special ordered. Dose is adjusted for patient weight if ≤45 kg or ≥90 kg.

**Therapy administration:** Before administration, the therapy data sheet is completed (Fig. 30-14). It establishes the need for this therapy and compliance with the institutional requirements regarding prior assessment and follow-up. Oral consent is obtained and documented on that sheet. The department's QMP is followed.

Therapy setup: When the patient arrives in NM, a package insert is provided for the patient to read before being interviewed by the NM physician who will fill in the data sheet. The technologist then places a 22-gauge Intracath and connects a short IV line, then a three-way stopcock and one 20-ml syringe of sterile saline. The area will be covered with adsorbable material, in case of a spill.

Administration: After informed consent is obtained, the NM faculty personally confirms the correct dose for the patient and identifies the patient by two specific procedures (e.g., birth date and medical record number), then administers the dose. This is done by slow IV infusion, checking constantly that the line is patent and that extravasation is unlikely. The shielded syringe is flushed three times to ensure that the entire dose is administered.

When the therapy is given:

- Disconnect the 20-ml syringe, cap it and the three-way stopcock, and enclose them in a glove for counting in the dosimeter with the dosimeter cradle removed.
- Disconnect the dose syringe and IV line, cap the end, withdraw the syringe from the shield, and count the line and syringe.
- Remove the Intracath and three-way stopcock, and measure the residuum.

The patient's arm is then surveyed to establish that extravasation has not occurred. If extravasation occurs, then warm compresses are used to hasten absorption (venous and lymphatic); the count rate is documented, and appropriate additional therapy or follow-up arranged.

At the completion of the injection the QMP prescription form is completed for full NRC compliance (see Chapter 28).

**Discussion:** The Sm-153 lexidronam was approved in mid-1997 and, with a shorter half-life (46.7 hours vs. 50.5 days), the onset of action is sooner, although of shorter duration. Sm-153 lexidronam also has a 103-keV gamma ray (28% abundant) that allows imaging.

## NONTHYROID THERAPY 2: INTRA-ARTICULAR THERAPY

CPT code: 79440

**Indications:** In inflammatory arthritis, synovial granulation tissue results in increased secretion of synovial fluid, degradation of cartilage and bone, and results in functional loss. Surgery can be used to treat these abnormalities, but simpler (and less expensive) alternatives, such as radiation synovectomy, should be considered. Indicated diseases include:

- Hemophilic arthropathy
- Rheumatoid arthritis
- Villonodular synovitis

**Patient preparation:** In hemophilia, factor VIII is usually given before therapy (50 U/kg) and at 24 and 72 hours after treatment (20 U/kg). This is required in factor IX deficiency, too. Laboratory and x-ray data are jointly reviewed to ensure

**Table 30-2.**

| Patient weight | Joint | Dose |
|---|---|---|
| 10–25 kg | Knee | 0.500 mCi |
| | Elbow/ankle | 0.250 mCi |
| 25–40 kg | Knee | 0.750 mCi |
| | Elbow/ankle | 0.375 mCi |
| >40 kg | Knee | 1.000 mCi |
| | Elbow/ankle | 0.500 mCi |

optimal procedure (lesser grades of joint damage respond best) in nonhemophilic disorders. Before the procedure, patients or their guardians are required to provide informed consent.

**Scheduling:** Allow 30 minutes of imaging performed before and after injection of therapeutic colloid (associated Tc-99m SC allows imaging) and GM counting at 24 and 72 hours after injection (optionally at 7 days) to detect nodal uptake of therapeutic colloid in draining nodes and liver.

**Radiopharmaceutical and dose**

- P-32 chromic phosphate as a colloid (size 0.6 to 2.0 μm). Dose: See Table 30-2.
- 1 mCi of Tc-99m SC for pre- and postinjection imaging

P-32 is a pure beta emitter with a maximum energy of 1.7 meV and a maximum tissue penetration of 7.9 mm. P-32 delivers approximately 8,000 to 10,000 rads/mCi to the synovium at a depth of 0.1 mm.

Significant tracer localization in the regional lymph nodes may occur (usually <1%).

**Imaging device:** Gamma camera with LEAP collimation for imaging to confirm dispersal of Tc-99m SC (and therefore therapeutic agent) through the joint.

**Protocol:** The procedure is done with fluoroscopy guidance.

1. Scrub injection site with povidone-iodine (Betadine).
2. Anesthetize area with 1% lidocaine. Enter joint.
3. Leave a stopcock valve in place after joint is entered.
4. Instill Conray (iothalamate) through the needle into the joint space to make sure that the needle is in the joint space.
5. Inject 1 mCi of Tc-99m SC into the joint space for imaging to ensure that the therapeutic agent will not loculate, but rather disburse through joint.
6. Inject the therapeutic P-32 chromic and remainder of the radiocolloid. Move the joint to ensure distribution of therapeutic tracer. Confirm this distribution with Tc-99m SC scan.
7. Inject dexamethasone 1 ml (4 mg) by flush through the same needle. Optionally, more lidocaine can be injected.
8. Place joint in a protective splint for 2 days to immobilize joint.

**Imaging procedure:** Anterior, posterior, and lateral images are obtained of the joint during and after injection. Tc-99m is imaged immediately before and after injection of the therapeutic agent.

## NONTHYROID THERAPY 3: INTRACAVITARY P-32 THERAPY

CPT code: 79200

**Rationale:** When tumor seeding of the peritoneal or pleural cavity occurs, serosal irritation results in excess cavity transudate. The fluid collections can be an important source of discomfort to the patient and may require palliative treatment. P-32 is a pure beta emitter; therefore, only the fluid-producing surfaces are irradiated, and, because a colloid is used, little systemic absorption occurs.

**Indications**

- P-32 chromic phosphate suspension for malignant effusions not successfully treated with sclerosing agents, such as tetracycline
- Treatment of malignant ascites (especially ovarian source)
- Adjunctive therapy of ovarian cancer (limited role)

**Patient preparation:** No patient preparation

**Scheduling:** A planning session with instillation of Tc-99m SC via the planned administration route is required before the therapy, for example, intrapleurally or intraperitoneally. The therapeutic intrapleural administration follows thoracentesis to remove the effusion. Two to 3.0 mCi of Tc-99m SC is instilled, and dispersal of the radiopharmaceutical is confirmed. Therapies are not given if the test dose is loculated because this results in inadequate dispersal and the possibility of local radiation necrosis.

A 2-hour time period is scheduled, with an hour of gamma camera time (to image test dose).

**Radiopharmaceutical and dose:** A dose of 10 to 20 mCi of P-32 as chromic phosphate suspension with 500 ml saline is given.

**Therapy administration:** Follow the general administration procedure as described in protocol Strontium 89 Therapy (CPT 79400, Nonthyroid Therapy 1) using intracavitary injection rather than the IV route. The check and disposal of the injection paraphernalia is similar to protocol Strontium 89 Therapy.

Post-therapy maneuvers: The patient is repositioned repeatedly in the first hour, then several times each hour for the next day. This is done to ensure widespread dissemination of the therapeutic dose (right decubitus, left decubitus, head up, head down).

Post-therapy precautions: The pure beta emitter does not represent a hazard while contained in the patient. Any body fluids leaking from the therapy site (abdominal cavity or pleural space) are treated as radioactive.

In the event of a leak, NM or Radiation Safety personnel will tend to the patient. Staff should initially stem any continued loss of fluid by gentle pressure using gloved hand and absorptive pads taped onto the patient. Spilled fluid should be mopped up with absorptive pads backed with plastic (Chux) and then stored. *Note:* Drainage tubes and dressings will be radioactive, so special precautions are required for these. In the event of patient death, the NM physician attending and Radiation Safety must be called before removing the body.

**Side effects:** These relate to local radiation effects and are more common with loculated doses.

**Efficacy**

- 50% to 80% response rates occur in malignant effusions and ascites.
- Maximum response occurs at 3 months.
- Repeated doses may be necessary.

## NONTHYROID THERAPY 4: POLYCYTHEMIA THERAPY

CPT code: 79100

**Indications:** This therapy is used in the treatment of polycythemia rubra vera and may be used in other marrow proliferative disorders. In all cases, the patient arrives with a prescription from an authorized and qualified hematologist (with the suggested dose included).

**Patient preparation:** No patient preparation

**Scheduling:** The patient is scheduled for 15 minutes of time. The P-32 sodium phosphate must be special ordered for the patient.

**Radiopharmaceutical and dose:** The prescription must be countersigned by an NM faculty physician, who will ensure that the referring physician is qualified to refer the patient for therapy. The QMP is followed.

The NM faculty physician verifies the dose before administration by two methods: calculation of the dose and volume of therapy from the manufacturer's specifications and by measurement. These must coincide within 10%. The radiopharmacist must be involved in this therapy dose preparation because pure beta emitters are poorly counted in a dosimeter.

**Therapy:** The radiopharmaceutical is administered by the NM staff via IV injection using the technique described in the protocol Strontium 89 Therapy (CPT 79400, Nonthyroid Therapy 1), making sure that extravasation does not occur. This can be checked by passing a GM tube with window open from the lower arm over the injection site to the upper arm. There should be no significant change in the dose rate in this sweep of the arm. The NM physician staff are required to inject this agent and to comply with the QMP.

# Laboratory Test Protocols

## LABORATORY TESTS: RBC AND PLASMA VOLUME

CPT code: 78122

**Indications:** This examination is performed to quantitate the volume of the patient's RBCs. It is used to screen patients suspected of having polycythemia vera, which is characterized by an elevated RBC volume and normal plasma volume. This is a study in which the technologist needs to fulfill the CLIA-88 requirements of training and continued proficiency, including pipetting and measuring requirements.

**Patient preparation**

- Verify that the patient has not had large volumes of blood drawn within the past month nor any recent transfusions: both will invalidate the study.
- Check the availability of the radiopharmaceutical (it often has to be special ordered).
- Recommend prior administration of Lugol's solution or SSKI to block the possible accumulation of I-125 in the thyroid gland resulting from the catabolism of iodinated I-125 albumin. This precaution is particularly important when the dosage given is >50 μCi.
- Instruct the patient to be NPO for 4 hours before the study.
- Obtain the height and weight of the patient and recent hematocrit value.

**Scheduling:** Schedule the patient for 2 hours; allow the technologist 4 hours. Only one technologist performs this procedure, so this individual must be available on the day the study is planned.

**Radiopharmaceutical and dose:** 40 to 60 μCi of Cr-51 $Na_2CrO_4$ and 8 to 12 μCi of I-125 human serum albumin (HSA). Cr-51 dose is adjusted for patient weight if ≤45 kg or >90 kg. Radioiodinated serum albumin dose is not adjusted for patient weight.

### Plasma Volume

1. Draw one purple background tube of blood for Cr-RBC labeling (save 5 ml for background).
2. Inject the entire contents of the iodinated HSA I-125 (Isojex) syringe intravenously. Rinse the syringe at least twice with the patient's blood while the needle remains in the vein.
3. After 5 to 10 minutes, withdraw 30 ml of blood from arm opposite the injection arm. Use purple top tubes.
4. Remove a large sample for a microhematocrit determination.
5. Pipette 4 ml of whole blood into a counting vial or test tube.
6. Centrifuge the remaining blood, and pipette 4 ml of plasma into another counting vial or test tube.

7. Count the standard, whole blood, and plasma sample for 5 minutes each or a minimum of 10,000 counts.
8. Count background for an equivalent time, as in previous step, and subtract from the plasma, whole blood, and standard counts.

### RBC Volume

Note: Check the calibration of the analytical balance before starting this test.

1. Prepare the sterile vial:
   a. Aseptically add 4 ml anticoagulant citrate phosphate dextrose (ACD) solution. Make sure there is air behind the solution in the syringe to express all the ACD out of the needle and into the vial.
   b. In the same manner, add the Cr-51 to the vial. *Caution:* Do not add ACD and Cr-51 together more than a minute or two before the patient's blood is added because ACD can reduce the chromium and hinder the tagging process.
2. Withdraw 25 to 30 ml of the patient's blood into the syringe using a 19-gauge needle. Add 5 to 10 ml into a purple-topped Vacutainer labeled "bkg." Add 20 ml into the sterile vial containing ACD and Cr-51.
3. Mix vial gently every 5 minutes for 30 minutes. During this time, obtain a hematocrit from the background sample. Use two capillary tubes and centrifuge over 4 minutes. Apply the appropriate correction factor from the table provided and then transfer 4 ml volumetrically into a counting tube. Label this tube #1.
4. At the end of 30 minutes add the 50 mg of ascorbic acid and mix well. Use air to expel all the ascorbic acid from the needle.
5. Draw the contents of the vial into a clean syringe using a 19-gauge needle. Put 3 to 5 ml into a red-topped Vacutainer tube labeled "standard." Put a clean needle on the syringe and weigh on the Mettler balance. Record the weight and volume of blood in the syringe.
6. Inject the contents of the syringe into vein of the patient, and note which arm was used. Weigh the empty syringe and needle after injection. Record the weight.
7. Allow the chromated cells to be thoroughly distributed throughout the patient's total blood volume. Allow at least 25 minutes.
8. Collect a 25-minute post dose injection sample from the opposite arm into two purple-top Vacutainer tubes.
9. a. Volumetrically pipette 1 ml of patient's standard into a test tube. Pipette slowly so that RBCs are not left on the walls of the pipette. Centrifuge 10 minutes. Remove the plasma.

Patient name _____  MR number _____

Date _____  Height (in inches) _____

Weight (in lb) _____ ÷ 2.2 = _____ kg

Hct _____ % × 0.92 (constant) TB$_c$ × _____ Df = HCT$_c$ _____

ACD _____ ml + Cr-51 _____ ml + Ascorbate _____ ml = Total _____ ml

I-125 IHSA: Lot # _____  Dose _____

NaCr-51: Lot # _____  Dose _____

Syringe Wt.  Full _____ g – Empty _____ g =

Net _____ g ÷ 1.057 g/ml = _____ ml

Observed volume in syringe _____ ml

| Plasma volume | CPM | Net CPM | RBC volume | CPM | Net CPM |
|---|---|---|---|---|---|
| 1. Pt. RISA Bkg* | | _____ | 6. Pt. Cr-51 Bkg* | | _____ |
| 2. I-125 Rm. Bkg* | | _____ | 7. Cr-51 Rm Bkg* | | _____ |
| 3. 10 min. IHSA | _____ | _____ | 8. Cr-51 STD* | | _____ |
| 4. Whole Blood | _____ | _____ | 9. Cr-51 STD* | | _____ |
| 5. STD* | | _____ | STD Ave. | | _____ |
| | | | 10. 25 min PT | _____ | |
| | | | 11. 25 min PT | _____ | |
| | | | Avg 25 min PT | _____ | _____ |

*Counter does automatically.

| Plasma volume (PV) | RBC volume (RBCV) |
|---|---|
| $PV\ (ml) = \dfrac{\text{Net standard count} \times 4{,}000}{\text{Net plasma count}}$ | RBCV = (Vol Inj Bld) (Corr HCT) (Cr-51 STD) (100) = (25 min PT) |
| | RBCV = (____) (____) (____) (100) = _____ ml |
| $\text{Whole blood volume (ml)} = \dfrac{\text{Net standard count} \times 4{,}000}{\text{Net whole blood count}}$ | |
| RBCV (ml) = WBV – PV = _____ ml | |
| $\text{Radioactive hematocrit} = \dfrac{RBCV}{WBV} = $ _____ | |

RBC volume = _____ ml ÷ weight _____ kg = _____ ml/kg

Total BV = PV + RBCV = _____ ml ÷ weight _____ kg = _____ ml/kg

Technologist signature _____

FIG. 30-15. Worksheet for RBC plasma volume

b. • Add 3 ml of sterile saline. Mix well. Centrifuge. Aspirate supernatant and discard. Repeat twice more. This process removes excess Cr-51 not tagged to the RBCs.

• What remains is the number of red cells contained in 1 ml of the chromated cells injected into the patient. It is necessary to dilute this sample 100-fold because the disparity in count rate between standard and patient samples would introduce an electronic counting error. The count rates should be similar.

c. After the third washing, add distilled water instead of saline. Transfer to a 100-ml volumetric flask using several water washes. Dilute to mark etched on flask. Mix well.

d. Volumetrically pipette two 4-ml samples into counting tubes. Label these tubes #2 and #3.

10. Volumetrically pipette two 4-ml samples of patient's 25-minute postinjection whole blood into counting tubes. Label these #4 and #5. Again, be careful to pipette slowly. Mark the volume. Centrifuge for 10 minutes. Carefully aspirate plasma off and discard. Using deionized water, return volume to mark. This removes Cr-51 not tagged to the RBCs.

## Calculations

1. Count all tubes for 10 minutes.

2. Fill in all spaces on the worksheet (Fig. 30-15).
3. Calculate volumes using the formulas provided on the worksheet.
4. Have all calculations checked by another technologist and countersigned.

**Interpretation:** This test was the primary means of diagnosing polycythemia vera, but when the hematocrit is high, a low serum erythropoietin can provide sufficient documentation. The values obtained are compared with normals (provided by sex and body surface area) to determine if there is a significant difference. In general, one standard deviation is 11% of the value, so the normal range is ±22%. Normal RBC volume range in men is 25 to 35 ml/kg and 20 to 30 ml/kg in females. The normal plasma volume is 40 ml/kg in both men and women.

Polycythemia rubra vera demonstrates an increased RBC mass with normal plasma volume. Other causes of increased hematocrit usually have a decreased plasma volume and normal RBC mass.

## LABORATORY TEST 2: RBC PROFICIENCY TEST

### Labeling of cells

1. Weigh the empty polyethylene bottle.
2. Transfer blood from blood bag into bottle. Weigh the filled bottle.

---

**Calculations for RCV in bottle**

Volume of original blood in bottle:

Full bottle _____ g

Empty bottle _____ g

Full bottle – empty bottle = _____ g ÷ 1.057 = _____ ml    **A**

Blood withdrawn from bottle:

Full syringe _____ g

Empty syringe (prior to filling) _____ g

Full syringe – empty syringe = _____ g ÷ 1.1057 = _____ ml  **B**

Blood reinjected into bottle:

Full syringe _____ g

Empty syringe (postinjection of blood) _____ g

Full syringe – empty syringe = _____ g ÷ 1.057 = _____ ml   **C**

Calculation for actual RCV in bottle

Total ml in bottle – (ml withdrawn from bottle) + (ml reinjected into bottle)

A – B + C = ml blood in bottle

ml blood in bottle × Hct = actual RCV in bottle

**FIG. 30-16.**

3. Subtract weight of empty bottle from weight of full bottle to obtain grams of blood in bottle. Then divide by 1.057 (specific gravity of blood) to obtain the correct number of milliliters of blood in bottle (Fig. 30-16).

4. Express 5 μCi of Cr-51 into evacuated sterile vial. Draw air into Cr-51 syringe. Use the air as a plunger so that all the Cr-51 is expressed into the vial.

5. Weigh empty syringe. Mix blood in bottle and remove 20 ml of blood. Weigh full syringe. Transfer 5 ml to one purple-top tube for a background sample. Then add the remaining blood to the vial containing Cr-51.

6. Incubate Cr-51 blood at room temperature for 30 minutes with occasional mixing.

7. Run a hematocrit from the background sample. Pipette 4 ml into a counting vial.

8. After the 30-minute incubation, add 50 mg ascorbic acid to vial using air as a plunger to remove all ascorbic acid from syringe. Mix well.

9. Subtract weight of full syringe from weight of empty syringe. Divide by 1.057 (specific gravity) to obtain milliliters of blood withdrawn from bottle.

### Reinjection of labeled cells

1. Draw entire contents of vial into a 20-ml syringe.
2. Put 2 to 3 ml of the chromated cells into a red-top tube labeled "standard."
3. Weigh the syringe on the Mettler balance. Note how many milliliters of blood are in the syringe.
4. Inject the chromated cells back into the polyethylene bottle containing blood.
5. Reweigh the syringe. Subtract empty weight from full weight to arrive at grams of blood injected. Divide grams of blood by 1.057 (specific gravity) to obtain milliliters of blood injected.
6. Allow chromated cells to equilibrate with blood in bottle for 30 minutes. Gently swirl every 5 minutes for thorough mixing.
7. Withdraw 10 ml of blood (patient test sample) and transfer into two purple-top tubes.

### Preparation of standard

1. Pipette 1 ml of standard sample into a red-top tube.
2. Centrifuge for 10 minutes at 2,000 to 2,500 rpm. Remove supernate.
3. Add 3 ml of saline, mix well, and repeat centrifugation. This will wash any Cr-51 not inside RBCs.
4. Aspirate supernate and discard.
5. Using deionized water, transfer all the RBCs to a 100-ml disposable volumetric flask. Dilute to 100-ml mark. Mix well.
6. Pipette two 4-ml samples of the diluted standard solution into counting vials. Standard samples are ready to count.

### Preparation of test sample

1. Pipette two 4-ml test samples into counting vials. Put a line on the counting vial at the level of the meniscus.

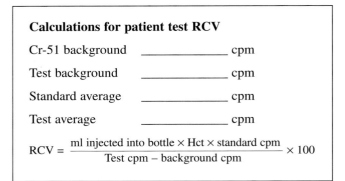

**Calculations for patient test RCV**

Cr-51 background _____ cpm

Test background _____ cpm

Standard average _____ cpm

Test average _____ cpm

$$RCV = \frac{ml\ injected\ into\ bottle \times Hct \times standard\ cpm}{Test\ cpm - background\ cpm} \times 100$$

**FIG. 30-17.**

2. Centrifuge test sample vials for 10 minutes at 2,000 to 2,500 rpm. Aspirate off supernate. Replace supernate with deionized water to meniscus line.

3. Now test samples are ready to count.

4. Use Figs. 30-16 and 30-17 to determine actual and calculated test RCV.

## LABORATORY TEST 3: RBC SURVIVAL AND SEQUESTRATION

**CPT code:** 78130 RBC Survival, 78135 Sequestration

**Indications:** This examination determines how long the patient's RBCs remain in circulation. It can be an important measurement in patients with faulty RBC production or abnormal splenic function. RBC survival studies are useful in determining the survival of RBCs in hemolytic anemias and the effects of therapy in patients with hemolytic anemia.

**Patient preparation:** This study should be scheduled to start on a Monday, when the patient will have an RBC volume measurement done. The patient will return Tuesday, Wednesday, and Thursday of that week; then on Monday, Wednesday, and Friday for each of the following 2 to 4 weeks.

**Scheduling**

• Check the availability of the radiopharmaceutical (needed only for first visit).
• Day 1: Schedule patient for 1 hour. Allow technologist 2 hours.
• All other days: Allow 1 hour.

**Radiopharmaceutical and dose:** 80 to 120 μCi, Cr-51 $Na_2CrO_4$.

**RBC survival procedure:** Perform a Red Cell Volume Determination (CPT code 78122) as described above. Draw a 30-minute postinjection sample (instead of 25 minutes, as in Red Cell Volume Determination). This sample is used as a standard against subsequent samples for determining RBC survival.

Blood samples

1. At 24, 48, and 72 hours after injection, and three times a week for approximately 2 more weeks, draw a blood

sample from the patient using a Vacutainer tube (lavender top, EDTA).

2. Determine the hematocrit for each sample. Correct for total body hematocrit and plasma trapping.
3. Volumetrically pipette a 4-ml aliquot of whole blood from each sample into a counting tube labeled with patient name, history number, and date. Mark the meniscus of the fluid on the tube.
4. Centrifuge the sample. Remove the plasma using a Pasteur pipette. Discard the plasma.
5. Add water to the original volume line to "lake" the RBCs. Cap the tube. Mix well.
6. Preserve the samples in a refrigerator until the end of the study.

At the conclusion of the study all samples are counted in the well counter, and the cpm per ml is calculated for each sample. This value is used to determine RBC survival. Using semilog graph paper, plot cpm per ml on the log scale versus time on the linear scale. The survival time of the cells is determined from a straight line drawn through these points extrapolated back to time zero.

The binding of the Cr-51 to the cells is relatively tight, and when labeled cells are handled carefully they will circulate in the body until they live out their normal life span and are sequestered in the spleen. If the time pattern of loss of radioactivity is followed, a measure of the life span of red cells within the body is obtained. The period of analysis is the time for the activity to fall to one-half the original level in the blood.

**RBC sequestration procedure:** RBCs are labeled with Cr-51 ($Na_2CrO_4$) in a manner similar to that described for Cr-51 ($Na_2CrO_4$) labeled blood volume studies except that a larger dose of Cr-51 ($Na_2CrO_4$) is used. The labeled blood is injected intravenously. Sequestration is decided by external monitoring of the heart, liver, and spleen.

Organ counts: With the uptake probe correctly peaked for counting Cr-51 and a 10-minute room background count done, 10-minute organ counts are taken over the heart, liver, and spleen beginning 30 minutes after injection. Record the counts. These counts are repeated at 24, 48, and 72 hours, then three times a week for approximately 2 more weeks. An NM physician should be consulted to determine completion of the study.

Marking the patient: With the patient in a supine position, mark the following areas with indelible ink. An NM staff physician should be consulted for marking the areas initially.

1. Heart (precordium): Place the center of the collimator over the fourth interspace approximately 4 cm to the left of the sternum, angling 15 degrees medially.
2. Liver: Place the center of the collimator over the ninth and tenth ribs on the right between the midclavicular and anterior axillary line angling 15 degrees cephalad.
3. Spleen: With the patient in a prone position, place the center of the collimator over the ninth and tenth ribs on the left at post axillary line, or when splenomegaly is marked the Nuclear Medicine physician will instruct the technologist on the correct position.

Calculations: At the conclusion of the study the following ratios should be calculated for each day:

1. $\frac{\text{Net cpm spleen}}{\text{Net cpm heart}}$

2. $\frac{\text{Net cpm liver}}{\text{Net cpm heart}}$

3. $\frac{\text{Net cpm spleen}}{\text{Net cpm liver}}$

Plot the ratios against the day of study on linear graph paper. Note: All calculations must be checked by another technologist and countersigned.

**Limitations of the procedure**

- A falsely shortened survival time due to careless handling of cells during the labeling process
- A falsely shortened survival time due to GI blood loss, urinary tract blood loss, or surgical procedures
- A falsely increased survival time due to transfusions during the procedure, effectively diluting the label

**Interpretation**

RBC survival: The chromium RBC half-time is about 25 to 35 days in normal subjects. This is because the labeling is of a mixture of RBCs of all maturities (zero through 120 days, mean 60 days) and the label elutes off the RBCs with time (~1%/day).

RBC sequestration: Even though the major site of removal of sequestered cells is the spleen, the liver also accumulates Cr-51 released from the normally dying senescent cells. Due to the large mass of the liver, the ratio of the liver-to-spleen distribution is almost equal. When the spleen accumulates more counts, hypersplenism may be present. When the liver accumulates more counts, intravascular hemolysis may be indicated.

In normal subjects the spleen-to-liver ratio is about 1:1. In patients with active splenic sequestration, the ratio varies from 2:1 to 4:1. The spleen-to-precordium ratio, however, provides a better index of the degree of splenic sequestration, because some patient livers may also be sequestering erythrocytes. Spleen-to-precordium ratios >2:1 are considered abnormal. An initial elevation of the spleen-to-precordium ratio reflects an increased splenic blood pool, whereas a progressive and gradual increase indicates sequestration of labeled cells.

## LABORATORY TEST 4: VITAMIN B$_{12}$ ABSORPTION STUDY WITH INTRINSIC FACTOR (DICOPAC KIT)

CPT code: 78270 vitamin B$_{12}$ absorption, 78271 vitamin B$_{12}$ absorption-intrinsic factor
**Indications:** Evaluation of suspected vitamin B$_{12}$ deficiency
**Patient preparation**

- The test should not be initiated within 24 hours of a therapeutic dose (1,000 µg) of vitamin B$_{12}$.
- Bone marrow examinations should precede the administration of the dose for this test. The flushing parenteral

dose of vitamin B$_{12}$ will alter the bone marrow picture and may suggest alternative incorrect diagnoses.

### Scheduling

- Patient fasts for 12 hours before test and for 2 hours after test dose.
- A 12-hour preadministration urine sample for background radioactivity is collected.

**Dosage and administration:** A single patient test unit dose consists of the following:

- One purple and white capsule containing 0.25 μg cyanocobalamin Co-57 (normal activity 0.5 μCi at calibration date) bound to human gastric juice for oral administration.
- One red and ivory capsule containing 0.25 μg cyanocobalamin Co-58 (normal activity 0.8 μCi at calibration date) for oral administration.
- One ampule of unlabeled cyanocobalamin (1 mg) for intramuscular injection.

### Procedure

1. One single test unit is used. Both capsules (one purple and white and one red and ivory) are given to the patient at the same time.
2. The cyanocobalamin injection (1 mg) is given IM by a physician, either immediately after oral administration of the capsules or within the next 2 hours.
3. Urine excreted during the 24 hours after oral administration of the capsules is collected for counting.
4. Preparation of samples
   a. Measure the total urine volume of the 24-hour urine collection.
   b. Mix the urine to ensure homogeneity.
   c. Accurately pipette an aliquot of urine for counting.
      - 10-ml 12-hour background urine
      - 10-ml 24-hour postdose urine
   d. 1.0-ml aliquot of the Co-57 standard solution brought up to 10 ml with water for counting
   e. 1.0-ml aliquot of the Co-58 standard solution brought up to 10 ml with water for counting
5. Counting procedure
   a. All samples and standards are counted in the auto-gamma counter in scintillation vials.
   b. Order of placement
      - Background urine
      - Co-57 standard
      - Co-58 standard
      - 24-hour urine
6. All calculations must be checked by another technologist and countersigned.

**Interpretation:** Vitamin B$_{12}$ (cyanocobalamin) is a trace vitamin found in foods of animal origin, such as milk, eggs, and meat, but virtually absent in vegetables and fruits. Humans are unable to synthesize the vitamin, so they must obtain it from ani-

mal or bacterial sources. An exclusively vegetarian diet will eventually result in a nutritional vitamin B$_{12}$ deficiency.

Vitamin B$_{12}$ is absorbed in the GI tract in humans, then stored in the liver and eventually excreted in the urine. The normal human small intestine is >7 m long. Vitamin B$_{12}$ is absorbed over the last 2 to 4 m. Before absorption can take place in the ileum, the vitamin must be bound to the glycoprotein known as *intrinsic factor,* which is secreted by parietal cells in the gastric mucosa. Specific receptors in the terminal ileum facilitate the absorption of the vitamin-intrinsic factor complex. The number of such receptors limits the amount of vitamin B$_{12}$ that can be absorbed at any one time. The intrinsic factor slowly becomes separated from the vitamin B$_{12}$ in or on the epithelial cells lining the ileal villi. The vitamin B$_{12}$ molecule reaches the blood in the portal veins in approximately 3 to 4 hours, attaining a maximum blood level 8 to 12 hours after its ingestion.

The package insert contains the normal result and abnormal result interpretations.

### LABORATORY TESTS: CLIA-88 ASSOCIATED 5: (RUSSELL 2-POINT) ABSOLUTE GFR

CPT code: 78725
**Indications:** To determine global GFR
**Patient preparation:** It is necessary that the patient be well hydrated.
**Scheduling**

- Schedule the patient early in the morning (8 AM) because this test takes about 4 hours to complete. Timing: The first 30 minutes are used for IV hydration, then 60- and 180-minute blood samples are obtained, then 60 minutes is required for counting and processing of samples.
- Obtain the patient's height and weight.
- Nondiabetic: NPO 12 to 16 hours
- Diabetic: NPO 10 hours
- The patient must drink 500 to 800 ml (about three 8-oz glasses) of fluid within 3 hours before the study.
- Two patients may be scheduled per day at 20-minute intervals (but check with supervisor for all studies).

**Radiopharmaceutical and dose:** 2.4 to 3.6 mCi Tc-99m DTPA in 1.0 ml. Dose is adjusted for patient weight if ≤45 kg or ≥90 kg. Two equal doses (within ±5%) are required: one for injection and one for a counting standard. If multiple patients are done the same day, the same standard can be used for all of them. The purity of the Tc-99m DTPA must be >98%, as determined by ITLC chromatography within 1 hour of injection.
**Procedure**

1. Insert a 22-gauge Angiocath IV line and infuse at least 250 ml normal saline for hydration.
2. Count dose in dose calibrator just before injection. Start the stopwatch at injection. Flush the injection syringe with saline at least 3 times. Assay the complete apparatus in dose calibrator for postinjection reading.

3. Time the blood samples in relation to the time of injection: Timing is critical. Draw the blood samples at approximately 60 and 180 minutes after injection. Accurately note the stopwatch time (SWT) for each sample.
   a. Blood should not be hemolyzed. If blood is hemolyzed, redraw and spin. If a nonhemolyzed sample cannot be drawn, discontinue the test. Check with NM staff physician as to when to reschedule.
   b. Label all samples with time and patient name.

Blood processing: Mix the blood well with the anticoagulant after drawing. Immediately centrifuge at 1,000$g$ to 2,000$g$ for 10 minutes. The plasma should not have any red color, indicating lysis of RBCs: If the plasma is red, draw another sample. Record time. Pipette duplicate 1.0-ml plasma aliquots into Centrifree ultrafiltration devices, ensuring that both devices have equal amounts of plasma. Centrifuge in a fixed angle head centrifuge for 15 minutes at 1,000$g$ to 2,000$g$; a swinging bucket head results in inadequate ultrafiltration. When the centrifuge stops, carefully retrieve the Centrifree apparatus. Remove filtrate cup containing the clear, colorless ultrafiltrate. Pipette accurately 100 µl from each cup into scintillation tubes. Cap tube, label, and save for counting.

Standard preparation: Use a 1:10,000 serial dilution for making the counting standard. Assay the standard dose in dose calibrator; record activity and time. It should be ±5% of the patient dose (decay corrected). Carefully inject the standard into a 100-ml volumetric flask containing 50 to 75 ml deionized water. Rinse the syringe three times with deionized water; add to the flask. Reassay the syringe, including the needle cap. If >2% remains, rinse again and reassay. Calculate the decay-corrected difference; record along with assay time. Add water to fill the flask to the mark, and mix thoroughly. Accurately pipette 1.0 ml of this 1:100 dilution into a second 100-ml volumetric flask labeled 1:10,000 dilution, which contains 50 to 75 ml deionized water, fill to mark, and mix thoroughly. Accurately pipette 100 µl of this 1:10,000 dilution into each of two scintillation tubes. Cap the tubes, label, and save for counting.

Counting procedure: Count the tubes (two standards and two patient tubes) in the autogamma counter with 140 keV ±20% window and background correction. Record the starting time. There should be at least 10,000 counts per tube.

Computer processing: Calculate the GFR by the Russell 2-point method. Normalize the results to 1.73 m² body surface area using the formula:

$$BSA \ (cm) = [wt \ (kg)]^{0.245} \times [ht \ (cm)]^{0.725} \times 71.84$$

**Interpretation:** Normal GFR is 125 ml per minute per 1.73 m².

## LABORATORY TEST 6: SMALL BOWEL TRANSPLANT

CPT code: 78299

**Indications:** To determine rejection of a small bowel transplant. The study is performed after small intestine transplantation, routinely postoperatively, then every 7 days as clinically indicated.

**Patient preparation:** NPO 2 hours predose and 2 hours postdose. Foley catheter in place for pediatric patients.

**Scheduling:** Wait 48 hours after any prior administration of Tc-99m. This is a laboratory test, so no gamma camera time is required.

1. Schedule the patient to arrive at 8:30 AM for the dose administration of Tc-99m DTPA through J-tube.
2. Instruct the ward to collect the patient's urine at two timed intervals:
   a. *For the next 6 hours.* Discard any urine collected prior to tracer administration. Collect all urine until ~2:30 PM; send this to NM to arrive by 3:00 PM. The 6-hour collection is processed so that immediate results are available.
   b. *From 6 to 24 hours after tracer administration.* The 6- to 24-hour collection must arrive promptly in NM at 24 hours after tracer administration. Two 5-ml aliquots of urine will be counted, and the total urine volume measured.

Note: It is imperative that **all** urine be collected.

**Radiopharmaceutical and dose:** Tc-99m DTPA, 400 to 600 µCi in 10 ml followed by up to 300 ml water. Dose and volume are adjusted for children only.

**Dose preparation:** Prepare a Tc-99m DTPA dilution containing about 1.0 mCi in enough purified water to yield 50 µCi/ml at administration. The DTPA % binding should be >98%.

1. Place 1 mCi DTPA (calibrated at the time of administration) in a scintillation vial. Assay in dose calibrator and note volume ($V_{DTPA}$).
2. Add purified water (~20 ml) to make a dose concentration of 50 µCi/ml at administration time, mix well. The calculation of added water is made: [(assay from step 1 decay corrected to the administration time in mCi)/0.05 (mCi/ml)] – $V_{DTPA}$
3. Dispense a 500-µCi patient dose into scintillation vial (~10.0 ml).
4. Use remaining 500 µCi to make counting standard (~10.0 ml).
5. Use a pipette for all manipulations in lieu of a syringe; the accuracy of the test depends on accurate volume measurements.

### Standard preparation

1. Assay the counting standard (S) and accurately pipette 500 µl into a 250-ml volumetric flask.
2. Add purified water to the fill line of the flask. Mix well.
3. Dispense two 5-ml aliquots of the dilution for use as counting standards.

### Administration

1. Assay dose (D) and record activity and time.
2. Administer the dose through J-tube (sometimes via a G-tube) with piston syringe. Rinse syringe several

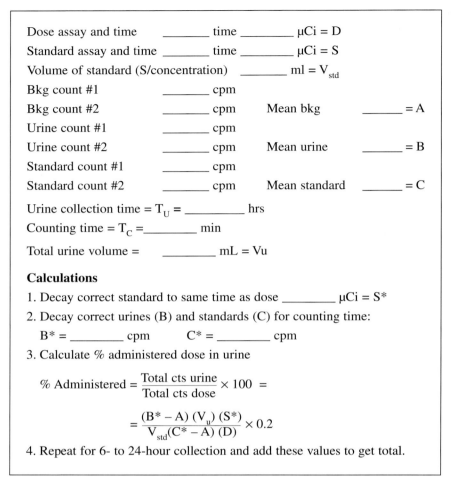

Dose assay and time _____ time _____ μCi = D

Standard assay and time _____ time _____ μCi = S

Volume of standard (S/concentration) _____ ml = V$_{std}$

Bkg count #1 _____ cpm

Bkg count #2 _____ cpm     Mean bkg _____ = A

Urine count #1 _____ cpm

Urine count #2 _____ cpm     Mean urine _____ = B

Standard count #1 _____ cpm

Standard count #2 _____ cpm     Mean standard _____ = C

Urine collection time = T$_U$ = _____ hrs

Counting time = T$_C$ = _____ min

Total urine volume = _____ mL = Vu

**Calculations**

1. Decay correct standard to same time as dose _____ μCi = S*

2. Decay correct urines (B) and standards (C) for counting time:

    B* = _____ cpm     C* = _____ cpm

3. Calculate % administered dose in urine

$$\% \text{ Administered} = \frac{\text{Total cts urine}}{\text{Total cts dose}} \times 100 =$$

$$= \frac{(B^* - A)\,(V_u)\,(S^*)}{V_{std}(C^* - A)\,(D)} \times 0.2$$

4. Repeat for 6- to 24-hour collection and add these values to get total.

**FIG. 30-18.** Small bowel worksheet.

times with 20 ml normal saline to ensure quantitative administration of dose.

3. Clamp or cap off the J-tube for 6 hours.
4. Assay the residual activity and record result. If >10 μCi (2%) remains, subtract this amount from administered activity.

## Counting

1. Measure total urine volume and record (V$_U$).
2. Mix well and place two 5-ml aliquots in scintillation vials.
3. Prepare two 5-ml blanks of water for background correction.
4. At 6 hours, use the thyroid uptake probe or MCA (the count rate is too high for the autogamma counter). Set on the 140-keV photopeak using one of the standards. Turn the probe upright and set the vials directly on the center of the crystal and count for 60 seconds ensuring that there are no dead-time losses.
5. At 24 hours, count the eight vials (two background, two standard, four urine) for 5 minutes in the autogamma counter.
6. If the urine count rate is <2,000 cpm, count all tubes for long enough to get 10,000 counts (T = 10,000 counts per urine count rate).

**Data:** Use the Small Bowel Worksheet (Fig. 30-18) to do the calculations.

**Interpretation:** Normally <1% of the administered dose is excreted in the first 6 hours and <2% total at 24 hours. For transplant rejection, >2% excretion is suggestive in the first 6 hours, >5% for 24 hours.

## LABORATORY TEST 7: PREVENTING BLOOD-BORNE PATHOGENS

### Labeling blood elements (WBCs, RBCs, platelets)

- Only one labeling procedure will be done in an area at one time to avoid mixing of patient samples and doses.
- The entire labeling procedure will be done by the same person, that is, the same person draws the blood, labels the product, and reinjects the labeled product.
- All used syringes, needles, and tubes are discarded in sharps (needle) disposal boxes immediately after use.
- Sharps disposal boxes are kept in each camera room, injection area, wet lab, and radiopharmacy.
- Surgical gloves will be worn when labeling blood elements.
- New needles and syringes will be used as needed.

- All employees are encouraged to get hepatitis B vaccine.
- RBC labeling for MUGA and GI bleeding studies will be done either in the laminar flow hood or in the patient room (one patient at a time). The modified in vivo technique will be done in the patient imaging room.

## LABORATORY TEST 8: LABELING TECHNETIUM RBCS

### Indications and CPT codes

To evaluate:

- Heart function: Rest MUGA Scan (CPT code 78472), Rest-Stress MUGA Scan (CPT code 78476)
- GI bleed: GI Bleeding Scan (CPT code 78278)
- Hepatic hemangiomas: Liver Scan with Flow (CPT code 78216)
- Any other abnormalities of vasculature.

**Patient preparation:** NPO for 4 hours for MUGA scan only
**Radiopharmaceutical and dose** Tc-99m $TcO_4^-$, up to 30 mCi, depending on procedure. Dose is adjusted for patient weight if ≤45 kg or ≥90 kg.
### UltraTag RBC technique

1. Collect 1 to 3 ml of blood using heparin (preferred) or ACD.
2. Transfer this via a 19- or 21-gauge needle to reaction vial supplied with UltraTag kit. Mix by inversion, allowing 5 minutes.
3. Add contents of UltraTag RBC syringe I. Gently invert four or five times.
4. Add contents of syringe II. Gently invert four or five times. Then allow reaction to continue for 20 minutes. Gently invert the vial containing the blood every 5 minutes to ensure adequate mixing and optimal tagging.
5. Shield vial. Add up to 3 ml of Tc-99m $TcO_4^-$.
6. Mix by gentle inversion four or five times. Then allow reaction to continue for 20 minutes.
7. Inject labeled RBCs into patient from which cells were taken. Use cells within 30 minutes of preparation after assaying.
8. Labeling efficiency is >95%.

**Modified in vivo:** *Optional procedure only if cold PYP is made, or no UltraTag is available*

1. Inject the patient with 10 µg/kg = 0.015 ml/kg cold PYP reconstituted with 3 ml normal saline (provides stannous ion).
2. Wait 10 to 20 minutes.
3. Draw 1 ml ACD into a 10-ml syringe.
4. Withdraw 5 ml of the patient's blood into the 10-ml syringe, which contains 1 ml of ACD.
   a. Use a 21-gauge butterfly attached to a three-way stopcock.
   b. Flush the system with saline at the end of the blood withdrawing.

5. Inject the Tc-99m $TcO_4^-$ with a 3-ml syringe into the blood-ACD 10-ml syringe via three-way stopcock.
6. Gently invert the syringe containing the blood every minute for 10 minutes to ensure adequate mixing and optimal tagging, or exchange blood between the shielded 3- and 10-ml syringes with the stopcock.
7. Inject the patient's tagged RBCs back into the patient.
8. Labeling efficiency is >85%.

## LABORATORY TEST 9: LABELING LEUKOCYTES WITH TC-99M HMPAO OR IN-111 OXINE

**Introduction:** This entire procedure is carried out in the laminar flow hood. Ensure that the hood is turned on at least 30 minutes before procedure is started. Hydroxyethyl starch (hetastarch) should be removed from refrigerator and HSA and ACD removed from the freezer when the laminar flow hood is turned on. All reagents, tubes, pipettes, syringes, and so forth are sterile. Use only plastic (polypropylene) sterile pipettes.
**Blood harvesting procedure:**

1. Withdraw 40 ml whole blood from the patient into a 50- to 60-ml syringe containing 6 ml citrate, phosphate, dextrose (CPD) anticoagulant (1.5 to 10 ml whole blood). An 18-gauge needle should be used. Total volume of blood and anticoagulant should be 46 ml.
2. Aliquot the blood equally into each of four "A" tubes (approximately 12 ml in each tube) in the laminar flow hood. It is imperative that the "contaminated" syringe does not touch the inner walls of the sterile tubes during the transfer.
3. Add 3 ml of 6% hydroxyethyl starch, at room temperature, to each of the four tubes. Total volume should now be approximately 15 ml per tube.
4. Mix well by inverting the tubes several times. Remove caps, and wipe away excess blood from inside of tube and cap using a sterile cotton-tipped swab. Replace cap. Allow the sample to sediment for 60 minutes at a 45-degree angle in predrilled wooden block.
5. After the sedimentation period, use a sterile plastic pipette to transfer the leukocyte-rich plasma into four "B" tubes. Care must be taken not to include RBCs. Each "B" tube should have a volume of approximately 7 ml.
6. Centrifuge the "B" tubes at 150 × G for 8 minutes. Before centrifuging, ensure that the tubes and metal holders are balanced. Pour or pipette off the supernatant plasma (the leukocyte-poor plasma) and discard (or save for labeling with Tc-99m HMPAO). The plasma should be cloudy due to the presence of platelets. A pellet or button of WBCs should remain at the bottom of the tube. This pellet may be pink if there is RBC contamination.
7. Holding the test tube by the top, tap the bottom of the tube to begin loosening the pellet. Resuspend the leukocyte pellets by gentle agitation with 2 ml of HSA/saline

(0.2 ml of 25% HSA in 40 ml normal saline; at room temperature). Avoid vigorous agitation.

8. Combine the resuspended pellets into one of the original "B" tubes. Bring the volume up to 10 ml by adding HSA/saline. Gently invert the tube several times to ensure uniform mixing.

9. Centrifuge at 150 × G for 8 minutes. Pour or pipette off and discard the supernatant. Resuspend the leukocyte pellet in 2 ml of HSA/saline. Gently mix the suspension and bring up to 10 ml with HSA/saline.

10. Centrifuge at 150 × for 8 minutes (925 rpm on IEC, ~40 on IEC setting). Pour or pipette off and discard supernatant.

11. Resuspend the leukocyte pellet in 5 ml 0.9% saline **without HSA**. If desired, the leukocyte pellet can be resuspended in 1.0 ml leukocyte-poor plasma for Tc-99m HMPAO labeling. Centrifuge at high speed (450 to 2,000$g$) to eliminate platelets and provide a cell-free plasma.

**Labeling:** Start with 600 µCi In-111 oxine *or* 30 mCi of Tc-99m TcO$_4^-$ in 1 ml and vial of HMPAO.

1. Run either In-111 oxine or Tc-99m HMPAO down the side of tube with leukocyte suspension. Rinse syringe with saline several times. Incubate at room temperature for 30 minutes on test tube rotator to ensure optimum labeling.

2. Centrifuge the labeled cells at 150 × G for 8 minutes (setting at ~40 for 1,000 rpm). Pour off the supernatant and save in a "B" tube (to maintain identical geometry when checking for % bound).

3. Resuspend the pellet in 3 to 5 ml 0.9% saline. Be sure the suspension of WBCs is uniform, with no gross clumps visible. If there are gross clumps, check with NM staff physician before proceeding.

### QC, reinjection, and viability

1. a. Assay the 5-ml supernatant in the "B" tube in dose calibrator.
   b. Assay the 5-ml resuspended WBCs in "B" tube in dose calibrator. Calculate the % bound.

$$\% \text{ Bound} = \frac{\mu\text{Ci in WBCs}}{\mu\text{Ci in WBCs} + \mu\text{Ci in supernatant}} \times 100\%$$

   c. Record % bound on request form. If 90% (less with Tc-99m HMPAO) tag is not achieved, check with an NM physician before injecting cells.

*If there is a question of cell viability, do step 2. If not, proceed to step 3.*

2. Using sterile technique, remove 0.2 ml of the cell suspension using a tuberculin syringe. In a 12 × 75–mm test tube prepare a 5:1 suspension of cells to trypan blue (0.5% solution). Mix well and incubate for 30 seconds. Transfer 20 µl or less of the stained cell suspension to a hemocytometer and check for viability of cells. Record results on request form.

3. In the laminar flow hood, using a 20-gauge spinal needle, draw the entire contents of the tube containing the resuspended WBCs into a 20-ml syringe and assay the radioactivity in the dose calibrator. Maximum dose for reinjection is 500 µCi for In-111, 30 mCi for Tc-99m.

4. The labeled cells are now ready to be reinjected into the patient. Reinjection should be accomplished within 1 hour of completion of the labeling procedure.

# SECTION IV

## Appendices

*Textbook of Nuclear Medicine,*
edited by Michael A. Wilson.
Lippincott–Raven Publishers, Philadelphia © 1998.

# APPENDIX A

# Système Internationale Units

The U.S. Trade Act of 1988 includes a provision establishing federal policy to designate the metric system as the preferred measurement system for U.S. trade and commerce. Système International (SI) units are now being used in many countries as the primary measurement system of radioactive materials. The system is slowly coming into use in the United States. Many journals (including those published by the American Medical Association) now require the use of SI units, and U.S. regulatory agencies are beginning to use SI units as well as conventional units in regulations. It is the policy of the U.S. government that regulations should not impede the transition to SI units. The government also required all federal agencies to adopt the metric system for business-related activities by 1992, except where it proves impractical. Recently, the Department of Transportation has required the use of SI units in transport of radionuclides.

The U.S. Council for Energy Awareness Committee on Radionuclides and Radiopharmaceuticals is seeking to familiarize users of radioactive materials with SI units and to facilitate their use in the United States. The SI unit for radioactivity is the becquerel (Bq), and is defined as one nuclear transformation per second. It is a small unit when compared to the curie (Ci), but it does have the convenience of relating directly to count rate once corrections have been made for counting efficiency.

Most suppliers of radioactive materials, including the National Institute of Standards Technology (NIST) have been using dual units (curies and becquerels) in catalogs, product literature, and labeling for some time and plan to do so for the foreseeable future. The European Economic Community (EEC) has stated that it will accept only SI units for radioactivity after 1999, and it is anticipated that all suppliers of radioactive products will be using only SI units at that time. In Canada, Atomic Energy Control Board documents produced since 1985 have been in SI units only, and conversion of regulations is in progress.

## SI UNITS

1 becquerel (Bq) = 1 disintegration per second
1 becquerel = $2.7027 \times 10^{-11}$ curie or ~27 picocuries (pCi).

Source: Modified from the U.S. Council for Energy Awareness, Committee on Radionuclides and Radiopharmaceuticals

**TABLE A-1.** *Conversions for radioactivity*

| Curie units | | Becquerel units |
|---|---|---|
| μCi | to | kBq |
| mCi | to | Mbq |
| Ci | to | GBq |
| 0.1 | | 3.1 |
| 0.25 | | 9.25 |
| 0.5 | | 18.5 |
| 0.75 | | 27.75 |
| 1 | | 37 |
| 2 | | 74 |
| 3 | | 111 |
| 5 | | 185 |
| 7 | | 259 |
| 10 | | 370 |
| 20 | | 740 |
| 25 | | 925 |
| μCi | to | MBq |
| mCi | to | GBq |
| Ci | to | TBq |
| 50 | | 1.85 |
| 60 | | 2.22 |
| 100 | | 3.7 |
| 200 | | 7.4 |
| 250 | | 9.25 |
| 500 | | 18.5 |
| 800 | | 29.6 |
| 1,000 | | 37 |

To convert becquerels to curies, divide the becquerel figure by $37 \times 10^9$ (alternatively, multiply the becquerel figure by $2.7027 \times 10^{-11}$).

1 curie (Ci) = $3.7 \times 10^{10}$ disintegrations per second or 37 gigabecquerels (GBq). To convert curies to becquerels, multiply the curie figure by $37 \times 10^9$ (Table A-1).

To convert from one unit to another, read across from one column to the other ensuring the units are in the same line of the column headings. For example:

From top of Table A-1:

0.1 mCi = 3.7 MBq
0.1 Ci = 3.7 GBq

From bottom of Table A-1:

50 mCi = 1.85 GBq
50 Ci = 1.85 TBq

## OTHER SI RADIATION MEASUREMENT UNITS

### Absorbed Dose

This is the amount of energy imparted to matter, and the rad has been the unit of measurement. The SI unit for absorbed dose is the gray (Gy).

1 Gray (Gy) = 100 rad
1 centiGray (cGy) = 1 rad
1 rad = 0.01 Gy (1 cGy)

1 mrad = 0.01 mGy

One roentgen of x-radiation in the energy range of 0.1 to 3.0 MeV produces 0.96 rad (0.96 cGy) in tissue.

## DOSE EQUIVALENT

The dose equivalent is the absorbed dose multiplied by modifying factors, such as a quality factor (accounts for the biological effect of different types of radiation) and the dose distribution factor. The rem is the unit of measurement that has been used, and the SI unit is the sievert (Sv).

1 Sv = 100 rem
1 rem = 0.01 Sv
1 mrem = 0.01 mSv (10 μSv)

*Textbook of Nuclear Medicine,*
edited by Michael A. Wilson.
Lippincott–Raven Publishers, Philadelphia © 1998.

# APPENDIX B

# Dose Adjustment Nomogram

| Weight (kg) | Fraction of normal adult dose | Weight (kg) | Fraction of normal adult dose |
|---|---|---|---|
| 1 | 0.059 | 105 | 1.310 |
| 2 | 0.093 | 110 | 1.352 |
| 3 | 0.122 | 115 | 1.392 |
| 4 | 0.148 | 120 | 1.432 |
| 5 | 0.172 | 125 | 1.472 |
| 6 | 0.194 | 130 | 1.511 |
| 7 | 0.215 | 135 | 1.549 |
| 8 | 0.236 | 140 | 1.587 |
| 9 | 0.255 | 145 | 1.625 |
| 10 | 0.273 | 150 | 1.662 |
| 11 | 0.291 | 155 | 1.699 |
| 12 | 0.309 | 160 | 1.735 |
| 13 | 0.326 | 165 | 1.771 |
| 14 | 0.342 | 170 | 1.807 |
| 15 | 0.358 | 175 | 1.842 |
| 20 | 0.434 | 180 | 1.877 |
| 25 | 0.503 | 185 | 1.912 |
| 30 | 0.568 | 190 | 1.946 |
| 35 | 0.630 | 195 | 1.980 |
| 40 | 0.689 | 200 | 2.014 |
| 45 | 0.745 | 205 | 2.047 |
| | | 210 | 2.080 |
| **46–89** | **1.000** | 215 | 2.113 |
| 90 | 1.182 | 220 | 2.146 |
| 95 | 1.226 | 225 | 2.178 |
| 100 | 1.268 | 230 | 2.210 |

*Textbook of Nuclear Medicine,*
edited by Michael A. Wilson.
Lippincott–Raven Publishers, Philadelphia © 1998.

# APPENDIX C

# Abbreviations

| | | | |
|---|---|---|---|
| AAA | abdominal aortic aneurysm | BERT | Background Equivalent Radiation Time |
| AACC | American Association of Clinical Chemistry | BGO | bismuth germanate |
| AB | antibody | BKG | background |
| ABNM | American Board of Nuclear Medicine | BMC | bone mineral content |
| ACD | anticoagulant-citrate-dextrose | BMD | bone mineral density |
| ACE | angiotensin-converting enzyme | BP | blood pressure |
| ACGME | American College of Graduate Medical Education | BR | bilirubin |
| ACNP | American College of Nuclear Physicians | BRBPR | bright red blood per rectum |
| ACP | American College of Physicians | BRH | Bureau of Radiological Health |
| ACR | American College of Radiology | BRIDA | mebrofenin (generic name) |
| ACS | American College of Surgeons | BUA | broad-band ultrasound attenuation |
| ACTH | adrenocortical trophic hormone | | |
| AD | Alzheimer's disease | CABG | coronary artery bypass graft |
| ADA | American Dental Association | CAD | coronary artery disease |
| ADR | adverse drug reaction | CAMH | Comprehensive Accreditation Manual for Hospitals |
| AFB | acid-fast bacillus | CAP | College of American Pathology |
| AFP | alpha-fetoprotein | CAS | coronary artery stenosis |
| Ag | antigen | CASS | Coronary Artery Surgery Survival |
| AGES | age, tumor grade, extent and size | CAT | computerized axial tomography |
| AHA | American Hospital Association | CBD | common bile duct |
| AIDS | acquired immunodeficiency syndrome | CCK-8 | terminal octapeptide of cholecystokinin, Kinevac (trade name) |
| ALARA | as low as reasonably achievable | CDC | Center for Disease Control |
| ALND | axillary lymph node detection | CDR | complementary determining region |
| AMA | American Medical Association | CFOV | central field of view |
| AMES | age, metastasis, tumor extent and size | CFR | Code of Federal Regulations |
| AMI | acute myocardial infarction | CHF | congestive heart failure |
| AP | anteroposterior | CI | confidence interval |
| APhA | American Pharmaceutical Association | CLIA-88 | Clinical Laboratory Improvement Act of 1988 |
| APUD | amine precursor uptake and decarboxylation | CPB | competitive protein binding |
| ARC | AIDS related complex | CBF | coronary blood flow |
| ARDS | acute respiratory distress syndrome | CEA | carcinoembryonic antigen |
| ARF | acute renal failure | CMV | cytomegalovirus |
| ARL | AIDS-related lymphoma | CNS | central nervous system |
| ATA | American Thyroid Association | COPD | chronic obstructive pulmonary disease |
| ATD | antithyroid drug | COR | center of rotation |
| ATPase | adenosine triphosphatase | CPA | costophrenic angle |
| ATN | acute tubular necrosis | CPR | cardiopulmonary resuscitation |
| AV | arteriovenous | CQI | continuous quality improvement |
| AVN | avascular necrosis | CSF | cerebrospinal fluid |
| | | CT | computed tomography |
| BAL | bronchoalveolar lavage | CXR | chest x-ray |
| BATO | boron adducts of technetium dioximes | | |
| BCD | benign cortical defect | | |

| | |
|---|---|
| CV | coefficient of variation |
| DAR | differential absorption rate, dose absorption rate |
| DE | dose equivalent |
| DEXA | dual-energy x-ray absorptiometry |
| DISIDA | disofenin (generic name) |
| DIT | diiodotyrosine |
| DMSA | dimercaptosuccinic acid |
| DOPA | dihydroxyphenylalanine |
| DOT | Department of Transportation |
| DPA | dual-photon absorptiometry |
| DTPA | diethylenetriaminepentaacetic acid |
| DUR | differential uptake rate, dose uptake rate |
| DVT | deep venous thrombosis |
| EC | electron capture |
| ECD | ethylcysteinate dimer |
| ECF | extracellular fluid |
| ECG | electrocardiogram |
| ECT | emission computed tomography |
| ED | end-diastole (end-diastolic) |
| EDE | effective dose equivalent |
| EDTA | ethylenediaminetetriacetic acid |
| EDTMP | ethylenediaminetetramethylenephosphonate |
| EF | ejection fraction |
| EHDP | ethylenehydroxydiphosphonate |
| EKG | electrocardiogram |
| ELISA | enzyme linked immunosorbent assay |
| EMIA | enzyme multiplied immunoassay |
| EPA | Environmental Protection Agency |
| ER | emergency room |
| ERPF | effective renal plasma flow |
| ES | end-systole (end-systolic) |
| ESR | erythrocyte sedimentation rate |
| ETT | exercise treadmill test |
| FA | fatty acid |
| Fab | antibody fragment (papain cleavage of MOAB) |
| $F(ab')_2$ | antibody fragment (pepsin cleavage of MOAB) |
| FBP | filtered backprojection |
| Fc | antibody fragment (papain cleavage of MOAB) |
| FDA | Food and Drug Administration |
| FDC | Food, Drug, and Cosmetic Act |
| FDG | fluorodeoxyglucose |
| $FEV_1$ | forced expiratory volume in 1 second |
| FFT | fast Fourier transform |
| FN | false negative |
| FNA | fine-needle aspiration |
| FNH | focal nodular hyperplasia |
| FOV | field of view |
| FP | false positive |
| FTI | free thyroxine index |
| $FT_4$ | free thyroxine |
| $FT_4E$ | free thyroxine estimate |
| 5-FU | 5-fluorouracil |
| FUO | fever of unknown origin |

| | |
|---|---|
| Fv | variable portion of antibody |
| FWHM | full width at half maximum |
| GB | gallbladder |
| GBM | glioblastoma multiforme |
| GE | gastroesophageal |
| GFR | glomerular filtration rate |
| GH | glucoheptonate |
| GHA | glucoheptonate |
| GI | gastrointestinal |
| GIT | gastrointestinal tract |
| GM | Geiger-Mueller |
| GMP | good manufacturing practice |
| GSD | genetically significant dose |
| GUR | glucose uptake rates |
| H | heavy chain of antibody |
| HAA | hepatitis associated antigen |
| HAHA | human anti-human antibody |
| HAM | human albumin microspheres |
| HAMA | human anti-mouse antibody |
| HAP | hydroxyapatite |
| HAT | hypoxanthine aminopterin thymidine |
| HCFA | Health Care Financing Agency |
| HCG | human chorionic gonadotropin |
| HCl | hydrochloric acid |
| HCT | 1. half-clearance time |
| | 2. hepatic clearance time |
| HD | Hodgkin's disease |
| HDP | hydroxymethylene diphosphonate |
| HED | hydroxyephedrine |
| HEDP | hydroxyethylene diphosphonate |
| HEF | hepatic extraction fraction |
| HIPDM | hydroxymethyliodobenzylpropanediamine |
| HIV | human immunodeficiency virus |
| HMDP | hydroxymethylene diphosphonate |
| HMPAO | hexamethyl propyleneamineoxime |
| HPLC | high performance (pressure) liquid chromatography |
| HPOA | hypertrophic pulmonary osteoarthropathy |
| HSA | human serum albumin |
| HSC | Human Subjects Committee |
| HVL | half-value layer |
| IBD | inflammatory bowel disease |
| ICP | Institute of Clinical PET |
| ICRP | International Commission on Radiation Protection |
| IDA | iminodiacetic acid |
| IDC | Investigational Drug Committee |
| IDDM | insulin dependent diabetes mellitus |
| IF | intrinsic factor |
| IMP | iodoamphetamine |
| IND | investigational new drug |
| IOM | Institute of Medicine |
| IRMA | immunoradiometric assay |
| IT | isomeric transition |

| | | | | |
|---|---|---|---|---|
| ITLC | instant thin layer chromatography | | MMI | methimazole |
| ITLC-SA | instant thin layer chromatography with solid phase silicic acid | | MNG | multinodular goiter |
| | | | MOAB | monoclonal antibody |
| ITLC-SG | instant thin layer chromatography with solid phase silica gel | | MPI | myocardial perfusion imaging |
| | | | MRI | magnetic resonance imaging |
| IVP | intravenous pyelogram | | MRSC | medical radiation safety committee |
| | | | MRU | molecular recognition unit |
| JCAH | Joint Commission on Accreditation of Hospitals | | MTC | medullary thyroid carcinoma |
| | | | MUGA | multiple gated acquisition at rest |
| JCAHO | Joint Commission on Accreditation of Health-care Organizations | | MUGX | multiple gated acquisition with stress |

| | | | | |
|---|---|---|---|---|
| K | equilibrium constant | | NaI | sodium iodide |
| $K_a$ | affinity constant | | NCA | nonspecific cross-reacting antigen |
| $K_d$ | dissociation constant | | NCCLS | National Commission for Clinical Laboratory Standards |
| KS | Kaposi's sarcoma | | | |
| | | | NCRP | National Council on Radiation Protection & Measurement |
| L | light chain of antibody | | | |
| LAD | left anterior descending | | NDA | New Drug Application |
| LAO | left anterior oblique | | NE | norepinephrine |
| LBBB | left bundle branch block | | NEMA | National Electronic Manufacturers Association |
| LCP | Legg-Calvé-Perthes disease | | NG | nasogastric |
| LCX | left circumflex coronary artery | | NHL | non-Hodgkin's lymphoma |
| LDL | low-density lipoprotein | | NIH | National Institutes of Health |
| LEGP | low-energy general purpose | | NIST | National Institute of Standards Technology |
| LEHR | low-energy high resolution | | NM | nuclear medicine |
| LET | linear energy transfer | | NPH | normal pressure hydrocephalus |
| LI | large intestine | | NPO | nil per os (nothing by mouth) |
| LIP | lymphocytic interstitial pneumonitis | | NPV | negative predictive value |
| LLQ | left lower quadrant | | NRC | Nuclear Regulatory Commission |
| LOR | line of response | | NSB | nonspecific binding |
| LPO | left posterior oblique | | NV | nausea and vomiting |
| LRP | leukocyte rich plasma | | | |
| L/S | liver/spleen | | OH | hydroxyl ion |
| LV | left ventricle, left ventricular | | OIH | orthoiodohippurate |
| LVEF | left ventricular ejection fraction | | OSEM | ordered subsets expectation minimization |
| LVH | left ventricular hypertrophy | | OSHA | Occupational Safety and Health Administration |

| | | | | |
|---|---|---|---|---|
| MAA | macroaggregated albumin | | PAH | para-aminohippuric acid |
| MACIS | metastasis, age, completeness of resection, invasion and size | | PAP | prostatic acid phosphatase |
| | | | PBI | protein bound iodine |
| MAG3 | mercaptoacetyltriglycine | | PCP | Pneumocystis carinii pneumonia |
| MAI | mycobacterium avium intracellular | | PDA | posterior descending artery |
| MDP | methylene diphosphonate | | PDCA | plan, do, check, act |
| MDR-1 | multiple drug resistant gene | | PE | pulmonary embolism |
| MEGP | medium-energy general purpose | | PER | peak ejection rate |
| MEIA | microparticle enzyme immunoassay | | PET | positron emission tomography |
| MEK | methylethylketone | | PFIA | polarized fluorescence immunoassay |
| MEN | multiple endocrine neoplasm | | PFR | peak filling rate |
| METS | metabolic equivalent test units | | P-gp | permeability glycoprotein |
| MI | myocardial infarction | | PHA | pulse height analyzer |
| MIBG | meta-iodobenzylguanidine | | PIOPED | Prospective Investigation of Pulmonary Embolism Diagnosis |
| MIBI | methoxyisobutylisonitrile (generic name sestamibi) | | | |
| | | | PMT | photomultiplier tube |
| MIRD | Medical Ionizing Radiation Dosimetry | | PPV | positive predictive value |
| MIT | monoiodotyrosine | | pQCT | peripheral quantitative computed tomography |
| MLEM | maximum likelihood expectation minimization | | PS | permeability-surface |

| | |
|---|---|
| PSA | prostate-specific antigen |
| PSF | point spread function |
| PTA | percutaneous transluminal angioplasty |
| PTCA | percutaneous transluminal coronary angioplasty |
| PT | proficiency testing |
| PTH | parathyroid hormone |
| PTT | parenchymal transit time |
| PTU | propylthiouracil |
| PVD | peripheral vascular disease |
| PYP | pyrophosphate |
| | |
| Q | quality factor |
| QA | quality assurance |
| QC | quality control |
| QCT | quantitative computed tomography |
| QI | quality improvement |
| QMP | quality management plan |
| Qp/Qs | pulmonary to systemic flow ratio |
| | |
| RAID | radioimmunodetection |
| RAIU | radioactive iodine uptake |
| RAO | right anterior oblique |
| RAS | renal artery stenosis |
| RBBB | right bundle branch block |
| RBC | red blood cell |
| RBF | renal blood flow |
| RCA | renal cortical activity |
| RCA | right coronary artery |
| RDRC | Radioactive Drug Research Committee |
| RE | reticuloendothelial |
| REAL | Revised European American Lymphoma |
| RES | reticuloendothelial system |
| RIA | radioimmunoassay |
| RIND | reversible ischemic neurologic deficit |
| rCBF | regional cerebral blood flow |
| RIS | radioimmunoscintigraphy |
| RIT | radioimmunotherapy |
| RLQ | right lower quadrant |
| ROC | receiver operator curve |
| ROI | region of interest |
| RP | radiopharmaceutical |
| RPF | renal plasma flow |
| RPG | radiation protection guide |
| RPO | right posterior oblique |
| RRA | radioreceptor assay |
| RSC | Radiation Safety Committee |
| RSD | reflex sympathetic dystrophy |
| RSO | radiation safety officer |
| $rT_3$ | reverse $T_3$ |
| RV | right ventricle |
| RVG | radionuclide ventriculography |
| | |
| SA | silicic acid |
| SC | sulfur colloid |
| SD | standard deviation |

| | |
|---|---|
| SDAT | senile dementia of Alzheimer's type |
| SEXA | single-energy x-ray absorptiometry |
| SFV | single chain binding protein |
| SG | silica gel |
| SI | small intestine |
| SNM | Society of Nuclear Medicine |
| SOD | sphincter of Oddi |
| SOS | speed of sound |
| SPA | single-photon absorptiometry |
| SPECT | single photon emission computed tomography |
| SPN | single pulmonary nodule |
| SRF | split renal function |
| SSN | suprasternal notch |
| STEP | simultaneous transmission emission protocol |
| sTg | serum thyroglobulin |
| sTSH | sensitive thyroid stimulating hormone |
| SUR | standardized uptake rate |
| SUV | standard uptake value (specific uptake value) |
| SVC | superior vena cava |
| | |
| $T_3$ | total triiodothyronine |
| $T_3U$ | $T_3$ uptake |
| TAA | tumor-associated antigen |
| TAC | time activity curve |
| TAG-72 | tumor associated glycoprotein 72 |
| TB | tubercle bacilli, tuberculosis |
| TBG | thyroxine binding globulin |
| $TcO_2$ | hydrolyzed (reduced) technetium |
| $TcO_4$ | pertechnetate |
| TCT | transmission computed tomography |
| TER | tubular excretion rate |
| TEW | triple-energy window |
| TF | transmitted fraction |
| TG | triglyceride |
| TIA | transient ischemic attack |
| $T_{max}$ | time to peak activity |
| TMBIDA | mebrofenin (generic name) |
| TMJ | temporomandibular joint |
| tPA | tissue plasminogen activator |
| TPBS | triple-phase bone scan |
| TPER | time to peak ejection rate |
| TPFR | time to peak filling rate |
| TPN | total parenteral nutrition |
| TQM | total quality management |
| TRH | thyroid-releasing hormone |
| TSAb | thyroid-stimulating antibody |
| TSH | thyroid-stimulating hormone |
| TTP | time to peak |
| | |
| UBT | urea breath test |
| UGI | upper gastrointestinal |
| UNOS | United Network for Organ Sharing |
| US | ultrasound |
| USAN | United States Adopted Names |
| USP | United States Pharmacopeia |

| | | | |
|---|---|---|---|
| UV | ultraviolet | VUR | vesicoureteral reflux |
| UWHC | University of Wisconsin Hospital and Clinics | | |
| VCUG | voiding cystourethrogram | WBC | white blood cell |
| $V_L$ | variable light chain | WPW | Wolf-Parkinson-White |
| $V_H$ | variable heavy chain | $W_T$ | weighting factor |
| VMA | vanillylmandelic acid | XRT | x-ray therapy |
| VPCs | ventricular premature contractions | | |
| V/Q | ventilation/perfusion | | |

# Subject Index

false-negative results in, 199–200, 262

metaphyseal equivalent regions in, 261–262

triple-phase, 25, 198–204, 524–525

vertebral, 199, 203–204

in diabetes mellitus, 199, 202–203

gallium 67 scans in, 192, 200

indium 111 white blood cell scans in, 25, 194, 198, 200–202, 524–525

in diabetes mellitus, 202

postoperative, 203

vertebral, 203–204

technetium 99m white blood cell scans in, 25, 202–203, 524–525

Osteonecrosis, bone scan in, 26–27

in children, 264, 267

Osteopenia, bone densitometry in, 284

Osteopoikilosis, 28

Osteoporosis

bone densitometry in, 279, 280, 284

bone scan in, 10

Osteosarcoma, bone scan in, 20, 28

Ovarian cancer

monoclonal antibodies in, 228, 231, 232, 313–319

radiation-induced, 494

Oxygen 15, in positron emission tomography, 376, 458

in perfusion imaging, 332, 333, 458

myocardial, 342, 343

P

Paget's disease of bone, bone scan in, 28

Pain

in back, 24–25

SPECT imaging in, 24, 25, 30

in bone tumors, 15, 16, 17, 579

strontium 89 therapy in, 354

in chest, myocardial perfusion imaging in, 535

in cholecystitis, 61

in goiter, 169

in hip, bone scans in, 24

in pulmonary embolism, 90

scrotal, scrotal scintigraphy in, 132, 134

in thyroiditis, 159, 169

Pair production in radiation-matter interactions, 381, 416

Palmitate, carbon 11, in metabolic imaging, 334, 335

Palsy, progressive supranuclear, 248

Pancoast syndrome, bone scan in, 17

Pancreas

transplant imaging, 293–294, 575

cystography in, 294, 575–576

protocol in, 293–294, 575

radiopharmaceuticals in, 293, 575

tumors of, indium 111 pentetreotide in, 309–310

Panda sign in gallium 67 scans, 190, 216

Para-aminohippuric acid in renal plasma flow measurement, 118, 120

Paragangliomas, 306–307

Parathyroid gland, 299–304

adenoma of, 221, 299–304

clinical protocol in, 576–577

immunoassay in, 484

bone scan in disorders of, 28, 29

embryology of, 299

hypoparathyroidism after thyroidectomy, 171–172, 175–176

parathyroid hormone immunoassays of, 484

tumor localization, 576–577

Parent-daughter radioisotopes, decay of, 379

Parkinson's disease, 341

Parotid salivary gland scans, 86, 533

Partial volume effects

in positron emission tomography, 460

in SPECT imaging, 448

Particulate radiations, 380–381

Parzen filters, 444, 472

Pediatric imaging, 259–276. See also Children

Peer review of quality improvement efforts, 502–504, 505

Pentagastrin, in gastric mucosa studies, 85

Pentetreotide, 233

indium 111. See Indium 111, pentetreotide

Peptide agents

in infection imaging, 198

in thrombosis detection, 233, 361–362

in tumor imaging, 232–233

Perchlorate discharge test, 551

thyroid uptake of radioiodine in, 157

Perfusion

cerebral, 239–248, 570

positron emission tomography of, 332, 333

radiopharmaceuticals in scans of, 399

hepatic arterial, 85

myocardial, 33–54, 533–536. See also Myocardial perfusion imaging

in pancreas transplantation, 294

positron emission tomography of, 332–333

in dementia, 340, 341

of heart, 332, 333, 342–344

quantitation methods in, 332–333, 342

tracers used in, 332

pulmonary, 92–95, 105, 539–541

in cancer of lung, 112

in heart failure, 111–112

in intracardiac shunts, 112–113

in intrapulmonary shunts, 113–114

in transplantation of lung, 112

and ventilation/perfusion scans, 89–114. See also Ventilation/perfusion scans

renal, in transplantation, 289

Pericarditis in HIV infection and AIDS, 328

Periodic table, 372

Periosteal reaction, bone scans in, 22

Periostitis, bone scans in, 22

Peritoneal shunt surgery, evaluation of, 85–86, 532–533

Pertechnegas in ventilation scans, 96, 100, 110

Pertechnetate

free, and soft-tissue uptake of bone tracers, 6, 11

technetium 99m. See Technetium 99m pertechnetate

PET. See Positron emission tomography

Pharmaceutical, definition of, 385

Phase images, 442, 465, 467–469

in Fourier transformation, 442

in radionuclide ventriculography, 143–144, 467–469

Pheochromocytoma, 212, 306–307

indium 111 pentetreotide in, 310

iodine 123 MIBG in, 308

compared to indium 111 pentetreotide, 310

iodine 131 MIBG in, 212, 233, 304, 308

compared to indium 111 pentetreotide, 310

indications for, 578

interpretation of, 578

therapeutic uses of, 212, 309

Phosphorus 32

decay of, 375–376

therapeutic uses of, 355, 390, 581

intra-articular, 581

intracavitary, 582

in polycythemia, 582

in skeletal metastatic disease, 353

Photodisintegration, 416

Photoelectric effect, 381, 387, 415

Photomultiplier tubes, 423, 425

number of photons reaching, 426

Photons, 373

and Compton scattering, 381, 387, 415–416

energy of, in diagnostic radiopharmaceuticals, 387–388

number reaching photomultiplier tube, 426

and photoelectric effect, 381, 387, 415

in production of electron-positron pair, 381, 416

Physician orders in radioiodine therapy, 557

Physics of nuclear medicine, 371–383

elementary particles in, 372–373

forces and stability in, 373

historical aspects of, 371–372

radioactive decay in, 373–380

Pick's disease, 248, 341